The Biologic & Clinical Basis of
Infectious Diseases

The Biologic & Clinical Basis of Infectious Diseases

Fourth Edition

Stanford T. Shulman, M.D.
Professor of Pediatrics
Northwestern University Medical School
Chief, Division of Infectious Diseases
The Children's Memorial Hospital
Chicago, Illinois

John P. Phair, M.D.
Professor of Medicine
Northwestern University Medical School
Chicago, Illinois

Herbert M. Sommers, M.D.
Professor of Pathology
Department of Pathology
Northwestern University Medical School
Chicago, Illinois

W.B. SAUNDERS COMPANY
Harcourt Brace Jovanovich, Inc.
Philadelphia London Toronto Montreal Sydney Tokyo

W. B. SAUNDERS COMPANY
Harcourt Brace Jovanovich, Inc.

The Curtis Center
Independence Square West
Philadelphia, Pennsylvania 19106

Library of Congress Cataloging-in-Publication Data

The biologic and clinical basis of infectious diseases / [edited by]
Stanford T. Shulman, John P. Phair, Herbert M. Sommers.—4th
ed.

  p. cm

Includes bibliographical references and index.

ISBN 0–7216–3066–9

1. Communicable diseases.   I. Shulman, Stanford T.
   II. Phair, John P.   III. Sommers, Herbert M.

[DNLM: 1. Communicable Diseases. WC 100 B615]

RC111.B47 1992

616.9—dc20

DNLM/DLC   91-19125

Cover photos: Three-dimensional structure of rotavirus-anti(VP4)Fab complex determined
using electron cryomicroscopy and computer image processing techniques (Prasad et al.,
Nature 343:476–479, 1990). Photo Courtesy: Dr. B.V.V. Prasad, Baylor College of
Medicine, Houston, Texas.

Editor: Martin Wonsiewicz
Designer: Susan Hess Blaker
Production Manager: Linda R. Garber
Manuscript Editor: Linda Davoli
Illustration Coordinator: Cecelia Roberts
Indexer: Nancy Weaver

The Biologic and Clinical Basis of
Infectious Diseases, 4th Edition   ISBN 0–7216–3066–9

Printed in Mexico.

Last digit is the print number: 9   8   7   6   5   4   3   2

The editors wish to dedicate this work to the pioneering efforts of the previous editors, Dr. Phil Paterson and the late Dr. Guy Youmans; to our wives, Claire Shulman, Nancy Phair, and Carolyn Sommers, who provide continuing support; and to our children. A special acknowledgment goes to Esther and Sam Levitt for their love and encouragement.

Contributors

Moshe Arditi, M.D.
Assistant Professor of Pediatrics, University of Southern California Medical School, Los Angeles, California; Division of Infectious Diseases, Children's Hospital of Los Angeles, Los Angeles, California
Introduction to Infections of the Central Nervous System; Common Etiologic Agents of Bacterial Meningitis

Ellen Gould Chadwick, M.D.
Assistant Professor of Pediatrics, Northwestern University Medical School, Chicago, Illinois; Attending Physician, Division of Infectious Diseases, Children's Memorial Hospital, Chicago, Illinois
Human Immunodeficiency Virus Infection and AIDS

John W. Corcoran, Ph.D.
Professor Emeritus of Biochemistry, Northwestern University Medical School, Chicago, Illinois
Molecular Biology of Sensitivity and Resistance to Antimicrobial Agents

A Todd Davis, M.D.
Professor of Pediatrics, Northwestern University Medical School, Chicago, Illinois; Chief, Division of General Academic and Emergency Pediatrics, The Children's Memorial Hospital, Chicago, Illinois
Temperature Regulation, the Pathogenesis of Fever and the Approach to the Febrile Patient; Zoonoses; Exanthematous Diseases

James L. Duncan, D.D.S., Ph.D.
Associate Professor of Microbiology-Immunology, Northwestern University Medical and Dental Schools, Chicago, Illinois
Dental Infections and Other Diseases of the Oral Cavity

Betsy C. Herold, M.D.
Research Associate, Department of Microbiology-Immunology, Northwestern University Medical School, Chicago, Illinois; Clinical Associate, Department of Pediatric Infectious Diseases, University of Chicago Medical School, Chicago, Illinois
Virus-Host Interactions

Robert L. Murphy, M.D.
Associate Professor of Clinical Medicine, Northwestern University Medical School, Chicago, Illinois; Medical Director, Sexually Transmitted Diseases and AIDS Clinics, Northwestern Memorial Hospital, Chicago, Illinois
Sexually Transmitted Diseases; Infection in the Compromised Host

John P. Phair, M.D.
Samuel J. Sackett Professor of Medicine, Northwestern University Medical School, Chicago, Illinois; Chief of Infectious Disease, Northwestern Memorial Hospital, Chicago, Illinois
Host-Bacteria Interactions; Temperature Regulation, the Pathogenesis of Fever and the Approach to the Febrile Patient; Laboratory Assessment of Immunocompetence; Infections of the Lower Respiratory Tract: General Considerations; Bacterial Pneumonias; Fungal Infections of the Respiratory Tract; Syndromes of Host Immunoincompetence; Human Immunodeficiency Virus Infection and AIDS; Nosocomial Infections; Infective Endocarditis; Antimicrobial Therapy

Boris Reisberg, M.D.
Assistant Professor of Medicine, Northwestern University Medical School, Chicago, Illinois; Northwestern Memorial Hospital, VA Lakeside Hospital, Chicago, Illinois
Common Intestinal Parasitic Infections; Malaria

Anthony J. Schaeffer, M.D.
Professor and Chairman, Department of
Urology, Northwestern University Medical
School, Chicago, Illinois; Attending,
Northwestern Memorial Hospital, Children's
Memorial Hospital and Veterans
Administration Lakeside Hospital, Chicago,
Illinois
*Urinary Tract Infections: Cystitis and
Pyelonephritis*

Nehama Sharon, Ph.D.
Associate Professor of Pathology,
Northwestern University Medical School,
Chicago, Illinois; Senior Attending, Evanston
Hospital, Evanston, Illinois
Laboratory Diagnosis of Infections

Stanford T. Shulman, M.D.
Professor of Pediatrics and Associate Dean for
Academic Affairs, Northwestern University
Medical School, Chicago, Illinois; Chief,
Division of Infectious Diseases, The Children's
Memorial Hospital, Chicago, Illinois
*Introduction to Infectious Diseases; The
Indigenous Microbiota of the Human Host;
Host-Bacteria Interactions; Microbe-Induced
Autoreactive Host Responses and Autoimmune
Disease; Laboratory Diagnosis of Infections;
Bacterial Infections of the Upper Respiratory
Tract; Infectious Diarrhea; Viral Hepatitis;
Infections Caused by Anaerobic Bacteria;
Rickettsial Diseases; Infective Endocarditis;
Staphylococci, Staphylococcal Disease, and
Toxic Shock Syndrome; Molecular Biology of
Sensitivity and Resistance to Antimicrobial
Agents; Antimicrobial Therapy; Principles of
Immunization*

Herbert M. Sommers, M.D.
Professor of Pathology, Department of
Pathology, Northwestern University Medical
School, Chicago, Illinois
*The Indigenous Microbiota of the Human
Host; Laboratory Diagnosis of Infections;
Infectious Diarrhea; Infections Caused by
Anaerobic Bacteria; Drug Susceptibility Testing
in vitro and Monitoring of Antimicrobial
Therapy*

Patricia G. Spear, Ph.D
Guy and Anne Youmans Professor and
Chairman of Microbiology-Immunology,
Northwestern University Medical and Dental
Schools, Chicago, Illinois
Virus-Host Interactions

Michele Till, M.D.
Clinical Instructor of Medicine, Division of
Infectious Diseases, Northwestern University
Medical School, Chicago, Illinois
Viral Infections of the Central Nervous System

John Warren, M.D.
Professor of Pathology, Northwestern
University Medical School, Chicago, Illinois;
Attending Staff in Pathology, Northwestern
Memorial Hospital, Chicago, Illinois; Chief of
Laboratory Service, VA Lakeside Medical
Center, Chicago, Illinois
Mycobacterial Infections; Sepsis

Steven M. Wolinsky, M.D.
Assistant Professor of Medicine, Division of
Infectious Diseases, Northwestern University
Medical School, Chicago, Illinois; Attending
Physician, Northwestern Memorial Hospital,
Chicago, Illinois
Viral Infections of the Central Nervous System

Ram Yogev, M.D.
Professor of Pediatrics, Northwestern
University Medical School, Chicago, Illinois;
Attending Physician, Division of Infectious
Diseases, The Children's Memorial Hospital,
Chicago, Illinois
*Introduction to Infections of the Central
Nervous System; Common Etiologic Agents of
Bacterial Meningitis*

Margaret Yungbluth, M.D.
Assistant Professor of Clinical Pathology,
Department of Pathology, Northwestern
University Medical School, Chicago, Illinois;
Attending Staff, Northwestern Memorial
Hospital, Chicago, Illinois
*Infectious Mononucleosis and Viral Infections
of the Upper Respiratory Tract; Viral Infections
of the Lower Respiratory Tract*

Preface to the Fourth Edition

This fourth edition of *The Biologic and Clinical Basis of Infectious Diseases,* prepared under substantially changed editorial leadership, represents a thoroughly revised and updated version of this textbook. As before, this text owes its existence to the annual infectious diseases course for sophomore medical students that has been taught at Northwestern University Medical School since 1966. The course continues to teach the core concepts of microbiology, immunology, and infectious diseases within an integrated biologic and clinical context. The infectious diseases course spawned the first edition of this text and has prompted each of the subsequent three editions. The individuals selected to revise or to author chapters in this text are all faculty members at Northwestern.

The editors continue to be committed to the view that microbial infection is important etiologically and/or pathogenetically in most human disease and that disorders of very wide diversity have a primary or secondary relationship to microbial infection. We believe that, as increasing numbers of patients survive with primary or secondary impairments of their host defenses, the core concept that the microbe–host relationship underlies the biologic and clinical expression of infectious disease increasingly will influence the practice of medicine. This remains the theme of Northwestern's infectious diseases course and of the previous and current editions of this text. An understanding of microbe–host interaction and of the linkage of basic microbiology to clinical infectious diseases facilitates effective diagnosis and patient care.

As in previous editions, we have focused particularly but not exclusively on those infectious diseases that are of major importance in the United States. All chapters have been revised and updated (most very substantially) to reflect the rapid progress that has been made since the last edition, and discussions of "new" infectious diseases have been added (e.g., Lyme disease, Kawasaki disease, toxic-shock syndrome). The Case Histories have been retained, for we believe them to be an important and effective way for medical students to begin to develop their analytic skills in using historical data, physical examination findings, and laboratory results to arrive at a differential diagnosis and to organize a treatment plan.

STANFORD T. SHULMAN, M.D.

Contents

I

Host-Microbe Interactions

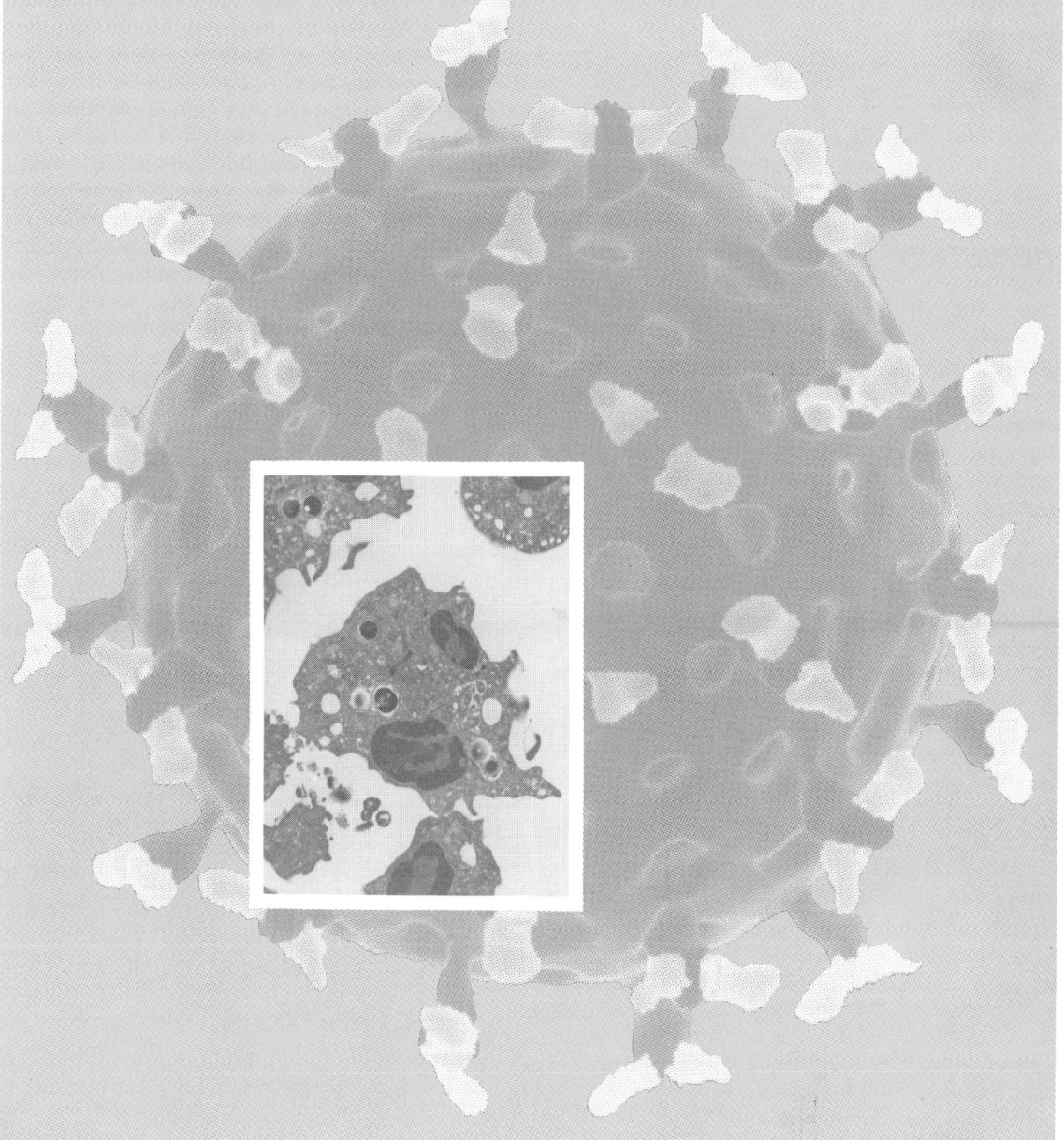

Introduction to Infectious Diseases

DEFINITION

The study of infectious diseases is a clinical specialty of medicine that is concerned with the diagnosis and management of illnesses directly caused by infectious microorganisms. This ever-widening variety of microorganisms includes bacteria, viruses, fungi, protozoa, helminths, and even algae. The specialty of infectious diseases rests firmly upon a broad scientific foundation of microbiology and immunology. Indeed, historically, the development of microbiology and more recently immunology spawned the discipline of infectious diseases. In recent years, advances in the fields of molecular biology, including molecular genetics and molecular virology and bacteriology, have contributed to improving our understanding of the mechanisms of host–parasite interactions in ways that were unthinkable even a few years ago. Consequently, tremendous advances have occurred, for example, in elucidating the precise molecular basis of the surface structures of an organism that allow the organisms to adhere to a specific surface receptor on a eukaryotic host cell.

VIRULENCE

All animals coexist with an indigenous microflora (see Chapter 2). We are each heavily colonized by, and live in a state of peaceful coexistence with, countless microorganisms that colonize our skin and most of our mucosal surfaces. We live in a veritable sea of microbes. The mouth, pharynx, gastrointestinal tract, and other areas are heavily colonized by many different bacterial species. A classic symbiosis appears to have been established between host and parasite. This relationship is so close that it has been suggested that, from an evolutionary perspective, mitochondria (the important energy-generating intracytoplasmic organelles) evolved phylogenetically from intracellular bacterial forms, representing actual fusion of microbe and host.

Under normal circumstances, a large number of host factors operate to maintain the delicate host–microbe balance. These include the normal physical barriers of intact skin and mucosal surfaces, as well as both nonspecific and highly specific aspects of the immune system (see Chapter 3). Any of a wide range of circumstances can disrupt this delicate balance between host and microbe. Examples include burns that disrupt the skin barrier, antibiotic therapy that alters the complex balance of microorganisms colonizing a mucosal surface, surgery that breaches normal anatomic barriers or leaves behind foreign bodies such as sutures or tubes, malnutrition, physical and/or emotional stress, and countless others.

When the delicate balance between eukaryotic host and prokaryotic microorganism becomes disrupted in these or in other ways, infection of the host may ensue. The relative ability of a microorganism to produce infection is termed *virulence* and is related to a variety of complex mechanisms of disease induction. However, it is imperative to recognize that virulence is a *relative* term. That is, some organisms are highly virulent in that most or all normal hosts who become exposed to and colonized by them develop clinical illness. Examples may include organisms like *Yersinia pestis,* the cause of plague, or *Salmonella typhi,* the agent of typhoid fever. On the other hand, if the normal host defenses are compromised, microorganisms that usually coexist symbiotically with the normal host can induce serious infections. In this way, a normally harmless microorganism can demonstrate its virulence, or its potential to cause clinically apparent infection opportunistically. Examples are the coagulase-negative staphylococci that opportunistically cause infection of implanted foreign bodies such as shunts or prosthetic heart valves. Clearly the apparent virulence of a microorganism depends upon the host setting and the status of the host's normal defenses, which ordinarily hold microorganisms in check.

Thus, infection is generally a consequence of the interaction between a relatively highly virulent microorganism and a normal intact host, or between a relatively less virulent microbe and a host with some degree of transient or permanent impairment of host defense mechanisms.

In general, most of the striking modern advances in medical therapy have resulted in the undesired effect of impairing the ability of the host to withstand infection. Examples include corticosteroid and cytotoxic medications that directly affect both specific and nonspecific components of the immune system, antimicrobial agents that modify the normal delicately balanced indigenous microflora, and drugs or procedures that lessen the gastric acidity that serves to kill ingested microorganisms. Common respiratory viral infections can reduce transiently the respiratory tract's mucosal surface receptors for normal bacterial microflora, facilitating replacement of these normal flora by potentially more invasive, more virulent bacterial agents.

The 1980s saw the astonishingly dramatic worldwide emergence of a "new" infectious disease caused by the human immunodeficiency virus (HIV), an infection that, ultimately, debilitates host immune mechanisms, leading to vulnerability to an incredible array of opportunistic infections. Most of these infections are caused by agents that uninfected individuals (those whose immune systems are intact) coexist with peacefully. HIV infection and its resultant acquired immune deficiency syndrome (AIDS) have become so widespread in certain areas of the world and of the United States that they have created a crisis in health care delivery. AIDS, even more than other illnesses, epitomizes the importance of understanding the balance between host and microbe and of recognizing the consequences of disruption of this balance.

HISTORIC BEGINNINGS OF THE STUDY OF INFECTIOUS DISEASES

The medical specialty of infectious diseases has its earliest beginnings in the descriptions by the Greeks, Romans, and Hebrews of epidemic afflictions—epidemics that reached particularly impressive proportions in the Middle Ages. Thucydides, a contemporary of Hippocrates, recognized the transmission of infection from one person to another, as occurred in the plague of Athens. Although Aretaeus in the second century A.D. was the first to allude to a doctrine of invisible infecting organisms, a variety of supernatural explanations were offered in the ancient and medieval worlds for smallpox and other epidemic disorders. The two great scourges of the Middle Ages were syphilis and bubonic plague; the latter was responsible for the Black Death, which appeared in Europe about 1348 and annihilated one fourth of the earth's population. Rather than being attributed to the crowded living conditions and poor sanitation of the walled medieval towns, these illnesses were blamed on comets or other astrologic features, crop failures, droughts or floods, or upon poisoning of wells by Jews.

The spread of syphilis through Europe, which began around 1495, was recognized early on to effect its contagiousness by direct contact. Girolamo Fracastoro, a classmate of Copernicus and the man who gave syphilis its name in the 16th century, came impressively close to proposing a germ theory of disease, long before the existence of microorganisms was known. Reflecting upon his clinical experience with plague in Italy, Fracastoro wrote in 1546 that the disease is not caused by a "mysterious shadow or miasma, nor by obstructed humors but by a kind of seed." He indicated that these substances were so minute that they were invisible and that when transmitted from one person to another, they multiply and propagate themselves, soon producing in the second person the disease seen in the first. He proposed that spread occurred in three ways: by direct bodily contact, by fomites, and at a distance through the air.

After the invention of the microscope by Antony van Leeuwenhoek in the late 17th century and its further refinements, active speculation began regarding a possible relationship between disease states and the microorganisms visualized with the microscope. Such speculation became even stronger by the 1830s when it was shown that both alcoholic fermentation and the process of putrefaction were the direct consequence of the activity of microscopic organisms. Both Fracastoro in the 16th century and Henle in 1840 emphasized the similarity between disease and putrefaction or decay. Robert Koch's isolation of the bacterial agent of anthrax in 1877, his development of techniques to culture microbes on solid media, and his most famous discovery of the tubercle bacillus in 1882 (an organism at that time responsible for one of every seven deaths) laid the groundwork for a flood of research aimed at the isolation and identification of the causative agents of many infectious diseases.

Two great landmarks in the *prevention* of infectious diseases were Jenner's demonstration, at the end of the 18th century, of the efficacy of vaccination against smallpox and Pasteur's production and utilization of a successful vaccine against rabies in 1885. On May 14, 1796, Jenner, a country physician in Gloucestershire, inoculated the arm of a lad named James Phipps with matter obtained from a cowpox lesion on the hand of a dairymaid, and on July 1, 1796, he challenged the boy with matter from a pustular smallpox lesion. In this scientific fashion, he demonstrated that a serious infection could be prevented after a previous infection with an attenuated strain of the causative agent. Similarly, beginning on July 6, 1885, Pasteur's successful development and use of attenuated rabies virus to immunize a youngster named Joseph Meister, who had been bitten by a rabid dog, quickly revolutionized the approach to the prevention of infectious diseases. In fact, almost 2500 individuals were immunized against the previously invariably fatal rabies in the year following.

Therapeutic advances that truly established the study of infectious diseases as a medical discipline date to von Behring's and Kitasato's discoveries in 1890 that animal antisera prepared by prior injection of toxins into the animal were useful in treating diphtheria and tetanus, classic toxin-mediated diseases. In 1909, Ehrlich produced the "magic bullet" salvarsan (arsphenamine), or 606, an arsenical that was highly effective in the treatment of syphilis. This ushered in the era of chemotherapy for treating infectious diseases. Of course, one of the key advances of this chemotherapeutic era was Fleming's serendipitous discovery in 1929 of the antibacterial effect of penicillin and the subsequent development of this material for human use by Chain and Florey in the early 1940s.

The accelerating pace of microbiologic discoveries and advances in prevention and therapy has now extended into the 1990s, with the application to problem solving of such modern molecular biologic techniques as gene manipulation. The discipline of infectious diseases has moved far beyond the descriptive stage, with the continuing promise of rapidly paced advances.

CURRENT STATUS OF THE DISCIPLINE

Despite the major technologic advances that influenced (and will continue to influence) the field of infectious diseases, major concerns persist regarding the implementation of simple preventative and therapeutic measures. For example, as discussed in Chapter 40, 70 million cases of measles still occur annually, producing considerable morbidity and 1.5 million deaths, mostly in underdeveloped areas of the world. These illnesses are preventable but occur because of economic and logistic factors that hamper the successful implementation of immunization programs. Only 5% of the world's health research resources are devoted to the problems of developing countries, even though those countries suffer 93% of the early mortality among the world's population. Shockingly, there were large outbreaks of measles in the United States in the late 1980s and early 1990s, with most cases occurring in the underimmunized, primarily African-American and Hispanic school-aged children of the inner cities (particularly Los Angeles, Houston, Dallas, and Chicago). The interplay between infectious diseases and malnutrition must also be noted, as it accounts for the approximate 10% mortality from measles and excess mortality from other infections in some areas. Thus, in the United States and elsewhere, the translation of the fruits of scientific progress and modern technology to the poorer segments of society remains a tremendous challenge. That is, the public health aspects of infectious diseases continue to be a challenge that requires much effort. Until this challenge can be met, children will continue to succumb to preventable diseases like measles. That success in these endeavors is possible with the proper commitment was demonstrated by the complete worldwide eradication of smallpox, achieved in 1977, and by the almost complete eradication of paralytic poliomyelitis from the entire Western Hemisphere by 1990.

In addition to focusing on improved control of the infectious diseases of childhood, the clinical practice of infectious diseases in Western society is increasingly involved with the prevention, diagnosis, and management of infections in the immunocompromised host. This patient population has increased dramatically as a consequence of increasing numbers of organ transplant recipients, AIDS patients, and individuals receiving immunosuppressive therapies for oncologic or other disorders. There is every indication that these populations will continue to increase. These immunocompromised individuals are highly susceptible to opportunistic infections caused by a very wide array of infectious agents (see Chapter 27), a fact that continues to stimulate the development of innovative preventative and therapeutic strategies.

A particularly exciting aspect of infectious diseases has been the recognition of "new" clinical syndromes during the past one to two decades, including AIDS, toxic-shock syndrome, Lyme disease, Kawasaki disease, and Legionnaires' disease. At the same time, other disorders have disappeared or are disappearing. Thus, there is a changing menu of problems that demand the attention of physicians who specialize in the exciting clinical field of infectious diseases. Indeed, all of clinical medicine is concerned with infectious diseases in some way, making this specialty one that is central to the entire discipline of medicine.

2 *HERBERT M. SOMMERS, M.D. • STANFORD T. SHULMAN, M.D.*

The Indigenous Microbiota of the Human Host

INTRODUCTION

Present-day infections more often result from host interaction with bacteria that comprise the normal flora of the host than from exogenous microorganisms. This is in sharp contrast to the infectious epidemics of the past—plague, cholera, and smallpox—which involved diseases associated with microorganisms capable of causing infection in any susceptible host and were thus the scourges of the human race. Today, the most serious threat of infection is posed by our own microbiota.

The virulence of parasites in the normal host microbiota may change rapidly, depending on the acquisition of new phage or serotypes of bacteria. Episomes coding for genetic resistance to antimicrobial agents can be transferred to one bacterium by another within the gastrointestinal tract. Bacterial populations previously sensitive to numerous antimicrobial agents can rapidly become resistant to many by episome transfer. Although bacteria such as *Mycobacterium tuberculosis* and *Yersinia pestis* (plague) are capable of inducing disease in well-nourished, vigorous young adults, the serious infections seen in today's hospitals are more commonly caused by *Escherichia coli, Klebsiella pneumoniae, Staphylococcus aureus,* and *Proteus mirabilis,* and others. All these organisms can be recovered from one site or another from the normal human host. Inasmuch as most humans live in harmony with these bacteria without signs of infection, physicians have come to regard them as normal flora. However, with tissue necrosis following surgery, suppression of immune responses associated with viral infection, or modification of host defense mechanisms, the nonpathogen may quickly become a pathogen.

INDIGENOUS MICROBIOTA

There are several reasons that the study of the normal human microbiota is helpful:

1. A knowledge of the different types of organisms in or on a surface of the body at various locations gives greater insight into the kind of infections that might occur following tissue injury at these sites (Fig. 2–1).

2. Knowledge of bacteria native to any one

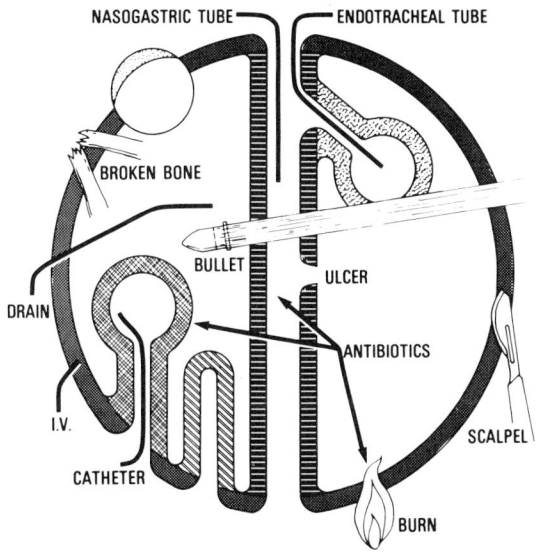

Figure 2–1. The epithelial disruptions induced by trauma, disease, and therapy, which permit microbial invasion. (Reproduced by permission from Meakins, J. L. Host defenses. In Howard, R. J., and Simmons, R. L.: Surgical Infectious Diseases, 2nd ed. New York: Appleton Century Crofts, 1988.)

part of the body helps the physician place in perspective the possible source and significance of microorganisms isolated from clinical infections. *Enterococcus faecalis,* normally found in the gastrointestinal tract, may be associated with urinary tract infections in middle-aged men. The incidence of prostatic enlargement and partial urinary tract obstruction in this group is thought to be one of the reasons that *E. faecalis* is one of the major causes of infective endocarditis in this population (see Chapter 35).

3. Knowledge of the indigenous microbiota is important in understanding the consequences of overgrowth by microorganisms normally absent at that site. One such example is the heavy growth of yeast in the oral cavity that may occur in conjunction with intensive, broad-spectrum antimicrobial drug therapy or profound depression of host immune defenses, for example, AIDS (see Chapters 26 and 27). Another example is the extensive yeast growth seen in the gastrointestinal tract of some patients given large doses of neomycin. Although neomycin is effective in suppressing bacteria in the Enterobacteriaceae family, it has no effect on yeast, and administration of this drug is frequently followed by an annoying diarrhea associated with an almost pure growth of *Candida albicans.*

4. Finally, there is increasing awareness that indigenous microbiota play a role in stimulating the host immune responses to provide protec-

tion from organisms that might otherwise cause serious disease. *Neisseria lactamica* is an organism closely related to *Neisseria meningitidis*, although it is much less likely to be associated with overt disease. Recent studies have shown that increased colonization in children with *N. lactamica* is associated with an increased incidence of bactericidal antibodies against *N. meningitidis*. These findings suggest that *N. lactamica* is able to stimulate production of cross-reacting antibodies to provide at least partial protection against all capsular types of *N. meningitidis*. A similar finding in experimental animals has shown that certain strains of *Escherichia coli* contribute to production of bactericidal antibodies providing protection against serious infections from *Haemophilus influenzae*.

INTERACTION AMONG INDIGENOUS MICROBIOTA

Little is known of the overall significance of the microbial flora in the human body. One reason for this is that the study of the microbial flora in the past has been primarily directed toward the isolation, enumeration, and classification of microbial species. Although procedures for enumerating bacteria on exposed surfaces such as the skin are not difficult, considerably more effort is necessary to study the microbial flora in different segments of the gastrointestinal tract. Investigations of this type require specialized sampling equipment and culture media as well as specialized technical training for personnel. Although the enumeration and identification of bacterial species make up a necessary first step, they do not provide information about the interaction between one bacterial species and another. *Bacteroides melaninogenicus*, for example, a strict gram-negative anaerobic bacillus, requires the presence of three other anaerobic bacteria to produce severe necrotizing infections of the mouth. None of these four microorganisms in itself is capable of causing infection. One of these microorganisms, a diphtheroid, is necessary for the synthesis of vitamin K, a substance *B. melaninogenicus* needs for growth. The interaction among the other two bacterial species, the bacteroides and the diphtheroid, that leads to a necrotizing infection is unknown. It is likely that many similar and complex interactions occur between or among different bacterial species within both diseased and normal regions of the body.

TABLE 2–1. Mechanisms by Which Indigenous Microorganisms Inhibit Potential Pathogens

Direct Effects

Production of bacteriocin	Depletion of essential nutrients
Production of toxic metabolic end products	Suppression of adherence
Induction of low oxidation–reduction potential	Inhibition of translocation
	Degradation of toxins

Indirect Effects

Enhancement of antibody production	Augmentation of interferon production
Stimulation of phagocyte production	Deconjugation of bile acid
Stimulation of clearance mechanisms	

Reproduced by permission from Mackowiak, P. A. The normal microbial flora. *N. Engl. J. Med. 307*:83, 1982. Adapted from Savage, D. C. Colonization by and survival of pathogenic bacteria on mucosal surfaces. In Britton, G., and Marshall, K. C., eds. *Adsorption of Microorganisms to Surfaces.* New York: John Wiley and Sons, 1980.

Mechanisms of Colonization

Colonization of epithelial surfaces can be divided into two general categories: (1) those that are associated with adherence to epithelial surfaces, and (2) those that enable microorganisms to survive in the surface environment.

The adherence of one species of bacteria to epithelial cells can be quite specific owing to binding of bacteria to lectins (adhesins) on epithelial surfaces. Structures extending from bacteria, termed *pili,* or *fimbriae,* are active in attachment of certain bacteria to epithelial surfaces; for example, glycolipids of the globoseries are the specific receptors for *Escherichia coli* associated with pyelonephritis in human beings.

In addition to the highly specific adhesins necessary for attachment of certain bacteria to specific epithelial surfaces, a number of obstacles must be overcome by pathogenic bacteria before they become attached or are able to invade the host. These include competition for food, oxygen, or vital nutrients; local immune systems; a continual flow of body fluids, usually sweeping the organisms out of the body; and a continual turnover of epithelial cells. Some of the mechanisms by which indigenous organisms are able to inhibit the growth of organisms considered likely to cause disease in humans are listed in Table 2–1. A much more complete discussion of the interactions between the indigenous flora and potential pathogens can be found in the review article by Mackowiak.

BACTERIAL NOMENCLATURE

One of the annoying problems facing the practicing physician is the constant reclassification and changing names of microorganisms. One example is the renaming of the bacterium associated with pneumococcal pneumonia. Until 1967, this microorganism was officially known as *Diplococcus pneumoniae* in the United States. Although taxonomists recognized for many years that there were similarities between the streptococci and pneumococci, microbiologists in the United States preferred to separate the two by continuing to use a different genus name even though scientists in other parts of the world had decided that these microorganisms were related. In 1967, microbiologists in the United States agreed to reclassify this organism within the Streptococcaceae by approving a change in the name from *D. pneumoniae* to *Streptococcus pneumoniae.*

Although the reasons for changing the names of microorganisms are usually not relevant to the medical significance of the microorganism, physicians should be aware that nomenclature for microorganisms is constantly changing—that one should be able to recognize an old friend (or enemy) in new clothes. Three recent examples of nomenclature changes are the following: *Enterococcus faecalis* (formerly *Streptococcus faecalis*), *Helicobacter pylori* (formerly *Campylobacter pylori*), and *Morganella morganii* (formerly *Proteus morganii*).

The change in the name of a microorganism usually reflects a better understanding of genetic similarities or the recognition of taxonomic characteristics not previously appreciated. Perhaps the best method of judging relatedness between two closely related bacteria is to compare the similarities between their DNA content. When the similarity between two organisms is 80% or greater, the organisms are considered to be of the same species. Proposals for the change in names of bacteria are made to the International Commission on Microbial Taxonomy, which after careful consideration and in accordance with accepted rules and precedents gives an opinion. The decision of the commission to change a name is reflected in a report explaining the reasons for the change.

A large group of medically significant gram-negative bacteria is composed of the *nonfermenters,* so called because of their inability to ferment glucose anaerobically. A similar group of gram-negative bacteria is distinguished by its inability to oxidize glucose. Organisms in this group are usually less virulent for humans than the Enterobacteriaceae, although the infections they cause can be very difficult to treat owing to their resistance to many of the commonly

TABLE 2–2. *Nonfermentative Glucose-Oxidizing and Nonoxidizing Bacteria*

Glucose-Oxidizing Bacteria	Glucose-Nonoxidizing Bacteria
Pseudomonas aeruginosa	*Pseudomonas maltophilia*
cepacia	*denitrificans*
fluorescens	*diminuta*
pseudomallei	*alcaligenes*
stutzeri	*putrifaciens*
putida	*Alcaligenes facecalis*
vesicularis	*odorans*
Acinetobacter calcoaceticus	*denitrificans*
var. *anitratus*	*Acinetobacter calcoaceticus*
(*Herellea vaginicola*)	var. *lwoffi*
Flavobacterium meningosepticum species	(*Mima polymorpha*)
Kingella kingii	*Moraxella phenylpuruvica*
	Flavobacterium odoratum

used antimicrobial agents. The organism most frequently associated with infection in this group is *Pseudomonas aeruginosa,* which differs greatly from the Enterobacteriaceae in the types of infection it causes in humans and in the drugs needed for successful therapy. Many of the other members of this group of organisms are found in the indigenous microbiota. A partial list of the organisms in this group is given in Table 2–2.

INDIGENOUS MICROBIOTA BY ANATOMIC REGION

In this section, information about host–parasite characteristics and the indigenous microbiota related to various anatomic regions of the body are presented. No attempt is made to list all factors relevant to establishing the characteristic indigenous microbiota. Knowledge of the microorganisms normally found at different regions of the body is helpful in the interpretation of reports from the clinical microbiologic laboratory.

Skin

The skin shows wide variation in structure and function from one site of the body to another. For example, differences in the thickness of the epidermis and number and type of dermal appendages among the eyelid, axilla, and sole of the foot determine differences in the numbers and types of microbial populations. Ecologic factors vary greatly between the desquamating surface epithelial cells and the lumen of sebaceous glands deep in the dermis. Most skin bacteria are found on the superficial squamous epithelium, colonizing keratinized, dead cells.

Viruses such as varicella–zoster (chickenpox), require living cells for hosts and, therefore, infect cells found in or near the basal germinal layers of the epidermis. Lipophilic anaerobic bacteria, such as *Propionibacterium acnes,* live in the deep sebaceous glands and are not exposed to surface decontaminating solutions used prior to venipuncture. For this reason, it is not unusual to find propionibacteria in blood and cerebrospinal fluid cultures and cultures of bone marrow after 5 to 7 days of incubation, presumably as a result of skin contamination of the aspirating needle at the time of specimen collection (see Table 2–3).

As discussed earlier, normal skin has several mechanisms to control overgrowth and infection by resident bacteria. Sweat glands excrete lysozyme (muramidase), which may be effective in lysing *Staphylococcus epidermidis* and other gram-positive bacteria. Sebaceous glands secrete complex lipids, which may be partially

TABLE 2–3. *Microorganisms Found on the Skin*

Microorganism	Range of Incidence (%)
Staphylococcus-epidermidis (albus) (coagulase-negative)	85–100
S. aureus (coagulase-positive)	5–25
Streptococcus pyogenes (group A)	0–4
Propionibacterium acnes (anaerobic corynebacteria)	45–100
Aerobic corynebacteria (diphtheroids)	55
Lactobacilli	55
Candida albicans	Uncommon
Other *Candida* species, particularly *C. parapsilosis*	1–15
Clostridium perfringens (especially lower extremities)	40–60
Enterobacteriaceae	Uncommon
Acinetobacter calcoaceticus	25
Moraxella species	5–15
Mycobacterium species	Rare

degraded by specific enzymes from certain gram-positive bacteria. These bacteria can change the secreted lipids to unsaturated fatty acids with strong antimicrobial activity against gram-negative bacteria and certain fungi. Some of the resulting unsaturated fatty acids from bacterial degradation are volatile and may be associated with a strong odor. For this reason, deodorants have been formulated containing antibacterial substances that selectively act against gram-positive bacteria. Suppression of gram-positive bacteria may result in a shift of the skin bacterial population to predominantly gram-negative bacteria. Such a shift of flora, although reducing the amount of aromatic unsaturated fatty acids and presumably making deodorant users more socially acceptable, may also predispose them to colonization and possible infection by gram-negative bacteria.

Some important pathogens commonly found on skin are really transient residents that contaminate the area around orifices. The best example is *S. aureus,* which resides in the nostrils and perianal region but survives poorly elsewhere on the skin. Similarly, *Clostridium perfringens* usually contaminates only the perineum and thighs. In this location, however, it can cause gas gangrene in as many as 1% of the patients undergoing above-the-knee amputations for diabetic vascular insufficiency. One effort to control this threat involved application of iodophor compresses for 15 min before surgery and resulted in failure to isolate the organism from 60 patients who had previously yielded *C. perfringens* on skin culture.

Prior colonization of the skin by one bacterial species may prevent or retard colonization by another. This phenomenon has been termed *bacterial interference* and may result from preferential attachment to specific receptors of the bacterium and epithelial cells (see Chapter 3). During the early antibiotic era, infection by penicillin-resistant *S. aureus* strains of phage type 80/81 frequently appeared in newborn nurseries, where spread from mothers to infants and from infant to infant often occurred with frightening speed and disastrous results. In an attempt to reduce this threat, newborn infants were deliberately colonized with a strain of *S. aureus* designated 502A, which seemed to prevent or at least delay colonization of the infant by a more virulent *Staphylococcus*. The use of *S. aureus* 502A to produce bacterial interference by intentional colonization was of help in selected situations, but occasional infections appeared in susceptible infants.

Nose and Nasopharynx

The most common bacteria found in the nose are staphylococci, usually in highest numbers just inside the nares. In this location, both *Staphylococcus aureus* and *S. epidermidis* are considered to mirror the microbiota of the skin of the face at the nasolabial fold. Obtaining a culture of the posterior nasopharynx is difficult owing to the problem of passing a swab or wire through the nasal passages without contamination. Although special swabs are available for this purpose, they are used infrequently because of the decreased need for such cultures. Cultures of the posterior nasopharyngeal region are indicated when one is surveying suspected carriers or contacts of patients with diphtheria. Diphtheroids, a large, poorly classified group of gram-positive bacteria rarely associated with infection, are commonly found in the nose as well as in the nasopharynx (see Table 2–4).

Anaerobic bacteria may cause infection in the nasal sinuses, but systematic surveys to determine the incidence and species of different types of anaerobic bacteria in normal subjects have been difficult to obtain. For this reason, the normal anaerobic bacterial flora of the nasal passages, sinuses, and the nasopharynx are not well defined. Many of the anaerobic bacterial species found in the oropharynx are probably present within the nasal passages and the nasopharynx.

Although small numbers of *Streptococcus pneumoniae, Neisseria meningitidis,* and *Haemophilus influenzae* may be found in the nasopharynx, most are not encapsulated with the polysaccharides usually present in strains causing clinical infection. However, nonencapsu-

TABLE 2–4. *Microorganisms Found in the Nose and Nasopharynx*

Microorganism	Range of Incidence (%)
Staphylococcus aureus	20–85
S. epidermidis	90
Aerobic corynebacteria (diphtheroids)	5–80
Streptococcus pneumoniae	0–17
S. pyogenes (group A)	0.1–10
Alpha- or nonhemolytic streptococci	Uncommon
Branhamella catarrhalis	12
Haemophilus influenzae	12
H. parainfluenzae	35–65
Neisseria meningitidis	0–10
Enterobacteriaceae	Uncommon
Moraxella nonliquefaciens	5–10

lated, nontypable *H. influenzae* are very important in the pathogenesis of acute, suppurative otitis media (see Chapter 9). The significance of these organisms in the patient without infection is not clear, but no attempt should be made to eradicate such organisms by antimicrobial drug therapy.

Oropharynx

Like the nose, the oropharynx contains large numbers of both *Staphylococcus aureus* and *S. epidermidis*.

The most important group of microorganisms native to the oropharynx are the alpha-hemolytic streptococci. Although the commonly used term for alpha-hemolytic streptococci,. *Streptococcus viridans*, is still used erroneously in many texts and by clinicians with the implication that it refers to a single bacterial species, the term actually applies to a large group of poorly classified streptococci that have in common the ability to produce alpha-hemolysis on sheep blood agar. Careful identification procedures can assign many of these alpha-hemolytic streptococci to well-defined species, including *S. mitis*, *S. mutans*, *S. milleri*, *S. sanguis*, *S. salivarius*, and others. Many laboratories do not speciate the alpha-hemolytic streptococci, but use simple identification kits now available. Speciation of alpha-hemolytic streptococci can be helpful when establishing the initial site of infection in patients with infective endocarditis.

Cultures from the oropharynx usually show large numbers of diphtheroids and *Branhamella catarrhalis*, small gram-negative cocci that are related in part to *Neisseria*. Although previously not considered to be capable of initiating infection in humans, *B. catarrhalis* has been well established as an infrequent cause of pneumonia and is an important microorganism in suppurative sinusitis and otitis media (see Chapter 9).

Cultures from patients with sore throat may show various types of bacteria associated with acute pharyngitis; Lancefield group A streptococci and *N. gonorrhoeae* are among them. Although *S. pneumoniae* and *Haemophilus influenzae* are occasionally recovered from patients with acute pharyngitis, they do not contribute to the signs and symptoms in these patients. In most instances, when these strains are studied further, they lack virulence factors such as serologically distinct capsules or other surface structures that characterize similar strains causing severe infectious disease (see Table 2–5).

TABLE 2–5. *Microorganisms Found in the Oropharynx*

Microorganism	Range of Incidence (%)
Staphylococcus aureus	35–40
S. epidermidis	30–70
Aerobic corynebacteria (diphtheroids)	50–90
Streptococcus pyogenes (group A)	0–9
S. pneumoniae	0–50
Alpha- and nonhemolytic streptococci	25–99
Streptococcus mutans	25–75
S. milleri	25–75
S. mitis	25–75
S. sanguis	25–75
S. salivarius	25–75
Branhamella catarrhalis	10–97
Neisseria meningitidis	0–15
Haemophilus influenzae	5–20
H. parainfluenzae	20–35
Gram-negative bacteria (e.g., *Klebsiella pneumoniae*)	Uncommon
Acinetobacter calcoaceticus	5–30
Anaerobic micrococci	Common
Anaerobic streptococci	Common
Bacteroides fragilis	Common
B. melaninogenicus	Common
B. oralis	Common
Fusobacterium necrophorum	Common
Campylobacter sputorum	5

One of the most interesting aspects of the microbial flora of the pharynx is the relationship of alpha-hemolytic streptococci to other bacteria in this region. A series of clinical studies has suggested that certain constituents of normal throat flora, antagonistic to group A streptococci *in vitro*, may provide a defense mechanisms against group A streptococcal infections. Strains of *S. salivarius* were among the most active antagonists and were found more often in the throat cultures of children who did not become colonized following exposure to epidemic strains of group A streptococci than from children who did become colonized. It was found that cell-free filtrates of *S. salivarius* inhibited the growth of group A streptococci but that this inhibition could be reversed by pantothenate. The activity was apparently not due to a simple depletion of the vitamin but rather to the presence of a substance that interfered with the utilization of pantothenate.

Factors such as the administration of antibiotics or the length of hospital stay may also be associated with modification of the pharyngeal flora. Several studies have suggested that the most important factor in pharyngeal colonization by gram-negative bacilli is the severity of the patient's underlying illness. Seriously ill or moribund patients are more likely to have gram-negative bacteria in the pharynx than those less seriously ill. Severity of illness was more highly correlated with colonization than was length of hospital stay or the history of antibiotic administration. Colonization of the pharynx was also found to be associated with an increased risk of pneumonia by gram-negative bacteria. The reason for colonization by gram-negative bacteria in this group of patients is not yet known. One suggestion is a change in the bacterial adhesins on pharyngeal epithelial cells from those favoring gram-positive bacteria to those favoring gram-negative organisms.

Mouth

The microbial flora of the mouth show marked individual variations, depending on the presence or absence of teeth and the presence or absence of caries. With the development of teeth in the child, different strains of streptococci appear. Some strains have a predilection for tooth surfaces (*Streptococcus sanguis* and *S. mutans*), whereas others attach to the buccal and gingival epithelial surfaces *(S. salivarius)*. Dental manipulation and tooth extraction, in particular, result in transitory bacteremia due to these streptococcal species and are important in the development of infective endocarditis (see Chapter 35). The presence of these streptococci and other oral bacteria contributes to the formation of dental plaque, which in turn results in a low oxidation–reduction potential on the surface of the tooth. The reduced oxidation–reduction potential supports the growth of strict anaerobic bacteria such as *Bacteroides melaninogenicus,* *B. oralis,* and *Veillonella alcalescens,* particularly between opposing teeth and in the dental–gingival crevices. *S. mutans,* one of the bacterial strains showing a predilection for attachment to tooth surfaces, is commonly associated with dental caries. The presence of a cavity in a tooth permits increased bacterial colonization and growth with further reduction in the oxidation–reduction potential. In this manner, uncontrolled dental caries predispose to large numbers of anaerobic bacteria and oral treponemes. Patients with advanced dental caries are at particular risk of incurring anaerobic pulmonary infections should they inadvertently aspirate oral–pharyngeal secretions. Upon extraction of carious teeth and removal of protected sites for bacterial colonization and growth, the number of anaerobic bacteria and treponemes in the mouth falls rapidly (see Table 2–6).

TABLE 2–6. *Microorganisms Found in the Mouth (Saliva—Tooth Surfaces)*

Microorganism	Range of Incidence (%)
Staphylococcus epidermidis (coagulase-negative)	75–100
S. aureus (coagulase-positive)	10–35
Streptococcus mitis and other alpha-hemolytic streptococci	100
S. sanguis	100
S. salivarius	100
S. mutans	100
Enterococci	5–20
Peptostreptococci	Prominent
Anaerobic micrococci	100
Veillonella alcalescens	100
Lactobacilli	95
Actinomyces israelii	Common
Enterobacteriaceae	65
Eikenella corrodens	0–5
Bacteroides fragilis	Common
B. melaninogenicus	Common
B. oralis	Common
Fusobacterium nucleatum	15–90
Mycobacteria	0–3
Candida albicans	6–50
Treponema denticola and *T. refringens*	Common / Common

Stomach

Under ordinary circumstances, the stomach does not contain many viable microorganisms because of the very acid pH of gastric contents. Most bacteria are either inactivated or killed when swallowed and exposed to a pH of 2 to 3 for even a short time. Exceptions may occur if there is rapid passage of microorganisms through the stomach or if the microorganisms are particularly resistant to gastric acidity (e.g., mycobacteria). Following ingestion of food, the number of bacteria increase, only to fall with gastric emptying. Changes in the gastric microflora also occur if there is an increase in gastric pH following high intestinal obstruction, thus permitting reflux of alkaline duodenal and jejunal secretions into the stomach. In addition, the acid barrier of the stomach is not intact in neonates or in those who have undergone gastrectomy. The bacterial content of the stomach is then likely to reflect that of the oropharynx and in addition includes both gram-negative aerobic and anaerobic bacteria (see Table 2–7).

Small Intestine

The upper portion of the small intestine contains few bacteria because of the combined influence

TABLE 2–7. *Microorganisms Found in the Stomach and Small Intestine*

Microorganism	Range of Incidence (%)
Stomach—usually sterile, owing to gastric pH of 2–3	
Jejunum—gram-positive facultative bacteria (enterococci, lactobacilli, diphtheroids)	Small numbers
—strict anaerobic bacteria	Uncommon
Ileum—distal portion may show small numbers of Enterobacteriaceae and anaerobic gram-negative bacteria	
—*Candida albicans*	40

of the strongly acid environment in the stomach and the inhibitory action of bile on many microorganisms. Of the bacteria present, gram-positive cocci and bacilli compose the majority. *Enterococcus faecalis* (group D streptococci), lactobacilli, and diphtheroids are occasionally found in the jejunum, representing organisms that best withstand the inhibitory effect of both bile and pancreatic secretions (see Table 2–7). The presence of diverticula of the duodenum or small intestine may create blind pockets and be associated with the proliferation of large numbers of bacteria, which can modify the microbiota of the intestine at that level. Occasionally, a duodenal diverticulum has been associated with such large numbers of bacteria as to impair the absorption of vitamin B_{12}.

The indigenous microbiota of the biliary tract are not known; however, in patients without biliary disease the bile is commonly sterile. Bacteria may be found in the bile ducts and gallbladder as the result of transphincteric reflux or of occasional invasion of the portal blood system from the intestinal tract and excretion by the liver. The antibacterial activity of bile limits the types of bacteria that can survive. Organisms that can tolerate bile salts include the *Salmonella* species (especially *S. typhi*), *Enterococcus faecalis*, *Clostridium perfringens*, and *Bacteroides fragilis*. Conversely, susceptibility of pneumococci to the surface-active properties of bile makes infection with these organisms uncommon in the hepatobiliary tract.

Candida albicans can be recovered from the distal small intestine in 40% of healthy people. Although colonization with *C. albicans* is not a problem for the normal person, patients receiving immunosuppressive therapy or those with lymphomas or leukemias that involve lymphoid tissue in Peyer's patches of the distal ileum are at special risk of developing either local or disseminated candidiasis. Antitumor chemotherapy can result in necrosis of the involved submucosal lymphoid tissue, providing a portal of entry for *Candida*. Because many of these patients also have defects in their humoral and cellular immune systems, they are at high risk for candidemia and disseminated *Candida* infection.

Occasionally, the administration of antibiotics to patients in preparation for intestinal surgery results in the overgrowth of large numbers of yeast. This can result from suppression of the facultatively anaerobic Enterobacteriaceae.

In the distal portion of the small intestine, the indigenous flora begin to take on the characteristics of the colonic flora. Increasing numbers of anaerobic bacteria appear, along with Enterobacteriaceae and enterococci. Modification of the normal small-intestinal motility pattern or anatomic relationships following surgical procedures for obstruction or intestinal bypass can result in bacterial overgrowth, producing a number of clinical syndromes.

Large Intestine

The colon has by far the largest microbial population in the body. The number of microorganisms in stool specimens approaches 10^{12} organisms per gram. This tremendous number of colonic microorganisms consists primarily of anaerobic, gram-negative, non–spore-forming bacteria, and gram-positive, spore-forming, and non–spore-forming bacilli. Not only are the vast majority of the microorganisms anaerobic, but there are also large numbers of different species involved. Several investigators have calculated the ratio of strictly anaerobic to facultative anaerobic (Enterobacteriaceae) bacteria at approximately 300:1. Less than 0.3% of all bacteria in the stool are members of the family Enterobacteriaceae or related species.

In elaborate studies to determine the qualitative and quantitative fecal microbiota, 93% of the bacteria estimated to be present by direct Gram's stain of serial dilutions of fecal specimens were recovered by culture. One hundred thirteen separate species of microorganisms were found, each representing at least 0.05% of the flora. The frequency of bacterial species and their relative percentage of fecal population are listed in part in Table 2–8.

Variability in the virulence of the different microorganisms in the colon is illustrated by the

TABLE 2–8. Relative Frequency of Bacterial Species in Fecal Flora

Rank	Percent	Organism(s)
1	12	Bacteroides vulgatus
2	7	Fusobacterium prausnitzi
3	6.5	Bacteroides adolescentia
4	6	Eubacterium aerofaciens
5	6	Peptostreptococcus productus II
6	4.5	Bacteroides thetaiotaomicron
7	3.6	Eubacterium eligens
8	3.3	Peptostreptococcus productus I
9	3.2	Eubacterium biforme
10	2.5	Eubacterium aerofaciens III
11	2.3	Bacteroides distasonis
28	0.7	Bacteroides ovatus
29	0.6	Bacteroides fragilis
59–75	0.13	Enterococcus faecalis
76–113	0.06	Escherichia coli, Klebsiella pneumoniae, and 37 other bacterial species

Adapted from Moore, W. E. C., and Holdeman, L. V. The human fecal flora of 20 Japanese-Hawaiians. *Appl. Microbiol.* 27:916, 1974.

several species of *Bacteroides* and their incidence of recovery from clinical sites of infection (Table 2–9). The number of infections yielding *B. vulgatus,* which comprises approximately 12% of the fecal flora, is much lower than those associated with *B. fragilis,* the organism ranked twenty-ninth in fecal flora, constituting only 0.6% of the flora. The reasons for this difference in virulence are not entirely clear but are considered to be related in part to the capsule on *B. fragilis* that is not present on other *Bacteroides* species.

The incidence of *Escherichia coli* in the flora of the colon is also at variance with its presence in clinical infection, where it is the most common agent in urinary tract infection and is frequently found in infections complicating abdominal surgery. The factor or factors that predispose to infection with this organism, in contrast to *B. vulgatus* or other more commonly found bacteria, are not known.

One of the most common microorganisms associated with gas gangrene, *Clostridium perfringens,* has been found in low numbers in the stools of 25 to 35% of normal subjects (see Table 2–10). *C. perfringens* appears on the skin and in the biliary tract as a result of organisms present in the colon. This organism, as well as other *Clostridium* species, is available for growth and production of toxic enzymes whenever trauma or surgery involves the contents of the colon with a decrease in the local E_h. Similarly, the presence of *C. perfringens* within the biliary tract without evidence of gas-producing infection suggests that the organism is readily available but has not yet caused disease.

The recovery of certain species of bacteria from blood cultures can be associated with a previously inapparent, ulcerating malignant lesion of the colon. Examples include *C. septicum* and *Streptococcus bovis,* a member of the Lancefield group D streptococci. With *S. bovis,* the patient may have infective endocarditis, but carcinoma of the colon is present in many cases. The incidence of *S. bovis* in the colon is not clearly established.

Table 2–10 lists a few representative species of the bacterial flora of the colon. In many instances, it is likely that the ability of these bacteria to invade tissues and cause infectious disease may be related to complex interactions among species, such as that referred to previously between *Bacteroides melaninogenicus* and the anaerobic diphtheroids.

Factors associated with establishing colonization of certain strains of bacteria at different sites in the body are discussed above and in Chapter 3. Briefly, indigenous microorganisms in the gastrointestinal tract can inhibit or pre-

TABLE 2–9. Anaerobic Bacterial Isolates, Northwestern Memorial Hospital, Chicago, Illinois

			Source of Isolates					
	Rank Frequency	Blood	Blood Culture— Autopsy	GI Tract	TTA-* PULM	GU Tract	Wounds	Abscess
Bacteroides vulgatus	1	4	5	1	2	1	7	7
B. thetaiotaomicron	6	3	2	4	1	1	6	6
B. distasonis	11–12	1	0	2	0	2	6	2
B. ovatus	25–28	1	1	0	0	0	5	1
B. fragilis	29	28	4	9	3	3	32	13
B. melaninogenicus		0	0	1	3	3	10	21
Bacteroides species†		14	6	15	21	15	72	37
Fusobacterium nucleatum		0	0	5	2	1	5	8
Fusobacterium species		1	4	3	1	2	9	10

*Transtracheal aspiration.
†To include *Bacteroides oralis,* ruminicola subsp. *brevis,* and clostridiformis subsp. *clostridiformis, capillosis, corrodens,* and *amylophilus.*

TABLE 2–10. *Microorganisms Found in the Large Intestine*

Microorganism	Range of Incidence (%)
Anaerobic Bacteria (300 Times as Many Anaerobic Bacteria as Facultative Aerobic Bacteria [e.g., Escherichia coli])	
Gram-Negative Bacilli (non–spore-forming)	
Bacteroides fragilis	100
B. melaninogenicus (3 subspecies)	100
B. oralis (2 subspecies)	100
Fusobacterium nucleatum	100
F. necrophorum	100
Gram-Positive Bacilli (with and without spores)	
lactobacilli	20–60
Clostridium difficile	0–3
C. perfringens	25–35
C. innocuum	5–25
C. ramosum	5–25
C. septicum	5–25
C. tetani	1–35
Eubacterium limosum	30–70
Bifidobacterium bifidum	30–70
Gram-Positive Cocci	
peptostreptococci (anaerobic streptococci)	Common
peptococci (anaerobic staphylococci)	Moderate
Facultative Aerobic and Anaerobic Bacteria	
Gram-Positive Cocci	
Staphylococcus aureus (associated with nasal carriage)	30–50
enterococci (group D streptococcus)	100
streptococci (group B, C, F, and G)	0–16
Gram-Negative Bacilli	
Enterobacteriaceae	100
Escherichia coli	100
Shigella (group A–D)	0–1
Salmonella enteritidis (2200 serotypes)	3–7
S. typhi	0.0001
Klebsiella species	40–80
Enterobacter species	40–80
Proteus mirabilis and other *Proteus* and *Providencia* species	5–55
Pseudomonas aeruginosa	3–11
Candida albicans	15–30

vent infections by *Vibrio cholerae, Shigella,* or *Salmonella.* Mechanisms for such interference include the production of antibiotics or bacteriocins by one group of organisms against a second, microbial competition for nutrients in one environment as compared with another, or susceptibility of one strain of bacteria to toxic substances produced by a second strain. An example of the third mechanism is the inhibitory effect of volatile, short-chain, fatty organic acids produced by anaerobic bacteria on the growth of *Salmonella typhimurium.* Similar susceptibility by other bacteria to short-chain fatty acids—produced in large quantity by anaerobic bacteria—signficantly inhibits growth and viability of *Shigella, Pseudomonas aeruginosa,* and *Klebsiella pneumoniae.*

The role of bacterial–epithelial attachment has recently been recognized as a factor in establishing infection in the gastrointestinal tract. Attachment of *V. cholerae* to epithelial cells in the small intestine can be prevented by specific IgA (see Chapter 19). Motility of the intestinal tract can also influence the composition of the intestinal microbiota. Rapid peristalsis is of significant value in maintaining low levels of indigenous flora in the small intestine (see also Table 2–1). Intestinal obstruction may quickly result in bacterial overgrowth in the proximal segment.

Genitourinary Tract

In the normal human, the kidneys, ureters, and urinary bladder do not have a microbial flora. In both the male and female, there may be a few bacteria present in the distal portion of the urethra; however, these are confined to short segments near the meatus, and the numbers of bacteria near the sphincter of the urinary bladder are usually negligible (see Table 2–11). In contrast, the adult female genital tract has very complex microbial flora, constantly changing with the variation of the menstrual cycle. Shortly after birth, the vagina becomes populated with lactobacilli (Döderlein's bacilli). As the infant loses the effect of maternal progesterone stimulation, lactobacilli disappear but return with menarche and the development of endogenous endocrine stimulation. Lactobacilli are so named because they produce lactic acid. A large population of lactobacilli helps maintain the pH of the vagina and external cervical os at approximately 4.4–4.6. Lactobacilli are characteristic of the menarcheal female and are not present in the prepubertal or postmenopausal periods. At this pH, many of the gram-negative bacteria found in the gastrointestinal tract do not grow. *Escherichia coli* may be inhibited from active growth at a pH of less than 5.0, although some strains can grow, albeit poorly, in more acid environments. In addition to lactobacilli, microorganisms capable of proliferating at this low pH include the enterococci, *Candida albicans,* and large numbers of anaerobic bacteria, including *Clostridium perfringens.*

TABLE 2–11. *Microorganisms Found in the Genitourinary Tract*

Microorganism	Range of Incidence (%)
Kidneys and Urinary Bladder (Normally Sterile)	
Female and male urethra usually sterile except for short anterior segment	
Vagina and Uterine Cervix	
Lactobacillus	50–75
Bacteroides	60–80
Clostridium	15–30
Peptostreptococcus	30–40
Bifidobacterium	10
Eubacterium	5
Aerobic corynebacteria (diphtheroids)	45–75
Staphylococcus aureus	5–15
S. epidermidis	35–80
enterococci (group D streptococcus)	30–80
streptococci (usually group B)	5–20
Enterobacteriaceae	18–40
Moraxella osloensis	5–15
Acinetobacter	5–15
Candida albicans	30–50
Trichomonas vaginalis	10–25

Soluble products from certain of the Enterobacteriaceae and lactobacilli can be inhibitory to the growth of *Neisseria gonorrhoeae*. In one study, a significant relationship was demonstrated between lactobacilli and *N. gonorrhoeae* in which inhibitory lactobacilli were recovered less often from women infected with *N. gonorrhoeae* than from uninfected women. Similarly, among women having contact with an infected partner, those who subsequently developed gonorrhea were less likely to have inhibitory lactobacilli than those who did not become infected. Recovery of inhibitory lactobacilli on culture was highest during the 2 weeks following menses, while the recovery of *N. gonorrhoeae* was lowest. These observations suggest a protective effect against infection from *N. gonorrhoeae* by indigenous lactobacilli related in part to changes associated with the menstrual cycle.

The vagina is subject to cyclic fluctuations with normal hormonal variation. Progesterone tends to increase the content of glycogen in the epithelial cells, which in turn increases the amount of carbohydrate available for microbial growth. During the early development of birth control pills, vaginal candidiasis (moniliasis) was an annoying problem for many patients taking pills containing relatively large amounts of progesterone. It should be noted that a pH of 5.0–6.0 may be selective for *Candida* and other yeasts.

The cervicovaginal canal has large numbers of anaerobic gram-positive cocci, gram-negative bacilli, and clostridia, outnumbering aerobic bacteria by at least 5:1. Most of these organisms are capable of growth in the low pH of the vagina and ordinarily are not of much medical significance. They represent a considerable threat and may produce a serious infection, however, as a complication following induced abortion. Contamination of traumatized, devitalized, and partially necrotic endometrium with *Clostridium perfringens* can lead to serious and even fatal sepsis (see the Case History).

SELECTIVE ANTIMICROBIAL MODULATION

Since about 1970, increasingly aggressive treatment of leukemia including bone marrow transplantation has resulted in patients with severe granulocytopenia. The result of prolonged granulocytopenia is usually infection that is difficult to treat and often progresses to death. Infection in these patients often results from *Pseudomonas aeruginosa*, members of the Enterobacteriaceae (e.g., *Escherichia coli*, *Klebsiella pneumoniae*, and *Proteus* species), *Staphylococcus aureus*, and *Candida albicans*, but seldom from anaerobic bacteria. Initial efforts to control infection in such patients involved placing them in laminar-airflow rooms to reduce, if not eliminate, exogenous organisms. In addition, attempts were made to achieve near total suppression of the normal endogenous microbial flora by the use of antimicrobial agents in ointments, gels, and suppositories and by the oral administration of multiple nonabsorbable antibiotics selected to eliminate aerobic, facultative anaerobic, and anaerobic bacteria and yeasts. These rather heroic efforts accomplished some reduction in the infection rate, usually 50% or greater, but were associated with considerable expense of the laminar-flow isolation room and psychologic trauma to the patient because of separation from family members during the isolation period.

In 1972, van der Waaij described a phenomenon while working with germ-free animals. He found that if *E. coli* was introduced by mouth to germ-free animals, as few as 10 to 100 organisms could colonize the gastrointestinal tract, whereas the conventional animal required 10^7 or more organisms. He termed the capacity of the microbial flora to prevent colonization by new organisms "colonization resistance." In further studies, he noted that when a normal animal had its aerobic flora suppressed while the anaerobic flora flourished, about 10^6 organisms were needed to cause colonization; colonization resistance was effectively intact. It was theorized that since organisms that cause infection in the granulocytopenic patient are primarily the aerobic bacteria and yeasts, application of the concept of colonization resistance might be of clinical value. Antibiotics capable of reducing the aerobic flora of the colon without reducing the anaerobic flora protected the patient in large part from new organisms acquired from the hospital environment, many of which were resistant to antibiotics and likely to cause hospital-acquired infection.

This approach to infection control in severely granulocytopenic patients has been termed *selective antimicrobial modulation (SAM)* and may reduce significantly their incidence of infections and obviate the need for reverse isolation, eliminating the consequent psychologic trauma and expense.

Evaluation of various oral antimicrobial agents useful for SAM is still underway. Trimethoprim/sulfamethoxazole combined with nystatin or gentamicin and nystatin have been used. The recognition that SAM can substantially reduce the incidence of infection in the granulocytopenic patient is an important observation but should be tempered with the knowledge that naturally resistant organisms may overgrow the anaerobic bacterial flora and lead to serious infection.

SUMMARY

The objective of this chapter was to provide an overview of the bacterial organisms native to different regions of the body and to introduce nomenclature of the type seen on culture reports. Many microorganisms associated with clinical infection are those constituting the patient's indigenous microbiota. This host-derived source of microbial infectious agents again emphasizes the role of host defenses in the development of infection. As defined in Chapter 3, the terms *pathogen* and *nonpathogen* are relative terms and are better replaced by a concept of continual variation of factors constituting the host defense. This complex interaction may be influenced by antimicrobial agents, normal cyclic hormonal changes, acute and chronic disease, as well as by many other factors still to be recognized.

CASE HISTORY

From August 8 to October 14, five women with septic complications following abortion were admitted to a south Texas hospital. One died from septicemia and renal failure; *Clostridium perfringens* grew from a blood culture.

Hospital records at the 270-bed community facility revealed that only one patient with septic complications following abortion had been admitted during the previous year; two more women had such complications but were not admitted. Further investigation indicated that all five women had abortions in Mexico. All were of Hispanic descent; four were U.S. citizens.

Endometrial or blood cultures or both from three of the women grew *C. perfringens;* a fourth patient had tetanus. Details of the fatal case follow.

A 27-year-old woman was hospitalized September 26, with fever, knee pain, and lower abdominal pain. In the previous 4 years, she had one previous live birth and one abortion. On September 1 and September 19, she had consulted her physician about sternal pain. On the second visit, when she indicated that she might be pregnant, he informed her that Medicaid no longer paid for abortions. She subsequently obtained an induced abortion in Mexico. On September 26 she was hospitalized with admission temperature of 101.8°F (38.8°C), blood pressure of 110/80, and pulse of 110. Her uterus was markedly tender and was not easily examined because of abdominal guarding. *C. perfringens* was grown from blood and endometrium. On September 27 a hysterectomy was performed to remove the focus of infection. Her condition continued to deteriorate, however, and she died October 3 from renal and cardiac failure.

REFERENCES

Book

Rosebury, T. *Microorganisms Indigenous to Man.* New York: McGraw-Hill Book Co., 1961.

Skinner, F. A., and Carr, J. G., eds. *The Normal Microbial Flora of Man.* London: Academic Press, 1974.

Review Articles

Mackowiak, P. A. The normal microbial flora. *N. Engl. J. Med. 307:*83, 1982.

Savage, D. C. Survival on mucosal epithelia, epithelial penetrations and growth in tissues of pathogenic bacteria. In: Smith, H., and Pearce, J. H., eds. *Microbial Pathogenicity in Man and Animals.* New York: Cambridge University Press, 1972.

Original Articles

Crow, C. C., Sanders, W. E., and Longley, S. Bacterial interference II. Role of the normal throat flora in prevention of colonization by group A *Streptococcus. J. Infect. Dis. 128:*527, 1973.

Gold, R., Goldschneider, I., Lepow, M. L., et al. Carriage of *Neisseria meningitidis* and *Neisseria lactamica* in infants and children. *J. Infect. Dis. 137:*112, 1978.

Gorbach, S. Intestinal microflora. *Gastroenterology 60:*1110, 1971.

Johanson, W. G., Pierce, A. K., and Sanford, J. P. Changing pharyngeal bacterial flora of hospitalized patients. Emergence of gram-negative bacilli. *N. Engl. J. Med. 281:*1137, 1969.

Johanson, W. G., Jr., Blackstack, R., Pierce, A. K., et al. The role of bacterial antagonism in pneumococcal colonization of the human pharynx. *J. Lab Clin. Med. 75:*946, 1970.

Liljemart, W. F., and Gibbon, R. J. Suppression of *Candida albicans* by human oral streptococci in gnotobiotic mice. *Infect. Immunol. 8:*846, 1973.

Marples, M. J. Life on the human skin. *Sci. Am. 220:*108, 1969.

Moore, W. E. C., and Holdeman, L. V. Human fecal flora: The normal flora of 20 Japanese-Hawaiians. *Appl. Microbiol. 27:*961, 1974.

Noble, W. C. Skin microbiology. *J. Med. Microbiol. 17:*1, 1984.

Ochman, H., and Wilson, A. C. Evolutionary history of enteric bacteria. In: Neidhardt, F. C., ed. *Escherichia coli* and *Salmonella typhimurium.* Washington, D.C.: American Society for Microbiology, 1987: 1649.

Pedersen, M. M., Marso, E., and Pickett, M. J. Nonfermentative bacilli associated with man. III. Pathogenicity and antibiotic susceptibility. *Am. J. Clin. Pathol. 54:*178, 1970.

Robbins, J. B., Schneerson, R., Argaman, M., et al. *Haemophilus influenzae* type b: Disease and immunity in humans. *Ann. Intern. Med. 78:*259, 1973.

Roszak, D. B., and Colwell, R. R. Survival strategies of bacteria in the natural environment. *Microbiol. Rev. 51:*365, 1987.

Saigh, J.H., Sanders, C. C., and Sanders, W. E. Inhibition of *Neisseria gonorrhoeae* by aerobic and facultatively anaerobic components of the endocervical flora: Evidence for a protective effect against infection. *Infect. Immunol. 19:*704, 1978.

Sanders, C. C., and Sanders, W. E. Enocin: An antibiotic produced by *Streptococcus salivarius* that may contribute to protection against infections due to Group A streptococci. *J. Infect Dis. 146:*683, 1982.

Savage, D. C. Colonization by and survival of pathogenic bacteria on intestinal mucosal surfaces. In Britton, G., and Marshall, K. C., eds. *Adsorption of Microorganisms to Surfaces.* New York: John Wiley and Sons, 1980, pp. 175–206.

Schimpff, S. C. Infection prevention during prolonged granulocytopenia. *Ann. Intern. Med. 93:*358, 1980.

Sprunt, K., and Redman, W. Evidence suggesting importance of role of interbacterial inhibition to maintaining balance of normal flora. *Ann. Intern. Med. 68:*579, 1968.

Valenti, W. M., Trudell, R. G., and Bentley, D. W. Factors predisposing to oropharyngeal colonization with gram-negative bacilli in the aged. *N. Engl. J. Med. 298:*1108, 1978.

van der Waaij, D., Berghuis, J. S., and Lekkerkirk, J. E. C. Colonization resistance of the digestive tract of mice during systemic antibiotic treatment. *J. Hyg. (Camb.) 70:*605, 1972.

Verghese, A. and Berk, S. L. Is normal throat flora causing pneumonia in your patients? *Am. Rev. Resp. Dis. 125:*783, 1982.

Wells, C. L., Maddaus, M. A., and Simmons, R. L. Proposed mechanisms for the translocation of intestinal bacteria. *Rev. Infect. Dis. 10:*958, 1988.

3

STANFORD T. SHULMAN, M.D. • *JOHN P. PHAIR, M.D.*

Host–Bacteria Interactions

INTRODUCTION

This chapter is concerned particularly with host–bacteria interactions. Very little attention is given to the interactions of other infectious agents with the host. Many host–parasite or host–fungus interactions involve mechanisms basically similar to those for host–bacteria interactions. Chapter 4 deals separately with host–virus interactions. In this chapter we emphasize certain basic principles with which all medical students should become familiar.

Bacteria are traditionally divided into two broad categories: *pathogenic,* referring to disease-producing bacteria, and *nonpathogenic,* referring to those which are non–disease-producing. Classically pathogens have been thought to possess certain characteristics that empower them with disease-producing capacity. For example, *Clostridium tetani,* which causes tetanus, is capable of doing so by virtue of its ability to elaborate and release a potent exotoxin which then induces disease by directly affecting the nervous system. *Streptococcus pneumoniae* produces infection primarily because it is protected from phagocytosis by the presence of a large polysaccharide capsule. Although other examples of this kind exist, it should be emphasized that special disease-producing characteristics of bacteria and fungi, such as exemplified by *C. tetani* and *S. pneumoniae,* probably represent the exception rather than the rule. Increasingly, we recognize that many bacteria not ordinarily regarded as pathogens in fact are capable of producing infection and disease, particularly in circumstances in which the host's defense mechanisms are less than intact. Consequently, the distinction between a *pathogen* and a *nonpathogen* or between *virulent* and *nonvirulent,* or *avirulent,* microorganisms has rather blurred. It is perhaps more useful to think of *parasites,* defined as organisms living at the expense of other organisms, and *nonparasites,* which are defined as saprophytes that live on dead or decaying matter. All microorganisms that are human parasites may potentially produce infection and/or disease in humans and, therefore, can be considered potentially pathogenic in many instances, provided that the host defense mechanisms are impaired in some way. Nevertheless, it is common practice to use the terms *pathogen* and *nonpathogen* or *virulent* and *avirulent* to indicate the *relative* capacity of parasites to cause disease. It should be apparent that there exists a continuum of disease-producing capability.

Human hosts with impaired immunologic or impaired nonimmunologic defense systems are increasingly commonly encountered in medicine, particularly as a result of organ transplantation, immunosuppressant regimens for the treatment of a variety of disorders, and the increasing prevalence of acquired immunodeficiency syndrome (AIDS) (see Chapter 26). Consequently, in the study of host–parasite interactions, emphasis is shifting from the more traditional consideration of only parasitic factors to those that affect host defenses and the ability of the host to react to an infecting agent. The development of an infection, as well as its eradication, very frequently comes down ultimately to issues that are defined more by the host than by the microbial parasite.

MICROBIAL ENVIRONMENT AND RESERVOIRS OF INFECTION

All animals, including man, live in a polymicrobial environment. We are all inhabited by huge numbers of diverse types of microorganisms that constitute our indigenous *microbiota,* or our *normal microbial flora.* These microorganisms are all parasites because they live on the skin or mucous membranes or within the lumen of the gut at the expense of the host, or, occasionally, within cells in tissues. All of these indigenous microorganisms are potentially disease-producing, depending upon the state of the host's defenses (see Chapter 2).

In addition, man is also in contact with a large exogenous population of microbes. This consists of the vast array of bacteria, fungi, and other microorganisms in soil and water, in air, in dust particles, and in our food. Most of these exogenous microbes are saprophytes that do not produce disease under ordinary circumstances. However, some are important disease-producing bacteria, such as *Clostridium tetani; C. botulinum,* which produces food poisoning; and *Bacillus anthracis,* which causes anthrax.

Lower animals possess another large microbial population. Many of these microbes can produce disease not only in the lower animals themselves but also in humans under appropriate circumstances when contact with an infected lower animal occurs. In some circumstances transmission of microorganisms from animal to man occurs by a vector such as an insect or arthropod. An entire group of human infections are classified as *zoonoses,* that is, diseases of animals that are transmissible to man. Several of the most important zoonoses are described in Chapter 31.

When considering these three general reservoirs of microorganisms (human beings, exogenous environmental microbes, and animal microbes), the most important by far is the human being. When host resistance is lowered, the normal microbial flora may invade and multiply, producing opportunistic infections (see Chapter 27). In addition, certain bacteria or fungi with great capacity to produce disease may be harbored by only a few individuals and then transmitted from these individuals to other more susceptible hosts, who may then develop infection and disease. Persons who harbor potential disease-producing microorganisms are frequently termed *carriers.* Carriers may be *diseased,* such as an individual with active pulmonary tuberculosis who is excreting large numbers of tubercle bacilli in the sputum, or *healthy.* An example of the latter is an individual who has recovered from typhoid fever but retains *Salmonella typhi* as a chronic low-grade infection in the gallbladder and subsequently asymptomatically excretes *S. typhi* in the stool, thus serving as a source of infection to others.

TRANSMISSION OF MICROORGANISMS

Because people are a major source of microorganisms capable of producing disease in humans, conditions that increase the rate of contact among humans promotes transmission of microorganisms from person to person and, therefore, increases the chance of development of disease. Crowding encourages respiratory transmission of microorganisms through coughing and sneezing, processes in which mucous droplets laden with bacteria are expelled from the respiratory tract into the air. These are called *droplet nuclei* and may remain suspended in the atmosphere for a considerable time, thereby available for inhalation by other individuals. This is a relatively efficient means of transmission of microorganisms from person to person. Excellent examples of diseases that are promoted by crowded conditions include tuber-culosis and streptococcal pharyngitis (see Chapters 9 and 15).

The hands of medical care workers are very important in the transmission of microorganisms, particularly within the hospital environment. Therefore, handwashing represents the best and most effective preventive measure against the presence of nosocomial (hospital-acquired) infections.

More intimate forms of contact, such as kissing and sexual intercourse, promote transfer of microorganisms that have disease-producing potential. Epstein-Barr virus infection is facilitated by kissing, and the increasing problems related to venereal diseases, including acquired immunodeficiency syndrome (AIDS), demonstrate the efficiency of sexual contact in transmission of infectious agents, including bacteria.

Person-to-person spread by more indirect means also occurs. Excellent examples of this kind of bacterial transmission are shigella or salmonella spread through food contaminated by a food handler who is shedding these organisms fecally, and water-borne epidemics of diseases such as typhoid fever. Adequate sewage disposal and water purification systems are essential for the prevention of water-borne epidemics of typhoid fever and many other infections spread by fecally contaminated water supplies. The development of modern sewage systems has contributed very significantly to the decreased prevalence of epidemic infectious diseases that ravaged the Western world in the Middle Ages.

Humans may acquire infection from nonhuman sources by contamination of wounds from soil or from soil contaminated by animal or human excreta. Neonatal tetanus is an example of this kind of infection in the Third World, where the umbilical cord is often deliberately or accidentally contaminated by bacteria-containing materials such as soil. Another mechanism for the spread of infection is direct human contact with infected lower animals. An example of this is the rabbit hunter who kills and skins a rabbit infected with tularemia and then acquires this zoonosis as the result of direct contact with the microorganisms. Additionally, transmission of infection to humans from other humans or from infected lower animals may occur by means of arthropod vectors, including mosquitos, mites, flies, and ticks. This mechanism is particularly important in the transmission of many viral and protozoal diseases.

ATTRIBUTES OF PATHOGENIC BACTERIA

The term *pathogen* means that a microorganism can, at least under certain circumstances, produce disease. The degree of pathogenicity of a microorganism is referred to as its *virulence.* Therefore, two pathogenic bacterial strains may differ in virulence in that one strain requires fewer microorganisms to produce infection under a given circumstance. It is common to treat the terms *pathogenicity* and *virulence* as synonymous, indicating that a microorganism is more or less pathogenic or more or less virulent under particular circumstances.

Different species differ widely in their capacity to produce progressive infection and disease. On one end of the spectrum, a single viable microorganism may be sufficient to produce disease (e.g., *Rickettsia tsutsugamushi*), whereas for other microbes, a million or more organisms may be required to produce disease (e.g., *Salmonella typhi*).

Only two general attributes are required for a parasite to produce disease. First, it must be able to metabolize and multiply in or on host tissues. That is, the microorganism must be able to find an oxygen tension, pH, temperature, and nutritional milieu appropriate for its growth. Second, assuming that the conditions are suitable for metabolism and multiplication, a pathogen must possess the ability to resist host defense mechanisms long enough to reach the critical numbers required to produce overt disease. Any existing impairment of host defense mechanisms clearly aids the establishment of a microbial infection.

CLASSIFICATION OF DISEASE-PRODUCING MICROORGANISMS

Extracellular Parasites

Extracellular parasites (Table 3–1) are microorganisms that produce infection after multiplying primarily or exclusively outside phagocytic cells. These microbes are generally readily destroyed when phagocytized by phagocytic cells such as neutrophils. These extracellular parasites produce disease in humans when they can resist ready phagocytosis, as is seen with the encapsulated bacteria such as *Streptococcus pneumoniae* or *Haemophilus influenzae*, in which the polysaccharide capsule is antiphagocytic, or in circumstances where impairment of

TABLE 3–1. *Classification of Pathogenic Microorganisms*

Genus	Species	Extracellular Parasite	Facultative Intracellular Parasite	Obligate Intracellular Parasite
Bacteria				
Actinobacillus	actinomycetemcomitans	+		
Actinomyces	israelii		+	
Bacillus	anthracis	+		
Bordetella	pertussis	+		
Brucella	(all species)		+	
Clostridium	(all species)	+		
Corynebacterium	diphtheriae	+		
Escherichia	coli	+		
Francisella	tularensis		+	
Haemophilus	(all species)	+		
Klebsiella	pneumoniae	+		
Legionella	pneumophila		+	
Listeria	monocytogenes		+	
Mycobacterium	(all species except *leprae*)		+	
Mycobacterium	leprae			+
Mycoplasma	pneumoniae	+		
Neisseria	gonorrhoeae	+		
Neisseria	meningitidis	+		
Nocardia	(all species)		+	
Pasteurella	multocida	+?		
Proteus	(all species)	+		
Pseudomonas	aeruginosa and others	+		
Salmonella	(all species)	+?	+?	
Serratia	(all species)	+		
Shigella	(all species)	+		
Staphylococcus	aureus and epidermidis	+		
Streptococcus	(all species)	+		
Vibrio	cholerae	+		
Yersinia	pestis		+	
Chlamydiae				
Chlamydia	psittaci and trachomatis			+
Fungi				
Blastomyces	dermatitidis		+	
Candida	albicans		+	
Coccidioides	immitis		+	
Cryptococcus	neoformans		+	
Epidermophyton	(all species)	+?		
Histoplasma	capsulatum		+	
Microsporum	(all species)	+?		
Monosporium	apiospermum	+?		
Sporothrix	schenckii	+?		
Trichophyton	(all species)	+?		
Rickettsiae				
Coxiella	burnetii			+
Rickettsia	(all species)			+
Spirochaeta				
Borrelia	(all species)	+		
Leptospira	(icterohaemorrhagiae interrogans)	+		
Treponema	pallidum	+	+	
Treponema	pallidum subsp. pertenue	+		

phagocytic mechanisms exist, such as in the quantitative (neutropenia) or qualitative (chronic granulomatous disease) deficiency of phagocytic cells.

Facultative Intracellular Parasites

Facultative intracellular parasites are generally readily phagocytosed but are resistant to intracellular killing by the phagocytic cells. Most of the organisms in this category are those which infect reticuloendothelial cells and lead to granuloma formation. The classic example of a facultative intracellular parasite is *Mycobacterium tuberculosis*.

Obligate Intracellular Parasites

Obligate intracellular parasites cannot multiply at all unless they are within host cells. Generally they utilize some of the metabolic apparatus of the host cell for their nutritional and/or energy supply. Some of these microbes are found in reticuloendothelial cells but others, such as rickettsiae, are found primarily in the endothelial cells of blood vessels. The pathogenesis of a particular infectious disease of course depends in large part upon the type of parasite producing the disease. All viruses and virtually all rickettsiae are obligate intracellular parasites, whereas bacteria and fungi tend to be extracellular or facultative intracellular parasites.

EXTERNAL BARRIERS TO INFECTION

The human host, although colonized or in contact with many bacteria, fungi, protozoa, or viruses usually does not develop clinical disease. This resistance to disease is due both to external barriers and complex systemic defense mechanisms that protect against invasion by microbes. External defenses include skin and mucous membranes and their secretions. It is necessary to understand that systemic mechanisms interact with these structures and their secretions so that discussing host defenses separately from one another is an artificial oversimplification.

This external system obviously is not totally protective, and infection, defined as tissue invasion, is favored by circumstances which interfere with these protective barriers. Examples of defects include achlorhydria, penetrating wounds from trauma or surgery, smoking (which alters the respiratory epithelium), or urinary bladder catheterization (which allows introduction of bacteria and fungi into the bladder).

Skin

The skin presents a mechanical barrier to invasion from organisms colonizing its external layers. Its outer layer, the cornified epithelium or epidermis is constantly shed, carrying with it surface bacteria. In addition, the pH of the skin is acidic, inhibiting many disease-producing microorganisms. Long-chain fatty acids secreted by sebaceous glands also inhibit replication of many bacteria. Finally, the resident normal flora have evolved mechanisms favoring their ability to colonize the skin and they compete successfully with pathogenic bacteria for living space on human skin.

Respiratory Tract

The upper respiratory tract is exposed constantly to inspired microorganisms on particulate matter and droplets. The nasal hairs create turbulence of the inspired air, which favors the trapping of such particles by the mucous membranes of the air passages. The nasal turbinates present a large surface for trapping inhaled particulate matter. The trapped particles are transported by the ciliated epithelium to the oropharynx and these secretions are periodically swallowed. Small particles can pass into the lower airways, and a similar transport system, the mucociliary elevator, again directs a flow of secretions to the oropharynx where it is swallowed. The smallest particles, 10 μm in diameter, can reach the alveoli, where they are phagocytosed by alveolar macrophages. The mucous secretions of the respiratory tract contain antibacterial substances such as lysozyme and phagocytes which aid in defending the host against infection. In addition, as discussed below, these secretions contain specific antibody which can prevent adherence of bacteria to the epithelial cells, neutralize specific viruses, and aid in phagocytosis. Finally, the resident normal flora of the upper respiratory tract plays a role in protecting the host from colonization by pathogenic organisms.

Alimentary Tract

The first line of defense of the gastrointestinal tract is constant swallowing, which acts to flush great numbers of organisms into the stomach. The normally acid stomach then eliminates the majority of ingested microbes. Achlorhydria, either due to disease or induced by therapy designed to prevent or treat peptic ulcer disease, is associated with enteric infection. An example of such an enteric infection is typhoid fever, which can be induced in achlorhydric volunteers with a much lower inoculum of ingested *Salmonella typhi* compared with subjects with normally acid gastric secretions. The upper small bowel contains few bacteria, but at the distal end of the ileum the small intestine normally is heavily colonized with colonic flora. With normal peristaltic activity the colonic and terminal ileal flora are evacuated in the feces. Fifty percent or more of dry fecal material consists of microorganisms. This mechanical activity represents a normal defense mechanism. Augmented peristalsis resulting in diarrhea induced by enteric infection is a further example of this protective host response.

Genitourinary Tract

Except for the terminal urethra, the urinary tract is sterile. The flushing associated with urination aids the antibacterial effects of urea, prostate secretions in men, and pH in maintaining sterile urine. In women the genital tract is colonized by lactobacilli which provide an acidic medium in the vagina, inhibitory to pathogenic microorganisms.

Eye

The flushing produced by tears serves to protect the eye from infection. Tears also contain lysozyme, an effective antibacterial substance.

ATTACHMENT OF BACTERIA TO EPITHELIAL SURFACES

From the preceding discussion of external host defenses, it is clear that if microorganisms encountered by a host are eliminated by these mechanisms, infection and disease do not occur. Infection does occur, however, when one or more defense mechanisms fail or even in the presence of apparently normally functioning defense mechanisms. In either circumstance, microorganisms must become attached to epithelial surfaces for infection to occur. The exception to this relates to skin where only *Staphylococcus aureus* and certain fungi appear to attach to epithelial surfaces as an important early step in infection. However, in infections of the respiratory tract, the gastrointestinal tract, or the genitourinary tract, mucosal surfaces are very important as sites of attachment for infection-producing microorganisms. It appears that most bacterial pathogens that infect humans or animals by way of mucosal surfaces preferentially attach to certain epithelial cells as an early step in the induction of disease.

This attachment of microorganisms to epithelial cells appears to occur usually through amazingly specific surface interactions. For example, studies of the attachment of streptococcal strains that are normal mouth inhabitants indicate that certain species of alpha-hemolytic (viridans) streptococci readily adhere to epithelial cells of the cheek and tongue, but not to the teeth. However, other alpha-hemolytic streptococci, such as *Streptococcus mutans*, preferentially attach to tooth surfaces, but not to the mucosal cells of cheek and tongue. It is likely that the specific attachment or adherence of bacteria to mucosal surfaces actually accounts for the characteristic distribution of the indigenous microbial flora in the upper respiratory tract and intestinal tract. The indigenous microbial flora of the intestinal tract appear to vary markedly from one anatomic site to another but are relatively constant at a given level of the intestinal tract from animal to animal. The basis for this constancy is also probably specific attachment to specific cell receptors. In general, more pathogenic strains of bacteria appear to attach more firmly to epithelial surfaces than less pathogenic strains do.

CONSEQUENCES OF ATTACHMENT

The normal bacterial flora appear to be of some importance regarding the prevention of infection. For example, penicillin therapy may suppress the normal bacterial flora of the upper respiratory tract, particularly alpha-hemolytic streptococci, and fungi such as *Candida albicans* may then attach, colonize the oral and pharyngeal mucosae, and produce disease. Similarly, therapy with broad-spectrum antibiotics can suppress the normal bacterial flora of the gut and lead to colonization and overgrowth of the gut by *Clostridium difficile*, resulting in severe exudative enteritis that may be fatal. These examples demonstrate the important role of the indigenous bacterial flora in preventing disease and point out an important reason why good judgment in the administration of antibiotics is always important.

The mechanisms by which the normal bacterial flora prevent infection by other bacteria are incompletely understood. Normally, the determinants include bacterial competition for nutrients and maintenance by the normal flora of conditions, such as pH and oxidation—reduction potential, that are unsuitable for the multiplication of certain other microorganisms. In addition, an important factor appears to be that nonpathogenic normal flora secrete *bacteriocins,* antimicrobial factors that exert direct inhibitory effects upon the growth of other bacteria. One example of this antimicrobial factor shows that alpha-hemolytic streptococci, which constitute a major portion of the normal flora of the oropharynx, secrete factors that inhibit the growth of gram-negative microorganisms that normally inhabit the intestinal tract. When antibiotic therapy reduces the density of alpha-hemolytic streptococci, the resultant decreased production of bacteriocins may explain the frequent emergence of gram-negative bacteria in the oral pharynx within a few days of therapy.

The nature of the normal flora depends upon the capacity of certain bacteria to attach firmly to epithelial cells. Following attachment, these bacteria must find conditions suitable for their metabolic activity and multiplication to become a significant part of the normal microbial flora. In addition, these bacteria must be harmless to the extent that they do not significantly affect the normal existence of the animal host. It is possible that these relatively innocuous bacteria on the surface of epithelial cells may prevent attachment of disease-producing bacteria by blocking specific attachment sites required by the pathogenic microorganisms. Thus, the initiating events of infection by highly pathogenic bacteria are prevented. Although blocking attachment is not the only factor involved in the normal bacterial flora's prevention of infection, it may be one of the more important mechanisms. Nevertheless, certain disease-producing bacteria may produce infection even in the presence of an apparently adequate indigenous bacterial flora. In these circumstances, the requirements for initiation of infection are not known, but again, attachment of the pathogens to the epithelial cells is the first step. Following attachment, three different disease-producing processes can be recognized.

1. The pathogenic microorganism may multiply on the surface of the epithelial cell without penetrating the cell or going into deeper tissues. Disease may be produced in this instance by the elaboration of a soluble toxic substance by the infecting organism that is absorbed through the mucous membrane, producing local and/or distant tissue damage. One classic example of this process occurs with *Corynebacterium diphtheriae,* the causative agent of diphtheria. This organism attaches to the pharyngeal epithelium and elaborates a potent toxin that is absorbed and then transported systemically to other areas (heart, nervous system) where major manifestations of the disease occur. *Bordetella pertussis,* the cause of whooping cough, is another example of an organism that multiplies in the mucociliary blanket of the bronchi without entering the epithelial cells but induces disease mediated by toxins. Similarly, *Vibrio cholerae,* the causative agent of cholera, attaches to epithelial cells at the base of the villi in the small intestine and elaborates a potent exotoxin. The cholera organism rarely, if ever, penetrates into or through the epithelial cells of the gut.

2. Alternatively, pathogenic bacteria may attach to epithelial cells, penetrate into these cells, multiply, and produce disease by destroying the epithelial cell layer. An excellent example are organisms of the genus *Shigella* which produce dysentery in humans by causing epithelial cell damage, but generally without penetrating into the submucosal tissues. The manner by which bacteria of this type penetrate into epithelial cells is not clearly understood, but it appears to involve a process that resembles phagocytosis by these epithelial cells which are not generally actively phagocytic. Thus, attachment of the pathogenic organisms somehow stimulates or activates a phagocyticlike process by the epithelial cells.

3. Some pathogenic bacteria, after attachment to epithelial cells, enter the cells and pass through them into the submucosal tissues, often without producing damage to the mucosal cells themselves. The mechanisms of this transport of bacteria through epithelial cells are not clearly known. However, electron microscopic studies indicate that a phagocytic vacuole containing the disease-producing microorganism may actually pass directly through the epithelial cell and into the lamina propria. From this submucosal site, bacteria may spread to other organs in the body. There are a large number of examples of disease-producing bacteria of this type, some being extracellular parasites, some facultative intracellular parasites, and some obligate intracellular parasites.

MULTIPLICATION OF BACTERIA IN VIVO

Once a pathogenic bacterium has escaped the defense mechanisms and gained access to subepithelial tissues, the organism must multiply in order to produce disease since the number of pathogenic bacteria ordinarily infecting humans is too small to result in disease immediately. Bacteria multiply by binary fission, so that the increase in bacterial numbers in the tissues of the host is approximately exponential.

When carefully measured in experimental animals, the rate of bacterial multiplication *in vivo* is usually somewhat less than the maximal rate that can be achieved in artificial culture media in the laboratory. It is important to understand that the observed exponential multiplication is independent of the size of the initial infecting inoculum. That is, whether a single viable cell gains access to subepithelial tissues in those situations where infection can result after only a single cell infection, or a very large number of viable bacterial cells represents the initial inoculum, the rate of *in vivo* bacterial multiplication is the same. In experimental animal models infected with highly virulent bacteria, death or initial clinical manifestation of infection occurs when the size of the bacterial population in the infected animal reaches a certain threshold value. This is termed the *lethal number* of bacteria when death is the parameter. Those animals receiving smaller inocula require the longest time for this threshold number of bacteria to be reached, whereas animals receiving the largest inocula live a shorter time (see Fig. 3–1). Therefore, it appears that the primary effect of various infecting doses in natural infection of human beings is to lengthen or shorten the incubation period between the time of initial infection and the onset of clinical symptoms. This is compatible with what is generally observed in certain infectious diseases of humans.

With most bacteria, considerably more than a single viable cell is necessary to produce infection and disease in humans or lower animals. In experimental situations it is possible to measure accurately the number of organisms required to produce disease or fatal infection. This is usually carried out by injecting a suitable susceptible species of animals with graded doses of a culture of the pathogenic bacterium and recording, for example, the number of animals dying at each infecting dose. It is then possible to calculate from these data the number of bacterial organisms required to kill 50% of the

experimental animals, a term called the *lethal dose 50* (LD_{50}). Thus, it can be shown that various strains of the same bacterial species may vary widely in their capacity to produce disease, that is, in their virulence. One strain of *Salmonella typhimurium* may have an LD_{50} for mice of 100 cells, whereas another strain has an LD_{50} of 5,000; thus, the first strain is 50 times more pathogenic or virulent than the second. Generally, the relative virulence of different species of bacteria can also be compared in this way. It is also possible to compare the inherent resistance of different species of animals to a given bacterial strain by determining their bacterial LD_{50}s. Studies of this kind have yielded valuable data concerning the relative virulence of microbial species, the nature of bacterial virulence, the effectiveness of various interventions such as antibiotics for the treatment of infection, factors involved in host resistance, and the effectiveness of vaccines for the prevention of infection.

Obviously, these methods cannot be employed to study the response of humans to microbial infection. However, data related to the response of humans to natural infection demonstrate that human response parallels that of lower animals. Different strains of a bacterial species may vary in virulence for humans. An example is that the mortality rate for humans from lobar pneumonia caused by type 3 *Streptococcus pneumoniae* is greater than that for lobar pneumonia caused by other pneumococcal serotypes. In addition, the susceptibility of humans to different species of bacteria also varies greatly: death may result in 50–70% of those infected with *Yersinia pestis* (bubonic plague) but in only 5–10% of those infected with *Brucella abortus*. Thus, bacteria may vary in their virulence for humans, and individuals may vary in their capacity to resist infection.

There remains a very important question. Among individuals infected with the same strain of the same bacterium, why do some individuals die but others recover? The factors involved in recovery from an infectious disease are complex and multiple. However, one factor plays a major role in determining the outcome of an infectious disease, that is, whether the infected individual is capable of mounting a specific immune response in time to bring the infection under control by humoral and/or cellular immune processes. In most circumstances, even in the presence of potent antimicrobial agents, ultimate cure of an infectious process depends on the immune mechanisms generated by the infected individual. In infectious diseases that are associated with a high mortality rate, the micro-organisms may multiply so rapidly that they reach a lethal number before an adequate immune response can be generated. In addition, an individual unfortunate enough to receive a very large infecting dose of a less lethal pathogen may succumb to the infection because a lethal number of microorganisms is achieved prior to the 5–10 days that may be required for an adequate immune response to develop, as illustrated in Figure 3–1. Circumstances that slow or prevent the development of specific immune responses contribute to an unfavorable outcome. Conversely, situations that result in slower multiplication of bacteria *in vivo* tend to favor recovery because more time is allowed for the development of the specific acquired immune mechanisms. Many antimicrobial agents function in this capacity. Throughout this book the importance of the development of host immunity for the control of infectious processes is emphasized.

It should be apparent that an individual may become infected with a small number of bacteria, develop a vigorous immune response, and control the infection before the number of bacteria necessary to produce symptoms is reached. Thus, an infection by bacteria that multiply in the tissues can occur but not result in apparent disease. These infections are referred to as *subclinical,* or *inapparent,* infections. All of us experience numerous inapparent infections with a wide variety of bacteria during our lifetime. In many circumstances these subclinical infec-

tions lead to immunity which, in some circumstances, may be long-lived and highly effective in preventing subsequent clinically apparent infections. The phenomenon of subclinical infection emphasizes the distinction between an infection (which is inapparent or apparent) and the development of an infectious disease.

SPREAD OF INFECTION

Depending upon the effectiveness of the host defense mechanisms, an infection may remain localized or may spread. Such spread may occur by direct extension to contiguous tissues or by way of the lymphatics and ultimately by way of the bloodstream via the thoracic duct. Occasionally, hematogenous spread occurs when bacteria enter the blood directly through a blood vessel that has been damaged by the necrotizing effect of the infection and its accompanying inflammatory process. Lymphatic spread, however, is the most common method of spread of infection, not only for bacteria but also for viruses and fungi.

FATE OF PATHOGENS IN THE HOST

When recovery occurs from most infections caused by extracellular parasites, all the pathogenic bacteria are killed and the patient is rendered free of the invading organisms. Notable exceptions to this rule do exist, however. In some infections caused by facultative intracel-

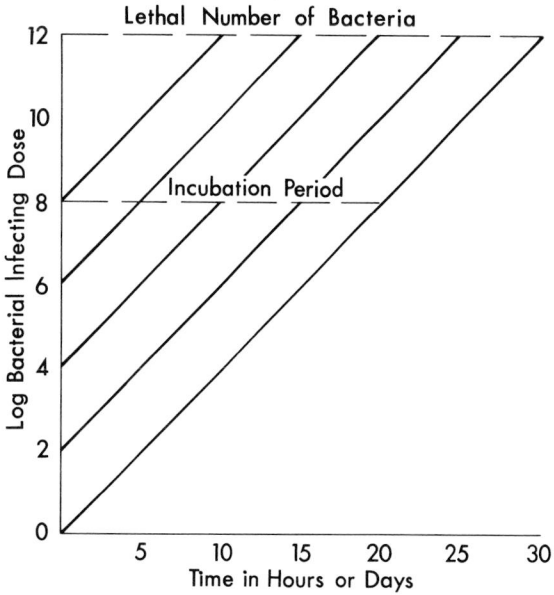

Figure 3–1. The rate of multiplication of bacteria producing infection. Note that the area between Incubation Period and Lethal Number of Bacteria represents symptomatic infection. Both the symptomatic period and death theoretically are reached sooner when there has been a larger infecting dose.

lular parasites, such as tuberculosis, it is the rule that not all the microorganisms are killed. Although the multiplication of the parasite may be inhibited strikingly by cellular immunity, small numbers of tubercle bacilli characteristically remain viable but dormant within tissues (usually within macrophages) for many years. These microorganisms may subsequently produce disease if the (T-cell) immune forces that hold them in check become depressed. This is discussed fully below.

SYSTEMIC RESPONSE TO INFECTION

Nonspecific Immune Mechanisms

An invasive microorganism induces a host reaction consisting of both an inflammatory and a specific immune response which generally are capable of killing or localizing the organism so that disease does not result. Disease is the consequence of signs and symptoms produced by this reaction, by a large inoculum of the invading microorganism or a virulent agent which overwhelms the host defenses, or by infection of a host with impaired defenses.

Inflammatory Response

The *inflammatory reaction* is the primary response to microbial invasion. This response is complex, involving a number of cells and humoral substances which interact in an attempt to localize and control the infection. The cellular response is modified over time depending upon the organism and the chronicity of the infection. The cells which constitute the inflammatory reaction include first, the polymorphonuclear leukocytes or segmented neutrophils. Secondarily, especially with intracellular pathogens such as *Mycobacterium tuberculosis*, monocytes/macrophages, lymphocytes, and plasma cells are involved. In the postcapillary venules in the area of microbial invasion, white cells adhere to and migrate between endothelial cells into tissue. Neutrophils appear initially, and move toward the microorganisms attracted by chemoattractants. These are produced by the organism or by complement products resulting from interaction of the organism and complement components (see next section for a discussion of complement). Neutrophils adhere to the microorganism and begin the process of engulfment, or *phagocytosis*. Some organisms, either due to

size as in the case of hyphal elements of fungi or characteristics of the microbial surface, are resistant to attachment and/or phagocytosis in the absence of opsonins. Opsonins, complement, and/or antibody facilitate attachment and phagocytosis by cells which have receptors for complement components or the Fc (crystalizable) fragment of antibody molecules (see below).

Once the neutrophil attaches to the microbe, the cell engulfs the organism by sending out pseudopods which surround it. These fuse forming a phagosome. This process requires energy, which is furnished by glycolysis. The granules of the neutrophils or granulocyte surround the phagosome, fuse with it, and discharge their contents into the structure now called a *phagolysosome*. This process, known as *degranulation*, releases hydrolytic enzymes and other bactericidal substances into the phagolysosome. In addition to the enzymes, which include cathepsin, acid hydrolase, and lysozyme, lactic acid, polypeptides, and lactoferrin are released into this structure. Simultaneously, through activation of oxidases located in the membrane of the neutrophil, hydrogen peroxide, peroxidase, oxygen radicals, and chlorine, which have microbicidal activity, are released into the phagolysosome. This is accompanied by an oxidative burst which can be measured as an assay of neutrophil function. This burst fails to occur following phagocytosis by neutrophils of individuals with chronic granulomatous disease. This illness is manifested by failure to kill catalase-producing microorganism such as *Staphylococcus aureus*, aerobic gram-negative bacilli, and fungi. The affected individual is subject to recurrent acute and chronic infections. Organisms which do not produce catalase (such as pneumococci) are readily killed by neutrophils of these patients.

It should be noted that the other major phagocytic cell, the monocyte/macrophage, utilizes the same oxidative enzyme systems for killing ingested organisms. These mononuclear phagocytes enter the inflammatory focus after neutrophils and predominate if the infection is due to an intracellular pathogen such as *M. tuberculosis*. Macrophages form the granuloma, the hallmark of infections with such organisms. Other phagocytic mononuclear cells are resident in a number of organs and systems, and are called *tissue histocytes*. Examples are the Kupffer cells of the liver, the macrophages of the spleen and lymph nodes, the microglial cells of the central nervous system, and the alveolar macrophages. The origin of the monocyte/macrophage is the bone marrow. These cells are long-lived; in contrast to the short (5–8 h) half-life of neutrophils in the circulation, monocytes migrate from the vascular system into tissue in response to inflammation and persist there for weeks or longer.

A number of tissue substances, generally polypeptides, have bactericidal properties. Whether or not they play a role *in vivo* in defense against infection, however, is unclear.

The inflammatory response is nonspecific, but interfaces with the specific immune responses as outlined below. This interaction serves to amplify and enhance the function of the phagocytic cells through the effects of specific antibody and cytokines released by the cells of the immune system, the lymphocytes and macrophages.

Complement

The complement system is an important component of both the humoral immune response and the inflammatory reaction, acting to amplify and/or augment the cellular reaction to microbial invasion (Fig. 3–2). The complement sys-

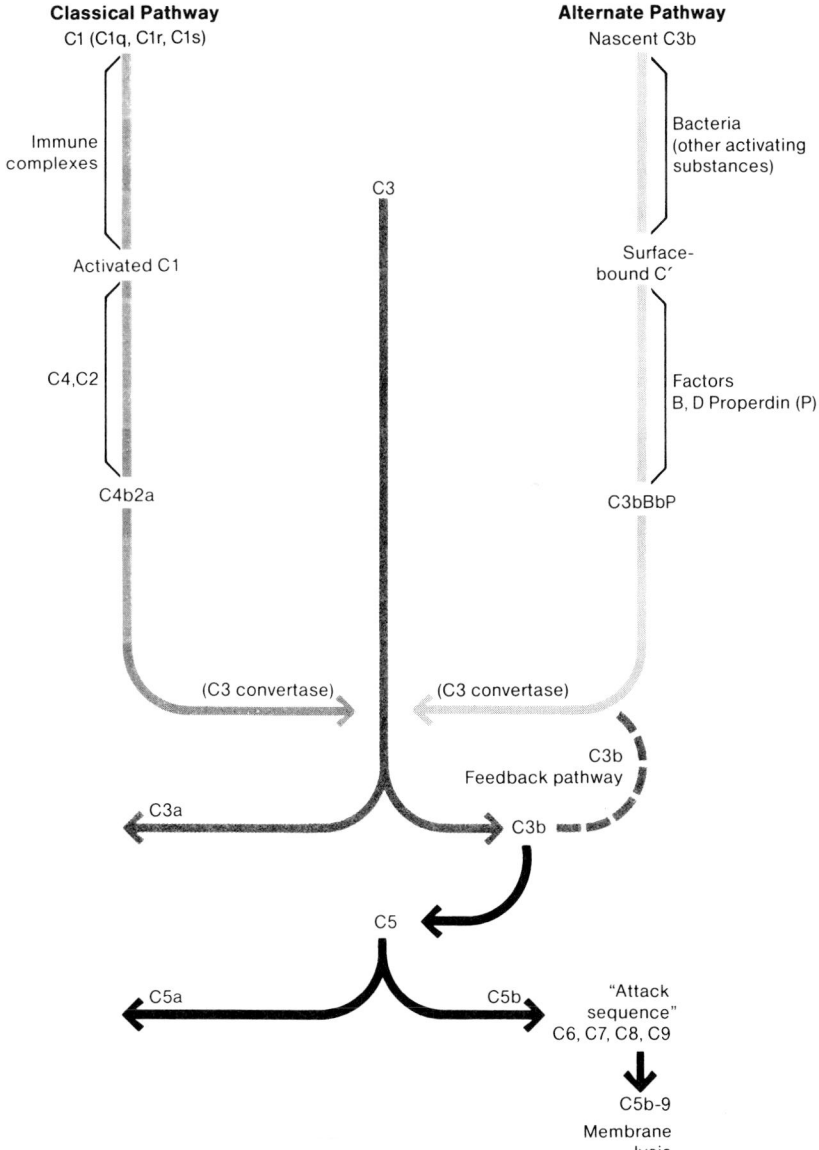

Figure 3–2. Pathways of complement activation. (From Goldstein, I. M.: Complement in Infectious Diseases. Current Concepts. Kalamazoo, MI: The Upjohn Company, 1980.)

tem consists of approximately 19 serum and 9 membrane proteins (Table 3–2) which participate in a series of active enzymatic reactions. These proteins are produced by the liver and monocytes/macrophages. Other cells, such as intestinal epithelium, cells of the urinary tract, and fibroblasts, may also synthesize various components of the system during infection. In general, the complement proteins exist in an inactive form, and the cascade is activated by the complexing of C1q with the Fc portion of antibody combined to antigen (the classic pathway), or through the alternative pathway. This latter pathway is initiated by the third component (C3) of complement interacting directly with the surface of a microorganism or other activating surfaces.

The first complement component C1 is a complex protein consisting of C1q, which binds to antibody, C1r and C1s. The second (C1r) and third (C1s) components released from C1 enzymatically activate C4 and C2. These act to convert C3 to its active form C3b, which combines with activated products of C4 and C2, C4b, and C2a, to activate the terminal components of complement, C5 through C9, after being fixed to the surface of microorganisms. C3b also amplifies the cascade by interacting with components of the proteins of the alternative loop, D, properdin, and B, and C3 itself. This results in the formation of C3bB3b convertase which also generates the active forms of the membrane-attached terminal complement components. These components, C5–C9, mediate cell lysis and death of specific "serum-sensitive" bacteria. Activation of C3, independent of antibody, thus can result in production of the membrane-lytic complex (Table 3–3).

Other components of the system are involved in down-regulating or slowing the cascade. C1 esterase inhibitor binds to C1, preventing spontaneous disassociation into its active components. A complex of C1 and this inhibitor also inactivates C1r and C1s, preventing cleavage of C4 and thus controlling the initiation of the classic pathway. In addition, the C3 convertases decay rapidly, limiting the activation of C3. The convertases also bind to C4 binding protein (C4bp) and to factor A, which inhibits formation of C3b. The active components C3b and C4b on the cell surface also are rapidly cleaved by factor I. Cofactors involved in this cleavage process include factor H and membrane cofactor protein (MCP). A third cell-bound protein, decay-accelerating factor (DAC), inactivates C3b.

In addition to activating the membrane-lytic complex, a number of biologically important fragments are released by the system which act as important amplifiers of the inflammatory response. Among these fragments are the anaphylatoxins (C4a, C3a, C5a) which induce release of histamine, cause vascular dilation, increase

TABLE 3–2. *Proteins of the Complement System*

Component	Molecular Weight (in thousands)	Approximate Serum Concentration (μg/mL)	Chromosome
Classic Pathway			
C1q	410	70	1p
C1r	168	34	12p
C1s	83	31	12p
C2	117	25	6p
C3	200	1300	19p
C4	209	600	6p
Membrane Attack Complex			
C5	180	80	9q
C6	128	60	?
C7	120	55	?
C8	150	65	1p
C9	79	60	?
Regulatory Proteins			
C1 inhibitor	105	200	11q
C4 binding protein	550	250	1q
Factor H	150	500	1q
Factor I	90	34	4
Anaphylatoxin inactivator (carboxypeptidase B)	280	35	?
S protein (vitronectin)	80	500	?
Properdin	220	25	Xp
Alternative Pathway			
Factor B	100	200	6p
Factor D	25	1	?

TABLE 3–3. *Principal Activities of Activated Complement (C) Proteins and Their Fragments*

Activity	C Protein or Fragment
Anaphylatoxin: Histamine release from mast cells and increased permeability of capillaries	C3a; C5a
Chemotaxis: Attract polymorphonuclear leukocytes and monocytes	C5a
Immune adherence and opsonization: Adherence of Ab-Ag-C complexes to leukocytes, platelets, etc., increasing susceptibility to phagocytosis by leukocytes and macrophages	C3b; iC3b
Platelet activation	C3a
Membrane damage: Lysis of red cells; leakiness of plasma membrane of nucleated cells; lysis of gram-negative bacteria	C5–9 attack complex

capillary permeability, and augment chemotaxis, intracellular killing, and neutrophil adhesiveness to endothelium. Other complement functions include solubilization of immune complexes, clearance of antigen–antibody immune complexes by interaction with complement receptors on tissue macrophages, and enhancement of leukocytosis by a fragment of C3. A major function of complement is to facilitate phagocytosis of microorganisms by *opsonization*. The phagocytic cells recognize C3b on the surface of microbes through the interaction with their membrane receptor for complement CR1, which enhances attachment, engulfment, and ultimately killing. Opsonization thus can be achieved by the activation of the classic or the alternative complement pathway.

Specific Immune Mechanisms

Humoral Immune Responses

Humoral immune responses can be induced by infection or by active immunization (see Chapter 40), with toxoids (altered toxins), with killed bacteria or virus, or with attenuated live virus vaccines. Passive immunization can be achieved by administration of IgG intramuscularly or intravenously (see Chapter 40). IgG or serum obtained from normal or hyperimmunized human donors is utilized to prevent disease after infection with *Clostridium tetani* or exposure to hepatitis B. Hyperimmune gamma globulin harvested from immune adult volunteers is used to provide prompt protection to the exposed nonimmune patient.

Immunoglobulins

Specific antibody is the product of plasma cells which are the progeny of the B lymphocytes (Fig. 3–3). The B lymphocytes can be identified by immunoglobulin or other cell surface markers. This class of lymphocyte was originally delineated in avian species and was shown to originate in the bursa of Fabricius, an appendage of the cloaca of birds. In mammals there is no strictly analogous structure to the bursa. B lymphocytes in man and other mammals derive from stem cells found in the fetal liver and adult bone marrow, and they are produced throughout life.

Antibodies, the secretory products of B lymphocytes and plasma cells, are glycoproteins (termed the *immunoglobulins*), with specific recognition sites for antigens. There are five classes of immunoglobulin, IgG, IgA, IgM, IgD, and IgE. IgG consists of four subclasses, IgG$_{1-4}$, circulates as a monomer, and accounts for the majority of immunoglobulin in serum. IgA also circulates in serum primarily as a monomer, and is found in bodily secretions in a dimeric form. All the forms of immunoglobulins have the same basic structure: two light or L chains, which contain part of the antibody binding site, and two heavy or H chains which also contribute to the antigen binding site on the Fab fragment. The Fc or crystalizable fragment of the heavy chain binds complement and interacts with Fc receptor on cell surfaces. Secretory IgA consists of two monomeric units bound by a 15-kd protein, the J chain, along

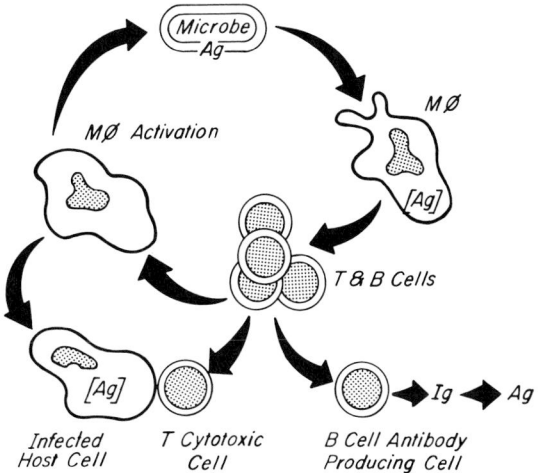

Figure 3–3. Major pathways of acquired immune responses to microbial antigens involving macrophages, T-cell, and B-cell populations.

with a secretory component synthesized by epithelial cells. The secretory component facilitates transport of IgA onto mucosal surfaces. IgM exists as a pentamer of five monomeric units bound together by J chains. IgD and IgE circulate in serum in low concentrations in a monomeric form.

The diversity of antibodies, which are estimated to be capable of recognizing 10^8 possible antigens, is the result of genetic recombination of immunoglobulin genes. The recognition site for specific antigens is structurally within the "variable regions" of the L and H chains. The genes encoding the L chains are found on chromosome 22 (κ L chains) and chromosome 2 (λ L chains). The process of recombination of the various DNA sequences, assembly of immunoglobulin, and somatic mutations results in the necessary variety of specific antibodies.

The stimulus for production of antibody is exposure to a "foreign" protein or polysaccharide. All B cells have cell-surface-bound immunoglobulin IgM and IgD, but with a single antigen specificity. Binding of antigen to the surface immunoglobulin results in activation and later to B cell proliferation, antibody secretion, and differentiation into plasma cells. This process is augmented by cytokines produced by a subset of thymic, or T, helper cells and mononuclear phagocytes. A second set of T suppressor cells acts to inhibit antibody secretion and thus modulate or turn off antibody production (Fig. 3–4).

Antibodies possess multiple functional capabilities relevant to the host's defense against infectious agents or products of microbes. In general, as stated above, the Fab end of immunoglobulins combine with antigen, but following antigen binding the Fc component of IgM, IgG_1, IgG_2, and IgG_3 interacts with the first component of the complement system, C1q. The Fc component of immunoglobulins also binds to Fc receptors on phagocytic cells to augment engulfment of microorganisms. Thus, a major function of antibody is to act as an opsonin that facilitates phagocytosis and the killing of a microorganism by phagocytic cells. The role of the complement system in this process and direct lysis of microorganisms will be discussed below. In addition to facilitating phagocytosis, antibody can *neutralize toxins* produced by bacteria by binding toxins, preventing interaction with cellular receptors, and blocking effects upon cells.

As noted previously, adherence of microorganisms to mucosal surfaces involves interaction

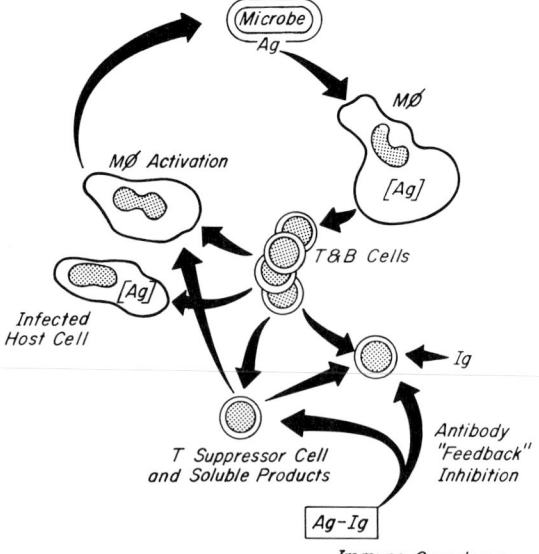

Figure 3–4. *Diversity of pathways of immunosuppression involving macrophages, T cells, B cells, and their products, collectively serving to inhibit active host immune responses to microbial antigens.*

of microbial surface adhesions with mucosal cell receptors. This colonization can be prevented by secretory IgA, which combines with the adhesion and blocks adherence. This represents an important (and for some infectious agents the primary) mechanism for preventing infection.

Antibodies of IgG, IgA, and IgM specific for surface proteins of viruses also inhibit infection of target cells. This form of *virus neutralization* represents an important defense against agents which have a cell-free phase, such as the etiologic agents of the childhood exanthems. With intracellular agents such as herpesvirus, "neutralizing" antibodies play a much less important role in combating infection. In addition, certain viruses induce alterations on infected cell surfaces, which results in antibody directed at these "new" cell-surface components. Cell lysis results from the lytic effect of complement bound by such antibody interacting with the cell surface. Alternatively, antibody can bind effector cells which destroy the virus-infected cell. Cytotoxic lymphocytes, neutrophils, or macrophages can participate in this *antibody-dependent, cell-mediated cytotoxicity* (ADCC).

IgE, or reaginic antibody, mediates immediate hypersensitivity reactions and may play a role in mediating cellular responses to protozoan and helminthic infections. Serum IgE concentrations are increased in chronic infections with these microorganisms. Mast cell–bound IgE following interaction with specific antigen induces the release of potent amines which mediate hypersensitivity reactions. It has been postulated that this reaction may result in expulsion of enteric parasites from the gastrointestinal tract.

The role of IgD in host defense has not been elucidated. The immunoglobulin does not opsonize microorganisms or participate in complement-mediated lysis and is not known to inhibit the adherence of a microorganism to cells or to neutralize virus. Its major role may be on the B cell surface, where it facilitates antigen binding.

It is worth noting that the only immunoglobulins which can cross the placenta and passively immunize the fetus are specific subclasses of IgG. The lack of IgM in the newborn may underlie the vulnerability of the infant to infection by aerobic gram-negative bacilli. In addition, premature infants do not receive much transplacental IgG and are often severely deficient. Nursing infants receive some antibody, primarily IgA, from maternal colostrum.

Cell-Mediated Immunity

Cell-mediated immunity (CMI) involves a complex interaction of lymphocytes and mononuclear phagocytes. The function of CMI is controlled by specific cell surface structures which regulate the interaction of these cells. This interaction can involve cell-to-cell contact or is mediated through the cytokines, which are secreted by these cells and act as hormones to activate and/or modulate the inflammatory and immune response.

CMI is especially relevant for prevention and control of infection due to intracellular pathogens such as brucella, listeria, mycobacteria, the herpesviruses, fungi such as *Coccidioides immitis*, intestinal parasites, and possibly to some extracellular agents such as *Pseudomonas aeruginosa*. Defects in this system are present in patients with Hodgkin's disease or acquired immunodeficiency syndrome, and these conditions are marked by infection with intracellular pathogens.

The early investigations of CMI began with the attempt to dissect the delayed hypersensitivity (DH) response. DH reactions are induced by intradermal challenge with an antigen such as purified protein derivative (PPD) of *Mycobacterium tuberculosis* in infected persons and are manifest 24–72 h after injection of PPD. Histologic examination of such dermal reactions reveals infiltrates of lymphocytes and mononu-

clear cells. In experimental animals delayed reactivity can be transferred by living lymphocytes but not by serum harvested from immune donors. In some experimental animal infections, resistance to a challenge inoculation with an intracellular pathogen correlates with DH responses, and resistance can be transferred with lymphocytes. With the recognition that lymphocytes could be identified as B cells and thymic-derived or T cells, the knowledge of this complex system began to increase exponentially. The thymic lymphocytes are produced in the bone marrow and migrate to the thymus in fetal life, where differentiation takes place under the influence of the thymic epithelium. The process of maturation and differentiation of the T cells in the thymus is complex and beyond the scope of this discussion. Mature T cells, however, can be grouped as $CD4^+$ cells and $CD8^+$ cells (Table 3–4). They are identified by the self-surface proteins CD4 and CD8; a third protein, CD3, identifies T cells of both classes. T cells also bear on their surface a receptor, the T cell antigen receptor, which functions in a manner analogous to membrane-bound immunoglobulin on B cells and is responsible for antigen specificity of T cells.

Antigen recognition by T cells requires that the antigen be presented in conjunction with a specific human leukocyte antigen, or HLA, molecule on the surface of a macrophage or other cell. There are two classes of HLA molecules involved in this cellular recognition. HLA class I surface proteins are found on most nucleated cells. Class II molecules are expressed on B cells and antigen processing/presenting cells, the macrophage. Antigen recognition by $CD4^+$ helper T lymphocytes requires that the antigen be displayed with the class II surface molecules. $CD8^+$ cells recognize antigens only in conjunction with class I surface proteins. These requirements for antigen recognition serve to restrict recognition and modulation of cellular responses. The specific antigen receptor, or TCR (T cell receptor), on T cells consists of two polypeptide chains. Similar to immunoglobulin these chains have a variable region which generates the diversity of receptors necessary for antigen recognition. The CD4 and CD8 surface molecules serve an accessory function in antigen recognition, interacting with the TCR and the class I and II major histocompatibility complex (MHC) molecules to stabilize antigen binding to the lymphocyte.

With binding of antigen, the T cell is activated resulting in production of lymphokines and cel-

TABLE 3–4. *Immunologic Functions of Regulatory T-Cell Subsets*

Function	T Helper/Inducer Cells (CD3+, CD4+)	T Cytotoxic/Suppressor Cells (CD3+, CD8+)
Proliferative responses		
to soluble antigen	+	−
to mixed lymphocyte culture	+	+
to concanavalin A	+	+
to phytohemagglutinin	+	±
Cytotoxic effector function	−	+
Regulatory events		
Help (induction)		
T–T	+	−
T–B	+	−
T-macrophage	+	−
Suppression		
T–T	−	+
T–B	−	+

From Reinherz, E. L., and Schlossman, S. F. Regulation of the immune response: Inducer and suppressor T-lymphocyte subsets in human beings. *N. Engl. J. Med. 303*:371, 1980.

lular proliferation. It is important to note that the antigens recognized by CD4+ cells are sequences of amino acids presented in association with the class II molecules. The original antigen is processed by macrophages which digest protein antigen to smaller peptides. Processed antigens recognized by CD8+ cells are bound to the class I HLA molecule within a cell and then transported to the cell surface.

CD4+ cells, restricted to recognizing antigen presented in conjunction with a class II HLA molecule, help in the production of antibody by B lymphocytes, and are termed *helper T cells*. A subclass of CD4+ cells subsequently develops that induces suppression of antibody production. CD8+ cells are cytotoxic, capable of killing virus-infected cells, tumor cells, or allogenic graft cells which present class I molecules and also suppress antibody production. They are generally termed *cytotoxic suppressor T cells*.

This interaction of macrophages, CD4+, and CD8+ T cells, is largely coordinated by the *cytokines,* including *lymphokines* produced by lymphocytes and *monokines* produced by monocytes/macrophages. These cytokines both amplify and down-regulate the immune response. Monocytes/macrophages produce interleukin-1 (IL-1), interferon-alpha, tumor necrosis factor (TNF), granulocyte-monocyte-colony stimulating factor (GM-CSF), granulocyte-colony stimulating factor (G-CSF), monocyte-colony stimulating factor (M-CSF), and IL-6. IL-1 causes fever, catabolism of muscle proteins, synthesis of acute-phase reactants, T cell activation, B cell proliferation, and release of neutrophils from the bone marrow. IL-6 induces immunoglobulin production, fever, and production of acute-phase reactants. Interferon-alpha in-

creases natural killer (NK) cell function and induces fever, in addition to having antiviral effects and decreasing cell proliferation. TNF has effects similar to IL-1 and also enhances macrophage release of the other monokines and itself. The colony stimulatory factors promote proliferation of neutrophils and/or monocytes and enhance their function.

The lymphokines include IL-2, which mediates T cell proliferation, production of other lymphokines, augments cytotoxic T cell differentiation, enhances NK activity and is a cofactor for B-cell function. IL-3 induces proliferation of bone marrow stem cells, IL-4 functions in a manner analogous to IL-1 and is a cofactor for colony stimulating factors, and IL-5 induces IgA and IgM synthesis. Interferon-gamma enhances macrophage function.

Attenuation of the immune response occurs through production of prostaglandins induced by TNF and IL-1. Prostaglandin E_2 specifically inhibits IL-1 activation of T cells. IL-1 also augments release of ACTH and glucocorticoids which down-regulate the inflammatory response and inhibit release of the colony stimulating factors as well as interferon and interleukins.

In addition to B and T lymphocytes, a third class of lymphocytes, NK cells, are found in the peripheral blood. On the surface of NK cells are receptors for sheep erythrocytes. This receptor is also on T cells but only a small subset of NK cells expresses the CD3 marker which identifies T cells. NK cells are large granular lymphocytes capable of recognizing the abnormal surface of a tumor cell or a virus-infected cell which lacks class I HLA antigens. Those cells expressing class I or II molecules are not lysed. NK cells thus are capable of lysing cells infected with virus directly and can participate in antibody-dependent cell mediated cytotoxicity.

Monocytes/macrophages act as the effector cells of CMI in its killing of intracellular pathogens. Macrophages exist in either a resting or activated state. The resting cells have receptors for IgG-Fc and C3b and can ingest microorganisms which gain access to tissue. Killing is dependent upon the organism (for example, *Mycobacterium tuberculosis* can replicate intracellularly and is relatively resistant to killing) and the state of activation of the macrophage. Macrophage activation is a consequence of the effects of interferon-gamma and TNF. Activation is characterized by increased microbicidal activity; chemotaxis; glucose metabolism; antigen presentation; and secretion of cytokines, complement components, and enzymes. Infection with specific organisms such as *M. tuberculosis* is associated with macrophage proliferation and the formation of a granuloma. Granulomatous macrophages are activated and the finding of granulomata is associated with the control of infection.

In summary, the cellular immune response to infection involves a variety of types of lymphocytes and mononuclear phagocytes, as well as the production of cytokines which amplify and modulate the response. These cytokines and other cellular products such as antibody and complement also enhance the function of neutrophils, the primary cell of the inflammatory reaction. This manifests as increased production of neutrophils by the bone marrow, increased adhesiveness of these cells to endothelial cells, enhanced chemotactic responses directed to foci of infection, and up-regulation of phagocytosis and killing of microorganisms. The inflammatory and immune responses thus linked act in concert to provide a systemic response to microbial invasion.

REFERENCES

Books

Brostoff, J. *Clinical Immunology.* Philadelphia: Lippincott, 1991.

Davis, B. D., et al. *Microbiology,* 4th ed. Philadelphia: Lippincott, 1990.

Galasso, G. J., Whitley, R. J., and Merigan, T. C.: *Antiviral Agents and Viral Diseases of Man.* 3rd ed. New York: Raven Press, 1990.

Golub, E. S., and Green, D. *Immunology. A Synthesis.* 2nd ed., Sunderland, MA: Sinauer Assoc., 1991.

Mims, C. A. *The Pathogenesis of Infectious Disease,* 3rd ed. London: Academic Press, 1987.

Roitt, I. *Essential Immunology.* 6th ed. Oxford: Blackwell Scientific Public., 1988.

Sell, S. *Basic Immunology.* New York: Elsevier Science Publ., 1987.

Sherris, J. C. *Medical Microbiology.* 2nd ed. New York: Elsevier Science Publ., 1990.

Wilson, G., Miles, A., and Parker, M. T. *Topley and Wilson's Principles of Bacteriology, Virology, and Immunity.* 7th ed. Baltimore: William & Wilkins Co., 1984.

Review Articles

Beachy, E. H. Bacterial adherence. *J. Infect. Dis. 143*:325, 1981.

Brubaker, R. R. Mechanisms of bacterial virulence. *Ann. Rev. Microbiol. 39*:21–50, 1985.

Cassell, G. H., ed. Microbial surfaces: Determinants of virulence and host responsiveness. *Rev. Infect. Dis. 10*(suppl.):S273–456, 1988.

Claman, H. N. The biology of the immune response. *JAMA 258*:2834–2840, 1987.

Cooper, M. D. B lymphocytes. *N. Engl. J. Med. 317*:1452–1456, 1987.

Dinarello, C. A., and Mier, J. W. Lymphokines. *N. Engl. J. Med 317*:940–945, 1987.

Finlay, B. B., and Falkow, S. Common themes in microbial pathogenicity. *Microbiol. Rev. 53*:210–230, 1989.

Middlebrook, J. L., and Darland, R. B. Bacterial toxins: Cellular mechanisms of action. *Microbiol. Rev. 48*:199–221, 1984.

Nossal, G. J. V. The basic components of the immune system. *N. Engl. J. Med 316*:1320–1325, 1987.

Roger, H. D., and Reinherz, E. L. T lymphocytes. *N. Engl. J. Med. 317*:1136–1142, 1987.

Urbaschek, B., ed. Perspectives on bacterial pathogenesis and host defense. *Rev. Infect. Dis. 9*(suppl. 5)S431–659, 1987.

4   *BETSY C. HEROLD, M.D. • PATRICIA G. SPEAR, Ph.D.*

Virus–Host Interactions

INTRODUCTION

The past few decades have been characterized by intense activity in the field of virology. Many previously unrecognized viral pathogens have been discovered. Previously unrecognized viral diseases, such as AIDS, have also been identified. The decade has seen the development of new techniques, especially in molecular biology, which may potentially serve as tools for diagnosis as well as a means for unraveling the mysteries of viral pathogenesis. There have been advances in the development of antiviral therapies and immunization strategies. Viruses, however, remain a major cause of human disease and continue to challenge scientists and clinicians.

Viruses are obligate intracellular parasites. They differ in fundamental ways, however, from bacterial, fungal, and protozoan intracellular parasites. Viruses are inert in their extracellular forms but have the capacity to invade cells. In the intracellular environment, the nucleic acid component of the virus is released to redirect the biosynthetic activities of the cell toward production of progeny virus particles. The virus contributes the genetic instructions for this process, such as genetic information for the viral enzymes, regulatory proteins and structural proteins needed for its replication, but otherwise must use the host cell machinery for its replication.

Every step of viral replication from entry into the cell, to the expression of viral genes, to the egress of progeny virus requires functional interactions between viral and cell proteins and nucleic acids. This means that a particular virus is suited for (has evolved for) replication in some cell types and species but not in others. Even if a cell is not permissive for viral replication (because it lacks one or more components required for that replication), the virus may still be able to invade the cell and, through the expression of a subset of viral genes, alter the properties of the cell. For example, the virus may induce cell proliferation under conditions that would normally not be conducive to cell proliferation.

Virus-induced pathology in the intact animal or human depends on the effects of the virus on each cell type it can invade and on the immune responses provoked by viral antigens. Infected cells may be killed by the virus, especially if the cells are permissive for viral replication. Infected cells may also be killed by cytotoxic immune responses, provided viral antigens are appropriately expressed. Finally, infected cells can survive and evade the immune response. Rarely are the cells permissive for viral replication under this latter condition. More often, the cells are latently infected, that is, a subset of viral genes may be expressed but virus is not produced. Latently infected cells can be important in pathogenesis because they harbor a reservoir of virus that is not eliminated on recovery from disease and that can later be reactivated to cause a recurrence of disease. Finally, by inducing cells to proliferate in the absence of the normal signals for cell proliferation, as mentioned above, viruses can be one of the multiple factors that contribute to the induction of cancer.

Following a brief discussion of virus structure and classification, attention will be focused first on describing the various kinds of virus–cell interactions, and considering the consequences to the virus and the cell. Viral pathogenesis in the intact host will then be addressed, with discussion of the factors that influence host resistance and susceptibility to viral disease.

VIRUS STRUCTURE AND CLASSIFICATION

Viruses are composed of nucleic acid, a capsid or protein coat and, in some instances, an outer membranous envelope. Viruses are quite small (10–300 nm) and cannot be visualized with the light microscope, making rapid clinical diagnosis difficult. With the advent of electron microscopy in the 1940s, viral particles could be visualized. Electron microscopy has since played a major role in studies of the etiology of viral disease, in diagnosis, and in the delineation of viral structure. Most recently, x-ray crystallography and electron microscopic analyses combined with computer-assisted image reconstructions have enabled researchers to produce very detailed images of virus particles, also called *virions* (Fig. 4–1).

Virus classification depends on properties of the viral genome and of the particle in which it is packaged. The differentiating properties of the viral genome include the nature of the nucleic acid (DNA or RNA), the number of strands to the nucleic acid (single- or double-), its shape (linear or circular), and size of the genome. Most DNA viruses associated with human disease have genomes of double-stranded DNA. RNA viruses are usually single-stranded, except for reoviruses, which have a double-stranded RNA genome. For single-stranded RNA viruses, the genome may be either positive sense (the same polarity as messenger RNA [mRNA]), negative sense (antipolar to the mRNA), or rarely, ambisense (part of the genome has the same polarity as mRNA

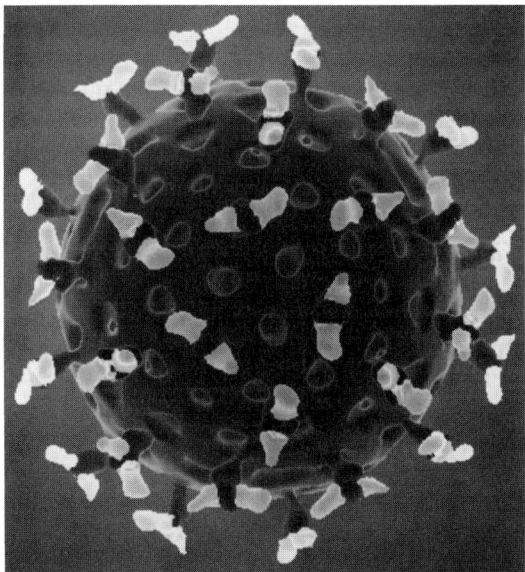

Figure 4–1. Three-dimensional structure of a rotavirus–Fab complex reconstructed by computer analysis from multiple electron-microscopic images of frozen, hydrated specimens. The virus particle has a diameter of 76 nm. The icosahedral surface of the virion is perforated by 132 aqueous channels. Sixty spikes, which are dimers of the viral protein VP4, extend from this surface. Two Fab fragments from a neutralizing monoclonal antibody against VP4 are shown (in lighter tone) at the distal end of each spike. (Photograph courtesy of B. V. V. Prasad, Baylor College of Medicine, Houston, TX; reprinted by permission from Prasad, B. V. V., Burns, J. W., Marietta, E., Estes, M. K., and Chiu, W. Localization of VP4 neutralization sites in rotavirus by three-dimensional cryoelectron microscopy, Nature *343:476–479; copyright © 1990 Macmillan Magazines Limited.)*

and the rest serves as template for producing other mRNAs).

The differentiating properties of the virus particle include the size, morphology, and symmetry of the protein coat, or capsid, and the presence or absence of a membranous envelope as an outer coat. The viral genome can be coated with proteins in a helical array (especially for single-stranded RNA viruses) or surrounded by an icosahedral protein shell. The arrangement of the capsid proteins in the helical nucleocapsid or in the icosahedral shell is characteristic for each distinct family of viruses. Some viruses also possess a viral envelope composed of a lipid bilayer and various proteins or glycoproteins specified by the virus. These viruses acquire their envelopes by budding through a virus-modified patch of host cell membrane. Thus, the envelope is composed of host cell lipids and viral membrane proteins and may contain small amounts of host membrane proteins in addition. The structural proteins and envelope (if present) of the virus particle serve at least two roles.

They protect the viral genome from degradation in the extracellular environment and provide the vehicle required to dock with and invade a cell. The outer surface of the virus particle, whether this is the protein capsid or the viral envelope, mediates attachment of the virus to a host cell, initiating the process that leads to penetration of the viral genome into the cell.

VIRUS–CELL INTERACTIONS

Viral infection of an animal or human being requires the invasion of individual cells at the portal of entry and replication of virus in at least some of these cells. Virus may then spread to cells in other tissues. If an infected cell has all the factors required for viral replication, a productive infection occurs. Otherwise, an abortive or latent infection occurs. These nonproductive infections can also have profound effects on the individual cell and on the natural history of the disease. Following a discussion of viral entry into cells, the various kinds of productive and nonproductive infections will be described.

Entry of Virus into a Cell

Specific attachment or adsorption of a virion to a cell precedes virus penetration into the cell and is mediated by binding of a viral protein (antireceptor) to a cell-surface receptor. Recently, receptors for several clinically important viruses have been identified, including the CD4 molecule for the human immunodeficiency virus (HIV), the CR2 complement receptor for Epstein-Barr virus (EBV), I-CAM for rhinoviruses, and heparan sulfate proteoglycans for herpes simplex virus (HSV).

It is coming to be recognized that presence of a cell-surface receptor appropriate for the attachment of virus may be necessary but not sufficient to allow penetration of the virus into the cell. A possible explanation is that penetration may require specific molecular interactions between the virion surface and the cell membrane, in addition to the interaction required for attachment of the virus to the cell. Various kinds of indirect evidence imply the necessity for these additional interactions, but they have not yet been well defined in any instance.

There are fundamental differences in the way enveloped and nonenveloped viruses penetrate into cells. For enveloped viruses, penetration results when the virion envelope fuses with a

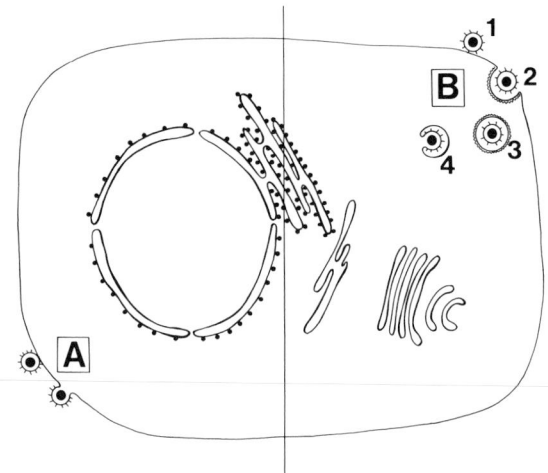

Figure 4–2. Pathways by which enveloped viruses can enter cells to initiate infection. The virion–cell fusion required to release the nucleocapsid into the cytoplasm may occur at the plasma membrane (A) or with the membrane of an endosome (B), depending upon the virus. The temporal sequence of events in the endocytic pathway (B) is thought to be similar to that defined for receptor-mediated endocytosis of other ligands. These events include attachment of virus to the cell surface (1), lateral movement to a clathrin-coated pit (2), ingestion by the cell in a coated vesicle (3), transition of the vesicle from coated to uncoated (endosome), and fusion of the virion with the membrane of the endosome (4). (Reprinted with permission from Spear, P. G. Virus-induced cell fusion. In Sowers, A. E., ed. Cell Fusion. New York: Plenum Publishing Corporation, 1987, p. 6.)

cell membrane (Fig. 4–2). The virion envelope may fuse directly with the cell-plasma membrane, following attachment of the virus to the cell surface. Alternatively, the virion envelope may fuse with an endosome membrane, after the entire virion has been taken into the cell by receptor-mediated endocytosis. For nonenveloped viruses, the virion is either translocated across the plasma membrane or translocated across an endosome membrane following endocytosis. The pathway of entry is characteristic for each virus family and may also be influenced by the host cell.

Viral Replication

The stages in a viral replicative cycle (following adsorption and penetration of virus) include uncoating of the viral genome, viral gene expression, replication of the viral genome, assembly of progeny virus, and egress of the progeny virus from the infected cell.

Penetration of virus into a cell is accompanied by and followed by disassembly of the virus particle and release of the viral genome. The viral genome is then translocated to the compartment of the cell where viral gene expression can occur (either the nucleus or cytoplasm, depending on the virus). The strategies for expressing the genetic information encoded in each viral genome are different for each virus family. Figures 4–3 and 4–4 outline the strategies of gene expression and replication for the major families of viruses that cause human disease.

A few general observations are pertinent. First, DNA viruses can use cell RNA polymerases for transcribing their genes and cell DNA polymerases for replicating their genomes.

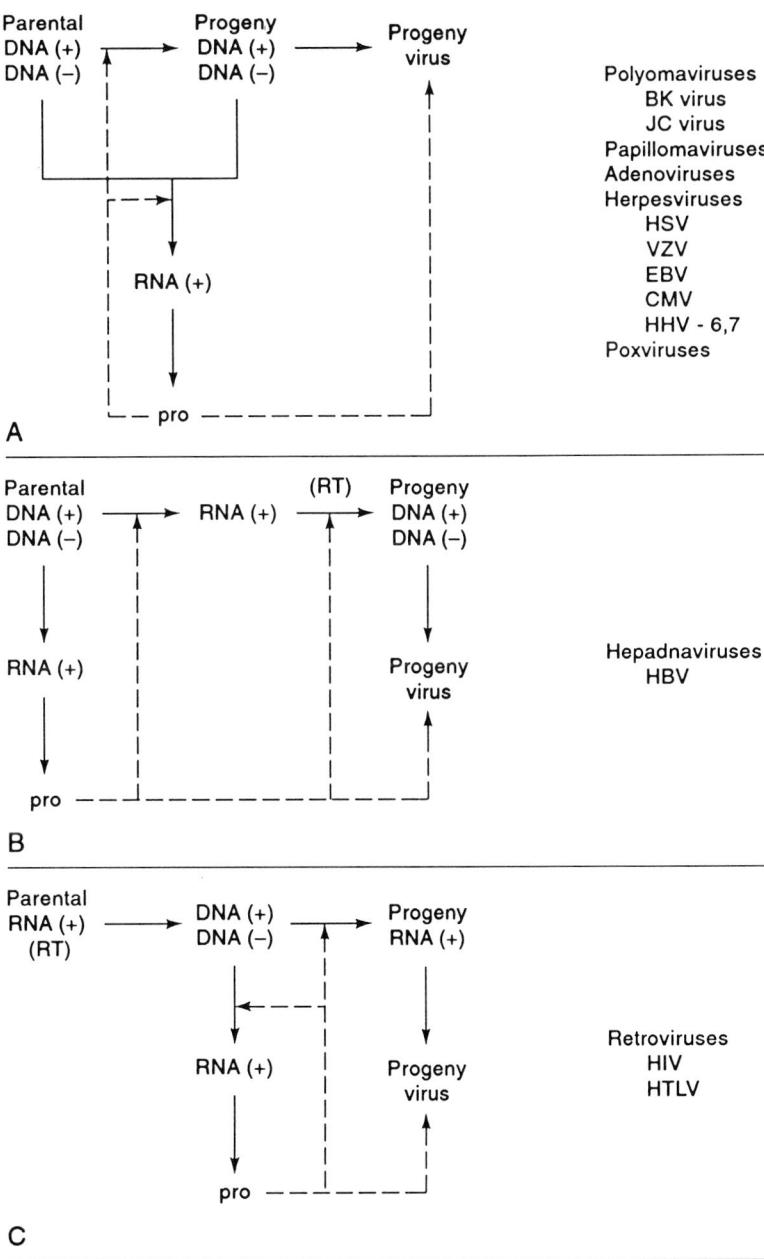

Figure 4–3. Strategies for gene expression and viral replication by selected DNA viruses and retroviruses. For all the DNA viruses listed in A, except poxviruses, the viral DNA is transported to the cell nucleus where it is transcribed into mRNA (RNA(+)) by cell RNA polymerase. The mRNA goes to the cell cytoplasm where it is translated into protein (pro). Viral proteins regulate transcription of the viral genome, participate in replication of the viral genome, and package the progeny viral genomes into virions, as indicated by the dotted lines. Adenoviruses and herpesviruses encode their own DNA polymerases, whereas polyomaviruses and papillomaviruses use the cell DNA polymerase. Poxviruses replicate entirely in the cell cytoplasm. These viruses encode all the enzymes required for transcription and replication of the viral genome. A viral RNA polymerase packaged in the virion mediates initial transcription of the viral genome. For hepadnaviruses (B), the viral genome is also transported to the cell nucleus where it is transcribed by cell RNA polymerase. Some of the transcripts produced serve as mRNA. A special full-length transcript is packaged into immature virus particles, along with a viral reverse transcriptase (RT). During the final stages of virion morphogenesis, the packaged RNA is transcribed into double-stranded DNA (the RNA is degraded subsequent to the reverse transcription; some nicks and gaps remain in the DNA). Viral proteins regulate transcription of the viral genome, mediate reverse transcription, and package the viral genome. For retroviruses (C), the viral RNA genome is introduced into cells along with a RT that was also packaged in the virion. This RT immediately transcribes the viral RNA genome into a double-stranded DNA, which is then integrated into the cell genome. A viral integrase catalyzes this integration. Cell RNA polymerase transcribes the integrated viral DNA (proviral DNA). Differential splicing of the transcripts yields several mRNAs needed for the production of the viral proteins. Full-length transcripts can be packaged into virions along with RT. Viral proteins regulate transcription and splicing, mediate reverse transcription and integration, and package progeny RNA into virions.

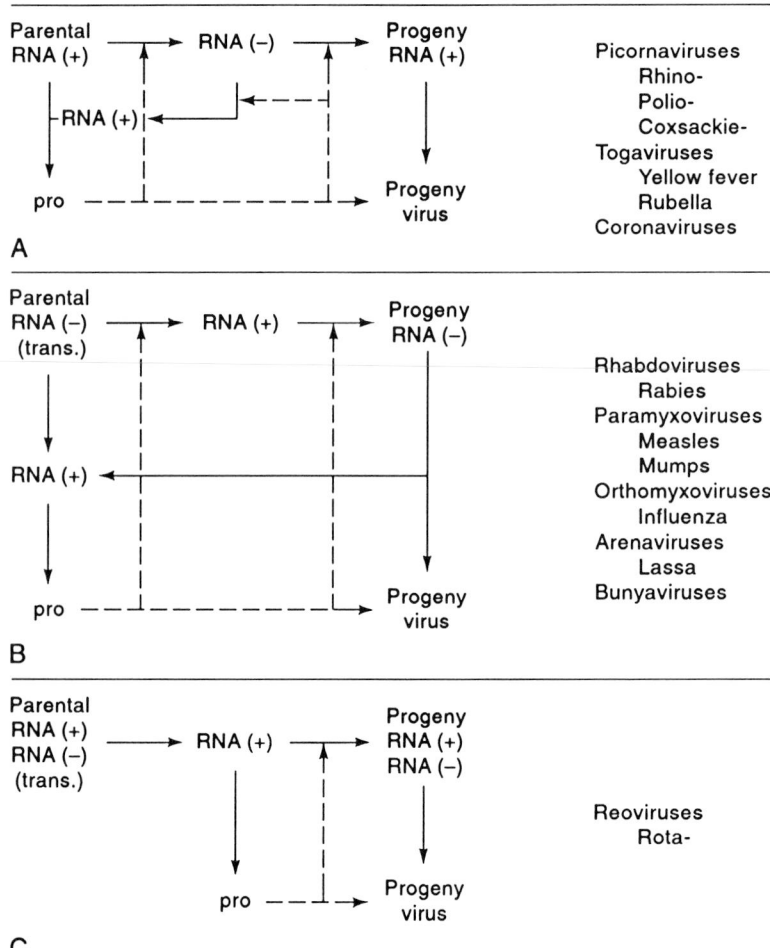

Picornaviruses
Rhino-
Polio-
Coxsackie-
Togaviruses
Yellow fever
Rubella
Coronaviruses

Rhabdoviruses
Rabies
Paramyxoviruses
Measles
Mumps
Orthomyxoviruses
Influenza
Arenaviruses
Lassa
Bunyaviruses

Reoviruses
Rota-

Figure 4–4. Strategies for gene expression and viral replication by selected RNA viruses. The RNA genomes of the viruses listed in A serve as mRNA immediately on entry into the cell cytoplasm. Newly synthesized viral proteins serve as transcriptase–replicase, first to transcribe the viral genome to produce a negative-polarity template. This template is then transcribed to produce positive-polarity RNA. Some of the RNA(+) serves as mRNA to make more viral proteins, including the virion proteins, and the remaining RNA(+) is packaged into virions. The RNA genomes of the viruses listed in B are of negative-polarity and are introduced into cells along with a viral transcriptase (trans.). This transcriptase immediately transcribes the viral genome to produce mRNAs that are translated to produce viral proteins. These proteins include a replicase that transcribes the viral genome to yield a positive-polarity copy and then transcribes this copy to yield progeny viral genomes. Reoviruses (C), have segmented genomes of double-stranded RNA. On entry into a cell, the virion is converted to a protein core containing the RNA genome and a viral transcriptase. The transcriptase transcribes the RNA genome to yield mRNA, which is released from the core and translated to produce viral proteins. These proteins include a replicase that produces double-stranded RNA segments from each mRNA. These segments are packaged into progeny virions.

DNA viruses, however, always encode their own regulatory proteins required to direct transcription and replication to the viral genome. Many DNA viruses also encode their own DNA polymerases and some of the other enzymes and factors required for replication of the genome.

Second, RNA viruses must encode their own RNA polymerases because there appear to be no cell enzymes capable of transcribing genetic information from RNA to RNA or replicating RNA using RNA as a template, at least not for viral RNA genomes. These viral RNA polymerases (often called *transcriptases/replicases*) are usually highly specific for the homologous RNA viral genome. In cases where the input parental RNA genome is not of positive polarity and therefore cannot serve as mRNA, a viral transcriptase must be packaged with the viral genome in the virion. This is to permit production of mRNA, using the parental genome as template, as soon as the virus penetrates into the cell.

Third, retroviruses and hepadnaviruses (hepatitis B virus) both encode reverse transcriptases (RTs) which are packaged in virions and are required for replication of the genome. Their strategies for use of the RTs (which transcribe RNA to produce a double-stranded DNA copy) are quite different, however, as outlined in Figure 4–3.

Fourth, a common strategy for the production of functional viral proteins is synthesis of viral polyproteins, followed by proteolytic cleavage of the polyproteins to yield the individual viral proteins. This strategy is especially important for RNA viruses, including retroviruses. The proteases required are usually encoded by the virus. The proteolytic cleavages may accompany, and may be required for, dynamic processes such as the assembly of progeny virus particles.

Assembly of progeny virions takes place in the cell compartment where replication of the viral genome occurred. Most RNA viruses are assembled in the cell cytoplasm, whereas most DNA viruses are assembled in the cell nucleus. For enveloped viruses, the final step in assembly is acquisition of the envelope by budding of the nucleocapsid through a patch of cell membrane modified to contain viral membrane proteins and glycoproteins. This envelopment can occur at the inner nuclear membrane, endoplasmic reticulum, Golgi apparatus, or the plasma membrane, depending on the virus (Fig. 4–5).

For an enveloped virus that acquires its envelope from the plasma membrane, the final step in assembly releases the virus from the cell. For other enveloped viruses, an exocytic process is required to transport the virions from cisternae of the endoplasmic reticulum or Golgi apparatus to the outside of the cell. For nonenveloped viruses, the progeny virus must escape from the nuclear or cytoplasmic compartment of the cell. It has been thought that this escape might depend upon lysis of the cell. More recent evidence suggests, however, that specific mechanisms may exist for the secretion or extrusion of nonenveloped virions. In general, the mechanisms governing the egress of viruses from infected cells are not well understood.

Death of the infected cell is the usual, but not invariant, consequence of viral replication. The precise mechanisms by which viruses kill cells are not very well understood. Many viruses produce specific inhibitors of cell macromolecular syntheses, presumably to provide a selective advantage for viral gene expression. For example, poliovirus produces a protease that inactivates a cap-binding protein required for the translation of capped-cell mRNAs but not for the uncapped viral mRNA. Viruses that can replicate without killing the host cell include retroviruses.

Many of the stages of each viral replicative cycle can be exploited in the development of antiviral drugs. The intense research effort to produce drugs effective against HIV provides some examples of promising new (but not yet proven) approaches. Soluble forms of the CD4 receptor have been shown to neutralize HIV infectivity in cell culture (presumably by blocking the binding of virus to the cell surface form of CD4) and are now being tested in clinical trials. In addition, the search is on for drugs that can inhibit the HIV protease. The structure of this protease and its active site have been defined at the atomic level in order to predict the properties of drugs that could potentially inhibit the proteolytic activity and therefore inhibit viral replication. The principal drug currently in use against HIV is azidothymidine (AZT), which specifically inhibits the viral reverse transcriptase (see Chapter 26).

Latent and Persistent Infections

A nonproductive infection results when a virus invades a cell that does not possess all the factors required for virus replication. The replicative cycle can be blocked at whatever stage requires the missing cell factor or factors. If the block occurs early in the replicative cycle, the parental viral genome may gradually be lost or diluted out by cell division. If the block occurs late in the replicative cycle, the cell may be killed but without releasing any progeny infectious virus.

Certain viruses, particularly DNA viruses, have evolved mechanisms for the long-term maintenance of viral genomes in cells that are nonpermissive for viral replication. This usually requires the controlled expression of a particular subset of viral genes and repression of most other viral genes, along with controlled replication of the viral genome. This type of virus–cell interaction is akin to lysogeny of bacteria by bacteriophage and, in eukaryotic systems, is called a *latent infection*. In latently infected cells, maintenance of viral genomes depends on cell viability, whereas in productively infected cells virus replication is usually incompatible with

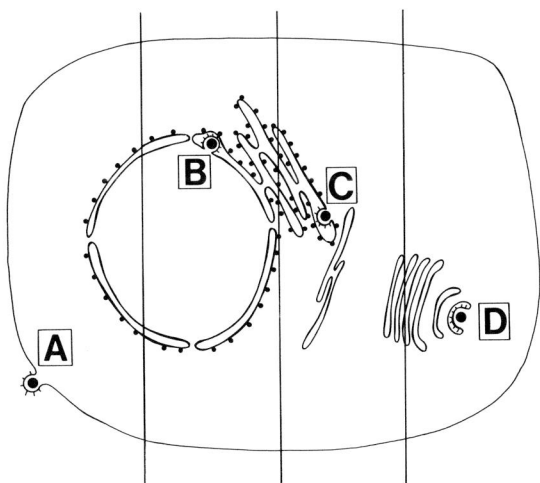

Figure 4–5. Envelopment of nucleocapsids by modified patches of cell membrane during the final stages of virion morphogenesis. Members of different virus families characteristically acquire their envelopes by budding through the plasma membrane (A), the inner nuclear membrane (B), membrane of the endoplasmic reticulum (C), or the Golgi apparatus (D). (Reprinted with permission from Spear, P. G. Virus-induced cell fusion. In Sowers, A. E., ed. Cell Fusion. New York: Plenum Publishing Corporation, 1987, p. 5.)

cell survival. Latent infection appears to be an alternative to productive infection, and not just an aborted productive infection. Under appropriate conditions, however, latently infected cells can be induced to produce virus, which means that the state of the cell governs whether latent or productive infection occurs.

Latent infections are central to the pathogenesis of certain viruses, such as members of the herpesvirus family. Molecular details of the virus–cell interaction in latency are best understood for EBV, principally because latently infected B lymphocytes can be cultured and studied *in vitro*. EBV maintains a few copies of its genome, as circular episomes, in latently infected cells. It does so by expressing a viral protein that binds to an origin of DNA replication in the viral genome, thereby directing cell DNA polymerase to replicate the genome in a controlled fashion during each S phase of the cell cycle. If the latently infected B cell is induced to produce virus, then viral DNA polymerase is expressed and catalyzes the exponential replication of viral genomes, using a different origin of DNA replication. Latently infected B lymphocytes can be isolated from EBV-positive individuals long after primary infection with this virus, whether or not the infection was symptomatic.

Retroviruses present a special case with regard to latency. These viruses have evolved the enzymatic machinery required to produce a double-stranded DNA copy of the RNA genome and then to integrate this DNA (called *proviral DNA*) into the cell genome. As described in Figure 4–3, this integration of proviral DNA is required for viral replication. Viral replication depends upon transcription of the integrated proviral DNA by cell RNA polymerase to produce progeny RNA genomes. Perhaps because maintenance of the template required for production of viral genomes depends upon cell viability, retrovirus replication usually does not result in cell death and is compatible with cell proliferation. Moreover, integration of proviral DNA ensures that an infected cell and its daughter cells are permanently altered genetically and can rarely if ever be "cured" of the infection. Whether cells carrying proviral DNA will be productively or latently infected depends upon whether the appropriate cell factors are present for transcribing the proviral DNA and for producing virus particles. Theoretically, cells can remain latently infected with a retrovirus for a long time and then begin to produce virus only when the cell is stimulated by external events

to produce the factors required for virus production. This possibility has been invoked to explain the variable, but often long, incubation period of AIDS.

Most RNA viruses do not transcribe their genetic information into DNA and do not have any known mechanisms for establishing latent infections of the kinds just described. Persistent, chronic infections with RNA viruses and at least one DNA virus (hepatitis B virus) do occur, however, both *in vivo* and, in some instances, in cultured cells. In persistently infected populations of cultured cells, virus replication and spread of infection may occur at reduced rates and levels so that cell proliferation can outpace cell death resulting from cytotoxic effects of the virus. Some of the factors that enable the establishment of persistent, chronic infections include the generation of defective viruses and the induction of interferon, both of which can modulate the replication of wild-type virus. Certain RNA viruses have the capacity to persist for long periods in individuals who have recovered from the primary disease and then perhaps to cause a different kind of secondary disease. For example, long after recovery from measles, a condition called subacute sclerosing panencephalitis (SSPE) may occur. SSPE is due to the abortive replication of persistent measles virus in cells of the central nervous system.

Virus-Induced Proliferation of Cells

Many DNA viruses encode proteins that can stimulate cell division or other cell processes. An important role of these proteins is to induce the production of cell enzymes and other factors required for viral DNA replication. If these viral stimulatory proteins, sometimes called *viral oncogenes,* are expressed in the absence of other viral proteins, the cells may be immortalized (converted from cells that can divide only a finite number of times to cells that can divide indefinitely) or may even be transformed from normal to malignant. A number of DNA viruses (including polyomaviruses and adenoviruses) can cause tumors in animals other than the natural host. Abortive infection of nonpermissive cells allows the viral oncogenes to be expressed in the absence of viral replication (illegitimate recombination between the viral genome and the cell genome is required to permanently alter the genotype and phenotype of the transformed cells).

Some DNA viruses can induce the proliferation of latently infected cells. The subsets of viral genes expressed under these conditions are those encoding the proteins that induce cell division and those that ensure replication of the viral genome in concert with the cell genome. Virus-induced cell proliferation is an important aspect of pathogenesis in diseases caused by viruses such as papillomaviruses and EBV.

Papillomaviruses can induce the proliferation of latently infected cells in the basal layers of epidermis, resulting in a benign tumor or wart. When the cells in the basal layer move toward the outer surface and differentiate, viral replication is activated. EBV can induce the proliferation of latently infected B lymphocytes, immortalizing the cells and enabling them to proliferate indefinitely in the absence of the antigenic stimulus usually required. Practical use is made of this phenomenon to isolate permanent cell lines from individuals for genetic studies or for use of the cells as autologous antigen-presenting cells in *in vitro* assays of immune function.

The cells that are induced to proliferate in response to virus infection express viral antigens and are usually highly immunogenic. The normal immune system, once primed for attack, can readily contain or eliminate these latently infected, proliferating cells. The consequences of deficiencies in this immunity will be discussed below. For EBV, and perhaps for other DNA viruses, there may be two kinds of latent infection—one in which cell proliferation is induced and another in which it is not. The kind in which cell proliferation is induced can explain the *in vitro* results observed and certain aspects of the pathology of infectious mononucleosis (this self-limiting lymphoproliferative disease appears to be due to the virus-induced proliferation of B lymphocytes and to the even more pronounced proliferation of T lymphocytes in response to the latently infected B cells) (see Chapter 10). Latently infected cells which do not express the viral genes required for cell proliferation may not be very immunogenic (due in part to the more limited expression of viral genes) and could persist for long periods in the infected individual. This kind of latent infection could explain the long-term persistence of EBV in the lymphocytes of asymptomatic individuals.

VIRUS–HOST INTERACTIONS

The signs and symptoms of disease caused by a particular virus depend in part on the virus–cell interactions that govern the portal of entry, the rate of viral replication and spread, the route of

spread of infection, the target organs or tissues, and the site from which virus is shed into the environment. The nature of the disease is also dependent on the vigor and nature of the immune response, in part because immune responses can contribute to the pathology of disease as well as to the containment of virus spread and the reduction in severity of disease.

The severity of viral disease is quite variable in animal or human populations. The consequences of virus infection for the individual may include no clinically evident disease, mild or severe acute disease, or chronic or persistent disease. The outcome depends on a variety of factors, including the properties and virulence of the virus, the innate susceptibility of the individual, and the efficacy of various induced responses to the virus, such as the production of interferon and viral antigen-specific antibodies and T cells. As more is learned about molecular mechanisms of disease and the genetics of virus and host, it should become possible to predict the relative risks to various genetically typed individuals of serious disease caused by a particular virus.

Innate Properties of the Virus and Host Cell That Influence Disease

Viral requirements for interactions with specific cell components (such as cell-surface receptors, cell factors required for gene expression and genome replication, etc.) can explain some of the known features of viral pathogenicity. For example, the very different kinds of disease caused by two of the human herpesviruses can be explained in part by their utilization of different cell-surface receptors. HSV requires the presence of cell-surface heparan sulfate for adsorption to and infection of cells, whereas EBV requires the presence of CR2. HSV can cause cutaneous lesions on any part of the body surface (mucosa or skin), presumably because the target cells in the epithelium or epidermis have cell-surface heparan sulfate and other factors required for replication of the virus. Disease caused by HSV is principally a consequence of virus-mediated cytopathology. HSV lesions often remain localized to the body surface (except that the virus can enter nerve endings in the epidermis and can be transported intraneuronally to the nerve cell bodies to set up a latent infection). There is some barrier to the spread of HSV infection from the epidermis to the dermis. This barrier has not yet been identified but could be composed in part of heparan-sulfate-rich basement membrane.

EBV, on the other hand, uses cell-surface receptors expressed on a more limited set of cell types. EBV usually infects only certain specialized epithelial cells and B lymphocytes in the oropharynx. Although the exact nature of the viral receptor(s) on the epithelial cells is as yet unknown, there is evidence to suggest that receptors related to the CR2 receptors of B lymphocytes are utilized by EBV for infection of the cells. The virus can replicate in cells of the oropharynx, providing the infectious agent needed for transmission of the disease. The pathology of EBV-induced disease, however, is due almost entirely to the latently infected B lymphocytes and the immune responses they provoke and is not due to cytotoxic effects of virus.

For other viruses as well, most notably HIV, research focused on characterization of the cell-surface receptors has provided information needed to understand some aspects of the pathology of the disease. It is clear that HIV utilizes the CD4 molecule for infecting T4 lymphocytes and macrophages. Moreover, much of the pathology is dependent on the effects of HIV on these two cell types that have critical roles in protective immune responses. Questions remain about whether and how the virus infects other cell types and about the importance of these other virus–cell interactions in the disease process. One very important aspect of HIV pathogenesis has nothing to do with cell-surface receptors, however. The fact that proviral DNA becomes integrated into the cell genome means that elimination of virus from an infected individual is virtually impossible without the ability to identify and eliminate all latently or productively infected cells.

Individuals may differ markedly in their susceptibility to virus infection and in their propensity to develop serious disease once infected. Presumably this is due in large part to polymorphism of the human genes that control immune responses and that encode many of the cell factors required for viral infection and replication. Because susceptibility or resistance to viral disease is influenced by multiple genetic loci of the host, identifying even the most important determinants has been difficult, for inbred strains of animals as well as for humans. In some cases, however, one genetic determinant may be dominant. For example, some inbred strains of mice are resistant to infection by mouse hepatitis virus (a coronavirus) because

their cells lack the correct form of the cell-surface receptor required for viral entry. In addition, there are some hereditary defects of humans that result in extreme susceptibility to disease caused by a particular virus. One is an X-linked defect that manifests itself when the individual is exposed to EBV. As many as 75% of people with this X-linked defect develop a fatal lymphoproliferative disease as a result of EBV infection. Another genetic defect results in the condition called epidermodysplasia verruciformis, in which the individual suffers throughout life from multiple, disseminated warts caused by papillomaviruses. Apparently, resistance to the development of warts and the ability to resolve the lesions are greatly impaired. The precise genetic defect is not yet known for either one of these diseases.

Interferon and Natural Killer Cells

Both interferon (IFN) and natural killer (NK) cells are important to the first line of defense against viral pathogens. IFN was first described in 1957 when Issacs and Lindenmann found that chick chorioallantoic membranes infected with influenza virus or heat-inactivated influenza virus produced a soluble factor capable of protecting other cells from viral infection. Normal cells do not usually produce IFN but can be induced to do so by various stimuli, including virus infection, double-stranded RNA (often produced in virus-infected cells), and the induction of immune responses. IFN does not itself have antiviral activity, but it induces cells to produce various factors that interfere with viral infection and replication. IFN is relatively species-specific in that it is most active on cells of homologous species. The effects of IFN are not virus-specific inasmuch as most viruses are susceptible to the antiviral activities induced.

IFN is not a single protein but rather a family of proteins encoded by three distinct subfamilies of genes. The multiple forms of IFN-α are expressed, principally by leukocytes, as the products of about 15 different nonallelic genes. Different forms of IFN-β are encoded by at least two nonallelic genes and are expressed principally in fibroblasts. Finally, there appears to be only one genetic locus for IFN-γ, which is produced by activated T lymphocytes.

In addition to interfering with viral replication, the various forms of IFN have a plethora of other activities, including modulation of cell growth and differentiation, enhancement of the expression of histocompatibility antigens (which can potentiate antigen recognition), and enhancement of NK cell activity. It is not clear how interferon exerts its antiviral effect. Two of the cell products known to be induced by IFN could act to inhibit viral protein synthesis, provided double-stranded RNA is present. One of these products is a protein kinase that, when activated by double-stranded RNA, phosphorylates and inactivates a factor required for the initiation of protein synthesis. The other is a synthetase of 2,5-oligoA (an unusual polyadenylic acid); the synthetase is activated by double-stranded RNA to produce the 2,5-oligoA, which in turn activates a latent RNase capable of degrading mRNA. Whatever the mode of action of IFN, its physiologic importance (not necessarily for its antiviral activity alone) is underscored by the number of genes encoding the various forms. The importance of the antiviral effects of IFN is evident from findings that anti-IFN antibodies, capable of neutralizing IFN activity, can greatly increase the severity of viral disease in experimental animals.

Intensive efforts have been and continue to be made to utilize IFNs clinically both for their antiviral effects and their cell regulatory properties. Recombinant IFN-α has proven effective in the treatment of hairy cell leukemia and refractory genital warts. In addition, intranasal administration of IFNs can reduce the incidence of disease after natural exposure to various respiratory viruses; the clinical utility of IFNs in this latter situation is limited, however. There may be a role for IFN in life-threatening viral illnesses such as rabies or in the treatment of chronic viral hepatitis (see Chapter 21). Current research efforts are directed at testing combination therapies using IFNs and other cytokines.

As mentioned above, one of the activities of IFN-γ is to stimulate NK cell activity. NK cells are large granular cells of the lymphoid lineage, but are differentiable from B cells and T cells bearing the typical markers of CD4 and CD8 cells. NK cells have the capacity to kill various kinds of "abnormal" target cells, including tumor cells and virus-infected cells. It is not clear how the target cells are recognized by the NK cells.

Antigen-Specific Immune Responses to Viruses

The immune response to viruses, as to other antigens, results in the production of antibodies, cytotoxic T cells, delayed-type hypersensitivity (DTH) T cells, and so forth. The antibodies can neutralize viral infectivity, either by blocking the adsorption of virus to cells or by blocking the penetration of virus into cells. Antibodies (with the participation of complement or cells that mediate ADCC) and cytotoxic T cells can kill virus-infected cells, thereby limiting the production of progeny virus and the spread of infection. T cells mediating DTH can direct the attack of activated macrophages to virus-infected cells.

The devastating consequences of viral infections in immunocompromised individuals demonstrate the importance of the immune response in the normal virus—host interaction. Interestingly, patients with agammaglobulinemia can respond adequately, if not optimally, to many viral infections, with the exception of enterovirus infections. This suggests that antibodies may not be as important as cell-mediated immunity for many viral diseases, except for those caused by enteroviruses.

The immune response is, to some extent, a double-edged sword in many viral diseases. Some antiviral antibodies may actually enhance the spread of infection. These include antibodies that can bind to virions without neutralizing infectivity. These antibodies can block the binding of neutralizing antibodies or can facilitate the infection of cells that are devoid of virus receptors but express Fc receptors. In addition, some of the pathology observed in viral infections can be due principally to immune effector mechanisms. This immunopathology may be of negligible consequence or it may be the major cause of distress, particularly in chronic viral diseases. For example, the liver damage in hepatitis caused by hepatitis B virus is due primarily to immune responses to the persistently infected cells. The virus itself may not cause much cytopathology (see Chapter 21).

Another aspect of the interaction between viruses and the immune system is crucial to pathogenicity. A number of viruses can infect cells of the immune system and thus modify the activities of these cells. HIV is the most prominent example. Presumably as a consequence of infecting CD4$^+$ T lymphocytes and macrophages, HIV impairs the immune system to the extent that opportunistic infections invariably occur and result in fatal disease. EBV induces the proliferation of B lymphocytes, thereby abrogating the normal controls of B cell function and proliferation. A number of viruses, most notably measles virus, can suppress certain aspects of the immune system, by mechanisms that are not yet understood. This immuno-suppression can explain, for example, the association of measles virus infection with the reactivation of tuberculosis.

In addition to interacting directly with cells of the immune system, viruses can express products that perhaps permit evasion of immune reactions directed against infected cells. For example, some of the herpesviruses express glycoproteins that can function, on the surfaces of infected cells and of virions, as Fc receptors and complement receptors. One of the HSV glycoproteins binds to C3b and accelerates the decay of this pivotal component of the alternative pathway for complement activation. Poxviruses produce a C4b binding protein that inhibits the classic pathway of complement activation. Viruses can also down-regulate the expression of cell MHC antigens on the surfaces of infected cells. Inasmuch as T cells recognize foreign antigens only in association with cell MHC antigens, this can render the infected cells "invisible" to T cells. Cytomegalovirus encodes a glycoprotein with homology to the heavy chain of MHC class I antigens. This viral glycoprotein competes with cell MHC antigen for interaction with β_2-microglobulin in infected cells, thereby reducing the transport of the cell MHC antigen to the cell surface. Adenovirus can reduce the cell surface expression of cell MHC antigens by two mechanisms. First, the virus represses expression of the cell MHC gene, and second, it encodes a protein that sequesters cell MHC antigen in the endoplasmic reticulum.

Despite the foregoing excursion into the complications of immune response to viruses, recovery from infection is usually a consequence of developing immunity, and specific immune responses can be exploited to prevent viral disease. Vaccination has been an effective means of preventing certain viral diseases despite our ignorance of the particular antigens and effector mechanisms that provide the protection. The diseases for which effective vaccines are currently available are, for the most part, those caused by viruses that are antigenically stable and in which recovery from primary infection is accompanied by the development of long-lasting immunity to disease. In general, the vaccines currently in use are either live attenuated viruses that can cause asymptomatic infection or inactivated whole viruses that include most or all viral antigens (see Chapter 40).

Live attenuated or killed whole viral vaccines may not be suitable or effective for certain viral diseases for a variety of reasons, including the possibility that the live vaccine virus could induce a latent infection with consequences that might not be evident for many years. In addition, the dominant epitopes for viruses that exhibit antigenic variation are often the most variable epitopes, such that vaccination with the whole virus induces variant-specific, but not cross-reactive, immunity. Given that it is now technically feasible to produce genetically engineered subunit vaccines, considerable attention is being focused on identifying for particular viruses the few antigens and epitopes, among many, that can induce effective cross-reactive immunity. Because T cells as well as B cells must be able to respond to the vaccine and because T cells recognize peptide fragments that can associate with MHC antigens, considerable attention must also be focused on determining how to formulate and administer the vaccine so that the antigens are processed and presented properly to T cells and B cells.

Viruses and Cancer

Several viruses are probably cofactors in the causation of human cancers, including papillomaviruses, EBV, human T-cell lymphotropic virus (HTLV) and hepatitis B virus (HBV). Establishing a causal role for these viruses in cancer is complicated by the relatively low incidence of cancer compared with incidence of virus infection, the long interval between virus infection and detection of the cancer, and the occasional appearance of similar cancers in the absence of virus infection.

The first three of the viruses mentioned above, and possibly the fourth, share the ability to induce the proliferation of infected cells under certain conditions. Papillomaviruses and EBV can stimulate the proliferation of latently infected cells, whereas productively infected cells are probably killed as a consequence of viral replication. For HTLV, virus-induced proliferation of cells may occur either in productively or latently infected cells. This virus-induced cell proliferation is not synonymous with malignant transformation, but possibly predisposes the dividing cells to mutations caused by carcinogens that act during DNA replication. In any event, the development of one of the cancers associated with these viruses probably depends upon multiple contributory factors, which may usually, but not always, include virus infection.

Certain of the many serologic types of papillomavirus appear to have a causative role in cancers of the urogenital tract, particularly cervical carcinoma. DNAs of types 16 or 18 are found in most of the cervical carcinomas screened. Expression of viral gene products known to be involved in inducing cell proliferation and immortalization is also regularly detected in the cancer cells.

EBV has been associated with Burkitt's lymphoma and with a nasopharyngeal carcinoma that occurs predominantly in people of Chinese extraction. More is known about the genetic basis for the lymphoma than the carcinoma. A chromosomal translocation that brings the c-*myc* oncogene under the control of the immunoglobulin locus is invariably found in cells of Burkitt's lymphoma. The possibility exists that this chromosomal translocation occurs more readily in B lymphocytes that have been stimulated to divide by EBV gene products, but the translocation and Burkitt's lymphoma can also occur in the absence of EBV infection. The EBV-positive Burkitt's lymphoma cells do not express the EBV proteins required to induce cell division in normal B lymphocytes. This implies that the translocation is the key event in the malignant transformation. Possibly cancer cells that express these EBV proteins are eliminated by the immune system inasmuch as B lymphocytes that express these proteins are highly immunogenic.

EBV can cause fatal lymphoproliferative disease or lymphoma in immunodeficient individuals. In early stages, the proliferating B cells may be polyclonal, suggesting that nonmalignant immortalized B cells may simply be dividing continually, as they would in cell culture, without the usual constraints supplied by the immune system. In later stages of disease, one or a few clones of proliferating B cells may predominate, suggesting that these clones have acquired mutations conferring a selective advantage for proliferation.

Just as EBV can immortalize B lymphocytes *in vitro*, HTLV-1 can immortalize T lymphocytes *in vitro*. Human infections with HTLV-1 are largely asymptomatic, indicating that the normal immune system can control the proliferation of the HTLV-1 infected cells *in vivo*. A small percentage (about 1%) of infected individuals eventually become ill with the malignant disease called adult T-cell leukemia. A dominant clone of HTLV-1-infected, malignant cells is present in most cases, indicating that the malignant transformation required a genetic event, as yet unidentified, subsequent to HTLV-1 infection.

The evidence that HBV has a role in hepatocellular carcinoma is largely based on epidemiologic studies. The incidence of this type of carcinoma is highest in populations where HBV infection is most prevalent. Integrated hepatitis B virus DNA and viral gene products have been detected in cancer cells. The molecular linkage between HBV infection and the carcinoma is not understood, however.

SUMMARY

The consequences of virus–host interactions are determined by the multiple kinds of virus–cell interactions that can occur and the immune responses provoked by the expression of viral antigens. As the molecular details of the virus–cell interactions and the immune responses are revealed, new approaches to preventing and curing viral diseases will also be revealed. This is a time of accelerating progress in this area of medical research.

REFERENCES

Books

Fields, B. N., and Knipe, D. M., eds. *Fields Virology.* 2nd ed. New York: Raven Press, 1990.

Notkins, A. L., and Oldstone, M. B. A., eds. *Concepts in Viral Pathogenesis III.* New York: Springer-Verlag, 1989.

Articles

Burgert, H.-G., Maryanski, J. L., and Kvist, S. E3/19K protein of adenovirus type 2 inhibits lysis of cytolytic T lymphocytes by blocking cell-surface expression of histocompatibility class I antigens. *Proc. Natl. Acad. Sci. USA* 84:1356, 1987.

Cheng-Mayer, C., Seto, D., Tateno, M., et al. Biologic features of HIV-1 that correlate with virulence in the host. *Science 240:*80, 1988.

Dalgelish, A. G., Beverly, P. C. L., Clapham, P. R., et al. The CD4 (T4) antigen is an essential component of the receptor for the AIDS retrovirus. *Nature 312:*763, 1985.

Douglas, R. M., Albrecht, J. K., and Miles, H. B. Intranasal interferon-α2 prophylaxis of natural respiratory viral infection. *J. Infect. Dis. 151:*731, 1985.

Fingeroth, J. D., Weiss, J. J., Tedder, T. F., et al. Epstein-Barr virus receptor of human B lymphocytes is the C3d receptor CR2. *Proc. Natl. Acad. Sci. USA 81:*4510, 1984.

Fries, L. F., Friedman, H. M., Cohen, G. H., et al. Glcyoprotein C of herpes simplex virus 1 is an inhibitor of the complement cascade. *J. Immunol. 137:*1636, 1986.

Gregory, C. D., Murray, R. J., Edwards, C. F., et al. Down regulation of cell adhesion molecules LFA-3 and ICAM-1 in Epstein-Barr virus-positive Burkitt's lymphoma underlies tumor cell escape from virus-specific T cell surveillance. *J. Exp. Med. 167:*2811, 1988.

Gregory, C. D., Rowe, M., and Rickinson, A. B. Different Epstein-Barr virus-B cell interactions in phenotypically distinct clones of a Burkitt's lymphoma cell line. *J. Gen. Virol. 71:*1481, 1990.

Greve, J., Davis, G., and Meyer, A. The major human rhinovirus receptor is ICAM-1. *Cell 56:*839, 1989.

Higgins, P. G., Al-Nakib, W., Willman, J., et al. Interferon-Bser as prophylaxis against experimental rhinovirus infection in volunteers. *J. Interferon Res. 8:*591, 1988.

Ho, D. D., Pomerantz, R. J., and Kaplan, J. C. Pathogenesis of infection with human immunodeficiency virus. *N. Engl. J. Med. 317:*278, 1987.

Holland, J.J. Receptor affinities as major determinants of enterovirus tissue tropism in humans. *Virology 15:*312, 1961.

Issacs, A., and Lindenmann, J. Virus interference: I. The interferon. *Proc. R. Soc. Lond. 147:*258, 1957.

Kotwal, G. J., Isaacs, S. N., McKenzie, R., et al. Inhibition of the complement cascade by the major secretory protein of vaccinia virus. *Science 250:*827, 1990.

Maddon, P., Dalgleish, A. G., McDougal, J., et al. The T4 gene encodes the AIDS virus receptor and is expressed in the immune system and brain. *Cell 47:*333, 1986.

Marsh, M. The entry of enveloped viruses into cells by endocytosis. *Biochem. J. 218:*1, 1984.

Mellerik, D. M., and Fraser, N. W. Physical state of the latent herpes simplex virus genome in a mouse model system: Evidence supporting an episomal state. *Virology 158:*265, 1987.

Mendelsohn, C., Wimmer, E., and Racaniello, V. Cellular receptor for poliovirus: Molecular cloning, nucleotide sequence, and expression of a new member of the immunoglobulin superfamily. *Cell 56:*855, 1989.

Palese, P., and Young, J. F. Variation of influenza A, B, and C viruses. *Science 215:*1468, 1982.

Quesada, J. R., and Gutterman, J. U. Interferons in the treatment of human neoplasms. *J. Interferon Res. 7:*575, 1987.

Redfield, R. R., Markham, P. D., and Salahuddin, S. Z. Genetic variation in HTLV-III/LAV over time in patients with AIDS or at risk for AIDS. *Science 232:*1548, 1986.

Rice, G. P. A., Schrier, R. D., and Oldstone, M. B. A. CMV infects human lymphocytes and monocytes: Virus expression is restricted to immediate-early gene products. *Proc. Natl. Acad. Sci. USA 81:*6134, 1984.

Sattentau, Q. J., and Weiss, R. A. The CD4 antigen: Physiologic ligand and HIV receptor. *Cell 52:*631, 1988.

Schrier, P. I., Bernards, R., Vaessen, R. T. M. J., et al. Expression of class I major histocompatibility antigens switched off by highly oncogenic adenovirus 12 in transformed rat cells. *Nature 305:*771, 1983.

Webster, R. G., Laver, W. G., Air, G. M., et al. Molecular mechanisms of variation in influenza viruses. *Nature 296:*115, 1982.

Wechsler, S., and Meissner, H. C. Measles and SSPE viruses: Similarities and differences. *Prog. Med. Virol. 28:*65, 1982.

Weinberg, R. A. Oncogenes, antioncogenes, and the molecular bases of multistep carcinogenesis. *Cancer Res. 49:*3713, 1989.

Weis, W., Brown, J., Cusack, S., et al. Structure of the influenza virus hemagglutinin complexes with its receptor, sialic acid. *Nature 333:*426, 1988.

Weismann, C., and Weber, H. The interferon genes. *Prog. Nucleic Acid Res. Mol. Biol. 33:*251, 1986.

WuDunn, D., and Spear, P. G. Initial interaction of herpes simplex virus with cells is binding to heparan sulfate. *J. Virol. 63:*52, 1989.

Microbe-Induced Autoreactive Host Responses and Autoimmune Disease

INTRODUCTION

The tools of modern molecular biology have enabled the recent explosion in our knowledge of how host immune responses are directed or misdirected toward constituents of our own tissues or cells. This increase in knowledge will, it can be predicted safely, continue to clarify the complex issues related to these phenomena. It has been known for decades that host immune responses that are directed against self-antigens may be associated with certain microbial infections. However, the precise relationship between those cellular and/or humoral responses and the pathogenesis of tissue damage has been difficult to establish. For example, establishing the fact that heart-reactive antibody is present in certain cardiac conditions does not, of course, confirm that that particular case of heart disease is a direct consequence of such antibodies.

Nevertheless, there are a number of examples of microbe-induced immune responses that are in fact central to disease pathogenesis. These include the development of acute rheumatic fever after group A streptococcal upper respiratory tract infection, acute poststreptococcal glomerulonephritis following skin or throat in-

fection (see Chapter 9), acute encephalomyelitis in humans receiving certain viral vaccines, and the so-called reactive arthropathies that occur in selected individuals recovering from acute gastrointestinal infection caused by salmonella, shigella, yersinia, or other agents.

The precise mechanisms by which microbe-stimulated immune responses may become "misdirected" toward host antigens remain somewhat mysterious. This relates in large measure to continuing uncertainty about the etiology and pathogenesis of autoimmune diseases in general, such as systemic lupus, which is associated with a particular proliferation of humoral immune responses that are directed against self-antigens. This uncertainty is in turn related to the broader (and even more complex) issue of the distinction between self- and non–self-antigenic determinants and the recognition process by which this discrimination is achieved.

SELF–NON-SELF RECOGNITION

The immune system is highly efficient in its ability to mobilize responses to an extraordinarily diverse range of foreign (that is, *non–self-*) antigenic stimuli. Under normal circumstances, by striking contrast, the host's *self* antigenic determinants are in large part ignored by the immune system. This ability to selectively avoid developing immune responses against self-epitopes is found even in primitive forms of life, suggesting that there is parallel acquisition of both immune responsiveness and selective self-nonresponsiveness. Clarifying the mechanisms by which this is accomplished holds the key to understanding many of the nuances of the immune system.

The immune response is initiated after foreign

antigen is processed by antigen-presenting cells (macrophages, among others), and peptides derived from that antigen are presented on the cell surface in a complex that includes a class II major histocompatibility complex (MHC) molecule (Fig. 5–1). This antigenic peptide–MHC II complex is recognized by the alpha-beta T-cell receptor (TCR) on CD4+ T cells. The alpha-beta TCR is physically associated with the CD3 complex that is expressed on the surface of all mature T cells and is necessary for membrane expression of the alpha-beta heterodimer. Histocompatibility between the antigen-presenting cell and the CD4+ T cell is necessary for this interaction to occur.

B and T lymphocytes each bear receptors (surface immunoglobulin molecules and T-cell receptors, respectively) that confer the ability to discern fine antigenic differences. These receptors mediate the distinction between recognition or nonrecognition of antigens. The diversity of the immunoglobulin molecules that serve as B-cell receptors results from somatic recombination of hundreds of variable (V) gene segments, dozens of diversity (D) gene segments, and several joining (J) gene segments. When soluble antigen binds to surface immunoglobulin on a B lymphocyte, it triggers cell division and results in clonal expansion and secretion of

antibody molecules. T-cell antigenic recognition differs in that soluble antigen is not recognized but rather antigenic determinants are recognized when presented to the T cell on the cell surface of antigen-processing cells only in conjunction with MHC molecules, as described above. Utilizing monoclonal antibodies and techniques for establishing T-cell clones and hybrids, the antigen-specific alpha-beta TCR complex was found to be composed of a 40–50 kd acidic alpha glycoprotein covalently linked to a 40–45-kd basic beta glycoprotein and to be non-covalently associated at the cell surface with the CD3 complex, which is itself composed of five protein chains. The TCR alpha and beta glycoproteins are transmembrane and contain extracellular variable and constant domains analogous to immunoglobulins, as well as a connecting segment, a transmembrane segment, and a short intracytoplasmic tail. The antigenic diversity of the TCR is generated by the combination of 50–100 V-beta and 6–7 J-beta gene segments, and in the alpha chain by 50–100 V-alpha and 30–100 J-alpha segments.

The interaction of the TCR-alpha-beta-CD3 complex with foreign-processed antigen and MHC leads to activation of the TCR-alpha-beta helper CD4+ lymphocytes. The most critical determinant of whether an immune response will occur is conferred by the TCR alpha-beta heterodimer that recognizes the complex of processed foreign peptide and MHC molecule being presented. Presumably nonrecognition of self-antigens occurs at this level. That is, T lymphocytes with TCR alpha-beta heterodimers that could recognize presented self-antigens do not exist in the normal T-cell repertoire, thus preventing the initiation of an immune response. This failure of T cells to recognize self-antigens is termed *tolerance*.

TOLERANCE

At least three mechanisms have been suggested to explain how tolerance, or nonresponsiveness to self-antigens, may develop. These include the concepts of (1) *elimination* of autoreactive T-cell clones early in development; (2) *nonresponsiveness* of such clones; and (3) active *suppression* of autoreactive T-cell clones. Attempts to elucidate these issues in experimental animal models have been difficult because a number of artifacts can interfere with the functional assays used to measure autoreactive cells. However, the following recent developments have clarified this picture: (1) construction of transgenic mice

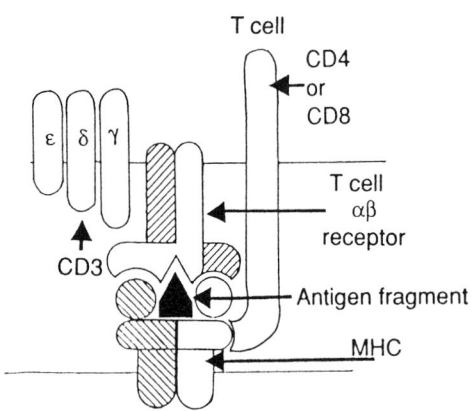

Antigen-presenting cell

Figure 5–1. Diagrammatic structure of the αβ TCR complexed to antigen plus MHC. The T cell αβ receptor has a combining site for antigen-MHC. The antigenic peptide (represented by the black pentagon) is bound by an MHC molecule on the surface of an antigen-presenting cell in a groove created by two α helices (circles) and a β-pleated sheet (platform). Other molecules involved in T-cell recognition and activation, the γ, δ, and ε chains of CD3, and the "accessory" or "costimulatory" molecules, CD4 and CD8, are shown. (Reprinted with permission from Blackman, M., Kappler, J., and Marrack, P. The role of the T-cell receptor in positive and negative selection of developing T-cells. Science 248:1335, 1990.)

that express specific T-cell receptors, (2) the demonstration that some TCR beta-chain-variable domains preferentially confer reactivity to specific self or to foreign antigens, and (3) the use of monoclonal antibodies to identify T cells that bear TCRs for a specific antigen. These studies have enabled direct demonstration that cells bearing autoreactive TCRs are selectively eliminated during early development within the microenvironment of the thymus gland. Thus, *intrathymic clonal deletion* is now considered a major mechanism for induction of tolerance to self-antigens. Apparently within the thymus of the developing animal, high avidity interactions between autoreactive T cells and the hematopoietic components of the thymus result in the deletion of those T cells. This results in tolerance to autoantigens.

Some of the studies clarifying these issues are impressively elegant. For example, the gene for hen-egg lysozyme was microinjected into the egg of a mouse, resulting in life-long tolerance of this molecule as a self-antigen; other mice received genes for antilysozyme antibodies and later had many B cells with lysozyme-specific immunoglobulin receptors. When cross-mated, the double transgenic offspring possessing both genes did not respond to lysozyme but had detectable B cells bearing lysozyme receptors that were functionally impaired; after transfer of these lysozyme-specific B cells to non-transgenic mice, no antilysozyme response could be induced, indicating that these B cells had been rendered functionally silent.

Tolerance to non–self-antigens also occurs but appears to be of less clinical relevance, except as pertains to its desirability in transplant recipients. Mechanisms of induction of tolerance to non–self-antigens are varied and complex, and they are beyond the scope of this chapter.

AUTOREACTIVE RESPONSES IN HUMANS

In general, humans remain tolerant of self-antigens, a fact that contributes to the healthy state. However, a large number of pathologic conditions are characterized by the development of autoimmunity, or the failure of self-tolerance.

It has been pointed out that autoimmune *responses* are rather common, whereas autoimmune *disease* occurs relatively rarely. That is, the quality and magnitude of the autoimmune mechanisms triggered may determine whether clinically apparent disease develops. The development of disease is dependent upon the anti-

genic properties of the inducing autoantigen, the mode of antigen presentation, the genetic make-up of the host, and the accessibility of the target antigen to immune effector mechanisms.

The clinical autoimmune disorders can be the result of a variety of effector pathways that may result in cell dysfunction, damage, or death. Autoreactive helper T-cell clones facilitate proliferation of autoreactive B-cell clones, producing autoantibodies which can participate in complement-mediated cell damage, immune-complex-mediated injury, or antibody-dependent cellular cytotoxicity (ADCC). Autoantibodies can also block cell receptors or act as false transmitters.

For example, the group of classic systemic autoimmune diseases, including systemic lupus erythematosus (SLE), rheumatoid arthritis, scleroderma, Sjögren's syndrome, dermatomyositis, and mixed connective tissue disease (MCTD), are characterized by spontaneous production of autoantibodies that react with cellular proteins and/or nucleic acids. It has recently been established that each of these disorders is characterized by its own distinctive set of autoantibodies. SLE is associated with several autoantibodies including anti-DNA (both single-stranded and native double-stranded DNA), anti-Sm (antibodies against complexes of small nuclear RNAs and proteins that are important for splicing of precursor mRNA), anti-PCNA (proliferating cell nuclear antigen, involved in DNA replication and repair), among others. In scleroderma, autoantibodies to centromere proteins involved in cell mitosis and spindle function are very common, as is anti-Scl-70, which is antibody to DNA topoisomerase I. Careful study of the patterns of autoantibodies in various disorders suggests that *in vivo* the immunogens may be subcellular particles in structurally distinct cellular compartments rather than individual proteins. Certain autoantibodies are directed against autoepitopes that are important in certain cellular functions, for example, those that are at a catalytic site. In fact, these autoantibodies are being utilized to aid in studies of the molecular structure of intracellular molecules and to clarify their biologic function.

Autoantibodies serve as convenient markers for autoimmunity, and perhaps the most important aspect of these phenomena relates to speculation regarding the nature of the triggering event that leads an antigen to become autoimmunogenic. For the most part, the role of specific exogenous factors remains unclear. Certain chemical agents, such as mercuric chloride in mice and rats and the drug procainamide in humans, clearly initiate autoantibody formation. Physical alteration of self-antigens, for example, by tissue injury, has been proposed as a possible mechanism by which an autoimmune response might be triggered. The role of infectious agents is clear in a few circumstances (see below) but is primarily speculative in many others.

MICROBE-INDUCED AUTOREACTIVE RESPONSES

There are several proposed mechanisms by which microbes might trigger autoreactive immune responses and thus lead to development of autoimmune clinical disorders. In some circumstances, infectious agents may induce in host tissues expression of a new epitope that is not present on uninfected tissue nor on the infecting agent. Coxsackie B–induced myocarditis/myocardiopathy in mice is associated with an early acute phase directly related to viral infection and with a later phase mediated by a T-cell autoimmune response directed against a new epitope on myocardial fibers and unrelated to viral antigen. A similar example of neoantigens related to experimental nervous system autoimmunity has been well studied.

Nowhere has the impact of modern molecular biologic techniques and modern computer capabilities been greater than in the study of *molecular mimicry* between immunodeterminants of microbial agents and those of host tissues. This is particularly striking in studies related to the so-called *reactive arthropathies* (including Reiter's syndrome) and to ankylosing spondylitis. Reactive arthropathy is of acute onset and occurs 2–6 weeks after a preceding gastrointestinal or genitourinary tract infection has subsided. This is an episodic disease that primarily involves peripheral joints. The implicated infectious agents include *Shigella, Salmonella, Yersinia, Campylobacter, Clostridia,* and *Chlamydia* species. These illnesses are considered to be reactive rather than infective because no viable organisms are detectable in the inflammatory sites, and antibiotic therapy is completely ineffective. In a recent study, evidence of salmonella lipopolysaccharide was found in synovial cells from patients with reactive arthritis but not from controls.

There is a strong association between these arthropathies and carriage of the histocompatibility antigen HLA-B27, particularly in Caucasians. For example, approximately 90% of patients with ankylosing spondylitis, about 80% of those with Reiter's syndrome, and 60–80% of those with reactive arthropathies are B27-positive; this contrasts with about 6–8% B27-positivity in the general Caucasian population. Several hypotheses have been proposed to explain how HLA-B27 and the bacteria noted above might interact to induce reactive arthropathy. One is that HLA-B27 is somehow quite important in the presentation of bacterial antigens in the form of peptides to putative disease-causing T lymphocytes. However, it has not been established that reactive arthropathies are T-cell mediated, nor have disease-inducing bacterial peptides been identified. A second hypothesis is that HLA-B27 molecules serve as cell-surface receptors for certain factors elaborated only by arthritis-inducing organisms, and that the genes encoding these factors are on plasmids and become integrated into the host cell genome. Few experimental data support this concept.

Another hypothesis, that of *molecular mimicry,* is supported by exciting new data and will be discussed in some detail here. The mimicry hypothesis implies that cross-reactive antigens exist between HLA-B27 and components or products of the disease-triggering bacteria, so that a B27-restricted response to bacterial determinants initiates the disease. The structure of HLA-B27 molecules, like other HLA class I cell-surface glycoproteins, includes a polymorphic heavy chain and a non-covalently associated light-chain peptide, beta$_2$-microglobulin. The HLA class I (HLA-A, B, and C alleles) genes have an exon–intron structure, and the exons encode a leader peptide and three extracellular domains (alpha$_1$, alpha$_2$, alpha$_3$), as well as transmembrane and cytoplasmic portions. Polymorphism among the class I alleles reflects amino acid substitutions mainly in the N-terminal alpha$_1$- and alpha$_2$-domains. Six HLA-B27 alleles have been defined by isoelectric-focusing gel electrophoretic differences, and they differ by 1–4 amino acid substitutions in eight variable positions in the alpha$_1$- and alpha$_2$-domains. X-ray crystallographic studies of HLA class I molecules indicate that the alpha$_3$ and beta$_2$-microglobulin domains have tertiary structures resembling immunoglobulin constant domains and that the alpha$_1$- and alpha$_2$-domains form a platform of eight beta strands topped by two alpha helices, with a long groove between the helices. The polymorphic residues of HLA class I molecules such as B27 tend to be clustered in this groove and are the sites at which peptide antigens are bound and serve as the TCR recognition site. All eight of the B27 variable positions point into this groove and thus appear functionally important.

The development of monoclonal antibodies was essential for studies evaluating possible cross-reactivity or mimicry between HLA antigens and bacterial determinants, because studies with polyclonal sera result in a great deal of background reactivity. One group of investigators produced a monoclonal antibody against *Yersinia enterocolitica* that also reacted exclusively with HLA-B27. Others raised a monoclonal antibody directed against B27 and found cross-reactions with a 16-kd component of a strain of *Y. enterocolitica* and two strains of *Klebsiella pneumoniae;* another anti-B27 monoclonal antibody reacted with a 20-kd molecule on a strain of *Shigella flexneri.* Cross-reactivity between B27 and a 19-kd component of *Y. pseudotuberculosis* has also been reported. Others have developed monoclonal anti-B27 antibodies that react with 23-kd and 36-kd envelope components in strains of *Shigella flexneri, S. sonnei, Salmonella typhimurium, K. pneumoniae,* and *Escherichia coli.*

Utilizing a somewhat different approach, other investigators compared the amino acid sequence of HLA-B27 with a computer bank of known protein sequences in order to identify a bacterial protein with close sequence homology. The most homologous were six consecutive amino acids shared by B27 (residues 72–77 in the hypervariable region) and *K. pneumoniae* nitrogenase (residues 188–193). Antibodies raised against the B27 peptide reacted not only with the peptide used for immunization, but also with peptides from *Klebsiella* nitrogenase containing the six consecutive amino acids. Peptides with single amino acid substitutions demonstrate substantially less cross-reactivity. Thus, amino acid homology between HLA-B27 and *Klebsiella* nitrogenase results in immunologic cross-reactivity. Sera from HLA-B27-positive patients with Reiter's syndrome or ankylosing spondylitis frequently react to these peptides, whereas sera from B27-positive normals do not. Therefore, it may be possible that many patients with these disorders have antibodies against self–HLA-B27 which are induced during an infection with *Klebsiella.* Sections of articular tissue from B27-positive patients with ankylosing spondylitis showed strong staining of the cells of the synovial lining and vascular endothelium after exposure to antibodies raised against peptides derived from B27 or from nitrogenase; this was not found in control articular tissues. These studies appear to show that an-

kylosing spondylitis patients clearly express the epitope shared by HLA-B27 and *Klebsiella* nitrogenase, such that it is accessible to a cross-reactive immune response. Thus, a possible sequence of events related to this molecular mimicry is as follows: *K. pneumoniae* infection or colonization induces an immune response that also recognizes self–B27-specific antigens; the shared antigen has enhanced expression in articular tissues, and the result is an autoimmune disorder such as ankylosing spondylitis or Reiter's syndrome.

Another instance of molecular mimicry relates to group A streptococcal M proteins and myosin, a relationship that may contribute to the pathogenesis of the carditis of acute rheumatic fever (see Chapter 9). Although several cross-reactive systems between streptococcal and mammalian antigens have been described, the best characterized system is that involving myosin. Sera from patients with acute rheumatic fever or chronic rheumatic heart disease contain elevated levels of antimyosin antibodies that cross-react with M protein, especially M types 1, 5, 6, and 19. Pepsin treatment of M protein leads to removal of its amino-terminal half (referred to as Pep M protein), and the epitope cross-reactive with myosin was localized to this Pep M protein. Using synthetic-overlapping peptides that copy the entire sequence of the Pep M5 molecule, the Pep M5 epitope recognized by human and murine cross-reactive antibodies was localized to a 14-amino acid sequence in the carboxy region of Pep M5, and a pentameric sequence (positions 184–188) was found to be essential for inhibiting the cross-reactive antibodies. Understanding the exact relationship of this kind of precisely determined molecular mimicry to the pathogenesis of human disease requires further studies.

Similar instances of molecular mimicry have been investigated that involve homologies between other important mammalian proteins, such as alpha-gliadin, insulin, and acetylcholine receptor, and a variety of microbial proteins. Mimicry between a major surface glycoprotein of *Streptococcus mutans* (an oral streptococcus) and human IgG heavy chains has recently been demonstrated. Considerable additional study is required to elucidate the significance of these and other instances of cross-reactivity between host and microbial antigens and their ultimate relationship to autoimmune disorders.

CASE HISTORY

In 1985, contaminated dairy milk led to the largest outbreak of acute salmonellosis in the

United States, with over 16,000 well-documented cases occurring in the greater Chicago area alone. Following resolution of their acute gastrointestinal illnesses, a number of individuals developed additional symptoms. A 45-year-old woman complained of the onset of acute right-knee swelling, pain, and tenderness 6 weeks after her acute salmonellosis that had been characterized by 3 days of fever, diarrhea, and vomiting. The knee complaints regressed after 1 week but recurred 2 months later. Physical examination was negative except for swelling, redness, and tenderness of the right knee. At that time, laboratory investigation yielded an erythrocyte sedimentation rate of 60 mm/h (Westergren method), WBC = 14,000/mm^3, HLA-B27 was positive, rheumatoid factor and antinuclear antibody were negative, and stool culture was negative. Treatment with nonsteroidal antiinflammatory agents was instituted with prompt response. Three months later, another episode of arthritis of the right knee necessitated additional therapy.

REFERENCES

Books

Dupont, B., ed. *Immunology of HLA*. Vol. I and Vol. II. New York: Springer-Verlag, 1989.

Rose, N. R., and MacKay, I. R., eds. *The Autoimmune Diseases*. New York: Academic Press, 1985.

Schumacher, H. R., Jr., Klippel, J. H., and Robinson, D. R., ed. *Primer on Rheumatic Diseases*. Atlanta, GA: Arthritis Foundation, 1988.

Review Articles

Blackman, M., Kappler, J., and Marrack, P. The role of the T-cell receptor in positive and negative selection of developing T-cells. *Science 248*:1335–1341, 1990.

Marrack, P., and Kappler, J. The T-cell receptor. *Science 238*:1073–1079, 1987.

Rose, N. R. Pathogenic mechanisms in autoimmune diseases. *Clin. Immun. Immunopathol. 53*:S7–16, 1989.

Schattner, A., and Rager-Zisman, B. Virus-induced autoimmunity. *Rev. Infect. Dis. 12*:204–222, 1990.

Sinha, A. A., Lopez, T., and McDevitt, H. O. Autoimmune diseases: The failure of self-tolerance. *Science 248*:1380–1388, 1990.

Tan, E. M. Antinuclear antibodies: Diagnostic markers for autoimmune diseases and probes for cell biology. *Adv. Immunol. 44*:93–151, 1989.

Tan, E. M. Interactions between autoimmunity and molecular and cell biology. *J. Clin. Invest. 84*:1–6, 1989.

Yu, D. T. Y., Choo, S. Y., and Schaak, T. Molecular mimicry in HLA-B27-related arthritis. *Ann. Intern. Med. 111*:581–591, 1989.

Zauderer, M. Origin and significance of autoreactive T-cells. *Adv. Imm. 45*:417–433, 1989.

Articles

Bjorkman, P. J., Sapier, M. A., Samraouri, B., et al. Structure of the human class I histocompatibility antigen, HLA-A2. *Nature 329*:506–512, 1987.

Bjorkman, P. J., Sapier, M. A., Samraouri, B., et al. The foreign antigen binding site and T cell recognition regions of class I histocompatibility antigens. *Nature 329*:512–518, 1987.

Chen, J-H., Kono, D. H., Young, A., et al. A *Yersinia pseudotuberculosis* protein which cross-reacts with HLA-B27. *J. Immunol. 139*:3003–3011, 1987.

Cunningham, M. W., McCormack, J. M., Fenderson, P. G., et al. Human and murine antibodies cross-reactive with streptococcal M protein and myosin recognize the sequence Gln-Lys-Ser-Lys-Gln in M protein. *J. Immunol. 143*:2677–2683, 1989.

MacDonald, H. R., Mechanisms of immunological tolerance. *Science 246*:982, 1989.

Morel, P. A., Erlich, H. A., Fathman, C. G. A new look at the shared epitope hypothesis. *Am. J. Med. 85*(suppl. 6A):20–22, 1988.

Oldstone, M. B. A. Molecular mimicry: Immunologic cross-reactivity between dissimilar proteins (microbial and self) that share common epitopes can lead to autoimmunity. *Cell 50*:819–820, 1987.

Schlosstein, L., Terasaki, P., Bluestone, R., et al. High association of HLA antigen W27 with ankylosing spondylitis. *N. Engl. J. Med. 288*:704–706, 1973.

II

Clinical and Microbiologic Diagnostic Considerations

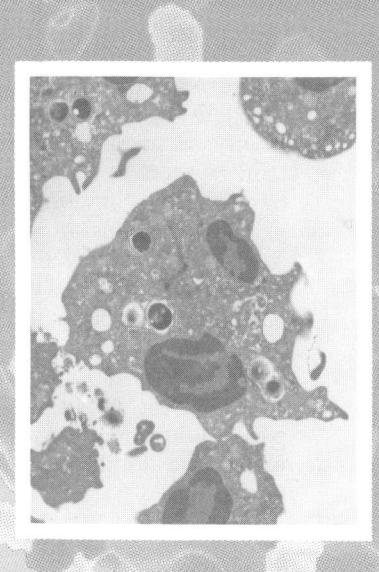

6
A TODD DAVIS, M.D. • *JOHN P. PHAIR, M.D.*

Temperature Regulation, the Pathogenesis of Fever, and the Approach to the Febrile Patient

INTRODUCTION

Fever, or an elevated body temperature, is the hallmark of infection; however, patients seriously ill with infection can be afebrile or have lower than normal temperature. In addition, there are many causes of fever other than infection. This chapter will briefly review regulation of body temperature, the pathogenesis of fever, and an approach to the febrile adult and pediatric patient.

REGULATION OF BODY TEMPERATURE

Body temperature in humans is the net result of heat production by metabolic processes and/or muscle activity and heat loss, mediated by the delivery of blood to the subcutaneous and cutaneous structures and dissipated by sweating. Obviously the ambient temperature plays a role in achieving this balance, and in the perception of heat by the individual. Body temperature usually varies slightly around 37°C (98.6°F) in most individuals, with a diurnal variation from a low of 35°C in the early morning hours at the end of sleep to a high of 37.5°C in the evening. The central regulator of body temperature is located in the anterior hypothalamus, which acts as a thermostat, directly controlling the autonomic nervous system and indirectly affecting the delivery of blood to the periphery. Thus, when heat needs to be conserved when ambient temperatures are low, peripheral vasoconstriction occurs. Shivering acts to augment heat production in this situation. During intense muscle activity, produced by exercise such as sustained running or swimming, internal body temperature is dissipated through diversion of blood to the skin. Sweating enhances heat loss through cooling by evaporation. The thermoregulatory center in the hypothalamus interacts with the partially independent spinal cord reflexes but is in fact the dominant control of body temperature.

FEVER

An elevation of body temperature occurs in a number of physiologic and pathophysiologic settings. As mentioned above, exercise can raise the body temperature. Long-distance runners at the finish of a race can record temperatures of 38°–38.5°C. Heat stroke is a pathologic and dangerous elevation of body temperature which can be the consequence of such exercise and of dehydration due to inadequate fluid intake or to the failure, due to disease or debility, of the heat-dissipation mechanisms in conditions of extremely high ambient temperature. Malignant hyperthermia is a rare hereditary disease occurring in association with general anesthesia. It appears to result from an inappropriate release of calcium from muscles upon exposure to an anesthetic agent and is accompanied by muscle rigidity, rhabdomyolysis, and acidosis. Another uncommon cause of excessive elevation of body temperature (41°C and greater) is associated with antipsychotic drugs, such as haloperidol, phenothiazines, and thioxanthenes. This condition, known as neuroleptic malignant syndrome, is characterized by fever, muscular rigidity, autonomic dysfunction, and changes in mental status. This syndrome results from blockage of central dopamine receptors, which leads to uncontrolled muscular contractions in association with peripheral vasoconstriction. Thus, heat is generated which cannot be dissipated.

The majority of fevers, however, are the result of conditions which produce alteration in the thermoregulatory center through the effects of cytokines produced by macrophages. Beeson in the 1940s performed experiments which demonstrated that stimulated phagocytic cells released a factor(s) which produced fevers in rabbits. One classic stimulant of this and other responses is endotoxin, or lipopolysaccharide (LPS) from gram-negative cell walls (see Chapter 34). Atkins, Wood, and coworkers in a series of elegant experiments proved that the "endogenous pyrogen" was distinct from endotoxin or other bacterial products. Bodel showed that the source of endogenous pyrogen was the mononuclear phagocyte, or macrophage. It is now established that interleukin-1 (IL-1), a product of stimulated mononuclear phagocytes, is a cytokine that stimulates release of the arachidonic acid product prostaglandin E_2, which apparently up-regulates the functioning of the thermoregulatory center. The result, as described above, is peripheral vasoconstriction often accompanied by shivering, which can be manifested as a shaking chill or rigor, leading to heat production, heat conservation, and elevation of temperature. Other cytokines, such as tumor necrosis factor, also produced by macrophages, appear capable of increasing body temperature, presumably through the same pathway. A newly discovered mediator, macrophage inflammatory protein-1 (MIP-1), acts independently of the prostaglandin pathway, and the mechanism by which it induces fever is unknown.

IL-1 has a wide variety of effects in addition to inducing hypothalamic up-regulation of body temperature (Fig. 6–1). It can stimulate hepatic production of acute-phase reactants such as fibrinogen. Elevated fibrinogen levels are the primary cause of more rapid than normal erythrocyte aggregation and sedimentation, which explains the elevated sedimentation rate seen in patients with infectious or inflammatory diseases. Other serum proteins, such as C-reactive protein, also increase in concentrations. The source of this increased protein production by the liver are amino acids derived from muscle breakdown or proteolysis which is mediated by IL-1. The low serum iron and serum zinc and rises in serum copper also appear to be induced by IL-1 and/or the other cytokines released by stimulated or phagocytosing mononuclear cells. Finally, leukocytosis, the other characteristic manifestation of infection, occurs as a consequence of release of these cytokines. In addition to mediating these characteristics of inflammation, IL-1 up-regulates the immune system. An elevated body temperature is associated with a more efficient response by thymic-derived (T cells) lymphocytes, which play a central role in the induction of the immune response.

With the accumulated knowledge of the augmented inflammatory and immune responses associated with fever, the febrile response has been viewed as conferring an advantage to the host. The primary cell defending the host against bacteria, the polymorphonuclear leukocyte, is released from the marrow, and is more adherent to endothelial cells, thus enhancing diapedesis into tissue. Lowered serum iron is thought to

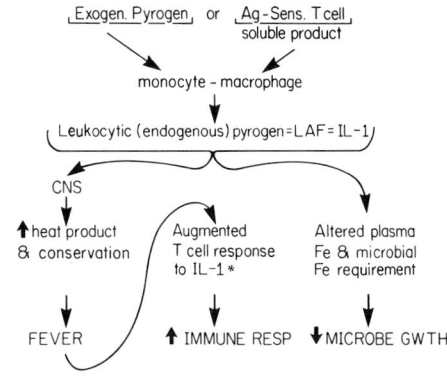

Figure 6–1. Pathways of endogenous pyrogen production with resulting fever and associated effects on host immune responses and iron metabolism.

provide a less favorable milieu for iron-dependent organisms. The augmented T-cell function may facilitate the specific immune response to microbial invasion. The beneficial effect of elevated temperature in infected cold-blooded animals has been amply documented, but this has not been demonstrated definitively in humans. Lowering the fever associated with influenza with salicylates prolongs viral shedding, and those elderly patients with bacteremia who do not mount a fever have a poorer prognosis than similarly aged individuals who develop a febrile response. However, this latter finding may reflect the association of debility, poor prognosis, and failure to respond with the normal inflammatory response, rather than a poorer prognosis because of the muted response. Furthermore, there is a physiologic cost associated with the febrile response. Heart rate increases, possibly straining a damaged heart, and the muscle proteolysis results in negative nitrogen balance, which persists for prolonged periods following resolution of the fever.

Approach to the Febrile Adult

The basic approach to the febrile patient should focus upon establishing the cause of the fever and then instituting appropriate therapy. Treatment of the temperature elevation itself is generally unnecessary except in special situations, for example, the patient who cannot tolerate a tachycardia, the child who has seizures, or the elderly patient who becomes disoriented with fever. Salicylates or nonsteroidal antiinflammatory agents are generally quite adequate to control fever, but have the adverse effects of inhibiting platelet aggregation, thus inhibiting clotting, and producing gastric irritation, erosions, and often bleeding. With extreme temperatures above 40°C, as in patients with heat stroke or malignant hyperthermia, cooling blankets are used to help control fever.

Except for malaria, the pattern or the fever curve provides little information about the etiology of the underlying condition. It has been suggested that fevers secondary to drug hypersensitivity are continuously elevated, whereas those associated with an abscess resemble a picket fence. However, most patients with drug fever demonstrate a diurnal variation in temperature with a return to the normal range in the morning, and many infected patients are constantly febrile.

The diagnosis of the cause of fever in most patients can be established by obtaining a thorough history and performing an adequate physical examination. Basic and necessary laboratory studies include a complete blood count, with differential count; examination of the urine; a chest x-ray; and culture of appropriate specimens including blood, urine, or sputum. These studies usually suggest whether or not the fever is due to infection or to some other cause.

Fevers that persist without explanation for several weeks despite such an evaluation are termed *fevers of unknown origin,* or FUOs. They represent one of the most challenging problems for a diagnostician. In general, FUOs are the result of common diseases presenting in an uncommon manner or uncommon conditions presenting typically (Table 6–1). The physician, when approaching a patient with FUO, must devise a diagnostic plan which can distinguish between a disease which is generalized, such as miliary (disseminated) tuberculosis, endocarditis, or noninfectious conditions such as sarcoidosis or a neoplastic, lymphoproliferative disease, and a localized process such as an abscess or other occult infections or tumors. The patient's history should be reevaluated, specifically to search for potential exposure to unusual infections. Examples of such exposure include travel to areas of endemic infection, exposure to certain wild animals through hunting, to pets, to drugs, or possible distant exposure to persons with tuberculosis. The physical examination bears repeating on several occasions, emphasizing a search for the changing murmur of endocarditis, the bony tenderness of chronic osteomyelitis, or right upper quadrant tenderness associated with a liver abscess or cryptogenic cholecystitis. Potential exposure to fungal infections, as might occur for individuals who explore caves, work with soil, or who have traveled for the first time to the Ohio/Mississippi Valley or the Southwest, warrants serologic assays for fungal antibody.

Cryptogenic localized infections which are commonly missed include abscessed teeth, pyelonephritis (occasionally), hepatic abscess, or pelvic tuberculosis. A diagnostic procedure which is often useful is examination and culture of the bone marrow in the presence of unexplained neutropenia, anemia, or thrombocytopenia. Specific diseases which are readily identified by bone marrow culture include disseminated histoplasmosis and other fungal infections, tuberculosis, or lymphoma. Computerized tomography and ultrasonography can be extremely helpful in searching for localized infections or tumors. The recent introduction of

TABLE 6–1. *Categories of Fever of Unknown Origin**

Diagnostic Categories	Petersdorf & Beeson 1961 Series (*n* = 100)† (%)	Jacoby & Swartz 1973 Series (*n* = 128) (%)	Larson et al. 1982 Series (*n* = 105) (%)
Infection	36	40	30
Neoplastic disease	19	20	31
Connective tissue diseases	15	15	9
Granulomatous and miscellaneous diseases	23	15	18
Undiagnosed	7	10	13

*Adapted from Petersdorf, R. G., and Beeson, P. B., *Medicine 40*:1, 1961; Jacoby, G. A., and Swartz, M. N., *N. Engl. J. Med. 289*:1407, 1973; and Larson E. B., Featherstone, H. J., and Petersdorf, R. G., *Medicine 61*:269, 1982.
†Number of patients indicated within brackets.

scans using indium 111-labeled polymorphonuclear leukocytes can aid in the discovery of localized abscesses. Laparoscopy and peritoneoscopy in persons with pelvic or abdominal symptoms, in combination with the new radiologic techniques, have obviated almost entirely the use of diagnostic laparotomy in the management of FUOs. Finally, there are increasingly useful serologic tests which can screen for and ultimately identify antibodies found in specific collagen vascular diseases, such as systemic lupus erythematosus, or mixed connective tissue disease. This group of conditions represents a large proportion of diseases reported in all series of adult patients with unexplained fever.

Other specific laboratory studies which can be useful include seeking polymorphonuclear leukocytes in the stool, which can be the earliest sign of inflammatory bowel disease, especially in patients with atypical abdominal complaints. Abnormalities of the serum concentrations of hepatic enzymes indicate a liver biopsy is in order. Histologic examination and culture of liver tissue can be extremely helpful, often diagnosing miliary tuberculosis, sarcoidosis, or granulomatous hepatitis. In the presence of normal liver enzyme levels the yield from liver biopsy is disappointing.

Occult neoplasms are almost as common as occult localized or disseminated infections as a cause of prolonged fever. In addition to non-Hodgkin's and Hodgkin's lymphoma, renal cell carcinoma is a common cause of fever. Therefore, radiologic or ultrasound examination of the kidney is often part of the evaluation of these patients. The availability of computerized tomography and gallium scans allows for examination of the retroperitoneum and can define enlarged lymph nodes, suggesting lymphoproliferative disease.

The evaluation of a patient with an unexplained fever is always easier in the absence of previous antimicrobial therapy. In general, therapeutic trials of antibiotics are not useful in this situation unless there is strong evidence of abacteremic endocarditis or occult tuberculosis. Finally, it must be recognized that the most well organized and thorough evaluation can fail to establish a cause of the fever. Reappraisal at a later time sometimes is successful but, more than occasionally, fever disappears and is never explained or, less happily, the underlying disease is diagnosed only at autopsy.

The Febrile Child

Fever is not always a presenting sign in children with infections. Neonates (children <28 days of age) may be seriously ill with an acute or chronic infection and yet be afebrile. In infants and older children, there is no necessary correlation between the height of the fever and seriousness of the infection. Among neonates, there are two general classifications of infections that occur: first, congenital or perinatally acquired infections such as TORCH infections; and second, acute bacterial sepsis and meningitis.

CONGENITAL INFECTIONS

TORCH is an acronym often used when discussing intrauterine or perinatally acquired infections: T stands for toxoplasmosis; O for other agents; R for rubella; C for cytomegalovirus; and H for herpes simplex. Originally, the "O" stood principally for syphilis (congenital lues). In recent years, the list of "other agents" has grown to include human immunodeficiency viruses (HIV-1 and -2), parvovirus, enterovirus, varicella–zoster virus (VZV), influenza virus, Epstein-Barr virus, plasmodia, and *Listeria*.

The acronym not only helps one to remember the etiologic agents, but serves the important function of emphasizing the overlapping clinical manifestations of the TORCH illnesses in neonates. As a consequence, it is not always possible to establish specific etiology on clinical grounds (Table 6–2). Rather, one must often depend on isolation of the agent or serologic testing.

Rubella

Maternally acquired rubella infections only pose a threat to the fetus during the first half of pregnancy. The risk is highest within the first few weeks of pregnancy, perhaps approaching 85%. By the 16–20th week of pregnancy, there is less than a 5% chance of spread to the fetus from its infected mother. Because fetal rubella infection occurs during organogenesis in the first trimester, this infection is uniquely able to cause congenital abnormalities such as cataracts, peripheral pulmonic stenosis, and other cardiac lesions.

The pathophysiology of fetal damage is not clearly understood, although several factors probably interact. First, vascular involvement leading to ischemia seems to play a major role. Second, immature fetal cells readily support the growth of rubella virus, which may lead to cell death. Third, little maternal IgG is transferred across the placenta during the first half of pregnancy. Fourth, fetal antibody production is nonexistent or minimal during the first trimester of pregnancy. And fifth, fetal cellular immune functioning does not begin until late in the first trimester.

Toxoplasmosis

In contrast to congenital rubella, the frequency of maternal toxoplasmal infection leading to fetal disease increases during pregnancy. Thus, 20% of first-trimester, but 65% of third-trimester primary maternal infections result in fetal infections. This, obviously, is the reverse of that seen in congenital rubella syndrome. However, as is the case in congenital rubella syndrome, the earlier in gestation that fetal infection occurs, the more serious the disease process. Thus, approximately 65% of fetuses infected in the first trimester develop serious disease, whereas third-trimester maternal infections rarely, if ever, result in severe disease, 90% being subclinical in the child.

As shown in Table 6–2, infections occurring early in pregnancy can lead to severe multisystem involvement. However, even those children who are born with subclinical infections may not escape damage. Because of the persistence of bradyzoites (small, comma-shaped forms) in many parts of the body, the child is always at risk for reactivation of the infection and consequent complications. This may explain the development of chorioretinitis years after birth.

French investigators, utilizing intrauterine blood sampling, have been able to make prenatal diagnoses of congenital toxoplasmosis infections and to institute treatment. Happily, treatment does seem to result in fewer babies who are symptomatic at birth. Further follow-up is necessary to determine the long-term outcome in treated infants.

Cytomegalovirus Infections

Cytomegalovirus (CMV) is a ubiquitous virus seen in many populations throughout the world. Fortunately, most women have had CMV infection prior to pregnancy. However, an unlucky

TABLE 6–2. *Clinical Manifestations of Generalized Congenital (TORCH) Infections*

	Rubella	Cytomegalovirus	Toxoplasmosis	Herpes Simplex	Treponema pallidum
Hepatosplenomegaly	+	+	+	+	+
Jaundice	+	+	+	+	+
Petechiae	+	+	+	+	+
Meningoencephalitis	+	+	+	+	+
Chorioretinitis	+ +	+	+ +	+	+
Microcephaly	−	+ +	+	+	−
Hydrocephalus	+	−	+ +	−	−
Intracranial calcifications	−	+ +	+ +	−	−
Myocarditis	+	−	+	+	−
Bone lesions	+ +	−	+	−	+ +

(−) Absent or rare.
(+) Occurs regularly in infected infants.
(+ +) Somewhat characteristic for a given kind of infection.
From Remington, J. S., and Klein, J. O., eds. *Infectious Diseases of the Fetus and Newborn*. Philadelphia: W. B. Saunders Co., 1976.

few escape cytomegalovirus during childhood, but become infected during pregnancy. A primary infection may lead to a generalized fetal infection with symptoms as described in Table 6–2. More than half of the survivors have sequelae such as psychomotor retardation, hearing loss, or microcephaly. Even infants who are infected but asymptomatic at birth have a 5–15% risk of hearing impairment. Unlike the previously discussed intrauterine infections, the risk of fetal infection with CMV appears to be constant throughout pregnancy in the mother undergoing a primary infection.

Only a small minority of CMV infections are acquired during gestation. Rather, most of these infections occur perinatally as a consequence of colonization of the birth canal. Some infants may become infected from breast milk laden with the virus. For the most part, infants infected perinatally appear to suffer few, if any, consequences.

Syphilis

Treponema pallidum spirochetes can probably be transmitted across the placenta at any time during pregnancy. However, no inflammatory response is evident until the second half of pregnancy. A vigorous fetal host response leads to the signs and symptoms outlined in Table 6–2.

Maternal syphilis acquired late in pregnancy may not cause any clinical symptoms in the baby at birth. Indeed, it may take several weeks or months before such symptoms develop, such as "snuffles" (a mucopurulent nasal discharge), a copper-colored large macular rash or plaquelike lesions around the mouth and anus, hepatosplenomegaly, or periosteal inflammation. The latter is a particular hallmark of congenital lues.

Herpes Simplex

Unlike the previously discussed congenital infections, herpes simplex is almost invariably a perinatally acquired disease. A maternal genital herpes type 2 lesion may serve as the source of infection. During a long labor, virus particles may ascend through the ruptured membranes to infect the fetus. During a short labor, infection occurs by direct exposure during the birth process. Cesarean section within 4 h of membrane rupture greatly decreases the risk of infection to the infant.

Symptoms in neonatal infection usually occur during the first week of life, although they may occasionally be delayed until 2–3 weeks of age. Symptoms may begin with typical vesicular lesions on skin or as undefined constitutional symptoms reflecting encephalitis, hepatitis, or symptoms attributable to multiple organ involvement. The diagnosis can be particularly difficult to establish in the absence of the skin lesions which occur in only about 50% of infants with disseminated organ infection.

The factors underlying the extreme susceptibility of infants to disseminated infection are somewhat unclear. Lessons from older children suggest that cellular immune responses are particularly important in the host response to herpes viruses. Newborns' relatively immunodeficiency vis-à-vis cellular immune mechanisms may explain the frequently devastating nature of these infections.

ACUTE CHILDHOOD INFECTIONS

After birth, the neonate's immune system continues to mature slowly, a fact which modifies the presentation and severity of illness compared with that of the older child and adult with fully intact immune systems.

For example, only about 60% of neonates respond with fever during an episode of meningitis or bacterial sepsis. The other 40% are either afebrile or hypothermic. Although irritability and lethargy may be seen in virtually all children with bacterial meningitis, systemic symptoms such as respiratory distress, apnea, and jaundice are uniquely found in meningitic neonates as opposed to older children (Table 6–3).

Newborn infants are at particular risk, for a short time, for some viral pathogens. If the mother develops varicella (chickenpox) from 4 days before delivery to 48 h afterward, her child is at particular risk to develop serious and potentially fatal varicella. However, if the mother develops chickenpox more than 5 days before delivery, her offspring is at little risk. The immunologic factors underscoring these phenomena are currently unknown. Some coxsackie B or echovirus infections which may be asymptomatic or cause mild constitutional symptoms in the mother, may result in devastating encephalitis and myocarditis (coxsackie) or hepatitis (echo) in the newborn.

On the other hand, some viral illnesses are milder in infants than in adults. For example, poliomyelitis occurring early in infancy (defined

TABLE 6–3. *Comparison of Symptoms in Neonates with Bacterial Infections and Metabolic or Central Nervous System Disorders*

	Irritability	Lethargy	Poor Feeding or Vomiting	High-Pitched Cry	Tremors	Convulsions	Cyanosis
Sepsis	+ +	+ +	+ +	+	+	+	+ +
Meningitis	+ +	+ + +	+ + +	+ +	+	+ +	+
Hypoglycemia*	+ +	+ +	+ +	+ +	+ + +	+ +	+ +
Hypocalcemia*	+ +	+ +	+ +	+ +	+ + +	+ +	+
CNS abnormalities	+ +	+ +	+ +	+ +	+	+ +	+

	Respiratory Distress	Apnea	Jaundice	Fever
Sepsis	+ +	+ +	+ +	+ + +
Meningitis	+ +	+ +	+ +	+ + +
Hypoglycemia*	+	+ +	+	+
Hypocalcemia*	+	+ +	+	+
CNS abnormalities	+	+	+	+

(+) Incidence 0–10%.
(+ +) Incidence 11–50%.
(+ + +) Incidence 51–100%.
*The majority of infants with these conditions are asymptomatic. When symptoms occur, tremulousness is most frequent.

as <2 years of age) rarely results in permanent paralysis. In populations with poor hygiene and sanitation, contact with the virus early in life, when the risk of paralysis is low, confers life-long immunity. Hepatitis A in children younger than 2 years of age presents either with vague constitutional symptoms or gastrointestinal complaints such as vomiting and diarrhea. Jaundice rarely occurs. By age 5 or 6, jaundice much more frequently accompanies this infection. The changes in the maturing immune system that underlie these changing responses to infection are not well understood.

In the child older than 3 months with sudden onset of a fever, the diagnosis is usually evident from the associated symptoms. Thus, those viruses causing upper respiratory infections usually present with cough and/or coryza. Stridor and/or wheezing occasionally occur. In later childhood, the child is able to complain about a sore throat. An erythematous pharynx or exudative tonsillitis points to the diagnosis. Gastrointestinal disease, exanthems with febrile diseases, and enanthems are all readily diagnosed. Urinary tract infections, particularly in young children, do not have any characteristic clinical findings. Indeed, some children with urinary tract infections present only with fever. Some may have some gastrointestinal symptoms as well. Because of the nonspecific nature of the symptoms of urinary tract infections in early childhood, it is important to obtain a urine specimen, particularly in girls, when a source of fever is not readily apparent.

There are, of course, some viral illnesses during the neonatal period and early infancy which present with no abnormal physical findings. In those circumstances, the careful physician must simply assure himself or herself that no serious, treatable pyogenic disease is being overlooked.

There are a few acute pediatric infectious diseases which present subtly and for which a diagnosis is rarely made unless the possibility of their occurrence is considered. Two important examples of such diseases are retropharyngeal abscess and suppurative pericarditis. Other diseases must be diagnosed rapidly because they are life-threatening or they may cause long-term disability if not promptly treated. Included among these are bacterial meningitis, herpes encephalitis, epiglottitis, and septic arthritis of the hip.

FEVER OF UNKNOWN ORIGIN IN CHILDREN

Like adults, children occasionally present with fever of unknown origin. FUO is considered when a fever has been present for 2 to 3 weeks without any apparent cause. Happily, most of these fevers resolve in time without a diagnosis being established. Nonetheless, a careful search for an etiology is imperative, beginning by considering four large categories of disease entities: infectious diseases, neoplasia, inflammatory bowel disease and other rheumatologic conditions, and other entities.

With this conceptual framework, a careful history sometimes points to a diagnosis. Useful clues include recent foreign travel, exposure to psittacine birds (psittacosis), ingestion of imported cheeses (listeriosis, brucellosis), close contacts with someone with a chronic cough (tuberculosis), abdominal pain and diarrhea (inflammatory bowel disease), and fleeting macular rashes with fever, swelling or redness of the joints, or morning stiffness (juvenile rheumatoid arthritis).

If history and physical examination fail to yield a diagnosis, then a number of imaging studies should be undertaken to exclude occult neoplasms or infections. Useful tests include a chest x-ray, nuclear bone scintigraphy, abdominal CT scan, and gallium scintigraphy. If these tests are normal, a bone marrow examination should be considered.

Diagnosing the child with a fever of unknown origin remains one of the most challenging intellectual exercises in medicine despite the increased diagnostic tools now available. The answer, however, usually yields to clinical insight.

CASE HISTORY 1

A 4-day-old infant was born 36 h after the premature rupture of membranes and weighed 2000 gm. The child had fed normally until the fourth day of life, when he vomited on early-morning feeding. The child was difficult to arouse 4 h later, suckled poorly, and took only half an ounce of formula. Four hours later, when the child was still lethargic and feeding poorly, a physician was summoned. The child was afebrile, but was noted to have somewhat elevated respiratory rate, with slight flaring of the alae nasi and slight retractions of the intercostal spaces; he also appeared "jittery." He suckled poorly and demonstrated no Moro reflex. Sepsis, hypoglycemia, and hypocalcemia were included in the differential diagnosis. Specimens of blood, cerebrospinal fluid, and urine were obtained. Blood glucose and calcium were normal. CSF glucose and protein were within normal limits. Only five white blood cells were present in the spinal fluid, all mononuclear, and Gram's stain was negative. Antibiotics were administered empirically. However, over the next 48 h, respiratory distress worsened and apnea developed, which necessitated mechanical ventilation. The child continued to be lethargic and irritable, with jaundice and hepatomegaly noted 24 h after the institution of antibiotic treatment. The child died from *Escherichia coli* sepsis 2 days after the institution of antibiotic therapy.

CASE HISTORY 2

An 8-year-old girl with a known polymorphonuclear chemotactic defect presented with a fever but no other symptoms of infection. A spinal tap revealed fewer than 10 polymorphonuclear leukocytes, but the culture yielded *Streptococcus pneumoniae*. The child continued to have a low-grade fever for the next 8 days while receiving penicillin intravenously at therapeutic doses. At the end of 8 days, a spinal tap was repeated, with essentially the same findings demonstrated as before therapy, including a positive culture. Again, the child had no symptoms of headache or meningismus. Bacteria were cleared from the spinal fluid only after the dose of penicillin was increased to twice the usual dose. She recovered without any sequelae.

CASE HISTORY 3

A 38-year-old housewife previously in good health developed fever (as high as 103°F, or 39.5°C), frontal headache, intense generalized muscular aching, and an intermittent nonproductive cough on January 4. She took to bed and over the next 5 days slowly improved as her symptoms were treated. On January 9 (the sixth day of illness) she suddenly experienced severe right-sided pleuritic chest pain, a sharp rise in fever to 104°F (40°C), a marked increase in cough, and increasing breathlessness. A few hours later in the emergency room, she appeared acutely ill, tachypneic, and cyanotic, and was noted to be coughing up traces of purulent sputum.

Physical examination revealed a temperature of 103.8°F (39.9°C); pulse, 110/min; blood pressure, 90/60; and respirations, 32/min. The nail beds were dusky; the skin reflected dehydration. Coarse inspiratory rales and impaired resonance were noted over the lower right lateral-posterior chest.

Laboratory data: Hemoglobin, 14.5 gm/100 mL; white blood count, 16,000 with 82% segmented neutrophils. Urinalysis was within normal limits. Sputum smear showed many polymorphonuclear leukocytes and many gram-positive cocci with occasional gram-positive rods and rare gram-negative coccobacilli. **Chest roentgenogram revealed a nondescript density in the right lower lung. Arterial blood gases were: pO_2 43 mm Hg and CO_2 13 mm Hg, with pH 7.48.**

CASE HISTORY 4

A 46-year-old female with a diagnosis of systemic lupus erythematosus established 6 months previously entered the hospital on February 15, with a 3-day history of shaking chills and fever spiking to 105°F (41°C) in association with attempts to decrease her daily prednisone dose from 60 to 20 mg per day. She appeared chronically ill and was weak and anorexic.

Physical examination revealed a temperature of 102°F (38.8°C); pulse, 100/min; blood pressure, 110/70; and respirations, 28/min. The patient had pale mucous membranes, a scaly erythematous maculopapular rash over both cheeks and the bridge of her nose, and patchy bitemporal alopecia. The remainder of the examination was within normal limits.

Laboratory data: hemoglobin, 10.5 gm/100 mL; leukocyte count, 4700 with normal differential. Urinalysis revealed 2+ proteinuria and a normal sediment. One of four blood cultures taken during the first 2 days of hospitalization was reported positive for a gram-positive coccus, tentatively identified as *Staphylococcus epidermidis*. Urine cultures were negative. Chest roentgenogram was within normal limits.

On the third hospital day, the patient's temperature approached 105°F (41°C) and she showed signs of clinical deterioration.

CASE 3 DISCUSSION

The type of initial illness and its setting, the winter season, point to influenza. The abrupt departure from an otherwise uneventful convalescence strongly suggests complicating secondary bacterial pneumonia, namely, preceding respiratory infection, purulent sputum, pleuritic chest pain, and leukocytosis. The sputum smear is consistent with pneumococcal or staphylococcal infection. Staphylococci and pneumococci are among the most common causes of bacterial pneumonia complicating influenza. Nafcillin, a semisynthetic and penicillinase-resistant derivative of penicillin, is administered, since a

beta-lactamase (penicillinase)–producing strain of staphylococcus could be present. This particular semisynthetic penicillinase-resistant antimicrobial agent is highly effective against the pneumococcus and against penicillin-resistant as well as penicillin-susceptible staphylococci. Therapy is initiated only after sputum has been collected and cultured and two blood cultures drawn in rapid succession from two separate venipuncture sites have been secured.

During the next 3 days, the patient showed gradual clinical improvement, even though there was an increase in the right lung infiltrate based on physical findings and chest roentgenograms. Sputum culture revealed a heavy growth of Staphylococcus aureus, *resistant to penicillin. Blood cultures were sterile. Serologic tests using paired sera showed a greater than fourfold antibody rise against influenza virus, "Asian" A_2 strain. On the fourth hospital day, defervescence occurred, with improvement in the chest physical examination.*

CASE 4 DISCUSSION

This patient was known to have a primary disease, systemic lupus erythematosus, associated with defective immunity. This fact, plus her corticosteroid therapy, should alert the physician to an increased likelihood of infection. There is no evidence of an infectious process to explain the single blood culture yielding a common microorganism constituting part of the normal flora of the skin. Therefore, the isolated microorganism is considered a contaminant. For these reasons, no antimicrobial therapy is prescribed, even though a strong plea to "cover the patient" with an antimicrobial agent was made by the house staff. The patient's prednisone dosage was increased on the premise that the fever and chills were due to increased activity of the autoimmune disease process in the face of decreased prednisone therapy.

The patient became afebrile, and marked clinical improvement occurred after the daily dose of prednisone was increased to 60 mg for 3 days. Two additional blood cultures taken during this period were sterile.

Another reason for withholding antimicrobial therapy in this patient is the propensity for antimicrobial drugs to alter the normal bacterial flora of the host. In an already debilitated host receiving an antiinflammatory drug such as prednisone, microbial "opportunists" may induce serious pneumonia or invade the bloodstream to cause systemic infection involving many different organ systems, that is, life-threatening "superinfections." The occurrence of superinfection is an important reason for not prescribing antimicrobial therapy unless clear evidence exists for doing so.

REFERENCES

Books

Feigin, R. D., and Cherry, J. D. *Textbook of Pediatric Infectious Diseases.* Vols. I and II. 2nd ed. Philadelphia: W. B. Saunders Co., 1987.

Remington, J. S., and Klein, J. O. *Infectious Diseases of the Fetus and Newborn Infant.* 3rd ed. Philadelphia: W. B. Saunders Co., 1990.

Stiehm, E. R. *Immunologic Disorders in Infants and Children.* 3rd ed. Philadelphia: W. B. Saunders Co., 1989.

Review Articles

Alford C. A., Stagno, S., Pass, R. F., et al. Congenital and perinatal cytomegalovirus infections. *Rev. Infect. Dis. 12:*S745, 1990.

Cairo, M. S. Neonatal neutrophil host defense: Prospects for immunologic enhancement during neonatal sepsis. *Am. J. Dis. Child 143:*40, 1989.

Dinarello, C. A., Cannon, J. G., and Wolff, S. M. New concepts on the pathogenesis of fever: *Rev. Infect. Dis. 10:*168, 1988.

Editorial. TORCH syndrome and TORCH screening. *Lancet 335:*1559, 1990.

Jaffe, D., and Davis, A. T. The febrile child. In Schwartz, M. W., Charney, E. B., Curry, T. A., and Ludwig, S., eds. *Principles and Practice of Clinical Pediatrics.* Chicago: Year Book of Medical Publications, Inc., 1987: 394.

Kasper, D. L. Bacterial capsule—old dogmas and new tricks. *J. Infect. Dis. 153:*407, 1986.

Koskiniemi, M., Lappalainen, M. and Hedman, K. Toxoplasmosis needs evaluation: An overview and proposals. *Am J. Dis. Child. 143:*724, 1989.

Original Articles

Albrecht, P., Ennis, F. A., Saltzman, E. J., et al. Persistence of maternal antibody in infants beyond 12 months: Mechanism of measles vaccine failure. *J. Pediatr. 91:*715, 1977.

Allsop, P., and Twigley, A. J. The neuroleptic malignant syndrome. Case report with a review of the literature. *Anesthesia 42:*49, 1987.

Atkins, E., and Bodel, P. Clinical fever: Its history, manifestations and pathogenesis. *Fed. Proc. 38:*57, 1979.

Bodel, P. Spontaneous pyrogen production by mouse histiocytic and myelomonocytic tumor cell lines in vitro. *J. Exp. Med. 147:*1503, 1978.

Centers for Disease Control. Rubella vaccination during pregnancy—United States, 1971–1988. *MMWR 38:*289, 1989.

Centers for Disease Control. Congenital syphilis—New York City, 1986–1988. *MMWR 38:*826, 1989.

Cluff, L. E., and Johnson, J. E., III Drug fever. *Prog. Allergy 8:*149, 1964.

Corey, L., Stone, E. F., Whitley, R. J., et al. Difference between herpes simplex virus type 1 and type 2 neonatal encephalitis in neurological outcome. *Lancet 1:*1, 1988.

Cornblath, M., Joassin, G., Weisskopf, B., et al. Hypoglycemia in the newborn. *Pediatr. Clin. North Am. 13:*905, 1966.

Davatelis, G., Wolpe, S.D., Sherry, B., et al Macrophage inflammatory protein-1: A prostaglandin-independent endogenous pyrogen. *Science 243:*1066, 1989.

Dinarello, C. A., Cannon, G. G., Wolff, S. M., et al. Tumor necrosis factor (cachectin) is an endogenous pyrogen and induces production of interleukin-1. *J. Exp. Med. 163:*1433, 1986.

Horstmann, D. M. Poliomyelitis—severity and type of disease in different age groups. *Ann. N. Y. Acad. Sci. 61:*946, 1955.

Koppe, J. G., Loewer-Sieger, D. H., and DeRoever-Bonnet, H. Results of 20-year follow-up of congenital toxoplasmosis. *Lancet 1:*254, 1986.

Miller, E., Cradock-Watson, J. E., and Ridehalgh, M. K. S. Outcome in newborn babies given anti–varicella-zoster immunoglobulin after perinatal maternal infection with varicella-zoster virus. *Lancet 2:*371, 1989.

Musher, D. M., Fainstein, V., Young, E. J., et al. Fever patterns: Their lack of clinical significance. *Arch. Intern. Med. 139:*1225, 1979.

Petersdorf, R. G. Fever of unknown origin. *Ann. Intern. Med. 70:*864, 1969.

Prober, C. G., Sullender, W. M., Yasukawa, L. L., et al. Low risk of herpes simplex virus infections in neonates exposed to the virus at the time of vaginal delivery to mothers with recurrent genital herpes simplex virus infections. *N. Engl. J. Med. 316:*240, 1987.

Roberton, N. R. C., and Smith, M. A. Early neonatal hypocalcemia. *Arch. Dis. Child. 50:*604, 1975.

7 *STANFORD T. SHULMAN, M.D. • HERBERT M. SOMMERS, M.D.*
NEHAMA SHARON, Ph.D.

Laboratory Diagnosis of Infections

WHY MAKE A DIAGNOSIS?

There are a number of reasons for establishing a specific diagnosis of an infectious disease. First, there is the advantage to the patient. Once a diagnosis has been established, further steps to determine the cause of the illness need not be taken, saving the patient expense and discomfort. Therapy is more easily determined and usually more specific. The prognosis for an illness of known cause is usually clearer than for an illness of unknown cause. Second, a diagnosis contributes to the education of the physician. This should result in earlier recognition and treatment for the next patient with the same illness. Third, after it is established that the cause of an illness is the microbial agent, the information can be used in preventive medicine. In many instances, vaccines can be developed. Recognition of specific causative agents can stimulate a search for new or modified antimicrobial agents or can indicate the need for other types of control measures, such as mosquito extermination for eradication of malaria. The early recognition of specific microorganisms also can serve as a warning of epidemics, thereby providing time for control measures to be taken.

The definitive diagnosis of an infectious disease is accomplished by the isolation and identification of a specific infectious agent. Frequently, however, isolation of the agent is not possible, and the diagnosis must be established by noting an increasing titer of antibody to a specific infectious agent or by finding an antigen, a cellular component, or a metabolic product unique to a specific organism.

Although the isolation and identification of bacteria and viruses usually are not difficult, the student should become familiar with certain general concepts related to the collection and transport of clinical specimens. In the following section, principles governing these steps are stressed, but no attempt is made to list the details associated with different procedures for isolation and identification. These and other aspects of the laboratory identification of infectious agents can be found in recent texts and manuals devoted to the subject (see References in this chapter).

RECOVERY OF BACTERIAL AND FUNGAL MICROORGANISMS BY CULTURE

Culture Media and Incubation

Bacteria and fungi are usually recovered by inoculation to artificial culture media. Most culture media are in either liquid or solid form, with agar acting as an inert solidifying agent. Liquid culture media usually are preferable to solid media for some purposes (e.g., blood cultures) in that they support growth of smaller numbers of microorganisms, but if more than one species is present, fastidious microorganisms may be rapidly overgrown. The advantage of a solid culture medium is that it allows isolation of individual microorganisms from mixed cultures. Enrichment or inhibitory agents may be added to either type of culture medium to enhance or suppress growth of different microorganisms.

Specimens for culture of bacteria or fungi may be collected either from sites normally sterile, such as blood and cerebrospinal fluid (CSF), or from sites that have a mixed normal bacterial flora, such as the oropharynx, gastrointestinal tract, and cervicovaginal canal. Most often, a single microorganism is present when infectious agents are found in normally sterile sites or fluids. In contrast, cultures of throat, gastrointestinal tract, or female genital tract may show many different bacterial species. Isolation of disease-producing agents from regions with mixed microbial flora may require selective culture media and specialized isolation procedures. To recover certain fastidious bacteria, it may be necessary that specimens be collected in a special manner. Different types of bacteria and fungi may need specific culture media or unique incubation conditions, or both, for growth. Failure to provide these conditions will result in failure to recover the microorganism, even though it may be present in large numbers. One such bacterium, *Neisseria gonorrhoeae,* is very sensitive to sudden changes in temperature. If the specimen to be cultured is inoculated to a cold agar plate just removed from a refrigerator, the organisms may not grow, even though many bacteria are present in the specimen. Other kinds of bacteria, such as *N. meningitidis,* grow very poorly unless incubated under an increased atmosphere of CO_2. Even under "ideal conditions," this bacterium is not isolated from cerebrospinal fluids of all patients with meningococcal meningitis (see Chapter 23). Many species of bacteria show growth stimulation when incubated in increased CO_2; for example, mycobacteria grow more rapidly with more and larger colonies when incubated in 8 to 11% CO_2. However, increased CO_2 tension should not be used for all specimens, as the change in surface pH of the culture medium can alter growth or antibiotic interactions with bacteria. The aminoglycosides and macrolide antibiotics can cause inhibition or potentiation of antibacterial activity, depending on slight changes in pH. Pneumococci *(Streptococcus pneumoniae)* may be recovered in only 45–55% of sputum specimens from patients with pneumococcal pneumonia who also have blood culture findings that are positive for *S. pneumoniae.* There is strong evidence that pneumococci may be inhibited by products of the oropharyngeal flora that contaminate sputum obtained for culture (Fig. 7–1). One approach to this problem has been to include gentamicin in the blood agar plates used to culture sputum. Gentamicin inhibits the growth of many of the bacteria in the oropharynx but permits the growth of pneumococci, improving the recovery of the organism from patients with pneumococcal pneumonia. Anaerobic bacteria also need a special environment for culture. These microorganisms do not grow in the presence of oxygen, and failure to provide an adequate oxygen-free environment may result in a culture negative for growth despite the presence of large numbers of anaerobic bacteria in the initial specimen.

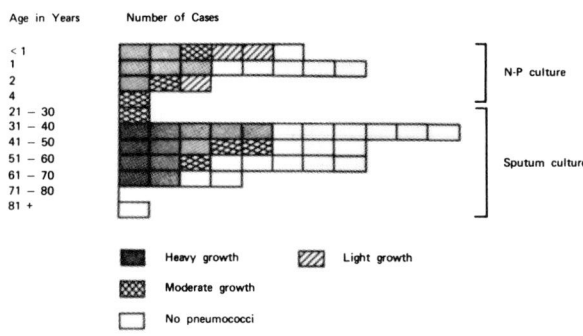

Figure 7–1. Recovery by culture of pneumococci from the respiratory tract of 51 patients with bacteremic pneumococcal pneumonia. N-P, nasopharyngeal. (From Barrett-Conner, E. The non-value of sputum culture in the diagnosis of pneumococcal pneumonia. Am. Rev. Resp. Dis. 103:845, 1971.)

Many microorganisms have specific temperature requirements for growth that can affect recovery. *Mycobacterium marinum* and *M. ulcerans* both cause ulcerating skin infections in humans. Both microorganisms have an optimal temperature range of 30°–33°C, growing slowly or not at all at 37°C, probably related to the fact that skin temperature is closer to 30°C than to 37°C. The same temperature preference is shown by fungi that inhabit skin (dermatophytes). Although most bacteria associated with disease in humans grow well at 35°–37°C, occasional strains grow better at higher temperatures. Examples are *Campylobacter jejuni,* an organism that causes acute enterocolitis and that grows more rapidly at 42°C than at 37°C, and *Mycobacterium xenopi,* an infrequent cause of pulmonary infection that grows better at 42°C.

COLLECTION AND PROCESSING OF SPECIMENS

Recovery of Microorganisms at Various Intervals during Infection

The type of specimen and the stage during an illness when a culture is obtained determine if the microorganism can be isolated. In typhoid fever, the bacillus can be isolated first from the blood and shortly afterward from the urine. Although a few typhoid microorganisms can be found in the stool early in the disease, large numbers do not appear until 10–20 days after the patient first ingests the microorganisms (Fig. 7–2). Isolation of *N. meningitidis* from patients with acute meningitis may be erratic when the CSF has large numbers of neutrophils.

For the diagnosis of tuberculosis, it is recommended that specimens be collected daily for a minimum of 4–6 days. Because of the slow, chronic course of the disease, there may be irregular shedding of *Mycobacterium tuberculosis,* resulting from sporadic ulceration and

discharge of bacilli from submucosal bronchial foci. The intermittent release of these microorganisms explains the clinical pattern of positive and negative cultures collected on successive days and emphasizes the need to collect specimens for at least several days (see Chapter 15).

Collection of cultures after initiation of antimicrobial therapy may also affect recovery of bacteria. Although small amounts of certain agents do not have a bactericidal effect, they may cause suppression of bacterial growth. One example is the inhibition of bacterial growth from patients with meningitis who have been given subtherapeutic doses of an oral antibiotic prior to lumbar puncture. This may prevent or

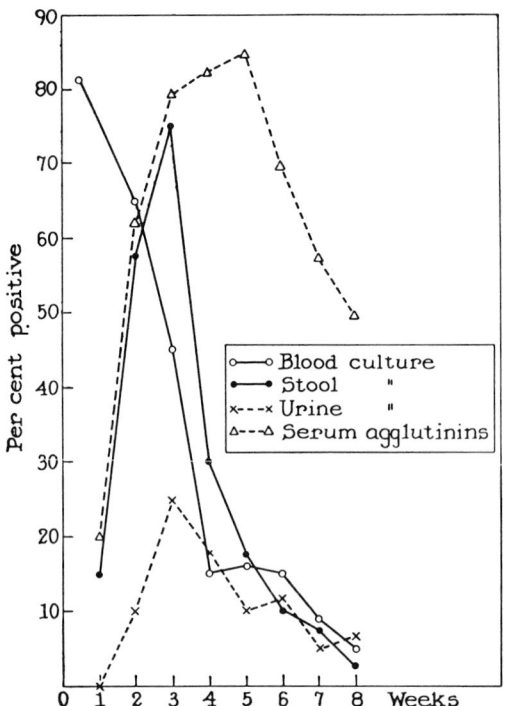

Figure 7–2. Results of serum agglutination tests and of blood, stool, and urine cultures on patients during the course of typhoid fever. (From Morgan H. The Salmonella. In: Dubos, R., ed. Bacterial and Mycotic Infections of Man. *3rd ed.* Philadelphia: J. B. Lippincott Co., 1958.)

delay culture recovery of the organism without curing the infection (see Chapter 15).

A method of removing antibiotics from blood culture specimens involves the use of a mixing vial containing neutral and polyanionic resins. The blood sample is rotated with the resins; after an appropriate period blood is withdrawn from the resin-containing vial and transferred to standard blood culture bottles. Some blood culture methods include resins for the entire incubation period. The theory is that this procedure removes inhibitory or subinhibitory amounts of antibiotic from cultured blood. Clinical trials in which blood exposed to antibiotic-absorbing resins was used have yielded variable results.

Isolation of Infectious Agents from Mixed Bacterial Populations

The challenge of isolating a disease-producing microorganism from a mixed microbial population may be met in several ways. Specimens can be inoculated directly onto agar plates and streaked to obtain isolated colonies. The isolates are then studied for differential colonial and metabolic characteristics. When large numbers of contaminating bacteria are present, inhibitory agents can be included in the culture plating medium. These inhibiting agents may be of many types: aniline dyes in small amounts inhibit gram-positive bacteria; increased sodium chloride content is selective for *Staphylococcus aureus* and *Vibrio parahaemolyticus;* increased agar content reduces the spreading motility of *Proteus mirabilis;* finally, antimicrobial drugs can be used either alone or in combination for the selective inhibition of growth of different types of microorganisms.

Need for Prompt Inoculation

The more rapidly the specimen is inoculated onto culture media, the better the chance of recovery of the suspected agent. Bacteria in urine specimens may show rapid growth, depending on pH, osmolality, and urea content. *Escherichia coli* in urine specimens at optimal conditions may show a generation time of 30–40 min. A large volume of urine for culture remains at body temperature for some time if neither refrigerated nor inoculated and incubated. Failure to inoculate the urine to culture media promptly or to refrigerate the specimen

may result in doubling and quadrupling the number of viable bacteria within 40–60 min of voiding.

Culture Swabs

There are a large variety of methods for collecting specimens for culture, and unfortunately no one method is best for the recovery of all infectious agents. Swabs made of differing types of material are useful, and cotton is commonly used. Although cotton swabs are inexpensive and readily available, some contain small amounts of lipoproteins that may be inhibitory to fastidious bacteria. To avoid the presence of inhibitory materials culture swabs made of polyester fibers are recommended. Polyester swabs are particularly effective in the recovery of group A beta-hemolytic streptococci in throat culture surveys when mailed to laboratories in envelopes containing a dehydrating agent. Another type of culture swab uses a fiber of calcium alginate, a material that is nontoxic to bacteria and has the added advantage of dissolving in sodium hexametaphosphate. By dissolving the calcium alginate, the microorganisms drawn into the fibers by capillary action are released and more easily recovered on culture. Despite the potential advantage of calcium alginate, this material is not widely used, perhaps because of its high cost and the extra effort required to dissolve the fibers. Calcium alginate swabs on thin aluminum wires are especially useful in obtaining cultures from small orifices such as the urethra, nasopharyngeal passages, nasal sinuses, and the external ear canal. Calcium alginate is not acceptable for collecting specimens for recovery of viruses.

Transport Media

A transport medium should be used for sending cultures to the laboratory when the specimen cannot be inoculated within a few minutes after collection. Transport media do not contain carbohydrate or nitrogen sources necessary for replication, thereby preventing overgrowth of fastidious organisms by contaminating flora. Transport media are buffered, and most have sufficient agar to be semisolid and may contain compounds designed to favor the survival of specific microorganisms. The main purposes of the medium are to protect the microorganisms from death by drying and to inhibit overgrowth by contaminants. Charcoal has been used in certain types of transport media to neutralize the possible effect of toxic lipoproteins on cotton swabs. Several similar types of transport media are in common use, and one, Cary-Blair, has been used successfully to recover shigellae from stool specimens after a 3-week journey from Thailand to Washington, D.C. The use of polyester culture swabs in plastic tubes containing a small ampule of a transport medium has improved the recovery of bacteria from cultures.

The transport of material to be cultured anaerobically poses a special problem. Exposure of these microorganisms to even small quantities of oxygen may kill or severely injure fastidious anaerobes, preventing or delaying their recovery and identification. Several systems for transport of such specimens have been proposed. These include the use of oxygen-free vials, a modified transport medium containing strong reducing agents, oxygen-free tubes for transporting culture swabs, and small, plastic oxygen-impermeable envelopes containing catalysts to convert hydrogen and oxygen to water (see Chapter 29).

Blood Cultures

Although recovery of bacteria from blood during episodes of septicemia is usually not difficult, an understanding of certain concepts is helpful. The skin must be thoroughly prepared at the anticipated venipuncture site with an antiseptic like iodine, using a saturated sponge, starting at the point of the anticipated venipuncture and moving in enlarging circles toward the periphery. The skin should then be further cleaned with 70% alcohol. Care must be taken not to allow prolonged contact with iodine, which may result in skin burns, particularly in the semicomatose patient. The fingers used for palpation of the anticipated venipuncture site should be disinfected to prevent contaminating the venipuncture site. Binding of iodine to the macromolecular polymer polyvinylpyrrolidone yields an antiseptic that significantly reduces toxicity while maintaining the antimicrobial activity of iodine. These *iodophors* are very effective as skin antiseptics prior to venipunctures, to the administration of parenteral medications, or to surgery. When using an iodophor, one should be careful that the compound dries on the skin completely before venipuncture. Alcohol should not be used as a second cleansing agent when an iodophor is used, as it may inactivate the compound.

For each blood culture, a minimum of 10 mL

of blood should be removed in a syringe when feasible. Culture of less than 10 mL of blood for each set of two culture bottles is associated with a significant decrease in recovery of certain bacteria, particularly the Enterobacteriaceae and *Pseudomonas aeruginosa*. Some studies have suggested improved recovery of bacteria and yeasts when amounts of up to 10 mL are drawn for each set of blood culture bottles. Smaller amounts should be taken from children, depending on their size. One blood culture bottle should be used for the recovery of aerobic and facultatively anaerobic bacteria, and the second bottle for the recovery of strictly anaerobic and nutritionally variant streptococci. The culture medium should include an anticoagulant, and in recent years there has been an increasing preference for sodium polyanetholesulfonate (SPS). SPS has, in addition to its anticoagulant action, an anticomplement and antiphagocytic effect that prevents further intracellular killing of microorganisms by neutrophils following injection of the blood into the culture bottle. SPS may inhibit recovery of some anaerobic bacteria and occasional strains of *Neisseria meningitidis*.

A culture positive for bacteria or fungi frequently indicates a serious infection. It must be emphasized, however, that blood culture data, like all laboratory information, must be evaluated in the context of the clinical setting. In most instances, bacteria and yeast grow promptly, allowing rapid identification. In some cases, however, recovery of the organism may take longer, since early or incomplete antibiotic therapy may have injured the microorganism, resulting in either a delay in recovery or interruption of growth. Reversible injury to the cell wall or plasma membrane may be caused by antimicrobial therapy, exposure to complement–antibody interactions or white blood cell effects in the host, or transient exposure of strict anaerobes to the oxygen contained in the arterial blood. Recovery may occur more rapidly if the organism is placed in a hypertonic, osmotically buffered culture medium containing 10–15% sucrose. Once the injured organisms have made several divisions, subculture to standard medium results in rapid growth. Culture media containing 10–15% sucrose may also promote the recovery of yeasts, which, like staphylococci, have a special propensity for infecting foreign implants of all kinds, for example, prosthetic heart valves or indwelling intravascular plastic catheters (see Chapter 28).

Rapid dilution of the blood sample in culture

media reduces humoral and cellular host defense mechanisms active at the time blood is taken for culture. Some bacteria are still inhibited from growth by human serum after a 20-fold dilution of blood with culture broth, as shown in Table 7–1, in which only 14 of 18 inoculated bottles yielded positive results after 1:20 dilution. Frequently, blood cultures are diluted only 10-fold, and this may be insufficient to prevent continued complement–antibody interaction with susceptible organisms. A 1:20 dilution of blood in culture broth may be sufficient to eliminate the effect of small amounts of antimicrobial agents present in the blood at the time of culture. Additionally, penicillinase or cephalosporinase can be added to the culture to enhance bacterial recovery if the patient had received one of these agents before the blood culture was taken.

The recognition that neutrophils, opsonins, specific antibodies, and other antibacterial substances in the blood can decrease the recovery of microorganisms from blood cultures has stimulated interest in alternative methods of demonstrating bacterial or fungal sepsis. One promising concept is based on the lysis of both red and white blood cells, with separation of any microorganisms in the blood by small-pore cellulose or polycarbonate filters. Following lysis and removal of the blood cells and serum, the filters are washed to remove any residual antibacterial substances present in the blood. The filters are then placed in a suitable culture medium, and growth is detected by conventional procedures or by the production of $^{14}CO_2$ from metabolites such as ^{14}C-glucose. The filtration–lysis procedure involves a number of processing steps that increase the time necessary to handle each culture and enhance the risk of contamination.

TABLE 7–1. *Growth from Small Inocula of Alpha-Hemolytic Streptococci in Blood–Broth Mixtures**

Blood–Broth Ratio	Positive/Total Bottles Inoculated
1:60	17:18
1:50	18:18
1:40	18:18
1:30	18:18
1:20	14:18
1:10	9:18
1:5	9:18
1:2	4:18
1:1	7:18

*Average number of organisms inoculated per experiment varied from 2 to 14.
From Roome, A. P. C. H., and Tozer, R. A. Effect of dilution on the growth of bacteria from blood cultures. *J. Clin. Pathol.* 21:719, 1968.

Another approach to the separation and rapid removal of bacteria and fungi from the antimicrobial activity of blood is the blood cell lysis–centrifugation procedure. This method requires a lysing agent to destroy both red and white blood cells. SPS is added as an anticoagulant and anticomplement factor. In addition, 0.3 mL of high-density hydrophobic cushion with an antifoaming solution is added. The mixture of blood, lysing agent, and microorganisms is centrifuged to precipitate the bacteria or fungi onto the high-density hydrophobic cushion. Following centrifugation, the lysing agent, hemolyzed blood, and serum are aspirated and the remaining fluid with any sedimented microorganisms is then withdrawn and inoculated directly to primary isolation culture media for bacteria and fungi. Preliminary evaluation has shown significantly reduced times for the isolation of yeasts and gram-positive cocci.

Another method for rapid isolation of bacteria and fungi from blood cultures involves preparation of a bottle containing both liquid and solid media. These "diphasic" bottles allow for easy isolation of microorganisms on solid agar slants. Following inoculation of 10 mL of blood into the laboratory's preferred liquid blood culture medium, the culture is incubated for 6–18 h, and a plastic paddle containing three different agar culture media is then attached to the primary blood broth bottle. Subculture can be easily performed by inversion of the primary blood culture bottle with its attached plastic paddle. Daily subculture can be carried out by inversion of the unit and observation for growth on the agar. This procedure provides isolated colonies after relatively short incubation periods and reduces the inhibition of growth of microorganisms by cellular and humoral elements in the original blood specimen.

An alternative approach to demonstrating the presence of bacteremia is the use of an instrument that detects the production of $^{14}CO_2$ by metabolizing bacteria from ^{14}C-glucose in a blood culture medium. Although this radiometric technique works well with microorganisms that rapidly ferment glucose, non–glucose-utilizing bacteria require other types of labeled substrates. One disadvantage to the $^{14}CO_2$ technique is that the commercially available culture bottles provide only 30 mL of medium, thereby restricting the amount of blood that can be cultured per bottle to 3 mL if a 1:10 dilution is to be maintained. Polyanionic resins for the adsorption and removal of antibiotics from blood are also available for use with the radiometric procedure.

Urine Cultures

One of the most common sites of clinically significant infection is the urinary tract (see Chapter 17). Infection may occur within the renal parenchyma, in the tubules or pelvis, or at any point along or within the ureters, urinary bladder, or urethra. Studies relating clinical infection to the number of bacteria in voided urine indicate that the best way to identify infection in the upper urinary tract (e.g., renal involvement) is to demonstrate at least 100,000 viable bacteria per milliliter of urine on culture (Fig. 7–3).

The microorganism associated most frequently with urinary tract infection is *Escherichia coli,* which *in vitro* may double in number every 20–30 min. Generation times may not always be as short as 20 min in urine, but bacteria may divide every 40–50 min. Factors influencing growth of bacteria in urine include pH, which is significantly higher in women than in men and therefore more conducive to bacterial growth in females; osmolality, which is lower in females than in males and again more likely to support bacterial growth in women (Fig. 7–4); and urea content, with higher values inhibitory to bacterial growth.

Although the replication rate following collection of a urine specimen is reduced by refrigeration, it is best to inoculate the specimen onto a culture medium promptly.

Collection of the urine specimen should minimize the possibility of external contamination, which may result in bacterial counts higher than those in the bladder at the time the specimen was voided. The procedure least likely to result in contamination of bladder urine is suprapubic puncture of the distended urinary bladder with a long aspirating needle. Because suprapubic aspiration does not appeal to most patients (or physicians), alternative methods of collecting urine are commonly used. The simplest and most practical method is the collection of a midstream urine sample during voiding.

Collection of the midstream urine from men involves starting the urine stream to wash out bacterial growth that may have developed in the urethra since the last voiding. Five to 10 mL is then collected in a sterile container prior to voiding of the latter part of the urine. Urine collected during the terminal phase of voiding should be avoided because prostatic secretions or urethral sphincter contractions may dislodge small clumps of bacteria and artificially increase the bacterial count. Although it may not be possible to exclude all contamination during collection—with the exception of suprapubic aspiration—midstream urine specimens usually accurately reflect the number of bacteria in the bladder.

Collection of urine specimens from females poses a special problem because of the increased possibility of contamination. The patient should be instructed in how to carefully clean the labia and external urethral meatus and how to prevent labial contamination of the urine stream during voiding (Fig. 7–5). A midstream specimen with prompt inoculation to culture medium usually adequately reflects the number of bacteria in the urine.

Sputum Cultures

Success in collecting sputum for culture depends on the type and extent of pulmonary disease.

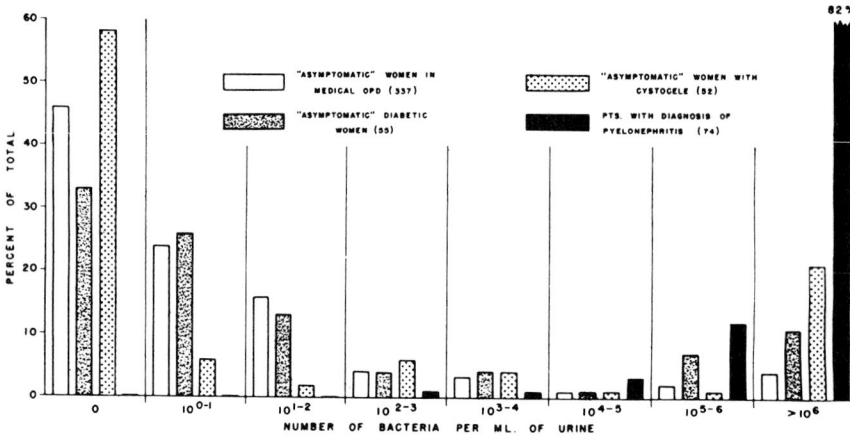

Figure 7–3. Bacterial counts in urines of various population groups. (From Kass, E. H. Asymptomatic infections of the urinary tract. Trans. Assoc. Am. Physicians *69:56, 1956.)*

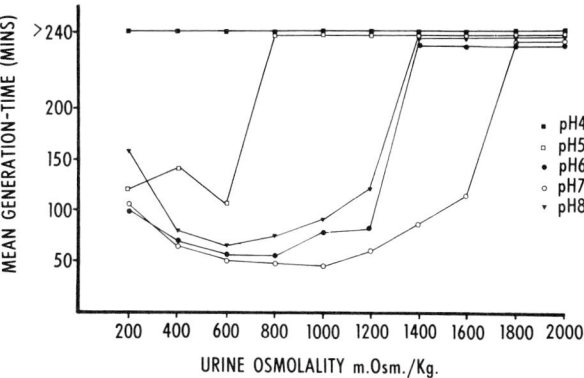

Figure 7–4. The effect of variation of urine pH and osmolality on the growth rate of Escherichia coli. *(From Asscher, A. W., Sussman, M., Walters, W. E., et al: Urine as a medium for bacterial growth.* Lancet 2:*1037, 1966.)*

Most sputum specimens are heavily contaminated with oropharyngeal secretions and bacteria and may contain only small amounts of secretions for the lower respiratory tract. Many sputum specimens contain *only* salivary and oropharyngeal secretions, representing an ineffective effort by the patient to raise secretions from the lower respiratory tract. Recovery of *Streptococcus pneumoniae* is poor, and there is evidence that interaction with other organisms or products from other organisms found in the oropharynx, such as the alpha-hemolytic streptococci, may suppress growth of pneumococci. Partial suppression of the endogenous flora using gentamicin-containing blood agar results in marked improvement in recovery of *S. pneumoniae* from sputum.

One method for collecting material for culture from the lower respiratory tract is inducting sputum by ultrasonic or heated-saline nebulization. Aerosolization increases the moisture content of the air reaching the lower respiratory tract and improves the ability of the tracheo-bronchial cilia to bring up otherwise thick, viscid, or partially dehydrated secretions. Nebulization is particularly well suited for the recovery of *Mycobacterium tuberculosis* but can also be used for inducing sputum in other patients.

To determine if a sputum specimen represents secretions from an acutely inflamed portion of the bronchopulmonary tree rather than merely salivary or oropharyngeal secretions, Gram staining of the specimen should be performed before it is cultured. If the majority of cells present are segmented neutrophils or other types of inflammatory cells, the specimen should be inoculated to culture media, but if most cells appear to be from squamous epithelium, the laboratory should request an additional specimen. Large numbers of segmented neutrophils indicate a cellular response to an acute injury, frequently associated with an acute bacterial infection. The different types and relative numbers of bacteria should also be noted, as well as whether there is evidence of bacterial phagocytosis.

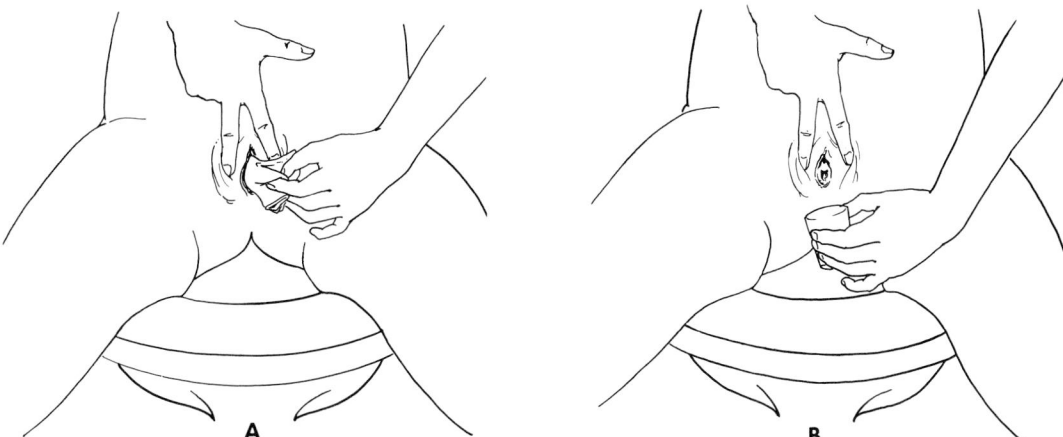

Figure 7–5. Collection of a urine sample from women. A, *With the labia held apart, washing is done from high up front toward the back with gauze soaked in soap.* B, *The cup is held so that it does not touch the body, and a sample is obtained only while the subject is urinating with the labia held apart. (From Kory, M., and Waife, S. O., eds.* Kidney and Urinary Tract Infections. *Indianapolis: Eli Lilly and Company, 1971.)*

Tracheal cannulation, bronchoscopy, bronchial brushing guided by fluoroscopy, and bronchoalveolar lavage are additional methods of collecting specimens from the lower respiratory tract. These procedures are all subject to variable degrees of contamination of lower respiratory tract secretions by the normal oropharyngeal microbial flora (see Chapter 12). Transtracheal aspiration, in which a needle is passed percutaneously between the cricothyroid and thyroid cartilages of the larynx, is infrequently used now.

Cerebrospinal Fluid Cultures

CSF from patients with suspected meningitis should be taken directly to the laboratory for prompt Gram staining, antigen detection, and inoculation to culture media. Certain strains of *Neisseria meningitidis* may be very sensitive to decreases in temperature below 35°C. Therefore, CSF must be kept warm during transportation to the laboratory, and culture media should be warmed to 37°C before inoculation. If the cerebrospinal fluid is not cloudy, microorganisms present should be concentrated by centrifugation. The supernatant spinal fluid should be saved in a sterile tube, and the sediment should be used to make smears for Gram staining and inoculation to culture media. All CSF not used for stains or culture inoculation or other tests may be incubated separately along with the inoculated media at 37°C under 5–10% CO_2. CSF can serve as a growth medium for a number of bacteria causing acute meningitis and may be stained again the following day for evidence of bacterial growth. If the bacterium invaded the meninges only shortly before the CSF was obtained and the microorganism is not found on the initial Gram's stain or culture, growth in the CSF following incubation may provide both a large number of microorganisms and an increased amount of bacterial polysaccharide that can be identified by counterimmunoelectrophoresis (CIE), latex agglutination, or other immunologic procedures.

Wound Cultures

For optimal recovery of microorganisms, specimens for culture from infection at different sites of the body may require a wide range of media, procedures, and techniques, depending on the body site involved and the type of infection suspected. Cultures of skin infections may require inoculation to only a few simple media, but drainage from postoperative wounds, from ascitic, pleural, and joint fluids, or from deep sinus tracts may harbor anaerobic bacteria. All such cultures should be obtained in a manner that minimizes or excludes exposure to oxygen. Recovery of organisms from thick pus is facilitated by dilution to reduce the antibacterial effect of inflammatory cells and serum factors. Dilution to 1:10 or 1:100 with normal saline (not containing bacteriostatic additives), or by adding one or two drops to a blood culture bottle, improves the yield. If infection with mycobacteria or fungi is suspected, portions of exudate or tissue should be collected for culture rather than merely using a swab. Few microorganisms are shed in these types of infection and the yield of microorganisms from a swab may be disappointing. Again, prompt delivery of the specimen to the laboratory reduces suppression by contaminating microorganisms and facilitates recovery of the organism or organisms causing the infection.

DIRECT STAINS OF CLINICAL SPECIMENS

Gram's Stain

One of the most useful and rapid procedures in the diagnosis of bacterial or fungal infections is Gram staining. A Gram's stain can be quickly and easily made on exudates, fluids, aspirates, and tissue impressions—in short, on any specimen suspected of being the site of bacterial, fungal, or, in some cases, viral infection. In the preparation and interpretation of Gram's stains, several points should be emphasized. Lack of familiarity with the staining procedure or with the appearance of Gram's stains may lead to errors in interpretation. Such errors can often be avoided by the simultaneous staining of previously prepared control slides containing both gram-positive and gram-negative bacteria that are readily found in saliva. Some gram-positive bacteria decolorize more easily than others and may appear gram-negative. Dead bacteria may also decrease in size, and this may lead the microscopist to the erroneous conclusion that there are two types of bacteria present when in fact there are both viable and nonviable cells of the same organism.

In addition to looking for bacteria in a Gram's stain, the presence and type of inflammatory cells should be noted. Segmented neutrophils in large numbers may denote an infection controlled primarily by phagocytosis and intracellular killing, such as infections caused by the obligate extracellular parasites (e.g., pneumococci, meningococci, gonococci, and *Haemophilus influenzae*). If segmented neutrophils are present, the presence or absence as well as the size and shape of phagocytosed intracellular bacteria can aid in the presumptive identification of pneumococci, meningococci, or gonococci. Smears from clinical specimens showing bacteria without accompanying inflammatory cells should be interpreted with caution, as they may represent colonizing microorganisms that are not associated with an invasive infection. Gram's stains may be helpful in the rapid, presumptive identification of a number of acute infections, such as gonorrheal urethritis, *Haemophilus* infections, meningococcal meningitis, nocardial abscesses, and other types of infections in which the shape and staining reaction of the microorganism, along with the type of inflammatory cell response, are consistent with a well-defined infectious disease. An exception is the watery diarrhea of cholera; this disease is caused by a toxin that does not incite an inflammatory cell response (see Chapter 19).

Gram staining should be performed as soon as a culture is taken from a wound. Correlation of the Gram's stain with the cellular and morphologic characteristics of the exudate and with the bacterial or fungal organisms recovered on culture may show a discrepancy, suggesting that other organisms, such as one or more anaerobic bacteria, had been present but were not recovered on culture.

Acid-Fast Stains

Mycobacteria are frequently called *acid-fast microorganisms* (see Chapter 15), meaning that they have a characteristically strong affinity for certain stains that allow them to resist destaining with strong acids. Classically, *acid-fast* refers to the ability of the microorganism to retain carbolfuchsin following decolorization with 3% hydrochloric acid in 95% ethyl alcohol, a procedure that readily decolorizes most other types of bacteria. The best known acid-fast stain is the Ziehl-Neelsen, which requires that the stain be applied to the smear or tissue section over a steaming water bath. Another carbolfuchsin acid-fast stain is the Kinyoun stain, comparable in reliability to but easier to prepare than the Ziehl-Neelsen stain. The Kinyoun stain does

not require steaming and can be used "cold." Acid-fast organisms appear red, leading to the slang term "red snappers."

Since the early 1960s, acid-fast fluorochrome stains for mycobacteria have been gaining popularity. Auramine, sometimes prepared in combination with rhodamine, is the most commonly used of the fluorochrome stains. Most laboratories employing auramine for identifying mycobacteria from smears or within tissues find it to be slightly more sensitive than the carbolfuchsin stains. Although auramine is no more specific for mycobacteria than is carbolfuchsin, the organisms are more easily seen when auramine is used, because they stain bright yellow to gold against a contrasting dark background. Because of this contrast, it is possible to screen larger areas of the slide using a lower magnification objective than the oil-immersion objective required for examination of carbolfuchsin acid-fast stains. Fluorochrome stains are *not* fluorescent antibody stains and should not be confused with them. Fluorescent antibody stains for different species of mycobacteria are of little practical use. For additional information regarding aids in establishing the diagnosis of tuberculosis, see Chapter 15.

Other Stains

Fluorescein-tagged or peroxidase-tagged antibodies to specific bacteria are used in both research and clinical microbiology laboratories to identify bacteria. Fluorescent antibody stains have been employed to identify enteropathogenic strains of *Escherichia coli*, *Neisseria gonorrhoeae*, group A streptococci, and a number of *Salmonella* species. The use of specific, fluorescein-tagged antisera provides a rapid, sensitive technique for identifying *Legionella pneumophila* in lung biopsies, pleural fluids, and other specimens.

Polychromatic stains for malaria and microfilaria are of great help in the rapid identification of protozoa and hemoflagellates in blood smears. Stains giving characteristic reactions for fungi include the periodic acid–Schiff (PAS) stain and the methenamine silver stain; the latter is particularly helpful in the identification of *Pneumocystis carinii*. Although the methenamine silver stain is almost specific for *P. carinii,* the staining procedure unfortunately is moderately complex and takes approximately 3 h. For a more rapid answer as to the presence or absence of pneumocystis cysts in a lung or bronchial biopsy, the polychromatic stain toluidine blue O (TBO) is quite sensitive and specific as well as rapid.

One can easily identify hyphal forms of fungi associated with infection in skin or nails after warming epithelial scrapings or nail clippings gently in 10% potassium hydroxide, which acts as a keratolytic agent. This is known as the KOH preparation. However, the use of potassium hydroxide for the identification of fungi from *non*keratinized specimens (e.g., sputum) is inappropriate. Phase microscopy is very helpful in the direct examination of sputum or other fluid specimens, because fungal spores and hyphae appear in sharp contrast to the background.

Negative staining techniques may be of great help in the visualization of organisms having translucent capsules (e.g., *Cryptococcus neoformans* and *Haemophilus influenzae*). A dilute solution of India ink or, in the case of *Streptococcus pneumoniae* and *H. influenzae*, methylene blue may be used. The presence of a capsule is indicated by a clear halo around the organism (Fig. 7–6). Reaction with specific anticapsular antisera increases the size of the capsule in

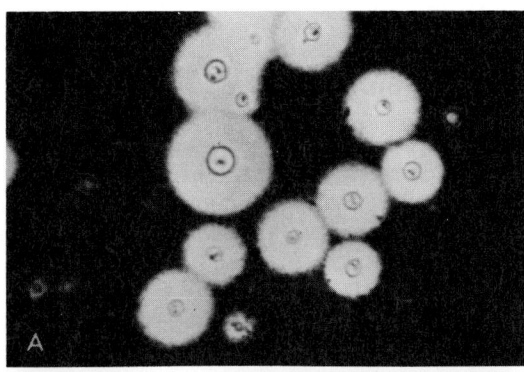
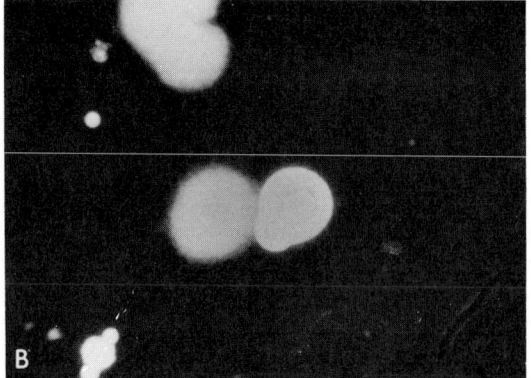

Figure 7–6. Cryptococcosis. A, India ink preparation of spinal fluid showing yeast cells surrounded by large capsule. B, Budding yeast cell within capsule. (From Rippon, J. W. Medical Mycology. Philadelphia: W. B. Saunders Co., 1974.)

pneumococci and *H. influenzae* and is the basis of the *quellung reaction* for serotyping of pneumococci. Care should be taken that the final solution of ink or methylene blue used is not so strong as to exclude all transmitted light. The India ink or other contrast material also should be checked on a regular basis to exclude the presence of any endogenous yeast or bacteria.

IDENTIFICATION OF ISOLATED MICROORGANISMS

Gram's Stain

Once a bacterial culture has shown growth, the first step in identification of the microorganism is Gram staining. Although it is usually not difficult to identify the staining reaction and the shape of the microorganism, occasionally microorganisms may best be described, for example, as "gram-variable coccobacilli." The shape of a microorganism may change slightly, depending on the culture medium used. A Gram's stain made from a broth culture may show microorganisms of one form, whereas a stain made from an agar medium may show organisms of a slightly different size and shape.

Biochemical Identification

With few exceptions, the identification of a bacterium is established by determining the presence or absence of various bacterial enzymes that are known to be characteristic of individual species. For example, *Proteus mirabilis* is oxidase-negative and urease-positive. In most instances, enzymes are assessed by bacterial inoculation to various culture media containing substrates for those enzymes found useful in taxonomic characterization. Most such reactions result in a decrease in pH from the production of varying amounts of weak or strong acids, although some cause an increase in pH (e.g., urease). For most such studies, standard acid–base indicators are incorporated into the culture media to indicate various end points. The number of metabolic characteristics necessary for accurate identification of microorganisms is variable, but samples for sufficient differential tests should be inoculated to separate closely related species. Identification of a species may require from 3 to 25 tests, depending on the microorganism. Highly successful automated instrumentation has been developed for the clinical microbiology laboratory. A number of different bacterial and yeast identification kits are now available, providing between 10 and 22 different identification characteristics for each isolate tested. Some of these kits require overnight incubation in small plastic cupules or microtiter trays, whereas others test for preformed enzymes available from bacterial colonies. Such kits have made a significant improvement in the ability of the small laboratory to identify accurately many, but not all, types of microbial isolates.

In addition to the packaged kits, there are now a number of instruments designed to provide 4–8 h identification of commonly isolated bacteria. The principle of operation of most of these instruments is based on the ability of the test organism to grow or to be inhibited from growth in the presence of a variety of substrates or antibiotics. Growth in broth culture (turbidity) is detected by optical sensors and changes in the scattering of light. Results are compared with previously programmed identification patterns of bacteria stored in either self-contained or reference computers. Microbial identification test results can then be stored in a file, printed on reports, or displayed in a variety of ways.

Gas Chromatography

In search for faster and more specific methods for separating bacteria with similar characteristics, gas chromatography has been used to detect short-chain volatile organic acids. This procedure has been found to be of significant help in identifying anaerobic bacteria. Propionibacteria produce propionic acid; lactobacilli produce lactic acid. The hope that this technique might have application for species identification of bacteria other than anaerobes has not been fulfilled, however, partially because of significant variability in the composition of different lots of culture media, which results in a wide variety of end products. Spontaneous bacterial mutants that show slightly different metabolic activity also cause variable production of different end products. Extraction of fatty acids from bacterial cell walls has been helpful in the early identification of mycobacteria and *Legionella*. Application of gas chromatography to all positive blood cultures as a means of rapid identification has not been successful for non-anaerobic bacterial isolates. Continuing efforts in detecting specific products (e.g., increased levels of ara-

binitol in patients with disseminated candidiasis) are resulting in some limited success.

DETECTION OF MICROBIAL PRODUCTS OR ANTIGENS

Immunodiffusion and Counterimmunoelectrophoresis

The recognition that soluble antigenic substances from microbial organisms can be detected in blood and tissue fluids opened a new approach to the diagnosis of infectious disease. One of the first applications of this principle was the demonstration of soluble polysaccharide from *Cryptococcus neoformans* in CSF of patients with cryptococcal meningitis. The same principle has been applied to other infectious agents in the central nervous system (e.g., the capsular polysaccharide antigens of pneumococci, meningococci, and *Haemophilus*, the three most common bacterial causes of meningitis). Soluble antigen may be present wherever the microorganism is replicating, for example, in serum, or where the antigen is cleared from the body, for example, in urine. Cryptococcal antigen can usually be found in serum as well as in the CSF in patients with cryptococcal meningitis. Cryptococcal polysaccharide in the urine may represent either renal infection or renal clearance of the antigen from blood. Similarly, type-specific pneumococcal polysaccharide may be found in CSF, serum, sputum, pleural fluid, or urine of patients with pneumococcal meningitis, pneumonia, or septicemia. The chemical composition of pneumococcal polysaccharide in urine may differ slightly from that found in serum, presumably as a result of partial degradation of the polysaccharide prior to clearance by the kidney.

Several different immunologic techniques are available for detection of microbial antigens in clinical specimens. Ouchterlony gel diffusion for antigen–antibody precipitin reactions was used originally, but the simplicity, speed, and increased sensitivity resulting from concentrating antigen and antibody in a small reaction zone have made counterimmunoelectrophoresis (CIE) preferable to the detection of precipitin reactions (Fig. 7–7). CIE has been useful in the rapid identification of antigens from bacteria associated with meningitis, septicemia, pneumonia, septic arthritis, and other serious infections. In some instances, the amount of antigen present in a specimen can be semiquantitated

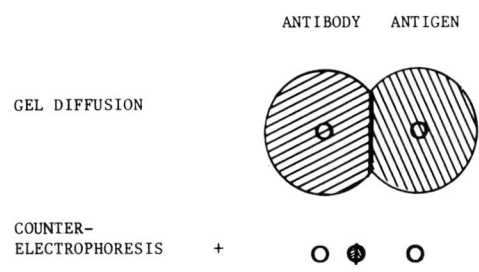

Figure 7–7. Schematic representation of precipitation in agar. Only small portions of the antibody and antigen are involved in the precipitin line in gel diffusion (double immunodiffusion), whereas all the antigen and antibody have an opportunity to participate in the precipitin reaction in counterimmunoelectrophoresis (immunoelectroosmophoresis). (From Kenney, G. E., and Foy, H. M. Detection and quantitation of circulating polysaccharide in pneumococcal pneumonia by immunoelectroosmophoresis [counterelectrophoresis] and rocket electrophoresis. In Schlessinger, D., ed. Microbiology—1975. Washington, DC: American Society of Microbiology, 1975.)

by comparison against purified polysaccharide. The rapid identification of microbial antigen in CSF or serum can provide important therapeutic and prognostic information, thereby giving the clinician early notice regarding the specific responsible infectious agent.

Latex Agglutination and Staphylococcal Coagglutination

A number of antibodies to antigens of various infectious agents (chiefly polysaccharide capsular materials) have been coupled to latex particles for use in the clinical laboratory. This provides simple agglutination tests for the identification of isolated colonies of bacteria (e.g., group A streptococci, *Neisseria gonorrhoeae,* the soluble polysaccharide capsular material of *Haemophilus influenzae* or *Streptococcus pneumoniae*). The ease of performance and rapidity of latex agglutination and its high sensitivity for many polysaccharide antigens suggest many applications for antigen detection. Latex agglutination has essentially replaced CIE in most clinical settings because of its greater ease in performing, its improved sensitivity, and its rapidity.

A similar approach involves attachment of the Fc fragment of an antibody molecule to protein A on the outer coat of certain strains of *Staphylococcus aureus*. This orients the antigen-binding end of antibody molecules outward from the staphylococcus, which then, in the presence of antigen, agglutinates in large clumps. Staphylococcal particles sensitized with specific antibody carry a short shelf life (30 days) compared with antibody-coupled latex particles, and both products are roughly equivalent in clinical application, sensitivity, and specificity. Antibody-tagged staphylococcal particles can also be used in detecting small quantities of antigens in body fluids. Both types of sensitized particles, when bound to appropriate antibodies, provide the clinical laboratory with valuable tools for both rapid and specific identification of microbial antigens directly from patient-derived fluids.

Radioimmunoassay and Enzyme-Linked Immunosorbent Assay for Detection of Antigen or Antibody

Two *in vitro* laboratory methods for detecting small quantities of antigens or antibodies to infectious agents have greatly increased the potential of the clinical laboratory to establish the diagnosis of infectious diseases. Both radioimmunoassay (RIA) and enzyme-linked immunosorbent assay (ELISA) procedures can be set up in a variety of configurations, using either antigen or antibody attached to a solid-phase support such as a plastic disc, plastic test tube, or plastic microtiter plate. Serologic tests using RIA are many times more sensitive than those using CIE. ELISA tests, such as those for the presence of rotavirus in the stool, are also much more sensitive than CIE tests.

There are advantages and disadvantages associated with both RIA and ELISA. These assays measure the total amount of antibody bound to the antigen in question rather than a specific subgroup of antibody, such as that which gives rise to agglutination, complement fixation, or precipitation reactions. Unfortunately, in both RIA and ELISA, IgM-specific tests may not always be capable of making a clear-cut distinction between a recent or past infection. A *prozone phenomenon* (high titer of one class of antibody obscuring lower levels of another class) should also be considered when one is screening for antibody. RIA, although sensitive, has not assumed a major role in the routine serologic laboratory because of the need for special handling and disposal of radioactive isotopes and the expense of monitoring devices. Reagents for RIA tests are expensive and usually have short shelf lives; therefore, tests should be performed in large volumes to make them cost-effective (e.g., the screening for hepatitis B surface antigen and antibody in serum). ELISA tests circumvent many of these disad-

TABLE 7–2. *Comparison between Viruses and Bacteria*

	Viruses	Bacteria
Size	20–300 nm	500–1000 nm
Nucleic acids	RNA or DNA	RNA and DNA
Growth requirement	Living cells	Artificial media
Energy source and enzymes	Host cells	Self-sufficient
Response to antibiotics	Not susceptible	Susceptible
Special staining	Giemsa, acridine orange	Aniline dyes

vantages, although some of the enzyme substrates are possibly carcinogenic. Fortunately, it is not necessary to use these substrates for all ELISA tests, and, when they are used, only small amounts are needed. ELISA procedures do not require expensive instrumentation, although if numerous tests are performed, automated spectrophotometers can facilitate the interpretation of results.

DEMONSTRATION OF CHANGE IN SPECIFIC ANTIBODY TITER

Often attempts to recover an infecting microorganism are unsuccessful. In many such instances, one can establish a diagnosis of infection by a specific infectious agent by demonstrating a rise in antibody titer against one or more antigens of that agent. This approach requires that patient serum be obtained early in the illness, with a second, or convalescent, serum collected after 10–21 days of illness. The objective of such studies is to demonstrate a significant antibody rise following an interval when the host can respond to antigenic stimulation. The antibody may be directed against a specific microorganism (e.g., group C *N. meningitidis*) or to a microbial product (e.g., streptolysin O, an extracellular protein produced by group A beta-hemolytic streptococci). For this reason, it is good practice to collect a serum

sample from patients with serious infections on admission to the hospital and retain it in a freezer for possible later use.

There are many immunologic procedures available for demonstrating changes in antibody titer, and the technique used varies depending on the type of antibody formed. Antibodies may be demonstrated by agglutination, precipitation, complement fixation, or hemagglutination, or by bactericidal or other methods. Total antibody formation, including all subgroups, can be determined by the RIA and ELISA procedures.

DIAGNOSIS OF VIRAL INFECTIONS

Viral diagnostic procedures differ from those for bacteria because of the properties listed in Table 7–2. Infectious virus particles (virions) can multiply only in cell cultures or in animals.

Use of Cell Cultures

Three types of cell culture systems are used for cultivating viruses in the laboratory:

1. Primary cell cultures, composed of cells from a single passage from an animal. Primary monkey kidney cells (PMK) are generally used, as well as various human embryonic organ cells. Primary cell cultures are morphologically heterogeneous and support the growth of entero-

TABLE 7–3. *Cell Cultures and Their Susceptibility to Multiplication of Viruses*

Cell Culture Type	Name	DNA Viruses Herpes Group	Adeno-viruses	Vaccinia Virus	RNA Viruses Enteroviruses	Myxoviruses	Measles/RSV
Primary	PMK	±	−	−	+	+	−
Primary	HEK	+	+	+	+	−	−
Strain	WI-38	+	+	−	±	−	−
Strain	IMR-90	+	+		±	−	−
Line	HEp-2	+	+	+	+	−	+
Line	HeLa	+	+		+	−	+

Abbreviations and symbols: PMK, primary monkey (Rhesus) kidney; HEK, human embryonic kidney; WI-38, Wistar Institute, human embryonic lung; IMR-90, Institute of Medical Research, human embryonic lung; HEp-2, human epithelial cells from carcinoma of larynx; HeLa, human epithelial cells from carcinoma of cervix; −, no growth of virus; +, growth of virus; ±, growth of some viral isolates (unpredictable).

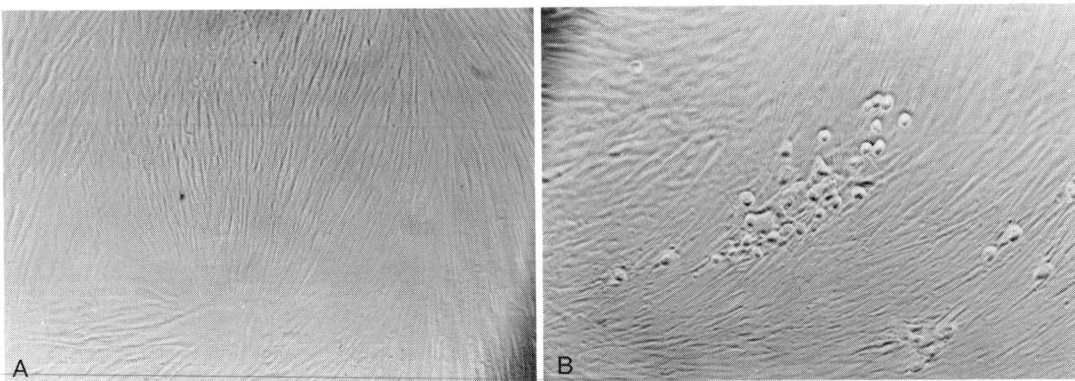

Figure 7–8. Cell cultures. A, *Uninfected WI-38.* B, *CMV-infected WI-38.*

viruses (polioviruses, coxsackieviruses, and echoviruses) and myxoviruses (influenza and parainfluenza viruses).

2. Semicontinuous diploid lines are cell strains derived from human placenta or embryonic lungs (IMR-90 and WI-38). The cells are homogeneous with fibroblast-like morphology; they support the growth of herpesviruses and adenoviruses.

3. Continuous cell lines. Assumed to be of cancerous origin, these heteroploid bodies resemble epithelial cells that multiply *in vitro* for an undetermined length of time (e.g., HEp-2). They support the multiplication of adenoviruses, herpesviruses, measles, and respiratory syncytial viruses.

Table 7–3 displays the three types of cell cultures and their susceptibility to infection by different types of viruses.

Most viruses interfere with cellular metabolism and produce visible changes in the infected cells. Cell destruction, or cytopathic effect (CPE), is the typical result of infection by viruses (Fig. 7–8). CPE is slow and mild in cytomegalovirus (CMV) and varicella–zoster virus (VSV) infections but rapid and generalized in enterovirus and herpes simplex virus (HSV) infections. Typical viral inclusion bodies in the nucleus or cytoplasm of infected cells can be seen after staining with specific stains. Some viruses cause chronic infections in cell cultures without CPE or obvious changes to the cells. These viruses can be detected by specific antigens that they introduce into the infected cells. Myxoviruses, for example, add to the cell surface a new hemagglutinin that binds erythrocytes, a phenomenon known as *hemadsorption*. They can also clump erythrocytes in suspensions, a reaction known as *hemagglutination*. Some viruses, such as rubella, may interfere with multiplication of a second virus in primary

green African monkey kidney cells. An interference test for rubella is not performed routinely in most laboratories. Oncogenic viruses accelerate mitosis and metabolism of cultured cells, cause loss of contact inhibition, and transform normal cells into cancer cells.

The smallest *in vivo* system for culturing viruses is the embryonated egg, since the embryo's membranes support viral growth. Today, this system is rarely used in the routine diagnostic laboratory; it is utilized more frequently in laboratories for isolating new strains of influenza virus for vaccine preparation. Another animal system, the mouse, although small and easily handled, is used only to a limited extent. Suckling mice are used for isolation of coxsackieviruses, and young mice are used for isolation of arboviruses. Large experimental animals are used in research centers for diagnosing special virus groups or as the source for virus-specific antisera. Monoclonal antibodies have largely replaced animal antisera for virus identification because of their uniformity.

BASIC APPROACH TO VIRAL DIAGNOSIS

Viruses are present in body fluids and cause symptoms in various locations. If the clinical picture is clear, diagnosis can be made with a minimum of laboratory assistance, as, for example, in the case of mumps, poliomyelitis with paralysis, or measles when Koplik's spots are detected. However, in most viral infections the clinical symptoms are not specific, and virus identification is necessary for specific diagnosis. There are four approaches to virus identification: (1) staining patient material for direct microscopic examination, (2) culturing body fluid or tissue for virus isolation, (3) polymerase

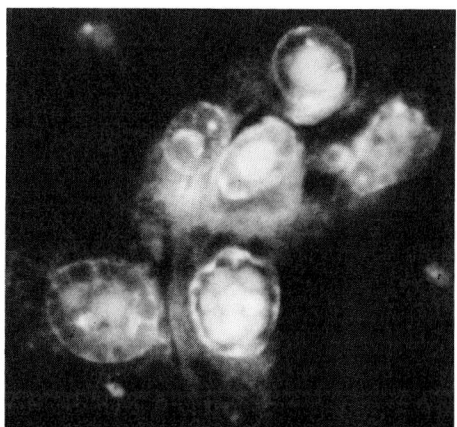

Figure 7–9. Acridine orange staining of intranuclear inclusion of adenovirus.

chain reaction and nucleic acid probes, and (4) identification of postinfection antiviral antibody by serologic methods.

Staining for Direct Microscopic Examination

Direct staining is useful if distinct, localized lesions are present and if the virus produces recognizable cellular changes. HSV and varicella–zoster virus cause skin vesicles, measles virus causes skin and lung lesions, and CMV can be detected in exfoliated cells in the urine. Scrapings from skin lesions, imprints from biopsied lung, or exfoliated cells from urine deposited on a glass slide are fixed with methanol and stained with Wright's, Giemsa, Feulgen's, or acridine orange stain. HSV is distinguished by multinucleated large cells, measles virus by syncytia, and CMV by large "owl type" cells with

intranuclear inclusions. Figure 7–9 shows intranuclear inclusions of adenovirus.

If necessary, the diagnosis is confirmed by application of labeled specific antiviral antisera to the specimen on the slide. Viral antigens bind the specific antibodies, the label serving as a marker for binding. The use of labeled specific antibody in a one-step procedure is called a *direct test,* for example, *direct immunofluorescent test* (DIF), and *direct immunoenzyme assay* (DIE), in which fluorescein and peroxidase, respectively, are utilized as labeling compounds. Since only a few viruses produce visible cellular changes, techniques other than traditional staining should be applied for identification of other viruses. For example, negative staining and electron microscopy (EM) can be used for identification of these virus groups. Samples are placed on EM grids, stained with 2% phosphotungstic acid, and examined. Virus particles remain unstained and visible against the stained dark background. They are identified by the morphology of their capsids. Virus particles in specimens can be aggregated by treatment with specific antiserum (immune EM).

Direct staining methods are rapid and practical and provide a diagnosis in 1–4 h. They are used mainly for identification of the herpesvirus group and rabies (see Chapter 24). The herpesvirus group includes HSV types 1 and 2, varicella–zoster virus (VZV), CMV, and Epstein-Barr virus and is associated with a number of clinical manifestations (Table 7–4). The sharp increase in cases of venereally transmitted HSV, which affects both young adults and newborn infants, and the prominence of CMV in AIDS patients and in other immunocompromised hosts makes rapid identification of the herpesvirus group important (see Chapters 18 and 26).

TABLE 7–4. *Clinical Manifestations of Herpesvirus Infections*

| Virus | Manifestations | |
	Common	*Less Frequent*
Herpes simplex virus	"Fever blisters" Pharyngitis, tonsillitis Keratoconjunctivitis Genital infections (type 2) Neonatal herpes (type 2)	Encephalitis Eczema herpeticum Hepatitis (infants)
Varicella–zoster virus	Chickenpox Shingles	Pneumonia Encephalitis
Cytomegalovirus	Infectious mononucleosis-like: Pneumonitis Hepatitis	Post-transfusion infection CID (cytomegalic inclusion disease) Guillain-Barré syndrome
Epstein-Barr virus	Infectious mononucleosis	Burkitt's lymphoma Nasopharyngeal carcinoma

TABLE 7–5. *Virus and Antibody Quantitation with Infections*

Stage of Disease	Amount of Virus	Titers of Specific Antibody
Prodrome	High	Absent to low
Acute	High to moderate	Low
Convalescence	Low to absent	High

The two following examples emphasize the desirability of rapid identification:

1. A young male patient entered the hospital for corrective surgery for a rectal fissure. Because the area looked suspicious, a slide was made for direct staining. Within 1 h, herpesvirus was identified. Surgery was avoided, in the hope that recovery from the rectal infection would result in disappearance of the fissure.

2. A pregnant woman came to the delivery room, and a lesion was detected on her cervix. The lesion was identified as containing herpes simplex virus. The newborn was delivered by cesarean section, thus escaping infection with the virus.

Rotavirus, the most common cause of non-bacterial childhood diarrhea throughout the world, can be detected by electron microscopy. Recently, an assay was developed for detection of rotaviruses that has largely replaced the EM technique. This is a direct immunoenzyme assay (ELISA) in which the virus binds to an antibody-coated plastic bead and is identified by specific antiserum labeled with peroxidase.

Isolation and Identification of Viruses

In viral infections with nonspecific symptoms, the direct staining methods are not helpful, and viruses should be isolated by cell culture. For successful virus isolation, remember the transitory presence of viruses in body fluids and the fragility of the viruses, as well as how to select a correct sampling. Since infectious virus is detected most readily during the prodromal and early acute stages of disease, any delay decreases the chances of detection. Virus is seldom isolated during convalescence (see Table 7–5). Specific holding media, immediate delivery of the specimens to the laboratory, and storage at −70°C until processing protect viruses from inactivation.

The clinical symptoms, as summarized in Table 7–6, are important in selecting appropriate specimens for virus isolation. The throat swab is generally the best single specimen, since it can be used in cases of encephalitis, meningitis, and respiratory and intestinal symptoms. Cultures inoculated with patient specimens are checked daily for development of CPE. Enteroviruses and myxoviruses are identified by this method. The enteroviruses, of the Picornaviridae family, include many of the important human pathogens of the gastrointestinal tract. They are divided into three subgroups—polioviruses, coxsackieviruses, and echoviruses (*En*teric *C*ytopathogenic *H*uman *O*rphan)—that can be identified by their growth characteristics, summarized in Table 7–7. The enteroviruses produce significant CPE within 18–24 h of infection. The intensity and timing of CPE in

TABLE 7–6. *Appropriate Specimens for Virus Isolation*

Clinical Syndrome	Likely Virus	Appropriate Specimens
Meningitis and encephalitis	Enteroviruses	Throat swab, stool, CSF
	Mumps	Throat swab, urine, CSF
	Herpes simplex	Throat swab, vesicle
Neonatal (TORCH) infections	Herpes simplex	Throat swab, vesicle
	Cytomegalovirus	Throat swab, urine
	Enteroviruses	Throat swab, stool
	Rubella	Throat swab, urine
Respiratory infections	Adenovirus, enteroviruses	Throat swab, stool
	Influenza, parainfluenza, rhinoviruses, respiratory syncytial	Throat swab
Skin and mucous membrane infections	Herpes simplex and poxviruses	Throat swab, vesicle
	Varicella–zoster	Throat swab
	Coxsackievirus A	Not applicable

TABLE 7–7. *Growth of Enteroviruses in Various Systems*

Propagation Media/Virus	Poliovirus	Coxsackievirus A	Coxsackievirus B	Echovirus
Mice	−	+	+	−
Primary cell culture	+	−	+	+
Cell strain	+	−	+	+
Cell line	+	−	+	−

Symbols: −, no growth; +, growth.

various cultures are used for subgrouping of the enteroviruses (Table 7–8).

Except for enteroviruses, viral agents rarely are isolated from CSF in instances of aseptic meningitis and are almost never recovered from the CSF of patients with acute encephalitis (see Chapter 24). Indeed when deciding whether to initiate antiviral therapy, the most rapid and accurate approach to diagnosing herpesvirus encephalitis is brain biopsy followed either by staining for inclusion bodies or by direct immunofluorescence using specific antiherpesvirus antibody conjugates (see Chapter 24). If enterovirus is isolated from CSF, identification proceeds in the usual way; that is, CPE is detected in tissue culture or the virus reacts with specific antibodies. In the case of aseptic meningitis the causative virus is much more often isolated from fecal specimens than from CSF. A diagnostic rise in titer of serum antibody to the fecal viral isolate is then looked for to implicate the fecal isolate as the cause of the meningitis. Precise identification of the fecal isolate can follow if necessary.

The second large group of viruses that is identified on cell cultures is the myxoviruses: orthomyxoviruses and paramyxoviruses. The group includes the influenza viruses A, B, and C; parainfluenza virus types 1 to 4; measles; mumps; and respiratory syncytial virus (RSV). Influenza, parainfluenza, and mumps viruses multiply in primary monkey (Rhesus) kidney (PMK); measles and RSV multiply in HEp-2. Multiplication of myxoviruses in PMK cells produces no CPE; instead, viral antigens are expressed on the surface of the infected cells and later released into the supernatant. One of the expressed antigens is the hemagglutinin that binds erythrocytes (guinea pig or human type O) and produces hemadsorption (HAd) or hem-agglutination (HA). Measles and RSV exhibit no HA or HAd activity with guinea pig erythrocytes. They produce typical giant cells or syncytium on HEp-2 cells. A rapid and sensitive immunoassay for detection of RSV in respiratory secretions has to a large extent replaced culture. Other virus groups can be isolated on cell cultures. Herpesvirus from generalized infections or from dry local lesions is isolated on human-origin cell strains and lines, as are the adenoviruses.

Polymerase Chain Reaction

Polymerase chain reaction (PCR) is a new molecular biologic tool that is expediting diagnosis of certain infectious diseases, primarily viral. It is so sensitive that a single DNA molecule can be amplified millions of times, thus yielding a detectable signal. PCR is based upon the use of polynucleotide primers that flank the sequence to be detected and requires a unique DNA polymerase. In addition to detecting HIV (Chapter 26), the PCR technique has been used to detect hepatitis B virus DNA in chronic hepatitis with low levels of virus, to identify HSV, CMV, and other agents. However, perhaps the most important role for the PCR technique has been in typing genital human papillomavirus (HPV) isolates. This group of viruses contains over 20 distinct types, two of which (16 and 18) are often found in cervical dysplasia and carcinoma. The typing of genital HPV in tissues may be important for differentiating benign lesions from carcinomas and has been valuable in epidemiologic studies of HPV infection.

Nucleic Acid Probe Technique

Another new technique for identification of infectious agents is the use of nucleic acid

TABLE 7–8. *Identification of Enteroviruses on Cell Cultures*

Virus	PMK	IMR-90	HEp-2
Polioviruses	+ + + +	+ + +	+ + + +
Coxsackieviruses A		−	−
Coxsackieviruses B	+ + + +	±	+ +
Echoviruses	+ + +	+ +	+

−, no CPE; +, mild CPE; + + + +, significant CPE; ±, may or may not be CPE.

probes. Their routine clinical use is limited at present by poor standardization, their expense, and their complexity. These probes are complimentary to a small portion of the viral nucleic acid. With amplification systems the technique can detect ≥50,000 nucleic acid molecules, a level insufficiently sensitive for detection of viruses. Studies are in progress to adapt this technique to the identification of CMV, HSV, and other large viruses, and to confirm viral identity after multiplication in cell cultures.

Identification of Viruses by Serologic Methods

In the later stages of infection, when viruses cannot be isolated, serologic methods of identification are used. For example, a 68-year-old woman complained of pleuritic chest pain. She had a slight cough a few weeks earlier but did not seek medical care at that time. Bacterial culture findings were negative, and it was too late to perform viral cultures. Antibody titer to influenza type A virus was very elevated, suggesting the identity of the infectious agent.

Viruses, like other foreign agents, elicit measurable antibody responses in the host. Complement-fixing (CF) antibodies appear early in the disease, increase in titer during the acute phase of illness, and decline within 6 months of recovery. A high titer of CF antibody to a specific virus in a single serum specimen is suggestive of recent contact with that virus. A fourfold or greater increase in CF antibody titer in two specimens over a 2–3 week interval is necessary for confirmation of the causative relation to the infection. The CF test is based on fixation of complement (C) by two different antigen–antibody systems used sequentially. One system, the *test system,* contains a selected viral antigen and dilutions of the patient's serum as a source of antibody. The second system, the *indicator system,* contains sheep RBCs as antigen and hemolysin as specific antibody. Fresh guinea pig serum is used as a source of complement. Complement is added to the test system, and the mixture is incubated at 4°C for 16–18 h. The indicator system is then added, and incubation continues for 30 min at 37°C. Sheep RBCs in the indicator system are lysed by complement; therefore, lysis in the indicator system indicates that complement was not consumed by the test system. Lysis thus suggests lack of fixation of

complement by the test system, or absence of antibody in the patient's serum.

CF antibody titer is reported as the reciprocal of the highest dilution of serum with no lysis. CF antibody is detected after recent contact with a virus but does not indicate immunity. Therefore, if immune status is to be examined, as is often done in cases of rubella or VZV infections in pregnancy, the CF test cannot be used. For example, a hospital clerk developed a fine rash on her face a few days after her daughter came home from school with chickenpox. The mother was not sure if she had the disease as a child. Were her coworkers in danger of contracting chickenpox? The answer to this question depends on her and their immune status. Immune status can be determined by neutralization, indirect immunofluorescence (IIF), ELISA, and RIA. Neutralization tests are very seldom done in the routine laboratory, as they present a high risk of infection to employees. They are used now only for determination of antitoxin titers. Rubella-neutralizing antibodies can be detected by the hemagglutination inhibition (HI) test, since both antibody types appear and disappear concurrently. Indirect tests, such as IIF, ELISA, and RIA, detect antibody by the sandwich technique. In these tests, the patient's serum is incubated with an antigen to allow antibody binding. Unbound globulins are washed away, and the bound antibody is detected by the addition of antiserum to human globulins, which has been labeled. Labels include fluorescein for the IIF, peroxidase for the ELISA, and ^{125}I for RIA. The titer of serum antibody is directly related to the quantity of the bound labeled compound. Fluorescein is detected by ultraviolet microscopy, peroxidase by a color reaction on a tissue section, and ^{125}I by a gamma counter. Antibodies detected by these indirect methods generally indicate earlier contact with an agent, and their presence therefore suggests immunity. In most cases, immunity is correlated with a minimum antibody titer. In the VZV/IIF and rubella HI tests, a titer of 1:8 or higher is generally considered protective. In the ELISA test for rubella, an index of 1.0 or higher is considered protective.

Coxsackievirus A cannot be identified by any of the aforementioned techniques. It can be isolated only by injection of the specimen into newborn mice, who if infected die within 24–48 h, after typical paralysis. This diagnostic method is not used in the routine lab. Pure antigens for coxsackievirus B are not available, and therefore serologic tests also cannot be performed.

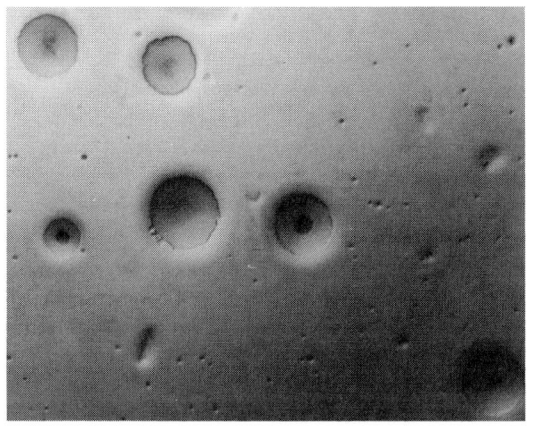

Figure 7–10. Mycoplasma pneumoniae *colonies on enriched agar.*

LABORATORY DIAGNOSIS OF MYCOPLASMA INFECTIONS

Mycoplasmas, also known as pleuropneumonia-like organisms (PPLO), are the smallest known free-living organisms. They multiply in highly enriched agar medium and produce very tiny (10–100 μm in diameter), poorly stained colonies that typically have a "fried egg" appearance (i.e., dark centers in which organisms have grown into the agar with lighter surroundings, Fig. 7–10). After being stained with Giemsa, they appear as tiny pleomorphic cocci, short rods, or hollow ring forms measuring approximately 0.3–0.5 μm in diameter. Mycoplasmas do not stain with Gram's stain. Human mycoplasmas include nine distinct species and a heterogeneous group of *T (tiny) strain* mycoplasmas that includes *Ureaplasma urealyticum* (Table 7–9).

Except for *Mycoplasma pneumoniae*, the pathogenic role of most mycoplasmas in humans is not yet clear. *M. pneumoniae* was identified by Eaton in 1962 ("Eaton agent"). Mycoplasmas can be isolated from respiratory and genitourinary tracts; however, most isolates are part of the normal flora of the throat and genitalia. *M. pneumoniae,* the best confirmed pathogen, is isolated from the respiratory tract. *M. hominis* and T-strain mycoplasmas (*U. urealyticum*), the prime suspects in genital diseases, are isolated from the urogenital tract. Vaginal, urethral, or cervical swabs and urine are suitable specimens for isolation of genital mycoplasmas. Sputum, throat swabs, and tracheal aspirates are acceptable specimens for isolation of *M. pneumoniae* and other respiratory mycoplasmas.

The mycoplasma transport medium contains penicillin to suppress bacterial growth, but not other antibiotics, such as aminoglycosides and tetracylines, that could kill or inhibit mycoplasma growth. Specimens in transport media cannot be stored, since most mycoplasmas are labile and will not survive; however, *M. pneumoniae* can survive for several days at 4°C and for months at 80°C with little loss of viability.

Identification of mycoplasmas depends on the specific substrates they metabolize, which can be glucose, arginine, or urea (Table 7–9). The typical colonies appear as early as 1 week or as late as 1 month after incubation at 37°C in 5% CO_2. Growth on glucose and not on arginine agar indicates *M. pneumoniae;* growth on arginine agar suggests only infection with commensal mycoplasmas. *U. urealyticum* colonies appear on urea agar, and *M. hominis* colonies are demonstrated on arginine agar.

Confirmation of results is complicated and is not performed in the routine laboratory. The difficulties in, and time required for, isolation of mycoplasma agents indicate the need for serologic diagnosis. Serologic tests are generally

TABLE 7–9. *Human Mycoplasmas*

Name	Site of Recovery	Associated Disease	Medium Requirements
M. pneumoniae	Oropharynx, middle ear	Upper and lower respiratory diseases	Glucose
M. hominis	Urogenital tract	Pelvic inflammation	Arginine
M. orale	Oropharynx	None yet known	Arginine
M. buccale	Oropharynx	None yet known	Arginine
M. faucium	Oropharynx	None yet known	Arginine
M. salivarium	Oropharynx	None yet known	Arginine
M. lipophilium	Oropharynx	None yet known	Arginine
M. fermentans	Oropharynx	None yet known	Glucose and arginine
M. genitalium	Urogenital tract	Urethritis?, pelvic inflammation	
T-strain mycoplasmas, *Ureaplasma urealyticum*	Urogenital tract, neonatal respiratory tract	Nongonococcal urethritis	Urea

available for *M. pneumoniae* only. Either the whole organism or a lipid extract can be used for the CF test. A fourfold increase in antibody titers within 3 weeks is indicative of recent infection. Antibody titers persist for 1 year or longer after infections. In the acute phase of *M. pneumoniae* disease and in some viral respiratory infections, a rise in cold hemagglutinin titer is also detected. The cold agglutinins react with the I antigen of human erythrocytes at 4°C, but confirmation by CF is required to make a specific etiologic diagnosis.

REFERENCES

Books and Laboratory Manuals

Balows, A., Hausler, W. J., and Hermann, K. L. *Manual of Clinical Microbiology*. 5th ed. Washington, D.C.: American Society for Microbiology, 1991.

Balows, A., Hausler, W. J., and Lennette, E. H. *Laboratory Diagnosis of Infectious Diseases*. Vol. I: Bacterial, Mycotic and Parasitic Diseases. Vol. II: Viral, Rickettsial, and Chlamydial Diseases. New York: Springer-Verlag, 1988.

Davidsohn, I., and Henry, J. B., eds. *Todd and Sanford's Clinical Diagnosis and Management by Laboratory Methods*. 17th ed. Philadelphia: W. B. Saunders Co., 1984.

Finegold, S. M., Martin, W. J., and Scott, E. G. *Baily and Scott's Diagnostic Microbiology*. 7th ed. St. Louis: C. V. Mosby Co., 1986.

Hoeprich, P. D., and Jordan, M. C., eds. *Infectious Diseases*. 4th ed. Philadelphia: J. B. Lippincott Co., 1989.

Holdeman, L. V., and Moore, W. E. C., eds. *Anaerobic Laboratory Manual*. Blacksburg, VA: Virginia Polytechnic Institute and State University Laboratory, 1977.

Jolik, W. K., ed. *Virology*. 3rd ed. Norwalk, CT: Appleton-Century-Crofts, 1988.

Koneman, E., Allen, S., Dowell, V., et al. *Color Atlas and Textbook of Diagnostic Microbiology*. 2nd ed. Philadelphia: J. B. Lippincott Co., 1983.

Lennette, D. A., Spencer, S., and Thompson, K. D. *Diagnosis of Viral Infections: The Role of the Clinical Laboratory*. Baltimore: University Park Press, 1979.

Notkins, A. L., and Oldstone, M. B. A., eds. *Concepts in Viral Pathogenesis*. New York: Springer-Verlag, 1984.

Rippon, J. W. *Medical Mycology*. 3rd ed. Philadelphia: W. B. Saunders Co., 1988.

Stanier, R. Y., et al. *The Microbial World*. 5th ed. Englewood Cliffs, NJ: Prentice-Hall, 1986.

Washington, J. A., II, ed. *Laboratory Procedures in Clinical Microbiology*. 2nd ed. New York: Springer-Verlag, 1985.

8 *JOHN P. PHAIR, M.D.*

Laboratory Assessment of Immunocompetence

INTRODUCTION

In concert with antibody and complement, leukocytes are the cells that determine a host's ability to defend against or control infection. Defective function or deficient numbers of segmented neutrophils, lymphocytes, phagocytic mononuclear cells, or complement components have been associated with infection (see Chapter 3). The purpose of this chapter is to present an approach to the laboratory evaluation of the patient whose resistance to infection may be defective.

The laboratory evaluation of host defenses begins with the determination of the total peripheral white blood cell count and differential count. Granulocytopenia is probably the most common definable host defect relevant to infection. Immunoglobulin levels and isohemagglutinin levels are easily obtained assays of the amount and function of the immunoglobulin-producing B cells. Specific antibody responses to common vaccines in adults are secondary measures of immune responses and can be helpful. Use of primary antigens often requires access to a research laboratory as do *in vitro* assays of B-cell function. In children responses to vaccines can often be used to assess primary antibody responses. The simplest and most available screening tests of cell-mediated immunity are skin tests using common antigens. Positive responses indicate that both thymic-dependent lymphocytes (T cells) and macrophages are competent. Enumeration of T cells and their subsets is available in many hospitals, as are assays of the lymphocyte response to such mitogens as phytohemagglutinin and to specific antigens.

The routine studies that should be carried out for every patient with recurrent infections are listed in Table 8–1. If there are abnormal pe-

TABLE 8–1. *Assessment of Host Defenses: Readily Available Assays*

Complete Blood Count	Normal Values (adults)
(number per mm³)	
Leukocytes	5,000–10,000
Neutrophils	2,000–6,000
Lymphocytes	1,000–3,500
Helper T cells	700–1,300
Suppressor T cells	350–700
Humoral Assays	
Immunoglobulins (mg/dL)	
IgG	600–1750
IgM	50–210
IgA	110–400
Complement components	
C3	70–176 mg/dl
C4	20–50 mg/dl
CH$_{50}$	25–50 units
Delayed Skin Tests (cell-mediated immunity):*	
Commonly Available Antigens	
Purified protein derivative	
Candida	
Trichophyton	
Mumps	
Histoplasmin	
Coccidioidin	

*One-tenth (0.1) mL should be injected *intradermally*. Reactions should be read at 48 h. Diameters of the area of induration should be measured.

ripheral white and differential counts, a lack of segmented neutrophils in inflammatory exudates, altered immunoglobulin levels, or negative delayed skin-test reactions (anergy), further work-up is required. In infants, a chest roentgenogram is useful in determining whether the thymus is present. If the results from these studies are normal, a well-defined defect in host defenses is unlikely. To determine specific defects in host resistance, studies of cellular function often must be carried out in research laboratories or teaching hospitals. The following is a brief description of the type of assays which are available.

THE SEGMENTED NEUTROPHIL

Neutrophils, to accomplish their task of killing microorganisms, must be produced in appropriate numbers and arrive at the site of invasion. The peripheral blood contains the majority of neutrophils available for delivery to tissue. Approximately one half of these cells are in the so-called marginal pool and are not enumerated by peripheral white counts. The cells in the marginal pool readily adhere to and migrate between the endothelial cells of postcapillary venules, thus entering the extravascular space. Lentnek and associates have demonstrated that adherence of neutrophils to endothelial cells and other surfaces is enhanced in inflammatory disease states and depressed with acute alcohol ingestion or when patients are receiving antiinflammatory agents. This phenomenon can be measured *in vitro* by determining adherence of neutrophils to plastic, nylon, wool, or monolayers of endothelial cells in culture.

Entry of neutrophils and mononuclear cells into a "skin window" produced by scraping the epidermis with a sterile scalpel assays the end product of adherence and determines motility *in vivo*. The entry of neutrophils into areas of inflammation is depressed in neutropenic states, with acidosis, and following alcohol ingestion. The normal migration of leukocytes into a skin window is sequential; after a latent period of 2 h neutrophils are noted, by 12 h this response peaks, and by 24 h the predominant cells are mononuclear.

Movement of neutrophils in tissue is dependent upon both the contractile elements in the cytoplasm of these cells and the cell's ability to respond to chemotactic stimuli. Such stimuli are generated by specific bacteria, direct bacterial activation of complement via the alternative complement pathway, or activation of the classic pathway by antigen–antibody reactions (see Chapter 3).

Assays of nondirected leukocyte motility and response to chemotactic stimuli usually are available only in research centers. However, only patients with unusual problems need to be studied, for example, the child with eczema and recurrent infections. It is usually sufficient for the physician to recognize that a patient has a disease which impairs leukocyte mobility and therefore is at an increased risk of infection and requires prompt therapy to prevent serious complications (see Chapter 27).

Neutrophils, after reaching the microorganisms in the extravascular space, must engulf and kill the invaders. Phagocytosis of encapsulated pyogenic organisms requires coating the bacteria with opsonins, specific antibody and complement, or both. Many hospital and commercial laboratories can measure the serum concentration of the complement components C3 and C4, but assays of opsonic activity are usually carried out in research settings. Severe opsonic defects have been reported in patients suffering from acute burns of greater than 20% of the body. This defect is associated with defective conversion of C3 to C3b by inulin. The observation that certain complement defects are associated with the failure of phagocytosis of *Staphylococcus aureus* but normal uptake of *Escherichia coli* emphasizes the complex relationship among opsonins, phagocytes, and bacteria. The measurement of functional activity of the classic pathway can be determined by assaying total hemolytic complement activity by the CH_{50} endpoint method. This test is available at most teaching hospitals, but should be reserved for patients with suspected congenital deficiencies or patients with infections such as recurrent disseminated gonococcemia or meningococcemia, who often lack functional terminal-complement components (C5–C9) (see Chapters 3 and 25).

The ability of neutrophils to engulf bacteria may be assessed by direct microscopy. Examination of inflammatory exudates can provide some indication of whether or not neutrophils are functioning normally, that is, pus that contains phagocytic cells with ingested organisms indicates normal phagocytosis. More sophisticated assays are required to measure phagocytosis directly and can be performed only by research facilities.

The prototypic example of the inability of neutrophils to kill ingested bacteria is seen in chronic granulomatous disease (CGD) (see

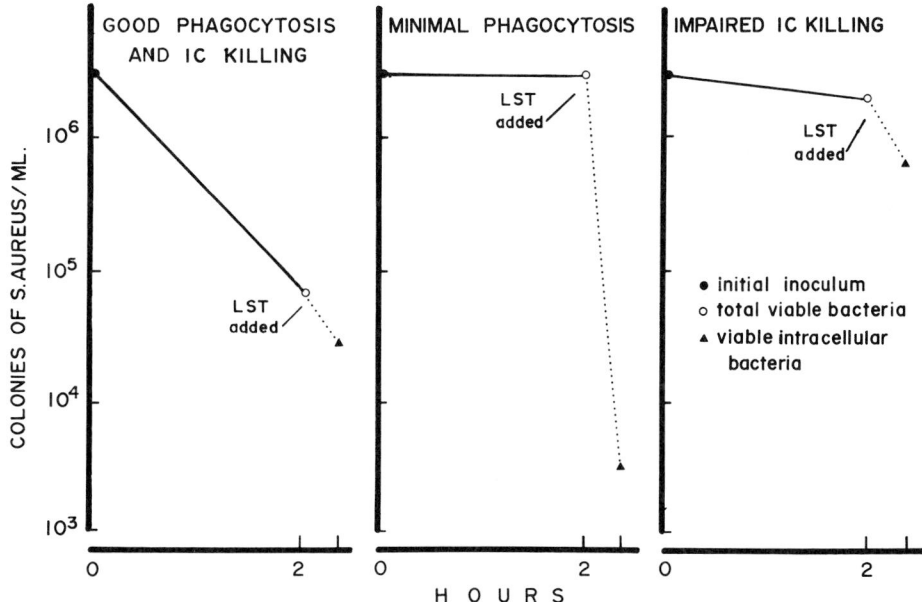

Figure 8–1. Examples of phagocytosis and intracellular (IC) killing of Staphylococcus aureus *by polymorphonuclear neutrophils. LST = lysostatin, a staphylocidal chemical. Patients with chronic granulomatous disease manifest impaired IC killing, as shown in the right panel.*

Chapter 25). Neutrophils harvested from a child with this disease cannot kill catalase-positive organisms such as *Staphylococcus aureus* (Fig. 8–1). In other diseases the difference in microbial killing between cells obtained from healthy volunteers and neutrophils from patients may vary, as is the case for the wide range of values produced by neutrophils obtained from individuals with diabetes (Fig. 8–2). Such bactericidal assays are research techniques and are not generally indicated in the routine evaluation of patients with recurrent infection.

Neutrophils kill bacteria both by oxidative bactericidal mechanisms and by releasing cationic proteins from cytoplasmic granules into the phagolysosome that contains bacteria (see Chapter 3). A number of tests have been developed that take advantage of the burst of oxidative metabolic activity which occurs with phagocytosis. A widely available assay measures either the quantitative or qualitative reduction of the dye nitroblue tetrazolium. This reduction is an indirect measure of hexose monophosphate shunt activity, which is responsible for the oxidative burst. Research assays utilize CO_2 production by cells incubated with radio-labeled glucose, or measure chemiluminescence occurring with the oxidative burst. It should be noted that increases in chemiluminescence can occur as a result of external perturbation of the neutrophil membrane in the absence of engulfment of particles. These assays are useful only when

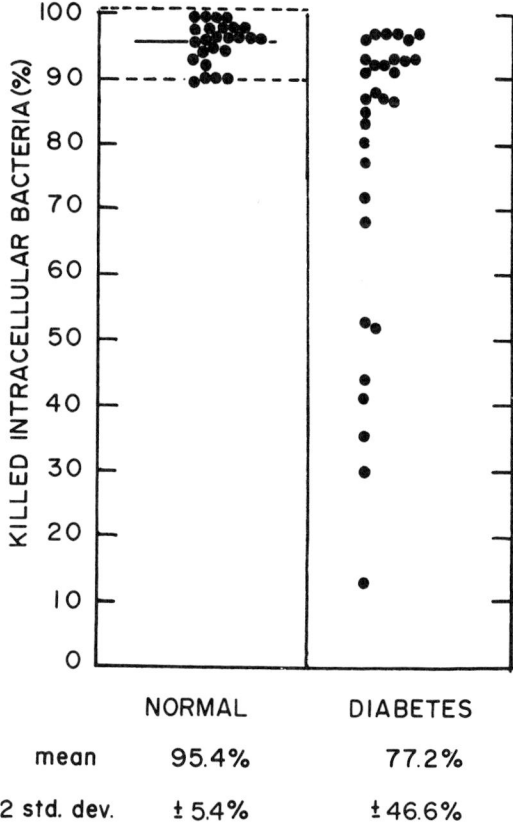

Figure 8–2. Killing of Staphylococcus aureus *by polymorphonuclear neutrophils obtained from diabetic patients and normal volunteers, demonstrating impairment in microbicidal mechanisms in diabetes.*

there is strong evidence of one of the congenital defects in neutrophil function, such as CGD, seen primarily in young children.

Finally, it should be reemphasized that the single most important assay relevant to the neutrophil and infection is the absolute neutrophil count. Neutropenia secondary to disease or cytotoxic therapy is the most common cause of infection due to defects in host resistance. If the cause of a deficient number of neutrophils is not readily discernible, examination of the bone marrow is the next step in evaluating the patient.

THE LYMPHOCYTE

The lymphocyte has been established as the major cellular element responsible for the immune response (see Chapter 3 for overview). Schematically, two populations of lymphocytes have been delineated: the antibody-producing B lymphocytes and the thymic-dependent lymphocytes (T cells). These subpopulations of human lymphocytes were recognized originally by the presence of surface immunoglobulins (B cells) or receptors for sheep erythrocytes (T cells). The most convenient method currently available for identifying the subsets of lymphocytes is to direct monoclonal antibodies at specific cell-surface antigens and use flow cytometry to count them. B lymphocytes, T lymphocytes (OKT3, CD3), and T-cell subsets [helper (OKT4, CD4) and suppressor (OKT8, CD8) cells] can be enumerated using this method (Chapter 3). These techniques are available at most medical centers and have supplanted older, more cumbersome assays. The usefulness of these assays in defining immunity or resistance remains to be assessed in all but a few situations. The normal ratio of one cell subtype to another is altered in many illnesses, both trivial and serious. The association between deficiency in helper T (OKT4) lymphocytes and disease is exemplified in infection with the human immunodeficiency virus (HIV). HIV infection is associated with depletion of OKT4 cells in the peripheral blood. The normal number of OKT4 cells varies between 700 and 1300/mm³. With advanced HIV infection, counts of OKT4 cells decrease to extremely low levels. In one study, the risk of developing pneumonia due to *Pneumocystis carinii* increased from zero in HIV-infected adults with more than 700/mm³ OKT4 cells to 18.4% for those with less than 200/mm³ over a 12-month period of follow-up. By 36 months, the comparable risks were 3.8 and 33.3%, respectively.

Immunoglobulins (Ig's), the secretory products of B lymphocytes, exist in a variety of classes and subclasses in serum and body secretions, as reviewed in Chapter 3. IgG and IgM mediate immune reactions against microorganisms by such means as complement fixation (IgM and IgG, subclasses IgG1 and IgG3), which is necessary for opsonization. Toxins are neutralized by IgG as well. Specific secretory IgA, produced as a result of infection or local immunization, prevents adherence of virus and bacteria to mucosal surfaces, the initial step required for colonization and, presumably, for tissue invasion. The function of IgD is unknown, but this immunoglobulin may act as a surface receptor on B lymphocytes that combines with antigen to trigger specific antibody production. IgE, or reagin, mediates immediate hypersensitivity reactions by activating release of vasoactive substances from mast cells following interaction of allergens with antigen-specific, cell-bound IgE.

The functional capacity of B lymphocytes is assessed by determining immunoglobulin concentrations in serum. This is accomplished using immunodiffusion techniques and appropriate specific antisera for the heavy chain of the specific immunoglobulin class. Automated nephelometric techniques are available for carrying out large numbers of assays. Specific immunoglobulin concentrations should be determined when a deficiency is suspected, even if no alteration is noted with paper electrophoresis of serum proteins. Paper electrophoresis does not determine concentrations of specific Ig classes.

Specific antibody increases following immunization with vaccines or "new antigens" (such as keyhole limpet hemocyanin or the bacteriophage φX19) are used to assess B-cell function *in vivo*. Failure to produce antibody can occur in the presence of normal serum immunoglobulin concentrations. B lymphocytes' spontaneous production of Ig or their response to stimulation by pokeweed mitogen can be studied *in vitro*. In addition, techniques are now available for assaying specific antibody production *in vitro*. These assays have been extremely useful in delineating B-cell dysfunction but are not required in the usual clinical evaluation.

The function of T lymphocytes can be evaluated using skin tests to determine responsiveness at 48 h to antigens to which the majority of individuals have been exposed. Induction of sensitivity to agents such as dinitrochlorobenzene also can be a useful means of determining cell-mediated immunity. The pitfalls of skin testing, however, are many. Variation in observer measurements of the degree of induration elicited by intradermal injection of antigen, failure to inject the antigens properly, and failure to use appropriate commercially available antigens or proper dilutions of antigenic preparations can obscure the assessment of response. Positive reactions indicate an intact system; a negative reaction to several antigens (anergy) is less easily interpreted (see Chapter 3).

In vitro, the functional capability of T lymphocytes is generally measured by determination of the response to mitogens or antigens. Incorporation of radio-labeled precursors, such as tritiated thymidine (^{3}H-TdR), into DNA or of ^{14}C or ^{3}H labeled amino acids into protein following exposure of cells to such agents (as determined by scintillation counting) is currently the most available method. Mixed lymphocyte cultures are also used to assess the system's ability to respond to antigens. The effector cells are mixed with lymphocytes, which serve as antigen. The antigenic cells are either irradiated or pretreated with the antibiotic mitomycin C to prevent them from responding. This assay is termed a *one-way reaction.* Soluble antigens used to assess T lymphocytes' responsiveness include purified protein derivative or *Candida.* Stimulation of mononuclear leukocytes in peripheral blood by plant lectins, such as phytohemagglutinin, usually reaches its peak following 72 h of culture. In contrast, responses to antigens are maximal at 5–6 days. Lymphocytes (separated from heparinized blood by density gradients), buffy coat cells, and whole blood have been used in such cultures. Cultures are run in triplicate with increasing concentrations of mitogen or antigen to determine a dose response. Cultures are also prepared without the antigen or mitogen. Results are expressed as the number of counts per minute or disintegrations per minute, representing DNA synthesis. Stimulated and control cultures are compared and expressed as a ratio (stimulation index) or as net counts (stimulated counts minus control counts per minute). To interpret accurately comparisons between normal individuals and a study population, the actual counts of control and stimulated cultures should be expressed because the effect of substantial alterations in background counts can be lost using only derived numbers (stimulation indices or net counts). Research laboratories also measure production of lymphokines.

In vitro assays of T-lymphocyte function are often difficult to interpret. Both T and B cells are known to respond to mitogens but B-lymphocyte proliferation requires the presence of T cells or soluble T-cell factors. Finally, correlation of the various *in vitro* assays with skin tests is poor. Patients with chronic mucocutaneous candidiasis have been described with positive skin tests and yet their lymphocytes fail to produce lymphokines. Conversely, patients with rubella are often skin test–negative and yet their *in vitro* lymphocyte responses to mitogen are intact.

THE MONOCYTE/MACROPHAGE

The mononuclear phagocytes are cells derived from bone marrow which exist in two distinct populations: the circulating monocyte and the tissue histiocyte, or macrophage. The tissue macrophages make up the reticuloendothelial system found in the liver, spleen, and pulmonary alveoli. The macrophages play a central role in the immune and inflammatory response. In their initial contact with foreign microorganisms, macrophages ingest, process, and present antigens to lymphocytes in order to stimulate a primary immune response and the production of cytokines, which modulate the immune and inflammatory response. In addition, monocytes produce specific components of the complement sequence. Laboratory evaluation of the function of this component of host defense is less well developed than the assessment of the cells discussed above.

Mononuclear cells from peripheral blood can be separated from lymphocytes by density gradient centrifugation or by adherence to plastic surfaces. Nonadherent lymphocytes are removed by washing. The phagocytic and bactericidal capacity of these cells can be assessed after establishment of monolayers in culture. Studies have demonstrated that monocytic phagocytosis and killing of microorganisms is slower than that by neutrophils. The function of the reticuloendothelial system, an indirect measurement of macrophage capacity, can be determined by uptake of radio-labeled particles and scanning of liver and spleen or by determining clearance rates of particles from blood. Currently, a major difficulty in assessing the contribution of mononuclear cells to host defense is the lack of a readily available, simple and specific test of function.

SUMMARY

The well-defined defects in host defense are usually readily identifiable; available methods of measuring host immunity are not sufficiently refined, however, to delineate subtle defects in resistance. The physician is often faced with whether or not to burden a patient with an expensive and often unproductive evaluation. On balance, the readily available tests rule out the majority of well-defined defects. The complete blood count determines if a patient is neutropenic, the positive skin test indicates an intact T-lymphocyte–macrophage system, and measurement of immunoglobulin concentrations assesses B-cell function. Of the defects discussed in Chapter 25, only hypogammaglobulinemia can be easily ameliorated by replacement of IgG. Since commercially available gamma globulin does not contain secretory IgA or IgM, its use will not reduce the number of viral upper respiratory infections which plague some individuals. At the current time, rather than searching for defects in "host resistance," a more productive therapeutic approach is to look for other means of correcting health problems. Examples include encouraging patients with chronic bronchitis to quit smoking, suggesting alterations in life styles for patients with recurrent sexually transmitted disease, and urging improvement in hygiene to eradicate *Staphylococcus aureus* in patients with recurrent furunculosis. A major contribution to patient well-being is ruling out serious disease by obtaining a thorough history, a complete physical examination, and the results of the readily available tests outlined in Table 8–1. Finally, it should be realized that advances in the knowledge of host defects underlying infection have not yet been matched by the ability to reconstitute defective individuals.

CASE HISTORY

Because of repeated infections, a 30-year-old woman was referred to an infectious disease specialist for evaluation for immunodeficiency. Her history included rheumatic fever as a child (but she had no knowledge of cardiac murmurs) and "rheumatoid arthritis" as an adult, which persisted for 6 months but improved during her pregnancy 7 years earlier. She had viral encephalitis following a camping trip 4 years before and "aseptic meningitis" the previous summer. She was able to work and maintain her house, had not lost weight, and had only occasional upper respiratory tract infections over the past 6 years. Specifically, there was no history of pneumonia, skin infections or rash, pelvic infection, or diarrhea.

She had had no surgery. Physical examination was completely within normal limits. Specifically, there was no evidence of lymphadenopathy or hepatosplenomegaly.

Laboratory studies, including a complete blood count, immunoglobulin concentrations, and CH_{50}, and antiglobulin (rheumatoid factor) determinations, were normal. She reacted to candida and trichophyton skin-test antigens with induration of 15-mm diameter at 48 h. Current knowledge regarding resistance to infection was explained to the patient and she was reassured. No further work-up was undertaken.

The history provided good evidence that the patient did not have deficient numbers of, or dysfunctional, neutrophils, low C_3, or an immunoglobulin deficiency. She had not been plagued with pneumonia or skin infections. The absence of a history of skin rashes associated with fever was evidence against deficiency of the terminal-complement components. She reacted to skin-test antigens, which indicated that lymphocyte–monocyte function was intact. The patient was intelligent and accepted the fact that she was not seriously susceptible to infections.

REFERENCES

Symposium Volume

Litwin, S. D., Christian, C. L., and Siskind, G. W., eds. *Clinical Evaluation of Immune Function in Man.* New York: Grune & Stratton, 1976.

Review Articles

Bentwick, A., et al. The use and abuse of immunological tests. Report of an IUIS/WHO working group on critical considerations of eight widely used diagnostic procedures. *Clin. Immunol. Newsletter* 2:178, 1981.

Densen, P., and Mandell, G. L. Phagocytic strategy versus microbial tactics. *Rev. Infect. Dis.* 2:839, 1980.

Elsbach, P. Degradation of micro-organisms by phagocytic cells. *Rev. Infect. Dis.* 2:106, 1979.

Farrar, J. J., and Hilfiker, M. L. Antigen-nonspecific helper factors in the antibody response. *Fed. Proc.* 41:263, 1982.

Fauci, A. S. Human B-lymphocyte function: Cell triggering and immune regulation. *J Infect. Dis.* 145:602, 1982.

Fauci, A. S. The syndrome of Kaposi's sarcoma and opportunistic infections: An epidemiologically restricted disorder of immunoregulation. *Ann. Intern. Med.* 96:777, 1982.

Gallin, J. T. Abnormal phagocyte chemotaxis: Pathophysiology, clinical manifestation and management of patients. *Rev. Infect. Dis. 3:*1196, 1981.

Haynes, B. F., Katz, P., and Fauci, A. S. Immune response of human lymphocytes *in vitro. Prog. Clin. Immunol 4:*23, 1980.

Oppenheim, J. J., Stadler, B. M., Siraganian, R. P., et al. Lymphokines: Their role in lymphocyte response: Properties of interleukin. *Fed. Proc. 41:*257, 1982.

Original Articles

Abdou, N. I., Napombejora, C., Sagawa, A., et al. Malaplakia: evidence for a correctable monocyte lysosomal abnormality. *N. Engl. J. Med. 297:*1413, 1977.

Bahner, R. C. Quantitative nitroblue tetrazolium test in chronic granulomatous disease. *N. Engl. J. Med. 278:*971, 1968.

Boyden, S. The chemotactic effect of mixing with antigen on polymorphonuclear leukocytes. *J. Exp. Med. 115:*453, 1962.

Cline, M. J., and Lehrer, R. I. Phagocytosis by human monocytes. *Blood 32:*423, 1968.

Dale, D. C., and Wolff, S. M. Skin window studies of the acute inflammatory response of neutropenic patients. *Blood 38:*138, 1971.

Gopal, V., and Bisno, A. C. Fulminant pneumococcal infections in 'normal' asplenic hosts. *Arch. Intern. Med. 137:*1526, 1977.

Lentnek, A. L., Schrieber, A. D., and MacGregor, R. A. The induction of augmented granulocyte adherence by inflammation. Mediation by a plasma factor. *J. Clin. Invest. 57:*1098, 1976.

MacGillen, J. J., and Phair, J. P. Adherence, augmented adherence and aggregation of polymorphonuclear leukocytes. *J Infect. Dis. 139:*69, 1979.

Rocklin, R. E., Myers, O. L., and David, J. An *in vitro* assay for cellular hypersensitivity in man. *J. Immunol 104:*95, 1970.

Tan, J. S., Watanakunakorn, C., and Phair, J. P. A modified assay of neutrophil function. Use of lysostaphin to differentiate defective phagocytosis from impaired intracellular killing. *J. Lab. Clin. Med. 78:*316, 1971.

III

Upper Respiratory Tract Infection and Sequelae

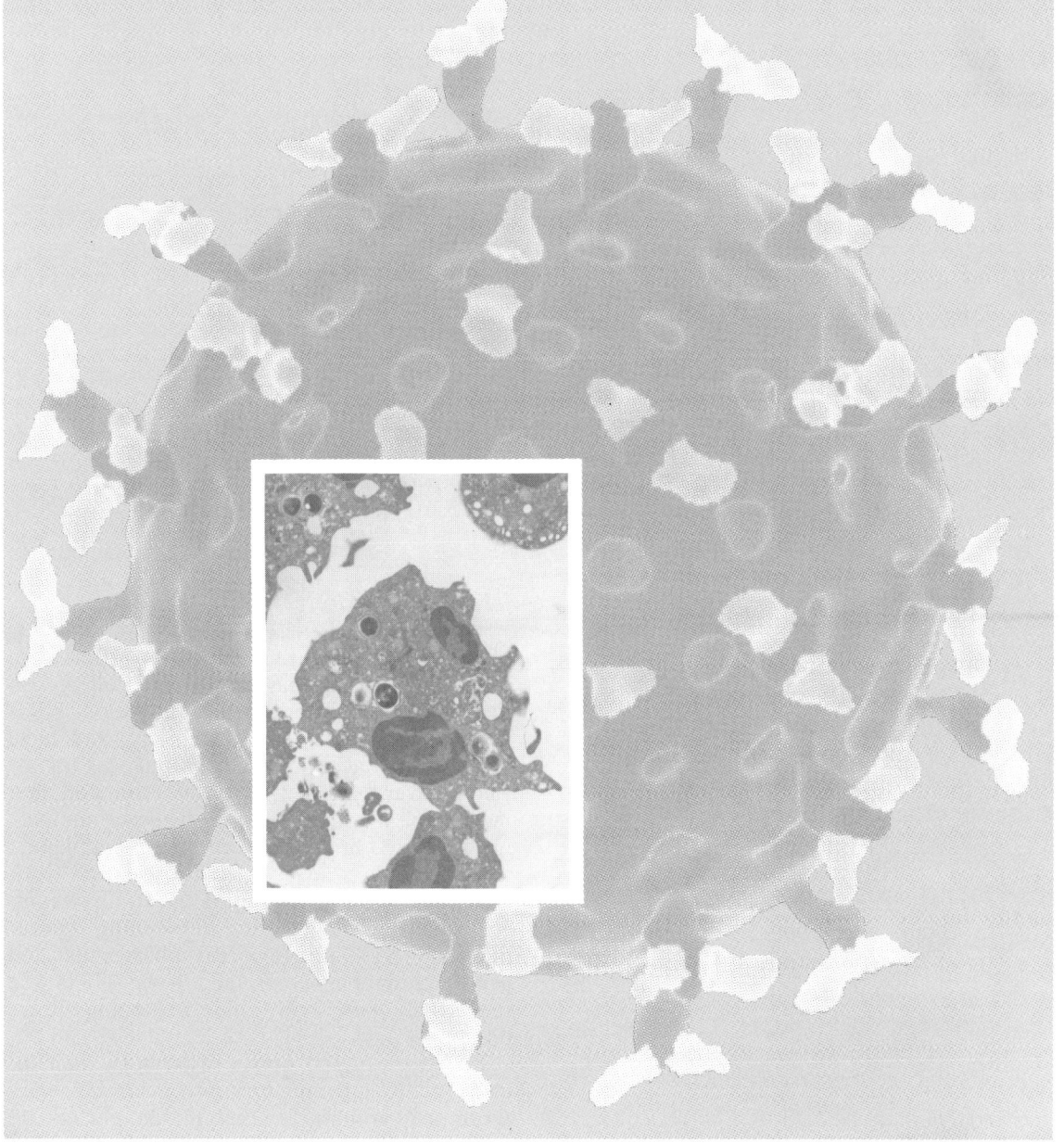

9

STANFORD T. SHULMAN, M.D.

Bacterial Infections of the Upper Respiratory Tract

INTRODUCTION

Upper respiratory tract infections (URIs) are one of the leading reasons people of all ages in the United States seek medical attention. URIs account for considerable morbidity, and have very substantial economic consequences for society. Several years ago it was estimated that more than 27 million office visits occur annually in the United States for sore throat complaints, and untold days are lost from school and work as a result of these infections. In certain circumstances, URIs have life-threatening consequences (e.g., streptococcal pharyngitis and acute rheumatic fever), and some URIs are themselves potentially life-threatening (e.g., diphtheria).

Infections of the upper respiratory tract include acute inflammatory processes involving the nose, paranasal sinuses, middle ear cavity, the oropharynx and tonsils, peritonsillar or retropharyngeal tissues, and the laryngeal–epiglottic region. Many URIs involve overlapping anatomic regions. However, it is important that physicians identify the primary sites of pathology in order to conclude accurately which are the most likely etiologic agents. There may be therapeutic implications to identifying the site of infection; for example, inflammation of the epiglottis (epiglottitis) in a child is virtually always due to *Haemophilus influenzae,* and laryngotracheobronchitis is almost always viral in etiology.

Considerable misinformation exists regarding infections of the upper respiratory tract, resulting in several important practical problems: (1) The large majority of URIs are viral in origin and do not respond to antibiotic therapy—a fact that is frequently ignored, resulting in patients receiving unnecessary and costly treatment with antibiotics; (2) it is often forgotten that "strep throat," acute pharyngitis/tonsillitis caused by group A streptococci (*S. pyogenes*), is the most important upper respiratory infection and should be treated with appropriate antibiotics; and (3) physicians often overlook the fact that it is impossible to differentiate reliably between viral and streptococcal pharyngitis/tonsillitis on clinical grounds alone. Such a differentiation requires a simple diagnostic test, such as a throat culture or a rapid antigen detection test. The diagnostic test is needed to avoid unnecessary overtreatment with antibiotics of the majority who have nonstreptococcal disease.

A simplified classification schema for clinically important streptococci (Table 9–1) is based primarily upon their typical hemolytic activity on sheep blood agar and upon the antigenic reactions of their cell-wall carbohydrates, as developed by Lancefield (see below).

ANATOMY OF THE UPPER RESPIRATORY TRACT

We will briefly consider the anatomy of the upper respiratory tract in order to appreciate the highly organized and extensive lymphoid structures of the region and the intimate relationship these structures have with the oral, nasal, and pharyngeal cavities. The great German anatomist, Wilhelm Waldeyer (1836–1921), described what is now known as *Waldeyer's ring,* the circular band of lymphoid tissue that guards the entrance to the respiratory and gastrointestinal tracts. Anteriorly, this ring is composed of submucosal lymphoid tissues of

TABLE 9–1. *Simplified Streptococcal Classification Scheme and Associated Clinical Conditions*

Beta-hemolytic streptococci (complete hemolysis)
  Group A *(S. pyogenes):* streptococcal pharyngitis, impetigo; acute rheumatic fever, acute glomerulonephritis (see text)
  Group B *(S. agalactiae):* neonatal and peripartum infections
  Group C *(S. equisimilis* and four others): pyogenic infections, probably pharyngitis
  Group G: probably pharyngitis

Alpha-hemolytic streptococci (incomplete hemolysis)
  S. pneumoniae (pneumococcus): pyogenic infections including pneumonia, meningitis, septicemia
  Viridans streptococci *(S. mutans* and many others): endocarditis, dental caries, dental infections

Gamma-hemolytic streptococci (no hemolysis)
  Anaerobic and microaerophilic streptococci *(Peptostreptococcus):* brain, liver abscesses
  Group D streptococci
    Enterococci (Enterococcus faecalis, E. faecium, E. durans): endocarditis, urinary infections
    Nonenterococci (S. bovis, S. equinus): endocarditis

*Enterococcal strains are occasionally alpha- or even beta-hemolytic, and some nonenterococcal group D organisms may be alpha-hemolytic.

the posterior part of the tongue; laterally, of the palatine tonsils, peritonsillar lymphatics, and adenoids adjacent to the pharyngeal orifices of the eustachian tubes; and posteriorly, of the submucosal lymphoid tissue of the posterior pharyngeal wall. Additionally, the ring has a rich network of lymphatics and regional cervical lymph nodes. These lymphoid structures often react to infection in proximate regions (hyperplasia, hypertrophy), generally contributing to control of the infection but occasionally resulting in symptoms. An example of such a symptom is the swollen, tender anterior cervical nodes most typically associated with acute streptococcal pharyngitis.

Anatomically, the upper respiratory tract may be envisioned as a passageway from the lips and nose to the trachea and bronchi, with a number of mucosally lined, narrow side passages that lead to somewhat larger mucosally lined cavities that are normally filled with air. These cavities (the middle ear, mastoid antrum and air cells, and paranasal sinuses) normally communicate with the oropharynx and nasopharynx. Obstruction of connecting passages, such as the eustachian tube or sinus ostia, contributes significantly to development of infection within these cavities. The intimate relationship among various lymphoid tissues, the mucosal surface, and the orifices of the communicating structures is remarkable and contributes to disease manifestations.

Normal Flora

The mucosal surfaces of the nose, mouth, and the remainder of the upper respiratory tract are normally colonized by a complex variety of bacterial species. The fascinating situation that exists in the oral cavity is outlined in Chapter 2. Under normal circumstances, the middle ear cavity and the paranasal sinuses are sterile. The pharynx, larynx, and trachea are colonized by anaerobic cocci and bacilli, as well as by aerobes, including *Streptococcus pneumoniae*, alpha-hemolytic streptococci, *Haemophilus influenzae*, neisseria, and coagulase-negative staphylococci. The character of the organisms that normally colonize the mucosae is important when examining and understanding organisms isolated in cultures of bronchoscopic specimens from ill individuals.

The normal flora appear to confer a certain degree of protection against infectious diseases originating at the mucosal surface. This protection manifests itself by providing *nonspecific* stimulation of the immune system, by providing *specific* immunization that leads to protection against pathogens with cross-reactive antigens, and by hampering colonization by other organisms through complex competitive mechanisms (collectively termed *bacterial interference*, or colonization resistance). The importance of the normal flora is readily apparent from studies of germ-free animals, which show deficient development of the immune system and excessive susceptibility to overwhelming infection.

Normal flora demonstrate a remarkable tropism for specific locations, the regions of the mouth, for example. Certain species of alpha-hemolytic streptococci characteristically colonize the anterior portion of the tongue, whereas other viridans species typically colonize the posterior portion, the gingivae, or the buccal mucosa. The precise determinants for these characteristic niches in the complex ecology of the oral cavity, for example, remain poorly defined but must depend at least in part upon specific mucosal receptors and binding molecules on the surface of microbes and epithelial surfaces.

PHARYNGITIS/TONSILLITIS

The most important bacterial cause of pharyngitis and tonsillitis is group A beta-hemolytic streptococci (*S. pyogenes*). The importance of this agent is due to its extreme frequency as a cause of pharyngotonsillar infection (with a great deal of associated morbidity), to its relatively infrequent complicating purulent infections (e.g., cervical lymphadenitis, sinusitis), and to its very important nonpurulent sequelae (acute rheumatic fever and acute glomerulonephritis) (Table 9–2). Because acute rheumatic fever and resultant rheumatic heart disease are major illnesses that are, for the most part, preventable by prompt diagnosis and treatment of acute streptococcal pharyngitis, clinical strategies for treating patients with acute pharyngitis focus on streptococcal pharyngitis in particular.

In 1868, Theodor Billroth coined the term *streptococcus* from the Greek (*streptos* = chain, *kokkos* = berry) for chain-forming cocci isolated from infected wounds. Ferdinand Widal in 1889 considered streptococci from all clinical sources to belong to a single species, *S. pyogenes*, and to be the primary cause of "septic sore throat" as well as of other illnesses. By 1923, A. R. Felty and A. B. Hodges had established sporadic acute pharyngitis as a specific entity related to beta-hemolytic streptococci.

Group A Streptococci

These organisms, all now classified as *S. pyogenes*, are characterized by the presence of a specific cell-wall carbohydrate, A carbohydrate, first defined serologically by Rebecca Lancefield around 1930 (see Table 9–1). The Lancefield serogrouping scheme distinguishes streptococcal groups on the basis of cell-wall carbohydrate antigenicity. Within group A streptococci, different cell-wall protein antigens (termed M, T, and R proteins) allow distinction of more than 80 serotypes. Although the group-specific cell-wall carbohydrate does not appear to be a virulence factor, M proteins are important determinants of virulence because of their antiphagocytic properties. M proteins stimulate the development of lasting type-specific immunity against strains possessing the homologous M protein.

Growth

Group A streptococci grow optimally at 34°–37°C and have complex nutritional requirements. Media containing brain and heart extracts, peptone, and glucose are most often utilized, frequently supplemented with whole blood. Solid media usually employ sheep blood for optimal growth and for visualization of the characteristic beta, or complete, hemolysis ad-

TABLE 9–2. *Biologic Differences between Poststreptococcal Glomerulonephritis and Rheumatic Fever*

Biologic Feature	Acute Glomerulonephritis	Acute Rheumatic Fever
Preceding infection	Pharyngeal or skin	Pharyngeal only
Geographic distribution	Uniform, more in tropics	More in developing countries
Age	Any age	Rare <4 yr, >30 yr
Sex incidence	Males predominate	Equal
Attack rate after streptococcal infection	Variable (to 28%)	Constant; pharyngeal strains only
Second attacks	Rare; may occur after skin infections	Common
Average latent period between infection and first attack	Pharyngeal: 10 days Skin: 3 weeks	18 days
Latent period between infection and later attack	Shortened as compared with latent period of first attack	Same as latent period of first attack
Relation of degree of ASO* increase to incidence of first attacks	No relation	Incidence proportional to degree of ASO increase
Serum complement and C3 levels	Decreased	Increased
M types of initiating group A hemolytic streptococcus	Pharyngeal: 1, 4, 6, 12, 18, 25 Skin: 2, 31, 49, 52, 55, 57, 60	Any pharyngeal type, particularly 1, 3, 5, 6, 18. Skin strains are *not* rheumatogenic

*Antistreptolysin O titer.

jacent to areas of bacterial growth. *S. pyogenes* is homofermentative, producing mainly L-lactic acid from glucose, and is catalase-negative. The organisms are nonmotile and are facultative, growing well under aerobic and anaerobic conditions.

Identification

Group A streptococci grow readily on standard laboratory media, forming discrete pinpoint colonies. On sheep blood agar they usually produce a large zone of beta (clear) hemolysis around each colony. Group A streptococcus (GAS) hemolysis is related to the extracellular elaboration of hemolysins: typically an oxygen-labile immunogenic protein, streptolysin O; and an oxygen-stable, nonimmunogenic protein, streptolysin S. Hemolysis on the surface of a blood agar plate is due primarily to streptolysin S, whereas subsurface hemolysis is due to streptolysin S and streptolysin O. Antibody responses to streptolysin O are important clinically (see below). Gram's stains show gram-positive cocci in short-to-medium chains, and group A may be differentiated from other streptococci by several methods, based generally on demonstrating the presence of specific reagents that utilize cell-wall A carbohydrate. These methods include agglutination of latex particles coated with anti–A carbohydrate antibody, reaction of acid-extracted or enzymatically extracted cell-wall carbohydrate with specific antisera in a capillary precipitin test, or counterimmunoelectrophoresis. A frequently employed presumptive test for group A streptococci is the determination of sensitivity or resistance to the antibiotic bacitracin, to which about 95% of

group A organisms (but only 5–10% of beta streptococci of other groups) are sensitive. Bacitracin impairs peptidoglycan synthesis and alters the membrane permeability of GAS.

Morphology

These gram-positive cocci are approximately 0.8 μm in diameter and grow in chains, particularly in purulent exudates. The organisms are composed of an outer capsule, a complex cell wall with attached fimbriae, a cytoplasmic membrane, a nucleus, ribosomes, and cytoplasmic granules (Fig. 9–1). The capsule, composed of hyaluronic acid, polymerized glucuronic acid, and *N*-acetylglucosamine, is more apparent early in growth; the later production of hyaluronidase removes the capsule. Infected individuals frequently respond with antihyaluronidase antibiodies following GAS infection. The capsule may play an antiphagocytic role. The fimbriae that project from the cell wall are composed, in part, of the M, T, and R proteins. The cell wall is a rigid structure that maintains the shape and osmotic integrity of the cell but is permeable to nutrients (Fig. 9–2). Enzymatic degradation of the cell wall leads to osmotic lysis of the streptococcal cell unless it is maintained in a hyperosmolar environment. Streptococcal cell-wall structure is complex, composed of a cross-linked *N*-acetylmuramylpeptide peptidoglycan, intercalated A carbohydrate (a polymer of rhamnose and terminal *N*-acetylglucosamine residues), lipoteichoic acid (LTA), and the M, T, and R proteins. The proteins, carbohydrate, and lipoteichoic acid extend outward to form the fimbriae. Enzymes located at or adjacent to the cell membrane at the base of

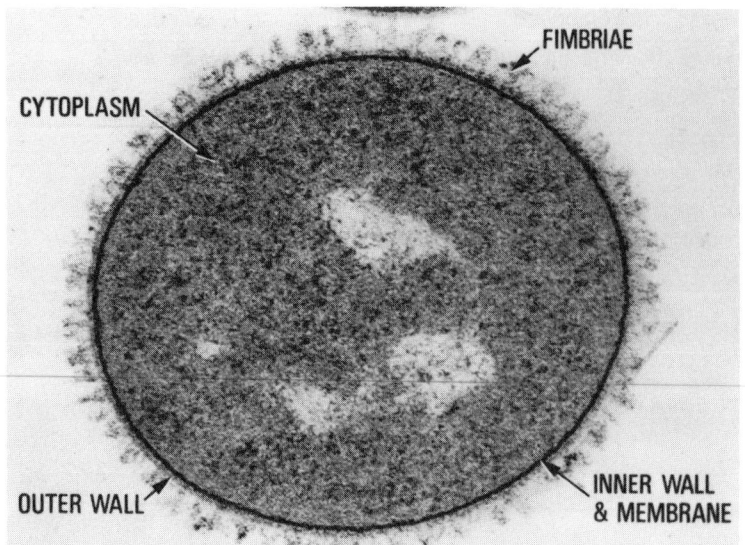

Figure 9–1. Cross-section of a group A streptococcus cell, type 23. Filamentous fimbriae are attached to the opaque outer cell wall. The inner wall is electron-dense. The thin protoplast membrane is forced against the inner surface of the wall by the internal osmotic pressure of the cell and is not clearly visible. In several places, a separation between the wall and membrane may be seen (× 126,500). (Courtesy of Dr. Roger Cole, National Institute of Allergy and Infectious Diseases, National Institutes of Health.)

the cell wall are responsible for synthesis of the cell-wall components.

The M proteins are among the most important components of GAS organisms because they are key virulence factors. Their antiphagocytic activity relates primarily to their ability to block alternative complement pathway activation. In experimental animals, increased quantity of M protein correlates with enhanced virulence, whereas anti-M protein is protective against GAS organisms of the homologous M type. Infection in man leads to the production of anti-M antibody, which is protective and long-lived. Subsequent GAS infections may occur but only from organisms that possess different M proteins. The structure of several M proteins has been characterized very thoroughly in recent years and homologies to mammalian myosin

have been found (see Chapter 5). Peptide sequences from conserved domains of several M proteins are being studied for possible vaccine development. T proteins, which are trypsin-resistant antigens generally associated with specific M proteins, are also found in GAS organisms. Like M proteins, T proteins are useful in serologically typing organisms—for epidemiologic purposes, for example. However, T proteins appear to be unrelated to virulence, and antibody to T proteins is not protective. Similarly, the R proteins, which share some sequence homology with M proteins, are unrelated to virulence or to protection. Another group of GAS surface structures are the serum opacity reaction (SOR) proteins, which possess lipoproteinase activity. These proteins correlate closely with M types of GAS strains and can be

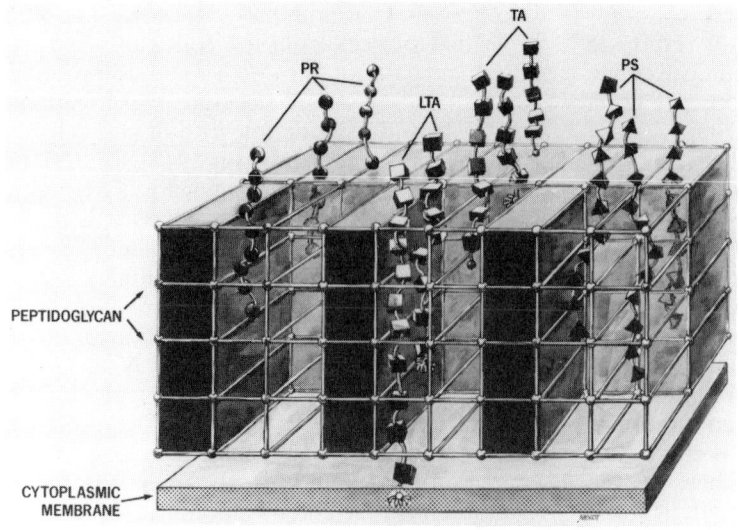

Figure 9–2. Model of the cross-section of a streptococcal cell wall. The peptidoglycan is "open" in several places in order to visualize the location of the antigenic polymers within the peptidoglycan. See pages 99–101 for a discussion of this model. PR, protein; PS, polysaccharide; LTA, lipoteichoic acid; TA, teichoic acid (deacylated form of LTA). (From Slade, H.D. Structural Model of Streptococcal Cell Wall in Secretory Immunity and Infection. New York: Plenum Press, 1978, pp. 761–763.)

utilized for typing purposes and for epidemiologic studies. In addition, certain surface proteins of GAS organisms have recently been recognized that nonspecifically bind the Fc end of immunoglobulin molecules. Lipoteichoic acids (LTAs), which are phosphate-diester-glycerol compounds found in many gram-positive bacterial cell walls, are covalently bound to cell-membrane lipids. In streptococci, LTA extends to the cell surface and serves as the major ligand for attachment of GAS to epithelial cell surfaces. LTA also functions in cation exchange reactions. The GAS cell-wall peptidoglycan is a rigid cross-linked polymer of N-acetylglucosamine—an N-acetylmuramic acid covalently bound to peptide bridges. Peptidoglycan is immunogenic, but its role in virulence and immunity is poorly defined. Peptidoglycan also possesses potent adjuvant, pyrogenic, and mitogenic activity. Interference with peptidoglycan synthesis is the major mechanism by which penicillins are bacteriocidal for GAS, which are universally sensitive to penicillin activity. The cell membrane of GAS is 60–70% protein and the remainder is composed of phosphatidyl lipids. The membrane serves as a permeability barrier and is rich in enzyme systems with synthetic and oxidative functions. Protoplasts, or L-forms, lack a cell wall, are enclosed by the cell membrane, and are osmotically fragile.

A variety of bacteriophages are commonly present within GAS, and it has become apparent that they encode for a number of extracellular products including erythrogenic (or pyrogenic) exotoxins A, B, and C, and streptolysin S, as well as antibiotic resistance. Erythrogenic toxin A is most likely responsible for the classic skin rash of scarlet fever and is encoded by a temperate phage.

Recent reports of severe GAS infections caused by strains that elaborate erythrogenic exotoxin A, a toxin that has otherwise been rarely observed in strains of GAS isolated in recent years, have generated considerable interest. Clinically, these illnesses resemble toxic shock syndrome, and it is noteworthy that streptococcal exotoxin A is similar in many respects to staphylococcal TSST-1, the mediator of toxic shock syndrome. GAS also produces several bacteriocins, small proteins of approximately 8000 D that kill a variety of other bacterial species and thus may be important in initiation or persistence of muscosal colonization or infection by GAS.

Extracellular Products

In addition to the previously mentioned hemolysins (streptolysin O and streptolysin S), GAS elaborates a wide variety of extracellular substances, most with enzymatic activity not toxic to mammalian or bacterial cells. These include hyaluronidase, which may facilitate tissue invasion by GAS; desoxyribonucleases A, B, C, and D, which are immunologically distinct and two of which possess RNAse activity as well; streptokinases, which activate the plasmin–plasminogen fibrinolytic system; nicotinamide adenine dinucleotidase (NADase); and others. The phage-related erythrogenic toxins noted above are pyrogenic, they enhance endotoxic shock, and they are neutralized by specific antibody. This is the basis of the classic Dick test to demonstrate lack of immunity to scarlet fever. A C5a peptidase that cleaves and inactivates the chemotactic complement activation product C5a has been described in GAS and has been shown to delay accumulation of polymorphonuclear neutrophils (PMNs) at foci of streptococcal infection.

Clinical Features of Streptococcal Pharyngitis/Tonsillitis

Streptococcal pharyngitis/tonsillitis is an exceptionally common clinical condition. Of the estimated more than 27 million visits to physicians each year in the United States for sore throat complaints, only approximately 15–20% represent GAS pharyngitis/tonsillitis, but this amounts to a very substantial number of cases. Most importantly, streptococcal pharyngitis/tonsillitis is the only common cause of pharyngitis that warrants antibiotic therapy because untreated GAS infection can lead to the development of acute rheumatic fever and chronic rheumatic heart disease.

Streptococcal pharyngitis is most typically an acute infection of school-aged children, although it may occur at any age. These patients manifest the relatively sudden onset of sore throat, fever, dysphagia, and tender anterior cervical lymph nodes. Rhinorrhea, cough, coryza, and hoarseness are absent. Examination reveals tonsillopharyngeal erythema, frequently with whitish exudates composed of fibrin, bacteria, white blood cells, and debris; petechiae may be present on the soft palate, and anterior cervical adenitis with tenderness is characteristic. Younger children with streptococcal infection typically manifest coryza, excoriated nares, general adenopathy, and a more chronic course. In contrast, in older children and young adults, abdominal pain and headache are frequently prominent symptoms, and tonsillopharyngeal exudates are a more constant feature. *Scarlet fever* is a GAS pharyngeal infection with an accompanying erythematous rash; it reflects an acute streptococcal infection caused by a lysogenized strain of GAS.

Unfortunately, the clinical features of streptococcal infection are quite variable and overlap with the signs and symptoms of other forms of pharyngitis. Thus, clinical assessment must be supplemented by laboratory testing to obtain an accurate diagnosis—either throat culture or rapid GAS antigen detection test (see below).

The primary importance of accurately identifying and promptly treating acute streptococcal pharyngitis is that untreated or inadequately treated patients are particularly likely to develop acute rheumatic fever (see below).

Epidemiologic Features

Streptococcal pharyngitis occurs primarily in endemic form, that is, sporadic cases, rather than in the epidemics prevalent prior to World War II in the United States. Food-borne epidemics or outbreaks in military populations are occasionally encountered, but streptococcal pharyngitis is most often endemic. Although it was once thought that streptococcal pharyngitis and acute rheumatic fever were diseases primarily of temperate climes, it is now apparent that they are worldwide in distribution. It has been suggested that urbanization of developing tropical countries has contributed to increases in acute rheumatic fever. The striking seasonality of acute streptococcal pharyngitis has been documented, particularly in temperate regions. Late winter and early spring peaks (January–April) with summer nadirs (July–August) are highly typical. Factors contributing to this cycle include the increased contact between children once they reach school age and the possible effect of intercurrent viral respiratory pathogens upon microbial flora–epithelial cell relationships and upon host immunologic factors. Age is also an important epidemiologic characteristic of streptococcal pharyngitis. Children between 5 and 10 years old experience the highest rates of infection; substantially lower frequencies occur in children 3 years old and younger and in those over 10 years old. Some researchers have observed a secondary peak at approximately 12 years of age and at 18–20 years (related to military recruits). The role of tonsillectomy in preventing streptococcal pharyngitis is controversial, with conflicting data in the literature. In general, removal of the tonsillar lymphoid tissue is not warranted on the basis of frequent episodes of streptococcal pharyngitis alone. It has also been established that pets rarely serve as a reservoir of GAS infection within a household.

GAS organisms are transmitted primarily by direct contact with large droplets or respiratory secretions rather than by air-borne spread or contamination of inanimate objects (fomites). Thus, spread within family groups or classrooms is common. Contagiousness appears maximal during the acute stage of illness and during the first 2 weeks after acquisition of the organism. Antibiotic therapy with an appropriate agent, especially penicillin, is associated with prompt suppression of contagiousness; children can therefore return to school after 24 h of therapy. Individuals who are chronically colonized in the pharynx with GAS (streptococcal carriers) pose little transmission risk. Spread of GAS infection and the frequency of poststreptococcal complications are clearly facilitated by crowded living conditions.

Diagnosis

The following is a profile of the classic patient with acute streptococcal pharyngitis: a 5–10-year-old child with sudden onset of fever, sore throat, and perhaps headache, nausea, malaise, and abdominal pain, whose examination shows moderate to severe tonsillopharyngeal erythema, tonsillar hypertrophy and exudates, palatal petechiae, and hypertrophied tongue papillae, with tender and enlarged anterior cervical nodes. When this classic picture is present, the clinician can expect a high degree of diagnostic precision based on clinical criteria alone. Unfortunately, however, most patients with acute streptococcal pharyngitis do not manifest this picture, but rather present with only some of these typical signs and symptoms. Thus, the clinician must rely upon laboratory studies for accurate diagnosis. This conclusion is confirmed by experience with scoring systems that attempt to differentiate those infected from those not infected by GAS. These systems ascribe point values to epidemiologic features (age, season), symptoms (sore throat, headache, absence of cough), signs (abnormal pharynx or cervical nodes, fever), and laboratory findings (leukocytosis). Even the best of these systems is unable to predict the presence or absence of GAS with sufficient accuracy to allow widespread use and to eliminate the need for adjunctive laboratory tests. However, it is possible to identify a subgroup of patients (about 20%) with an extremely low probability of streptococcal pharyngitis, particularly those with rhinorrhea and cough who appear to have viral infections. For the remaining 80% or so, the clinical impression must be confirmed by laboratory studies. Serum streptococcal antibody levels are *not* useful for diagnosis of acute streptococcal pharyngitis because demonstration of a significant increase (fourfold or greater) in antibody titer over 2–4 weeks is necessary—a procedure that is clearly impractical. In addition, there is evidence that prompt antibiotic therapy can abort the antibody responses following GAS infection.

The standard, time-tested, and most reliable method for diagnosing streptococcal pharyngitis is the performance of the throat culture. This entails obtaining a swab of the posterior pharyngeal and tonsillar region and streaking it on a plate containing sheep blood agar—a method in widespread practice in the United States since about 1960. This practice was pioneered by Burtis Breese and Frank Disney, Rochester, N.Y. pediatricians, who began to use this technique around 1953. After 18–24 h of incubation at 37°C, beta-hemolytic streptococci appear as small colonies surrounded by large zones of beta or complete hemolysis. Differentiation of group A from other serogroups of beta streptococci can be made on a presumptive basis by finding inhibition of growth of subcultured organisms using discs impregnated with the antimicrobial agent *bacitracin*. About 95% of bacitracin-sensitive (i.e., growth is inhibited) beta streptococci are group A organisms, whereas 99% of bacitracin-resistant beta streptococci belong to other serogroups, and are collectively referred to as non–group A beta streptococci, lacking the potential to lead to acute rheumatic fever. The blood agar plate is streaked from the site of initial application of the throat swab using a sterile wire loop. The procedure should include an agar stab to enable subsurface growth. The stab frequently enhances the beta hemolysis related to streptolysin O (oxygen-labile) production.

The throat culture is the standard against which other diagnostic tests for streptococcal pharyngitis are compared, even though it is associated with only approximately 90% accuracy. This culture is limited because it cannot distinguish reliably between patients with active streptococcal infection and those who are chronic pharyngeal carriers of GAS but who may have a coincidental acute viral pharyngitis. The former patients tend to have heavier growth of GAS on the culture plate than the latter

group, but sufficient overlap in the intensity of growth exists to render this distinction unreliable.

In the past 5 years, a large number of diagnostic tests, so-called rapid antigen detection tests, have been developed and marketed. These tests are performed using a patient's throat swab that is first subjected to a brief extraction step (usually with nitrous acid) to release cell-wall A carbohydrate from GAS organisms, followed by an immune reaction employing anti–A carbohydrate antibody. This reaction is then configured to be readily detectable—color change or agglutination is used to distinguish between specimens positive and negative for GAS. Results are generally available in 10–30 min. The marketed tests vary considerably in their *sensitivity* (the fraction of culture positives that are positive by the rapid test) and *specificity* (the fraction of rapid test positives that are culture-positive), when compared with simultaneous culture results. High specificity (i.e., few false-positives) but varying and frequently inadequate sensitivity (i.e., too many false-negatives) are usually seen. Thus, a positive test is usually valid and may serve as the basis for initiating treatment, but a negative test is less reliable and should be backed up by a culture. Rapid tests are also incapable of distinguishing between GAS carriage and active infection. They serve as a useful adjunct to the clinician but should not completely displace the throat culture in routine clinical practice.

Treatment

Acute streptococcal pharyngitis/tonsillitis is generally a self-limited illness. Over a period of days, symptoms spontaneously subside in the large majority of instances. A small minority of untreated patients develop suppurative complications (e.g., cervical adenitis, peritonsillar abscess) or nonsuppurative complications (e.g., acute glomerulonephritis, acute rheumatic fever). The primary reason that streptococcal pharyngitis should be identified and treated is *to prevent acute rheumatic fever and resultant rheumatic heart disease.* Older data point to certain features that correlate with increased risk for developing rheumatic fever (Table 9–3).

Despite almost five decades during which penicillin was used to treat streptococcal pharyngitis, group A streptococci have not developed resistance to penicillin; not a single penicillin-resistant strain has been reported. Thus, penicillin remains the drug of choice given either

TABLE 9–3. *Sore Throats and Risk of Initial Attacks of Rheumatic Fever (RF)**

Features of Sore Throat	Number of Patients†	Percent of Patients with RF
Fever and pharyngeal erythema	1293	0.15
Exudate present	310	0.65
Exudate and beta-hemolytic streptococci	216	0.90
Exudate, group A streptococci	186	1.0
Exudate, group A streptococci and diagnostic ASO titer	95	2.1
Exudate and group A streptococci in throat for 21 days	81	2.5

*Adapted from Siegel, A. C., Johnson, E. E., and Stollerman, G. H. Controlled studies of streptococcal pharyngitis in a pediatric population. I. Factors related to the attack rate of rheumatic fever. *N. Engl. J. Med.* 265:559, 1961.

†None of 1293 was treated with antimicrobial drugs.

orally for 10 days or as a single parenteral injection of a depot preparation (benzathine penicillin). Oral regimens have the practical problem of relying upon patient compliance, whereas parenteral penicillin is painful and may be associated with higher rates of significant allergic reactions. Individuals known or suspected to be allergic to penicillin should be treated with alternative, non–beta-lactam agents, such as erythromycin or clindamycin. Even though streptococcal pharyngitis is self-limited, antibiotic treatment is associated with somewhat accelerated clearing of fever and other signs and symptoms of streptococcal pharyngitis. In contrast to its response to penicillin, GAS resistance to erythromycin or clindamycin has been well documented and reflects, in general, the frequency of usage of the agent in a particular population. For example, in Japan, where erythromycin has been used very freely, up to 40% of GAS isolates have been found to be erythromycin-resistant. Antibiotics that cannot be recommended for treatment of streptococcal pharyngitis include sulfa drugs (which are useful for *prevention* but not for *treatment*), tetracyclines, and chloramphenicol.

Purulent Complications of Streptococcal Pharyngitis

Prior to the availability of antibiotics in the past four decades, purulent streptococcal complica-

tions were very common and greatly feared, having substantial associated mortality (Table 9–4). In the antibiotic era, purulent infections that represent extension of GAS infection from the pharynx to adjacent structures are much less common but still occur. These infections include (1) *peritonsillar abscess* ("quinsy"): presenting as fever, dysphagia, and referred ear pain, with asymmetry of the tonsils and a bulge in the peritonsillar area; (2) *retropharyngeal abscess:* presenting as fever, dysphagia, drooling, stridor, and extension to the neck, with a bulging mass in the posterior pharyngeal wall; (3) suppurative *cervical lymphadenitis:* presenting as tender swollen cervical nodes that may become fluctuant, representing lymphangitic spread from the tonsils; and (4) otitis media, sinusitis, and mastoiditis, all more commonly due to bacteria other than GAS but occasionally complicating streptococcal pharyngitis. Therapy to treat these purulent complications of course includes antibiotics effective against GAS. Peritonsillar and retropharyngeal abscesses require surgical drainage; each may present as a cellulitis that has not yet walled off to form an abscess. Drainage is not helpful until abscess has developed. Cervical adenitis may resolve with antibiotic therapy alone or may suppurate and require drainage.

Nonpurulent (or Nonsuppurative) Complications of Streptococcal Pharyngitis

Acute Rheumatic Fever

Acute rheumatic fever (ARF) is a major medical disorder that occurs in selected individuals following untreated upper respiratory tract infection with GAS. This systemic inflammatory illness involves connective tissue and produces *carditis* (which may lead to heart disease that is frequently permanent or at least long-standing), joint inflammation (*arthritis* or arthralgia, with transient involvement only), and neurologic in-

TABLE 9–4. *Complications of Group A Streptococcal Pharyngitis*

Purulent
Cervical adenitis, sinusitis, otitis media
Peritonsillar and retropharyngeal abscess
Sepsis, metastatic infection (rare)
Nonpurulent
Acute rheumatic fever
Acute glomerulonephritis

volvement (*chorea,* transient only). From 1925 to 1950, rheumatic fever and resultant rheumatic heart (valvular) disease (RHD) was the leading cause of death in American children and adolescents 5–19 years of age and was the leading cause of heart disease in those younger than 40. Although suspected as being related to streptococcal infection in the late 19th century, ARF was unequivocally linked to recent GAS pharyngitis around 1930, following Lancefield's identification of the cell-wall A carbohydrate that distinguishes GAS and following Todd's subsequent development of the antistreptolysin O serologic test that enabled documentation of recent GAS infection. It is clear that a steady decline in the frequency of ARF and RHD and in mortality from these illnesses had begun as early as 1900 or 1910, antedating Lancefield's work, the institution of effective control measures, and the development of antibiotic and corticosteroid therapy. The occurrence of ARF and RHD decreased markedly during the 1960s and particularly during the 1970s and early 1980s. Recent generations of U.S. medical students and house officers had been trained without encountering patients with ARF. In 1985, the Jones Memorial Lecture to the American Heart Association was entitled "The Virtual Disappearance of Rheumatic Fever in the United States," and the American Heart Association was prompted to support a symposium entitled "Management of Pharyngitis in an Era of Declining Incidence of Rheumatic Fever" (see Shulman in reference list). In addition to convincing evidence of a decline in the *incidence* of ARF in the United States, there is also a body of knowledge indicating that the *severity* of ARF had also decreased substantially even before penicillin or corticosteroids had become available.

It seems clear that the striking decline in ARF and RHD in the first half of this century was due, in large measure, to improved living conditions with less crowding and improved nutrition and sanitation. However, it is difficult to ascribe the more striking fall in ARF since 1950 to such nonspecific societal improvements. Thus, other possible explanations were sought for the near-disappearance of ARF by 1985 in the United States. One hypothesis was that there might have been a sharp decline in the frequency of acute streptococcal pharyngitis in children, but no data support this prospect. Some suggested that a decline in incidence of some other disorder like measles or rubella, resulting from successful vaccine programs,

might have contributed by the elimination of some necessary cofactor, but even fewer data support this hypothesis. Close analysis of patterns of access to health care suggests that this is at least an important contributing factor to the observed decline in ARF. In Baltimore, for example, the incidence of ARF in the inner city during the 1960s declined only in those populations living in proximity to comprehensive care clinics and not in those areas not served by such clinics. This suggests that accurate diagnosis and timely treatment of streptococcal pharyngitis contributed in a major way to the decline.

The epidemiologic picture changed course once again when, around 1985–1986, a completely unexpected substantial resurgence in ARF was noted in several areas of the United States, most dramatically in the intermountain region near Salt Lake City, but also in Pittsburgh, Columbus, and Akron, and several other locales. Although ARF had traditionally been an illness with greatest incidence in the lowest socioeconomic groups of our society, the recent outbreaks appeared to be focused on white, suburban, middle-class children. That this resurgence is not a true national phenomenon is suggested by survey data that fail to demonstrate an overall increase nationally in ARF but rather indicate focality of the outbreaks. Of great interest is the observation that highly mucoid, heavily encapsulated strains of GAS have been recovered on throat culture of family members, random community sources, and occasionally from ARF patients themselves in Salt Lake City, Akron, and several other areas during this recent resurgence of ARF. Unfortunately, the precise relationship between these mucoidal isolates, which represent several different M types (even within a single geographic area), and the increase in ARF is unclear. The application of the tools of modern molecular biology to study these GAS isolates may provide important insights into the pathogenesis of this major medical disease.

ARF characteristically demonstrates its peak incidence in children 5–12 years of age, being relatively rare under the age of 4 years and in adulthood. This parallels the age distribution of streptococcal pharyngitis. However, chronic rheumatic heart disease that represents the residua of earlier ARF is important in adults and accounts for a sizable fraction of those who require placement of prosthetic heart valves. ARF is characterized by a propensity to recur after subsequent GAS infections (see below). Table 9–2 contrasts certain features of ARF with those of acute poststreptococcal nephritis.

Clinical Features. A single diagnostic test for ARF does not exist, prompting T. Duckett Jones in 1944 to develop what have since become known as the Jones criteria for the diagnosis of ARF. The subsequently modified and revised Jones criteria stand as the worldwide standard for diagnosis of ARF (Table 9–5). These criteria are divided into five major criteria, several minor (or less specific) criteria, and an absolute requirement for evidence of a recent GAS infection, either by positive throat culture or serologic demonstration of elevated antibody to GAS or by history of scarlet fever. The diagnosis of ARF requires the combination of at least one major criterion and two minors, or two majors, plus evidence of recent GAS infection. The Jones criteria were designed specifically to decrease the overdiagnosis of ARF and to set some minimum requirements for diagnosis; not all patients who meet the Jones criteria necessarily have ARF. Individualized assessment is mandatory.

CARDITIS. The most important manifestation of ARF is cardiac inflammation since this leads to the only long-term sequelae of an episode (or an "attack") of ARF. Carditis is present in approximately 50% of ARF patients, manifested as tachycardia and murmurs of mitral and/or aortic valve insufficiency. Involvement of endocardium (valves), myocardium (myocarditis), or pericardium (pericarditis, effusion) may occur, with valvular involvement invariably present. Myocarditis or pericarditis without valvular involvement is rarely, if ever, related to ARF. When all three cardiac layers are involved, the term *pancarditis* is used, referring to a very serious, even life-threatening, acute disease. Clinical symptoms associated with acute

rheumatic carditis include dyspnea (and other features of congestive heart failure) and chest pain. Following ARF with carditis, patients are frequently left with chronic mitral and/or aortic valve insufficiency that may lessen in severity with time or may alternatively evolve to the development of stenotic valvular lesions, generally over at least 5–10 years. Recurrent episodes of ARF are frequently associated with increasingly severe rheumatic heart disease. Pathologically, the hallmark of rheumatic carditis is the Aschoff body, a perivascular aggregation of large cells with polymorphous nuclei and basophilic cytoplasm rosetting around an avascular core of fibrinoid necrosis. This Aschoff body is of uncertain origin and can probably be seen in other cardiac disorders, but it remains most characteristic of rheumatic carditis.

ARTHRITIS. The most common major manifestation of ARF is migratory polyarthritis, seen in about 75% of attacks. Typically, this involves the large joints, particularly the knees, ankles, wrists, and elbows, and rarely affects smaller joints. The involved joints are usually exquisitely tender, with even the friction of a bedsheet inducing pain; redness, heat, and swelling are also usually present. The degree of patient discomfort frequently seems disproportionate to the objective findings. Most characteristic is the migratory nature of the arthritis, so that without therapy an involved joint becomes normal within 1–5 days while other previously uninvolved joint(s) become inflamed. Untreated patients manifest an average of six joints involved over 1–2 weeks. Also highly characteristic is the dramatic response of the arthritis of ARF to even small doses of salicylate, a feature well known to clinicians of 100 years ago. There appears to be somewhat of an inverse relationship between the severity of arthritis and the incidence of cardiac involvement in ARF. The migratory arthritis of ARF does not lead to chronic or deforming joint disease.

CHOREA. Sydenham's chorea (or St. Vitus's dance) occurs in about 10% of ARF patients, manifesting as uncoordination, choreoathetoid movements, emotional lability, poor school performance, and facial grimacing. Symptoms are frequently exacerbated by stress. Sydenham's chorea usually develops weeks to months after the other manifestations of ARF; that is, the latent period between acute streptococcal infection and onset of chorea is substantially longer than the approximately 3 weeks between GAS infection and the other major manifestations of

TABLE 9–5. *Jones Criteria (Revised) for Guidance in the Diagnosis of Acute Rheumatic Fever*

Major Manifestations	Minor Manifestations
Carditis	**Clinical**
Polyarthritis	Fever
Chorea	Arthralgia
Erythema marginatum	Previous rheumatic fever or
Subcutaneous nodules	rheumatic heart disease
	Laboratory
	Acute-phase reaction
	(erythrocyte sedimentation
	rate, C-reactive protein,
	leukocytosis)
	Prolonged PR interval

Additional Criteria
Supporting evidence of preceding streptococcal infection (increased ASO or other streptococcal antibodies), or
Positive throat culture for group A streptococci, or
Recent scarlet fever

ARF. Even though chorea may last several months, it is not associated with persistent neurologic findings.

SUBCUTANEOUS NODULES. These are seen only rarely in ARF and are firm nodules approximately 1 cm in diameter palpable along extensor surfaces of tendons near bony prominences. Most patients with this finding have prominent rheumatic heart disease.

ERYTHEMA MARGINATUM. This is also a rare manifestation of ARF, a macular nonpruritic erythematous rash with irregular margins and clear center. The rash is evanescent, exacerbated by warming as with a warm wash cloth, and appears on the trunk and extremities but not on the face.

MINOR MANIFESTATIONS OF ACUTE RHEUMATIC FEVER. These features of ARF are more nonspecific than the major manifestations discussed above. They are divided into clinical manifestations (i.e., fever, arthralgia, and previous history of ARF) and laboratory manifestations (i.e., prolonged PR interval on ECG, and presence of acute-phase reactants, such as elevated sedimentation rate, C-reactive protein, and leukocytosis). Arthralgia can be used as a minor criterion only if arthritis is not used as a major.

EVIDENCE OF RECENT GROUP A STREPTOCOCCAL INFECTION. This is an absolute requisite in addition to the major and minor Jones criteria. Approximately 20% of ARF patients still harbor GAS on throat culture at the time of presentation; the other 80% are culture-negative, presumably after spontaneous clearing of their earlier pharyngeal infection. Therefore, alternative evidence of recent GAS infection must be sought, usually in the form of serum antibody against streptococcal products or antigens, for example, antistreptolysin O, anti-DNase B, anti-hyaluronidase, or anti–A carbohydrate. A single antibody test will be definitely positive in about 80% of patients with ARF; therefore, in clinically suspected cases, it may be necessary to obtain several streptococcal antibody assays to establish the diagnosis of ARF. A clear and unequivocal history of an episode of preceding scarlet fever also fulfills the Jones criteria for evidence of recent GAS infection. An exception to the requirement for recent GAS evidence can be made in patients with Sydenham's chorea as their sole major manifestation, because the long latency between GAS infection and onset of chorea may allow decline of antistreptococcal titers to near-baseline levels.

Recurrences. Probably the single most important feature of ARF is its propensity to recur in the same individual with subsequent acute GAS infections. This was emphasized almost 100 years ago by the great Sir William Osler. Recurrences tend to mimic the first attack in clinical manifestations, but there is a cumulatively increasing frequency (and severity) of cardiac disease as the number of recurrences increases. This is the basis for the recommendations for long-term antibiotic prophylaxis to prevent GAS infections and thus to prevent recurrences of ARF in individuals who have had at least one attack.

Pathogenesis of Acute Rheumatic Fever. The evidence that ARF is directly related to GAS infection can be summarized as follows:

1. One half to two thirds of ARF patients give a clear history of a recent upper respiratory illness, usually sore throat, and 20% still harbor GAS in the pharynx.
2. Streptococcal antibody tests provide serologic confirmation of recent GAS infection in those with or without clear clinical evidence.
3. Titers of antistreptococcal antibodies are higher in ARF than in those following uncomplicated GAS infection.
4. The age distribution of ARF parallels that of acute streptococcal pharyngitis.
5. Antibiotic therapy for acute streptococcal pharyngitis that is instituted within 9 days of the onset of symptoms appears highly effective in preventing ARF.
6. Long-term, continuous prophylactic administration of antibiotics is highly effective in preventing recurrent episodes of ARF in susceptible individuals.

The precise mechanism(s) by which GAS infection of the upper respiratory tract leads to ARF remains unclear despite many decades of intense investigation. The concept of the "susceptible host" with genetically determined susceptibility has become accepted even though the precise determinants of susceptibility have been difficult to define. In some, but not all, patient populations it appears that the presence of a specific HLA-D locus marker correlates with susceptibility to ARF (i.e., DR4 in those of European ancestry, DR2 in those of African ancestry). Family clustering of ARF supports a genetic predisposition, and a specific B-lymphocyte surface antigen has been claimed to be more common in rheumatic individuals. That only up to 3% of individuals with untreated streptococcal pharyngitis in epidemic circumstances, and a much lower percentage in endemic circumstances, go on to develop ARF also suggests that a host susceptibility factor is operative.

The proposed pathogenetic mechanisms that lead to the clinical manifestations that we recognize as ARF fall into three general categories: (1) persistent streptococcal infection; (2) reaction to a toxic streptococcal product or component; and (3) an aberrant immune response to group A streptococci. Essentially no evidence supports the likelihood of persistent GAS infection within tissues affected by ARF, as demonstrated by the failure of massive amounts of penicillin to alter ARF. A direct toxic effect of one of the many extracellular products elaborated by GAS, including streptolysin O (which is directly toxic to myocardial cells in tissue culture), seems unlikely. The latent period between acute streptococcal pharyngitis and onset of ARF makes it quite difficult to implicate a direct toxic effect.

By far, most attention has focused upon an immune-mediated pathogenesis of ARF. The following support the hypothesis that ARF is an immune-mediated disorder: (1) the striking clinical similarity of ARF to certain diseases that clearly have an immune pathogenesis; (2) the presence of the several-week latent period between acute streptococcal pharyngitis and the onset of ARF; (3) the antigenicity of such a variety of streptococcal products and constituents; and (4) the extensive immunologic cross-reactivity that exists between GAS constituents and human tissues (Table 9–6). The cross-reactivity existing between streptococcal cell membrane and cardiac sarcolemma and subsarcolemma, or between group A carbohydrate and cardiac valvular glycoprotein, suggests the possibility that GAS triggers an immune response that is misdirected against host "self" antigens, resulting in tissue damage that manifests clinically as ARF. In addition, serum heart-reactive antibodies can be demonstrated in patients with acute rheumatic carditis, and antineuronal antibodies are found in sera from those with chorea. However, a central role in pathogenesis of ARF for any specific reaction has been difficult to define, and the precise pathogenetic mechanisms are still unclear. The absence of an animal model for ARF has significantly hampered pathogenetic studies.

Central to pathogenetic considerations, of course, is the group A streptococcus. Although it had long been thought that all GAS strains were equally capable of triggering the events that lead to ARF, more recent evidence (primarily epidemiologic) suggests that a relatively limited number of M types are usually linked to ARF. These have been considered to be *rheumatogenic* strains, but it is not known what confers rheumatogenicity. As noted earlier, the recent resurgence of ARF in selected areas of the United States has been associated with the recovery of heavily encapsulated (mucoid) GAS strains of several serotypes that had been isolated earlier from patients in epidemics of ARF. Further analysis of such strains and identification of a "rheumatogenic factor" will be necessary to further our understanding of this fascinating disorder.

Although its full significance has not yet been clarified, a fascinating relationship between the structure of certain streptococcal M proteins and human myosin has been described. Antibodies reactive against M protein types 5 and 6, for example, cross-react with myosin and suggest a possible role in pathogenesis of acute rheumatic fever. The epitope responsible for this cross-reactivity has been localized to a specific short amino acid sequence of M protein. Additional studies of this epitope are necessary to clarify its possible involvement in pathogenesis of ARF.

Treatment

ACUTE EPISODES. *Acute* episodes of ARF are treated with *antiinflammatory* drugs, *antibiotics,* and *cardiac drugs* when needed. Antiinflammatory therapy comprises aspirin (50–100 mg/kg/day in four doses) for those without carditis or with mild carditis or corticosteroids (prednisone at 2 mg/kg/day in four doses) for those with significant cardiomegaly or congestive failure. Joint symptoms resolve extremely rapidly. Although acute cardiac manifestations resolve promptly with steroids, there is no evidence that the incidence of residual chronic rheumatic valvular dysfunction long after ARF is reduced by the use of steroids. When steroids are used, they are withdrawn gradually after 2–4 weeks, with salicylates phased in during the prednisone

TABLE 9–6. *Cross-Reactivity between Group A Streptococci and Human Tissues*

Cross-Reactive Streptococcal Constituent	Human Tissue Component
Cell wall	Sarcolemma and subsarcolemma
Cell membrane	Sarcolemma and subsarcolemma
M protein	Sarcolemma and subsarcolemma
Group A carbohydrate	Heart valve glycoprotein
Cell membrane	Neurons of caudate and subthalamic nuclei
Hyaluronic acid	Connective tissue protein-polysaccharide complex

taper. All patients with ARF should receive oral penicillin or erythromycin or an injection of depot penicillin to achieve at least 10 days of therapy to ensure eradication of any residual GAS. Cardiac medications such as diuretics and digoxin should be used as necessary in patients with congestive failure.

CHRONIC THERAPY. After the acute illness has subsided, *chronic therapy* for rheumatic fever includes long-term administration of prophylactic antibiotics to prevent further episodes. Acceptable regimens include intramuscular injections of benzathine penicillin (1.2×10^6 units for those over 60 lb, 0.6×10^6 units for those under 60 lb) every 3 to 4 weeks, or oral penicillin (250 mg) or oral sulfadiazine (500 mg). The oral regimens are slightly less effective than the parenteral regimen and they rely upon patient compliance, but they are more convenient. Benzathine penicillin is painful but does not require daily patient cooperation. The duration of rheumatic fever prophylaxis is somewhat controversial but should be maintained for at least 5 years from the last attack, at least until age 21 years, or, in the case of those with significant residual cardiac disease, perhaps for life. Clearly the greatest risk of recurrent ARF is in the first 5 years after an attack and in those with increased risk of GAS upper respiratory infection (school teachers, parents of young children, etc.).

Acute Poststreptococcal Glomerulonephritis

The other nonsuppurative complication of GAS infection is acute glomerulonephritis (AGN), described by Richard Bright in 1836. This important renal disorder contrasts with ARF in many respects. Examination of the epidemiologic, pathogenetic, and biologic differences between these illnesses should yield insights into our understanding of these diseases (Table 9–2).

The most striking epidemiologic differences between AGN and ARF relate to the fact that AGN develops following *either pharyngeal or skin infection* with GAS, whereas ARF occurs only following upper respiratory infection, never after streptococcal skin infection. The explanation for this is not at all clear. AGN is quite common in very young children, generally related to preceding streptococcal pyoderma or impetigo. These skin infections are most common in the warmer months, related to streptococcal superinfection of insect bites or sites of minor trauma. Males predominate in patients with AGN, perhaps because of their increased

frequency of minor trauma. Second episodes of AGN are unusual.

The M types of GAS frequently associated with AGN are limited in number and represent the so-called nephritogenic types (particularly types 1, 4, 6, 12, 18, and 25, in addition to some higher numbered pyoderma types). Even within a given nephritogenic M type, only certain strains of the nephritogenic types seem to be capable of initiating AGN.

Clinical Features. AGN is typically characterized by the sudden onset of edema, hematuria, and decreased urination. Hypertension, azotemia, hematuria, and proteinuria also occur. Although a large number of infectious agents, including group C streptococci, other bacteria, and some viruses, can lead to development of acute glomerulonephritis, GAS is the most common. There is usually evidence of previous pyoderma or streptococcal pharyngitis. The latent period between pharyngeal infection with GAS and onset of AGN is approximately 10 days, in contrast to a longer latent period of up to 6 weeks (usually 3 weeks) following streptococcal skin infection or pyoderma. AGN is generally a self-limited illness in children, rarely leading to chronic renal disease. By contrast, in adults, approximately 20% of episodes of AGN result in chronic renal disease, leading to renal insufficiency in 10–30 years.

Serologic or culture evidence of recent or active GAS infection usually confirms the diagnosis of AGN in acute hypocomplementemic nephritis with hypertension and azotemia.

Pathogenesis. AGN appears to be a classic immune-mediated disorder and is associated with generally profoundly depressed serum complement levels (total complement, C3, properdin). Proliferative or exudative glomerular changes with virtually all glomeruli being diffusely affected are characteristic (Fig. 9–3). Crescent formation may occur. Immunofluorescence studies demonstrate subepithelial humps of electron-dense material containing IgG, C3, and properdin, as well as several streptococcal antigens. Among the streptococcal antigens is a 45kD protein termed nephritic strain–associated protein (NSAP). NSAP is recovered from streptococcal cell extracts, induces an antibody response, and is chemically and immunologically similar to streptokinase C. NSAP-producing strains of GAS induce AGN in rabbits, but NSAP-negative strains do not. Purified NSAP infused into rabbits over 8 days induced renal lesions resembling AGN, and NSAP could be

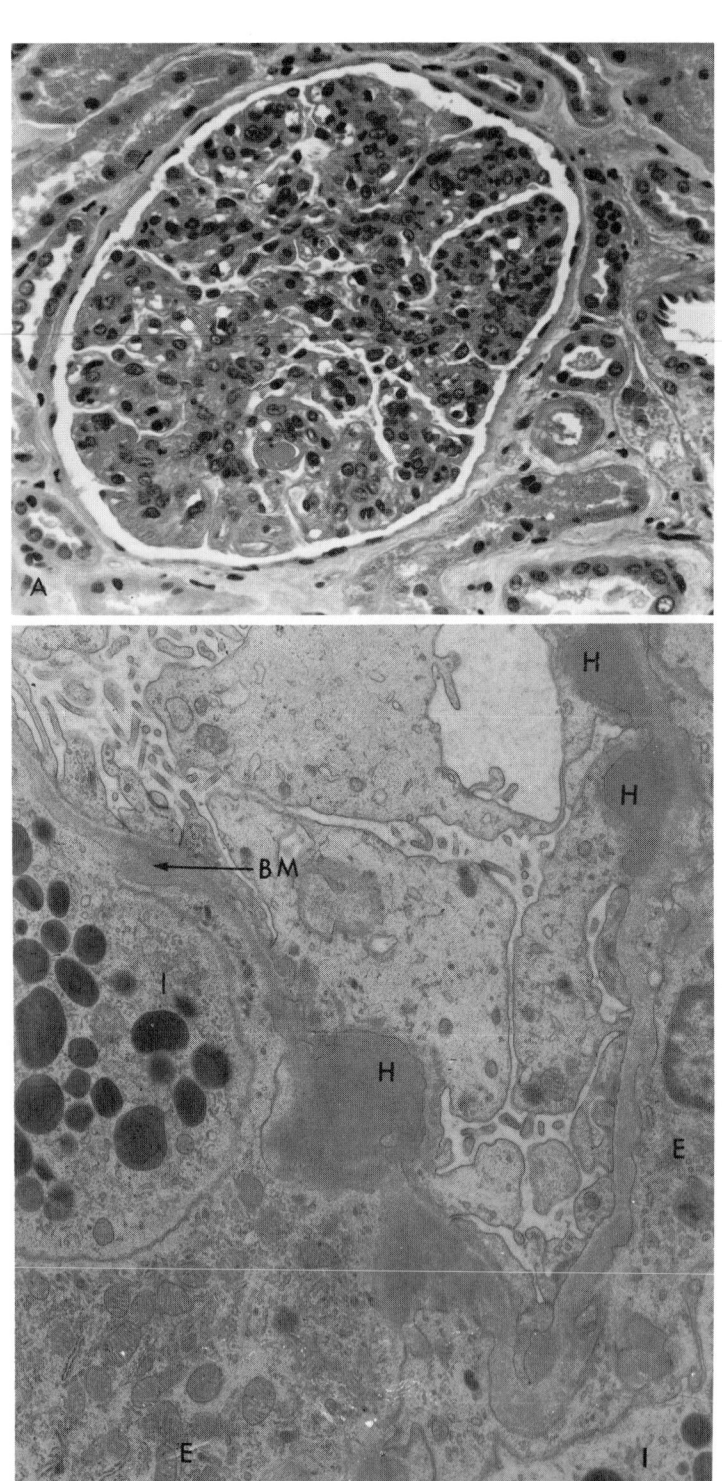

Figure 9–3. Poststreptococcal acute diffuse glomerulonephritis. A. Proliferation and exudation. Biopsy was obtained 30 days after onset of the condition. Hematoxylin and eosin stain (× 147). B. Characteristic electron-dense subepithelial "humps." BM, basement membrane; E, endothelial cell; H, hump (immune deposit); I, inflammatory cell; M, basement membrane–like material (in mesangium). Electron microscopy (× 12,000). (Both from Jennings, R. B., and Earle, D. P. In: Becker, E. L., ed. Structural Basis of Renal Diseases. New York: Harper & Row, 1968.)

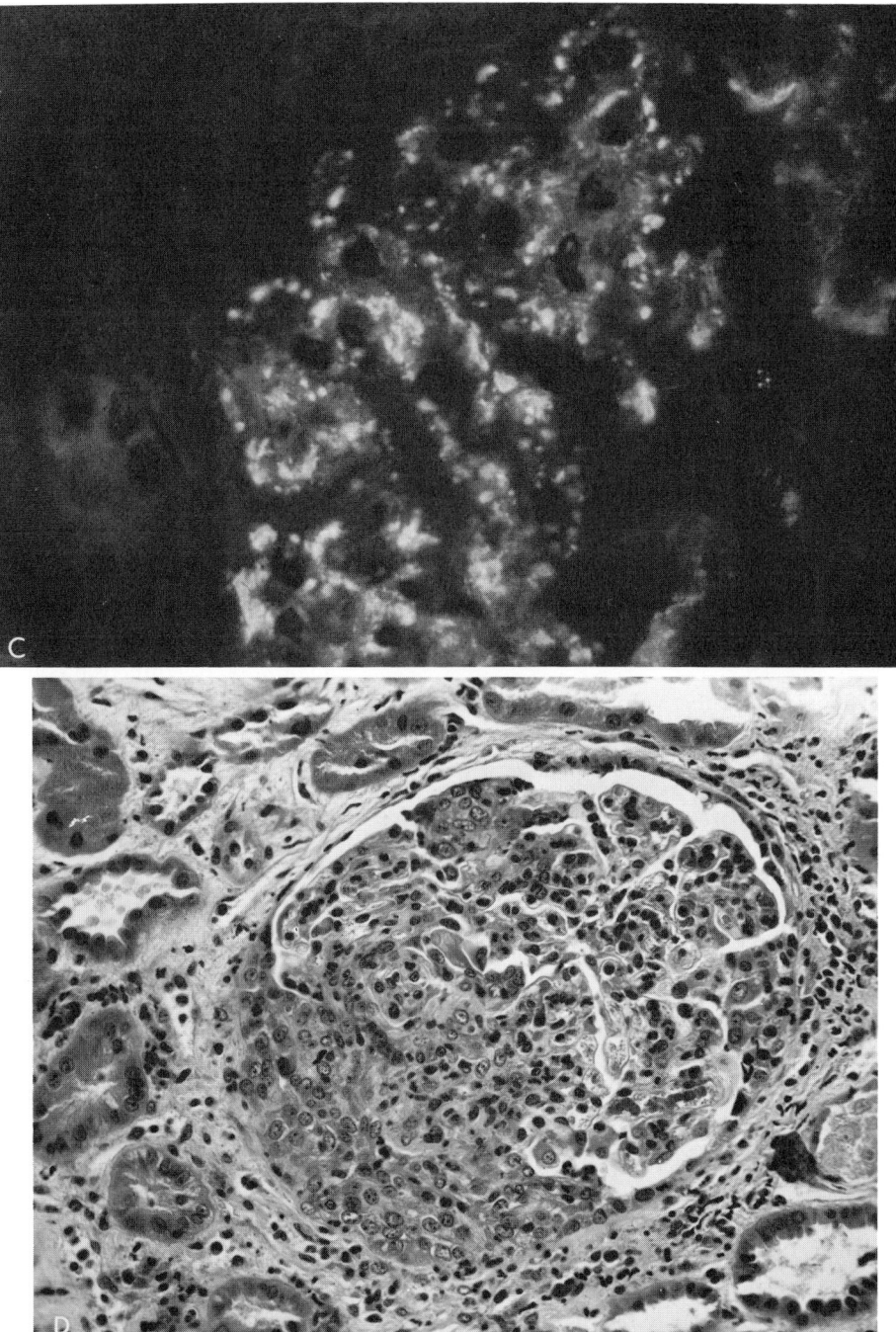

Figure 9–3 Continued C. *Characteristic deposition of IgG in a granular pattern along the glomerular capillary basement membrane. Immunofluorescent anti-IgG stain (× 25). (Courtesy of Dr. Elizabeth V. Potter.) D. Crescent formation characteristic of severe acute glomerulonephritis. Hematoxylin and eosin stain (× 276). (From Jennings, R. B., and Earle, D. P.* In: *Becker, E. L., ed.* Structural Basis of Renal Diseases. *New York: Harper & Row, 1968.)*

TABLE 9–7. *Possible Initiating Mechanisms in Poststreptococcal Acute Glomerulonephritis*

Deposition of circulating antigen–antibody complexes on glomerular capillary basement membrane
Fixation of streptococcal antigen in the glomerular capillary wall, followed by reaction with circulating free antibody
Autoantibody formation following alteration of host protein or glomerular antigens by streptococcal products or antigen
Cross-reaction between glomerular and nephritogenic streptococcal antigens
Direct toxic effect of streptococcal products on glomeruli

demonstrated in the lesions. Table 9–7 lists several proposed initiating mechanisms of renal injury in AGN, with most data supporting the first listed mechanism.

Therapy. Penicillin or erythromycin therapy is given to eradicate streptococci, and diuretics and antihypertensive agents are used as necessary. AGN tends to be a self-limited disorder, and immunosuppressive therapy is not warranted.

Prophylaxis. Effective prevention of AGN by prompt treatment of acute streptococcal infections is much less clearly documented than for ARF; indeed, most evidence suggests that it is not possible to prevent AGN effectively. Since recurrent attacks of AGN are quite rare (in direct contrast to ARF), long-term prophylactic antibiotics as used in ARF are not warranted or recommended.

DIPHTHERIA

A very important acute bacterial infection of the upper respiratory tract is diphtheria—the result of extracellular toxin production by toxigenic strains of *Corynebacterium diphtheriae*. This illness was described as a distinct entity by Pierre Brettonneau in 1821, who recognized its contagious nature. Around 1883, Theodor Klebs and Friederich Löffler observed the causative agent in smears of diphtheritic membranes, isolated the organism on artificial media, and produced fatal infection in guinea pigs. In 1923, a safe and effective vaccine composed of formalin-treated toxin was introduced by Gaston Ramon.

Corynebacterium diphtheriae is also known as the Klebs-Löffler bacillus, and is a gram-positive, nonmotile, nonsporulating, pleomorphic gram-negative rod, that sometimes has a club-shaped appearance. Media containing tellurite are best for recovery of *C. diphtheriae* because they inhibit other flora. Colonies may be rough or smooth in appearance, frequently classified as gravis, mitis, or intermedius. Toxin production does not correlate with colonial morphology and is present in strains of *C. diphtheriae* that are lysogenic for a prophage or phage encoding for diphtheria toxin. Toxin production *in vitro* is inversely related to the inorganic iron content of the medium.

Epidemiologically, diphtheria occurs worldwide, particularly in areas where immunization with diphtheria toxoid is not near-universal. In the United States only small numbers of cases are reported yearly (Fig. 9–4), primarily in unimmunized patients, and the fatality rate is about 5%. Transmission is the most efficient in crowded circumstances and occurs by droplets during coughing or sneezing by a carrier or a person with disease. Fomites appear unimportant. *C. diphtheriae* infection of skin may occur in the unimmunized, who thereby may be predisposed to respiratory colonization and infection.

The pathogenesis of diphtheria begins with *C. diphtheriae* mucosal colonization of the nose or mouth, with toxin elaboration by lysogenized strains occurring after an incubation period of several days. Tissue necrosis and local inflammation occurs in areas of colonization, eventually producing an adherent gray-black membrane that includes fibrin, blood, inflammatory cells, and epithelial cells and that bleeds on attempts to remove it. The membrane and underlying edema may compromise the airway, and the membrane may extend into the major bronchi. Elaborated toxin is absorbed through the damaged mucosa and carried to distant sites. Fragment B of the 63 kD polypeptide toxin is adsorbed by receptors on the cell membrane, and the smaller fragment A then enters the cell, interfering with protein synthesis by enzymatically inactivating elongation factor 2 by ADP ribosylation. Diphtheria toxin is particularly adept at binding to cardiac, neural, and renal cells. Antitoxin is effective in neutralizing circulating diphtheria toxin, but is ineffective once toxin is fixed to the cell membrane. Clinical manifestations appear some time after tissue fixation of toxin, with myocarditis appearing 10–14 days and peripheral neuritis 3–7 weeks after onset of disease.

Clinical Features

The result of the interaction between *C. diphtheriae* and the human host is determined by the

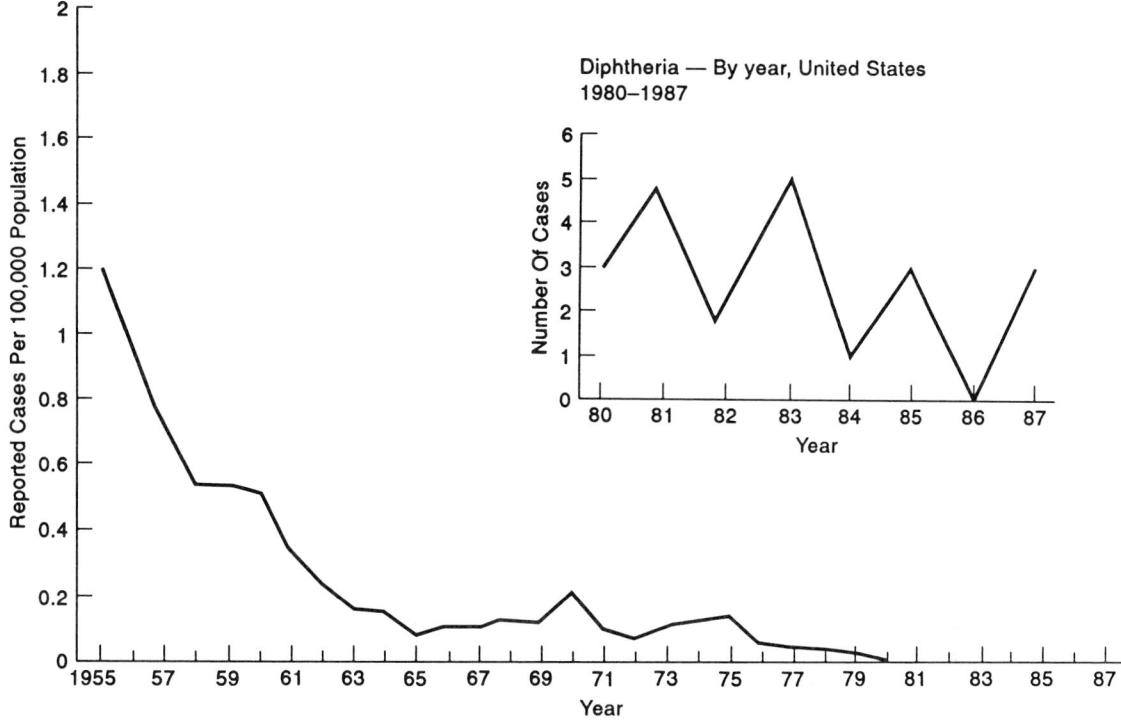

Figure 9–4. Diphtheria—by year, United States, 1955–1987. Data from Centers for Disease Control.

virulence of the specific organism (that is, its ability to adhere, to multiply, and to elaborate toxin) and by the immune status of the host (whether or not serum antitoxin is present). It appears possible for immune individuals to become colonized but not ill with *C. diphtheriae* and to serve as reservoirs of infection.

Diphtheria develops after an incubation period of 1–5 days and is conveniently classified by the anatomic location of the affected membrane (nasal, tonsillar, pharyngeal, laryngeal or laryngotracheal, and nonrespiratory). Tonsillar and pharyngeal diphtheria is characterized by the insidious onset of anorexia, malaise, low-grade fever, and sore throat. A membrane of varying extent forms within 1–2 days, depending upon the host's immune status. The grayish membrane can cover the tonsils and the pharyngeal walls and extend inferiorly to the larynx and trachea. Cervical adenopathy varies but may be associated with edema of the soft tissues of the neck, producing a "bull-necked" appearance. In milder cases the membrane sloughs after 7–10 days and recovery ensues. However, severe cases are associated with increasing toxemia followed by prostration, tachycardia, stupor, coma, and death within 6–10 days. Palatal paralysis, the most common manifestation of diphtheritic neuritis, may be noted, associated with difficulty swallowing. Ocular palsies and

diaphragmatic palsy may be seen. Severe diphtheria is also associated with diphtheritic myocarditis and with arrhythmias, congestive failure, and ECG changes.

Diagnosis

Because of the potential severity of the consequences of diphtheria, the diagnosis must be suspected on clinical grounds and therapy not withheld pending confirmation. Accurate confirmation of diphtheria requires isolation of *C. diphtheriae* on culture. Smears of the diphtheritic membrane are unreliable, and immunofluorescent studies are not routinely performed. After forewarning the microbiology laboratory so that appropriate tellurite media and a Löffler's slant can be prepared, material from beneath the membrane should be obtained for culture. Once isolated, recovered diphtheria organisms should be tested for toxin production, usually by intracutaneous inoculation of guinea pigs with a broth suspension of the organism, both with and without prior diphtheria antitoxin administration. The animal receiving no antitoxin should develop a necrotic skin lesion at the inoculation site in 72 h if the organism is toxigenic, but the other animal should develop no skin reaction.

Other laboratory tests are of little value: the WBC is normal to elevated, anemia from hemolysis is rare, CSF pleocytosis and protein elevation are mild, blood urea nitrogen will be elevated if acute tubular necrosis is present, and ST and T wave tracing patterns change on ECG in patients with myocarditis. A classic test of the immune status of a patient, little used today, is the Schick test, in which a small amount of diphtheria toxin is injected intracutaneously and, in the absence of antitoxin, a local inflammatory response occurs, peaking at 5 days. A toxoid control is necessary because some persons are sensitized to the toxin and develop a positive reaction despite the presence of neutralizing antitoxin.

Treatment

The best treatment of diphtheria, of course, is prevention by appropriate immunization. Once diphtheria is suspected, aggressive therapy to neutralize free toxin with antitoxin and to eradicate *C. diphtheriae* with antibiotics is essential. Antitoxin of equine origin must be given intravenously in a dose large enough to neutralize all free toxin but as a single dose to avoid reaction to the horse serum. Prior sensitivity to horse serum should be assessed with a test dose of 0.1 mL of 1:1000 dilution intracutaneously or into the conjunctiva; if positive, careful desensitization is necessary. The dose of antitoxin is 40,000–120,000 units depending upon the severity of illness. In addition to antitoxin, antibiotics such as penicillin or erythromycin are administered for about 7 days. The diphtheritic carrier state can be treated with an injection of benzathine penicillin or oral eythromycin. Additional therapy includes bed rest, hydration, and immunization following recovery, since at least 50% fail to develop immunity after natural infection.

OTHER BACTERIAL CAUSES OF PHARYNGITIS

Arcanobacterium haemolyticum

This organism (formerly Corynebacterium haemolyticum) has been reported to cause a scarlet fever–like illness with acute pharyngitis and a scarlatinal rash, particularly in teenagers and young adults. The peak age appears to be 15–20 years. Although well described in Scandina-via and Britain, this has been little studied in the United States. These patients fail to respond to penicillin therapy but have dramatic clinical responses to erythromycin. Clinical features exhibited by patients from whom *A. haemolyticum* has been recovered include tonsillitis or pharyngitis, and about 50% have an associated scarlatinal rash appearing several days after the onset of pharyngeal symptoms. Recovery of *A. haemolyticum* was 80-fold more common in those who were symptomatic than in normal, age-matched individuals.

Neisseria gonorrhoeae

Acute pharyngitis due to this agent is the result of oral–genital sexual contact and presents as an ulcerative, exudative tonsillopharyngitis. Culture on selective media for recovery of gonococci is necessary to establish the diagnosis. Therapy with penicillin resolves this infection.

OTITIS MEDIA

Infection of the middle ear is an extremely common infection in children, one associated with high morbidity but very low mortality. It has been shown by prospective cohort studies that by the age of 3 years two thirds of American children have experienced at least one episode of otitis media (OM), and one third of children have had three or more episodes. OM is the most frequent illness diagnosed and the most frequent reason for physician visits by children except for well-baby and well-child care. Middle ear effusion persists for weeks to months after an episode of acute OM: 40% still are present at 1 month and 10% at 3 months. Because conductive hearing impairment accompanies middle ear effusion and because many patients develop chronic effusions or chronic infections of the middle ear cavity and adjacent structures, OM is an extremely important disorder, particularly in childhood.

Anatomy and Physiology

Under normal circumstances the mucosa-lined middle ear cavity communicates with the nasopharynx via the mucosa-lined eustachian tube. The eustachian tube serves three functions: (1) to *ventilate* the middle ear cavity (i.e., equilibrate air pressure, replenish oxygen); (2) to facilitate *clearance* of secretions produced in the middle ear cavity; and (3) to *protect* the middle ear cavity from reflux of nasopharyngeal secretions. Under normal circumstances, the eustachian tube is functionally collapsed at rest but opens intermittently during swallowing by contraction of the tensor veli palatini muscle. Eustachian tube dysfunction can take the form of obstruction or of abnormal patency and is crucial to the pathogenesis of OM. Most simply, obstruction of the eustachian tube tends to prevent drainage of secretions, whereas excessive patency facilitates aspiration of pharyngeal organisms into the middle ear cavity. Both circumstances predispose to acute OM. In young children, the eustachian tube is more susceptible to functional obstruction because its cartilaginous support is less than in older children and adults. In addition, the tube is very short in infants and young children, making aspiration of nasopharyngeal flora somewhat easier. In effect, the dysfunction associated with a short floppy eustachian tube appears to account in large part for the frequency of OM in this population. Nasal allergy also contributes to the development of OM, presumably by leading to mucosal swelling that extends to the eustachian tube, where it can compromise the lumen.

Bacteriology

The microbiology of acute OM has been defined by middle ear fluid cultures obtained by tympanocentesis (needle aspiration through the tympanic membrane). Viruses and mycoplasmas are rarely recovered from middle ear fluid, but bacteria that are among the normal flora of the respiratory tract are very commonly isolated, particularly *Streptococcus pneumoniae* and *Haemophilus influenzae*. *S. pneumoniae* is the most important cause of OM at all ages, recovered from about 33% of middle ear aspirates in acute OM. *H. influenzae* is recovered from about 20% of aspirates, with 90% of those isolates nontypable (nonencapsulated) and only 10% representing type b strains (see Chapter 23). *Moraxella* (formerly *Branhamella*) *catarrhalis* (6–10%), *Staphylococcus aureus* (2%), GAS (2%), and mixed isolates (6%) represent the remainder of isolates. Approximately 30% of aspirates fail to yield pathogens; it has been shown that excellent anaerobic culturing technique decreases this category. Of importance is the observation that increasingly the isolates of *H. influenzae* and *M. catarrhalis* (as well as *S. aureus*) are beta-lactamase producers and therefore resistant to penicillin. This of course has

therapeutic implications. Chronic suppurative OM is associated with infection with organisms more difficult to eradicate, including *Pseudomonas aeruginosa, Proteus mirabilis,* and *S. aureus.*

Therapy

Decongestant and antihistaminic medications are of little or no value in treating acute OM. Antibiotic therapy with agents effective against the common pathogens clearly speeds resolution of symptoms and hastens clearance of middle ear effusions. Common choices include amoxicillin, cefaclor, erythromycin-sulfadiazine, and trimethoprim-sulfamethoxazole. In most circumstances, middle ear aspiration is not performed to determine the etiologic agent, but is generally used for patients who are treatment failures or compromised hosts for whom it is most important to establish a specific etiology because of the possibility of unusual pathogens.

Persistent middle ear effusion predisposes patients to recurrent acute episodes of OM. In addition, persistent effusion or infection leads to hearing impairment, usually conductive but occasionally sensorineural as well. Protracted hearing impairment in young children is thought to be associated with impaired speech development. Other untoward sequelae include perforation of the tympanic membrane, tympanosclerosis, adhesive fibrotic changes of the tympanic membrane with fixation of ossicles, chronic suppurative OM with chronic drainage through a perforated tympanic membrane, cholesteatoma formation within the middle ear, mastoiditis (see below), labyrinthitis representing spread of infection into the inner ear, facial nerve paralysis, and (rarely) suppurative intracranial complications (e.g., epidural or subdural empyema, brain abscess, meningitis). Mastoiditis is due to the same organisms that cause OM; indeed, the mastoid air cells are directly contiguous to the middle ear cavity.

SINUSITIS

Infection of the paranasal sinuses bears many similarities to infection of the middle ear cavity. The normal physiology of the sinuses depends upon: (1) patency of the ostia; (2) function of the ciliary apparatus; and (3) the quality of the mucosal secretions. Ostial obstruction or ciliary dysfunction predisposes to infection of the normally sterile paranasal sinuses. Sinus development varies: ethmoidal and maxillary sinuses are patent at birth, sphenoidal sinuses begin to develop at about 2 years of age, and frontal sinuses are usually very small until 5 or 6 years of age. Full sinus development may not be complete until about 20 years of age.

Ostial obstruction of the sinuses is facilitated by the small diameter of the ostia—maxillary sinus ostia are about 2.5 mm in diameter and ethmoidal air cell ostia are only 1–2 mm in diameter. Factors that predispose to sinus ostial obstruction include those related to mucosal swelling, including viral infection, allergy, immotile cilia, chemical irritation by medications (rhinitis medicamentosa), barotrauma (diving), and facial trauma. In addition, nasal polyps, foreign bodies, tumors, deviated nasal septum, and congenital choanal atresia may each lead to mechanical ostial obstruction. The most important of these factors that create mucosal swelling are clearly allergies and viral URIs. Sinusitis is an extremely common disorder, frequently subclinical and self-limited, but often requiring medical attention.

Microbiology

The paranasal sinuses are normally sterile. When sinusitis develops, the responsible bacterial organisms are the same that cause acute otitis media, that is, *H. influenzae* (nontypable) and *S. pneumoniae* most often, with lower frequencies of *M. catarrhalis, Staphylococcus aureus,* and *Streptococcus pyogenes.* In older children and adults, penicillin-sensitive anaerobes such as *Peptostreptococcus, Peptococcus,* and *Bacteroides* are recovered as well. Chronic sinusitis is characterized by a very similar distribution of pathogens.

Clinical Features

The clinical features of sinusitis are somewhat age-dependent, and the physician's challenge is to distinguish simple upper respiratory tract infection or allergy from secondary bacterial infection of the sinuses. Only the patients with secondary infection will benefit from antibiotic therapy. Young children most commonly manifest persistent rhinorrhea (serous or purulent), frequently with a cough that is worse at night. The examination of these children rarely demonstrates sinus tenderness, but periorbital edema may be seen, as well as postnasal drainage and foul-smelling breath. More commonly than younger children, older children and adults complain of headache and dental and facial pain, and show evidence of sinus tenderness to palpation. Transillumination of the sinuses with a bright light may be a useful adjunctive test for diagnosing maxillary or ethmoidal sinusitis, particularly in older children and adults. Laboratory studies that often facilitate diagnosis of sinusitis include radiographs that show air–fluid levels, complete opacification, or mucosal thickening of the sinuses, and possibly ultrasound studies of the sinus region. Nasopharyngeal and throat culture results do not correlate with the organisms within sinuses, and they thus should not be relied upon.

Treatment

The goals of antimicrobial therapy of acute sinusitis are to achieve clinical improvement and sterilization of sinus secretions, and to prevent chronic sinusitis as well as the intracranial and orbital complications of sinusitis. Based upon the spectrum of organisms isolated from infected sinuses, one can predict that antibiotics such as amoxicillin, ampicillin, cefaclor, or trimethoprim-sulfamethoxazole would be appropriate. Parenteral cephalosporins such as cefuroxime may be useful in hospitalized patients. Local or systemic administration of vasoconstrictive agents may contribute to reopening the sinus ostia, thereby improving the drainage of secretions. Occasionally, surgical drainage is necessary in a particularly ill patient with acute or chronic sinusitis or the patient with intracranial spread of infection from the sinuses.

CASE HISTORY 1

A 23-year-old school teacher (sixth grade) saw her physician in early March because of a persistent sore throat and low-grade fever of approximately 3 days' duration. When her symptoms first began she had taken an oral tetracycline preparation that a neighbor had given to her. Physical examination revealed several discrete white to yellow-gray patches of exudate over both tonsillar areas. Marked point tenderness at the angle of the right jaw coincided with enlarged palpable submandibular cervical lymph nodes.

A throat culture was obtained, and the patient was told that if she had streptococci in

her throat culture she would be notified and should then start penicillin therapy. Forty hours after this visit, the patient was contacted by telephone and told that a heavy growth of group A beta-hemolytic streptococcus was identified by culture. Although she reported that fever had subsided and that her sore throat was improved, she was strongly urged to take a full 10-day course of penicillin. A follow-up throat culture taken 10 days after starting therapy failed to reveal beta-hemolytic streptococci.

CASE 1 DISCUSSION

Several points about this case are worth emphasizing. First, the patient is an elementary school teacher and thus is almost constantly exposed to young children of an age (5–14 years) most prone to harbor group A streptococci in their respiratory tracts. Second, the time of year when her illness developed coincides with the peak occurrence of streptococcal pharyngitis. Third, close questioning is often necessary to elicit a history of self-medication. In some instances, this may be very important. For example, it may help explain delay in isolating a microorganism by culture. Note that the neighbor had some of her oral tetracycline preparation "left over," evidence that patients frequently do not consume all of an oral medication for the full course. Fourth, note that tetracycline, which is ineffective against group A streptococci, did not prevent heavy growth of the organism. Fifth, although the physician found clinical manifestations consistent with streptococcal disease of the oropharynx, the exudative process was minimal and the pharynx was not "beefy red," as is frequently the case. Perhaps the best indicator of streptococcal disease in this patient was the marked tenderness over the enlarged cervical lymph nodes beneath the right jaw. Sixth, note that when streptococci were isolated, the patient was instructed to take the eradicative 10-day course of penicillin, even though clinical features had begun to resolve spontaneously. Eradicative therapy was effective, as shown by the follow-up throat culture.

CASE HISTORY 2

A 10-year-old boy was seen by an intern at 6 P.M. on July 2 in an emergency clinic because of fever of several hours' duration, headache, and sore throat. Oral temperature was 102.4°F (39°C). The posterior pharynx was intensely erythematous; the tonsils were swollen, red, and partially covered with a skim milk–like exudate. The remainder of the physical examination was normal. A throat culture was obtained. Aspirin, fluids, and bed rest were recommended as supportive therapy and he was instructed to return the next day.

On July 3, he appeared to be less acutely ill, temperature was 101.6°F (38.7°C) and the tonsillar exudate was thicker, resembling cottage cheese in consistency. The original throat culture was reported to be free of beta-hemolytic streptococcal colonies. A second throat culture at this time was also found to be free of group A streptococci. In addition, throat and rectal swabs for viral culture and an acute-phase serum for baseline serologic studies were obtained.

The boy improved rapidly and felt well by July 6, and returned to his normal activities. A convalescent-phase serum was obtained 3 weeks later. The laboratory studies revealed the following: viral cultures—throat, adenovirus type 3; rectum, no virus isolated. Serologic studies:

Antigen	Antibody Titer of Sera Collected	
	July 3	July 24
Streptolysin O	1/100	1/100
Adenovirus (group-soluble antigen)	<1/4	1/16
Heterophil	<1/56	<1/56

CASE 2 DISCUSSION

The illness in this 10-year-old boy could have erroneously been considered to be streptococcal. The harried clinic staff could have simply given the patient a "shot of penicillin." However, the intern recognized that summer is not when group A streptococcal respiratory infection is prevalent and that a virus would more likely be responsible for this illness. Therefore, symptomatic measures were employed. The validity of this approach was verified by failure of each of two throat cultures to yield group A streptococci. Note that the probably well-informed and cooperative parents did not demand that an antimicrobial agent be given and brought the patient back for follow-up.

Further retrospective evidence that this infection was not streptococcal was provided by the lack of a rise in antistreptolysin O titer. Isolation of type 3 adenovirus from the throat and a diagnostic, greater than fourfold rise in antibody to adenovirus group antigens proved that this patient had an adenovirus infection. Such special laboratory procedures are not often available but provided instructive data in this instance.

Note that the emergency clinic staff was aware that infectious mononucleosis can simulate streptococcal pharyngitis, as evidenced by their request for a heterophil titer (see Chapter 10).

CASE HISTORY 3

A 10-year-old boy developed fever and sore throat in April. His physician diagnosed streptococcal pharyngitis, confirmed by a rapid strep antigen-detection test, and prescribed 10 days of oral penicillin. The patient rapidly improved, discontinued his medication after 3 days, and was well until 3 weeks after the onset of sore throat when he developed fever to 103°F and exquisite pain in the left knee. At this time the knee was mildly red and swollen but very painful to touch, he was unable to bear weight, and a loud apical systolic murmur radiating to the axilla was noted. He was hospitalized and confined to bed rest without medication. By the next morning, the left knee was much improved but the right wrist was very painful and slightly swollen. He was mildly tachypneic, quite tachycardic (pulse 140/min), and the liver was palpable 3 cm below the right costal margin. Laboratory studies indicated 1+ cardiomegaly on chest x-ray, WBC of 18,000/mm³ with 70% PMNs, 10% bands, 15% lymphocytes, ESR = 60 mm/hr (uncorrected), throat culture negative for *Streptococcus pyogenes*, prolonged PR interval, and antistreptolysin O titer = 1:1600. Echocardiogram showed a small pericardial effusion, mild left ventricular dilatation, and moderate mitral regurgitation. Therapy with prednisone, penicillin, digitalis, and diuretics was instituted. The patient was markedly improved by the next day from both the arthritic and cardiac perspectives. Prednisone was tapered over the next 2 weeks, and aspirin was instituted. When seen 6 months later, the patient had persistent evidence of mitral regurgitation without congestive failure. He was receiving monthly injections of benzathine penicillin prophylaxis and had been instructed regarding the importance of endocarditis prophylaxis. Five years later, no evidence of residual cardiac disease was detectable. He had been highly compliant with his monthly prophylaxis.

CASE 3 DISCUSSION

The failure to receive 10 days' treatment for acute streptococcal pharyngitis placed this child at risk for acute rheumatic fever (ARF). His clinical illness fulfilled the modified Jones criteria (Table 9–5) with two major and three minor (fever, acute-phase reactants, prolonged PR interval) criteria and evidence of previous streptococcal infection. The migratory nature of the arthritis is striking. Prompt suppression of the acute manifestations by antiinflammatory therapy (begun only after the diagnosis was established) is typical. Corticosteroids were chosen because of the evidence for congestive heart failure. This case demonstrates that in some patients healing of their cardiac lesions occurs if they are protected from recurrent attacks of ARF and from infective endocarditis.

CASE HISTORY 4

A 17-year-old high school student with no prior known renal disease developed sore throat and fever of 103°F on November 18, lasting 3 days. On November 28, he developed hematuria, puffy eyelids, and swollen ankles. A physician noted an inflamed pharynx, enlarged and reddened tonsils, and palpable cervical lymph nodes, as well as pitting edema of his feet and pretibial areas and blood pressure of 165/105 mm Hg. Urine contained 4+ protein, 20–30 erythrocytes and 25–30 leukocytes per high-powered field, some hyaline and granular casts, and one erythrocyte cast. The physician admitted the patient to a hospital where he was given bed rest and 10 days of oral penicillin. Throat culture revealed 4+ group A streptococci, antistreptolysin O titer was 1:500 (elevated), C3 level was 53 mg/dL (normal 110–160), and serum creatinine was 2.5 mg/dL (normal <1.5 mg/dL).

CASE 4 DISCUSSION

This teenager presents with typical postpharyngeal acute poststreptococcal glomerulonephritis. Oliguria and hypertension persist up to 1–2 months, and the disease process resolves spontaneously. Younger patients rarely develop chronic renal disease, but adults may develop evidence of progressive glomerulonephritis.

REFERENCES

Books

Bluestone, C. D., and Klein, J. O. *Otitis Media in Infants and Children.* Philadelphia: W. B. Saunders, 1988.

Breese, B. B., and Hall, C. B., eds. *Beta-Hemolytic Streptococcal Disease.* Boston: Houghton-Mifflin, 1978.

Read, S. E., and Zabriskie, J. M., eds. *Streptococcal Diseases and the Immune Response.* Orlando, FL: Academic Press, 1980.

Shulman, S. T., ed. *Pharyngitis: Management in an Era of Declining Rheumatic Fever.* New York: Praeger, 1984.

Taranta, A., and Markowitz, M. *Rheumatic Fever, 1981.* Boston: MTP Press, 1981.

Wannamaker, L. W., and Matsen, J. M., eds. *Streptococci and Streptococcal Diseases: Recognition, Understanding, and Management.* New York: Academic Press, 1972.

Review Articles

Ayoub, E. M., and Shulman, S. T. Streptococcal infections and their complications. In: Cluff, L. E., and Johnson, J. E., eds. *Clinical Concepts of Infectious Diseases.* 2nd ed. Baltimore: Williams and Wilkins, 1978.

Bluestone, C. D. Management of otitis media in infants and children: Current role of old and new antimicrobial agents. *Pediatr. Infect. Dis. J. 7:*S129–136, 1988.

Gordis, L. The virtual disappearance of rheumatic fever in the United States. *Circulation 72:*1155–1162, 1985.

Markowitz, M., and Kaplan, E. L. Reappearance of rheumatic fever. *Adv. Pediatr. 36:*39–66, 1989.

Stollerman, G. H. The relative rheumatogenicity of strains of group A streptococci. *Mod. Concepts Cardiovasc. Dis. 44:*35–40, 1975.

Stollerman, G. H. The return of rheumatic fever. *Hosp. Pract.* Nov. 15, 1988:100–113.

Articles

Banck, G., and Nyman, M. Tonsillitis and rash associated with *Corynebacterium haemolyticum. J. Infect. Dis. 154:*1037–40, 1986.

Bisno, A. L., Shulman, S. T., and Dajani, A. S. The rise and fall (and rise?) of rheumatic fever. *JAMA 259:*728–729, 1988.

Breese, B. B. A simple scorecard for the tentative diagnosis of streptococcal pharyngitis. *Am. J. Dis. Child. 131:*514–517, 1977.

Committee on Rheumatic Fever, Endocarditis, and Kawasaki Disease of the Council on Cardiovascular Disease in the Young. The American Heart Association. Prevention of rheumatic fever. *Pediatr. Infect. Dis. J. 8:*263–266, 1989.

Cunningham, M. W., McCormack, J. M., Fenderson, P. G., et al. Human and murine antibodies cross-reactive with streptococcal M proteins and myosin recognize the sequence Gln-Lys-Ser-Lys-Gln in M protein. *J. Immunol. 143:*2677–2683, 1989.

Kaplan, E. L., Johnson, D. R., and Cleary, P. P. Group A streptococcal serotypes isolated from patients and sibling contacts during resurgence of rheumatic fever in the United States in the mid-1980's. *J. Infect. Dis. 159:*101–102, 1989.

Lancefield, R. C. A microprecipitin-technic for classifying hemolytic streptococci. *Proc. Soc. Exp. Biol. Med. 38:*473–478, 1938.

Massell, B. F., Chute, C. G., Walker, A. M., et al. Penicillin and the marked decrease in morbidity and mortality from rheumatic fever in the United States. *N. Engl. J. Med. 318:*280–286, 1988.

Potter, E. V., Lipschultz, S. A., Abidh, S., et al. Twelve to 17 year follow-up of patients with post-streptococcal acute glomerulonephritis in Trinidad. *N. Engl. J. Med. 307:*725–9, 1982.

Stevens, D. L., Tanner, M. H., Winship, J., et al. Severe group A streptococcal infections associated with a toxic shock-like syndrome and scarlet fever toxin A. *N. Engl. J. Med. 321:*1–7, 1989.

Veasy, L. G., Wiedmeier, S. E., Orsmond, G. S., et al. Resurgence of acute rheumatic fever in the intermountain area of the United States. *N. Engl. J. Med. 316:*421–427, 1986.

Infectious Mononucleosis and Viral Infections of the Upper Respiratory Tract

INTRODUCTION

The majority of the viral infections in this chapter cause only minor, temporary departures from good health, with both society and many physicians often dismissing them as just another of life's unavoidable nuisances. Although viral upper respiratory disease is hardly the most serious medical problem, casual disregard of it is inappropriate and trivializes the cumulative burden these infections place on society—in terms of the direct costs of medical care, in lost productivity, and in more serious long-term sequelae such as hearing loss and learning disabilities linked to secondary cases of otitis media.

Three common clinical upper respiratory in-

fectious syndromes and their most frequent causative microbial agents are listed in Table 10–1. Viruses clearly have been shown to predominate in prospective epidemiologic surveys in which cultures were performed during acute illness to identify the infectious agent responsible. Studies designed to determine person-to-person transmission patterns using specific viral strains also have reinforced the dominant causative role of viruses in upper respiratory tract infections.

Unlike rhinovirus and coronavirus, the myxoviruses (particularly influenza, parainfluenza, and respiratory syncytial virus) and adenovirus are notable for their ability to produce disease at multiple sites in both the upper and lower respiratory tracts. Symptoms may be centered in the oropharynx, as is typical for adenovirus. However, with influenza and respiratory syncytial virus, more extensive inflammation of the entire respiratory tract is common, and the pulmonary features of infection often are more striking than upper airway involvement.

THE COMMON COLD

The common cold is aptly named since it is the most frequently occurring illness in pediatric and adult populations worldwide. Typically, children in the United States average six colds per year, and adults experience two to four infections annually. Colds are the most often cited medical reason for absenteeism from school or work and are linked to considerable losses in both industrial and academic productivity. Americans spend nearly $2 billion on

TABLE 10–1. *Principal Viral Causes of Upper Respiratory Tract Infections*

Common Cold	Acute Oropharyngitis	Mononucleosis
Rhinovirus	Adenovirus	Epstein-Barr virus
Coronavirus	Herpes simplex virus	Cytomegalovirus
Myxoviruses	Enteroviruses	*Toxoplasma
Respiratory syncytial	Coxsackievirus	Human herpesvirus 6
Parainfluenza	Echovirus	Human immunodeficiency virus
Influenza	Enterovirus	
Adenovirus	Myxoviruses	
	Parainfluenza	
	Respiratory syncytial	
	Influenza	
	*Mycoplasma pneumoniae	
	*Chlamydia pneumoniae	

*Nonviral.

over-the-counter cold remedies annually, and more than 10% of pediatric office visits are for evaluation of cold symptoms.

Colds occur in all parts of the world, in rural and urban environments. They are more frequent in damp, cold-weather months, although ambient temperature has never been proved to facilitate the spread of cold viruses or to depress host immune responses. On the other hand, the crowded conditions that exist in schoolrooms and day-care centers definitely promote transmission. School-aged children serve as the chief reservoir of cold viruses, and lateral spread classically takes place in the classroom as new strains are introduced. Young students circulate these strains to family members, who then help to spread them within the greater community. Adult smokers do not have more colds per year than their nonsmoking cohorts; nevertheless, tobacco users have more sustained and intense cold symptoms because the mucociliary damage caused by smoke inhalation compounds the tissue injury of viral infection.

The number of microorganisms which has been causally linked to the common cold now stands at nearly 200. Rhinoviruses account for about one third of all colds, and more than 110 antigenic types have so far been identified. Rhinoviruses are part of the Picornaviridae family, with an RNA genome surrounded by an icosahedral protein capsid. The lack of a fragile lipid envelope probably gives rhinoviruses a durability which enhances their survival on hands and fomites. Coronaviruses have also been demonstrated to cause colds and are responsible for at least 10–15% of total cases. As coronaviruses are fastidious and grow poorly in tissue culture, to date only three antigen strains have been identified, and the true impact of coronaviruses on the common cold is probably incompletely appreciated. Adenovirus and the myxoviruses also can produce typical cold symp-

toms and altogether are associated with about 10% of cases. Despite careful comprehensive cultures to isolate an infectious agent from patients with colds, no organism is recovered in up to 30% of cases. Nevertheless, it is reasonable to presume that the majority of these infections probably also are viral in origin.

There are three recognized routes for transmission of cold viruses. The most conspicuous involves virions suspended in *large-droplet aerosols* which are sneezed or coughed at close range onto unfortunate bystanders. However, such aerosols are largely composed of saliva droplets, and, as rhinovirus replication in the oral cavity is known to be poor, this method accounts for less transmission than gross appearances might imply. Low virus titers in saliva also explain why kissing generally is not responsible for the spread of colds. Rhinovirus can also survive in *small-droplet aerosols* which, because of their minute diameters, can remain airborne for long distances before inhalation and inoculation onto the nasal mucosa. Yet another important mechanism for spread is viral contamination of the hands of the infected individual with subsequent *hand-to-hand transfer*. Virions on the recipient's hand can then be easily self-inoculated into the nose or onto the conjunctival mucosa with subsequent extension of the organism down the nasolacrimal duct into the nose. Via either route, nasopharyngeal infection is easily established.

Study of both natural and experimental rhinovirus infection indicates that both aerosol and hand routes of spread are effective; mechanisms which facilitate transfer of other cold viruses have been studied less thoroughly and as yet are incompletely understood. Fairly close contact, however, seems essential for transmitting coronavirus, adenovirus, and the respiratory myxoviruses.

Cold viruses initiate a typical pathophysiologic sequence. Again, greater detail is available for rhinovirus infection, but the symptoms in most colds are sufficiently similar to presume that other cold viruses produce similar events. Rhinovirus adheres to specific receptors (intercellular adhesion molecule-1, or ICAM-1) on the ciliated columnar epithelial cells of the upper respiratory tract, is internalized, and begins actively replicating in the cell's cytoplasm. Ciliated epithelial cells are distributed liberally in the mucosa of the nose, sinuses, and pharynx, but not on the squamous epithelial surfaces of the gingiva, tongue, or buccal mucosa. When inoculated directly onto nasal mucosa with its high concentration of ciliated columnar cells, one (or fewer) median tissue culture infective dose ($TCID_{50}$) of rhinovirus is required to produce infection. However, when squamous surfaces such as the tongue or skin of the anterior nares are the portals of inoculation, a substantially higher dose of virus (at least 10,000-fold greater) is needed to establish infection. These data are summarized in Table 10–2.

Viral inclusions are usually lacking in rhinovirus-infected nasopharyngeal cells, and there is little cytonecrosis. Neutrophils accumulate in the lamina propria of the nasopharyngeal mucosa, and inflammatory mediators are released locally. High concentrations of bradykinin have been measured in nasal secretions and cause increased vascular permeability in the mucosal capillary bed, which leads to edema and nasal stuffiness. Stimulation of cholinergic nerves produces a dramatic increase in mucus production and profuse, watery nasal discharge. The mild degree of sore throat discomfort accompanying the common cold is due to local inflammatory mediators which stimulate pain-nerve fibers and to limited epithelial cell necrosis. Dependent drainage of mucoid secretions in the pharynx

(postnasal drip) is the chief cause of cough rather than pathology in the lower respiratory tract. Virus excretion, and therefore infectivity, parallels the intensity of clinical illness. The mean duration of rhinovirus and coronavirus colds is less than 1 week. The pathophysiologic sequence of a typical rhinovirus upper respiratory infection is outlined in Figure 10–1.

Within 1–2 days of onset of a rhinovirus cold, neutralizing secretory immunoglobulin A is detectable in nasal secretions; specific IgG then appears both in nasal mucus and serum. Specific serum IgG develops in up to 80% of patients and may persist for years. Adults eventually acquire antibody to several rhinovirus antigenic types, with a corresponding measure of immunity to reinfection by these particular serotypes. However, humoral defenses are probably inadequate to overcome a large viral challenge, providing yet another explanation for repeated rhinovirus colds.

Cold symptoms begin following an incubation period of 2–5 days, with symptoms so typical that the diagnosis is self-evident, even to children. There is abrupt onset of watery nasal discharge, nasal stuffiness, and modest sore throat, with brisk rhinorrhea persisting for 2–4 days and then gradually subsiding. Nasal discharge initially is mucoid and acellular but becomes thicker and purulent in character as inflammatory cells and detached epithelial cells accumulate in the mucoid secretions. Colds are generally afebrile infections, with temperature elevations limited to about 1°F.

Physical findings in a patient complaining of a cold are usually limited to hyperemia and edema of the nasal and pharyngeal mucosa. Skin around the nares can become red and swollen, particularly when rhinorrhea is intense. Physical examination should focus, however, on a careful search for findings that suggest a disease more serious than a simple cold. Marked pharyngeal injection or exudate, pseudomembrane formation, and palatal petechiae or vesicles shift consideration to acute viral or bacterial oropharyngitis. The nasal turbinates should be inspected for polyps, which suggest allergic rhinitis, and for foreign bodies in little children. Adults and adolescents should be questioned about cocaine-induced nasal congestion; patients who smoke should be reminded that tobacco smoke aggravates cold symptoms. Secondary bacterial infection of the middle ear and sinuses occurs in a minority of colds (1–2%); careful otoscopic examination of the tympanic membranes and transillumination of the sinuses

TABLE 10–2. *Infectivity of Rhinovirus for Human Volunteers by Different Routes of Inoculation**

Portal of Inoculation	No. of Subjects	Dose of Virus, in $TCID_{50}$, for Infection of 50% of Subjects[†]
Intranasal	38	0.28
Inside of anterior nares	13	1.39
Tongue	15	2,260
Outside of anterior nares	8	11,000

*Data adaptation from D'Alessio, D.J., et al. Short-duration exposure and the transmission of rhinoviral colds. *J. Infect. Dis.* 150:189, 1984.
†Dose of rhinovirus type 16 expressed in terms of amount of virus to infect 50% of WI-38 human diploid cells, i.e., $TCID_{50}$; infection of humans defined as recovery of virus from nasopharynx or antibody seroconversion.

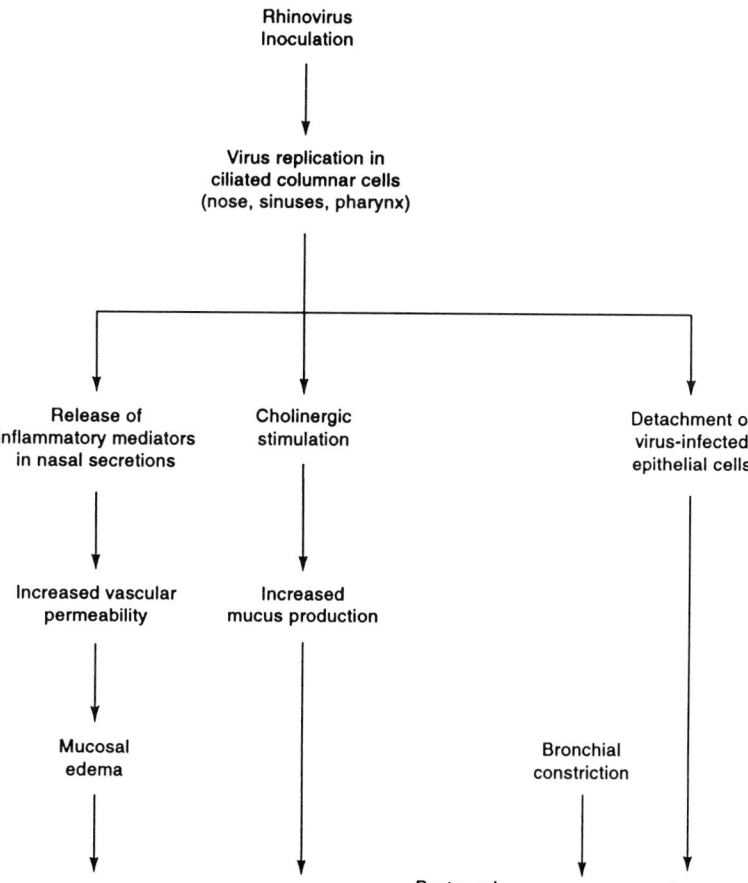

Figure 10–1. Pathophysiology of rhinovirus common cold. (Adapted from Szilagyi, P. G.: Viruses and the common cold. Pediatr. Virol. 5:1–4, 1990.)

are appropriate for patients with high fever, facial pain, or earache.

Although a focused physical examination is reasonable for the patient with a cold, laboratory work-up generally is not. Culture or serologic confirmation of the causative viral agent has no effect on management and is not usually cost-effective. The patient with acute oropharyngitis as the predominant feature of his illness, however, requires an antigen screen and/or culture for *Streptococcus pyogenes* infection. (See Chapter 9.)

Management of the typical cold centers upon two issues: minimizing the intensity of symptoms and preventing spread. Antibiotics have no antiviral activity and, unless bacterial superinfection has occurred, are unwarranted. There are several pharmacologic approaches for palliation of nasal mucosal congestion. Sympathomimetic amines, which imitate the function of the endogenous neurotransmitters of the sympathetic nervous system, produce vascular constriction and thus decrease local blood flow and mucus production. Phenylephrine, pseudoephedrine,

and the metazolines all exert these effects and differ from one another only in duration of action. Topical preparations produce almost immediate effects but rebound vasodilatation can be expected. Oral agents have less intense and more sustained results, but may cause such side effects as tachycardia, irritability, and wakefulness. Eosinophilia, tissue basophilia, and histamine release are not part of the host response to colds, so antihistamine drugs provide no direct help. The slight anticholinergic effect generated by antihistamines, however, may add a modest measure of benefit. In addition, most antihistamine preparations have a sedative effect, which may be beneficial at nighttime but often interferes with daytime activities.

The majority of over-the-counter cold medicines combine a sympathomimetic decongestant with an antihistamine for short-term palliation of rhinorrhea. Many preparations also include a nonnarcotic cough suppressant, dextromethorphan being the most commonly used agent. Such antitussive agents are generally unnecessary in cold preparations, as cough is not a major feature of the common cold; bothersome cough implies pathology in the lower respiratory tract and a causative organism other than rhinovirus. Another superfluous additive in combination cold preparations is the expectorant agent guaifenesin (glyceryl guaiacolate), since adequate expectorant action can be accomplished with good hydration. Likewise, analgesics such as aspirin and acetaminophen provide little palliation in an uncomplicated cold. High fever or severe headache suggests the development of secondary bacterial complications such as otitis media or sinusitis. Aspirin does not produce a statistically meaningful reduction in cold symptoms and in one study was shown to enhance the shedding of rhinovirus into nasal secretions, possibly increasing communicability.

Prevention of colds through vaccination seems as unlikely today as when the possibility was first raised over 20 years ago. The diversity of viral agents and the wide array of viral serotypes is a major drawback in formulating an effective cold vaccine. Also, the limitations inherent in using a parenteral inactivated vaccine to generate sustained, protective mucosal IgA immunity further complicates the design of a useful product. Avoiding contact with infected individuals is an unworkable tactic in preventing colds. Nevertheless, practical measures that can interrupt the transmission of cold viruses have been recognized for years and are worth repeating: the aesthetic importance of covering sneezes and coughs hardly needs emphasis, but both patients and physicians should be reminded that frequent handwashing is a simple and effective means for decreasing rhinovirus spread via hand-to-hand or hand-fomite-hand routes. Adults as well as children with colds inadvertently but unavoidably contaminate their hands with virus and should be aware that they can reduce viral transfer just as much by careful handwashing as by muffling sneezes. Frequent handwashing by physicians can help minimize virus spread among patients as well as reduce the likelihood of the health care provider's becoming infected.

Another hygienic measure reported to be of moderate value in reducing the spread of colds was the use of disposable tissues coated with virucidal agents. Iodine-impregnated tissues were studied initially and successfully reduced the number of secondary colds in a trial conducted in a group of workers at an Antarctic camp; however, these tissues had a disagreeable odor, stained the skin of the users, and held little promise of popular acceptance. Another germicidal tissue, formulated to exploit the known acid lability of rhinoviruses, was prepared by soaking disposable tissues in citric acid and malic acid. Sodium lauryl sulfate was also added to inactivate enveloped viruses. Use of these chemically stable, odorless, colorless virucidal tissues successfully interrupted transfer of rhinovirus in a study that used a prolonged card game to generate manual and aerosol spread. No predictions of the value of such a product for general use have been made, and germicidal tissues have not been commercially marketed.

Studies of topical intranasal interferon alfa-2 and interferon-inducing chemicals for prevention of colds have shown variable efficacy. Interferon alfa-2 topical nasal spray applied after exposure produced a 39% reduction in the number of secondary rhinovirus colds in household members and an 88% decrease in laboratory-induced rhinovirus colds. However, long-term prophylaxis with interferon is unreasonable, and even short-term use provoked local side effects, such as nasal stuffiness and minor bleeding, in up to 14% of users. Interferon-inducing compounds are generally regarded as failures in preventing colds. Intercellular adhesion molecule-1, the principal surface receptor on respiratory tract epithelial cells which binds most rhinovirus serotypes, has now been identified and its amino acid sequence determined. This molecule exhibits dose-dependent inhibition of rhinovirus *in vitro;* a soluble purified form is being tested as a possible prophylactic that could selectively and specifically bind rhinovirus and thus prevent infection. However, for the present, the only reasonable steps for managing colds are drugs for palliating acute symptoms and sensible hygienic measures to minimize spread.

ACUTE OROPHARYNGITIS

Pharyngitis is a common accompanying feature of several respiratory tract infectious syndromes, ranging from the common cold to infectious mononucleosis to influenza. Acute oropharyngitis, however, has features which help to distinguish it from the overlap involvement of the pharynx in these other infectious conditions. Inflammation of the mucosa in the mouth or throat is the patient's dominant complaint and may vary from limited hyperemia and edema to obvious epithelial necrosis with exudation. Because symptoms may be quite intense, patients are more likely to need and seek medical attention.

A wide variety of microorganisms can cause acute oropharyngeal infection, and although viruses are prominent causes (Table 10–1), bacteria also account for a substantial proportion of cases. Precise numbers and percentages vary, and the relative importance of each organism is still incompletely defined. Seasonal variations have been described for several types of pharyngitis, and epidemiologic patterns vary among adult, pediatric, and military populations.

Streptococcus pyogenes (beta-hemolytic streptococcus, group A) accounts for about 20% of all cases of acute pharyngitis. *Mycoplasma pneumoniae* and *Chlamydia pneumoniae* (formerly called *Chlamydia psittaci* TWAR strain) are also linked to acute oropharyngitis, and in industrialized nations outrank *Corynebacterium diphtheriae* and mixed anaerobic infections in numerical importance. Parainfluenza and respiratory syncytial virus in older children and adults may produce only modest sore throat or cold symptoms with no clinical evidence of lower respiratory tract involvement. Most cases of acute pharyngitis do not have specific physical findings that can predict reliably the causative agent. However, there are several distinctive pharyngitis syndromes which have been linked with specific viral agents.

Acute Herpetic Gingivostomatitis

Herpes simplex virus serotype 1 (HSV-1) is an endemic virus worldwide which infects as many as 75% of Americans by the age of 5. Humans are the only natural reservoir for HSV-1, so all infections represent person-to-person spread. Transmission is almost always salivary, typically through kissing or the drooling that occurs between children at play. HSV is a DNA virus with a fragile lipid envelope, so viability on fomites is quite limited. Squamous epithelial cells of the lips, oral cavity, and pharynx have surface receptors for herpes virus, and therefore are the principal sites of infection. Following an incubation period of 2–4 days, acute replication of HSV-1 in the squamous epithelium leads to a characteristic sequence of events: infected cells develop nuclear viral inclusions, adjacent infected cells fuse their cytoplasmic membranes to produce multinucleated syncytial giant cells, and intraepithelial vesicles form as the desmosomal junctures between squamous cells degenerate. Large amounts of virus accumulate in the saliva as infected cells undergo lytic disintegration. Because of constant friction, herpetic vesicles in the oropharynx rupture much more rapidly than similar lesions on the skin surface, so superficial ulcerations generally are apparent within 1–2 days. A healthy individual with intact cell-mediated immunity generates a clone of cytotoxic T lymphocytes capable of destroying cells infected with HSV-1; this specific cytolytic immune response is active within 5–7 days, and HSV-1 replication usually ends by 10–14 days. Mucosal ulcers heal completely without scarring, since the basal layer of the epithelium remains intact. Many cases of primary HSV-1 infection are mild, lack conspicuous vesicles and ulcers, and present only as nondescript oropharyngitis; seroconversion with acquisition of antibodies specific for HSV-1 is the only means for verifying the herpetic etiology of the pharyngitis. At the opposite extreme, some individuals, including those with impaired cell-mediated immunity, may experience a somewhat protracted infection with severe, painful, ulcerative stomatitis accompanied by high fever and anterior cervical lymphadenopathy.

All of the herpes viruses share the biologic property of persisting in a latent state and then episodically reactivating to produce acute recurrent infection. During acute primary infection in the oropharynx, HSV-1 virions travel retrograde along sensory nerve axons to the trigeminal ganglion neurons, where they become latent. The cell-mediated immune system is presumed to contribute the major force in maintaining this dormancy, but the means by which this is accomplished are unknown. Although the majority of people worldwide are seropositive for HSV-1 and probably harbor latent ganglionic virus, only a minority (10–20%) experience clinically obvious episodic reactivation. HSV-1 replication is initiated in the trigeminal ganglion, and virus travels antegrade along neurosensory axons to infect the mucocutaneous epithelium. Recurrent lesions are initially vesicular but quickly convert to ulcers as the infected squamous cells degenerate; complete healing is prompt, and often complete within 5–10 days. Recurrent herpetic eruptions are fairly mild and can appear at any squamous epithelial site in the pharynx, mouth, or face. However, most patients develop lesions on the lips or the adjacent facial skin, characteristic eruptions commonly called "fever blisters" or "cold sores." Patients often state that recurrences can be triggered by intense sunlight exposure, emotional stress, or coincident infection or fevers.

No conspicuous *in vitro* or *in vivo* defects in cell-mediated immunity can be identified in the HSV-1 seropositive individual who experiences recurrent lesions, but a subtle transient aberration in the surveillance function of cell-based immunity probably is responsible. The frequency of recurrence is unpredictable and may vary from one episode every few years to several per year. Acyclovir, used either topically or orally, is active against HSV, but circumstances are generally insufficient to justify its use. Several folk remedies have been proposed as prophylaxis or as treatment, but in controlled trials none significantly shortened the duration of viral shedding or promoted healing.

Patients with impaired cell-mediated immunity are at risk for recurrent HSV-1 infections with severe protracted mucocutaneous ulceration. Ulcers may progressively enlarge as virus spreads centrifugally across the squamous epithelium, unmodified by T-lymphocyte response. Painful coalescent ulcers can develop as well as extension into the lower respiratory tract and dissemination systemically. Parenteral acyclovir is a necessity in this setting, to control aggressive mucosal disease as well as viremic spread. Even with systemic antiviral therapy, visceral herpetic dissemination is frequently fatal.

Adenoviral Pharyngoconjunctival Fever

Several of the 41 known adenovirus serotypes can infect the respiratory tract. Although acute pharyngotonsillitis is the most common type of infection produced, adenoviruses can also cause simple colds and lower respiratory tract bronchitis and pneumonia. Receptors for adenovirus are also located on the anterior epithelial surface of the eye, so keratoconjunctivitis as an isolated infection or as an accompaniment of pharyngitis is a well-recognized form of adenovirus illness.

Adenoviral respiratory tract infections have no distinct seasonal distribution. The majority of illness occurs in young children, but acute upper respiratory tract epidemics have been described in adult military recruits. Adenovirus is easily spread in oropharyngeal secretions, particularly in the crowded situations in schools and army camps. Adenoviruses are nonenveloped, having only a protein capsid coat, and apparently can survive for short periods in the external environment. Contaminated swimming pool water is a classic vehicle for epidemic spread of pharyngoconjunctival fever, and several nosocomial outbreaks of adenovirus upper respiratory and conjunctival infections have been traced to the contaminated hands of health care workers.

Virus can be directly inoculated onto upper respiratory tract epithelial cells or introduced via the conjunctival sac with extension along the nasolacrimal duct onto the pharyngeal mucosa. Incubation periods of 2–4 days are typical, and acute pharyngitis with edema, hyperemia, and purulent mucosal exudate lasts 5–7 days. Fever is common, with temperature elevations often reaching 102°F. More so than with other viral upper respiratory tract infections, adenovirus induces lymphoid hyperplasia with prominent tonsillar and cervical lymph node enlargement; follicular lymphoid aggregates are easily visible through the injected conjunctival membrane and can occasionally produce cobblestone submucosal changes in the pharynx also. Adenovirus can persist in lymphoid tissue for several weeks after acute symptoms have resolved, serving as an ongoing source for further spread of infection.

A typical childhood is marked by several adenoviral infections, the majority of which are caused by the dozen serotypes classically linked to respiratory tract illness. Specific IgG characteristically develops following infection, but since neutralizing secretory IgA concentrations may vary and provide an incomplete mucosal defense, reinfection with a single serotype is not uncommon. The dwindling number of adenoviral respiratory infections seen in the adult years represents an accumulation of humoral antibodies as well as a more hygienic lifestyle.

Herpangina and Hand-Foot-Mouth Syndrome

Enterovirus infections are common in warm weather months, and the majority of the coxsackievirus, echovirus, and enterovirus serotypes can produce sore throat, either as a solitary febrile illness or as a symptom accompanying rash or meningitis. Pharyngitis in these cases is generally nondistinct with mucosal hyperemia and patchy or no exudate. High fever is typical, and the duration of symptoms in uncomplicated pharyngitis is usually only a few days.

However, two distinctive enterovirus infections with striking findings in the upper respiratory tract have been described: herpangina and hand-foot-mouth syndrome. Herpangina is an acute-onset febrile pharyngitis with characteristic discrete vesicular lesions distributed on the palatal, posterior buccal, tonsillar, and pharyngeal mucosa; these vesicles convert to open ulcers as the overlying squamous epithelium disintegrates. Fever can be as high as 104°F, and sore throat pain, as the name herpangina implies, may be so intense that swallowing is difficult. Symptoms usually resolve in less than 1 week. Coxsackie A enteroviruses are most frequently associated with herpangina, but coxsackie B and echoviruses can also produce this syndrome.

Hand-foot-mouth syndrome is generally linked to coxsackie A16 and also has fever as a prominent finding. Painful oral lesions follow the onset of fever, beginning as vesicles that subsequently erode to ulcers. Unlike herpangina involvement of the posterior pharynx, hand-foot-mouth oral vesicles are distributed on the buccal, palatal, and gingival mucosa as well as on the tongue and anterior tonsillar pillars. About 50% of patients develop discrete vesicles on the hands and feet as well; similar lesions can also be found elsewhere on the extremities and trunk in a minority of cases. This disease is self-limiting and also usually resolves within 1 week.

Laboratory Evaluation of Oropharyngitis

Physical findings are insufficiently distinct to separate viral from streptococcal oropharyngitis in most cases. Both culture and *Streptococcus pyogenes* antigen assay are widely available laboratory tests, so routine prompt confirmation of streptococcal pharyngitis is easily accomplished. However, verification of chlamydial or mycoplasmal pharyngitis requires expensive and complex culture, antigen assay, or nucleic acid probe assay; both cost and limited availability constrain the practical use of these confirmatory tests in guiding management.

Serologic diagnosis of viral oropharyngitis has limited clinical applicability in the evaluation of individual patients. The multiplicity of potential viral serotypes makes antibody assay with group antigen insensitive and nonspecific. Large reference laboratories or public health facilities have comprehensive sets of individual serotyping reagents which are valuable in the epidemiologic characterization of outbreaks, but this information adds little to the management of single cases.

Viral culture confirmation, although more rapid and precise than serologic diagnosis, generally is not needed for appropriate handling of uncomplicated acute pharyngitis. Nevertheless, the major viral pathogens (HSV, adenovirus, and several members of the enterovirus family) are not fastidious and can be grown easily in standard tissue culture cell lines. Specimens should be collected during the first few days of illness when virus replication is maximal. Vesicles, ulcers, or exudative mucosal lesions should be swabbed vigorously so that a liberal sample of virus-infected cells is recovered. Contamination of the specimen with unwanted normal microflora is unavoidable, so swabs should be placed immediately into a transport medium containing antibiotics and then brought to the laboratory as promptly as possible for tissue culture inoculation. The serotypic diversity of enteroviruses has made production of an antigen assay for rapid diagnosis an unrealistic goal. However, antigen assays, using both fluorescein-conjugated antibody and enzyme immunoassay, are available for HSV and adenovirus. Fluorescent-antibody-stained smears have limited sensitivity compared with culture (overall approximately 40–50%), since intact cells with abundant viral antigen are needed to yield a positive result. Enzyme immunoassays do not rely on intact virus-infected cells but still have a false-negative rate of 30–40%. Tissue culture virus isolation remains the most sensitive, widely available method for laboratory verification of viral oropharyngitis.

INFECTIOUS MONONUCLEOSIS

Infectious mononucleosis is a specific clinical entity caused by primary infection with Epstein-Barr virus (EBV). Although acute pharyngotonsillitis is a very prominent feature of infectious mononucleosis, it is only one manifestation of this systemic febrile lymphoproliferative disease, which also typically involves lymph nodes, spleen, liver, and peripheral blood, and, rarely, lungs, kidney, skin, myocardium, and central nervous system as well. The name *glandular fever* was applied in the past to infectious mononucleosis and aptly describes the principal clinical features of this illness.

EBV is another herpesvirus that infects the majority of the population worldwide. The virus is easily spread by saliva of an infected individual to susceptible persons, so initial EBV infection usually occurs in young children. In developing countries with crowding or suboptimal sanitation, EBV seropositivity rates of almost 100% are common by age 5. Primary EBV infection is usually an asymptomatic event in young children or produces minor symptoms which are indistinguishable from other causes of febrile pharyngitis. However, specific EBV antibodies are produced as a lifelong marker that subclinical infection had occurred.

In upper socioeconomic groups of the United States and other affluent societies, up to 50% of individuals entering adolescence are seronegative for EBV. However, the virus is still widely available in the saliva of many of their infected peers, so despite their sanitized childhoods, these seronegative adolescents easily encounter EBV during dating. By age 30, EBV seroprevalence approaches 100% in all social strata in all countries. Statistics extrapolated from physician-reported cases suggest that middle-income societies have about 100 cases of infectious mononucleosis per 100,000 population annually. Although symptomatic mononucleosis is an infrequent sporadic event in young children, in high school and college students case rates of 200–800/100,000 population have been estimated (Fig. 10–2). Overall, approximately 200,000 cases of infectious mononucleosis can be anticipated each year in the United States.

After a 2–4-week incubation period, at least one half of adolescents and young adults primarily infected with EBV develop a characteristic clinical illness that typically begins with abrupt onset of malaise, profound fatigue, fever (up to 103°F.), and headache, followed shortly thereafter by pharyngitis with tonsillar enlargement and patchy purulent exudate. Cervical lymph nodes which drain the pharynx are enlarged and usually tender, but EBV infection is not limited to the upper respiratory tract. Viral replication in oropharyngeal mucosal cells produces lytic destruction of pharyngeal epithelium early in infectious mononucleosis, but the virus is also strikingly lymphotropic and attaches to the C3d receptor located on the cytoplasmic membrane of mature B lymphocytes. This C3d complex also functions as the receptor (CR2) for the d fragment of the third component of complement. This binding of EBV to resting B lymphocytes activates cellular signals which trigger a polyclonal proliferative response, and it is this intense local and systemic lymphoproliferation which gives infectious mononucleosis its distinctive clinical features. Lymphoid hyperplasia of the tonsils is typical, and lymph node enlargement is invariably present in both anterior and posterior cervical chains. Anterior cervical lymph nodes drain the tonsils and pharynx and become enlarged in a wide variety of pharyngeal infections; therefore, this finding has limited diagnostic specificity. The presence of posterior cervical adenopathy, however, implies a systemic illness. Inguinal and axillary nodes often are modestly enlarged. Splenomegaly, which can vary from minimal to massive, occurs in at least 50% of patients and is apparent by the second week of illness. Mild hepatomegaly, from triadal and sinusoidal lymphoid infiltration, is seen in up to 25% of cases; modest elevation of liver enzymes, usually detected fortuitously on serum chemistry profiles, is almost universal, but jaundice is infrequent (less than 10%). Palatal petechiae can be found in one third of cases, and a diffuse, faint, transient morbilliform rash also develops in about 5% of patients. Visceral extension of the lymphoid infiltrate can produce such diverse complications as interstitial pneumonitis, aseptic meningitis, Guillain-Barré syndrome, cerebellar ataxia, polyneuritis, myocarditis, hemolytic anemia, and cytopenias (but each of these occurs in fewer than 1% of cases).

Fever and pharyngitis usually resolve over a 1–3-week period; lymphadenopathy and splenomegaly generally subside in 4–6 weeks. Malaise and weakness can linger for several weeks, accounting for impaired performance at work or school. Serious morbidity and mortality in

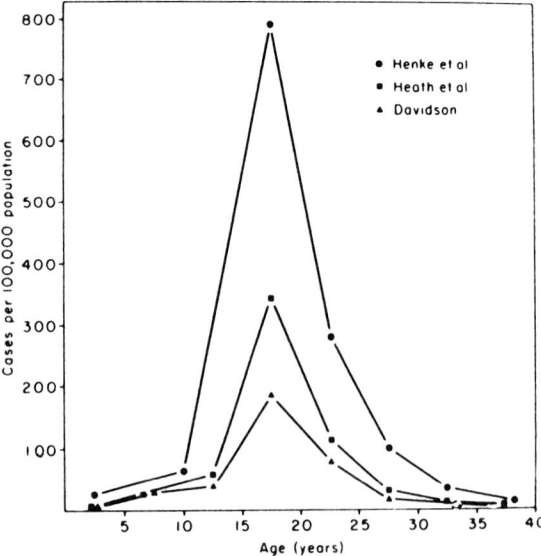

Figure 10–2. Incidence of infectious mononucleosis by age in the general population. Data compiled from three studies. (Reproduced from Straus, S., and Fleisher, T. Infective mononucleosis epidemiology and pathogenesis. In: Schlossberg, D.: Infectious Mononucleosis. 2nd ed., New York: Springer-Verlag, 1989.)

infectious mononucleosis are quite rare and generally are linked to severe hepatitis, encephalitis, or splenic rupture. Splenic enlargement can develop so rapidly that either spontaneous rupture or capsular tearing after minor trauma can occur. To minimize the likelihood of splenic injury, repeated palpation of the left upper quadrant is contraindicated, and mononucleosis patients should be cautioned to avoid strenuous sports until spleen size has normalized.

Patients with EBV mononucleosis are best treated with supportive measures only. Bed rest until fatigue subsides is needed, and patients are usually so tired that compliance is guaranteed. Aspirin or acetaminophen will control fever and headache. Antibiotics are not indicated unless a coincident bacterial infection, such as streptococcal pharyngitis, is documented. Corticosteroids can blunt the degree of lymph node enlargement, but do not shorten the duration of illness; steroids should be reserved for the rare patients with massive adenopathy that compromises the airway, severe cytopenias, or evidence of severe visceral damage. Acyclovir is active against EBV *in vitro,* but little effect *in vivo* beyond a transient reduction in the concentration of salivary virus. Following infectious mononucleosis, immunity to reinfection is established, so verified recurrent EBV mononucleosis is a rarity.

During acute infectious mononucleosis, absolute lymphocytosis with up to 20% atypical lymphocytes circulating in the peripheral blood is common. Despite active EBV production in infected B cells, however, virus can be detected only in 1–2% of circulating lymphocytes. The majority of the abnormal cells in the peripheral blood are a clone of EBV-specific cytotoxic T cells which emerge after several days of infection as the result of the host's cell-mediated immune response targeted against the EBV-infected B-lymphocyte population. Activated CD4 lymphocytes and natural killer cells also contribute to the circulating atypical mononuclear cell population (Fig. 10–3). Lymph node histopathology reflects this dramatic confrontation between infected B cells and cytotoxic T cells. Reactive follicular hyperplasia of nodal germinal centers indicates EBV-induced B-cell proliferation. The interfollicular and paracortical zones of the node also can be distorted by the expanding clone of cytotoxic T cells. Lymph nodes may contain cells with such cytologic atypia that histologic confusion with Hodgkin's lymphoma can arise.

Natural killer cells, which do not require prior sensitization to EBV antigen, also are part of the host response in infectious mononucleosis, and they contribute immediately and nonspecifically to the elimination of virus-infected cells. Synergistic activity between natural killer cells and interferon released by infected cells has been postulated, and antibody-dependent, cell-mediated cytotoxicity also is an accessory in curtailing acute infection. However, the cytotoxic T-cell population is the most important element in terminating EBV B-cell proliferation. Following a successful composite cell-mediated immune response, constitutional symptoms subside in parallel with the regression of lymphadenopathy, and memory T cells which specifically recognize EBV appear and persist.

The polyclonal B-lymphocyte proliferation of EBV mononucleosis generates a variety of odd autoantibodies, which for the most part are not linked to secondary clinical complications. Transient neutropenia and mild thrombocytopenia occur often, as does a positive direct Coombs' test. Cold-reacting, low-titer IgM anti-i antibody (cold agglutinin) is found in up to two thirds of mononucleosis patients, but hemolytic anemia is seen in fewer than 5%. Immune complexes, antinuclear antibody, rheumatoid factor, and several other low-titer autoantibodies can develop but have no consistent connection with rheumatic symptoms during the acute course of mononucleosis or with the secondary development of a persistent collagen vascular disease.

Since EBV is a herpesvirus, it also has the ability to persist as a latent infection, with its viral genome incorporated as an episome fragment in the nuclei of a small percentage of B lymphocytes. From this dormant state, episodic asymptomatic reactivation occurs; at any time as many as 20% of young healthy adults in the United States shed Epstein-Barr virions into their saliva, ensuring an ongoing supply of virus to infect the seronegative members of society. Transfusion-associated cases of EBV mononucleosis are also well recognized and have been traced to the presence of infectious virions in circulating white blood cells of healthy blood donors.

Individuals who have an impaired cell-mediated immune response to viral infection may experience especially severe primary EBV infection, exhibit an inability to maintain EBV in a latent state, or suffer uncontrolled malignant lymphoproliferative complications. X-linked lymphoproliferative syndrome (Duncan's syndrome) patients have a genetic aberration with a selectively defective response to EBV infection. Severe or fatal infectious mononucleosis is

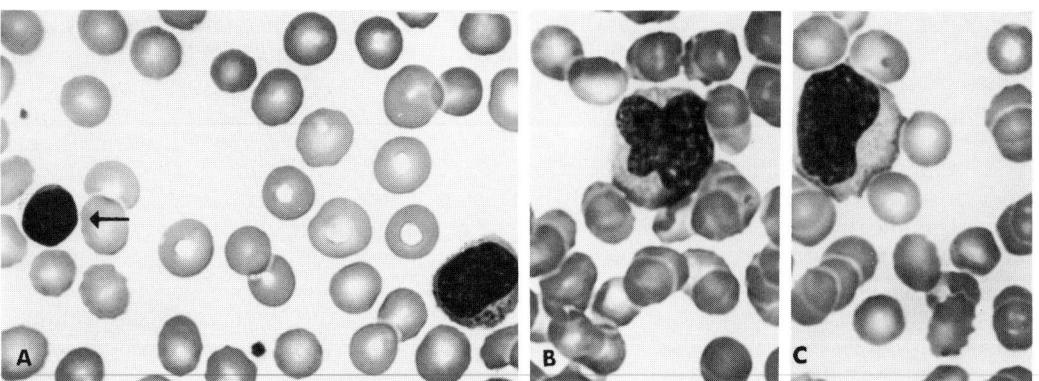

Figure 10–3. Atypical mononuclear cells from the peripheral blood of a patient with serologically proven EBV mononucleosis. White blood cell count 18,200/mm³, 26% atypical lymphocytes. Wright-Giemsa stain, 1000 × (oil) magnification. A. Lymphocyte with enlarged ovoid nucleus and prominent cytoplasmic granules. Normal small lymphocyte (arrow) for size comparison. B. Abnormal lymphocyte with irregular lobulated nucleus. C. Large atypical lymphocyte with irregular cell contour; cytoplasmic membrane is fragile and easily indented by adjacent erythrocytes.

seen in two thirds of these patients, and profound secondary hypogammaglobulinemia or B-cell malignancies occur in the remainder. Ataxia-telangiectasia patients, who have a combined T- and B-cell immunodeficiency, and patients being treated with immunosuppressives may develop EBV-associated B-cell proliferative disease. HIV-induced helper T-lymphocyte depletion has caused several EBV-linked diseases in AIDS patients, including hairy leukoplakia, lymphoid interstitial pneumonitis, malignant lymphoma, and colonic lymphoid hyperplasia. The oncogenic role of EBV in African (Burkitt's) lymphoma is well established, and its association with nasopharyngeal carcinoma continues to be actively investigated.

Serologic Diagnosis of Infectious Mononucleosis

EBV is not easily cultivated in standard tissue culture cell lines. Also, since recovery of virus by culture does not differentiate primary infection from latently reactivated EBV, serology is the only feasible laboratory approach for diagnosing mononucleosis.

The serologic response to EBV infection includes the production of antibodies to specific EBV antigens as well as the generation of a variety of heterophil antibodies. Heterophil antibodies can be detected in the serum of mononucleosis patients within 1 week of onset of symptoms and are IgM-class antibodies which recognize antigens found in sheep, horse, or beef erythrocytes. These heterophil antibodies are not directed against any of the known Epstein-Barr antigens and there is no prior sensitization with nonhuman red blood cells to explain their development. EBV-induced polyclonal B-lymphocyte proliferation is linked to production of these bizarre immunoglobulins. Heterophil antibodies are not unique to infectious mononucleosis; they can develop in serum sickness and occasionally in other viral infections. However, heterophil antibodies with strong affinity for beef erythrocytes unaffected by adsorption with guinea pig kidney antigen (the differential absorption test) can differentiate acute EBV infection from these other uncommon causes.

Heterophil antibodies associated with infectious mononucleosis can be rapidly and inexpensively identified by mixing patient serum with bovine or equine red blood cells and observing direct hemagglutination, or by a latex agglutination method with bovine erythrocyte membrane antigen bound to latex particles (the so-called mono-spot test). Both assays are highly specific as screening tools of EBV-induced heterophil antibody; false-positive results are encountered occasionally in leukemia, lymphoma, rheumatoid arthritis, and hepatitis, but represent less than 1% of positive assays. The major drawback with heterophil antibody testing, however, is its insensitivity; heterophil antibodies are found in only approximately 80% of adolescent and adult patients with primary EBV infection and are found in less than 25% of cases in young children. Therefore, more sensitive serologic assays are needed to evaluate mononucleosis cases which are heterophil antibody-negative.

The specific serologic response to EBV infection is complex but logical once the evolution of EBV antigens from the initial active lytic phase of infection through the latent stage of infection is understood. Immediately after EBV enters B lymphocytes, the synthesis of EBV nuclear antigen (EBNA) occurs, followed by EBV-induced antigen changes in the lymphocyte cell membrane (lymphocyte-detected membrane antigen, LYDMA). Shortly thereafter, EBV early antigen (EA) is expressed in the infected cell. EBNA, LYDMA, and EA are crucial elements in the synthesis of EBV; however, none are structural antigens found in the EB virion. As EBV begins DNA replication, viral capsid antigen (VCA) is also manufactured. VCA is a necessary structural component of the protein capsid which surrounds and protects the viral DNA. Lymphocyte membrane antigen (MA) then appears in the infected cell and facilitates the release of the newly assembled infectious EB virion. The entire cycle of lytic (i.e., virus-productive) infection culminates in the establishment of an immortalized, transformed, self-replicating population of proliferating B cells. Even with an effective natural killer cell and cytotoxic T-lymphocyte immune response, a small percentage of EBV-immortalized B lymphocytes escape destruction and retain the virus indefinitely in a latent (nonproductive) state. In this permanent carrier phase of infection, the EBV genome is present in the cell nucleus in an episomal fragment; it is replicated along with the host nucleus and is associated with the production of EBNA and Epstein-Barr LYDMA. Latency is a characteristic of all herpesviruses, but the cellular events which arrest virus in dormancy, maintain dormancy, or which allow latent virus to reemerge as active virus are not known. All latently infected healthy adults exhibit episodic asymptomatic shedding of EBV in the saliva from reactivated viral infection. In severely immunocompromised individuals, EBV can be recovered from saliva almost all of the time.

The complicated sequence of EBV antigens and the patient's immune response produce characteristic antibody profiles which help define the stage of infection. Individuals who have never been infected with EBV lack heterophil antibody as well as all EBV-specific antibodies. In acute infectious mononucleosis, by the time that symptoms and atypical lymphocytosis have developed, patients have IgM heterophil antibody as well as IgM antibody against VCA and high titers of IgG against VCA. IgG antibody to EA is also present but IgG antibody against

EBNA is absent while acute symptoms persist. Both heterophil and VCA IgM become undetectable shortly after symptomatic illness resolves; however, IgG against EBNA then develops and along with VCA IgG persists as a lifelong serologic marker of EBV infection.

Silent primary EBV infection may produce only weak, transient heterophil and VCA IgM titers; however, VCA IgG and EBNA IgG remain as serologic evidence of infection. Individuals who are immunocompromised, with poor T-cell performance and persistently reactivated EBV infections, may exhibit atypical antibody profiles which reflect these sustained episodes of active EBV synthesis. High titers of VCA IgG and EA IgG can develop and variably positive heterophil, VCA IgM, and EBNA antibody can also be seen. The antibody patterns encountered in EBV-associated disease states are summarized in Table 10–3.

Mononucleosis Syndromes

EBV is the most common cause of infectious mononucleosis and is responsible for up to 80% of cases. However, a significant minority of patients with a clinical illness typical of mononucleosis lack heterophil antibody or VCA IgM antibody to verify EBV as the cause. These non-EBV, febrile, lymphoproliferative illnesses are collectively classified as the mononucleosis syndrome and have been linked to a diverse list of infectious agents (see Table 10–1). *Primary cytomegalovirus (CMV) infection,* particularly when acquired after childhood, can produce a systemic illness with pharyngitis, widespread lymphadenopathy, and fever. Evidence of mild hepatocellular necrosis is not unusual, but atyp-

TABLE 10–3. *EBV Serologic Profiles*

	Heterophil Antibody IgM	VCA IgM	VCA IgG	EA IgG	EBNA IgG
Never infected	−	−	−	−	−
Silent primary infection	+/−	+	+	+/−	−
Infectious mononucleosis	+	+	+ +	+	−
Past infection	−	−	+	+/−	+
Immunodeficient patient, reactivated infection	+/−	+/−	+ +	+ +	+/−

−: No antibody +: Positive antibody + +: Elevated antibody titer

Data adapted from Okano M., et al. Epstein-Barr virus and human diseases: Recent advances in diagnosis. *Clin. Microbiol. Rev.* 1:300–312, 1988.

ical lymphocytosis is less dramatic than with EBV infection. CMV can usually be isolated from urine during acute illness, and serum contains IgM CMV-specific antibody. CMV mononucleosis follows a clinical course quite similar to EBV-induced disease, with complete resolution of symptoms by 3–6 weeks.

Acute *Toxoplasma gondii* lymphadenitis can also mimic EBV mononucleosis. Toxoplasma infection can be acquired from contact with infected domestic pets (almost exclusively cats) that are shedding oocysts from colonized intestinal mucosa or from the ingestion of improperly cooked meat, particularly lamb or pork, that contains toxoplasma bradyzoites encysted in skeletal muscle. Following ingestion of either the oocyst or bradyzoite form, toxoplasma invades the blood, proliferates as a facultative intracellular parasite, disseminates systemically, and produces fever and lymphadenopathy reminiscent of mononucleosis. Pharyngitis is not pronounced, however, and atypical lymphocytes are uncommon in the peripheral circulation. Toxoplasma culture requires inoculation of susceptible rodents with patient blood or tissue and is technically too complex for routine use, but acute toxoplasmosis can be accurately diagnosed by demonstrating a high specific IgM titer or a significant rise in IgG titer by either indirect immunofluorescent or ELISA assays.

Human herpesvirus 6 (HHV-6) is the most recently characterized member of the herpes family, and like EBV, is a lymphotropic virus which provokes cellular transformation of infected B lymphocytes. HHV-6 has been established as the cause of roseola infantum, a common childhood febrile maculopapular exanthem, and because of its ability to replicate in B cells, not surprisingly, a connection to mononucleosis has also been identified. Evaluation of patients with mild mononucleosis-like illness but no serologic evidence of acute EBV, CMV, toxoplasma, or hepatitis B virus infection shows that approximately one third have demonstrable IgM specific for HHV-6, often accompanied by a fourfold rise in specific IgG titer as well. In most cases, a 1–3-week-long febrile illness with mild pharyngitis and cervical adenopathy is described. Lymphocytosis with atypical lymphocytes in the peripheral blood is common, and abnormal liver function studies implying hepatocyte necrosis may also be present.

Acute infection with *human immunodeficiency virus 1* (HIV-1) has also been associated with an illness that has clinical features indistinguishable from EBV infectious mononucleosis. Although acquisition of HIV-1 is generally regarded as an asymptomatic event, there are now many reports of a multisystem illness with fever, lymphadenopathy, atypical lymphocytosis, mild hepatic necrosis, and, occasionally, meningoencephalitis that can be traced to acute HIV infection. Case reports in health care workers with specific exposure dates delineate a 3–8-week incubation period prior to the onset of mononucleosis symptoms. Standard ELISA HIV serology often is falsely negative in this early phase of illness. HIV antigen can be detected in serum, however, and ELISA, Western blot, and IFA serologic methods are invariably positive for HIV antibody upon repeat testing 2–3 months later. Mononucleosis seems to coincide with seroconversion, and with the exception of occasional neurologic deficits, patients usually become asymptomatic in 1–4 weeks. Although mononucleosis associated with acute HIV infection is not an AIDS-defining illness, it remains to be seen whether progression of disease in these patients differs significantly from that in patients whose seroconversion is asymptomatic.

Figure 10–4 shows an algorithmic approach for the serologic work-up of a patient with acute mononucleosis symptoms. Because heterophil antibody testing is widely available, well standardized, and inexpensive and can identify EBV as the cause of disease in at least 70–80% of cases, it is the logical first step in laboratory evaluation. In mononucleosis with a negative heterophil antibody, EBV is still found to be the cause in nearly half the cases, and VCA IgM is the serologic test of choice for verification. For mononucleosis patients who have no evidence of acute EBV disease, a variety of miscellaneous possibilities remain. Both toxoplasma and CMV IgM assays are widely available, but serologic testing for HHV-6 is limited principally to research laboratories. Antigen and antibody assays for acute HIV are appropriate only for patients with a reasonable history of exposure risk.

A minority of mononucleosis cases have no etiologic agent identified by the serologic procedures described, but symptoms subside over a 2–4-week period, suggesting an infectious cause. Rarely, rubella, adenovirus, and HSV are shown to cause heterophil-negative mononucleosis. Dilantin also has been linked to a benign febrile lymphoproliferative disease that clinically can mimic mononucleosis. Lymphoma, both Hodgkin's and non-Hodgkin's types, can

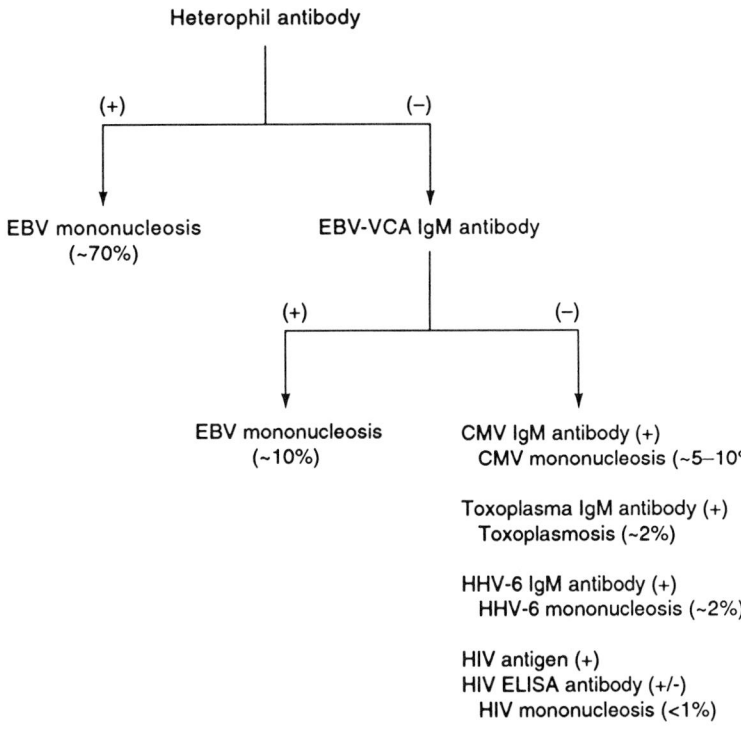

Figure 10–4. Algorithm for serologic evaluation of a patient with acute mononucleosis symptoms. Numbers in parentheses are the approximate percentages of patients who have a specific diagnosis established by serologic testing.

have features which resemble mononucleosis early in the course of disease before malignancy is verified by biopsy.

CHRONIC FATIGUE SYNDROME

In the past 5 years, considerable attention has been given in the medical and lay press to a chronic clinical entity characterized principally by disabling persistent fatigue. Fever, pharyngitis, tender lymphadenopathy, arthralgias, and myalgias are frequent accompanying complaints, but severe, almost incapacitating lethargy is the shared symptom in virtually all cases. The clinical aspects of this illness imply an infectious etiology, and initial reports suggested that EBV, either as a chronically persistent primary infection or as a reactivated infection, might be the cause, since afflicted patients had high titers to both EBV, VCA and EA.

Predictable confusion followed these preliminary studies due in part to difficulty reproducing serologic data and also due to wide variation in clinical criteria for defining this illness. Ultimately, a consensus was reached on a working case definition of chronic fatigue syndrome, a major criterion of which is new onset of debili-

tating fatigue sufficiently severe to reduce the patient's normal activity level by at least half for a period of at least 6 months. Thorough evaluation was also required to rule out occult malignancy, autoimmune disease, subacute or chronic infection, endocrine disease, or neuromuscular and psychiatric disorders. Fever, pharyngitis, adenopathy, myalgia and arthralgia, and neuropsychologic complaints were given minor criteria status. Diagnosis of this disorder, therefore, is defined entirely by signs and symptoms. No etiologic agent has been clearly identified and the choice of the name *chronic fatigue syndrome* underscores the fact that this illness may not necessarily be a single disease and may have several causes.

A study with EBV culture and EBV *in situ* hybridization on saliva and peripheral leukocytes showed no difference between chronic fatigue patients and normal controls. Acyclovir, which inhibits productive EBV replication, was no more effective than placebo in alleviating symptoms of chronic fatigue syndrome, further discounting the importance of EBV as the cause. When carefully performed with verified reproducibility and precision, serologic titers for EBV VCA, EA, and EBNA were similar for both chronic fatigue cases and controls. While several studies have suggested an etiologic role for CMV, toxoplasma, human herpesvirus-6, or human immunodeficiency virus, serologic findings have been inconclusive or have shown no significant differences between chronic fatigue patients and matched controls. To date, there is no agent accepted by consensus as the sole cause or even as a contributory cause for this syndrome.

Despite failures to identify a causative agent(s) for chronic fatigue syndrome, immunologic characterization of these patients has shown aberrations which imply a chronic viral reactivation state. Reports of increased numbers of natural killer cells but decreased natural killer cell function, decreased *in vitro* lymphoproliferative responses to phytohemagglutinin and pokeweed mitogen stimulation and depressed gamma interferon production do suggest suppressed cell-mediated immunity; however, there is widespread disagreement about absolute numbers, percentages, and ratios for helper T lymphocytes (CD4) and suppressor T lymphocytes (CD8) in chronic fatigue syndrome. Therefore, before any immunologic abnormalities are accepted as representative of this disorder, methodologic variability and problems with reproducibility should be resolved.

Patients who are disabled with chronic fatigue deserve a thorough evaluation to rule out the diagnosable and treatable disorders which may explain their incapacitated states. However, in the absence of neurologic, endocrine, autoimmune, or malignant disease, continued laboratory studies generate unnecessary medical bills but rarely a diagnosis.

CASE HISTORY 1

An 18-year-old college freshman was seen at the student health clinic on a Monday morning in early November complaining of malaise and fever. She stated that 5 days earlier, during a moderately strenuous physical education class, she first became aware of a marked reduction in her usual level of energy. During subsequent classes that day she felt quite tired and had difficulty staying alert and attentive. She returned to her dorm room for a late afternoon nap (an atypical event in her busy college routine) and ended up sleeping for 4 hours—right through supper and a planned evening study session. Upon awakening, she did not feel refreshed, and after reading for little more than 1 hour, went back to bed exhausted. The following morning she had little appetite for breakfast and still felt weary and inattentive despite two cups of strong tea. By evening a mild sore throat had developed, but no cough, rhinitis, or difficulty swallowing. A friend, who was in pre-med, took her temperature (100.6°F, oral) and then gave her Tylenol and cough drops. Over the subsequent 3 days she remained feverish and confined to bed, sleeping for up to 16 h daily.

She had no nausea, vomiting, diarrhea, or abdominal pain, and no dysuria or flank pain. She was not sexually active and none of her close friends had been ill. The patient grew up in rural South Dakota and was the second oldest in a family of nine children. She had experienced the usual childhood illnesses and had had a complete immunization series. She had had several episodes of "strep throat" during grammar school and high school, but never had "mono." She had no chronic medical problems and was taking no medications other than acetaminophen. She sporadically drank modest amounts of alcohol, but had never used recreational drugs.

Physical examination demonstrated a young female who did indeed appear tired and listless. Oral temperature was 100.4°F; other vital signs were normal. Inspection of the oropharynx showed modest enlargement of the tonsils with hyperemia of the pharynx; there were no petechiae, vesicles, ulceration, or mucosal exudates. There was moderate, nontender anterior and posterior cervical lymphadenopathy, with the largest detectable lymph node measuring about 1.5 cm in maximal dimension. Axillary and inguinal lymph nodes were nonpalpable. Lungs were clear to auscultation, and cardiac exam was normal. The abdomen was soft and nontender, and there was no appreciable hepatomegaly or splenomegaly.

The health service physician believed that this case exhibited many features consistent with infectious mononucleosis and obtained blood for a peripheral smear and heterophil antibody screen. A modified Giemsa-stained peripheral smear, however, did not suggest lymphocytosis or a left shift in the neutrophil series; atypical lymphocytes accounted for only 2% of the white blood cells present; RBCs and platelets were not remarkable. A rapid latex agglutination test for heterophil antibodies was negative. Results from both tests were available in 1.25 h.

At this point, the physician took a throat culture for *Streptococcus pyogenes* (beta-hemolytic strep, group A); he vigorously swabbed the posterior pharynx and tonsils, and then rolled the cotton swab tip across one quadrant of a blood agar plate. The blood agar plate was sent to a microbiology laboratory for further incubation.

The patient was asked to contact the health service office in 2 days for results of the throat culture, at which time antibiotics would be prescribed if *S. pyogenes* had been isolated. She was instructed to rest, maintain a good fluid intake and take acetaminophen for temperature elevations above 100°F. After 48 h of incubation, the throat culture showed only normal flora. The patient returned to the health service, still complaining of disabling fatigue. She had persistent low-grade fever and physical examination was unchanged. Urinalysis showed no pyuria, bacteriuria, or hematuria. An additional blood sample was obtained for a serology profile, which included tests for specific IgG and IgM antibodies for the most common causes of mononucleosis: Epstein-Barr virus VCA, cytomegalovirus, and toxoplasma.

Instructions for supportive care were repeated, and when the patient returned 5 days later, she stated that she had begun to improve somewhat: her sleep requirement had decreased to approximately 10 h/day, pharyngitis had resolved, her appetite had returned to normal, and although she still found studying difficult, she was able to attend several of her classes. Her physician then reviewed the serology results with her, which showed:

EBV VCA	IgG (+) and IgM (−)
CMV	IgG (+) and IgM (+)
Toxoplasma	IgG (−) and IgM (−)

The presence of EBV VCA IgG but the absence of IgM indicated remote infection with EBV, probably an asymptomatic event in early childhood. Lack of IgM antibody to toxoplasma demonstrated that her acute systemic febrile illness was not toxoplasmosis. Primary CMV infection with a mononucleosis-like illness, however, was verified by the presence of IgM antibody specific for CMV.

Her physician explained that she had probably been infected with CMV several weeks earlier in the semester, with exposure most likely via a salivary route. Since her initial CMV infection had occurred past childhood, it was not surprising that she developed a symptomatic illness; primary CMV infection in this setting commonly leads to mononucleosis. She was advised that her illness was benign and self-limiting and that no serious complications or sequelae were likely to occur. The patient continued to convalesce slowly and, following her return to college after Thanksgiving break, was back to her normal level of physical and academic activity.

CASE HISTORY 2

A pathology resident arrived at the ophthalmology clinic in May complaining of eye pain. He stated that 2 days earlier he noticed an irritating sensation of a foreign body in the left eye, which rapidly progressed to constant, severe pain that was accompanied by diffuse, conjunctival hyperemia and excessive tearing. The pain was sufficiently severe that he had difficulty sleeping, and the discomfort intensified in bright light. He was unable to identify a foreign body by self-inspection. Use of topical over-the-counter eyedrops had produced no relief. He was married and had two preschool-aged children who were quite healthy, and except for this illness, the patient had also been in excellent health.

He had a low-grade fever (100.2°F), and vital signs were otherwise normal. Ocular examination showed unilateral conjunctivitis; blood vessels were so congested that a diffuse reddening was apparent throughout the palpebral conjunctiva and extended to the entire bulbar conjunctiva. Faint, submucosal nodules were apparent through the conjunctival membrane of the lower lid, and there was a modest accumulation of thin, yellow exudate near the inner canthus. The cornea, anterior chamber, vitreous, and retina were unremarkable.

Scrapings of the conjunctival surface were obtained and were smeared onto two slides for Gram's and Giemsa stains. Many neutrophils were apparent; however, only an insignificant number of bacteria were seen, and the conjunctival epithelial cells lacked both chlamydial and viral inclusions. Additional scrapings were obtained for routine bacterial and viral cultures. No topical antibiotics were prescribed; the closed eye was covered with a gauze patch, and the patient was scheduled to return to the clinic in 3 days. He was told he most probably had an infectious conjunctivitis, and was reminded to wash his hands frequently to minimize the likelihood of spread.

The bacterial culture grew only a few colonies of *Staphylococcus epidermidis*. The specimen for virus culture had been inoculated into monolayer tubes for standard tissue culture as well as into shell vials with MRC-5 fibroblast monolayers. After 48 h, one MRC-5 shell vial monolayer that was stained with a fluorescein-conjugated antibody to adenovirus was positive for adenovirus antigen. Two days later, the fibroblast monolayer in the standard tissue culture tube also showed cytopathic changes consistent with adenovirus growth.

Reevaluation of the patient 3 days after the initial visit showed moderate improvement in the degree of conjunctivitis. However, the patient stated that he had also developed moderate sore throat and had remained febrile (temperature never exceeding 101°F.). He also mentioned that 3 days before the onset of his ocular symptoms he had performed an autopsy on an elderly patient who had died with a fulminant, poorly characterized pneumonia. He had not worn eyeglasses or protective goggles during the autopsy, and while dissecting the lungs he accidentally splashed his eye with water from the morgue table. Adenovirus was subsequently cultured from the autopsied lung, and pulmonary histopathology was quite consistent with adenovirus pneumonia. Serotyping was not performed on either the autopsy adenovirus isolate or on the patient's conjunctival isolate.

One week later, the patient's conjunctivitis had completely resolved, as had the pharyngitis and low-grade fever. This physician had an adenovirus infection which began with accidental inoculation of the eye; subsequent spread of the virus via the nasolacrimal duct also infected the pharynx. Although this patient had only upper respiratory tract involvement, this case also demonstrates the wide anatomic distribution of cells from the eye, through the pharynx and down into the lung, which can be infected with adenovirus.

REFERENCES

Books

Feigin, R. D., and Cherry, J. D., eds. *Textbook of Pediatric Infectious Diseases*. 2nd ed. Volumes I and II. Philadelphia: W. B. Saunders Co., 1987.

Mandell, G. L., Douglas, R. G. Gordon Jr., and Bennett, E., eds. *Principles and Practice of Infectious Diseases*. 3rd ed. New York: Churchill Livingstone Co., 1990.

Moffet, H. L. *Pediatric Infectious Diseases*. 2nd ed. Philadelphia: J. B. Lippincott Co., 1981.

Schlossberg, D., ed. *Infectious Mononucleosis*. 2nd ed. New York: Springer-Verlag, 1989.

Articles and Chapters

Britton, S., Andersson-Anvret, M., Gergely, P., et al. Epstein-Barr virus immunity and tissue distribution in a fatal case of infectious mononucleosis. *N. Engl. J. Med.* 298:89–92, 1978.

Buchwald, D., Sullivan, J. L., and Komaroff, A. L. Frequency of "chronic active Epstein-Barr virus infection" in a general medical practice. *JAMA* 257:2303–2307, 1987.

Cherry, J. D. Enteroviruses: Polioviruses (poliomyelitis), coxsackieviruses, echoviruses, and enteroviruses. In: Feigin R. D., Cherry J. D., eds. *Textbook of Pediatric Infectious Diseases*. 2nd ed. Philadelphia: W. B. Saunders Co., 1987: pp 1729–1790.

D'Alessio, D. J., Meschievitz, C. K., Peterson, J. A., et al. Short-duration exposure and the transmission of rhinoviral colds. *J. Infect. Dis. 150:*189–194, 1984.

D'Angelo, L., Hierholzer, J. C., Keenlyside, R. A., et al. Pharyngoconjunctival fever caused by adenovirus type 4: Report of a swimming pool-related outbreak with recovery of virus from pool water. *J. Infect. Dis. 140:*42–46, 1979.

Dick, E. C., Hossain, S. U., Mink, K. A., et al. Interruption of transmission of rhinovirus colds among human volunteers using virucidal paper handkerchiefs. *J. Infect. Dis.* 153:352–356, 1986.

Dick, E. C., Jennings, L. C., Mink, K. A., et al. Aerosol transmission of rhinovirus colds. *J. Infect. Dis.* 156:442–448, 1987.

Edwards, K. M., Thompson J., Paolini J., et al. Adenovirus infections in young children. *Pediatrics* 76:420–424, 1985.

Fleisher, G. R. Epstein-Barr virus. In: Belshe, R., ed. *Textbook of Human Virology*. Littleton, MA: PSG Publishing Co., 1984:853–886.

Fleisher, G. R., Collins, M., and Fager, S. Limitations of available tests for diagnosis of infectious mononucleosis. *J. Clin. Microbiol.* 17:619–624, 1983.

Forbes, B. A. Acquisition of cytomegalovirus infection: An update. *Clin. Microbiol. Rev.* 2:204–216, 1989.

Gold, D., Bowden, R., Sixbey, J., et al. Chronic fatigue:

A prospective clinical and virologic study. *JAMA 264*:48–53, 1990.

Grayston, J. T., Kuo, C., Wang, S., et al. A new *Chlamydia psittaci* strain, TWAR, isolated in acute respiratory tract infections. *N. Engl. J. Med. 315*:161–68, 1986.

Hayden, F., Albrecht J., Kaiser, D., et al. Prevention of natural colds by contact prophylaxis with intranasal alpha$_2$-interferon. *N. Engl. J. Med. 314*:71–75, 1986.

Hellinger, W. C., Smith, T. F., Van Scoy, R. E., et al. Chronic fatigue syndrome and the diagnostic utility of antibody to Epstein-Barr virus early antigen. *JAMA 260*:971–973, 1988.

Hendley, J. O., and Gwaltney Jr., J. M. Mechanisms of transmission of rhinovirus infections. *Epidemiol. Rev. 10*:242–258, 1988.

Holmes, G. P., Kaplan, J. E., Gantz, N. M., et al. Chronic fatigue syndrome: A working case definition. *Ann. Intern. Med. 108*:397–399, 1988.

Horwitz, C. A., Henle, W., Henle G., et al. Long-term serological follow-up of patients for Epstein-Barr virus after recovery from infectious mononucleosis. *J. Infect. Dis. 151*:1150–1153, 1985.

Huovinen, P., Lahtonen, R., Ziegler, T., et al. Pharyngitis in adults: The presence and coexistence of viruses and bacterial organisms. *Ann. Intern. Med. 110*:612–616, 1989.

Kesler, H. A., Blaauw, B., Spear, J., et al. Diagnosis of human immunodeficiency virus infection in seronegative homosexuals presenting with an acute viral syndrome. *JAMA 258*:1196–1199, 1987.

Kirov, S. M., Marsden, K. A., Wongwanich, S. Seroepidemiological study of infectious mononucleosis in older patients. *J. Clin. Microbiol. 27*:356–358, 1989.

Klimas, N. G., Salvato, F. R., Morgan, R., et al. Immunologic abnormalities in chronic fatigue syndrome. *J. Clin. Microbiol. 28*:1403–1410, 1990.

Levandowski, R. A., and Rubenis, M. Nosocomial conjunctivitis caused by adenovirus Type 4. *J. Infect. Dis. 143*:28–31, 1981.

Marlin, S. D., Stauton D. E., Springer T. A., et al. A soluble form of intercellular adhesion molecule-1 inhibits rhinovirus infection. *Nature 344*:70–72, 1990.

Matoba, A. Ocular viral infections. *Pediatr. Infect. Dis. 3*:358–368, 1984.

Naclerio, R. M., Proud, D., Kagey-Sobotka, A., et al. Is histamine responsible for the symptoms of rhinovirus colds? A look at the inflammatory mediators following infection. *Pediatr. Infect. Dis. 7*:218–222, 1988.

Okano, M., Theile, G. M., Davis, J. R., et al. Epstein-Barr virus and human diseases: Recent advances in diagnosis. *Clin. Microbiol. Rev. 1*:300–312, 1988.

Okuno, T., Takahashi, K., Balachandra, K., et al. Seroepidemiology of human herpesvirus 6 infection in normal children and adults. *J. Clin. Microbiol. 27*:651–653, 1989.

Pacini D. L., Collier A. M., Henderson F. W. Adenovirus infections and respiratory illness in children in group day care. *J. Infect. Dis. 156*:920–927, 1987.

Reed, B. D., Huck, W., Lutz, L. J., et al. Prevalence of *Chlamydia trachomatis* and *Mycoplasma pneumoniae* in children with and without pharyngitis. *J. Fam. Pract. 26*:387–392, 1988.

Steeper, T. A., Horwitz, C. A., Ablashi, D. V., et al. The spectrum of clinical and laboratory findings due to human herpesvirus 6 (HHV-6) in patients with mononucleosislike illnesses not due to EBV or CMV. *Am. J. Clin. Pathol. 93*:776–783, 1990.

Steeper, T. A., Horwitz, C. A., Hanson, M., et al. Heterophil-negative mononucleosis-like illnesses with atypical lymphocytosis in patients undergoing seroconversions to the human immunodeficiency virus. *Am. J. Clin. Pathol. 89*:169–174, 1988.

Straus, S. E., Dale J. K., Tobi M., et al. Acyclovir treatment of the chronic fatigue syndrome: Lack of efficacy in a placebo-controlled trial. *N. Engl. J. Med. 319*:1692–1698, 1988.

Sumaya, C. V., and Ench, Y. Epstein-Barr virus mononucleosis in children. II. Heterophil antibodies and viral specific responses. *Pediatrics 75*:1011–1019, 1985.

Szilagyi, P. G. Viruses and the common cold. *Pediatr. Virol. 5*(3):1–4, 1990.

Tindall B., Barker S., Donovan B., et al. Characterization of the acute clinical illness associated with human immunodeficiency virus infection. *Arch. Intern. Med. 148*:945–949, 1988.

Turner, B. R., Hendley, J. O., and Gwaltney, Jr., J. M. Shedding of infected ciliated epithelial cells in rhinovirus colds. *J. Infect. Dis. 145*:849–853, 1982.

11 *JAMES L. DUNCAN, D.D.S., Ph.D.*

Dental Infections and Other Diseases of the Oral Cavity

INTRODUCTION

The most common infections of the oral cavity are dental caries and periodontal disease, afflictions that are almost ubiquitous in civilized populations. Caries is a microbial attack that occurs directly on the teeth, whereas periodontal disease involves the supporting structures of the teeth. These diseases are unusual in several respects. First, they are usually long-lasting infections that progress very slowly, often over a period of years. Second, despite the recent emphasis on *Streptococcus mutans* in initiating dental caries, both diseases appear to be the result of mixed infections, with a variety of microorganisms contributing to the disease process. Third, the diseases are not the result of infection by organisms considered foreign to the oral cavity; the agents involved are, in general, found in the mouths of all humans. Fourth, some forms of the diseases are not self-limiting, and in the absence of treatment they often progress until the tooth or its supporting tissues are essentially destroyed.

Ecology of the Oral Cavity

No other area of the body illustrates so well the dynamic interaction occurring between microorganisms and host as does the human oral cavity. The situation is complex because the mouth is frequently exposed to environmental extremes with respect to temperature, pH, viscosity and osmolarity, and chemical composition of the materials taken in. Furthermore, a considerable number of saprophytic organisms enter each day, via food, water, and other substances. Despite these continuous assaults from without, the types of organisms constituting the indigenous microbial flora of the oral cavity generally remain relatively constant, varying, however, with the presence or absence of teeth, in certain oral diseases, and after the administration of certain drugs, such as antibiotics.

A variety of microbial ecosystems can be found in the oral cavity; for example, the composition of the microbial flora found in a deep periodontal pocket differs from that found in superficial dental plaque or on the surface of the tongue. Local environmental factors, such as pH, oxidation–reduction potential (Eh), and availability of appropriate nutrients, account in part for the types of organisms found. An additional characteristic that is important in microbial colonization of both hard and soft oral tissues is that of selective adherence of microorganisms. This phenomenon, as initially emphasized by Gibbons and his colleagues, indicates that organisms can persistently colonize the oral cavity only if they are able to attach to host tissues there; otherwise, they are washed away by the flow of saliva, then swallowed and destroyed. Certain oral microorganisms selectively colonize particular tissue surfaces. For example, *Streptococcus salivarius* is found in high concentrations on the dorsal surface of the tongue, but its numbers on the teeth are very low. *S. mutans,* however, an organism considered to be of prime importance in dental caries, is found in low numbers on the tongue and other mucosal surfaces, but it may constitute a significant proportion of the organisms adhering to the teeth, especially in dental plaque overlying carious lesions.

Most of the organisms that initially adsorb to oral surfaces are thought to desorb subsequently, and only a small proportion of the initially adherent organisms become firmly bound and result in persistent colonization. The adsorption and desorption processes occur continuously, and the number of microorganisms present in the saliva (up to 10^9 organisms per milliliter) is a reflection of the organisms that have become dislodged. In addition, epithelial cells of the oral mucosa containing adherent bacteria are continually desquamated, adding to the complexity of the colonization process. This does not occur on the nonrenewing hard surfaces of the teeth, and, as a result, large numbers of bacteria (up to 10^{11} bacteria per gram wet weight) may accumulate on these structures.

Streptococci are the most prominent group of organisms occurring in the oral cavity, but improvements in anaerobic culture techniques over the past few years have given increasing emphasis to the occurrence of obligate anaerobic bacteria in the mouth. Many of these organisms, including gram-negative rods and spirochetes, can be found in the gingival sulcus, where the oxidation–reduction potential is appropriate for their growth. These bacteria increase in number in periodontal disease, and they have been isolated with increasing frequency from dentoalveolar abscesses.

Host Defense Mechanisms

The oral tissues are continually bathed in a mixture of indigenous microorganisms, and foreign organisms enter the mouth many times each day. In addition, the integrity of the oral mucosa is not infrequently disrupted by traumatic injuries, which may occur during mastication or dental procedures or as the result of accidents. Despite these insults, however, acute infections of the oral tissues are relatively uncommon. This is undoubtedly a reflection of the host defense mechanisms that operate in the mouth.

Mechanical defense processes remove enormous numbers of microorganisms from the oral cavity. These include the flow of saliva, desquamation of the oral mucosa, and the motion of the lips, cheeks, and tongue. The latter process helps cleanse some of the surfaces of the teeth and moves the saliva, desquamated epithelial cells, and microorganisms to the back of the mouth where they are swallowed. Dental caries most frequently develop in areas that are inaccessible to these cleansing effects.

In addition to its physical properties, saliva contains a number of substances that contribute to the host's defenses. These include lysozyme, lactoferrin, an iron-binding protein that deprives some bacteria of essential concentrations of iron, and lactoperoxidase, an enzyme that inhibits the growth of a variety of bacteria, fungi, and viruses, in the presence of the cofactors hydrogen peroxide and thiocyanate. Salivary glycoproteins are known to bind to certain bacteria resulting in aggregation, and this process may prevent the initial attachment of some organisms to the teeth and oral mucosa. The predominant immunoglobulin present in saliva is secretory immunoglobulin A (IgA), produced by the major salivary glands and the numerous minor salivary glands present throughout the oral mucosa. Salivary IgA antibody is thought to contribute to immunity in the oral cavity primarily by interfering with the adherence of microorganisms to oral tissues. This effect, which can be readily demonstrated in *in vitro* models of bacterial adherence, is the basis of some of the vaccines against dental caries that have been tested in experimental animals. Two common inhabitants of the oral cavity, *Streptococcus sanguis* and *S. mitis,* produce a highly specific IgA protease that cleaves immunoglobulins of the IgA1 subclass to yield Fab and Fc fragments. The significance of this protease *in vivo,* however, is unknown.

An additional source of immune elements in the oral cavity is the gingival sulcus. The fluid that seeps into the sulcus from the gingival tissues contains IgG, IgA, and IgM immunoglobulins, complement and other serum proteins, and phagocytic cells, primarily segmented neutrophils. All these components are thought to contribute to normal host defense mechanisms within the gingival tissues and in the gingival sulcus. In addition, they enter the saliva from the sulcus; this process is enhanced when the gingival tissues become inflamed. Although segmented neutrophils as well as macrophages can be found in saliva, many appear to have undergone degenerative changes, and their ability to carry out phagocytic functions is uncertain.

The indigenous flora of the oropharynx may itself contribute to the host's defenses. Alpha-hemolytic streptococci, which are present in large numbers in the oral cavity, are thought to exert an antagonistic effect on the colonization of the oropharynx by *S. pyogenes, S. pneumoniae, Candida albicans,* and other organisms.

DENTAL CARIES

General Considerations

Dental caries is a commonly occurring microbial infection seen most frequently in children and young adults. Caries is usually not a self-limiting disease, and in the absence of treatment, the infection progresses to involve the dental pulp and, in some instances, the tissues surrounding the apex of the tooth. There is no evidence of actively acquired immunity to the disease itself, and recurrence of caries is very common.

Caries attacks the hardest, most calcified tis-

sues of the body, the enamel and dentin of the teeth, and is characterized by an initial demineralization of the inorganic material of these structures, followed by the destruction of their organic components. There have been a number of proposals over the years to explain the etiology of caries, but the most widely accepted theory is one originally proposed by W. D. Miller, a pioneering oral microbiologist. Basically, this view holds that the demineralization of the tooth structure is due to organic acids produced by the fermentation of dietary carbohydrates by bacteria found in the oral cavity. Miller isolated a number of different microorganisms from the oral cavity, many of which were capable of forming lactic acid in amounts sufficient to demineralize teeth. Nearly 100 years later, the bulk of scientific evidence can be said to support Miller's thesis.

Once initiated, caries progresses into the enamel layer of the tooth, where it can be visualized in histologic sections as consisting of an advanced zone of partial decalcification, followed by zones of more complete decalcification, with loss of tooth structure and the pres-

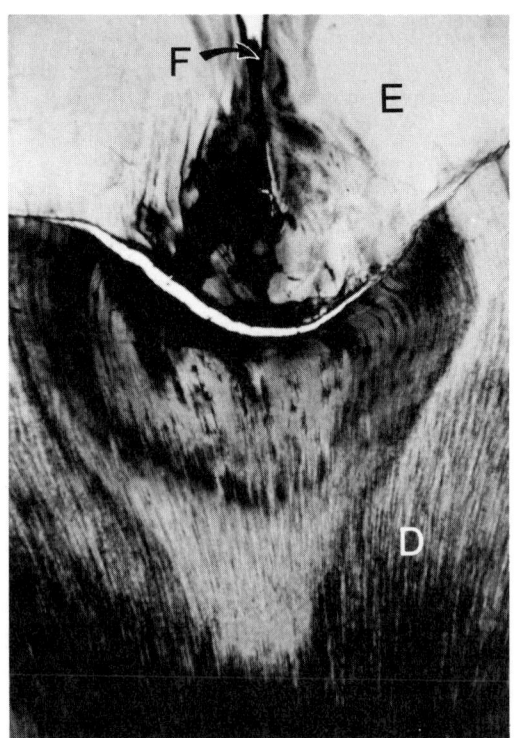

Figure 11–1. Histologic section of a tooth showing the progression of dental caries from an occlusal fissure (F) *through the enamel* (E) *into the dentin* (D). *The lesion spreads laterally at the dentoenamel junction, involving large numbers of dentinal tubules. Zones of decalcification can be seen in the dentin. (Courtesy of Dr. E. Stephen Smith.)*

ence of acidogenic microorganisms (Fig. 11–1). At the dentoenamel junction, the infection spreads laterally to involve large numbers of dentinal tubules. The lesion progresses through the dentin by decalcification of the inorganic components and proteolysis of the organic matrix of the tissue. Microorganisms are readily apparent in the dentinal tubules, and as the infection progresses, the microbial flora is thought to change from predominantly acidogenic organisms to more proteolytic forms, since dentin contains more organic material than does enamel. Dentin is a vital tissue, and in response to the insult and irritation of the advancing lesion, the dentinal tubules may become sealed off by calcification, and additional layers of dentin may be laid down in what might be described as an attempt to wall off the infection. Without treatment, however, the lesion usually progresses to the dental pulp.

Role of Diet and Tooth Morphology in Caries

For caries to occur, appropriate microorganisms, fermentable carbohydrates in the diet, and susceptible sites on the teeth must be present. The microorganisms involved in the caries process will be discussed later. The importance of dietary fermentable carbohydrates in the development of dental caries is supported by a large number of epidemiologic and laboratory studies. An increase in the consumption of sugar results in an increase in the incidence of caries. Sucrose has been found to be an especially important sugar in promoting the disease. It is readily fermented and makes up a large percentage of the carbohydrate consumed in this country. The cariogenicity of carbohydrates in the diet is related not only to the amount consumed but also to the frequency of ingestion and the physical and chemical forms of the sugar.

Caries does not attack the teeth in a uniform manner; rather, there appear to be certain regions on the teeth that are more vulnerable than others. The occlusal surfaces are most frequently affected, and the caries that occurs here is described as *pit and fissure caries* because the process is thought to be initiated as a result of the trapping of food debris and microorganisms in the pits and fissures that are characteristic of these surfaces. These fissures and faults are usually so deep and narrow that they cannot be effectively cleaned during tooth-brushing, and they are often covered by only a thin layer of enamel, so that once caries is initiated, it quickly progresses to involve the underlying dentin of the tooth. Caries also occurs at certain sites on the smooth surfaces of the teeth. *Smooth surface caries* is seen primarily on the interproximal surfaces of the teeth near the point at which they contact the adjacent teeth. Caries in this region is related to the formation of dental plaque, which holds certain microorganisms and their metabolic end products in close contact with the tooth enamel. Smooth surface caries is also found at the cervical region of the teeth, where the gingiva contacts the enamel. Dense, adherent plaque is important in the development of caries in this area as well. *Root surface caries* may develop in elderly people when a portion of the root may be exposed due to receding periodontal tissues. Carious lesions are not seen frequently on other smooth surface areas of the teeth which are more readily cleansed by the movement of lips, cheeks, and tongue and by the flow of saliva. Some teeth are more susceptible to caries than are others. When caries is present, the first and second molars are almost always affected. Caries is seen infrequently on cuspids and mandibular incisors.

Dental Plaque

Plaque is an aggregation of bacteria, extracellular bacterial products, and certain salivary constituents that adheres firmly to the surface of the teeth (Fig. 11–2). It is of primary importance in the development of caries, especially of the smooth surface variety. The accumulation of plaque allows continual contact between acidogenic microorganisms and the enamel surface, where the localized production of lactic acid initiates the destruction of the hydroxyapatite structure of the enamel. Plaque is also thought to be important in the initiation of periodontal disease.

Bacteria make up about two thirds of the bulk of dental plaque, and the number of organisms may be as high as 10^{10} to 10^{11} per gram wet weight of plaque. Intercellular material of bacterial or salivary origin makes up the plaque matrix. The salivary constituents of plaque matrix include acidic glycoproteins that interact with some oral bacteria and mediate their adherence to the teeth. About half the matrix consists of polysaccharides and includes glucans and fructans, products of sucrose metabolism by some of the plaque flora. These polysaccharides, especially the less soluble glucans, are

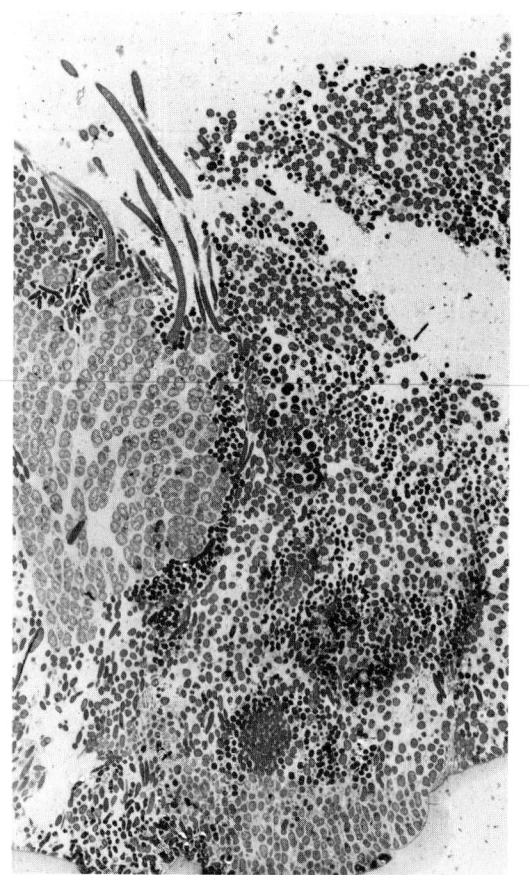

Figure 11–2. Electron micrograph of a thin section from dental plaque. The microbial flora is seen to consist primarily of cocci, although a few rods and filamentous forms are also present (× 1900). (From Lai, C.-H., Listgarten, M. A., and Rosan, B. Immunoelectron microscopic identification and localization of Streptococcus sanguis *with peroxidase-labeled antibody: localization of* Streptococcus sanguis *in intact dental plaque.* Infect. Immun. 11:200, 1975.)

the plaque, its location in the mouth, and even the site on an individual tooth from which it is taken. Plaque overlying carious lesions differs from plaque obtained from noncarious areas of the same tooth. Cariogenic plaque contains high levels of *Streptococcus mutans* compared with noncariogenic plaque, and can be shown to metabolize significantly more sucrose than noncarious plaque, consequently producing higher levels of metabolic end products, including lactic acid.

Bacteriology of Dental Caries

The critical role of microorganisms in dental caries was demonstrated unequivocally in experiments with germ-free rats during the 1950s. Such animals developed no caries even when they were maintained on a cariogenic diet; upon implantation of streptococci, however, dental caries appeared. Studies with gnotobiotic and conventional animals have shown that caries can be initiated by several *Streptococcus, Lactobacillus,* and *Actinomyces* species. The animal model studies as well as clinical and epidemiologic investigations over the past three decades, however, point to one organism as being of primary importance in the initiation of dental caries: *Streptococcus mutans.*

Streptococcus mutans

Over the past 20 years, a voluminous literature dealing with *S. mutans* and its role in caries has accumulated. The organism was first isolated from human carious lesions in 1924 by J. K. Clarke, who suggested that the ability of *S. mutans* to adhere to the surface of teeth was of great importance. Unfortunately, the organism was forgotten for four decades, only to be rediscovered in the 1960s. As the importance of this organism became more apparent, studies of isolates from various sources revealed antigenic differences which were used to separate the organism into eight serotypes (a–h). At the same time, base composition analyses and hybridization studies of DNA from various isolates revealed remarkable heterogeneity. This situation was resolved by designating different genetic groups as species. The mutans streptococcus group now includes seven species: *S. mutans* (serotypes c, e, f); *S. sobrinus* (d, g); *S. cricetus* (a); *S. rattus* (b); *S. ferus* (c); *S. macacae* (c); and *S. downei* (h).

The most common member of this group in

important in maintaining the physical integrity of the plaque.

Studies of plaque formation show that there is an initial adsorption of salivary glycoproteins to the enamel surface, forming a thin, amorphous film called the *acquired pellicle.* Certain oral microorganisms, including streptococci and actinomycetes, selectively adsorb to this material; other bacteria may specifically adhere to previously bound bacteria. Within a few hours, microcolonies and aggregates of bacteria can be observed. As the organisms continue to multiply, some produce extracellular polysaccharide polymers. The microcolonies eventually coalesce to form a continuous mass of bacteria and polysaccharides on the tooth enamel.

Plaque is a heterogeneous material, and the microbial flora and composition of the matrix differs considerably, depending on the age of the human oral cavity is *S. mutans,* serotype c. There is a strong positive correlation between the development of caries and the number of *S. mutans* in plaque; it is virtually always present in cariogenic plaque, often in high numbers, and is absent or present only in low numbers in plaque covering noncarious surfaces of the teeth. The second most common mutans streptococcus in the oral cavity is *S. sobrinus;* the role of this organism in dental caries is less certain. Some human populations harbor *S. rattus* and *S. cricetus,* but these are not common inhabitants of the mouth.

The strong correlation between *S. mutans* and dental caries has led to intensive investigation of the physiologic properties of this organism that may contribute to its virulence. One such property is the ability of *S. mutans* (and *S. sobrinus*) to synthesize polysaccharides. The organism elaborates several glucosyltransferase enzymes, which synthesize polymers of glucose, known as glucans, from sucrose. The glucosyltransferase enzymes are associated with the bacterial cell surface and produce both water-soluble and water-insoluble glucans. Both types of glucan contain branched chains of alpha 1,6- and alpha 1,3-linked glucose units, but the alpha 1,3 linkages predominate in water-insoluble glucan. The sticky, water-insoluble glucan molecules synthesized by *S. mutans* are thought to contribute to plaque development (Fig. 11–3)

and microbial colonization of the smooth surfaces of the teeth. In addition to glucosyltransferases, *S. mutans* also produces fructosyltransferase, which synthesizes fructose polymers from sucrose, and extracellular invertase, which hydrolyzes sucrose to free glucose and fructose.

Another characteristic of *S. mutans* that is thought to play a role in the initiation of caries is the acidogenic and aciduric nature of the organism. *S. mutans* consumes more sucrose than other organisms commonly found in plaque and consequently produces higher levels of lactic acid. In addition, *S. mutans,* unlike most plaque bacteria, remains metabolically active at pH values of 5 which are achieved when plaque is exposed to fermentable carbohydrates.

A third characteristic that may be important in caries is the ability of *S. mutans* to store large amounts of intracellular polysaccharides. These intracellular reserves of carbohydrate may be used as energy sources during times when dietary carbohydrates are not present.

Diagnosis and Treatment

The diagnosis of dental caries on occlusal surfaces of the teeth is made by visual inspection and the use of a sharp-pointed dental explorer, which tends to catch in grooves and fissures in which caries formation has begun. Caries of the

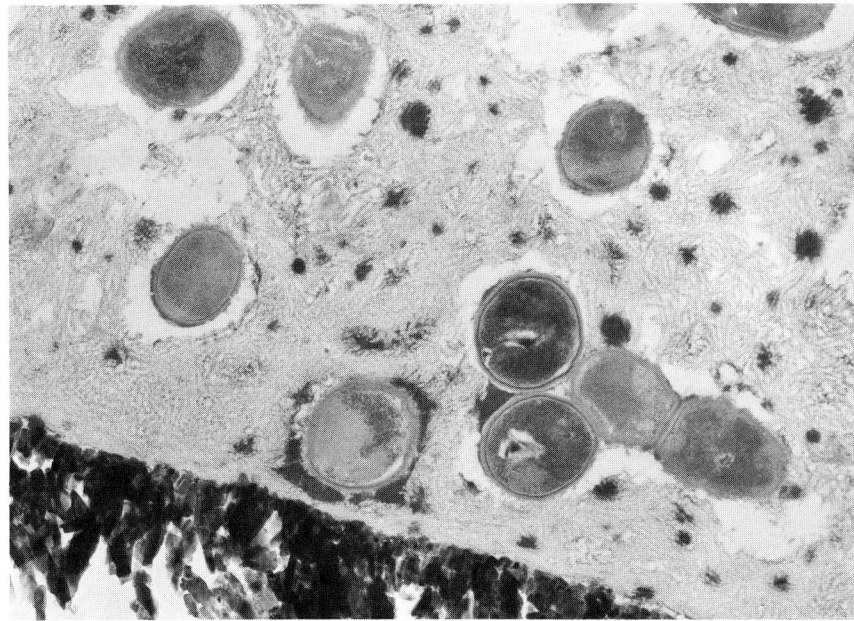

Figure 11–3. Electron micrograph of sectioned Streptococcus mutans *cells attached to extracted human enamel, after growth in a 5% sucrose medium. The microorganisms are enmeshed in an extensive fibrillar matrix of extracellular polysaccharide. (Courtesy of Dr. N. Tinanoff.)*

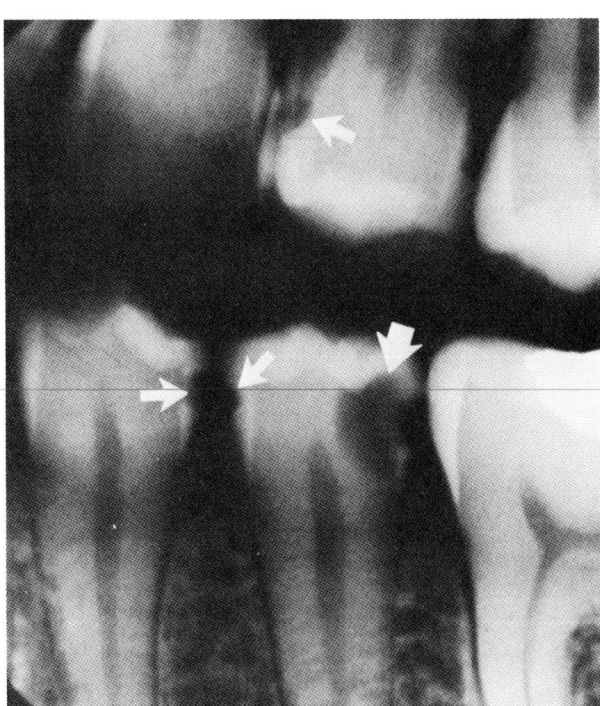

Figure 11–4. Characteristic radiolucent areas (arrows) produced by dental caries on the interproximal surfaces of the teeth. (Courtesy of Dr. E. Stephen Smith.)

interproximal surfaces is usually diagnosed by the characteristic radiolucency seen on radiographs (Fig. 11–4). The treatment of caries is radical in the sense that all the affected tissues are removed mechanically and the tooth structure is replaced by one of several types of inert filling materials.

Prevention

Billions of dollars are spent each year in the United States to restore and replace teeth lost to dental caries. Fortunately, a number of effective, low-cost procedures are available to prevent the disease. Many of these are based on the use of fluorides, either systemically in public water supplies or in topical applications of fluoride in toothpastes, or in gels applied in the dental office. In addition, the use of inert polymers to seal pits and fissures is very effective in preventing caries on occlusal surfaces of the teeth.

The prevalence of dental caries has dramatically declined in the United States and other industrialized countries over the past 20–30 years. Surveys carried out in 1987 indicated that 50% of all children between the ages of 5 and 17 years had no decay in their permanent teeth. Although this decline has been attributed to the increasing availability of fluoride in water and processed foods and in topical applications, large reductions have also occurred in unfluoridated areas in several countries. The reasons for this substantial reduction in tooth decay, which cannot apparently be attributed to fluoridation, are unknown.

INFECTIONS OF THE DENTAL PULP AND PERIAPICAL TISSUES

The dental pulp is a loose connective tissue lined at its periphery by a layer of odontoblasts, specialized cells that are responsible for the formation of dentin. With the exception of the foramen at the apex of the roots of the teeth, the pulp is completely enclosed by the dentin. Cementum overlies the dentin on the root surface, and enamel covers the dentin on the crown of the tooth (Fig. 11–5). Although these calcified tissues protect the pulp, they are unyielding structures and therefore indirectly contribute to the pressure, pain, and tissue necrosis that may be associated with an inflammatory response in the pulp.

The healthy, vital pulp of an intact tooth is nearly always free of microorganisms. There are several routes by which bacteria can infect the dental pulp, but by far the most important is the extension of caries through the enamel and dentin into the pulp chamber. When bacteria

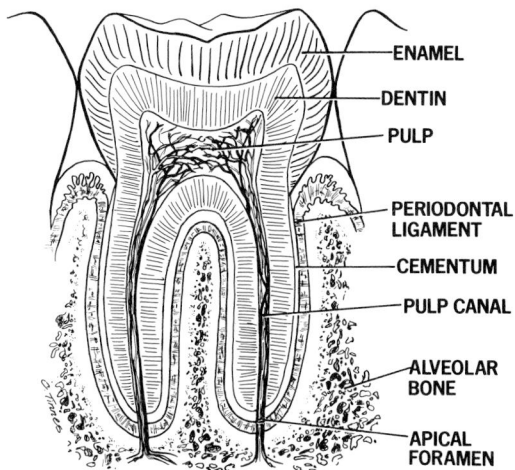

Figure 11–5. Diagrammatic representation of a mandibular molar, illustrating the tooth structures and periodontal tissues.

break through into the pulp chamber, an acute inflammatory response is elicited at the exposure site, and a small abscess, surrounded by segmented neutrophils, develops in the pulp tissue beneath the exposure. The infectious process may then spread so that the entire pulp becomes acutely inflamed, and partial or total necrosis of the pulp tissue may occur. The inability of the pulp to tolerate edema and the lack of significant collateral blood circulation severely limit the ability of the pulp to cope with bacterial invasion and tissue necrosis.

Bacterial infections with degeneration and necrosis of the pulp are sometimes found in teeth that are completely intact, with no evidence of dental caries. This situation is most frequently encountered in adolescents and young people who have suffered a traumatic blow to their anterior teeth. The infection in such cases is thought to occur by a hematogenous route, in which blood-borne bacteria become localized and fixed in the irritated and inflamed pulp tissue. Another possible pathway to the pulp is through the apical foramen at the tip of the root. Bacteria present in periodontal pockets (see further on) may be able to make their way to the apical foramen via the periodontal ligament.

There appears to be little reliable correlation between the histologic status of the pulp and the clinical symptoms that are present (e.g., pain, sensitivity to heat or cold). The determination of whether the pathologic condition of the pulp is reversible is based on clinical findings. A frank, carious exposure of the pulp requires that the pulp tissue be removed and

the pulp chamber and root canals filled with an inert material.

As might be expected, the microorganisms that can be cultured from infected pulps and periapical abscesses consist of bacteria that are found in the oral cavity. In virtually all cases, these are mixed infections. Alpha-hemolytic (viridans) and nonhemolytic streptococci are prominent, but more recent studies carried out under strict anaerobic conditions have emphasized the presence of anaerobes, especially the "black-pigmented" *Bacteroides*. These organisms, which produce black colonies on blood agar, include *B. intermedius, B. endodontalis,* and *B. gingivalis*.

The inflammatory and degenerative processes that occur in the infected pulp may extend through the apical foramen into the surrounding bone of the periapical region (Fig. 11–5). The involvement of the periapical tissues may take several forms. *Chronic apical osteitis* is a relatively asymptomatic condition characterized by the presence of a radiolucent area in the periapical region of a nonvital tooth (Fig. 11–6). Histologically, the lesion may appear as a granuloma, chronic abscess, or cyst. An *acute apical*

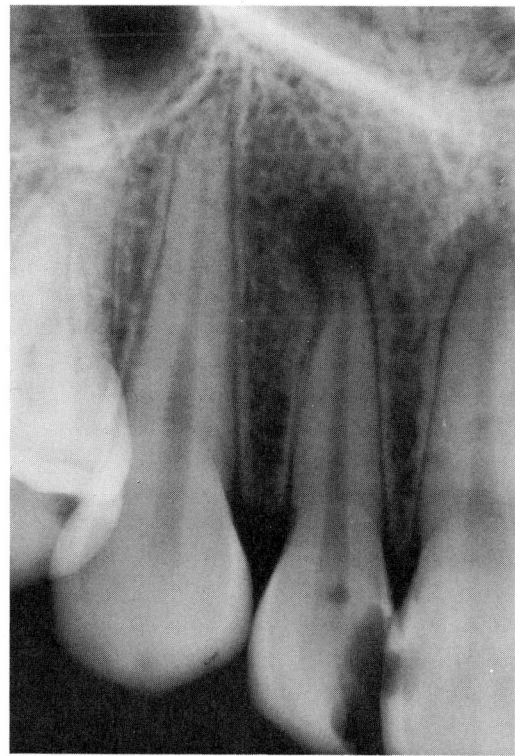

Figure 11–6. Dental radiograph showing a pathologic lesion at the apex of a maxillary lateral incisor. A large carious lesion is present in the crown of the tooth. (Courtesy of Dr. E. Stephen Smith.)

abscess is characterized by an acute inflammatory response with cell destruction and pus formation. Swelling is often present, the pain may be severe, and the tooth is extremely sensitive to percussion and palpation. Often there is no radiographic evidence of pathology; erosion of periapical bone, sufficient to produce a radiolucency in the area, may not have occurred owing to the rapid formation of the abscess.

Apical abscesses may occasionally penetrate the cortical plate of the maxillary or mandibular bone and drain through a fistula into the oral cavity or to the face. On rare occasions, however, the infection extends into fascial spaces of the head and neck. The rapid spread of infection with attendant airway obstruction often makes such an extension a life-threatening situation. Anatomic considerations relative to the affected teeth determine the route of spread along fascial planes. The submaxillary and parapharyngeal spaces are most frequently involved.

PERIODONTAL DISEASE

General Considerations

Diseases of the periodontium affect those tissues that support and anchor the teeth (Figs. 11–5 and 11–7). These include the *gingiva*, the coral-pink-colored mucous membrane that covers and is attached to the alveolar bone and the cervical regions of the teeth; *periodontal ligament*, composed of collagen fibers that are attached to the cementum of the tooth and are inserted into the gingiva, alveolar bone, and cementum of the adjacent teeth; *cementum*, the calcified bonelike structure that covers the dentin of the roots of the teeth; and *alveolar bone*, ridges of maxillary and mandibular bone into which the roots of the teeth are embedded. Although acute infections of the periodontium occur, the disease that is most common and of greatest concern is a chronic inflammatory condition known as periodontal disease. Two forms of this syndrome are recognized; the first, known as *gingivitis*, is seen as an inflammation of the more superficial soft tissues of the periodontium. Gingivitis may remain as a stable, chronic condition for many months or years without further affecting the function of the other periodontal tissues. A more serious form of the disease occurs in some individuals in which the inflammatory process involves not only the gingiva but also the periodontal ligament and alveolar bone. In this

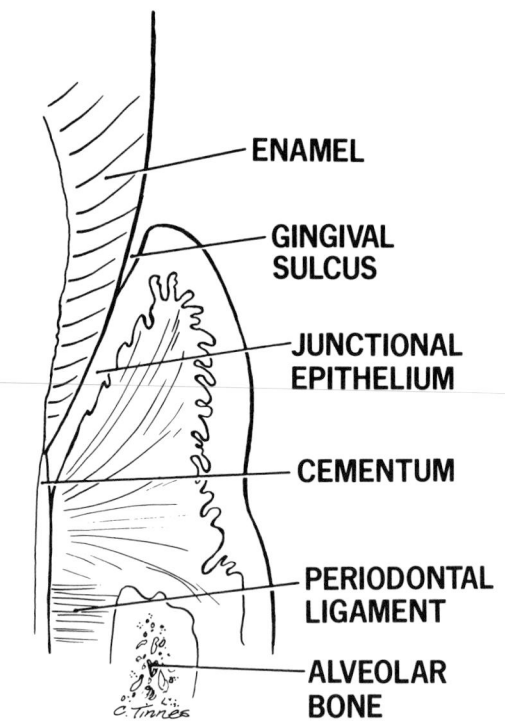

Figure 11–7. Diagrammatic representation of the gingival sulcus region.

condition, known as *periodontitis*, the periodontal ligament is destroyed and alveolar bone is progressively resorbed, resulting in increased mobility and eventual loss of the affected teeth. Periodontitis in adults has traditionally been thought to be a slow but continuous process. However, more recent data suggest that the progression of the disease may be discontinuous, with episodic and relatively brief bursts of tissue destruction at a given site, followed by longer periods of remission and repair.

Periodontal disease involves the gingival sulcus (or crevice) and surrounding tissues; the sulcus and marginal gingiva are unusual because of the unique interface between the humoral and secretory immune systems in this region. The tissues are bathed in crevicular fluid, which contains cellular and soluble humoral immune elements, as well as saliva, which contains secretory IgA. This immunologic feature may be responsible for the relatively low incidence of advanced, destructive periodontitis in the population.

Periodontal disease is said to be a widespread and common affliction, but this statement is a reflection of the common occurrence of gingivitis. Serious, advanced periodontitis is much less frequently seen. Several epidemiologic factors appear to be correlated with risk of periodontal disease, the most important being age and oral hygiene. With increasing age, there is an increase in the number of individuals affected, and a worsening of preexisting periodontal conditions. Microbial plaque, lying in close proximity to the gingival tissues, is thought to be an important factor in the initiation of gingivitis, and clinical studies have shown that after the interruption of oral hygiene measures and the formation of microbial plaque, the clinical manifestations of gingivitis can be observed in about 10 days.

Pathogenesis of Periodontal Disease

Gingivitis

Histopathology. The progressive histopathologic changes that lead to clinically apparent gingivitis (Fig. 11–8) have been described as *initial, early,* and *established* stages, which occur sequentially over a period of 2–3 weeks after the accumulation of microbial plaque. During this process, neutrophils, which are normally present in gingival tissues, are seen to increase in number. Later, macrophages become apparent, and lymphocytes and plasma cells infiltrate into the area. Perivascular collagen loss and alterations in fibroblasts have also been noted. In the established stage of gingivitis, the junctional and crevicular epithelium may begin to migrate toward the apex of the teeth, deepening the gingival sulcus.

Microbial Flora. The flora that can be isolated from the normal gingival sulcus region is com-

TABLE 11–1. *Microbial Flora of the Gingival Sulcus*

Condition	Characteristic Features of the Microbial Flora
Normal	Complex flora, with *Streptococcus, Actinomyces,* and *Veillonella* present in greatest numbers.
Gingivitis	Increased numbers of microorganisms, especially gram-positive, filamentous actinomycetes. Some gram-negative organisms (*Fusobacterium, Bacteroides*) may increase in number.
Advanced periodontitis	Predominantly gram-negative rods, including *Bacteroides, Fusobacterium, Wolinella, Eikenella, Selenomonas, Capnocytophaga, Actinobacillus;* and *Spirochaeta.*

plex, consisting of gram-positive species, primarily *Streptococcus* and *Actinomyces,* as well as some gram-negative species, including *Veillonella.* When plaque formation begins in the area of the marginal gingiva, gram-positive bacteria, mostly streptococci, are observed in a thin layer adhering to the tooth enamel. As the plaque develops over a period of days or weeks, there is an increase in the number of organisms present, reflected primarily as an increase in the numbers of gram-positive filamentous *Actinomyces* species (Table 11–1). With the development of clinical gingivitis, there is also an increase in the number of certain gram-negative organisms in the gingival sulcus, including *Fusobacterium, Bacteroides,* and *Eikenella.* Spirochetes are also present. The complexity of the flora found in the gingival sulcus is illustrated by a study of experimental gingivitis in four subjects, in which 166 bacterial species and subspecies were isolated. The flora became

Figure 11–8. Gingivitis. The marginal gingiva is dark red and inflamed, and its normal regular contour has been lost. Dental plaque and debris are present on the teeth. (Courtesy of Dr. E. Stephen Smith.)

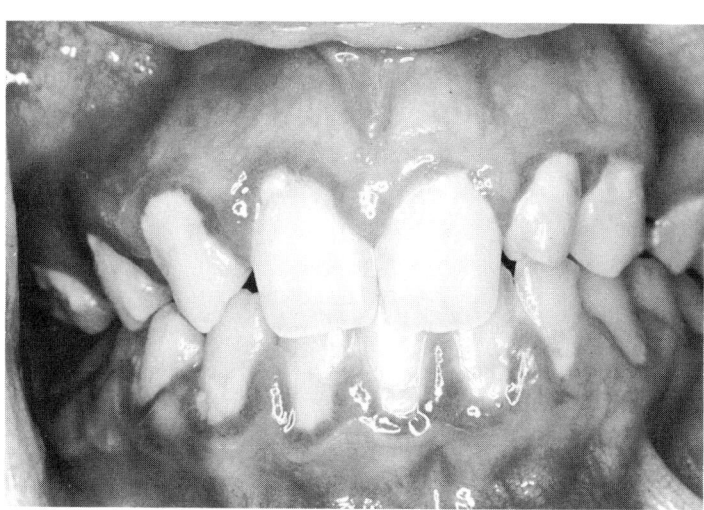

more diverse as gingivitis developed, and sequential colonization by certain species was observed.

Advanced Periodontitis

Histopathology. In a few individuals, gingivitis progresses to the destructive *advanced lesion* of overt periodontitis. Characteristics of chronic inflammatory and immunopathologic damage are seen throughout the tissues. A dense infiltrate of plasma cells, lymphocytes, and macrophages is present, and high concentrations of immunoglobulins and complement are found in the crevicular fluid. The junctional and sulcular epithelium continues to migrate toward the apex of the root of the tooth, forming a *periodontal pocket* between the cementum and the surrounding tissues. These pockets allow a greater accumulation of debris, plaque, and calculus, and suppurative periodontal abscesses may be produced. The periodontal ligament is destroyed, and resorption of alveolar bone is seen (Fig. 11–9). Unless halted, these events result in the loss of the tooth. The microbial and host factors that may contribute to these processes will be discussed later.

Microbial Flora. In contrast to the situation seen in gingivitis, as much as 75% of the bacterial population found in the gingival sulcus region in periodontitis consists of gram-negative organisms, many of which are obligate anaerobes (Table 11–1). Various organisms, including *Bacteroides, Fusobacterium, Wolinella, Eikenella, Selenomonas,* and *Capnocytophaga,* have been isolated from periodontal pockets. Recent studies have emphasized the possible role of black-pigmented *Bacteroides* species, especially an asaccharolytic species, *B. gingivalis.* Spirochetes, including *Treponema denticola,* are also present in greatly increased numbers. The gram-negative organisms appear as a loosely attached band of cells that extends to the apex of the pocket. Spirochetes localize on the outer surface of the plaque, in intimate contact with the epithelium of the gingival sulcus.

Juvenile Periodontitis

Juvenile periodontitis, or *periodontosis,* is an uncommon form of periodontal disease found primarily in young people, especially females. It is a separate disease entity characterized by reduced numbers of bacteria (compared with those observed in adult periodontitis), minimal plaque formation, and less severe inflammation. Nevertheless, the destruction of periodontal tissues that occurs has the same consequences as periodontitis. *Actinobacillus actinomycetemcomitans* (Fig. 11–10), a facultative, gram-negative coccobacillus, may be of particular importance in juvenile periodontitis. This organism is invariably present in relatively high numbers in the disease, and it is known to produce several substances, such as leukotoxin and endotoxin, that may contribute to pathologic processes.

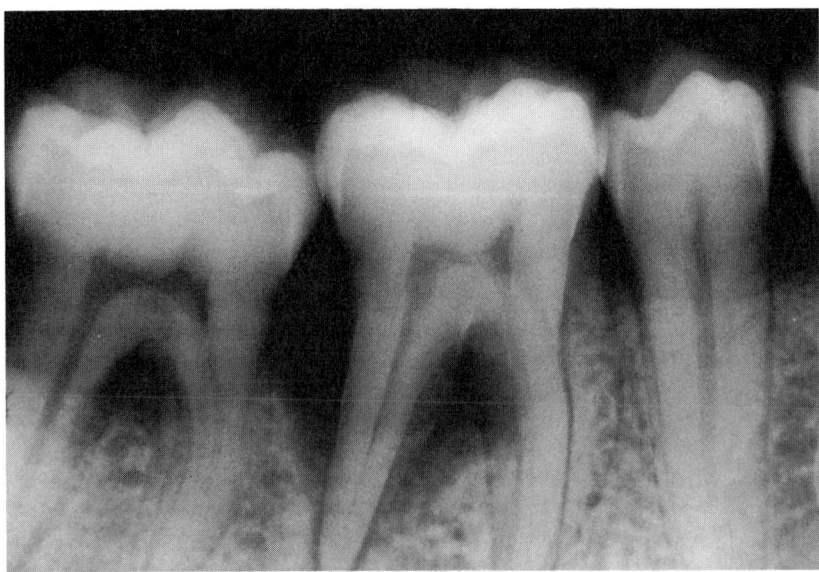

Figure 11–9. Advanced periodontitis. Extensive loss of alveolar bone around the first and second molars can be seen. (Courtesy of Dr. E. Stephen Smith.)

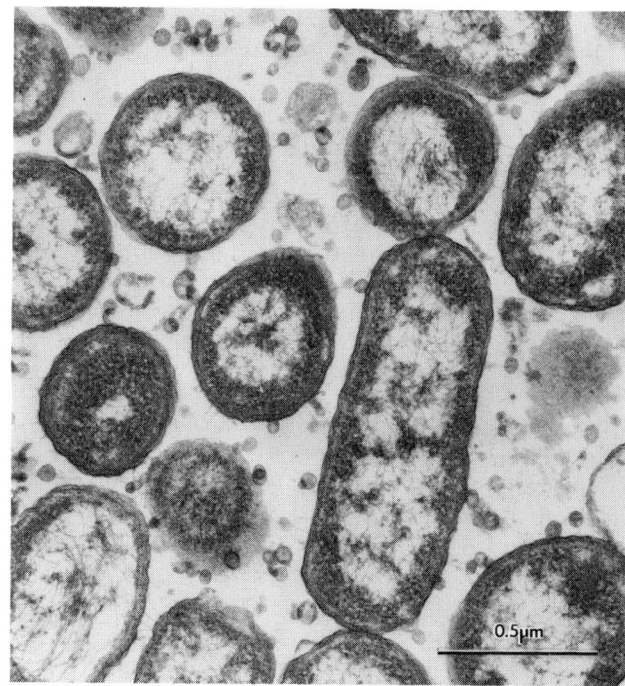

Figure 11–10. Thin sections of Actinobacillus actinomycetemcomitans *strain Y4. Large numbers of extracellular lipopolysaccharide-containing vesicles originating from the outer membrane are present. (Courtesy of Dr. C.-H. Lai.)*

Microorganisms as Initiating or Contributing Factors in Periodontal Disease

A considerable amount of evidence indicates that oral microorganisms play a role in the initiation of marginal gingivitis and in the more destructive forms of periodontal disease. Clinicians have long noted the direct relationship between the microbial plaque burden in the cervical regions of the teeth and the presence and severity of gingivitis, and that gingival inflammation can be reduced or eliminated by procedures that remove the plaque and by antibiotics and other antimicrobial agents.

The most provocative evidence relating microorganisms to periodontal disease has been the use of isolates from the human mouth to produce the periodontal disease syndrome in experimental animals. Several gram-negative organisms, including *Bacteroides, Fusobacterium, Capnocytophaga,* and *Actinobacillus,* which are found to increase in number in periodontitis and periodontosis, are capable of producing some of the pathologic features (e.g., alveolar bone destruction) associated with periodontal disease when they are implanted into the oral cavity of gnotobiotic rats or nonhuman primates. These experiments can be criticized because they represent an artificial situation in which pure cultures of a single organism are implanted in gnotobiotic animals and because

the histologic alterations seen in the periodontium of the animals are not always typical of those found in human periodontitis. Nevertheless, they indicate that certain members of the human oral flora do have the potential to produce tissue damage of a kind similar to that found in periodontal disease.

Mechanisms of Tissue Destruction in Periodontal Disease

Microbial Products

Although the issue has recently become controversial, histologic studies have generally demonstrated that even in the most destructive cases of periodontal disease, the bacteria usually remain confined to the periodontal pocket and seldom are found in large numbers in the underlying connective tissues. For this reason, the possibility that microbial products penetrate the highly permeable junctional epithelium and act directly or indirectly to initiate or contribute to the tissue destruction seen in periodontal disease has been investigated.

A number of studies suggest that endotoxin, that is, lipopolysaccharide derived from the outer membrane of gram-negative bacteria, may contribute to the tissue damage. The availability of endotoxin may occur as the result of shedding of outer membrane vesicles during growth (Fig.

11–10). The amount of endotoxin found in crevicular fluid correlates with the severity of periodontal inflammation, and endotoxin preparations from cultures of the gram-negative bacteria that dominate the microbial flora in periodontitis have been shown to be highly destructive to gingival tissues. There are a number of ways in which the lipopolysaccharide endotoxin molecules could cause tissue damage in the periodontium. Endotoxin is known to induce the production of cytokines, including interleukin-1, tumor necrosis factor, and interferon gamma. Some of these host cell products are now known to be responsible for the biologic effects ascribed to the endotoxin molecule. For example, lipopolysaccharide from *B. gingivalis* stimulates bone resorption in organ cultures, an effect that appears to be due to the release of interleukin-1. The complement system is activated by endotoxin via the alternative pathway, resulting in the production of a variety of biologically active effector molecules. Endotoxin has also been shown to act on macrophages, enhancing their ability to produce oxygen radicals (which have been implicated as mediators of tissue damage in inflammation) and stimulating the production and release of collagenase.

In addition to endotoxin, a number of other bacterial products may stimulate destructive events in the periodontium. These include toxic metabolic products, such as H_2S, butyrate, or peptidoglycan, or bacterial enzymes such as collagenase.

Destructive Immune Mechanisms

The immune response in periodontal disease is extremely complex; in addition to providing protection, it also undoubtedly contributes to the destruction of periodontal tissues. The possibility that immune and inflammatory mechanisms are responsible for tissue damage in periodontal disease has received a great deal of attention, but the interaction and precise role of the various components of the immune system are not yet understood.

Interest in the possibility that immune elements might contribute to the tissue destruction seen in periodontitis was initially aroused by the work of Ivanyi and Lehner, who demonstrated that peripheral blood leukocytes from patients with periodontal disease underwent proliferative transformation and produced cytokines after incubation with dental plaque bacteria, whereas normal individuals were unresponsive. The histopathologic changes in periodontal disease, including infiltration of increased numbers of macrophages, lymphocytes, and plasma cells into the affected tissues, are compatible with a role for immune elements in the disease. For example, interleukin-1 (IL-1), a cytokine secreted primarily by macrophages that plays an important role in immunologic and inflammatory reactions, stimulates prostaglandin and collagenase release from connective tissue and induces bone resorption as measured by Ca^{2+} release from organ cultures of fetal rat bones. Significant levels of IL-1 activity have been detected in gingival crevicular fluid obtained from sites in patients with periodontitis, and peripheral blood mononuclear cells can be stimulated by antigens present in dental plaque to produce IL-1 (originally described as osteoclast-activating factor). Other cytokines, including tumor necrosis factor and lymphotoxin, may contribute to bone resorption.

The protective and/or destructive role of antibody in periodontal disease is uncertain. B lymphocytes and plasma cells increase and predominate in the periodontium in advanced disease; immunoglobulin-containing cells, primarily of the IgG isotype, are present; and IgG antibody, some of which is thought to be locally produced, is present in the periodontal tissues. In addition to this localized response, elevated serum levels of IgG to *B. gingivalis* and other organisms that are associated with periodontitis may be elevated. A destructive role for antibody in the pathogenesis of periodontal disease is entirely speculative, but could include complement fixation with the release of chemotactic factors, antibody-dependent cytotoxicity, and opsonization of tissue-associated antigens.

Acute Periodontal Infections

Acute Necrotizing Ulcerative Gingivitis

Various names have been used to describe the clinical entity known today as *acute necrotizing ulcerative gingivitis*. These include Vincent's infection, fusospirochetal disease, and a less delicate term, "trench mouth," which was coined by the troops in World War I, who developed the disease in epidemic proportions. Despite the increased incidence of acute necrotizing ulcerative gingivitis seen in certain populations, the disease is considered an endogenous infection in which certain bacteria normally found in the oral cavity initiate or contribute to the disease process.

A number of predisposing factors are thought

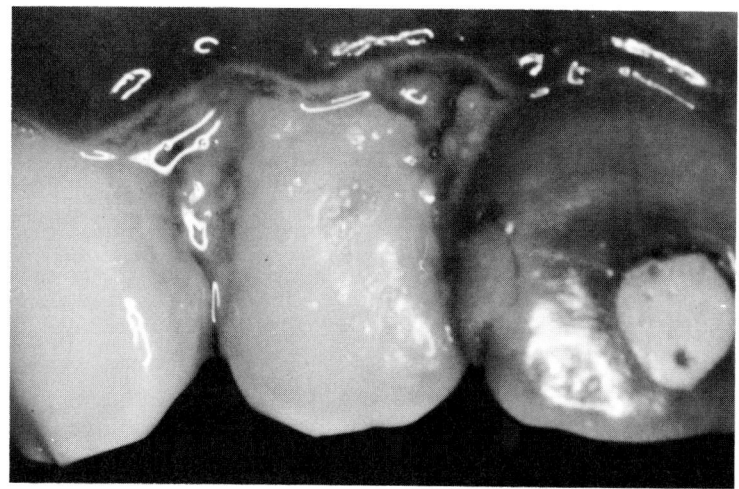

Figure 11–11. Acute necrotizing ulcerative gingivitis. The interdental papillae have eroded, and a grayish pseudomembrane is present on the marginal gingiva. (Courtesy of Dr. E. Stephen Smith.)

to be important, and these may account for the increased incidence seen in particular population groups, such as military recruits and college students. The disease is seen primarily in young adults in the 18–30-year age group, and epidemiologic studies suggest that emotional stress is an important predisposing factor, leading to diminished host immune responsiveness. In addition to psychologic factors, fatigue, malnutrition, neglected oral hygiene, and local trauma are thought to be contributing elements.

Clinically, the disease is characterized by the presence of painful, sore, bleeding gingivae. Necrosis and erosion of the gingival papillae between the teeth are usually seen, and in many cases, a grayish pseudomembrane covers the margins of the affected gingiva (Fig. 11–11). Increased numbers of spirochetes, which appear to invade the gingival tissues actively, and gram-negative anaerobes, including *Bacteroides intermedius* and *Fusobacterium* species are found, but their contribution to the pathogenesis of the disease is uncertain.

OTHER ORAL INFECTIONS

A large number of bacterial, mycotic, and viral infections may produce oral manifestations. The reader should consult an oral pathology textbook for a complete description of those lesions. The diseases described here are among the more important primary infections of the oral tissues.

Actinomycosis

Actinomycosis in the cervicofacial region is a chronic granulomatous infection characterized

by firm, nodular swelling and persistent, draining sinus tracts. Several species of *Actinomyces* are found in the oral cavity, where they are associated with dental plaque and carious lesions, the gingival sulcus, periodontal pockets, and tonsillar crypts. *A. israelii* is usually the causative organism, although other reports have also implicated *A. naeslundii*. There frequently appears to be a relationship between actinomycosis and previous trauma to the area, such as a blow to the teeth, fractures, or dental extractions. These events presumably allow the organisms to penetrate into the soft tissues or bone under anaerobic conditions. Actinomycetes are occasionally the predominant organism isolated from periapical lesions of the teeth. Actinomycosis of the cervicofacial area ("lumpy jaw") is thought to occur less frequently in the United States today than it did years ago. This probably reflects increased concern with dental health by the general population.

Venereal Infections of the Oral Cavity

It has been known for many years that syphilitic lesions can occur in and around the oral cavity. Chancres of the lip are the most common extragenital primary lesions, but they may also be found on the tongue, palate, and other oral tissues. In the secondary stage of syphilis, grayish white mucous patches may be found in the oral cavity, usually on the tongue or buccal mucosa, and the gumma of tertiary syphilis may involve the tongue or palate.

The frequency with which gonococci can be isolated from the oropharynx has only recently been appreciated. Data from a number of studies now suggest that the pharynx may be an important reservoir of *Neisseria gonorrhoeae.* Lesions within the oral cavity thought to be due to gonococcal infection have rarely been described.

Venereal transmission of herpes simplex type 2 virus has been reported to cause oral lesions or asymptomatic infections of the oral cavity.

Candidiasis

Oral candidiasis, or *thrush,* is the most common fungal infection of the mouth. *Candida albicans* is an opportunistic organism, normally found in the oral cavity, whose numbers are thought to be held in check by other members of the oral flora and by host defense mechanisms. Overgrowth of the organism is seen primarily in newborn infants, diabetics, or persons who have immunodeficiencies; the disease is uncommon in healthy adults who have not received broad-spectrum antibiotics or corticosteroids. Oral candidiasis is the most frequent opportunistic infection seen in patients with AIDS, and unexplained oral candidiasis in people belonging to groups at high risk for AIDS is an indicator that the development of severe opportunistic infections or Kaposi's sarcoma is likely.

Infection is characterized by the presence of white plaques or patches on the buccal mucosa, tongue, palate, and other mucous membrane surfaces. These lesions, which consist of masses of mycelial and yeast forms, may remain as discrete areas or coalesce to form a continuous white to gray pseudomembrane. Parts of the pseudomembrane may be stripped from the underlying tissue, revealing a red, bleeding surface. This characteristic is often useful in distinguishing candidiasis from other white plaquelike pathologic lesions of the oral cavity.

Herpes Simplex

The most important viral disease affecting the oral mucosa is infection by herpes simplex type 1 virus (HSV-1). Primary infections of HSV-1 most commonly occur in the mouth, usually in children between the ages of 6 months and 6 years. The majority of primary infections are thought to be subclinical, but in many individuals, a severe gingivostomatitis occurs. Initially, the gingivae become red and swollen, the mouth is sore, and, within a few days, vesicles appear, which progress to form ulcers. Although these lesions may be found throughout the mouth on any part of the oral mucosa, they tend to occur most often in the anterior regions of the oral cavity. Fever and lymphadenopathy may be present. In most individuals, the primary oral infection is self-limiting, and the lesions heal spontaneously in 1–2 weeks. Transmission of HSV-1 to patients from the hands of dental personnel with herpetic whitlow (a soft-tissue herpetic infection of the finger pulp) has been documented.

One of the most interesting features of herpes simplex is the tendency of the virus to persist in a latent state in nerve tissues, particularly sensory ganglia, and to cause localized recurrent infections, despite the presence of circulating neutralizing antibodies. Recurrent infections are often associated with certain stimuli, such as sunlight, menstruation, fatigue, and emotional stress, which are thought to trigger viral replication, resulting in clinical disease. It is estimated that up to one third of the population has recurrent episodes, the majority suffering more than one attack each year; many persons develop one or more recurrent lesions each month. Labial herpes infections, known as cold sores or fever blisters, are the most common form of the recurrent disease; usually the outer third of the lower or upper lip is affected. A prodromal period, characterized by a burning or tingling sensation, precedes vesicle formation at the site. The vesicles rupture, leaving a shallow ulcer, which becomes covered with a brownish crust, and the lesions heal within 7–10 days after their appearance.

Although labial herpes is far more common, recurrent herpetic lesions occasionally occur within the oral cavity proper. Intraoral lesions are virtually always found on oral mucosa that is tightly bound to the periosteum, most commonly on the hard palate.

Aphthous ulcers (canker sores) are painful, recurrent idiopathic lesions of the oral mucosa, which are far more common than intraoral recurrent herpes infections. They appear as shallow ulcers with a gray or yellow center, surrounded by a distinct erythematous halo. In contrast to intraoral herpetic lesions, with which they are frequently confused, aphthous ulcers are usually found on movable mucous membranes—the buccal mucosa and mucobuccal vestibule, lips, and tongue.

Recurrent herpetic lesions have been treated in a variety of ways over the years. However, no procedure has proved consistently effective in placebo-controlled trials. Oral acyclovir does not significantly affect recurrent herpes labialis in terms of reducing the duration of pain, time to complete healing, or area of the first lesion. Topical acyclovir has not been found to be clinically effective.

DISEASES BEARING A SPECIAL RELATIONSHIP TO THE ORAL CAVITY

Certain diseases, although they are not considered to be oral infections, are especially important in the practice of dentistry. Hepatitis B will be considered in this section from the standpoints of the increased risk of the disease for dentists, and of the potential role of dental health personnel in its transmission (see Chapter 21). The increasing prevalence of human immunodeficiency virus (HIV) in the population, the fact that HIV has been isolated from saliva as well as blood, and the presence of oral manifestations of disease in many AIDS patients make it crucial for dentists to be knowledgeable about HIV and AIDS (see Chapter 26). The importance of the alpha-hemolytic group of streptococci in infective endocarditis and the number of instances in which prior dental procedures are thought to initiate an endocarditis episode make it imperative for dentists to be fully aware of their responsibilities in the prevention of this disease as well.

Hepatitis B

The increased risk of hepatitis B in dentists has been documented in a number of epidemiologic studies. A study of 434 dentists in Dade County, Florida, revealed that 6.7% had a history of hepatitis during their years of practice. The attack rate for general dentists was 5%, but for oral surgeons it rose to 21%. Only 2.4% of a control group of attorneys had a history of clinical disease. The higher incidence of clinical hepatitis in this and other surveys of dentists is supported by serologic studies. Dentists in the United States have a higher carrier rate for the serologic markers HBsAg and anti-HBs (see Chapter 21) than do unpaid blood donors and other control groups. Furthermore, despite the finding that the prevalence of type B hepatitis in fourth-year dental students and second-year dental hygienists is no greater than in control populations, the proportion of practicing dentists who are seropositive markedly and pro-

gressively increases as the number of years in practice increases (Fig. 11–12). Taken together, the results suggest that dentists have a risk of hepatitis B virus infection about two to three times higher than that of people in the general population, and it appears that oral surgeons are at even greater risk.

Of additional concern is the possibility that a dentist who has contracted hepatitis B may transmit the disease to patients. At least nine outbreaks of hepatitis B traceable to dentists or oral surgeons have been reported in the United States since 1974. The number of clinically infected patients ranged from 3 to 55, and two patients died of fulminant hepatitis B. In each outbreak, the implicated dentist was seropositive for HBsAg and did not use gloves during dental or surgical procedures.

Although these reports demonstrate that HBsAg-positive dentists may transmit hepatitis B to their patients, it by no means follows that this happens in every instance. A prospective study of over 200 dental patients, who had been treated during a 6-week period prior to the onset of hepatitis in two dentists, showed that none of the exposed patients developed hepatitis or became positive for HBsAg.

The nature of dental practice offers a variety

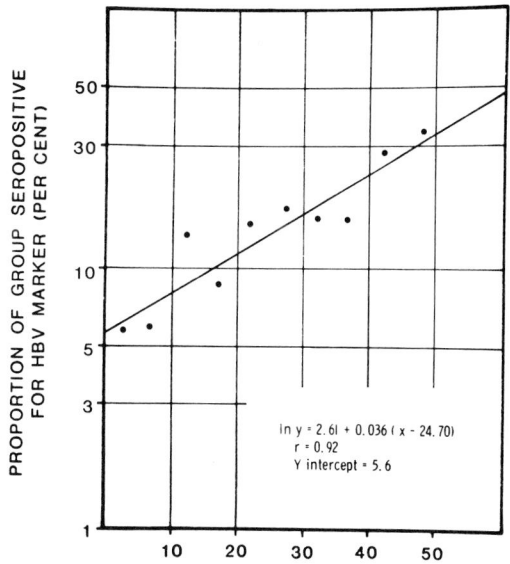

Figure 11–12. Proportion of dentists with a serologic marker (HB$_s$Ag or antibody) for hepatitis B virus in relation to average years of professional experience within 5-year groups from time of dental school graduation. (From Mosley, J. W., Edwards, V. M., Casey, G., et al. Hepatitis B virus infection in dentists. N. Engl. J. Med. 293:729, 1975. Reprinted by permission.)

of means for the transmission of hepatitis B virus. The dentist's hands are almost constantly in contact with the patient's saliva and frequently with the patient's blood. The presence of viral antigens in the blood of infected individuals is well known, but HBsAg is also known to be present in the saliva of a high proportion of persons who have acute hepatitis or who are chronic carriers. Surveys in the past have found that few dentists wear gloves routinely, and the presence of cuts and abrasions on the dentist's fingers might provide an appropriate portal of entry for the virus. The greater risk of hepatitis B for oral surgeons presumably reflects their more frequent contact with the patient's blood and blood-contaminated instruments, gauze, and so forth. The spread of hepatitis B virus in saliva-contaminated aerosols created by the use of high-speed drills may also occur, although this has not been proved.

There are widely recommended and easily available measures to protect dentists (and all health care workers) against hepatitis B and to prevent transmission of the virus from dentist to patient. These include vaccination with the safe and effective recombinant hepatitis B vaccine and the routine use of gloves when treating patients.

Acquired Immunodeficiency Syndrome

The HIV/AIDS public health crisis has important implications for the practice of dentistry, especially in the area of infection control and in the diagnosis and management of oral infections and pathologic lesions related to acquired immunodeficiency syndrome (AIDS). An estimated 1 million people in the United States are infected with HIV, and dental professionals are likely to be exposed repeatedly to persons infected with HIV before those persons know they have been infected or become ill. Nevertheless, a recent study showed that despite infrequent adherence to recommended infection control practices, frequent occupational exposure to persons at risk for AIDS, and frequent accidental parenteral inoculations with dental instruments, dental professionals are at low occupational risk for HIV infection. Recommended infection control precautions require that blood, saliva, and crevicular fluid from all patients be regarded as infective; gloves should be used for contact with oral mucous membranes of all patients, and surgical masks and

protective eyewear should be worn during dental procedures in which splashing or spattering of blood, saliva, or gingival fluids is likely.

Manifestations of AIDS are seen in the oral cavity of a significant number of AIDS patients, and indeed, oral lesions may be the first clinical expression of HIV infection. Oral tumors may be present in up to half of the patients with Kaposi's sarcoma, and in some patients the mouth is the only site involved. Candidiasis is the most common oral infection, present in 70% of AIDS patients in some studies. Other oral changes include a white hyperplasia of the epithelium, termed *hairy leukoplakia,* and recurrent herpetic lesions. In addition, changes in the periodontal tissues are present in many patients; these changes are seen as a generalized gingivitis and rapidly progressive periodontitis characterized by gingival recession and rapid and extensive alveolar bone loss.

Infective Endocarditis

Several observations combine to make infective endocarditis a disease of considerable importance for dentists and dental auxiliaries (see Chapter 35):

1. Streptococci are the most frequent cause of endocarditis, and, numerically, the viridans (alpha-hemolytic) streptococci are the most important organisms associated with the disease.

2. Large numbers of alpha-hemolytic streptococci colonize the oral cavity, including *S. salivarius, S. sanguis, S. mitis,* and *S. mutans.*

3. Dental procedures, especially extractions and manipulation of periodontal tissues, result in a transient bacteremia of alpha-hemolytic streptococci and other organisms in many individuals. Even less traumatic events, such as dental prophylaxis, brushing the teeth, and chewing hard wax and candy, are thought to provoke a bacteremia in some instances. In most individuals, the bacteria are rapidly and completely cleared from the blood without further incident. For individuals with rheumatic heart disease or congenital heart defects or for those who have prosthetic heart valves, however, the transitory bacteremia may have disastrous consequences; the organisms may lodge on and colonize damaged heart valves or other parts of the endocardium, initiating an episode of endocarditis. In a significant number of endocarditis episodes, the patient is found to have a history of recent dental work.

The role of the dentist and other dental

personnel in preventing episodes of endocarditis is straightforward. First, a medical history of each patient must be taken before any manipulative dental procedure is undertaken. Second, antibiotics must be used in patients at risk to prevent or reduce bacteremia and to eradicate bacteria that may implant on heart valves. The treatment schedule suggested by the American Heart Association (see Chapter 35) should be followed. Unfortunately, cases of infective endocarditis due to antimicrobial drug-susceptible streptococci occur despite vigorous adherence to this recommended prophylaxis regimen.

REFERENCES

Books

Genco, R.J., and Mergenhagen, S.E., eds. *Host–Parasite Interactions in Periodontal Diseases.* Washington, D.C.: American Society for Microbiology, 1982.

Grant, D.A., Stern, I.B., and Listgarten, M.A. *Periodontics.* 6th ed. St. Louis: C.V. Mosby Co., 1988.

Marsh, P., and Martin, M. *Oral Microbiology.* 2nd ed. Washington, D.C.: American Society for Microbiology, 1984.

Newman, M.G., and Nisengard, R. *Oral Microbiology and Immunology.* Philadelphia: W.B. Saunders Co., 1988.

Roitt, I.M., and Lehner, T. *Immunology of Oral Diseases.* 2nd ed. Oxford: Blackwell Scientific Publications, 1983.

Schluger, S., Yuodelis, R.A., Page, R.C., et al. *Periodontal Disease.* 2nd ed. Philadelphia: Lea & Febiger, 1990.

Schuster, G.S. *Oral Microbiology and Infectious Disease.* 3rd ed. Philadelphia: B.C. Decker, Inc. 1990.

Seltzer, S., and Bender, I.B. *The Dental Pulp.* 3rd ed. Philadelphia: J.B. Lippincott Co., 1984.

Shafer, W.G., Hine, M.K., and Levy, B.M. *A Textbook of Oral Pathology.* 4th ed. Philadelphia: W.B. Saunders Co., 1983.

Topazian, R.G., and Goldberg, M.H. *Oral and Maxillofacial Infections.* 2nd ed. Philadelphia: W.B. Saunders Co., 1987.

Review Articles

Burt, B. Public health implications of recent research in periodontal diseases. *J. Public Health Dent.* 48:252, 1988.

Corey, L., and Spear, P.G. Infections with herpes simplex viruses. *N. Engl. J. Med.* 314:686, 1986.

Cottone, J.A. Recent developments in hepatitis: New virus, vaccine, and dosage recommendations. *JADA 120:*501, 1990.

Coykendall, A.L. Classification and identification of the viridans streptococci. *Clin. Microbiol. Rev.* 2:315, 1989.

Diesendorf, M. The mystery of declining tooth decay. *Nature 322:*125, 1986.

Farber, P.A., and Seltzer, S. Endodontic microbiology. I. Etiology. *J. Endodont.* 14:363, 1988.

Hamada, S., and Slade, H.D. Biology, immunology, and cariogenicity of *Streptococcus mutans. Microbiol. Rev.* 44:331, 1980.

Hirsch, R.S., and Clarke, N. Infection and periodontal disease. *Rev. Infect. Dis. 11:*707, 1989.

Johnson, B.D., and Engel, D. Acute necrotizing ulcerative gingivitis. A review of diagnosis, etiology and treatment. *J. Periodontol.* 57:141, 1986.

Koch-Weser, J. Treatment .of herpesvirus infection. *N. Engl. J. Med.* 309:963, 1983.

Kolenbrander, P. Intergeneric coaggregation among human oral bacteria and ecology of dental plaque. *Annu. Rev. Microbiol. 42:*627, 1988.

Leverett, D.H. Fluorides and the changing prevalence of dental caries. *Science 217:*26, 1982.

Listgarten, M.A. Pathogenesis of periodontitis. *J. Clin. Periodontol.* 13:418, 1986.

Loesche, W.J. Role of *Streptococcus mutans* in human dental decay. *Microbiol. Rev.* 50:353, 1986.

Mayrand, D., and Holt, S.C. Biology of asaccharolytic black-pigmented *Bacteroides* species. *Microbiol. Rev.* 52:134, 1988.

McGhee, J.R., and Michalek, S.M. Immunobiology of dental caries: Microbial aspects and local immunity. *Annu. Rev. Microbiol.* 35:595, 1981.

Page, R.C. Gingivitis. *J. Clin. Periodontol.* 13:345, 1986.

Shaw, J.H. Causes and control of dental caries. *N. Engl. J. Med. 317:*996, 1987.

Original Articles

Dewhirst, F.E., Stashenko, P., Mole, J.E., et al. Purification and partial sequence of human osteoclast-activating factor: Identity with interleukin 1B. *J. Immunol. 135:*2562, 1985.

Gibbons, R.J., and van Houte, J. Selective bacterial adherence to oral epithelial surfaces and its role as an ecological determinant. *Infect. Immunol.* 3:567, 1971.

Haapasalo, M., Ranta, H., Ranta, K., et al. Black-pigmented *Bacteroides* spp. in human apical periodontitis. *Infect. Immunol.* 53:149, 1986.

Holt, S.C., Ebersole, J., Felton, J., et al. Implantation of *Bacteroides gingivalis* in nonhuman primates initiates progression of periodontitis. *Science 239:*55, 1988.

Ivanyi, L., and Lehner, T.: Stimulation of lymphocyte transformation by bacterial antigens in patients with periodontal disease. *Arch. Oral Biol.* 15:1089, 1970.

Kabashima, H., Maeda, K., Iwamoto, Y., et al. Partial characterization of an interleukin-1-like factor in human gingival crevicular fluid from patients with chronic inflammatory periodontal disease. *Infect. Immunol.* 58:2621, 1990.

Klein, R., Harris, C., Small, C., et al. Oral candidiasis in high risk patients as the initial manifestation of the acquired immunodeficiency syndrome. *N. Engl. J. Med. 311:*354, 1984.

Klein, R.S., Phelan, J.A., Freeman, K., et al. Low occupational risk of human immunodeficiency virus infection among dental professionals. *N. Engl. J. Med. 318:*86, 1988.

Lamont, R.J., and Rosan, B. Adherence of mutans streptococci to other oral bacteria. *Infect. Immunol.* 58:1738, 1990.

Larjava, H., Uitto, V.-J., Eerola, E., et al. Inhibition of gingival fibroblast growth by *Bacteroides gingivalis. Infect. Immunol.* 55:201, 1987.

Manzella, J.P., McConville, J.H., Valenti, W., et al. An outbreak of herpes simplex virus type 1 gingivostomatitis in a dental hygiene practice. *JAMA* 252:2019, 1984.

Millar, S.J., Goldstein, E.G., Levine, M.J., et al. Modulation of bone metabolism by two chemically distinct lipopolysaccharide fractions from *Bacteroides gingivalis*. *Infect. Immunol. 51:*302, 1986.

Minah, G.E., and Loesche, W.J. Sucrose metabolism in resting-cell suspensions of caries-associated and non–caries-associated dental plaque. *Infect. Immunol. 17:*43, 1977.

Moore, W.E.C., Holdeman, L.V., Smibert, R.M., et al. Bacteriology of experimental gingivitis in young adult humans. *Infect. Immunol. 38:*651, 1982.

Mosley, J.W., Edwards, V.M., Casey, G., et al. Hepatitis B virus infection in dentists. *N. Engl. J. Med. 293:*729, 1975.

Ogawa, T., Tarkowski, A., McGhee, M.L., et al. Analysis of human IgG and IgA subclass antibody-secreting cells from localized chronic inflammatory tissue. *J. Immunol. 142:*1150, 1989.

Roberts, M., Brahim, J., and N. Rinne. Oral manifestations of AIDS: A study of 84 patients. *JADA 116:*863, 1988.

Silverman, S., Migliorati, C., Lozada-Nur, F., et al. Oral findings in people with or at high risk for AIDS: A study of 375 homosexual males. *JADA 112:*187, 1986.

Socransky, S.S., Haffajee, A.D., Goodson, J.M., et al. New concepts of destructive periodontal disease. *J. Clin. Periodont. 11:*21, 1984.

Winkler, J., Murray, P., Grassi, M., et al. Diagnosis and management of HIV-associated periodontal lesions. *JADA 119:*25S, 1989.

IV

Lower Respiratory Tract Infection

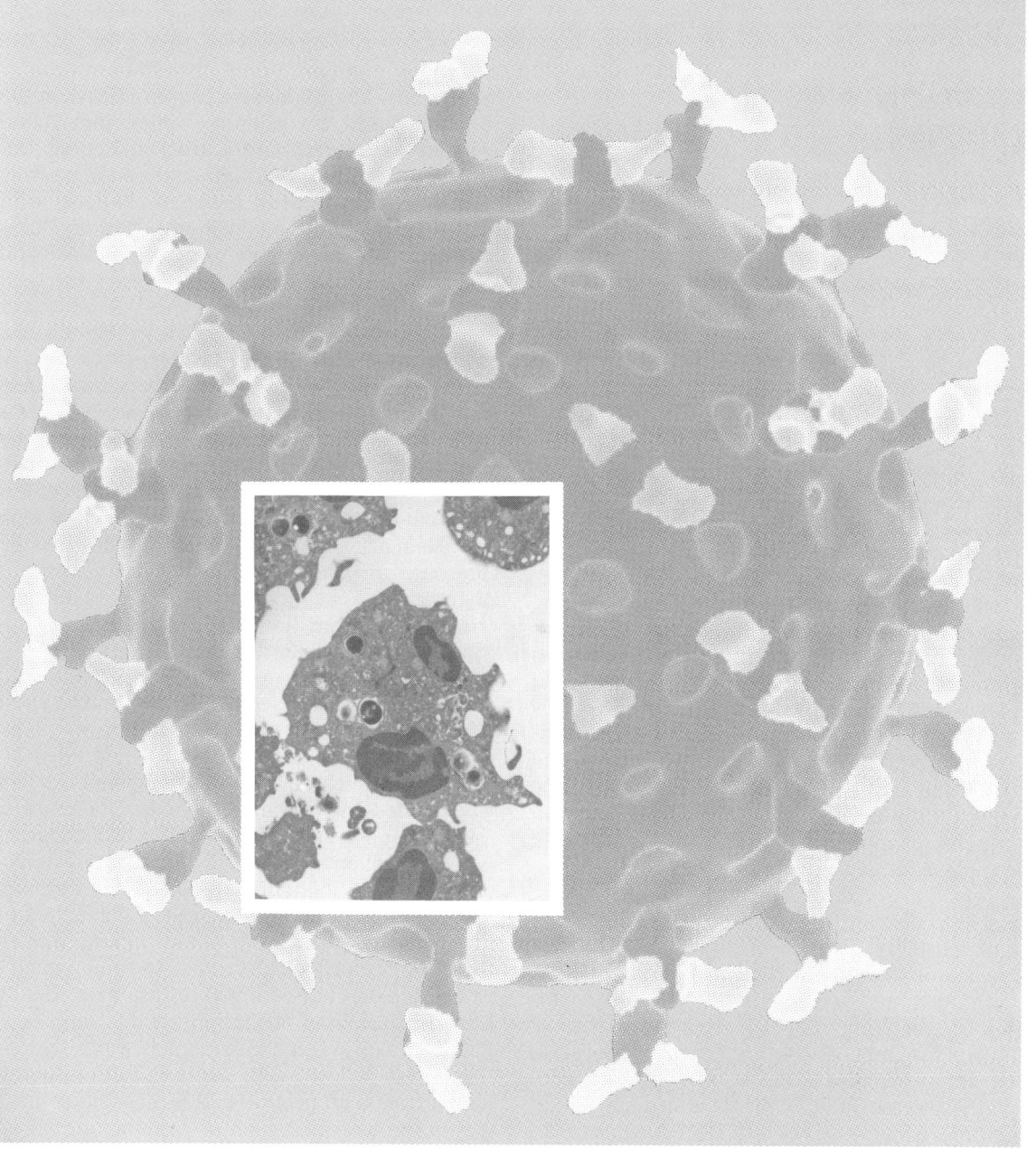

JOHN P. PHAIR, M.D.

Infections of the Lower Respiratory Tract: General Considerations

INTRODUCTION

The lower respiratory tract is vulnerable to infection by a wide variety of microorganisms because it is one of the organ systems which communicate directly with the environment. Its physiologic function, the exchange of gases, can result in exposure to bacteria, fungi, viruses, and other potentially pathogenic agents. In addition, the entire blood supply must pass through the pulmonary capillary bed, and bloodstream infections can produce secondary infection in the lower respiratory tract. The lower respiratory tract, comprising the bronchial tree, the pulmonary parenchyma, and the pleura, can be the locus of infection which presents as similar or quite distinct symptom complexes with a variety of physical findings.

Infections of the lower respiratory tract represent a constantly increasing cause of morbidity and mortality. This is in large part a consequence of smoking; it is estimated that 30% of both men and women in the United States smoke. Smoking results ultimately in chronic obstructive lung disease, which predisposes to infection, significant levels of disability, neoplastic disease, and death. It is estimated that chronic respiratory disease, including asthma,

represents the fifth leading cause of death in the United States. In addition, pneumonias and related lower respiratory tract infections acquired during hospitalizations are an increasing and extremely difficult problem. Patients with severe, debilitating medical and surgical illness are extremely vulnerable to such infections and much of the therapeutic intervention for such patients leads to an increased risk of lower respiratory tract infections. This problem is discussed more fully in Chapter 13.

The patient with lower respiratory tract infection usually presents with signs and symptoms referable to the chest. Fever and cough are the two most prominent complaints. With involvement of the pleura, chest pain is also present. Physical examination provides evidence of lung involvement, inflammation of bronchi, or the presence of pleural fluid. The cornerstones of diagnosis are chest radiography (x-ray) and microscopic examination and culture of expectorated sputum or pleural fluid if available.

The interpretation of Gram's stains and sputum culture is discussed in Chapter 7. The chest x-ray can demonstrate consolidation of a lobe or lobule of the lung caused by fluid-filled alveoli. An "air bronchogram," air-filled bronchi surrounded by fluid-filled alveoli, can be seen on a chest film. Absence of an air bronchogram suggests collapse of a lung segment or atelectasis. Diffuse interstitial processes, if chronic, usually represent granulomatous involvement of the alveolar septa or, if acute, edema due to heart failure or fluid overload. In these circumstances, pleural disease with effusions is usually found at the base of the lung and, if not loculated, moves when the patient is repositioned. An air–fluid level with a pleural effusion can result from a bronchopleural fistula. In the lung, an air–fluid level is seen in conjunction with a

TABLE 12–1. *Differential Diagnosis of Lower Respiratory Tract Infection*

Pulmonary embolism
Pulmonary tumor, primary or metastatic
Pulmonary hemorrhage
Congestive heart failure
Hypersensitivity pneumonitis
Vasculitis

partially fluid-filled emphysematous cyst or a lung abscess. The latter is usually thick-walled, whereas the former is thin-walled. The physician must evaluate the history, physical examination, and the chest radiograph to determine if the patient's complaints are related to upper (Chapter 9) or to lower respiratory tract disease. If lower tract disease is the most likely cause of the patient's complaints, infection must be distinguished from other causes of bronchial, lung, or pleural disease (Table 12–1). Pulmonary embolism, hemorrhage, lung tumors, congestive heart failure, hypersensitivity pneumonitis, or vasculitis can present with pulmonary symptoms, fever, and an abnormal chest film. An elevated white cell count in the peripheral blood can be helpful for diagnosis, as is careful examination of expectorated sputum. However, invasive procedures, such as bronchoscopy with lavage, transbronchial biopsy, and/or open lung biopsy, may ultimately be required to determine the cause of lower respiratory tract disease.

PATHOGENESIS OF LOWER RESPIRATORY TRACT INFECTION

The great majority of lower respiratory tract infections are the consequence of inhalation or aspiration of microorganisms. The upper airway is designed to warm, humidify, and screen inspired air to reduce the number of organisms or other foreign aerosolized particles reaching the bronchi. The nasal turbinates, mucus, and nasal hairs serve to trap such inhaled particles. Those organisms that traverse the nasal passages and reach the trachea are screened again by the cilia and mucus of this major airway. The cilia serve to carry particles trapped in mucus up to the pharynx (the so-called mucociliary elevator), thus providing a second barrier to colonization of the lower bronchial tree or alveoli, which in normal individuals remains sterile. Immunoglobulins, especially IgA, are contained in the mucus and provide another defense against microbial invasion.

The majority of organisms which produce lower respiratory infection first colonize the nasal and pharyngeal epithelium. Colonization is the result of an interaction of a surface molecule on the microorganism, an adhesin, interacting with a receptor on cells of the nasopharyngeal mucus membrane. In the healthy person, normal flora of the nasopharynx has an advantage in this ecology. As an example, in normal individuals, gargling of aerobic enteric organisms does not result in prolonged colonization of the pharynx. Cultures obtained 60 min after such exposure grow the usual flora of the oropharynx.

Certain pathogenic bacteria, such as *Streptococcus pneumoniae, Haemophilus influenzae,* and *Neisseria* species, however, can colonize the nasopharynx, and colonization rates with these organisms rise in the colder months of the year. In the setting of an intercurrent viral upper respiratory infection the defense mechanisms discussed above (normal ciliary function, for example) are altered, and inhalation of these organisms into the lower respiratory tract occurs, setting the stage for infection of the lungs.

Other pathologic situations which favor colonization of the oropharynx with organisms which can cause bronchitis and pneumonia include acute and chronic alcoholism and severe intercurrent illness. Alcohol ingestion, in addition to being associated with colonization of the upper airway by aerobic gram-negative bacilli, leads through its central nervous system effects to a diminished gag reflex and poor tracheobronchial ciliary function, thus altering important defenses of the lower respiratory tract. The pathogenic bacteria which colonize the upper airway in this situation gain access to the lower respiratory tract and produce pneumonia. Alcoholism is also associated with nausea and vomiting, and when coupled with loss of the gag reflex can lead to aspiration either of the oropharyngeal flora or stomach contents. When vomitus is aspirated, a chemical pneumonitis is produced which increases the susceptibility of the pulmonary parenchyma to bacterial infection.

Severe illness also is associated with changes in the surface secretions of the oropharynx which favor colonization by organisms capable of producing bronchial or pulmonary infections. For reasons that are not clear, severe illness is associated with an increase in salivary protease activity and a reduction of mucosal fibronectin that augment the ability of gram-negative bacilli to colonize these surfaces. Immobilization due to debility also favors aspiration of the organisms of the upper airway into the lower respiratory tract. In critically ill patients, antacids or H$_2$ blockers are used to prevent gastric ulceration (stress ulcers), resulting in a rise in stomach pH. The stomach, which is normally sterile, can then become colonized with bacteria. These bacteria are capable, especially with nasogastric intubation, of colonizing the pharynx and subsequently causing pneumonia.

Certain bloodstream infections lead to metastatic infection in the lungs. An example are the multiple foci of pneumonitis which occur in endocarditis involving the tricuspid and pulmonary valves (Chapter 35). Vegetations break off from the valves as septic pulmonary emboli, lodge in the pulmonary capillaries, and serve as foci for phlebitis and pneumonitis. Pelvic infections with anaerobic organisms such as *Bacteroides* species also cause thrombophlebitis and septic pulmonary emboli—infections seen most frequently as a complication of parturition or abortion.

Finally, inhalation of irritant gases, such as cigarette smoke, alter the bronchial epithelium, leading to a loss of the cilia-bearing columnar epithelial cells and ultimately to chronic inflammation, with or without microbial infection of the bronchi. Acute bronchitis, in contrast, can occur as a direct result of viral or bacterial infection independent of such irritant effects. Structural damage to bronchi due to chronic infection can produce saccular pockets in the bronchial wall, collecting mucus secretions which commonly become infected with oropharyngeal bacteria. This condition, known as *bronchiectasis,* results in further destruction of the bronchial tree. A common condition underlying severe bronchiectasis is cystic fibrosis, an autosomal recessive disorder, which is associated with mucus plugging of bronchi, chronic infection, and destruction of the integrity of the bronchial wall. The usual cause of infection of the pleural space is direct extension of infection from the lungs. Purulent infection of the pleural space is a closed space infection similar to an abscess and is termed *empyema.*

ETIOLOGY

Any microorganism, given the appropriate circumstances and host factors, can cause lower respiratory tract infection. However, among bacteria, the common causes of lower respiratory tract infection in normal adults include *Streptococcus pneumoniae, Mycoplasma pneumoniae,* and *Legionella* species—the usual causes of community-acquired pneumonia.

Group A streptococcus *(S. pyogenes)* causes outbreaks of pneumonia in such closed populations as recruit camps and boarding schools. *Staphylococcus aureus* and *Haemophilus influenzae* are uncommon causes of pneumonia in adults except in association with influenza epidemics. Lung infections with these organisms are more commonly seen in children. Children also commonly develop pneumococcal and mycoplasmal pulmonary infections. Among compromised hospitalized patients, *S. aureus* and aerobic gram-negative bacilli including *Legionella* are common causes of pneumonia (see Chapter 13). Aspiration pneumonia is usually due to the aerobic and particularly the anaerobic oropharyngeal flora. Mycobacterial infections are primarily lower respiratory tract infections and are discussed in Chapter 15.

Most of the deep mycoses, such as histoplasmosis, blastomycosis, coccidioidomycosis, and cryptococcosis, begin as lower respiratory tract infections following inhalation of the infecting form of these fungi. A more complete description of these infections is found in Chapter 16.

Viral infection is probably the most common cause of acute bronchitis and pneumonia in adults and children. It can be caused by any of the "respiratory viruses," including adenovirus, influenza, parainfluenza, and respiratory syncytial virus, as well as the enteroviruses. Coxsackievirus is the cause of epidemic pleurodynia, a form of pleuritis which, as its name implies, occurs in outbreaks. See Chapter 14.

SPECIFIC SYNDROMES

There are a variety of specific clinical syndromes due to infection of the lower respiratory tract (Table 12–2). *Pneumonia,* the most common lower respiratory tract infection, is discussed in Chapter 13 (community-acquired) and Chapter 28 (nosocomial pneumonia).

Acute bronchitis is usually a self-limited infection of the bronchial tree due to viral infection. Similar symptoms can be seen with infection due to *Mycoplasma pneumoniae.* Patients usually seek medical attention because of a persistent cough which can be paroxysmal. Often the cough is nonproductive, but purulent sputum may be expectorated even when the infection is due to viral infection. Patients complain of difficulty sleeping because of the cough and of tightness or discomfort in the anterior chest. Fever is not always present, but when it occurs it is usually low grade. Patients note chills but

TABLE 12–2. *Lower Respiratory Tract Infection*

Infection	Etiology
Bronchitis	
acute	Respiratory viruses
	Mycoplasma pneumoniae
chronic	Respiratory viruses
	Streptococcus pneumoniae
	Haemophilus influenzae
Pneumonia	
community-acquired	Respiratory viruses
	Streptococcus pneumoniae
	Legionella pneumophila
	Mycoplasma pneumoniae
hospital-acquired	Aerobic gram-negative bacilli
	Staphylococcus aureus
aspiration/necrotizing	Oropharyngeal flora
	(anaerobic/aerobic
	organisms)
	Oropharyngeal flora
Lung abscess	Oropharyngeal flora
Bronchiectasis	Oropharyngeal flora
	Pseudomonas aeruginosa
	Aerobic/anaerobic bacteria
Empyema	Group A streptococcus
	Streptococcus pneumoniae

not rigors. Acute bronchitis is often preceded by an upper respiratory tract infection. The physical examination generally reveals normal breath sounds upon auscultation of the chest, but occasionally wheezes and rhonchi are present. Therapy can be aimed at controlling symptoms, unless it is suspected that the infection is due to *M. pneumoniae.* Usually, mycoplasmal infections occur in outbreaks within a geographic locale, and in interepidemic years the most common cause of acute bronchitis is viral infections, which should not be treated with antibiotics.

Chronic bronchitis represents a condition of chronic inflammation of the bronchi most commonly due to prolonged cigarette smoking. Smoking the equivalent of 20 cigarettes per day for 20 years (20 pack-years) is associated with changes in the bronchi that predispose to chronic bronchitis and that are often found in association with emphysema. An increase in the prevalence of chronic bronchitis and emphysema is found in persons who are heterozygotic for alpha$_1$ antitrypsin deficiency, even with minimal smoking. The diagnosis of chronic bronchitis is made on the basis of the history of 3 consecutive months of productive cough, 2 years in a row. Acute exacerbations of chronic bronchitis occur secondary to intercurrent viral or

bacterial infection. Such exacerbations are associated with either increased sputum production or a marked reduction in sputum produced by cough. Usually, the patient seeks medical attention because of increasing shortness of breath. An emphysematous chest (hyperexpanded) with low diaphragms and diminished breath sounds is a common finding upon physical examination. The body temperature and white cell count usually are not elevated, and the chest x-ray commonly does not reveal pulmonary infiltrates. Evaluation of arterial blood gases reveals respiratory acidosis or compensated respiratory acidosis in severely ill patients with hypoxemia. Management usually includes antibiotics effective against *S. pneumoniae* and *H. influenzae,* such as ampicillin or sulfamethoxazole/trimethoprim. The chronic treatment for such patients includes cessation of smoking, bronchial hygiene, and in some patients prolonged antibiotic therapy. Antibiotics are often administered prophylactically in the winter months when respiratory infections occur with increased frequency.

Pneumonia following aspiration of vomitus, a foreign object, or oropharyngeal flora commonly results in a necrotizing process with destruction of pulmonary tissue and production of a lung abscess. Patients with a lung abscess complain of fever, foul-smelling, often fetid sputum, and chest discomfort. There is commonly a history of alcoholism, seizures, impaired swallowing or cough mechanisms, loss of consciousness, or aspiration of a foreign object; for example, symptoms develop following inhalation of food. Organisms isolated by invasive techniques such as transtracheal aspiration include both aerobic and anaerobic flora of the oropharynx. The fusobacterium and other anaerobic microbial species are the cause of the fetid odor of the breath and sputum. Physical examination often reveals an area of consolidation. Amphoric breath sounds (blowing across the top of a bottle) sometimes can be heard if the abscess cavity communicates with a bronchus. The peripheral white count is elevated and the chest x-ray reveals a fluid-filled, or partially filled, thick-walled cavity. Treatment is dependent upon drainage, which is achieved by bronchoscopy or by having the patient practice postural drainage (chest physical therapy). Postural drainage is accomplished with the patient lying across the bed with the arms upon a chair, placing the head lower than the thorax. Coughing, aided by chest percussion, usually results in expectoration of large amounts of sputum. Antibiotic therapy has greatly reduced the morbidity due to lung abscess and has largely eliminated the need for surgical drainage. The agents of choice must be active against the oropharyngeal flora. Penicillin G, ampicillin, first generation cephalosporins, or clindamycin are all effective against this infection.

Bronchiectasis can be managed in much the same fashion as a lung abscess. Stimulation of coughing to drain infected secretions and institution of similar antibiotics usually control acute exacerbations. Prolonged antibiotic therapy with the agents listed above can lead to superinfection with antibiotic-resistant gram-negative bacilli, such as *Pseudomonas aeruginosa,* which require treatment with an enhanced-spectrum penicillin or cephalosporin in combination with an aminoglycoside. These agents must be given parenterally. In general, lung abscess and bronchiectasis require a minimum of 2 weeks of parenteral antibiotic therapy. Follow-up oral antibiotic therapy of a lung abscess is usually continued, however, until there is evidence of a substantial decrease in size of the cavity on chest x-ray.

Empyema, or infection of the pleural cavity, is usually the result of extension of an underlying pneumonia to the pleural space. Although empyema can occur with any form of bacterial pneumonia, it is seen in a minority of cases of infection due to *S. pneumoniae.* In contrast, 50% of pneumonias due to group A streptococcus are complicated by empyema. This is presumably due to the multiplicity of enzymes produced by *Streptococcus pyogenes* which interfere with the inflammatory barriers that usually localize infection (see Chapter 9).

Necrotizing pneumonia following aspiration also is associated with empyema due to destruction of lung tissue and spread of infection to the pleural cavity. Pulmonary infections with actinomyces are also commonly complicated by empyema because of the predilection of infection with this organism to cross tissue barriers. Empyema can be suspected from physical findings compatible with the presence of fluid between the lung and outer chest wall. Breath sounds are distant and there is flatness or lack of resonance with percussion of the thorax of the affected side. Unless the infection is loculated, a chest x-ray will demonstrate pleural fluid that changes in position with the patient lying on the involved side. The diagnosis is established by needle aspiration of the empyema fluid, which is often viscous and contains many leukocytes, a high concentration of protein, and a low concentration of glucose. The concentration of the enzyme lactic dehydrogenase is much higher than in serum. A Gram's stain often can suggest the etiologic agent(s), but cultures provide the definitive evidence of the cause of the underlying pneumonia as well as the empyema. Treatment generally requires placement of a chest tube with suction to ensure drainage, and appropriate antibiotic therapy. The choice of antibiotics is dictated by the identity of the isolated organism(s) and the results of antibiotic susceptibility tests. Tube drainage is continued as long as fluid is draining. Antibiotic therapy is continued usually until the chest tube is removed or for a minimum of 3 weeks. A complication of empyema due to necrotizing pneumonia is the development of a bronchopleural fistula. In the preantibiotic era undrained empyema could dissect through the chest wall and drain spontaneously, producing empyema necessitans.

PREVENTION

Prevention of lower respiratory tract disease represents a major challenge to the medical profession. The single most important step is reduction in smoking. Additionally, reduction in excessive use of alcohol decreases the prevalence of bacterial pneumonias, aspiration pneumonia, and lung abscess. Recently, it has been suggested that administration of nonabsorbable antibiotics by mouth, to prevent colonization of the stomach when gastric acidity is reduced, will prevent hospital-acquired pneumonia. Finally, as discussed in Chapter 40, immunization to prevent influenza and pneumonia due to *Streptococcus pneumoniae* and *Haemophilus influenzae* in selected groups of the population can further reduce the prevalence of lower respiratory tract infections.

CASE HISTORY

A 52-year-old man with a long history of alcohol abuse and a 50 pack-year smoking habit is admitted with fever and cough productive of foul-smelling sputum. These symptoms have been present for 3 weeks following an alcoholic binge during which the patient lost consciousness. He had become anorectic, lost 5 lb, and noted a dull discomfort in his right chest. He had fetid halitosis, a temperature of 102°F, and was in moderate distress, with 20 respirations per

minute. His thorax expanded normally with inspiration, and breathing was not associated with pain. The right and left hemithoraces were equally resonant to percussion, but auscultation revealed crackles over the right posterior chest. Breath sounds were accentuated in this area. His white blood cell count was 12,200/mm³, with 70% neutrophils and 10% band forms. Gram's stain of the sputum revealed many neutrophils, gram-negative bacilli and coccobacilli, and gram-positive cocci. Forty-eight hours later, the laboratory reported the presence of "normal oropharyngeal flora" in the sputum culture. The chest x-ray demonstrated a thick-walled cavity in the upper segment of the right lower lobe with an air–fluid level surrounded by an infiltrate. The diagnosis of lung abscess was made, and therapy was initiated with intravenous penicillin G, 1×10^6 U every 4 h. Bronchial hygiene was established with postural drainage and chest percussion. This was productive of large amounts of sputum. Within 3 days the sputum no longer had a fetid odor and the daily temperature elevation was lower. In view of this response, penicillin V, 500 mg by mouth every 6 h, was substituted for intravenous penicillin G. After 10 days the patient was eating well, had gained 3 lb, and was afebrile. A repeat x-ray showed clearing of the infiltrate and a decrease in the size of the cavity. Sputum cytology did not demonstrate any malignant cells. The patient, after counseling, agreed to join Alcoholics Anonymous and to attempt to give up smoking. He was discharged with a prescription for penicillin V with instructions to return to the pulmonary clinic in 2 weeks.

CASE DISCUSSION

This is the typical presentation of a lung abscess which commonly develops following aspiration of vomitus during an alcoholic binge. The infection is polymicrobial, reflecting the aerobic and anaerobic oropharyngeal bacteria. Therefore, the culture of sputum does not grow a specific pulmonary pathogen such as Klebsiella *or* S. pneumoniae. *The bacteria constituting the oropharyngeal flora are generally susceptible to penicillin. Occasionally, infection with the beta-lactamase-producing* Bacteroides fragilis *occurs, requiring treatment*

with clindamycin or cefoxitin. Establishing drainage of the abscess is necessary and usually can be accomplished adequately by postural drainage. Surgical intervention is therefore not usually required.

Once the inflammatory response is decreased, it is necessary to determine if the abscess has developed in the necrotic center of a lung tumor. Cytologic examination of cells in the sputum can be helpful, as is the continued response to therapy. If repeat x-rays do not demonstrate improvement in the abscess, bronchoscopy is required to rule out the presence of bronchial carcinoma, especially in smokers. Prolonged antibiotic therapy for 4–6 weeks is advocated for treatment of lung abscess. Thus, it is important to provide for appropriate follow-up during convalescence after hospital discharge.

REFERENCES

Monograph

Pennington J. *Respiratory Tract Infections: Diagnosis and Management.* New York: Raven Press, 1983.

Articles

Bartlett, J., Gorbach, S., and Finegold, S. The bacteriology of aspiration pneumonia. *Am. J. Med. 56:*202–207, 1974.

Bartlett, J., and Finegold, S. Anaerobic infections of the lung and pleural space. *Am. Rev. Respir. Dis. 110:*56–77, 1974.

Bartlett, J., Gorbach, S., Tally, F., et al. Bacteriology and treatment of primary lung abscess. *Am. Rev. Respir. Dis. 109:*510–524, 1974.

Beachey, E. Bacterial adherence: Adhesion–receptor interactions mediating the attachment of bacteria to mucosal surfaces. *J. Infect. Dis. 143:*325–345, 1981.

Cameron, E., Applebaum, D., Pudefin, D., et al. Characteristics and management of chronic destructive pneumonia. *Thorax 35:*340–346, 1980.

Green, G. In defense of the lung. *Am. Rev. Respir. Dis. 102:*691–703, 1970.

Lebowitz, M., and Burrows, B. The relationship of acute respiratory illness history to the prevalence and incidence of obstructive lung disorders. *Am. J. Epidemiol. 105:*544–554, 1977.

Lees, A., and McNaught, W. Bacteriology of lower-respiratory tract secretions, sputum and upper-respiratory tract secretions in "normals" and "chronic bronchitis." *Lancet 2:*1112–1115, 1959.

Levison, M., Mangura, C., Larber, B., et al. Clindamycin compared with penicillin for the treatment of anaerobic lung abscess. *Ann. Intern. Med. 98:*466–471, 1983.

Monto, A., Ross, H. The Tecumseh study of respiratory illness. X relation of acute infection to smoking, lung function and chronic symptoms. *Am. J. Epidemiol. 107:*57–64, 1978.

Sherman, M., Subramenian, V., and Berger, R. Management of thoracic empyema. *Am. J. Surg. 133:*474–479, 1977.

Sprunt, K. Infection in chronic lung disease. *Bull. N.Y. Acad. Med. 48:*698–703, 1972.

Stott, N., and West, R. Randomized controlled trial of antibiotics in patients with cough and purulent sputum. *Br. Med. J. 2:*556–559, 1976.

Thorsteinsson, S., Musher, D., and Fagan, T. The diagnostic value of sputum culture in acute pneumonia. *JAMA 233:*894–895, 1975.

Wood, D. Role of fibronectin in the pathogenesis of gram-negative bacillary pneumonia. *Rev. Infect. Dis. 9:*S386–390, 1987.

13 *JOHN P. PHAIR, M.D.*

Bacterial Pneumonia

INTRODUCTION

Before the antibiotic era, bacterial pneumonia was a leading cause of morbidity and mortality in the United States, and it remains an important form of infection that is difficult to manage. Specific treatment currently available, however, has greatly altered the clinical approach to this disease. A wide variety of bacteria cause infection of the lungs both in previously healthy individuals and in those with underlying debilitating disease. This chapter discusses the causes of bacterial pneumonia and their differing clinical presentations and management. Bacterial pneumonia can involve an entire single lobe, multiple lobes, lobular segments, or can present as bronchopneumonia, defined as a patchy involvement of several lobes. It can develop explosively or have a more indolent onset. Multiple complications can arise due to either hematogenous or contiguous spread of the in-fecting organism. The frequency of such complications differs with the infecting organism.

DIAGNOSIS AND DIFFERENTIAL DIAGNOSIS

Bacterial pneumonia should be suspected in patients whose signs of infection include chills, fever, and symptoms referable to the lower respiratory tract. An elevated peripheral neutrophil count with early forms of neutrophils is common, although neutropenia can also be found, especially in patients with bacteremic pneumonia. A chest x-ray should demonstrate pulmonary infiltrates (Figs. 13–1a and b); however, early in the course of the infection or in dehydrated patients, the x-ray can be misleading. Although this constellation of findings is helpful in suggesting infection in the lungs, it does not establish the etiology of the pneumonia. The causative organism can be identified definitively only by isolation from cultures of sputum, pleural fluid (if available), or blood. Thoracentesis should be performed if pleural fluid is present, and a minimum of two blood cultures should be obtained from every patient in whom bacterial pneumonia is suspected. In some forms of pulmonary infection, such as that due to *Mycoplasma pneumoniae* or *Legionella,* serology can be extremely helpful in retrospect (Table 13–1).

It is important to collect sputum in an appropriate manner because bacteremia or pleural involvement does not occur in every patient. Culture of sputum obtained following a deep cough can establish the etiology of the infection. A Gram's stain of sputum is extremely useful in determining whether or not the specimen represents secretions from the site of infection or merely expectorated saliva. Culture of im-

TABLE 13–1. *Differential Diagnostic Features of Bacterial versus Nonbacterial Pneumonia*

Feature	Pneumococcal Lobar Pneumonia	Viral–Mycoplasmal Pneumonia
Onset	Sudden	Gradual
Rigors	Single chill	"Chilliness"
Facies	"Toxic"	Well
Cough	Productive	Paroxysmal; nonproductive
Sputum	Purulent (bloody)	Mucoid
Herpes labialis	Frequent	Rare
Temperature	103°–104°F	<103°F
Pleurisy	Frequent	Rare
Consolidation	Frequent	Rare
Gram's stain (sputum)	Neutrophils; cocci	Mononuclear cells; mixed flora
White blood cell and differential count	>15,000/mm³ Immature neutrophils	<15,000/mm³ Normal
Chest roentgenogram	Defined density	Nondefined infiltrate

properly collected sputum can be misleading about the cause of the infection. Expectorated sputum in bacterial pneumonia should contain neutrophils and not more than 10 epithelial cells per high-powered field. If a good specimen is obtained and a predominant organism is present, a skilled microscopist can provide a tentative etiologic diagnosis from the Gram's stain. Some patients cannot produce sputum spontaneously. For these patients, an appropriate sputum specimen can be induced using inhaled nebulized steam and gentle chest percussion. Children under the age of 7 or 8 rarely are capable of producing adequate sputum specimens. Invasive techniques such as transtracheal aspiration by needle, in which sterile saline is instilled and then aspirated, were utilized in the recent past to overcome difficulties in obtaining a high-quality sputum sample. Because this technique is associated with bleeding and other complications, it is now used less frequently. Bronchoscopy with bronchial lavage and brushings or transbronchial biopsy is now utilized in specific situations and can be extremely useful in determining etiology.

It is important to recognize that not all patients with fever, respiratory symptoms, and a pulmonary infiltrate have pneumonia. Other common causes of these signs and symptoms include pulmonary embolism (with or without infarction), primary or metastatic lung tumors, or, less commonly, pulmonary hemorrhage, among many other conditions. Thus, the physician is required to decide if the pulmonary symptoms are due to infection, and, if so, to establish a bacteriologic cause. At this point a decision regarding empiric antibiotic therapy is necessary. Once culture results are available, antibiotic treatment should be modified to use the safest, most conveniently administered, and least expensive effective agent.

ETIOLOGY

Of the bacterial causes of community-acquired pneumonia, *Streptococcus pneumoniae, Haemophilus influenzae,* and *Klebsiella pneumoniae* have been well recognized for many years. They are extracellular pathogens which are killed by phagocytic cells, neutrophils, and macrophages. *Staphylococcus aureus* and group A streptococcus are also extracellular pathogens but, in contrast to the three organisms listed above, are less frequent causes of pneumonia. Legionella, mycoplasma, and moraxella are more recently identified causes of pulmonary infections and raise specific issues relevant to diagnosis and treatment. The three most common bacterial causes of community-acquired pneumonia in adults are *Streptococcus pneumoniae, Mycoplasma pneumoniae,* and *Legionella pneumophila* (Table 13–2). In children *Haemophilus influenzae, S. pneumoniae,* and *Staphylococcus aureus* are also seen frequently, but legionella infection is very uncommon.

SPECIFIC FORMS OF PNEUMONIA

Pneumococcal Pneumonia

Streptococcus pneumoniae are gram-positive diplococci which require an enriched medium for growth *in vitro.* On blood agar plates colonies produce alpha, or green, hemolysis. When heavily encapsulated, the colonies appear mucoid. These organisms are facultative anaerobes which often are difficult to maintain in culture because of autolysis produced by an endogenous enzyme, muramyl-L-alanine amidase. This enzyme, activated by a variety of stimuli including

TABLE 13–2. *Etiologic Categories of Infectious Pneumonia among Hospitalized Patients at Yale–New Haven Medical Center**

Microbial Agent Isolated	July 1969–Jan. 1972		July 1979–Jan. 1982	
	Percentage		*Percentage†*	
Streptococcus pneumoniae	46.0		21.0	
Staphylococcus sp.	6.8		3.4	
Haemophilus influenzae	3.8		3.2	
Klebsiella sp.	1.8		3.0	
Other bacteria	9.5		22.0	
Total bacteria		67.9%		52.6%
Mycoplasma pneumoniae	5.6		3.4	
Fungi (*Candida* and others)	<7.2		13.2	
Influenza	1.0		3.4	
Cytomegalovirus	0		1.5	
"Unspecified virus(es)"	16.5		28.0	
Total viruses		17.5%		32.9%
Miscellaneous agents	2.1		4.4	
Total patient records reviewed		935		1175

*Adapted from Fick, R. B. Jr., and Reynolds, H. Y. Changing spectrum of pneumonia—news media creation or clinical reality? *Am. J. Med.* 74:1, 1983. Etiologic categories modified by the author of this chapter as follows: "Other bacteria" includes other streptococci, *Pseudomonas aeruginosa*, *Legionella pneumophila*, and *Mycobacterium tuberculosis*; "miscellaneous agents" includes *Pneumocystis carinii*, *Chlamydia* sp., and parasitic microorganisms.

†Cumulative total percentage exceeds 100% because more than one agent was isolated in some patients.

bile, is the basis of the bile solubility of these organisms, and distinguishes them from other alpha-hemolytic streptococci. *S. pneumoniae* is sensitive to optochin, and this characteristic is used to identify the organism when isolated in culture.

The serologic reactions of the capsular polysaccharide identify more than 80 separate serotypes of *S. pneumoniae*. The amount of capsular polysaccharide produced by an organism correlates roughly with virulence within a specific serotype. Thus, a type 3 *S. pneumoniae* with a large capsule is, in general, more virulent than a type 3 pneumococcus with less capsular polysaccharide. Normally, humans are resistant to this organism, which is a part of the normal nasopharyngeal flora. Those *S. pneumoniae* which bind well to respiratory epithelial cells appear to be more pathogenic than those that are less firmly bound. With aspiration or inhalation into the lower respiratory tract, in the absence of antibody in the alveoli specific for the capsular polysaccharide, the organism replicates and edema and neutrophils fill the alveoli. The mechanism of alveolar cell injury which leads to the inflammatory response is not clearly delineated. In contrast to group A streptococci, *S. pneumoniae* does not produce toxins. The capsule inhibits phagocytosis by neutrophils. In the presence of opsonins (specific antibody or complement), ingestion and killing of the organism by phagocytes is rapid. In the absence of antibiotic therapy, recovery is associated with production of specific antibody. Without therapy, the infection can spread via the lymphatics to the hilar nodes and contiguous organs as well as by hematogenously producing metastatic infection.

Pneumonia due to *S. pneumoniae* is the most common form of bacterial lung infection requiring hospitalization. It can occur in any age group and on a background of good health as well as in the presence of an underlying disease. In the colder months of the year, the "respiratory season," an increased number of normal individuals carry *S. pneumoniae* asymptomatically in the pharynx. Humans thus constitute the most important reservoir of this microorganism. Aspiration of *S. pneumoniae*, or the pneumococcus, into the lower respiratory tract is enhanced by a preceding viral upper respiratory illness which interferes with the normal upper respiratory tract defense mechanisms (Chapter 10). In addition, alcohol ingestion increases the risk of developing pneumococcal pneumonia. See Chapter 12 for a complete description of these defense mechanisms.

Classically, this infection has a sudden onset, heralded by a single severe rigor, and followed by a precipitous increase in body temperature and cough productive of rusty sputum. The patient usually is dyspneic and often complains of pleuritic chest pain. Examination of the chest reveals evidence of consolidation of a lobe, including limited expansion of the thorax on the affected side, increased tactile fremitus, dullness to percussion, bronchial breath sounds, and rales. Not uncommonly, the physical signs of consolidation are absent, especially if the patient is seen early in the course of the infection.

Furthermore, the classic history of the acute illness can be absent or greatly altered. For example, elderly individuals complain only of fever and shortness of breath and often are unable to produce sputum.

The laboratory usually provides adjunctive evidence of infection. The peripheral white count typically is elevated, and there are many young forms of neutrophils seen on smear, the so-called shift to the left. Acutely, arterial blood gases often reveal marked hypoxemia. The arterial oxygen can be disproportionately low in relation to the actual amount of lung involvement, reflecting marked shunting of blood within the pulmonary vasculature.

In the untreated patient, the temperature continues to remain high for 7–10 days. The "crisis" at the end of this period is marked by a rapid rise in fever to levels of 105°F and is associated with the appearance of detectable levels of serum antibody to the capsular polysaccharide of the infecting pneumococcus. Once the peak of the fever is reached, the temperature drops precipitously to normal or below. The crisis is sometimes associated with cardiopulmonary collapse but more often heralds the beginning of convalescence. Appropriate antibiotic therapy, with penicillin G or erythromycin, in the majority of young healthy individuals is associated with rapid defervescence. In older or debilitated patients, in contrast, the temperature often falls more slowly, requiring 5–7 days to reach normal levels. Complications which were prevalent in the preantibiotic era include empyema, pericarditis, pyogenic arthritis, endocarditis, and meningitis. Empyema and pericarditis are due to direct extension of the infection to the contiguous structure; the remaining complications represent metastatic infection following bacteremia. Antibiotic therapy has greatly reduced the prevalence of these complications except in patients who delay seeking medical attention or who have a defect in host defenses such as hypogammaglobulinemia. The initial response to antibiotic therapy can be followed by recrudescence of fever. This can be due to development of one of the complications of pneumococcal pneumonia noted above, or it can represent a hypersensitivity reaction to the antibiotic used in treatment. Less commonly, the development of a sterile nonpurulent pleural effusion, in reaction to the underlying pneumonia, is the cause of the new fever. Drug fevers can mimic fevers seen with infection. The temperature may rise daily so that the fever curve resembles a picket fence. In other patients

drug fever results in a constant temperature elevation marked by a dampened diurnal variation. This hypersensitivity reaction responds within 2–3 days to cessation of administration of the antibiotic. Drug fevers often occur without rash, eosinophilia, or other common manifestations of an allergic response.

The mortality rate for this form of pneumonia remains at 15–20% despite the availability of curative antibiotic therapy. Approximately one in five patients with pneumococcal pneumonia has positive blood cultures before initiation of treatment. Bacteremia, involvement of multiple lobes, advanced age, and metastatic infection all independently worsen the prognosis. Splenectomized individuals are also at great risk of developing fulminant infection with circulatory collapse and disseminated intravascular coagulation as a consequence of bacteremic pneumococcal infections (Chapter 27).

The polysaccharide capsule of *S. pneumoniae* inhibits phagocytosis of the organism by neutrophils. Antibody to the capsule serves as an opsonin and is protective. Immunization designed to induce specific antibody to capsular polysaccharide was shown to reduce the frequency of pneumococcal infection before the antibiotic era. With the widespread availability of penicillin G and other effective agents, further development of vaccines was discontinued after World War II. The realization that bacteremic pneumococcal infection continued to be associated with high mortality renewed interest in developing a means of preventing this often-lethal form of pneumonia. Although there are more than 80 serotypes, a limited number account for the majority of bacteremic pneumonias. Therefore, a vaccine containing the polysaccharides of the 23 serotypes most commonly associated with bacteremia has been developed for use in "high-risk" individuals, including those with immune deficiencies, postsplenectomy, chronic cardiac and pulmonary disease, and the elderly. Controversy about the usefulness of the vaccine has continued since its introduction to clinical use (see Felice in the references for a complete discussion of this issue).

Legionella Pneumonia

In August 1976, a pneumonic illness with a high fatality rate occurred among men and women who attended a state American Legion convention in Philadelphia. The majority of affected individuals had stayed at a single hotel and became ill within 2–3 days after returning home. Treatment with penicillin or cephalosporin antibiotics was not associated with improvement. Many of the individuals, in addition to pneumonia, were noted to have diarrhea, renal and hepatic dysfunction, or change in mental status.

The isolate associated with the outbreak in Philadelphia was initially identified by methods used for isolation of rickettsia, inoculation of embryonated eggs. It was later grown on artificial media containing a higher concentration of cysteine than is present in commonly used media. In addition, ferric pyrophosphate stimulates growth but is not necessary for primary recovery of the organism. Following isolation, the organisms can be identified by immunofluorescent stains. Six serotypes of the organisms, *Legionella pneumophila,* have been identified; type 1 caused the outbreak in Philadelphia. Closely related organisms, *L. bozemanii* and *L. micdadei,* first isolated in Pittsburgh, also have been isolated from patients with similar forms of pneumonia. *L. micdadei* is unique in that it does not produce a beta-lactamase and appears to be associated most commonly with infection in compromised hosts. With identification of the etiologic organism, stored specimens from previous outbreaks of unexplained febrile illnesses revealed that this aerobic gram-negative bacillus had been the cause not only of pneumonia but also of a febrile illness which was short in duration and less lethal. This latter illness was termed Pontiac fever. With the isolation of *Legionella,* an assay for antibody to the bacteria and a simplified culture technique were developed. It is now apparent that *Legionella* species are a relatively common cause of pneumonia in adults, accounting for a large proportion of the hospitalizations resulting from pulmonary infection. Serologic surveys have documented that approximately 5% of the population has antibody to these organisms.

The pneumonic form is by far the most common manifestation of this infection, and it occurs both in outbreaks and episodically. Individuals with chronic bronchitis or emphysema, cardiac disease, or immunodeficiencies are clearly more susceptible to this infection and have the highest morbidity and mortality. The organism is water-borne and can live in hot water systems as well as in air-conditioning ducts. This finding explains the outbreaks localized to a single building such as hotel or hospital. The organism, however, is ubiquitous and has been isolated from shower heads in homes and from the banks of rivers.

Legionella infections generally present with rigors, fever, and respiratory symptoms, but the onset is somewhat less explosive than pneumonia due to *S. pneumoniae.* The cough is often nonproductive and, in contradistinction to other forms of bacterial pneumonia, Gram's stains of sputum reveal mononuclear cells rather than neutrophils. A paucity of microorganisms is found in smears of sputum. A high peripheral white count is generally present. If there is renal and hepatic involvement, elevation of serum creatinine, blood urea nitrogen, and hepatic enzymes are noted. Hyponatremia and hypophosphatemia suggest this form of pneumonia. The findings on chest x-ray can vary. The pneumonia can be lobar, but more commonly presents as a bronchopneumonia involving multiple lobes with or without a pleural effusion. The infection can also produce cavitary disease.

Diagnosis of legionella pneumonia requires a high degree of suspicion by the physician. The clinical presentation, although generally different from that of pneumonia due to *S. pneumoniae* and *Mycoplasma pneumoniae,* can mimic these infections completely. Acutely, the diagnosis is suggested by a serum antibody titer, using an indirect immunofluorescent technique, of greater than 1:64. If the titer is greater than 1:256 the diagnosis can be made more confidently. A fourfold rise or fall in antibody titer over a 4–6 week period is diagnostic of infection with a species of *Legionella.*

The antibiotics shown to be effective are erythromycin, ciprofloxacin, and rifampin. Erythromycin has been the most widely used form of therapy, and it is generally administered intravenously, 1 gm every 6 h. The penicillins and cephalosporins are ineffective because these organisms, except for *L. micdadei,* produce a beta-lactamase which renders them resistant to beta-lactam agents.

Mycoplasmal Pneumonia

Pulmonary infection due to *Mycoplasma pneumoniae* is most commonly diagnosed in young adults and older children. In the late 1930s, an atypical form of lung infection which differed from classic "pneumococcal pneumonia" was first described. During World War II the clinical features of the illness were delineated and the association of serum antibodies which aggregated erythrocytes in the cold and agglutinins for the MG streptococcus were noted. Eaton produced pneumonia in rats and hamsters with filtered sputum obtained from infected patients and documented that serum from convalescent patients protected the animals. In the 1950s,

Liu identified the "Eaton agent" on bronchial epithelium of chick embryos using immunofluorescent techniques. Chanock and coworkers in the early 1960s proved that this agent caused "atypical pneumonia" and successfully cultured the organisms on artificial media.

M. pneumoniae requires supplemental enriched media for *in vitro* replication. It is slow-growing and has the typical properties of a mycoplasma. It is a small procaryotic organism, bounded by a cell membrane and lacking a cell wall. Mycoplasma are the smallest free-living organisms, distinct from viruses in that they can be grown on cell-free media. They grow under both aerobic and anaerobic conditions. The inability of this organism to synthesize a cell wall renders it resistant to antibiotics which inhibit cell-wall synthesis, such as penicillins, cephalosporins, and vancomycin. Erythromycin, tetracycline, and quinoline antibiotics which inhibit protein synthesis or DNA gyrase activity provide effective therapy.

Glycolipids in the cell membrane of *M. pneumoniae* induce both specific antibody responses and nonspecific antibody production. Thus, a positive serologic test for syphilis sometimes develops following infection with this organism. A specific mycoplasmal lipid sequence apparently interacts with the erythrocyte antigens I and i, and presumably this is the basis for the induction of the cold hemagglutinin antibody—the cold agglutinins. Occasionally, high titers of the cold hemagglutinin are associated with hemolysis.

The infection is documented in susceptible populations in the temperate climates throughout the year. Thus, in the warmer months pneumonia due to *M. pneumoniae* increases relative to the decreasing prevalence of *Streptococcus pneumoniae* infection. When epidemics occur, mycoplasma infection can account for 15–20% of pneumonic illness in a community. However, the infection is usually mild and accounts for a small number of hospitalized patients even in epidemic periods. Upper respiratory infection with the organism is common in children under 5 years of age; pulmonary infection occurs most commonly in school-aged children and young adults. It is common to obtain a history of upper respiratory infections spreading through children in the family of an adult patient with this form of pneumonia for weeks before the pulmonary infection occurred. Attack rates are estimated to be very high once one member of a family or a closed population, such as boarding school students or military recruits, is infected.

Respiratory secretions contain *M. pneumoniae* for a week before the onset of clinical symptoms, but the concentration is highest at the time of onset of disease. The organism can then be detected in respiratory secretions for weeks after convalescence. The organism attaches to respiratory epithelium through the interaction of a membrane protein termed P1 and a cell-surface receptor. It is thought that oxidants produced by *M. pneumoniae* damage cells. It has also been postulated that clinical symptoms are the result of the immunologic response by the host to the organism. This could account for more severe disease occurring in older children and young adults who had been immunized by exposure to the organism early in life and for the infrequent form of pneumonia due to this organism in immunocompromised patients. The characteristic cellular infiltrate induced by infection consists of lymphocytes and plasma cells. Patient recovery from infection is associated with detection of specific IgG and IgA antibody in respiratory secretions. Thus, the immune response may be involved in production of clinical manifestations as well as in recovery.

Mycoplasmal pneumonia is generally mild, with fever and cough being the prominent signs. The disease begins slowly with nonspecific symptoms such as headache, malaise, and fever. Symptoms increase over the course of a few days before a nonproductive cough is noted which is often associated with substernal discomfort. Symptoms of an upper respiratory infection can be present. Rigors are not commonly reported by patients, and fever can range from low grade to 40°C. Examination of the chest can reveal wheezing, rhonchi, or rales, or it can be negative. A minority of patients have myringitis and some patients complain of muscle tenderness and joint discomfort. Gastrointestinal symptoms include anorexia, nausea, and vomiting.

The chest x-ray usually demonstrates bronchopneumonia, which can involve multiple lobes, and a small pleural effusion is present in a quarter of the patients. The white blood cell count is often normal but can be moderately elevated. Few young neutrophilic forms are seen in the differential smears in contrast to results for pneumonococcal pneumonia. Sputum smears reveal phagocytic cells but usually contain mixed pharyngeal flora. The diagnosis is supported by the finding of cold agglutinins in serum usually within a week of the onset of the illness. The cold agglutinin is an IgM antibody directed against the I antigen on the red cell surface and can be detected at the bedside by cooling anticoagulated blood obtained from the patient to 4°C and observing red cell aggregation. When the antibody is present in very high concentrations, erythrocytic aggregation can be seen at room temperature. A rise in specific complement-fixing antibodies to the organism late in the infection establishes the diagnosis.

The pneumonic form of mycoplasmal infection is generally self-limited but on rare occasion can be fatal. The course is shortened by treatment with erythromycin or tetracycline therapy for 7 days, if initiated early in the infection. Complications include meningitis, encephalitis, pericarditis, myocarditis, and erythema multiforme or its more severe form, Stevens-Johnson syndrome. Patients with sickle cell anemia develop severe illness with mycoplasmal pneumonia, marked by a brisk leukocytosis and pleural effusions. Other causes of atypical pneumonia which resembles that caused by *M. pneumoniae* include psittacosis, Q fever, and infections with the TWAR (*Chlamydia pneumoniae*) agent as well as with legionella. Treatment with tetracycline is effective for pulmonary infection with these agents, but erythromycin more effectively treats Legionnaire's disease, a more common infection. Moreover, tetracycline should not be used in children under 8 years of age, as it stains the developing permanent teeth.

Pneumonia Caused by Haemophilus Influenzae

Haemophilus influenzae is a common cause of lower respiratory infection in children; but its most dramatic manifestations are epiglottitis or meningitis (Chapter 23). In adults serious infection with this small gram-negative coccobacillus is less frequent. In common with *Streptococcus pneumoniae,* most strains of *H. influenzae* are encapsulated by polysaccharide which inhibits phagocytosis by neutrophils in the absence of opsonic antibody.

Exposure in childhood to *H. influenzae* type b is thought to result in immunity and the lessened frequency of infection due to this encapsulated serotype in adults. In addition, cross-reactivity of the capsular polysaccharide with some pneumococcal types and with the *Escherichia coli* K1 antigen has been documented. Six antigenic types of capsular polysaccharide of *H. influenzae* have been distinguished: types a through f. Type b is by far the most frequent

cause of serious infection. The role of unencapsulated (nontypable) *H. influenzae* in disease is less clearly defined. Such organisms, as well as the encapsulated strains, are found in the normal pharyngeal flora. Frequent isolation of these bacteria from sputum specimens in patients with chronic bronchitis has led to the use of antibiotics to prevent and treat acute exacerbations of bronchitis. The role of *H. influenzae* in the pathogenesis of these acute episodes, however, remains problematic.

The pathogenesis of pulmonary infection due to *H. influenzae* is similar to pneumonia produced by the pneumococci. The organism, residing in the upper airway, reaches the lower respiratory tract when the normal defense mechanisms are altered, usually by a viral infection or alcohol ingestion. If the organism is encapsulated, phagocytosis by alveolar macrophages and neutrophils is inhibited. Bacterial replication occurs, followed by an inflammatory reaction and symptoms of pneumonia. In adults the onset is less dramatic than that of classic pneumococcal pneumonia, but severe dyspnea, cough, and fever are prominent features of the clinical picture. Lobar pneumonia is less frequently seen with *H. influenzae* than in pulmonary infection due to *S. pneumoniae*. The chest x-ray often demonstrates diffuse bronchopneumonia involving multiple lobes. In children, *H. influenzae* pneumonitis is frequently associated with bacteremia, but it is unclear whether the bacteremia is a primary or secondary event.

Treatment with ampicillin was previously effective. However, an increasing percentage of encapsulated (type b) and unencapsulated (nontypable) strains now produce beta-lactamase and are resistant to ampicillin and to first-generation cephalosporins. The extended spectrum second- and third-generation cephalosporins are the empiric treatment of choice for serious infection due to *H. influenzae*. If the laboratory demonstrates lack of beta-lactamase production by the clinical isolate, ampicillin can be substituted.

Klebsiella Pneumonia

Pneumonia due to the aerobic gram-negative bacilli of the *Klebsiella* species is an uncommon cause of community-acquired pneumonia. Pulmonary infection with the low-numbered serotypes of these organisms was formerly called Friedländer's pneumonia. These organisms were first isolated in the late 19th century by Karl Friedländer, a clinician and microbiologist. The low-numbered serotypes are encapsulated by a polysaccharide capsule which is antiphagocytic and, therefore, a virulence factor.

The pneumonic form of infection with *Klebsiella* is most common among alcoholics and debilitated or elderly patients. The clinical onset is sudden, but a rigor is not a component of the classic picture. Fever and leukocytosis are usually present, but, as in many severe infections due to gram-negative bacilli, hypothermia and neutropenia may occur and are associated with a poor prognosis. The sputum produced by patients with Klebsiella pneumonia is usually thick and tenacious. The chest x-ray can reveal either lobar or lobular infiltrates. Often with lobar involvement the volume of the affected lobe is expanded, marked by a convex bowing of the interlobar fissure. It is not uncommon to find cavity formation as a consequence of this necrotizing infection. The Gram's stains of the sputum should demonstrate neutrophils in abundance and many short, thick, gram-negative bacilli. Failure to recognize this form of pneumonia and to begin appropriate treatment can result in rapid death. In the preantibiotic era mortality rates reached 80%.

At the present time the most effective antibiotics used to treat Klebsiella pneumonia are the extended-spectrum second- and third-generation cephalosporins. Many isolates are now resistant to the first-generation cephalosporins, cephalothin, and cefazolin. It has been suggested that the addition of an aminoglycoside such as gentamicin enhances these patients' odds of survival. However, except for patients with neutropenia due to cytotoxic therapy or a hematologic malignancy, there is little information to indicate that the addition of these potentially toxic agents is beneficial.

Staphylococcal Pneumonia

Pulmonary infection due to *Staphylococcus aureus* is a rare form of pneumonia except in immunocompromised patients and occasionally in infants and children. The pneumonia is generally a diffuse bronchopneumonitis which complicates a preceding viral upper respiratory infection and is especially common during community outbreaks of influenza. The clinical onset generally differs from that of pneumococcal infection in that staphylococcal pulmonary infections are insidious; chills are uncommon, but fever is high and the patient appears septic. Sputum can be purulent and is classically described as salmon-pink. However, in many patients, it is blood-tinged, and in some sputum production is scant, especially early in the course of the infection. If sputum is available, grapelike clusters of staphylococci are easily demonstrated by Gram's stain. As the disease progresses the chest radiograph often demonstrates multiple, small-cavitary lesions or abscesses or one or two large abscess cavities with air–fluid levels. Complications include spread of the infection to the pleura (empyema) or pericardium, and (with bacteremia) infection of cardiac valves (endocarditis), bone, kidneys, or meninges. Before the availability of effective antibiotic therapy, the prognosis was extremely poor, with mortality reaching 80–90% in some series. More recently, mortality is in the range of 5–10%.

Antibiotics of choice for treatment of severe staphylococcal infections are the penicillinase-resistant penicillins. At present the most commonly used forms of these antibiotics are nafcillin or oxacillin. The great majority (90%) of community-acquired, as well as hospital-acquired, *S. aureus* pneumonia are penicillin-resistant. An increasing number of these organisms are also methicillin-resistant (MRSA). The increased prevalence of MRSA infections is well documented in such epidemiologically restricted populations as intravenous drug users, but they are increasing in prevalence throughout society. Therefore, monitoring of the susceptibility pattern of *S. aureus* isolates, both hospital-acquired and community-acquired, is necessary. The antibiotic used to treat MRSA infection is vancomycin.

Endocarditis of the tricuspid and pulmonary valves due to *S. aureus* is diagnosed frequently among intravenous drug users and is seen in individuals with left-to-right shunts resulting from congenital cardiac disease. Septic emboli from these infected valves typically lodge in the pulmonary capillary bed and produce multiple scattered areas of bronchopneumonia. This is probably the most common form of hematogenously acquired pulmonary infection.

Group A Streptococcal Pneumonia

Pneumonia is an uncommon form of infection due to this organism; however, it can be an especially virulent clinical illness. Most often, pneumonia due to group A streptococcus occurs, epidemically, in closed populations following an outbreak of a viral upper respiratory infection. However, sporadic cases are seen. The details of the microbiology and pathogenic potential of this organism are presented in Chapter 9.

The pathogenesis of pneumonia due to this organism is similar to that for *Streptococcus pneumoniae*. Following alteration in the normal host defenses of the upper airway, thought sometimes to be a consequence of viral infection, the organism reaches the lower respiratory tract. The onset of signs and symptoms is explosive, and the patient is usually extremely toxic. The extracellular products which contribute to the virulence of this organism influence the clinical picture of pulmonary infection. The pneumonia spreads rapidly and empyema is documented in up to 50% of cases. Management requires early recognition and institution of therapy with penicillin. Mortality due to group A streptococcal pneumonia is low unless treatment is delayed.

Pneumonia Caused by Moraxella Catarrhalis

Although sinusitis and otitis media are the most common infections associated with *Moraxella catarrhalis* (formerly named *Branhamella catarrhalis*), bronchopulmonary infections have been reported with increasing frequency over the past decade. However, respiratory tract infections are most definitively documented in patients with a significant compromise of host defenses. In patients who are the recipients of organ grafts, *M. catarrhalis* pneumonitis can develop rapidly, be associated with moderate to severe toxicity, but respond rapidly to appropriate antimicrobial therapy. Beta-lactamase production has been increasingly documented in clinical isolates. Therefore, ampicillin, which had been universally effective, can no longer be used empirically. A broad-spectrum cephalosporin or the combination of a beta-lactamase inhibitor such as clavulanic acid plus ampicillin are the agents to be used when this organism is suspected.

The pathogenesis of pneumonia due to this member of the normal oropharyngeal flora closely mimics that of *Haemophilus influenzae* or *Streptococcus pneumoniae*—that is, aspiration from the usual locus of colonization, failure or absence of defense mechanisms, bacterial replication, and an inflammatory response in the alveoli.

CASE HISTORY 1

A 30-year-old lawyer was seen in the emergency room for fever, cough, and pain in the right side of the chest with breathing. He had been well until 7 days before when he had caught a "cold" which he thought was improving. Two nights before coming to the hospital he had "partied" with friends and become intoxicated. The day before he noted a severe chill, followed by fever, chest pain, and cough productive of yellow sputum.

Physical examination revealed a young man in moderate respiratory distress. He was febrile (39°C), breathing 20 times per minute, and had a tachycardia of 110/min. His blood pressure was 120/80. The positive physical findings were limited to a "fever blister" on his lower lip, limited expansion of the right thorax on inspiration, dullness to percussion over the right posterior lung fields, and bronchial breath sounds.

The white count was 12,000/mm³ with an increase in young neutrophils (30%), and the chest x-ray revealed right lower and middle lobe pneumonitis. Gram's stain of expectorated sputum revealed neutrophils and gram-positive, lancet-shaped diplococci. One sputum culture and two blood cultures were obtained.

The patient was hospitalized and penicillin G (600,000 U) was administered intravenously. This was followed in 4 h by procaine penicillin (600,000 U) given intramuscularly. The procaine penicillin was then given every 12 h for the next 48 h. At that point the patient was afebrile and felt subjectively much better. The sputum culture grew *Streptococcus pneumoniae*, but the blood cultures were sterile. With the clinical improvement the therapy was changed to 500 mg penicillin V by mouth every 6 h. He continued to improve and was discharged on the fourth hospital day to continue the oral penicillin for 3 more days at home. He was seen by his physician a week following discharge and requested to return to work because he felt well.

CASE 1 DISCUSSION

This is a typical presentation of pneumonia due to Streptococcus pneumoniae. *The lower respiratory signs and symptoms developed on the background of an upper respiratory infection and acute alcohol ingestion and were associated with an exacerbation of Herpes simplex infection. The initial sign was a rigor.*

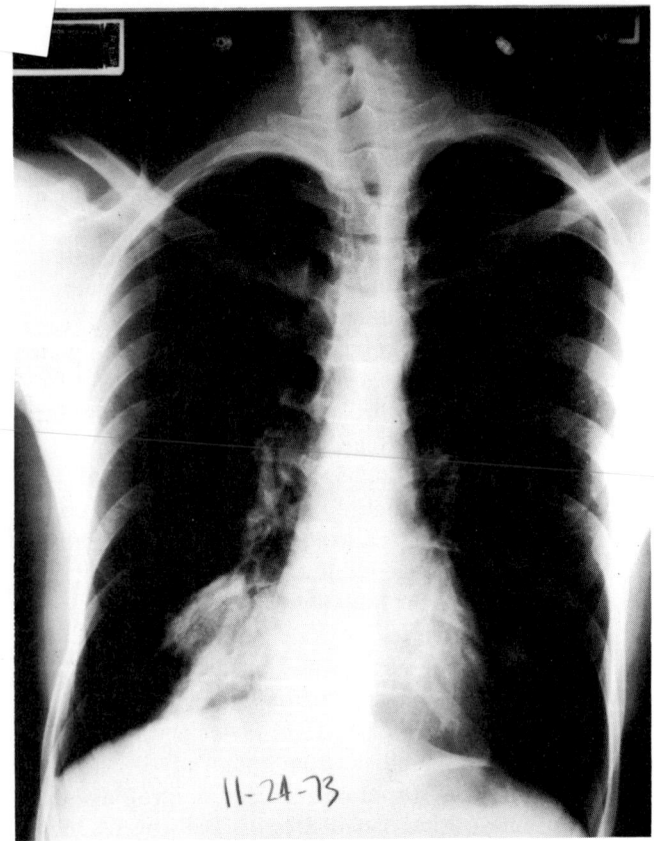

Figure 13–1. Posteroanterior chest roentgenogram of the patient discussed in Case History 1. Note the fairly well defined density in the lower right lung field. Without the right lateral roentgenographic projection (see Fig. 13–2), it would be impossible to know whether the pneumonic infiltrate occupies the right middle or right lower lobe of the lung.

11-24-73

Figure 13–2. Right lateral chest roentgenogram of the patient discussed in Case History 1. Although difficult to discern because of the cardiac shadow, the density noted in the right lung (Fig. 13–1) appears to be within the middle lobe and also the lower lobe of the right lung. The "stringy" densities confined to the hilar region are not uncommon in patients with bronchial asthma.

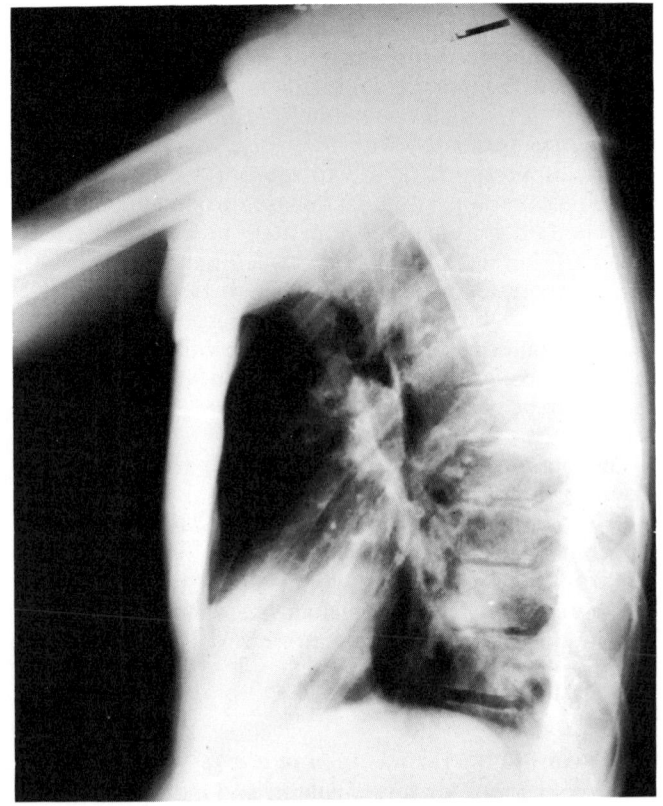

In this healthy young man the response to penicillin therapy was rapid. The organism's extreme susceptibility to penicillin allows for low parenteral and low oral doses of penicillin to be used in therapy. Early discharge was possible because the absence of documented bacteremia reduces the risk of arthritis, meningitis, or endocarditis which can complicate bloodstream infection. A follow-up chest x-ray would continue to demonstrate a pulmonary infiltrate, because x-ray findings commonly lag behind clinical improvement by several weeks.

CASE HISTORY 2

A 50-year-old air conditioner repair man was admitted to the hospital with pneumonia. He had noted onset of chills, fever, and cough 3 days before admission. At admission he was somewhat confused but able to give a complete history. He stated that he had had diarrhea for the past 2 days, as well as the respiratory symptoms. He was a heavy smoker but did not drink alcohol. He was febrile (39.5°C), breathing 25 times per minute, had a tachycardia of 120/minute, and his blood pressure was 90/60. Rales were heard over the left posterior lung fields, and a chest x-ray confirmed the presence of pneumonitis in the left lower lobe. He could not produce sputum. The white count was elevated (13,500/mm³), and there was a shift to the left. Serum chemistries revealed elevated levels of transaminases, bilirubin, blood urea nitrogen, and creatinine. The serum sodium value was below normal. Two blood cultures were obtained.

Therapy was initiated with erythromycin, 1 gm intravenously every 6 h, as empiric therapy for a community-acquired pneumonia. The history of diarrhea, liver function, and renal abnormalities on a background of good health suggested to a consultant the possibility of Legionnaire's pneumonia. Serologic studies for antibody to *Legionella* and *Mycoplasma* were obtained on the second hospital day. By the fourth hospital day, although the patient remained febrile, he was clear mentally and subjectively improved. The blood cultures were sterile, but the titer of antibody to *Legionella* type 2 was 1:64. There were no antibodies to *Mycoplasma*. Therapy was

continued with erythromycin. By day 7 he was afebrile, and asking to go home. The abnormal serum chemistries had improved. He was discharged to continue erythromycin (500 mg orally) every 6 h for 7 additional days.

CASE 2 DISCUSSION

The presence of mental status changes, diarrhea, and abnormalities in renal and liver function in association with pneumonia alerted the physician to the possibility of infection with Legionella pneumophila. *The patient's occupation exposed him to potentially contaminated aerosols in air-conditioning ducts. The antibody titer of 1:64 was suggestive but not diagnostic of this infection. Approximately 5% of the population has antibody to this organism. The diagnosis could be proved by obtaining a convalescent sera and demonstrating a significant (≥fourfold) rise or fall in the antibody titer.*

The three most common causes of community-acquired pneumonia in adults can be treated effectively with erythromycin. Legionella *and* Mycoplasma *are resistant to such beta-lactam antibiotics as penicillin, but* Streptococcus pneumoniae *is susceptible to both penicillin and erythromycin.*

REFERENCES

Books

Heffron, R. *Pneumonia*. Cambridge, MA: Harvard University Press, 1979.

Symposia

Balows, A., and Fraser, D. International symposium on Legionnaire's disease. *Ann. Intern. Med.* 90:491–703, 1979.

Articles

Austrian, R. Pneumococcal infection and pneumococcal vaccine. *N. Engl. J. Med.* 297:938–939, 1977.

Austrian, R., and Gold, J. Pneumococcal bacteremia with especial reference to bacteremic pneumococcal pneumonia. *Ann. Intern. Med.* 60:759–776, 1964.

Busk, M., Rosenow, E., and Wilson, W. Invasive procedure in the diagnosis of pneumonia. *J. Infect. Dis.* 155:855–861, 1988.

Carpenter, J. Klebsiella pulmonary infections: Occurrence

at one medical center and review. *Rev. Infect. Dis. 12:*672–682, 1990.

Fekety, R., Caldwell, J., Gump, D., et al. Bacteria, virus, and mycoplasma in acute pneumonia in adults. *Am. Rev. Respir. Dis. 104:*499–507, 1971.

Filice, G. Pneumococcal vaccine and public health policy. *Arch. Intern. Med. 150:*1373–1375, 1990.

Fraser, D., Tsai, T., Ornstein, W., et al. Legionnaire's disease. Description of an epidemic of pneumonia. *N. Engl. J. Med. 297:*1189–1197, 1977.

Gopal V., and Bisno, A. Fulminant pneumococcal infection in "normal" asplenic hosts. *Arch. Intern. Med. 137:*1526–1530, 1977.

Grayston, J., Alexander, E., Kenny, G., et al. *Mycoplasma pneumoniae* infections. Clinical and epidemiologic studies. *JAMA 191:*369–374, 1965.

Hahn, H., and Beaty, H. Transtracheal aspiration in the evaluation of patients with pneumonia. *Ann. Intern. Med. 72:*183–187, 1970.

Highman, J. Staphylococcal pneumonia and empyema in childhood. *Am. J. Roentgenol. 106:*103–108, 1969.

Murray, P., and Washington, J. Microscopic and bacteriologic analyses of expectorated sputum. *Mayo Clin. Proc. 50:*339–344, 1975.

Spencer, C., and Beaty, H. Complications of transtracheal aspiration. *N. Engl. J. Med. 295:*488–490, 1976.

Stover D., Zaman, M., Hajdu, S., et al. Bronchoalveolar lavage in the diagnosis of diffuse pulmonary infiltrates in the immunocompromised host. *Ann. Intern. Med. 101:*1–7, 1984.

Stout, J., Yu, V., Vickers, R., et al. Ubiquitous *Legionella pneumophila* in the water supply of a hospital with endemic Legionnaire's disease. *N. Engl. J. Med. 306:*466–468, 1982.

Tillotson, J., and Lerner, A. Pneumonias caused by gram-negative bacilli. *Medicine 45:*65–76, 1966.

Wallace, R., and Musher, D. In honor of Dr. Sarah Branham a star is born: The realization of *Branhamella catarrhalis* as a respiratory pathogen. *Chest 90:*447–450, 1986.

Wallace, R., Musher, D., Morton, R. *Hemophilus influenzae* pneumonia in adults. *Am. J. Med. 64:*87–93, 1978.

Warshauer, D., Goldstein, E., Akers, T., et al. Effect of influenza viral infection on the ingestion and killing of bacteria by alveolar macrophages. *Am. Rev. Respir. Dis. 115:*269–277, 1977.

Wilkenson, H., and Fikes, B. Detection of cell-associated or soluble antigens of *Legionella pneumophila* serogroups 1 to 6, *Legionella bozemanii, Legionella dumoffii, Legionella gormani,* and *Legionella micdadei* by staphylococcal coagglutination tests. *J. Clin. Microbiol. 14:*322–325, 1981.

Wimberly, W., Faling, L., and Bartlett, J. A fiberoptic bronchoscopy technique to obtain uncontaminated lower airway secretion for bacterial cultures. *Am. Rev. Respir. Dis. 119:*337–342, 1979.

14 *MARGARET YUNGBLUTH, M.D.*

Viral Infections of the Lower Respiratory Tract

INTRODUCTION

Nonbacterial lower respiratory tract infections are frequent occurrences in pediatric and adult populations worldwide. The majority of these infections occur in otherwise healthy individuals, and from an epidemiologic standpoint are community-acquired. Infections usually are abrupt in onset, follow an acute, short course of less than 1–2 weeks, and can be expected to resolve in most cases without any permanent sequelae. This chapter emphasizes lower respiratory tract infections, defined anatomically as infection below the level of the epiglottis; this section of the respiratory tract begins with the glottis and trachea and extends downward through the bronchial tree and into the alveolar

portion of the lung. Viral infections of the lower respiratory tract are subdivided into several syndromes, based principally on the anatomical segment that seems most involved. These categories were established primarily on clinical and radiographic grounds, and for the most part have been validated by tissue histopathology. The most common viruses associated with lower respiratory tract disease are listed in Table 14–1. The respiratory myxoviruses (respiratory syncytial virus, influenza, parainfluenza, and measles), as well as adenovirus, are the organisms most frequently linked to these syndromes, although enteroviruses and agents such as *Chlamydia pneumoniae* (formerly *Chlamydia psittaci*-TWAR) and *Mycoplasma pneumoniae* are also well-recognized causes. Because of the potential for compromise of ventilation, patients with viral infections of the lower respiratory tract tend to be sicker than patients with simple upper airway colds and pharyngitis, and thus are more likely to need medical intervention.

The tracheobronchial mucosa is a dense layer of ciliated columnar cells and mucin-secreting goblet cells. The mucosa changes abruptly at the level of the alveolus to a flattened, attenuated, gas-permeable epithelial monolayer quite similar to the endothelium of the capillary plexus in the lung. Ciliated cells are intermixed with the stratified squamous epithelium that predominates in areas of the nose, mouth, pharynx, and larynx; however, in the lower respiratory tract the ciliated cells represent a continuous, homogeneous mucosal surface. The ciliated columnar epithelial cells are rich in surface receptors which bind respiratory myxoviruses and adenovirus, and support the attachment of *Chlamydia pneumoniae* and *Mycoplasma pneumoniae*. These organisms can be expected to infect a wide distribution of epithelial cells in

TABLE 14–1. *Principal Viral Causes of Lower Respiratory Tract Infections*

Croup	Bronchiolitis/Pneumonia	Influenza
Parainfluenza virus, 1, 2, and 3	Respiratory syncytial virus	Influenza A virus
Respiratory syncytial virus	Parainfluenza virus, 1 and 3	Influenza B virus
Rhinovirus	Adenovirus	
*Mycoplasma pneumoniae**	Measles virus	
*Chlamydia pneumoniae**	Rhinovirus	
	*Mycoplasma pneumoniae**	
	*Chlamydia pneumoniae**	

*Nonviral

both the upper and lower respiratory tracts. Anatomic factors as well as the modifying influence of the host immune response often dictate at what site in the respiratory tract clinical symptoms will be most pronounced.

INFLUENZA

Virus Morphology and Epidemiology

Influenza is an acute, febrile respiratory illness that is caused exclusively by influenza type A or influenza type B virus. Although both of these viruses can also produce nondescript upper respiratory infections that clinically resemble ordinary colds and sore throats, influenza ("the flu") is a specific syndrome with a distinctive clinical presentation and epidemiologic pattern.

Influenza outbreaks occur almost annually during cold weather months in temperate climates. The conspicuous clustering of cases into a 1–2-month long epidemic is a characteristic feature of influenza, as is the increase in death rate from primary viral pneumonia combined with bacterial superinfections that usually accompany an influenza epidemic.

The influenza viruses (types A, B, and C) are the only members of the Orthomyxoviridae family, and all have the same structural and morphologic features (Fig. 14–1). Influenza virus may be either spherical or elongated into filamentous strands, and has a lipid bilayer envelope that encircles a single-stranded helical RNA nucleocapsid. The influenza virus envelope is acquired from the host cell's cytoplasmic membrane as the newly assembled viral nucleocapsid exits the cell. Two glycoprotein viral antigens, hemagglutinin (HA) and sialidase, or neuraminidase (NA), are located on this lipid envelope, and they play an essential role in initiating infection. The HA antigen is embedded by its hydrophobic end into the envelope's lipid bilayer and has a hydrophilic end which projects above the viral surface and functions as the ligand for attachment of the virion to receptors on the columnar epithelial cell of the respiratory tract. HA also can bind to chicken erythrocytes (a fortuitous observation that led to its name), but the pathogenesis of influenza begins when this antigen anchors the virus to the respiratory epithelium, initiating fusion of the viral envelope with the cytoplasmic membrane of the host cell so that the RNA nucleocapsid can be released into the cytosol for replication.

The other critical protein antigen located on the viral envelope is neuraminidase. NA is an enzyme which hydrolyzes the glycosidic linkage of sialic acid to glycoprotein, but its contribution to the pathogenesis of influenza is not entirely clear. It may partially denature respiratory mucin and thereby promote viral adherence to the epithelial surface, or it may be needed in the envelopment and final release of mature virions from the infected cell. Like HA, NA spicules are also anchored into the virion envelope and project above the viral surface.

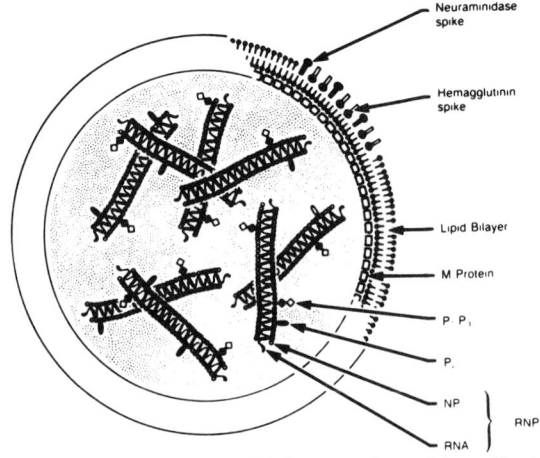

Figure 14–1. Diagram of influenza virus virion. Single-stranded RNA nucleocapsid is divided into eight segments. Lipid bilayer envelope has neuraminidase and hemagglutinin antigens. (From Ginsberg, H. S. Orthomyxoviruses. In: Davis, B. D. (ed), Microbiology. 4th ed. Philadelphia: Lippincott, 1990, p. 990)

The influenza virus genome is organized into eight helical segments of double-stranded RNA flanked by capsid polypeptides. This viral RNA encodes for all the synthetic enzymes needed for influenza replication, as well as for all the structural antigens of the nucleocapsid and envelope.

To date, three major HA and two NA antigenic types have been identified, and influenza virus strains can be precisely classified by the virus type, geographic site of first isolation, year of first isolation, and HA type and NA type (e.g., influenza A/Hong Kong/68/H3N2). A specific influenza strain has its antigen epitopes modified slightly year by year *(antigenic drift)* as a consequence of random point mutation in the RNA genome, but herd immunity characteristics remain fairly stable and annual wintertime influenza outbreaks are contained at relatively low levels.

Antigenic shift is a dramatic alteration in influenza virus antigenic composition, with the introduction into society of a "new virus" with novel antigens to which much of the population has either no immunity or inadequate antibody levels. This major change in the antigen profile of influenza virus is brought about by genetic reassortment rather than by point mutation. Notice in Figure 14–1 that the influenza genome is subdivided into eight sections. When a cell is simultaneously infected with two different influenza strains, the stage is set for the possible reshuffling of RNA segments into a hybrid virion which encodes for a new combination of HA and NA surface antigens, unlike that of either parent strain. In two recent severe influenza pandemics during the 20th century (1957 and 1968), novel virus was generated by human strains capturing exogenous RNA from avian influenza virus, most likely through simultaneous infection and genetic reassortment. The more dramatic the HA and NA antigenic alterations produced, the more susceptible the general population to infection, and the more severe the ensuing influenza outbreak.

Recent influenza pandemics in 1957 (influenza A, H2N2), 1968 (influenza A, H3N2), and 1977 (influenza A, H1N1) originated in mainland China from genetic reassortment and then spread in all directions to the rest of Asia, Australia, Europe, and the Americas. The severe 1957 and 1968 outbreaks each took between 1 and 2 years to extend globally. In interpandemic years there have been smaller, regional epidemics of influenza traced to antigenic drift in these new strains. Influenza B has a more stable genome than influenza A, less pronounced antigen alterations, a tendency to persist at lower infection rates year by year, and less likelihood for causing pandemic disease.

During an epidemic season, one influenza strain typically predominates, but two or more additional altered strains of influenza A and B can often be isolated from a minority of the infected population. Careful surveillance to identify prevalent strains is needed to ensure that annual vaccine reformulations include the most likely viral candidates for the upcoming flu season.

Influenza is spread easily from person to person. Respiratory tract secretions are rich in influenza virions during acute illness, and virus is incorporated into small-particle aerosol droplets by sneezing, coughing, and even by simply talking. The fragile lipid envelope and glycoprotein HA spicules make viral survival on inanimate objects very short, but low humidity and low ambient temperature do favor virus stability.

Pathogenesis and Clinical Illness

Once virus is introduced into the respiratory tract by aerosol inhalation, it attaches via its HA envelope antigen to a ciliated columnar epithelial cell, invades the cell, and promptly begins replicating. New virion synthesis is apparent in less than 24 h, spreading to nearby cells on the respiratory mucosal surface. The incubation period lasts only 1–3 days, after which enough virus has accumulated to produce symptoms. Individuals who have partial immunity to the infecting viral strain may develop only pharyngitis or cold symptoms. Nonimmune persons exposed to influenza virus develop classic influenza, with attack rates which may be as high as 70%. The diagnosis of influenza should be reserved for those patients who have a systemic febrile respiratory illness; severe upper airway illness without accompanying lower respiratory and systemic features, even if caused by influenza virus, should not be labeled as "the flu."

The systemic features of influenza are abrupt in onset and include fever (up to 104°F), chills, headache, myalgias, lumbosacral backache, and profound weakness. Headache and muscle aches are conspicuous complaints, and their intensity parallels the height of fever. Fever usually lasts 2–4 days. Dry cough, sore throat, and rhinorrhea are also present, are less intense at the outset, and become more prominent as fever subsides. Necrosis of infected respiratory epithelial cells is marked in influenza, and respiratory complaints reflect this damage. Viral shedding, and hence infectivity, is roughly proportional to the severity of pharyngitis, cough, and coryza.

Although the clinical features of acute influenza are usually distinctive enough to suggest the diagnosis, physical findings are often nonspecific. Physical examination is valuable more for ruling out other serious respiratory problems than for confirming a diagnosis of influenza. The pharyngeal mucosa is hyperemic but without exudate, and enlargement of tonsillar and anterior cervical lymph nodes is limited. The conjunctivae are somewhat inflamed and there is often a clear nasal discharge, but rhinorrhea is less than with a typical rhinovirus cold. Cough is usually nonproductive and often accompanied by substernal discomfort; however, pleural rubs are uncommon and the lung fields are clear to auscultation. Despite headache, myalgia, and low back pain, objective neurologic and musculoskeletal findings are lacking. Utter exhaustion is often the most pronounced early feature of influenza, and malaise is generally the symptom which resolves most slowly, usually taking about a week. Recovery from influenza is uneventful in the majority of cases without lingering or persistent symptoms. The clinical features of acute influenza are summarized in Figure 14–2.

Although society dwells upon the misery of influenza in adults, children also are easily infected, and during epidemic periods as many as one third of out-patient pediatric visits are for flu symptoms. Children often experience more sustained fever, shed virus longer than adults, and are more likely to develop primary viral pneumonia. Flu may provoke asthma in children with reactive airways and may precipitate febrile seizures. Reye syndrome, a rare complication of influenza exhibiting a sudden evolution of hepatocyte steatosis with mitochondrial damage and associated encephalopathy, has been linked with the use of salicylate antipyretics. Reye syndrome occurs even less frequently now that salicylate use in small children with influenza or chickenpox has been discouraged.

Like all viral infections, recovery from acute influenza requires an adequate cell-mediated immune response. CD4 lymphocytes exposed to viral antigen initiate clonal expansion of specific cytotoxic T8 lymphocytes which recognize and destroy host cells that contain influenza virus. This process promptly and efficiently terminates viral replication but also temporarily accelerates cytonecrosis of respiratory tract epithelium. Lymphocytic, rather than neutrophilic, infiltrates characteristically accompany the cellular damage, and the newly regenerated replacement epithelium has a metaplastic appearance (see Fig. 14–3).

Influenza antigen also stimulates a humoral B-lymphocyte response with the manufacture of specific IgM, IgG, and IgA antibodies. IgM antibody is detected approximately 1 week after the onset of influenza, but remains for only 2–3 months. IgG antibody can persist in the blood for up to several years. Secretory IgA antibody appears in nasal secretions in parallel with the development of humoral IgG but generally cannot be detected after 3–6 months. Protection against reinfection is the result of adequate concentrations of both serum and secretory antibody. Antibody directed against the hemagglutinin antigen stereotactically interferes with the binding function of this envelope structure and prevents viral attachment and infection. Antineuraminidase antibody modifies an existing viral infection, possibly by interfering with NA function in release of newly replicated virus from host cells. High levels of both types of antibody protect the host against reinfection; borderline or low antibody concentrations may only moderate the severity of illness.

Complications of Influenza

Although acute influenza is temporarily quite debilitating, most cases resolve within 1–2 weeks and leave no permanent damage. However, in a typical epidemic two types of complications predictably develop, compounding the morbidity of influenza and accounting for the vast majority of deaths: primary influenza virus pneumonia and secondary bacterial pneumonia. In every large outbreak, cases of viral pneumonia occur; overall, this severe form of influenza is seen in less than 1% of cases, but mortality rates as high as 30% can occur in this subset. Primary influenza virus pneumonia has classically been described in patients with underlying heart disease, particularly rheumatic mitral stenosis, but sporadic cases in otherwise healthy children and adults are also reported. Healthy pregnant women have an unexplainable but well-recognized higher risk for influenzal pneumonia. Involvement of the pulmonary parenchyma usually is apparent after a few days of typical influenza. Extensive viral-induced cellular damage is seen throughout the tracheo-

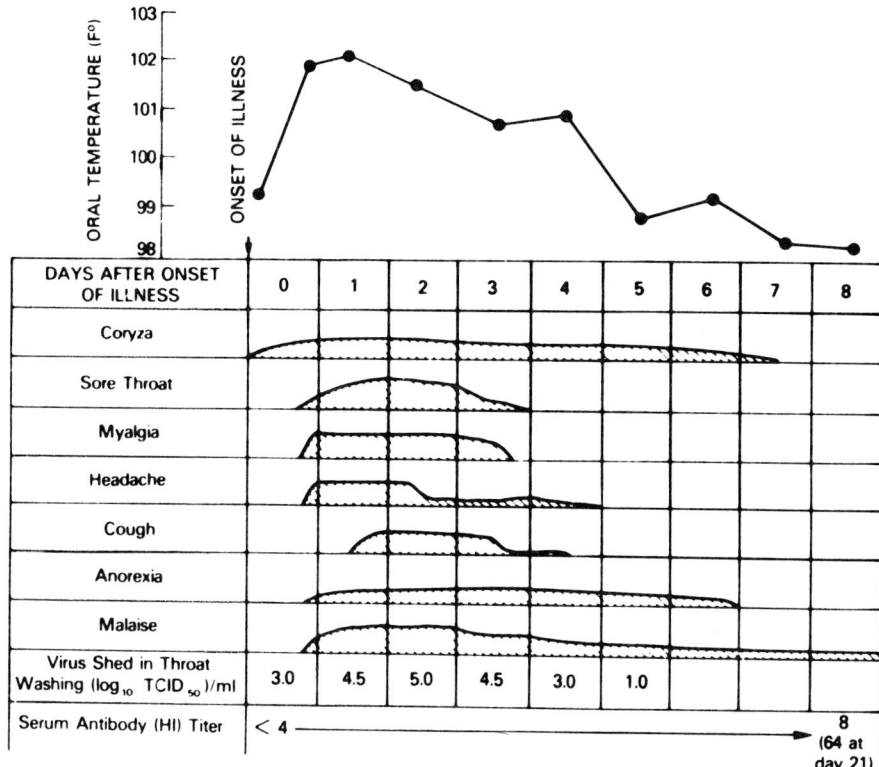

DAYS AFTER ONSET OF ILLNESS	0	1	2	3	4	5	6	7	8
Coryza									
Sore Throat									
Myalgia									
Headache									
Cough									
Anorexia									
Malaise									
Virus Shed in Throat Washing ($\log_{10}$ $TCID_{50}$)/ml	3.0	4.5	5.0	4.5	3.0	1.0			
Serum Antibody (HI) Titer	< 4								8 (64 at day 21)

Figure 14–2. Symptoms of naturally occurring influenza in a normal 28-year-old man. Shaded area height is proportional to the intensity of clinical complaint. (From Kilbourne, E. D. Influenza. *New York: Plenum, 1987.)*

bronchial mucosa and also involves the distal bronchioles and the alveolar epithelium. An acute interstitial pneumonitis then develops with a diffuse radiographic pattern. Gram's stain and bacterial culture show only normal flora, but influenza virus cultures are positive. Severe hypoxia from interstitial lymphocytic inflammation and edema follows, and despite intensive supportive care and ventilatory assistance, mortality rates are high. Figure 14–4 shows the histopathologic features of primary influenzal pneumonia.

The epithelial damage in the tracheobronchial tree seen in a typical case of acute influenza disrupts the mucociliary clearance function of the lung; in addition, neutrophil chemotaxis is impaired, and bacterial colonization patterns may be altered. These factors together predis-

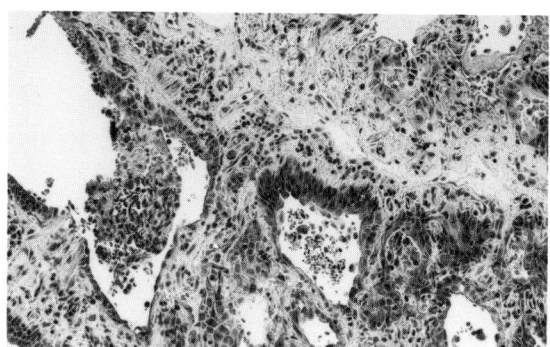

Figure 14–3. Acute influenza in a 34-year-old man; lung biopsy was performed during emergency replacement of aortic valve. Note necrotic epithelial debris in bronchial lumen and lymphocytic inflammatory infiltrate. Hematoxylin and eosin stain, 40× magnification.

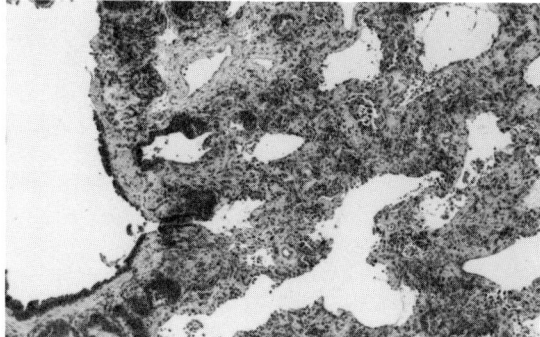

Figure 14–4. Fatal influenza A virus pneumonia in a 26-year-old woman. Bronchiolar mucosa has been destroyed and replaced by metaplastic epithelium. Alveolar walls are distorted and thickened by edema and dense lymphocytic infiltrate. Hematoxylin and eosin stain, 25× magnification.

pose influenza patients to secondary bacterial infection of the lower respiratory tract. Patients who develop secondary acute bacterial pneumonias often are elderly; have underlying chronic lung disease; or hypertensive, ischemic, or valvular heart disease. A biphasic pattern of illness is typical; after acute influenza begins to resolve, fever recurs and is accompanied by productive cough with purulent sputum from lobar or bronchopneumonia (see Fig. 14–5). In some cases viral and bacterial pneumonia overlap or progress almost simultaneously. *Streptococcus pneumoniae, Staphylococcus aureus, Haemophilus influenzae,* and *Neisseria* and *Moraxella* species are the usual secondary bacterial pathogens, and if promptly treated with antibiotics most patients respond favorably. Rare cases of toxic shock syndrome traced to staphylococcal superinfection have been described.

Other serious complications of acute influenza include encephalopathy, myopathy and rhabdomyolysis, and myocarditis; these are very unusual and account for very few of the fatal or nonfatal flu complications.

The disabling impact of influenza on society is most dramatic during a pandemic. However, during a local epidemic where partial herd immunity can be expected to limit the number of cases, influenza can still greatly disrupt a community. Figure 14–6 compares the influenza virus isolation rate in a typical outbreak with several measures of the accompanying morbidity

and mortality. School and industrial absenteeism paralleled the epidemic, as did total emergency room visits and the number of those visits for respiratory complaints. Hospitalizations for pneumonia showed that pediatric pneumonia admissions closely followed the viral isolation rate, but that adult pneumonia activity was maximal as the number of influenza isolates dropped; adult pneumonia, much of which was probably secondary bacterial superinfection, accounted for most of the mortality, and lagged behind the intensity of the influenza epidemic.

Treatment and Vaccination

Influenza is a preventable disease, but avoiding crowds and wearing masks in public places to reduce aerosol acquisition are unreasonable and impractical control measures. On the other hand, inactivated vaccines are quite effective in preventing infection or in modifying the severity of disease. Influenza vaccine is reformulated yearly and typically includes the three antigenic types felt to be the most likely to circulate through society. In recent years, two influenza A types and a single B type have been combined in a trivalent vaccine, which is recommended for use in early fall so that protective antibody levels are achieved before the predictable wintertime outbreak. Local irritation is a common side effect of vaccination with transient fever

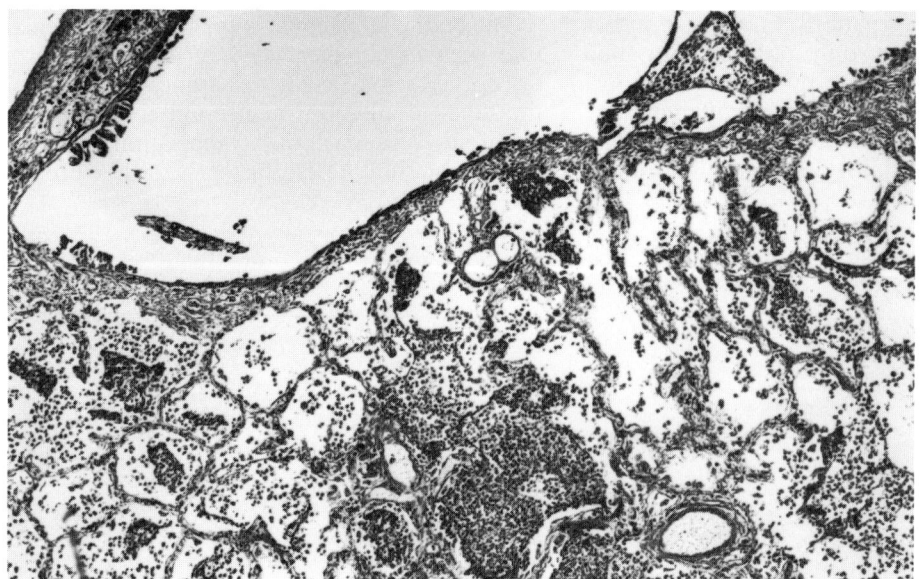

Figure 14–5. Fatal secondary bacterial bronchopneumonia in a 64-year-old woman with hypertensive heart disease. Bronchial epithelium still shows focal metaplastic change from prior influenzal damage. Alveolar walls are normal, but alveolar spaces are consolidated with neutrophils and fibrin from acute bacterial infection. Hematoxylin and eosin stain, 40× magnification.

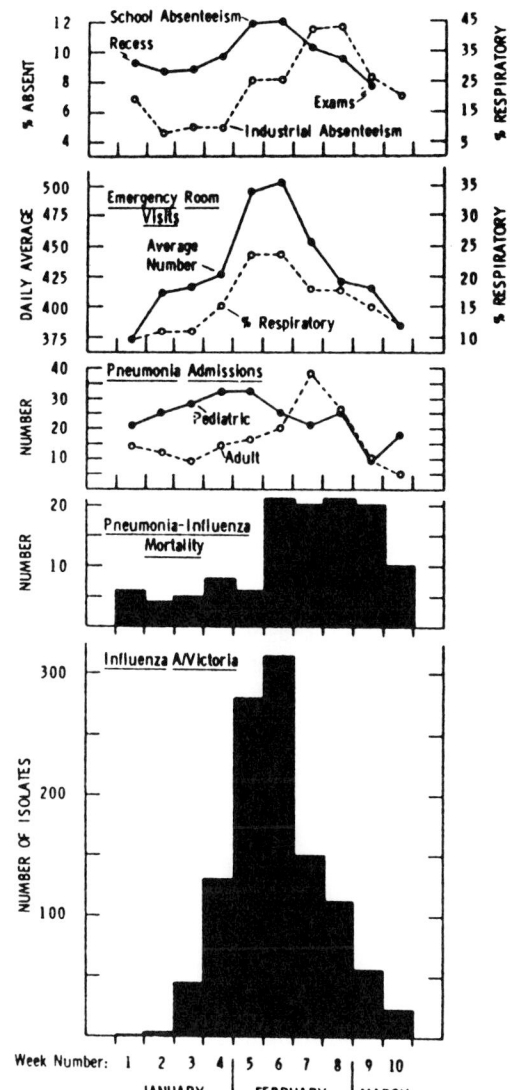

Figure 14–6. Correlation of nonvirologic indices with influenza virus isolation during outbreak. (From Glezen, W. P., and Couch, R. B. Interpandemic influenza in the Houston area, 1974–1976. N. Engl. J. Med. 298:587–592, 1978.)

seen in less than 5%. During 1976, a national immunization program to prevent an anticipated swine influenza epidemic was linked to several cases of Guillain-Barré syndrome, which had an associated 5% mortality rate. There has been no subsequent association of influenza vaccine with Guillain-Barré syndrome, and there have been no other recorded deaths linked to flu vaccination.

Influenza vaccination has traditionally been promoted for the elderly and for patients of any age with underlying chronic cardiac or pulmonary disease. Widened recommendations for immunization now include patients with noncar-

diopulmonary chronic illness such as diabetes, renal disease, collagen vascular disease, and malignancy. Individuals infected with human immunodeficiency virus also benefit from vaccination but frequently respond poorly. In addition to promoting annual vaccination for patients at high risk for influenza morbidity or mortality, health care workers have an obligation to also have themselves immunized. Physicians, nurses, and allied personnel working in hospitals, clinics, and chronic care facilities surely have a high probability of contact with influenza patients. Not only does efficient delivery of medical care suffer when critical personnel are unable to work because of influenza, but infected health care workers also serve as vectors for nosocomial spread of the virus. The only absolute contraindication to vaccination is hypersensitivity to hens' eggs, since immunizing virus strains are propagated in this medium. The overall risk-benefit ratio favors vaccination by several hundredfold. Nevertheless, the medical profession greatly underutilizes flu vaccination every year, and avoidable disease and associated deaths continue to occur.

Amantadine hydrochloride has shown a 70–90% efficacy in preventing influenza A when used for short-term prophylaxis. Unvaccinated high-risk individuals, household contacts of index cases, and health care workers may benefit from prophylactic administration of amantadine during periods of high influenza activity. Bothersome side effects of amantadine are largely confined to the gastrointestinal and central nervous systems, with insomnia, dizziness, anorexia, and nausea the chief complaints. Side effects occur in up to 15% of amantadine users, but are reversible once the drug is discontinued. Rimantadine, an analog of amantadine, also has antiviral activity; it is both safe and effective for influenza prophylaxis and has an overall lower risk of side effects (6–10%). Use of both amantadine and rimantadine has provoked the emergence of resistant influenza A virus strains *in vitro* and during rimantadine clinical trials, but the effect these resistant viral strains may have on the epidemiology and management of influenza is still unclear.

Management of uncomplicated, acute influenza remains largely supportive. Rest is a necessity and since most flu patients feel exhausted for the first few days of illness, compliance with bed rest recommendations is not a problem. Adequate hydration can usually be accomplished without the use of intravenous fluids. Acetaminophen or aspirin is adequate for fever and myalgias but salicylates should be avoided in children. Routine use of antibiotics is inappropriate and should be reserved for cases where secondary bacterial superinfection of the lower respiratory tract is suspected. Influenza virus is highly contagious so respiratory isolation of flu patients should be practiced in hospitals and nursing homes; handwashing is also important to minimize spread.

Laboratory Diagnosis

The presentation of influenza is often straightforward so that during an epidemic, diagnosis is usually made on clinical grounds alone. Nevertheless, laboratory verification of influenza does have distinct advantages. Influenza A and B are not fastidious viruses and grow easily in several standard tissue culture cell lines. Virus is abundant in cilliated columnar epithelial cells during the first few days of illness; a pharyngeal swab specimen recovers an adequate amount of virus for culture, and if the patient is coughing productively, sputum contains infected tracheobronchial cells. Either specimen needs to be placed in a viral transport medium that contains antibiotics to inhibit unwanted upper respiratory microflora and can be held (refrigerated) up to 24 h before tissue culture inoculation. If centrifugation-enhanced shell vial tissue culture is used, influenza can be readily identified in 24–48 h (the same approximate time frame as for routine bacterial culture). Early laboratory confirmation of influenza can encourage physicians to consider amantadine prophylaxis of contacts, discourage inappropriate use of antibiotics, and underscore the importance of respiratory isolation precautions for the index case. Viral recovery in tissue culture is the most efficient means for serotyping influenza strains—data that have considerable epidemiologic value in studying outbreaks. Positive laboratory identification also serves to remind physicians that influenza is an annually recurring problem, and may nudge distracted doctors to follow immunization guidelines for their high-risk patients.

Serologic diagnosis of influenza has considerable value for the epidemiologic investigation of outbreaks. In individual cases, however, results are usually not positive until convalescence, when a fourfold rise in antibody titer has developed.

CROUP: LARYNGOTRACHEOBRONCHITIS

Croup is the term used to describe several clinical illnesses with varying degrees of inflam-mation involving the larynx (resulting in hoarseness), trachea (producing stridor), and bronchi (characterized by cough). The relative degree of involvement of these anatomic regions varies considerably, but children with croup generally have some involvement in all three areas. In its classic forms, croup is almost invariably a viral disorder, although one must be careful to distinguish those patients with epiglottitis (due to *Haemophilus influenzae* type b) and those with bacterial tracheitis (usually related to *Staphylococcus aureus*).

Etiology and Epidemiology

Croup is characteristically seen in young children, about 75% of whom are younger than 3 years of age, with boys substantially outnumbering girls. Late fall–early winter peaks of illness are observed, corresponding to the viral respiratory illness season. The illness typically begins with upper respiratory symptoms of coryza, nasal irritation, and sore throat, as well as cough and fever. Shortly thereafter, signs of upper airway obstruction occur, with a "croupy" cough that sounds like a barking seal and gradually increasingly stridorous respirations. Symptoms usually begin to resolve after a few days but may progress to frank respiratory obstruction, with retractions, cyanosis, and restlessness. Duration of illness is typically 7–10 days.

Pathogenesis and Clinical Illness

Croup is characteristically a viral illness, with the large majority of cases caused by the respiratory viruses, particularly parainfluenza types 1, 2, and 3, and less often related to influenza, RSV, and adenovirus infection. Other agents including enteroviruses, herpes simplex virus, and rhinoviruses are rarely implicated.

The parainfluenza viruses include four serotypes (parainfluenza 1–4) of enveloped paramyxoviruses that contain single-stranded RNA and, like influenza virus, possess neuraminidase and hemagglutinin. They differ from influenza in that antigenic shift and drift do not occur and nucleocapsid assembly occurs in the cytoplasm rather than the plasma membrane. Parainfluenza 1, 2, and 3 are important causes of croup but also can cause pharyngitis, other upper respiratory tract infections, and bronchitis or pneumonitis. Parainfluenza 4 is much less common and generally causes only mild upper respiratory tract symptoms. These agents account for about 20% of nonbacterial respiratory infections leading to the hospitalization of young children. Transmission occurs from person to person through large-droplet spread or through self-inoculation.

Diagnosis

Following parainfluenza infection, immunity is only transient. When repeated infections occur in older children and adults, they are much milder than those seen in infancy and early childhood. Specific diagnosis can be established by virus isolation, usually in monkey kidney-cell culture, or by serologic demonstration of at least a fourfold increase in antibody titer (measured by complement-fixation, hemadsorption-inhibition, or neutralization) in paired sera. Rapid diagnosis can sometimes be established by demonstrating viral antigen directly in respiratory epithelial cells.

No specific therapy or prophylaxis exists for these infections. Treatment is supportive, including hydration and mist therapy.

BRONCHIOLITIS AND PNEUMONIA

Etiology and Epidemiology

Bronchiolitis is a common acute viral infection of the lower respiratory tract, which occurs principally in children under 2 years of age and accounts for most of the serious morbidity of viral lower respiratory tract disease in the pediatric population. Respiratory syncytial virus (RSV) is responsible for 45–55% of total cases of acute bronchiolitis and up to 75% of those cases severe enough to require hospitalization. Parainfluenza virus (PIV) types 3 and 1 each account for approximately 10% of cases of bronchiolitis, as does adenovirus. Rhinovirus, influenza virus, enteroviruses, and *Mycoplasma pneumoniae* are each responsible for a small number of cases. The epidemiology of bronchiolitis shows a striking peak annually in the winter months, primarily due to the contribution of RSV and PIV-1. Lower levels of activity are seen in the spring and summer from PIV-3; rhinovirus and adenovirus also account for a low percentage of bronchiolitis cases year round.

All of these respiratory viruses are spread from person to person, principally via droplet

aerosols but also on contaminated hands. As with influenza, the reservoir for the respiratory paramyxoviruses between epidemics is not obvious; humans are the only known host, however, and presumably low levels of infection must persist in the community. The factors which trigger explosive RSV bronchiolitis each winter are unknown (see Fig. 14–7).

Bronchiolitis is common during the first year of life with up to 12% of children under 1 year of age diagnosed. In the second year of life incidence drops by about half and becomes negligible thereafter. Although many cases of bronchiolitis are managed in an outpatient setting, approximately 4% of total pediatric hospitalizations are specifically for this diagnosis. RSV seems more virulent than PIV and produces less sustained immunity. Practically all primary infections occur in the first year of life and are symptomatic to some degree; symptomatic reinfection in early childhood is also common. Adult RSV infections identified in intra-family transmission studies and in health care workers also are not usually silent, and range from disease as trivial as a mild cold to an illness that resembles influenza.

RSV is a paramyxovirus with a lipid envelope similar to that of influenza virus, but only one glycoprotein surface antigen and a linear helical RNA nucleocapsid. The lack of a segmented genome (i.e., no possibility for genetic reassortment) and the single envelope antigen mean that the antigenic composition of RSV remains relatively stable year after year. Similar homogeneity is seen with the parainfluenza and measles viruses.

Pathogenesis and Clinical Illness

RSV adheres via its surface antigen to ciliated columnar epithelial cells throughout the respiratory tract. Viral replication, cytonecrosis, edema, and inflammation then occur in the respiratory epithelial surface from the nasopharynx to the terminal bronchioles, but the most severe complications are found in the most distal airways. Inflammation of small bronchi and bronchioles leads to luminal narrowing, and as necrotic debris accumulates, plugs of sloughed epithelial and inflammatory cells may actually block the smallest airways (see Fig. 14–8). Bronchospasm does not contribute significantly to the degree of obstruction. Bronchiolar inflammation produces the most dramatic obstruction in very young children whose small airways can only tolerate a modest degree of

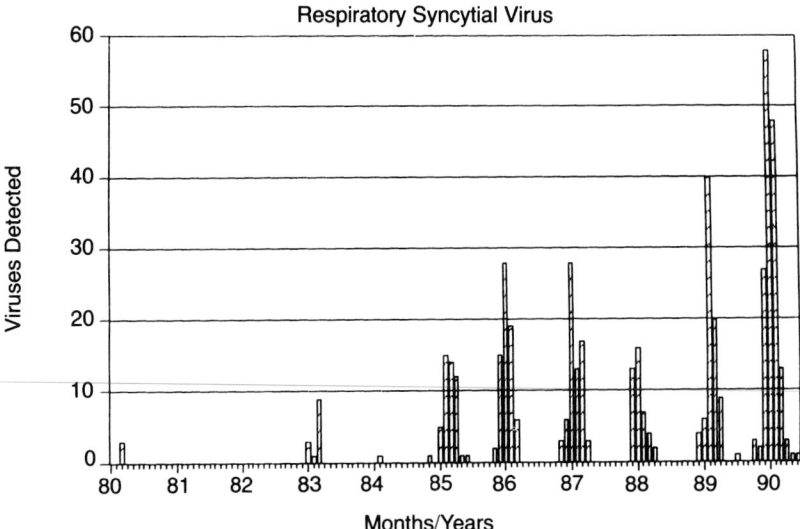

Figure 14–7. RSV identification by month. Annual wintertime epidemic pattern is seen. Sustained improvement in RSV recovery is noted since 1985 when nasopharyngeal wash collection procedure was standardized.

occlusion before symptoms are evident. The negative intrathoracic pressure created during inspiration allows air to flow through a partially obstructed bronchiole, but then air becomes trapped in the alveolar spaces as the cross-sectional area of the bronchiole naturally decreases with the positive pressure of expiration. Hyperinflation results, and eventually ventilation and oxygenation are impaired. Dyspnea, air hunger, and intense inspiratory effort develop. Hypoxia leads to restlessness, tachycardia, and tachypnea, and as the added work of ventilation becomes fatiguing, carbon dioxide is retained.

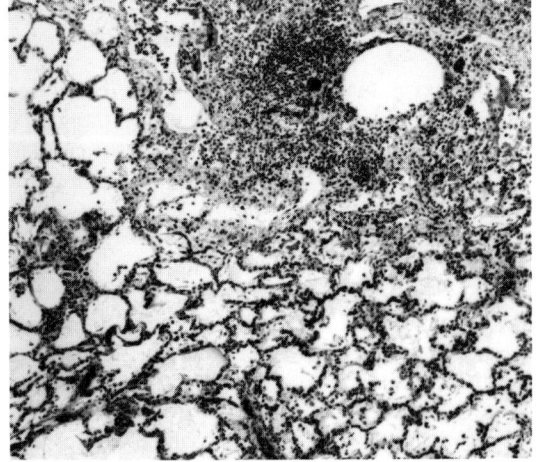

Figure 14–8. RSV bronchiolitis in an 18-month-old boy. There is acute necrotizing inflammation of terminal bronchiole with minimal focal extension into surrounding alveoli. Hematoxylin and eosin stain, 25× magnification.

Early in RSV infection a specific CD8 cytotoxic T-lymphocyte response is initiated which peaks in activity at approximately the fifth day of illness and is critical to the containment and elimination of virus. The inflammatory response in RSV bronchiolitis is primarily lymphocytic, and presumably the majority of these cells are part of this cytotoxic clone. A specific antibody response to RSV follows later; IgM is transient and appears too late to contribute to the pathogenesis of bronchiolitis. Specific IgG and IgA antibodies appear by the second week, but are so short-lived that patients are vulnerable to reinfection within 1 year. There is some concern that the severity of symptoms in subsequent infections may be greater in patients who have high concentrations of RSV-specific IgE. An alternative reason for the more serious degree of bronchiolitis seen in some patients is a deficiency in the function of the RSV antigen-specific suppressor cells.

Mucosal inflammation from RSV infection occurs up and down the respiratory tract; nondescript cold or pharyngitis symptoms may precede or parallel bronchiolitis, but the small size of the distal airways makes their involvement the most conspicuous. Physical examination of a patient with acute bronchiolitis shows accompanying coryza and pharyngeal hyperemia. Fever typically is mild. There are wheezing inspiratory breath sounds which shift somewhat in intensity and location with serial reauscultation of the lungs. Tachypnea is accompanied by intense inspiratory effort with grunting and nasal flaring. Because babies have such compliant chest walls, suprasternal and costal retractions are easily evident and the costal margin widens conspicuously with each breath in an effort to lower the diaphragm and increase tidal volume. Although hypoxemia is common, cyanosis is rare.

Physical examination should also include a quick look for alternative explanations for dyspnea and wheezing. Check for possible exudative obstructive debris in the pharynx and for a foreign body lodged in or near the larynx. Inquire about a history of allergies and look for signs of edema in the eyelids and face which might accompany laryngeal angioedema.

Laboratory Diagnosis

A complete blood count shows a modest elevation of the white blood cell count with or without a left shift in neutrophil maturation. Hypoxemia almost always is found in hospitalized babies, but the intensity of wheezing and retractions do not accurately predict the pO_2. Only the most severely ill show an elevated pCO_2, and serum electrolytes reflect the degree of accompanying dehydration. Chest x-ray often shows only signs of hyperinflation with hyperlucent lung fields and depressed symmetrical diaphragms. Trapped parenchymal air which is subsequently resorbed may produce zones of atelectasis, and foci of true pneumonia may also be present.

Virus isolation or antigen identification is now widely available to assist in diagnosis and management of pediatric viral lower respiratory diseases. Since RSV, PIV, adenovirus, and influenza virus infect ciliated epithelial cells throughout the respiratory tract, a nasopharyngeal wash specimen contains the same microorganisms producing bronchiolitis, croup, or influenza in the lower respiratory tract. One to two mL of saline introduced into one nostril and then promptly reaspirated with a suction catheter from the other nostril contain abundant epithelial cells for virus culture and a comprehensive panel of viral antigen assays as well. Nasopharyngeal and oropharyngeal swabs often are insufficient, and a true sputum specimen can rarely be collected from a baby. A good specimen is crucial for successful laboratory diagnosis. Figure 14–7 graphs RSV detection at a large, suburban community hospital. RSV recovery was meager prior to 1985, when a hospital policy was introduced which required that nasopharyngeal wash specimens be collected by properly trained respiratory therapy technologists, rather than by nurses, physicians, and medical students. The vast majority of specimens subsequently obtained by qualified personnel had ample epithelial cells for both virus culture and a viral antigen assay that included RSV; PIV-1, 2, and 3; adenovirus; and influenza A and B.

Antigen assays are quite sensitive and specific and can be completed in less than 4 h, providing almost immediate information. Virus culture, although endorsed as the "gold standard" laboratory diagnostic test, generally takes 3–7 days for positive results; and RSV unfortunately is the slowest and most fastidious of the pediatric respiratory viral pathogens in tissue culture. Serologic diagnosis provides little meaningful information since few IgM-specific assays are widely available, and since recurrent disease with the same respiratory virus is common in children.

Management of Bronchiolitis

Pediatric viral bronchiolitis can be expected to resolve after a 3- to 10-day period. Most babies are substantially improved by day 3 or 4 of illness and gradually recover over the next 1–2 weeks. Mortality is rare and usually linked to complicating pneumonias. Children sick enough to require hospitalization are usually hypoxic and need supplemental humidified oxygen. Mechanical ventilation is needed only in a minority of cases. Bronchodilator therapy is controversial and probably of little value. Intravenous rehydration is often needed. Antibiotics are not appropriate unless there is serious concern about a secondary bacterial pneumonia or otitis media.

Ribavirin, a synthetic nucleoside, has antiviral activity against RSV. When administered as a small-particle aerosol, ribavirin reaches the distal airways and inhibits RSV replication, thereby minimizing further tissue damage and ameliorating the severity of disease. Oxygenation is significantly improved and the duration of viral shedding is reduced. Ribavirin, however, cannot replace supportive measures and its practical value in babies with less severe cases of bronchiolitis has not been substantiated. Ribavirin is expensive and its use adds several hundred dollars to hospitalization costs, so indiscriminate and unnecessary use should be discouraged. Although ribavirin is teratogenic in several animal models studied, aerosol therapy has not been linked to any damage in either patients, health care workers, or their offspring.

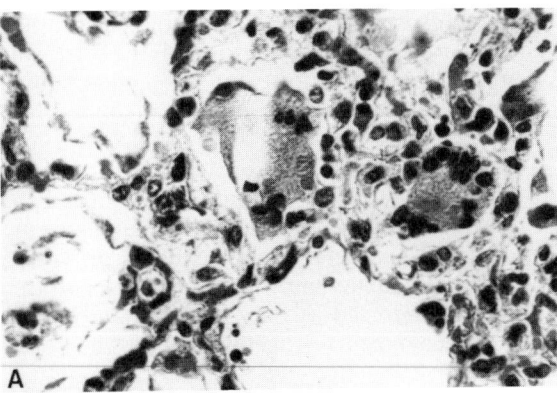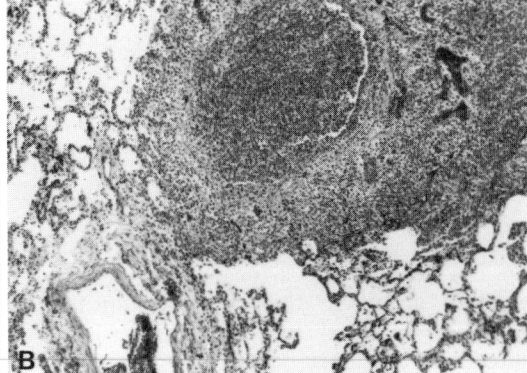

Figure 14–9. Measles pneumonia in an unvaccinated 2-year-old boy. A. Measles pneumonitis with multinucleated syncytial giant cells in the alveoli and lymphocytic alveolar wall infiltrate. 250× magnification. B. Suppurative bacterial broncho-pneumonia complicating measles. 25× magnification. Hematoxylin and eosin stain for both.

RSV is highly contagious and is the most common nosocomial infection in pediatric wards. RSV is spread person to person via aerosol, as are all other respiratory myxoviruses, and can be transmitted up to 6 ft in small-particle droplets. However, spread on the contaminated hands of children and health care workers is an important means of transmission that has traditionally been underestimated. Vigorous hand-washing practices and glove-and-gown precautions can substantially limit nosocomial transmission of virus by health care workers, and use of disposable, plastic eye–nose goggles further decreases spread from patients to hospital staff and subsequently to other patients. Cohorting of babies with respiratory tract infections into the same rooms or wards has been practiced for many years; hospitals rarely have sufficient patient rooms to accommodate all of the babies with contagious respiratory infection in private rooms, as recommended by the Centers for Disease Control for adults.

Pneumonia

Pneumonia can complicate any viral infection of the lower respiratory tract in either adults or children. This is especially well appreciated in influenza A pandemics but can also be seen with RSV and PIV infections. When bronchiolitis is the principal manifestation of respiratory tract infection, extension of virus into the adjacent alveolar epithelium and secondary bacterial bronchopneumonia are not infrequent complications.

Both measles and adenovirus have also been linked to severe distal airway infection and pneumonia. Measles is also a member of the paramyxovirus family. It characteristically produces a systemic febrile exanthem, but the virus initially invades via the respiratory tract, and cough, coryza, and conjunctivitis are common. Primary measles virus giant-cell pneumonia and bacterial superinfecting pneumonia account for more than half of the morbidity in infants dying of measles. Figure 14–9 demonstrates the histopathology of measles pneumonia and secondary bronchopneumonia; the giant-cell characteristic of this disease is in fact a syncytium of infected epithelial cells whose cytoplasmic borders have fused as a direct result of virus-induced changes on the plasma membrane. Accompanying interstitial edema and lymphocytic margination can severely impair alveolar gas exchange, but an associated bacterial superinfection is generally found at autopsy and presumably is the greater contributing factor in fatal cases.

Adenovirus, although generally recognized for its role in conjunctivitis and pharyngitis, also can produce lower respiratory tract disease. Outbreaks of acute pneumonitis in military camps, where crowding is a major factor in spread, have been described but rarely produce fatalities. Adenovirus pneumonia, with or without extrapulmonary dissemination, occurs rarely in immunocompromised adults and children, and occasionally also in elderly patients as a final, fatal complication of nonrespiratory tract diseases, such as stroke or myocardial infarction.

REFERENCES
Books

Feigin, R. D., and Cherry, J. D., eds. *Textbook of Pediatric Infectious Diseases.* 2nd ed. Volumes I and II. Philadelphia: W. B. Saunders Co., 1987.

Kilbourne, E. D. *Influenza*. New York: Plenum Medical Book Co., 1987.

Mandell, G. L., Douglas, R. G., and Bennett, E., eds. *Principles and Practice of Infectious Diseases*. 3rd ed. New York: Churchill Livingstone Co., 1990.

Stuart-Harris, C. H., Schild, G. C., and Oxford, J. S. *Influenza: The Viruses and the Disease*. 2nd ed. London: Edward Arnold, 1985.

Articles and Chapters

Centers for Disease Control, State and local influenza immunization program activities. *MMWR* 37:705–707, 1988.

Douglas, R. G. Prophylaxis and treatment of influenza. *N. Engl. J. Med.* 322:443–450, 1990.

Frank, A. L., Taber, L. H., Wells, C. R., et al. Patterns of shedding of myxoviruses and paramyxoviruses in children. *J. Infect. Dis.* 144:433–441, 1981.

Gala, C. L., Hall, C. B., Schnabel, K. C., et al. The use of eye-nose goggles to control nosocomial respiratory syncytial virus infection. *JAMA* 256:2706–2708, 1986.

Ginsberg, H. S. Orthomyxoviruses. In: Davis, B. D., ed. *Microbiology*. 4th ed. Philadelphia: J. B. Lipincott, 1990:990–1002.

Glezen, W. P., and Couch, R. B. Interpandemic influenza in the Houston area, 1974–76. *N. Engl. J. Med.* 298:587–592, 1978.

Grayston, J. T., Campbell, L. A., Kuo, C., et al. A New respiratory tract pathogen: *Chlamydia pneumoniae* strain TWAR. *J. Infect. Dis.* 161:618–625, 1990.

Guenthner, S. H., and Linnemann, C. C. Indirect immunofluorescence assay for rapid diagnosis of influenza virus. *Lab. Med.* 19:581–583, 1988.

Hall, C. B., McBride, J. T., Walsh, E. E., et al. Aerosolized ribavirin treatment of infants with respiratory syncytial viral infection: A randomized double-blind study. *N. Engl. J. Med.* 308:1443–1447, 1983.

Hall, C. B., Geiman, J. M., Biggar, R., et al. Respiratory syncytial virus infections within families. *N. Engl. J. Med.* 294:414–419, 1976.

Hayden, F. G., Belshe, R. B., Clover, R. D., et al. Emergence and apparent transmission of rimantadine-resistant influenza A virus in families. *N. Engl. J. Med.* 321:1696–1702, 1989.

Kilbourne, E. D. New viral diseases: A real and potential problem without boundaries. *JAMA* 264:68–70, 1990.

Kimball, A. M., Foy, H. M., Cooney, M. K., et al. Isolation of respiratory syncytial and influenza viruses from the sputum of patients hospitalized with pneumonia. *J. Infect. Dis.* 147:181–184, 1983.

Leclair, J. M., Freeman, J., Sullivan, B. F., et al. Prevention of nosocomial respiratory syncytial virus infections through compliance with glove and gown isolation precautions. *N. Engl. J. Med.* 317:329–334, 1987.

MacDonald, N. E., Breese Hall, C., Suffin, S. C., et al. Respiratory syncytial viral infection in infants with congenital heart disease. *N. Engl. J. Med.* 307:397–400, 1982.

Miotti, P. G., Nelson, K. E., Dallabetta, G. A., et al. The Influence of HIV infection on antibody responses to a two-dose regimen of influenza vaccine. *JAMA* 262:779–783, 1989.

Morse, S. S., and Schluederberg, A. Emerging viruses: The evolution of viruses and viral diseases. *J. Infect. Dis.* 162:1–7, 1990.

Sperber, S. J., and Francis, J. B. Toxic shock syndrome during an influenza outbreak. *JAMA* 257:1086–1087, 1987.

Stokes, C. E., Bernstein, J. M., Kyger, S. A., et al. Rapid diagnosis of influenza A and B by 24-h fluorescent focus assays. *J. Clin. Microbiol.* 26:1263–1266, 1988.

Stretton, M., and Newth, C. J. Croup and epiglottitis: The critical early diagnosis. *J. Respir. Dis.* 11:1087–1100, 1990.

Weingarten, S., Friedlander, M., Rascon, D., et al. Influenza surveillance in an acute-care hospital. *Arch. Intern. Med.* 148:113–116, 1988.

Welliver, R. C. Detection, pathogenesis, and therapy of respiratory syncytial virus infections. *Clin. Microbiol. Rev.* 1:27–39, 1988.

Mycobacterial Infections

Tuberculosis is an infectious disease of humans caused by the microorganism *Mycobacterium tuberculosis*. Most individuals infected with *M. tuberculosis* do not develop the disease tuberculosis. However, when it does occur, tuberculosis is marked by chronicity with tissue necrosis due to delayed-type hypersensitivity. Mycobacterial species other than *M. tuberculosis*, including the "atypical" mycobacteria and the causative agent of leprosy, also produce human disease. Diagnosis and effective treatment depend on awareness of the wide spectrum of mycobacterial disease.

TUBERCULOSIS

Microbiology

The *Mycobacterium tuberculosis* complex of organisms consists of five species: *M. tuberculosis*, *M. bovis*, *M. africanum*, *M. ulcerans*, and *M. microti*. In the past, *M. bovis* was a frequent cause of human tuberculosis, usually acquired by the ingestion of milk contaminated with *M. bovis*. However, with eradication of *M. bovis* mastitis in dairy herds and the pasteurization of milk, tuberculosis due to *M. bovis* has been largely eliminated. *M. africanum* is a rare cause of human tuberculosis in Africa. *M. ulcerans*, the causative agent of necrotizing cutaneous ulceration in Africa and Australia, grows only at cooler skin temperatures (30°–31°C). *M. microti* is an animal pathogen.

Essentially, *Mycobacterium tuberculosis*

causes all cases of human tuberculosis in the United States and in other developed countries. *M. tuberculosis* is a facultative intracellular parasite which produces disease by growth within macrophages, but can also proliferate in the extracellular spaces of infected tissue, and is able to grow *in vitro* in cell-free culture systems. Humans are the only natural reservoir of *M. tuberculosis*. However, monkeys in captivity can contract *M. tuberculosis* infection from human handlers or other infected monkeys, and can be a source of infection to personnel working with caged monkey colonies. *M. tuberculosis* is also highly virulent to the guinea pig, which has served as an experimental model for invaluable studies on the pathogenesis of tuberculosis. *M. tuberculosis* is an obligate aerobe whose growth is favored by 5–10% CO_2 tension, but is inhibited by pH below 6.5 and long-chain fatty acids. Tubercle bacilli grow only at temperatures of 35–37°C, which is consistent with their ability to infect internal organs, especially the lungs. This microorganism is a non–spore-forming, nonmotile bacillus measuring approximately 0.4 × 4.0 μm, whose cell wall has a very high content of lipid. Lipid constitutes 25–60% of the organism's dry weight, as compared with 0.5% for gram-positive bacteria and 3.0% for gram-negative bacteria. Tubercle bacilli grow very slowly: their doubling time is 12–20 h, as compared with less than 1 h for most other bacterial pathogens.

No exotoxins, endotoxins, or tissue-necrotizing enzymes of *M. tuberculosis* have been discovered. However, an array of glycolipids and peptides have been implicated in the virulence and hypersensitivity of tuberculous infection. *Cord factor* is a glycolipid which causes virulent strains of *M. tuberculosis* to grow as ropes, bundles, or serpentine cords in liquid media. Cord factor can be extracted from tubercle bacilli with organic solvents, and if cord factor is extracted, the bacilli become avirulent. At the present time the exact role of cord factor in the pathogenesis of tuberculosis is unknown. A primary component of host responses to infection with *M. tuberculosis* is the development of delayed-type hypersensitivity against mycobacterial proteins. Several constituents of the mycobacterial cell wall, especially the glycolipid *wax D* and *muramyl dipeptide,* enhance this hypersensitivity. Finally, tubercle bacilli ingested by macrophages in the nonimmune host reside in phagosomes that seldom provoke lysosomal fusion. Consequently, multiplication of tubercle bacilli is unimpeded within macro-

phages until immunity develops. The mycobacterial *sulfatides,* polyanionic trehalose glycolipids associated with virulence of *M. tuberculosis,* are readily taken up by lysosomes, and modify lysosomal membranes so that lysosome fusion with phagosomes is inhibited.

Pulmonary Tuberculosis

Pulmonary tuberculosis is a disease which results from infection of the lung with an *M. tuberculosis* complex organism—in the United States almost always *M. tuberculosis* itself. Essentially all pulmonary infections are due to inhalation of *droplet nuclei,* small (1–5 μm) particles of respiratory secretions containing a few (1–3) tubercle bacilli. Droplet nuclei are usually produced when an individual with respiratory tract disease due to *M. tuberculosis* coughs, sneezes, or talks. These secretions remain suspended in the air until inhaled; they can then reach the deep alveolar spaces of the lung because of their small size. *Secondary aerosols* are formed from respiratory droplets which fall to surfaces (floors, tables) or objects, such as bedding or clothing (fomites), where they become associated with particles of dust or lint, and dry. The association with dust or lint increases particle size (>5 μm), and secondary aerosols are not highly infectious since they are more efficiently cleared by the mucociliary apparatus of the respiratory tract. Consequently, the tuberculosis patient is the primary source for transmission of tubercle bacilli, and fomites are not important. Moreover, patients with extrapulmonary disease cannot form infected droplet nuclei and are, thus, noninfectious. Although tuberculosis is not highly contagious, it is estimated that 25–50% of close contacts of patients with sputum smears that are microscopically positive for mycobacteria become infected. To prevent transmission of tubercle bacilli, it is advisable to maintain "air control" by providing adequate ventilation or ultraviolet lighting, or by simply urging patients to cover their nose and mouth when coughing or to wear masks until their sputum smears are converted to negative by treatment.

A total of 5–15% of individuals infected with *M. tuberculosis* develop active tuberculosis. The likelihood of active disease varies with age, and is greatest in the very young, adolescents, and young adults, and in older individuals over age 60 (Fig. 15–1). Several decades ago, infection with *M. tuberculosis* was almost universal among children in the United States, and active tuberculosis was predominantly a disease of young

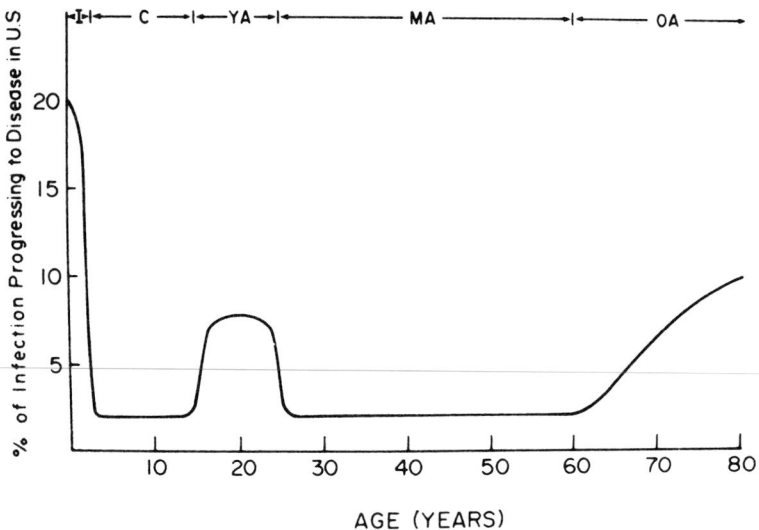

Figure 15–1. The risk of active disease due to M. tuberculosis *infection in different age groups. I, infancy; C, childhood; YA, young adulthood; MA, middle adulthood; and OA, old age. (From Des Prez, R. M., and Heim, C. R. Mycobacterium tuberculosis. In: Mandell, G. L., Douglas, R. G., Jr., and Bennett, J. E., eds.* Principles and Practice of Infectious Diseases. *3rd ed. New York: Churchill Livingstone, 1990: pp. 1877–1906.)*

adults. However, in the United States today, infection is the exception, not the rule, among children, and it occurs most frequently among adults. Individuals with poor nutrition or substandard, close living conditions, and patients with silicosis, cancer (especially bronchogenic carcinoma), diabetes mellitus, or HIV coinfection, and persons receiving immunosuppressive corticosteroids or cytotoxic drugs are particularly susceptible to tuberculosis. The number of tuberculosis cases declined steadily until the mid-1980s (Fig. 15–2), when that trend stopped. In fact, the number of new reported cases in the United States increased to 9.46/100,000 population in 1989 from 9.13/100,000 population in 1988, with cities such as New York and Newark, New Jersey, reporting increased case numbers. It is likely that this increase primarily involves individuals infected with HIV-1. It is estimated that HIV-1 infection increases the risk of tuberculosis by a factor of 200–300.

Primary Tuberculosis

Primary tuberculosis occurs in individuals who have no preexisting immunity to *M. tuberculosis*. Inhaled tubercle bacilli in droplet nuclei reach the alveoli, where they are ingested by alveolar macrophages. Since immunity is absent, tubercle bacilli proliferate within phagosomes, alveolar macrophages die and release their bacillary load, and the released bacilli are ingested by other alveolar macrophages. Also, tubercle bacilli escape via draining lymphatics and establish separate foci of infection in ipsilateral hilar lymph nodes of the lung. From the hilar lymph nodes, bacilli spread via the thoracic duct into the circulation, and seed multiple organs, including the bone marrow, liver, spleen, kidneys, the meninges, and (of particular importance in the development of chronic pulmonary tuberculosis) the posterior regions of the apices of the upper lung lobes and supe-

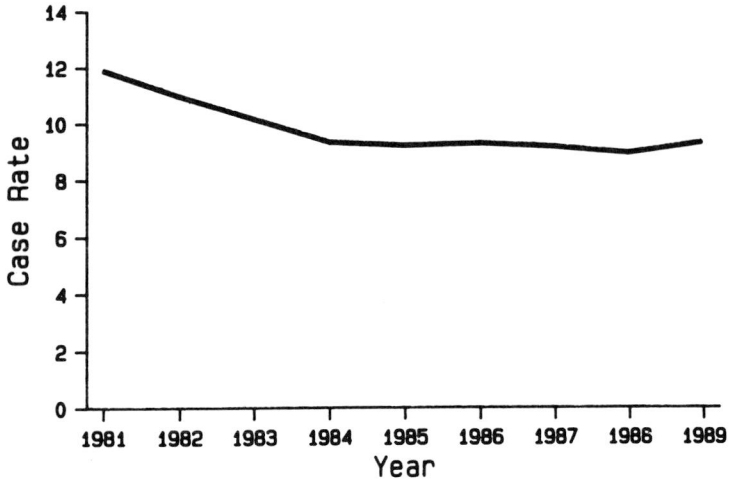

Figure 15–2. The case rates for tuberculosis in the United States for the period 1981–1989. The rate is per 100,000 population. (From MMWR, Centers for Disease Control, Vol. 38, No. 54, October 5, 1990.)

rior segments of the lower lobes. This bacillemic phase of infection is clinically silent. However, within 2–6 weeks the infected host develops *cellular hypersensitivity* to tubercle bacilli, which evokes a granulomatous inflammatory response at sites of tissue infection. Granulomas are produced consisting of focal aggregates of macrophages, Langhans' giant cells, lymphocytes, and granulation tissue (fibroblasts and capillaries) (Fig. 15–3), and which are referred to as *tubercles*. Granulomas in the lower lobes of lung and hilar lymph nodes enlarge and undergo central *caseation necrosis* (Fig. 15–4). Caseation necrosis is a manifestation of hypersensitivity to high concentrations of mycobacterial antigen. In caseation necrosis, dead tissue consists of gray to white granular debris with the appearance of a friable, cheesy material (hence the term *caseous*). Concomitant with hypersensitivity, immunity is expressed by differentiation of macrophages to *epithelioid cells*—enlarged and activated macrophages which assume the morphologic appearance of epithelial cells. Activated macrophages are able to suppress the proliferation of phagocytosed tubercle bacilli, and infection is contained. Also, cytolytic T lymphocytes are generated in the cellular immune response, which may attack and release tubercle bacilli from quiescent (unactivated) macrophages, with subsequent uptake of the released bacilli by activated macrophages.

The development of hypersensitivity and immunity occurs during primary infection, which for most individuals is subclinical; the only evidence that infection has taken place is the presence of cutaneous delayed hypersensitivity to mycobacterial protein *(tuberculin)*. Healing of granulomas occurs by fibrosis, and the fibrotic granulomas sometimes calcify to produce the *Ghon complex,* a complex of calcified pulmonary and hilar node granulomas.

Progressive primary tuberculosis, when it occurs, is observed most frequently in the young. Roentgenograms in primary tuberculosis frequently show dense infiltrates in a lower or midlung field, accompanied by large, occasionally massive hilar or mediastinal lymphadenopathy. Fever and lassitude may be present, and hilar or mediastinal lymphadenitis may compress a bronchus, causing a brassy cough. Less commonly, the bacillemic phase may result in life-threatening miliary–meningeal tuberculosis.

Chronic Pulmonary Tuberculosis

Chronic pulmonary (reactivation) tuberculosis occurs in individuals who have some degree of immunity to *M. tuberculosis.* The bacillemic phase of primary infection results in dissemination of tubercle bacilli to the posterior apical regions of the upper lung lobes or the superior segments of the lower lobes. The subsequent development of cellular immunity contains but does not always eradicate tubercle bacilli, and cavitary disease can develop in these pulmonary regions within a short time after the bacillemic phase of primary infection, or (more commonly) after a long latent period. Chronic pulmonary tuberculosis most often occurs in the posterior regions of the lung apex because of the relatively

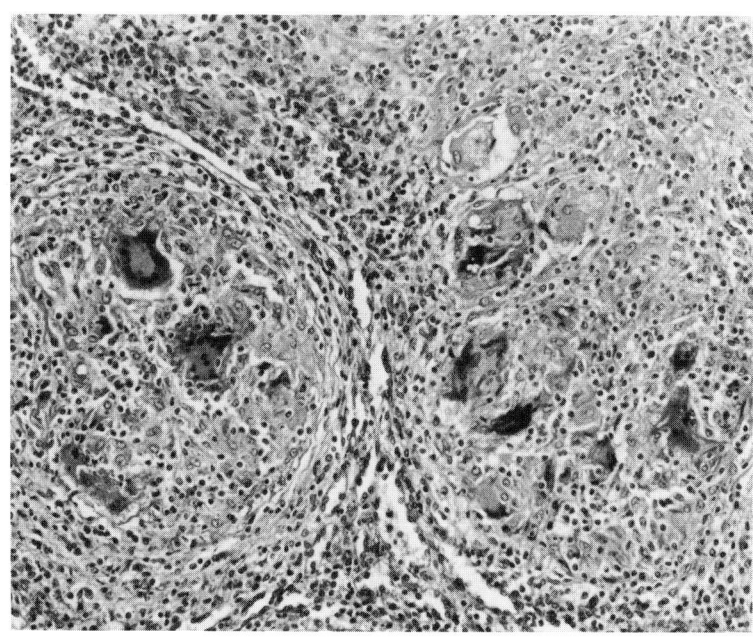

Figure 15–3. Tuberculous granulomas (tubercles). Two granulomas are shown, each consisting of a compact collection of large activated macrophages (epithelioid cells), multinucleated giant cells, and small dark lymphocytes. (From Warren, J. R., Scarpelli, D. G., Reddy, J. K., and Kanwar, Y. S. Essentials of General Pathology. New York, Macmillan Publishing Company, 1987.)

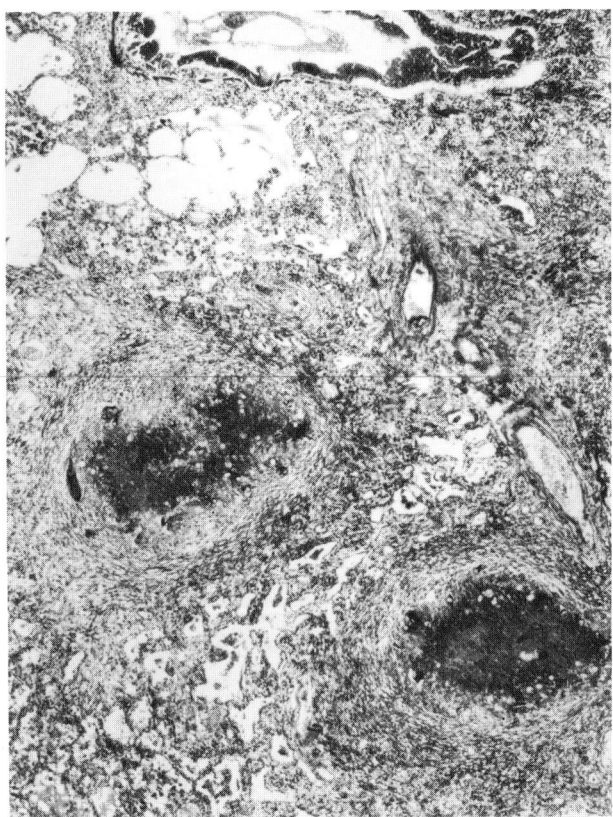

Figure 15–4. Caseating granulomas. Two areas of caseous necrosis are present in the central region of tuberculous granulomas (lower half of the field). (From Warren, J. R., Scarpelli, D. G., Reddy, J. K., and Kanwar, Y. S. Essentials of General Pathology. New York, Macmillan Publishing Company, 1987.)

high oxygen tension and low lymphatic drainage in these regions. Advanced age, HIV infection, diabetes mellitus, cancer, and immunosuppression for any reason, including that resulting from corticosteroids, can lower cellular immunity sufficiently to cause reactivation of latent organisms and chronic pulmonary tuberculosis. Because of the development of hypersensitivity, large areas of caseous necrosis are surrounded by a granulomatous rim of epithelioid cells and Langhans' giant cells (Fig. 15–4).

Accumulation of large concentrations of mycobacterial antigen results in severe hypersensitivity, and the caseous centers of tubercles become liquefied. Liquefaction necrosis is one of the most harmful host responses in tuberculosis. The liquefied caseum is an excellent culture medium for tubercle bacilli, which extensively multiply extracellularly and attain large numbers. Erosion of liquefied caseum into a bronchus results in drainage of necrotic material into the bronchial tree and cavitation of the lung. Cavity formation is the pivotal event in chronic pulmonary tuberculosis, since tubercle bacilli proliferate to enormous numbers in the ambient O_2 tension of air, and bronchial drainage of necrotic material establishes new exudative foci of infection within the lung *(broncho-*

genic spread). Pulmonary and systemic signs and symptoms are often pronounced, with hectic fever, night sweats, weight loss, dyspnea, cough, and hemoptysis. Cellular immunity slows the progression of pulmonary tuberculosis in most individuals, and healing of cavities ensues with fibrosis and dystrophic calcification. Apical calcified lesions present on chest roentgenogram in the region of the clavicle are referred to as *Simon's foci*. However, viable tubercle bacilli often persist within the "healed" fibrocalcific granulomas of chronic pulmonary tuberculosis, and there is *always* the potential for breakdown of these lesions with recurrence of active disease.

Extrapulmonary Tuberculosis

As described above, lymphohematogenous spread of tubercle bacilli occurs during primary infection of individuals who have no tuberculous immunity. In the very young child, the hematogenous phase may progress into *disseminated tuberculosis*. This phase is most often transient, since the acquisition of cell-mediated immunity prevents disseminated tuberculosis. However, the lymphohematogenous phase creates a situation in which most organs are seeded with tubercle bacilli. Extrapulmonary tuberculosis in adults is generally assumed to be the result of remote seeding rather than to occur with primary tuberculosis. Many of these patients have a predisposing condition, including immunosuppressive treatment (particularly the use of steroids), HIV infection, or chronic illness (especially renal failure, connective tissue disease, and diabetes mellitus), which permits reactivation of a tuberculous focus.

Miliary Tuberculosis

The pathologic lesions in disseminated tuberculosis are tiny caseous granulomas which resemble millet seeds—hence the term *miliary tuberculosis.* The presenting symptoms of miliary tuberculosis are nonspecific. Miliary tuberculosis evolves over several weeks with fever, anorexia, sweats, and weight loss. Abnormal laboratory findings are also nonspecific, and a mild anemia, elevated erythrocyte sedimentation rate, hyponatremia, and polyclonal gammopathy are typically present. In most patients, the discovery of a miliary or reticulonodular infiltrate on chest roentgenogram raises the suspicion of miliary tuberculosis. Despite its atypical presentation, prompt diagnosis and treatment of miliary tuberculosis are critical, since untreated miliary tuberculosis is almost uniformly fatal within 1 year.

Isolated Organ Tuberculosis

Isolated organ tuberculosis is an extrapulmonary disease due to hematogenous seeding of a particular organ system, especially the central nervous system, pericardium, genitourinary tract, and peripheral lymph nodes. Not infrequently, an asymptomatic latent period (sometimes years) follows the hematogenous seeding of extrapulmonary organ systems.

Tuberculous Meningitis. This disease most often results from rupture of a tubercle into the subarachnoid space, with development of granulomatous meningitis at the base of the brain. Low-grade fever, headache, and altered mental state in a patient with clinical evidence of tuberculosis—especially miliary lesions on a chest roentgenogram—suggest tuberculous meningitis. Meningeal inflammation can result in fibrous encasement of cerebral arteries with accompanying ischemia and infarction of dependent brain tissue, or obstruction of basilar cisterns and ventricular foramina leading to hydrocephalus.

Tuberculous Pericarditis. Tuberculous pericarditis most often results from rupture of a hilar or mediastinal caseous lymph node into the pericardial space. The pericardial effusion may or may not be accompanied by signs of infection (fever, pericardial pain). Fibrous organization of a caseous effusion can progress to pericardial constriction and cardiac failure.

Renal Tuberculosis. This disease reflects extension of cortical foci of infection to the medulla, where the hypertonic environment inhibits cell-mediated immunity. This form of extrapulmonary tuberculosis has an especially long latent period, generally greater than 5 years. Tuberculous bacilluria causes cystitis, and local urinary symptoms and signs, including dysuria with hematuria and pyuria, are frequent. The scarring of chronic renal tuberculosis may lead to obstructive uropathy.

Tuberculous Lymphadenitis. Mostly occurring in otherwise healthy individuals, tuberculous lymphadenitis initially appears as rapidly enlarging, firm lymph nodes, which later undergo caseation necrosis, may soften and become matted, and form draining fistulae.

Other forms of isolated organ tuberculosis include skeletal tuberculosis of the spine *(Pott's disease),* granulomatous hepatitis, and tuberculous peritonitis.

Cell-Mediated Immunity and Hypersensitivity

Max Lurie reported in 1942 that macrophages from rabbits immunized with tubercle bacilli greatly inhibited the intracellular proliferation of tubercle bacilli. The addition of immune serum to mixtures of mononuclear phagocytic cells and tubercle bacilli had no effect. Approximately 10 years after Lurie's report, Suter demonstrated that cultures of monocytes could be infected with tubercle bacilli, and intracellular multiplication of the bacilli was greatly inhibited within monocytes obtained from immune animals. The increased microbicidal activity of macrophages during infection with facultative intracellular parasites is referred to as *macrophage activation.* A number of important facts have emerged in studies on macrophage activation in mycobacterial disease. First, once established, macrophage activation is nonspecific, and enhanced bactericidal activity is directed not only toward the inducing mycobacterial species, but also against unrelated facultative intracellular bacteria. Second, induction of macrophage activation depends upon specific interaction between immune lymphocytes and the infecting organism. Lymphokines, peptides which act as intercellular signals between lymphoid cells, are secreted by specific lymphocytes upon contact with homologous mycobacterial antigen, and the lymphokines activate macrophages for intracellular killing. The lymphokine *interferon gamma* plays the major role in activating macrophages for inhibition of mycobacterial growth. Third, macrophage activation is under the control of T lymphocytes. Antibody against thymocytes or T cells ablates the ability of splenic lymphocytes to activate macrophages, and mice deficient in T lymphocytes develop persistent mycobacterial infections. Fourth, mycobacterial antigen is processed by macrophages and is displayed on the macrophage membrane in association with class II histocompatibility antigens. T lymphocytes become specifically sensitized by contact with mycobacterial antigen and, upon later exposure to mycobacterial antigen and the same class II antigens, release the inflammatory lymphokines responsible for macrophage activation.

Lymphocytes and macrophages exist side by side in granulomas, where macrophages become highly activated by local T-cell secretion of interferon gamma. In addition, T cells secrete *macrophage chemotactic factor* (MCF), which attracts macrophages to local sites of infection, and *migration inhibitory factor* (MIF), which holds macrophages at sites of infection. Consequently, macrophages are present within granulomas in large numbers. These macrophage recruitment mechanisms are of critical importance, since the mere presence of activated macrophages without granuloma formation is insufficient to control mycobacterial infection.

Role of T Cells in Immunity

In recent years, a great deal has been discovered concerning the roles of T-lymphocyte subsets in the cell-mediated immunity of tuberculosis. Quiescent CD4+ helper/inducer T cells are activated by mycobacterial antigen displayed on macrophage membranes with histocompatible class II antigen. Helper T-cell activation is supported by interleukin-1 produced by the macrophage. The activated CD4+ cell, in turn, both produces interleukin-2 (IL-2) and expresses large numbers of IL-2 receptors on its membrane. Consequently, IL-2 acts as an autocrine factor, producing clonal expansion of

the immunologically specific CD4+ lymphocytes, which secrete interferon gamma, MIF, and MCF. Recently, a possible role has become apparent for CD8+ cytolytic T lymphocytes in the cell-mediated immunity of tuberculosis. Thus, depletion of CD8+ cells in mice renders them more susceptible to infection with *M. tuberculosis,* and cloned CD8+ cell lines obtained from mice immunized with tubercle bacilli can destroy infected macrophages. Kaufmann proposed an interesting model for cell-mediated immunity in tuberculosis, in which both macrophage activation and target-cell lysis provide potent mechanisms for host defense (Fig. 15–5). This model is based on murine tuberculosis, and many questions remain. For example, are cytolytic T lymphocytes in mycobacterial infection equivalent to class I–restricted cytolytic T cells in viral immunity? Also, can cytolytic T cells recognize nonactivated macrophages as target cells in preference to activated macrophages, and if so, how? Nevertheless, the dynamic interplay of T-cell subsets and macrophages envisioned in this model is highly useful for analyzing human mycobacterial immunity.

Cell-Mediated Damage

Tissue injury (caseation necrosis, liquefaction) occurs in tuberculous lesions when mycobacterial protein antigens reach high local concentrations. This injury reflects cell-mediated damage due to lymphocytes and macrophages mobilized in the immune response to these protein antigens. Cellular immunity is usually sufficient to suppress the proliferation of tubercle bacilli, and caseation necrosis is limited to focal areas such as the upper lung lobes. However, if cellular immunity is depressed, bacillary proliferation produces a high concentration of tuberculoprotein, and extensive tissue destruction results from hypersensitivity to tuberculoprotein. Caseation necrosis and liquefaction are caused by many factors; they result from the release by activated macrophages of hydrolytic enzymes, reactive O_2 intermediates, and tumor necrosis factor (TNF). In addition, activated macrophages secrete procoagulant factors, which cause thrombosis of local blood vessels and ischemia. Destruction of host tissue also probably occurs through lysis of host cells by CD8+ T lymphocytes.

Cutaneous Tuberculin Reaction

Many years ago, Robert Koch recognized the hypersensitivity response induced by infecting

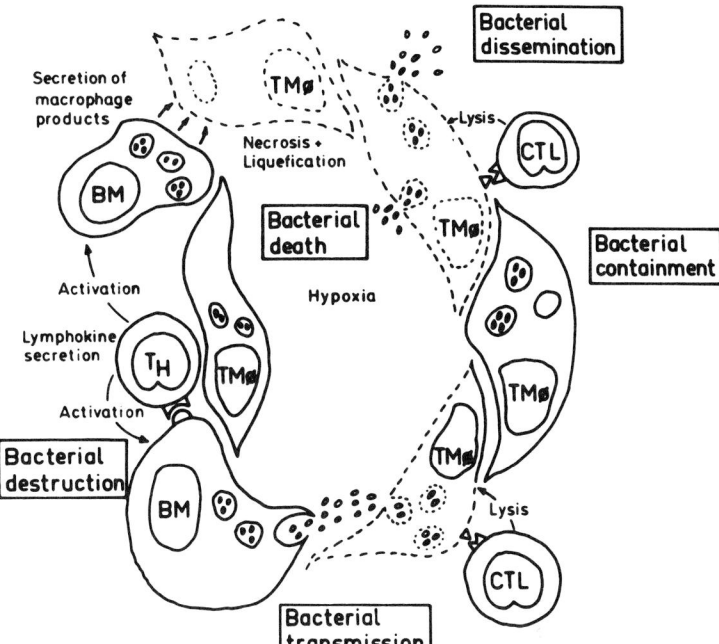

Figure 15–5. A proposed model for T lymphocyte–macrophage interactions in a tuberculous granuloma. BM, unactivated macrophage (blood-borne monocyte); T_H, CD4+ helper T cell; TMφ, activated tissue macrophage; and CTL, CD8+ cytolytic T cell. (From Kaufmann, S. H. E. In vitro analysis of the cellular mechanisms involved in immunity to tuberculosis. Rev. Infect. Dis. 11:S448, 1989.)

guinea pigs with *M. tuberculosis*. Subcutaneous infection by tubercle bacilli in a nonimmune guinea pig caused a persistently infected ulcer which failed to heal. In contrast, secondary infection by tubercle bacilli at another subcutaneous site in the infected animal elicited brisk formation of an indurated lesion, which ulcerated and then healed rapidly. In subsequent work, Koch demonstrated that a crude extract of a boiled culture of tubercle bacilli *(old tuberculin)* produced a similar secondary response when injected into an infected animal. The tuberculin hypersensitivity of infected individuals was initially thought to be of potential therapeutic usefulness. It was soon recognized, however, that the tuberculous patient is inordinately sensitive to tuberculin, and that hypersensitivity (allergy) can be deleterious in the presence of high tuberculin concentration. However, cutaneous tuberculin hypersensitivity is very important for the diagnosis of tuberculous infection.

In the early 1930s, F. B. Seibert prepared products from old tuberculin by fractionation with trichloroacetic acid, ammonium sulfate, and alcohol. These products were labeled *purified protein derivative* (PPD) of tuberculin, although in reality PPD consists of a heterogeneous mixture of mycobacterial cell-wall proteins and polysaccharides. In the early 1940s, a single lot of PPD (as PPD-S) was adopted as the biologic standard by which all clinical PPD preparations are standardized. A 5-tuberculin unit (TU) dose of PPD is equivalent to 0.0001 mg of PPD-S in 0.1 mL of solution. Extensive

clinical studies have demonstrated that 90% of individuals with at least 10 mm of induration 2–3 days following an intracutaneous 5-TU dose of PPD are infected with *M. tuberculosis*, and that essentially 100% of individuals with a 20-mm reaction are infected. The persistence of cutaneous tuberculin hypersensitivity requires the continued presence of tubercle bacilli, although in many individuals the bacilli are present in small numbers and in a slowly replicating, slowly metabolizing form without clinical disease. Histologically, the cutaneous indurated lesion of tuberculin hypersensitivity consists primarily of infiltrates of mononuclear cells in the superficial and deep dermis, and fibrin deposition in the interstitium. The induration is due mostly to fibrin.

A positive *tuberculin reaction* is generally defined as induration ≥10 mm 2–3 days following intracutaneous injection of a PPD dose equivalent to 5 TU *(intermediate-strength PPD)*. In certain situations (contact investigations, HIV-infected persons) the threshold for a positive test is reduced to 5 mm to enhance the sensitivity of the test. Also, *second-strength PPD* (equivalent to a 250-TU dose) can be utilized in individuals negative to intermediate-strength PPD and suspected of having low levels of tuberculin hypersensitivity. Conversely, for persons strongly suspected of active tuberculosis, use of *first-strength PPD* (equivalent to a 1-TU dose) is appropriate. A positive tuberculin reaction indicates probable clinical or subclinical infection by *M. tuberculosis*. However, both false-positive and false-negative reactions occur. False-positive reactions are due to infection with nontuberculous mycobacteria, especially *M. kansasii. False-negative reactions* (anergy) can occur in patients with active tuberculosis, but most of these patients become tuberculin-positive when their illness begins to resolve with antituberculosis chemotherapy. Cutaneous hypersensitivity to tuberculin in infected patients can also be lost due to suppression of cellular immunity by viral infections, lymphoreticular malignancies, AIDS, and corticosteroid therapy. Thus, the absence of a positive tuberculin test does not necessarily reflect absence of tuberculous infection.

Chemotherapy of Tuberculosis

Effective chemotherapy for tuberculosis is based on two fundamental principles. First, spontaneous genetic resistance is present in populations of tubercle bacilli not previously exposed to antituberculous drugs. The frequency of genetic drug-resistant mutants is estimated at 1 in 10^5 tubercle bacilli for isoniazid (INH), and 1 in 10^6 bacilli for streptomycin. Second, tubercle bacilli in the infected patient exist as three different bacterial populations: extracellularly in cavitary lesions, in closed caseous lesions, and intracellularly in macrophages (Fig. 15–6). *M. tuberculosis* is an obligate aerobe, and thus rapidly proliferates to large numbers (10^7–10^9 organisms) in the high oxygen tension of open cavities. However, in closed caseous lesions and within macrophages, where oxygen tension is

reduced, only low numbers (10^4–10^5) of slowly growing tubercle bacilli are present. Based on these principles, a combination of bactericidal drugs rather than a single drug is necessary in the chemotherapy for active disease when large numbers of tubercle bacilli are present, in order to prevent overgrowth by drug-resistant bacteria (Fig. 15–7). In addition, it is necessary to use drugs which are bactericidal not only for extracellular tubercle bacilli in cavities, but also for slowly growing bacilli in closed caseous lesions and in macrophages. These slowly metabolizing organisms are selectively killed by the drugs rifampin and INH. Rifampin and INH are also bactericidal against rapidly proliferating tubercle bacilli in cavitary lesions. Combination chemotherapy with rifampin and INH for a prolonged period (9 months) is sufficient to eliminate both rapidly growing cavitary organisms and slow-growing bacilli in noncavitary lesions. Most patients on this regimen convert to negative sputum cultures within 2 months, and relapse is infrequent.

Primary Drug Resistance

Primary drug resistance refers to the presence of a predominantly drug-resistant population of tubercle bacilli in a previously untreated patient. The occurrence of primary drug resistance reflects person-to-person transmission of drug-resistant strains. The prevalence of drug-resistant strains, in turn, reflects the degree of supervision of patients on antituberculous medication. In the United States, where supervision is generally good, the prevalence of pri-

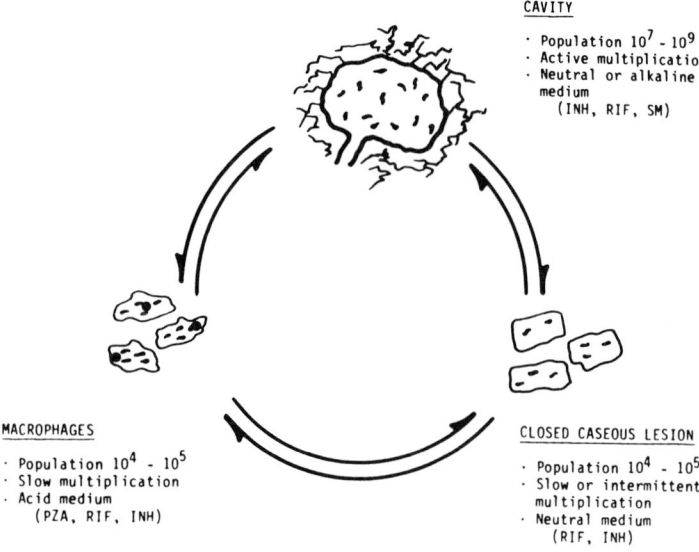

CAVITY
· Population 10^7 - 10^9
· Active multiplication
· Neutral or alkaline medium
   (INH, RIF, SM)

MACROPHAGES
· Population 10^4 - 10^5
· Slow multiplication
· Acid medium
   (PZA, RIF, INH)

CLOSED CASEOUS LESION
· Population 10^4 - 10^5
· Slow or intermittent multiplication
· Neutral medium
   (RIF, INH)

Figure 15–6. Three populations of tubercle bacilli in tuberculosis. Drugs active against each population are indicated as INH (isoniazid), RIF (rifampin), SM (streptomycin), and PZA (pyrazinamide). (From Dutt, A. K., and Stead, W. W. Present chemotherapy for tuberculosis. J. Infect. Dis. 146:698, 1982.)

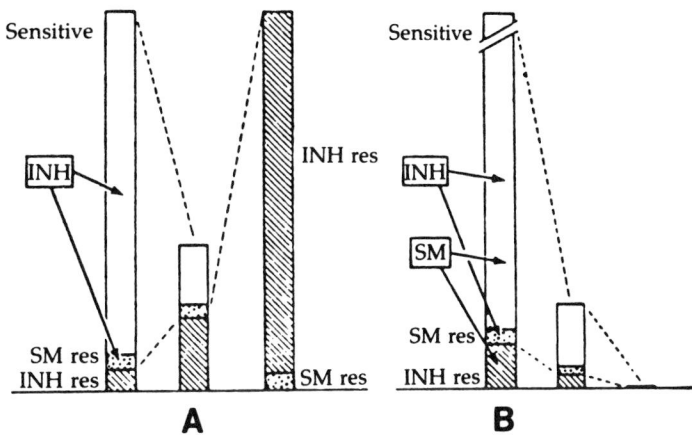

Figure 15–7. Emergence of drug-resistant bacteria in tuberculosis treated with a single drug. In panel A, the patient is treated only with isoniazid (INH). In active tuberculosis with 10^7–10^9 bacilli, INH-resistant mutants present at a frequency of 10^{-6} emerge, and soon constitute the majority of organisms. In panel B, the patient is treated with both INH and streptomycin (SM). Streptomycin suppresses the INH-resistant mutants, and INH suppresses the streptomycin-resistant mutants. Consequently, neither drug-resistant mutant can overgrow, and the combination drug therapy is successful where single drug therapy fails. (From Crofton, J.: Some principles in the chemotherapy of bacterial infections. Br. Med. J. 2:209, 1969.)

mary drug-resistant infection is approximately 7%. However, some areas in the United States, notably southern California, south Texas, and New York City, show a high prevalence of primary drug resistance (approximately 20%). Pockets of relatively high rates of primary resistance are also known to exist within areas of generally low resistance. In Southeast Asia, where antituberculosis drugs can be obtained without physician supervision, the prevalence of primary drug resistance is about 50%.

Secondary Drug Resistance

Secondary drug resistance is the emergence of a drug-resistant strain during antituberculous chemotherapy and among persons previously treated with such drugs. Secondary drug resistance occurs in a patient who fails to complete a full course of chemotherapy after initial improvement during early therapy, and then suffers a relapse with a drug-resistant strain. Obviously, such patients provide a source of infection for uninfected individuals, and the occurrence of secondary drug resistance promotes a high prevalence of primary drug resistance.

Isoniazid in Tuberculosis Chemotherapy

INH is the cornerstone of therapy. Streptomycin, pyrazinamide, and ethambutol, along with INH and rifampin, are considered "first-line drugs" in tuberculosis therapy. Streptomycin is active only against extracellular bacilli, whereas pyrazinamide has specific bactericidal activity against organisms in the acidic environment of phagosomes in macrophages. Ethambutol is not a bactericidal drug, but it penetrates both the extracellular and intracellular environments of

lesions and deters selection of resistant mutants. The addition of pyrazinamide to INH and rifampin for the first 2 months of therapy allows targeting of each of the three bacterial subpopulations (Fig. 15–6) and provides a maximally efficient regimen. Thus, these three drugs provide cure rates at 6 months that are equivalent to results achieved by any longer duration of therapy. A combination of pyrazinamide plus streptomycin or ethambutol, together with INH and rifampin, is indicated for patients with suspected or proven drug-resistant infection. In rare infections with multiple drug resistance, "second-line drugs" should be used (ethionamide, cycloserine, and capreomycin or kanamycin). The use of combination chemotherapy to kill both extracellular and intracellular tubercle bacilli is identical for extrapulmonary (miliary, isolated organ) tuberculosis.

Chemoprophylaxis with INH deserves special mention. Converting a skin test from negative to positive reactivity, especially in individuals who are close contacts of patients with active tuberculosis, mandates 1 year of INH chemoprophylaxis. Also, individuals with upper lobe fibrotic lesions of the lung and a positive tuberculin test, and younger individuals (<35 years of age) with positive tuberculin reactivity but without documented conversion, should have 1 year of INH prophylaxis. Chemoprophylaxis is a misnomer, however, since the real intent is therapy of subclinical, but active, *M. tuberculosis* infection. Since small numbers of tubercle bacilli are present in subclinical infection, use of the single drug INH is effective. In older individuals (>35 years) with a positive skin test, but without documented conversion, contact with active cases, HIV infection, fibrotic pulmonary lesions, or other circumstances known to increase the risk of progressive tuberculosis,

INH prophylaxis is not recommended because of the risk of INH hepatotoxicity in older age groups.

NONTUBERCULOUS MYCOBACTERIAL DISEASE

Overview

Mycobacteria other than *M. tuberculosis* (MOTT) are an important cause of human disease, including chronic pulmonary infection, lymphadenitis, skin and soft tissue infection, and disseminated mycobacteremia. Prior to their identification with species names, MOTT organisms were designated by early investigators as the "atypical" mycobacteria. This historical designation is no longer appropriate but it remains widely used. MOTT organisms differ from *M. tuberculosis* in a number of important respects. First, MOTT species are ubiquitous in the environment, being found in water, soil, and house dust. Most infections with MOTT are acquired from a natural reservoir. Person-to-person transmission of disease, if it occurs, is exceptional. In contrast, there is no natural reservoir of *M. tuberculosis,* and the spread of tuberculosis is by direct contact with infectious cases. Second, the human pathogenicity of MOTT varies greatly for different species, whereas *M. tuberculosis* is an obligate pathogen for humans. Third, MOTT organisms are commonly recovered in cultures of human secretions and fluids as contaminants, MOTT may colonize individuals without causing invasive disease, or MOTT may cause true invasive disease. Thus, growth of MOTT in culture may indicate a contaminant, a saprophyte, or a true pathogen. This circumstance differs sharply from that for *M. tuberculosis,* which when recovered in culture is *always* considered a pathogen. Because of the ubiquity and variable pathogenic potential of MOTT, it is necessary both to understand the disease-producing spectrum of the various MOTT species and to carefully consider the evidence for clinical disease in individual patients (presence of infiltrates on chest roentgenogram, enlarged lymph nodes, nonhealing wounds, skin abscesses or ulcers, or constitutional signs). Multiple isolates of the same MOTT organism and absence of other potential pathogens suggest disease due to the MOTT organism.

Runyon Method of Classification

The Runyon method for the classification of MOTT is based on pigmentation and growth rate. The *photochromogens* (Runyon group I) produce bright yellow to orange beta-carotene pigment when exposed to visible light, but are unpigmented when grown in the dark. The *scotochromogens* (Runyon group II) are pigmented in the dark, usually a deep yellow to orange, and the pigmentation darkens with prolonged exposure to light. The *nonphotochromogens* (Runyon group III) are unpigmented or light yellow and are not affected by light. *Rapid growers* (Runyon group IV) are unpigmented species which produce colonies in less than 7 days when isolated by subculture. The Runyon classification provides clinically relevant information when MOTT species are initially examined in patient cultures. Also, the major Runyon groupings provide a highly useful conceptual framework for understanding MOTT disease. However, definitive diagnosis of MOTT disease always requires complete microbiological identification of isolates to the species level.

Those MOTT species responsible for the majority of human disease are discussed individually in the following sections.

Photochromogens (Runyon Group I)

Mycobacterium kansasii is a photochromogenic acid-fast bacillus which characteristically produces chronic granulomatous pulmonary disease in older-aged white men with underlying chronic obstructive pulmonary disease. Chest roentgenograms typically show involvement of an upper lobe with one or more cavities. Most strains are susceptible to rifampin and slightly resistant to INH. Prolonged combination chemotherapy with rifampin, INH, and ethambutol (the latter to suppress emergence of rifampin and INH resistance) is generally adequate. Disseminated disease with *M. kansasii* has been observed in AIDS. *M. marinum* is a photochromogen which has an optimal growth temperature of 31°–32°C, and which grows poorly if at all at 37°C. Infection with *M. marinum* is confined to superficial cutaneous tissue, and is characteristically acquired from skin trauma while in contact with contaminated nonchlorinated fresh or salt water. Small skin papules develop within 2–8 weeks, often with progression to a verrucous or ulcerated lesion. Cutaneous lesions often resolve spontaneously, but persistent infection requires surgical excision or chemotherapy. Most strains of *M. marinum* are INH-resistant, but are susceptible to combination therapy with rifampin and ethambutol.

Scotochromogens (Runyon Group II)

The vast majority of scotochromogenic myco-bacteria do not produce human disease. They are ubiquitous organisms that frequently contaminate specimens or colonize patients. Consequently, it is important to recognize *M. scrofulaceum* and *M. szulgai,* because these two scotochromogenic species do produce disease. *M. scrofulaceum* is associated with cervical granulomatous lymphadenitis in children (most often in those 1–5 years old), which is unilateral and typically submandibular in location. Surgical excision of involved nodes is almost always curative. *M. szulgai* is an unusual scotochromogen in two regards. First, it is scotochromogenic when grown at 37°C but photochromogenic at 25°C. Second, although clinical isolates are infrequent, most are associated with disease. The predominant form of disease is chronic cavitary pulmonary infection in middle-aged men.

Nonphotochromogens (Runyon Group III)

The *Mycobacterium avium complex* (MAC) organisms *(M. avium* and *M. intracellulare)* are the nonphotochromogens most frequently associated with human disease. Four forms of disease due to MAC infection are commonly seen:

1. Chronic cavitary pulmonary disease occurs, typically in a middle-aged white man with preexisting lung disease, including chronic obstructive pulmonary disease, bronchiectasis, and silicosis. Clinical presentation of MAC pulmonary disease resembles tuberculosis, with a sputum-producing cough, fatigue, weight loss, fever, night sweats, and occasionally hemoptysis.
2. Chronic fibronodular disease with or without cavitation is caused by MAC especially in elderly white women, with cough and progressive respiratory symptoms over years.
3. MAC may cause cervical lymphadenitis in children and sometimes in adults, indistinguishable from adenitis due to *M. scrofulaceum.*
4. Disseminated MAC infection occurs in immunocompromised states, especially due to adrenocorticosteroid therapy or HIV infection.

Most immunocompromised patients with disseminated MAC infection present with fever;

weight loss; and, in many AIDS patients, gastrointestinal symptoms, including abdominal pain and diarrhea. In patients with gastrointestinal disease, aggregates of foamy macrophages are present in the small intestinal mucosa, which resemble those in Whipple's disease but (unlike in Whipple's disease) contain numerous intracellular acid-fast bacilli. The heavy mycobacterial load has led to the proposal that the gastrointestinal tract is the portal of entry for MAC in AIDS patients with a gastrointestinal syndrome. MAC is an environmental organism that can colonize individuals without causing disease. Thus, a diagnosis of MAC disease should be made only after repeated isolation of MAC in culture from a patient with signs and symptoms consistent with MAC disease.

Chemotherapy of MAC disease is difficult because of the prevalent resistance to first-line antimycobacterial drugs among clinical strains. Consequently, second-line antimycobacterial drugs must often be added to combination chemotherapy. In AIDS patients no combination of antimycobacterial drugs currently available eradicates MAC infection, and restoration of immune capacity is the only hope for these patients, but treatment with some multiple-drug regimens has been reported to improve symptoms.

Rapid Growers (Runyon Group IV)

The human pathogens in this group are *M. fortuitum* and *M. chelonae. M. fortuitum* and *M. chelonae* are environmental organisms present in water, soil, and dust, and most human infections are due to accidental inoculation of skin and soft tissue during surgery or with trauma. Median sternotomy in cardiovascular surgery, augmentation mammoplasty, peritoneal dialysis, hemodialysis, surgical insertion of a percutaneous catheter, and arthroplasty have been implicated in postsurgical infections. Patients present with failure of the wound to heal. Cutaneous infections due to trauma can resemble pyogenic infection with suppuration or may progress to chronic ulceration with sinus tract formation. Like other mycobacteria, treatment for *M. fortuitum* and *M. chelonae* infection is best done with a combination of drugs to avoid emergence of resistance. Unlike most other mycobacteria, however, these rapid growers are susceptible to drugs generally used in the therapy of infection due to facultative bacteria. The aminoglycosides are most active therapeutically, especially amikacin (preferably combined with cefoxitin, doxycycline, ciprofloxacin, or rifampin).

LEPROSY

Leprosy is a chronic infection of the skin, mucous membranes, and peripheral nerves by *M. leprae* (Hansen's bacillus). *M. leprae* is an acid-fast bacillus which grows very slowly. When injected into the footpads of mice, its doubling time is 11–13 days. It is an obligate pathogen for humans, and transmission of the bacillus is by direct and prolonged contact with individuals shedding large numbers of bacilli from open skin lesions or in nasal mucus. The leprosy bacillus does not grow in cell-free culture systems and can be detected only by acid-fast staining of infected tissue. The incidence of leprosy in the United States is increasing as a result of increased immigration from areas of the world where leprosy is common, especially India, Vietnam, Laos, and the Phillipines.

Tuberculoid Leprosy

The clinical spectrum of leprosy reflects the degree of cell-mediated immunity toward the leprosy bacillus. At one extreme of the spectrum, tuberculoid granulomas form in the skin and peripheral nerves of patients with T-lymphocyte responsiveness to *M. leprae*. This form of leprosy is designated *polar tuberculoid leprosy*. Only rare bacilli are present in the granulomas, and the tuberculoid form is not contagious. The tuberculoid granulomas result in raised erythematous plaques of the skin with flattened pale (healed) centers. These areas are *anesthetic* due to involvement of cutaneous nerve fibers by the granulomatous inflammatory response.

Lepromatous Leprosy

At the opposite extreme of the spectrum are patients who lack T-lymphocyte reactivity to leprosy bacilli, and who have huge numbers of acid-fast bacilli within macrophages *(lepra cells)*. There is no granulomatous inflammatory response, but instead nodular or diffuse aggregates of foamy macrophages appear in the skin, mucus membranes, and peripheral nerves. This form of leprosy is designated *polar lepromatous leprosy*. These aggregates are distributed bilaterally and symmetrically as erythematous nodular lesions of the skin, which often coalesce to impart diffuse thickening of the facial skin *(leonine facies)*. In severe disease, perforation of the nasal septum and destruction of nasal cartilages can occur. Lepromatous skin and mucus membrane lesions contain large numbers of bacilli, and the lepromatous form is contagious. Because of lack of host resistance, lepromatous leprosy is more extensive and more difficult to cure.

Forms intermediate between tuberculoid and lepromatous leprosy are variable in their tissue reactions and bacillary load, and there is a clinically silent phase which can last for many years during which the bacilli slowly proliferate and disseminate.

Diagnosis

As in tuberculosis, cutaneous hypersensitivity develops in leprosy. *Lepromin* is a crude preparation of bacillary antigens obtained from lepromatous nodules, which can be used as a skin-test antigen to gauge the intensity of delayed-type hypersensitivity in individual patients. Positive reactions are biphasic, consisting of transient induration at 48 h, followed by progressive nodule formation which is maximal at 3–4 weeks, sometimes with ulceration. Histologically, these nodules consist of tuberculoid inflammation. A positive lepromin test is typical in tuberculoid leprosy, but the lepromatous patient is anergic (nonreactive) to lepromin. However, patients with lepromatous leprosy characteristically have a polyclonal gammopathy with antibodies to *M. leprae*. These antibodies are not protective, but rather are deleterious since immune complex formation often leads to an Arthus-type vasculitis and *erythema nodosum leprosum* (ENL). ENL is associated with painful necrosis of skin nodules, fever, arthralgias, and sometimes even glomerulonephritis. ENL can be fatal.

Treatment

Infection with *M. leprae* tends to be persistent, especially in lepromatous leprosy, and prolonged chemotherapy is necessary to control, and hopefully, eradicate the leprosy bacilli. Dapsone (DDS) (4,4'-diaminodiphenyl sulfone) is the mainstay of therapy and is usually combined with clofazimine (a lipophilic drug which selectively concentrates in infected macrophages) and rifampin to suppress emergence of DDS resistance.

LABORATORY DIAGNOSIS OF MYCOBACTERIAL INFECTION

Although mycobacteria may infect almost any tissue or organ, they most frequently infect the lungs, urogenital tract, gastrointestinal tract, meninges, and blood. Pulmonary secretions are present in expectorated sputum, aerosol-induced sputum, gastric lavage (due to swallowing), and bronchoscopy washings. Voided urine specimens are useful for the laboratory diagnosis of urogenital infections and disseminated disease. The shedding of mycobacteria into the respiratory or urogenital tracts is irregular. Thus, a minimum of three early-morning sputum, gastric lavage, or urine specimens should be collected on three separate days. Fecal specimens are submitted for evaluation of enteric disease and blood specimens for disseminated disease, especially with MAC infection in AIDS patients.

Pulmonary, urogenital, and fecal specimens are contaminated by bacterial commensals (normal flora), and consequently the recovery of mycobacteria requires both decontamination and concentration. The "gold standard" for bacterial decontamination is brief treatment (15–20 min) of specimens with 2% NaOH solution containing *N*-acetyl-L-cysteine (NALC). NALC acts as a mucolytic agent, thereby releasing mycobacteria trapped in mucin strands for detection by acid-fast stain and culture. Following decontamination, hypotonic phosphate buffer is added to terminate NaOH decontamination and also to lower the specific gravity of the specimen. The high cell-wall lipid content of mycobacteria renders them buoyant during centrifugation. Thus, the specific gravity of the specimen must be low in order to concentrate mycobacteria by centrifugation. The specimen is subjected to centrifugation, and mycobacteria are concentrated in a pellet, which is retrieved for acid-fast staining and culture.

Specimens obtained from normally sterile sources (blood; cerebrospinal, pleural, peritoneal, or joint fluid; and tissue) do not require decontamination, and can be either processed directly by acid-fast staining and culture or first concentrated by centrifugation.

The laboratory detection and evaluation of mycobacteria are accomplished by (1) acid-fast staining; (2) growth in culture; (3) species identification by growth properties, pigmentation, and biochemical phenotype; and (4) nucleic acid hybridization. Although other procedures have been found useful, especially the analysis of cell-wall long-chain fatty acids by gas–liquid chromatography, they have yet to achieve general use in clinical mycobacteriology laboratories. Once isolated, the antimicrobial drug susceptibility of a mycobacterium must be carefully determined under strictly defined conditions.

Acid-Fast Staining

The *mycosides* are mycolic acid–containing glycolipids and glycolipid-peptide complexes, which imbue mycobacteria with *acid fastness*. To perform a *Ziehl-Neelsen acid-fast stain*, a smear is briefly heated to obtain deep penetration of carbolfuchsin into mycobacterial cell walls. In the *Kinyoun stain*, a higher carbolfuchsin concentration is utilized so that heating is not necessary. When the red dye fuchsin is combined with phenol (carbolic acid) as a mordant to intensify dye binding, the bound fuchsin resists decolorization with acid-alcohol solution (acid fastness). Avid binding of fuchsin to cell-wall mycolic acid forms a barrier which traps fuchsin inside the mycobacterial cell. Tubercle bacilli stained with carbolfuchsin appear as red, irregularly beaded, slim rods in oil immersion microscopy. Other mycobacteria stain similarly, but there are some notable variations. *M. kansasii* is strongly acid-fast with long rods which are banded, and MAC organisms appear as pleomorphic coccobacillary acid-fast forms. Rapid growers are acid-fast by carbolfuchsin staining, but unlike other mycobacteria (which do not stain with crystal violet of the Gram's stain), *M. chelonae* and *M. fortuitum* appear as gram-positive diphtheroids by Gram's stain. More sensitive fluorochrome stains are now available, in which fluorescent dyes (auramine O, rhodamine) bind in acid-fast fashion to cell-wall mycolic acid. Mycobacteria display a characteristic bright yellow to golden color by fluorescent microscopy. One limitation is failure of most rapid growers to stain with fluorochromes. Thus, negative fluorochrome stains should be confirmed by a carbolfuchsin stain, with specimens obtained from body sites where infection with rapid growers characteristically occurs (surgical wounds, percutaneous catheters, traumatic cutaneous lesions).

Acid-fast stains can detect mycobacteria when present in specimens at concentrations of at least 10,000 bacilli per milliliter. Patients with open cavity disease shed large numbers of mycobacteria, and acid-fast smears of sputum are highly sensitive for detection of disease in such individuals. However, in patients with less advanced disease, positive smears are present in only 25–50%. Tuberculous meningitis is particularly difficult to detect by acid-fast smear, since there may be very few organisms in the CSF. A minimum of 10 mL of CSF is recommended for recovery of mycobacteria, and prolonged centrifugation must be performed to concentrate bacilli in a pellet for acid-fast staining.

Growth in Culture

The most commonly used medium for the culture of mycobacteria is the *Löwenstein-Jensen* (LJ) *medium,* which is a solid, egg-based, heat-inspissated medium, containing the inhibitory agent malachite green to prevent overgrowth by normal bacterial flora. Also, defined *Middlebrook media* are available, in both liquid (7H9) and transparent (7H10, 7H11) agar-based forms. They contain salts, vitamins, oleic acid, albumin, catalase, glycerol, and dextrose to support mycobacterial growth. The 7H11 medium can be made selective for the growth of mycobacteria by the addition of antibiotics which suppress overgrowth by normal bacterial flora. In a significant improvement, ^{14}C-labeled palmitic acid has been incorporated into Middlebrook 7H9 broth as a metabolic substrate for mycobacteria. When present, mycobacteria convert ^{14}C-palmitic acid to ^{14}CO$_2$, and the presence of ^{14}CO$_2$ gas allows rapid detection of the mycobacteria *(radiometric culture systems).* Standard laboratory practice dictates use of at least two of the three different media (LJ, selective 7H11, radiometric broth) for clinical specimens. In general, growth of *M. tuberculosis* complex and MOTT organisms is initially detected in 1–3 weeks in radiometric broth, and after somewhat longer times with the solid media.

Species Identification

Following initial appearance in culture, it is necessary to determine whether an isolate is a member of the *M. tuberculosis* complex, or is a MOTT organism. A rapid way to accomplish this is by use of the NAP growth inhibition test. NAP (*p*-nitro-alpha-acetylamino-beta-hydroxypropiophenone) is an intermediate compound

in the synthesis of chloramphenicol, which selectively inhibits the growth of *M. tuberculosis* complex organisms (Fig. 15–8). The NAP test can be performed in just a few days and provides clinically relevant information. Most importantly, identifying an acid-fast bacillus from a respiratory specimen as *M. tuberculosis* complex indicates the need to isolate the patient since tuberculosis is communicable, whereas MOTT infection is not communicable.

MOTT organisms must be further characterized regarding pigmentation and growth rate, using subcultures prepared from the initial culture isolate. Photoreactivity is measured by brief

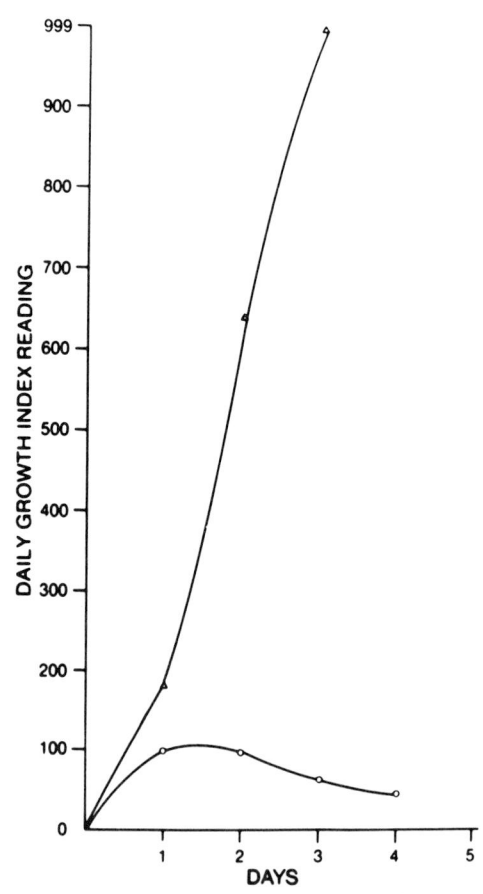

Figure 15–8. NAP inhibition test for the identification of M. tuberculosis *complex organisms. NAP (p-nitro-alpha-acetylamino-beta-hydroxypropiophenone) selectively inhibits the growth of* M. tuberculosis *complex organisms in Middlebrook broth containing* ^{14}C-labeled palmitic acid as substrate for mycobacterial metabolism. Growth in this radiometric system is measured by rate of appearance of ^{14}CO$_2$. Growth in absence of NAP is indicated by triangles (△ positive growth control), and inhibited growth in presence of NAP (5 µg/mL) is indicated by circles (○). (From Laszlo, A., and Siddiqui, S. H. Evaluation of a rapid radiometric differentiation test for the* Mycobacterium tuberculosis *complex by selective inhibition with* p-nitro-alpha-acetylamino-beta-hydroxypropiophenone. J. Clin. Microbiol. 19:694, 1984.)*

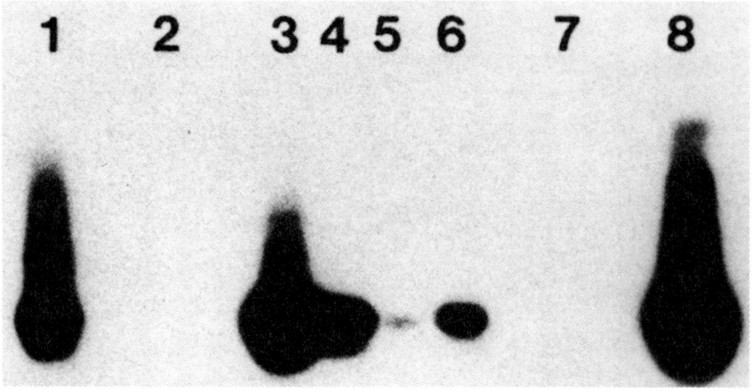

Figure 15–9. Direct detection of M. tuberculosis *in clinical specimens by polymerase chain-reaction (PCR) assay. A repetitive element in the* M. tuberculosis *genome was amplified by PCR and was then hybridized to a ^{32}P-labeled nucleic acid probe complementary to the chromosomal element for visualization by autoradiography after purification by agarose gel electrophoresis. DNA was directly isolated from CSF of a patient with tuberculous meningitis (lane 1), and lung biopsy tissue (lane 3) and pleural fluid (lanes 4 through 6) were strongly positive for presence*

of M. tuberculosis *DNA. CSF from a patient with pneumococcal meningitis (lane 2) and pleural fluid from a patient with a malignant effusion (lane 7) were negative. Lane 8 is an* M. tuberculosis *chromosomal DNA–positive control. (From DeWit, D., Steyn, L., Shoemaker, S., and Sogin, M. Direct detection of* Mycobacterium tuberculosis *in clinical specimens by DNA amplification.* J. Clin. Microbiol. 28:2437, 1990.)

(3–5 h) light exposure of young colonies previously grown in the dark, and growth is measured by the rate of colony formation on a solid medium inoculated with a broth culture of the organism, using the Runyon classification described earlier. Information on photoreactivity and growth rate can provide important preliminary information for patient evaluation and must be promptly reported to the patient's physician (see Case History). However, definitive diagnosis requires species identification, which can be accomplished by a variety of biochemical tests and, more recently, by nucleic acid hybridization assays (see below). Species identification is required since some MOTT species are facultative pathogens, whereas other species are common saprophytes or environmental contaminants.

Nucleic Acid Hybridization

Specific ribosomal RNA and chromosomal DNA of *M. tuberculosis* or MAC complex organisms growing in culture can be readily detected by hybridization of complementary nucleic acid probes. Nucleic acid hybridization analysis can be performed in a few hours, compared with the days or weeks required for identification by conventional biochemical techniques. Very recently, a polymerase chain-reaction (PCR) assay has been developed for the amplification of a repetitive base pair sequence unique to the chromosomal DNA of *M. tuberculosis*. This PCR assay is sensitive to fewer than 10 tubercle bacilli and can rapidly and directly detect tubercle bacilli in clinical

specimens (Fig. 15–9). Although still in its infancy, DNA probe analysis is powerful and specific and likely will become a mainstay in the laboratory diagnosis of mycobacterial disease.

Drug Susceptibility Testing

If more than 1% of a patient's tubercle bacilli are resistant to a drug, that drug is unlikely to be effective in therapy. Consequently, drug susceptibility assays have been established which quantitatively measure whether fewer or more than 1% of organisms in an isolate are drug-resistant. These assays are performed with the drug incorporated into transparent Middlebrook agar or broth (Fig. 15–10).

CASE HISTORY

The patient was a 62-year-old, barrel-chested white male who complained of increasing shortness of breath and fever. He was a heavy cigarette smoker, and his shortness of breath was attributed to chronic obstructive pulmonary disease. However, the dyspnea had considerably worsened in the preceding 3 weeks. Physical examination revealed a temperature of 100°F, pulse rate of 90/min, respiration of 24/min, and a blood pressure of 110/80 mm Hg. Chest roentgenogram revealed small, scattered pneumonic infiltrates in both upper lobes, accompanied by several small cavities. Sputum Gram's stain performed the first hospital day showed numerous neutrophils

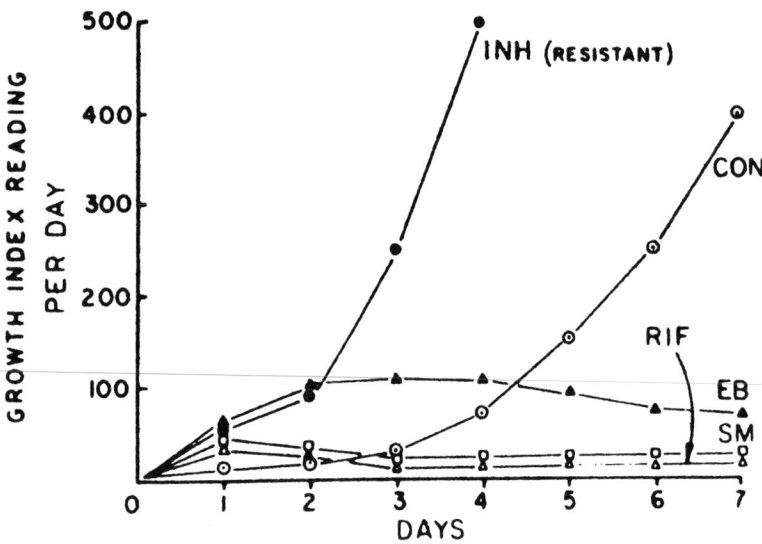

Figure 15–10. A 1% threshold as determinant of drug resistance for M. tuberculosis. *Growth of* M. tuberculosis *in drug-containing radiometric broths is directly compared with growth in control broth in which the inoculum of organisms is only 1/100th that used for drug-containing broths. As can be seen, growth in isoniazid (INH)-containing broth is greater than growth in the control broth, indicating more than 1% of organisms are resistant to INH. Hence, this isolate is considered INH-resistant. In contrast, growth in the presence of rifampin (RIF), streptomycin (SM), and ethambutol (EB) is less than in the control broth, indicating that fewer than 1% of the organisms are resistant to these drugs. Therefore, this isolate is considered susceptible to RIF, SM, and EB. (From Siddiqui, S. H.,*

Libonati, J. P., and Middlebrook, G. Evaluation of a rapid radiometric method for drug susceptibility testing of Mycobacterium tuberculosis. J. Clin. Microbiol. 13:908, 1981.)

(>25 per low-power field), only occasional oropharyngeal epithelial cells (<10), and scattered gram-positive cocci and a few gram-negative cocci and rods. Routine bacterial culture of the sputum showed a mixed flora of alpha-hemolytic streptococci, coagulase-negative staphylococci, diphtheroids, and *Haemophilus* species. Three sets of blood cultures submitted the first day were negative after 1 week's incubation. Because of the appearance of the chest roentgenogram, three early-morning sputum specimens obtained on three different days were submitted for auramine O-rhodamine acid-fast stain and mycobacterial culture. The first two sputum specimens were negative by acid-fast stain, but the third specimen revealed golden-colored acid-fast bacilli present in small numbers (10 bacilli per entire smear). Thus, the patient was masked to prevent possible transmission of acid-fast bacilli to other individuals, and combined therapy was instituted with INH and rifampin. Within 5 days of inoculation with the acid-fast-positive sputum of radiometric BACTEC 12B broth, a positive growth index (GI) was recorded (GI>10), and by the next day the GI value exceeded 100. After confirmation by Kinyoun stain that organisms growing in the radiometric broth were indeed acid-fast bacilli, the broth was reinoculated to fresh radiometric broth for a NAP test. The broth was also subcultured to a selective

Middlebrook 7H11 agar plate which was incubated in the dark at 35°C. Within 5 days, positive growth was recorded for the isolate in the presence of NAP, and preliminary identification as a mycobacterium other than *M. tuberculosis* complex (MOTT) was reported to the patient's physician. Since communicability of infection was no longer a possibility, the patient was advised that it was no longer necessary for him to mask. As a preliminary test of pigmentation, the selective 7H11 plate (which showed many nonpigmented colonies) was exposed for 3 hours to light from a 100-W tungsten bulb, and returned to the incubator. Within 1 day all colonies demonstrated bright yellow-orange pigmentation, and thus further identification as a photochromogenic MOTT species was reported to the patient's physician. Because *M. kansasii* is by far the most common photochromogenic species which produces pulmonary disease and because it can demonstrate increased resistance to INH, ethambutol was added to the patient's drug combination. Within 6 weeks, formal biochemical identification of the isolate as *M. kansasii* (strong heat-stable catalase, positive Tween 80 hydrolysis, positive nitrate reduction, negative niacin accumulation) had been accomplished. By this time, however, the patient had been discharged from the hospital and was doing well at home.

REFERENCES

Review Articles

Berlin, O. G. W. Mycobacteria. In: Baron, E. J., and Finegold, S. M., eds. *Bailey & Scott's Diagnostic Microbiology*. 8th ed. St. Louis: C. V. Mosby Company, 1990: 597–640.

Bullock, W. E. Mycobacterium leprae (leprosy). In: Mandell, G. L., Douglas, R. G., Jr., and Bennett, J. E., eds. *Principles and Practice of Infectious Diseases*. 3rd ed. New York: Churchill Livingstone, 1990: 1906–1914.

Dannenberg, A. M., Jr. Immune mechanisms in the pathogenesis of pulmonary tuberculosis. *Rev. Infect. Dis. 11:*S369, 1989.

Hahn, H., and Kaufmann, S. H. E. The role of cell-mediated immunity in bacterial infections. *Rev. Infect. Dis. 3:*1221, 1981.

Kim, J. H., Langston, A. A., and Gallis, H. A. Miliary tuberculosis: Epidemiology, clinical manifestations, diagnosis, and outcome. *Rev. Infect. Dis. 12:*583, 1990.

Sanders, W. E., Jr., and Horowitz, E. A. Other mycobacterium species. In: Mandell, G. L., Douglas, R. G., Jr., and Bennett, J. E., eds. *Principles and Practice of Infectious Diseases*. 3rd ed. New York: Churchill Livingstone, 1990: 1914–1926.

Wallace, R. J., Jr., Swenson, J. M., Silcox, V. A., et al. Spectrum of disease due to rapidly growing mycobacteria. *Rev. Infect. Dis. 5:*657, 1983.

Woods, G. L., and Washington, J. A., II. Mycobacteria other than *Mycobacterium tuberculosis:* Review of microbiologic and clinical aspects. *Rev. Infect. Dis. 9:*275, 1987.

Original Articles

Anargyros, P., Astill, D. S. J., and Lim, I. S. L. Comparison of improved BACTEC and Löwenstein-Jensen media for culture of mycobacteria from clinical specimens. *J. Clin. Microbiol. 28:*1288, 1990.

Eisenach, K. D., Crawford, J. T., and Bates, J. H. Repetitive DNA sequences as probes for *Mycobacterium tuberculosis. J. Clin. Microbiol. 26:*2240, 1988.

Flesch, I., and Kaufmann, S. H. E. Mycobacterial growth inhibition by interferon-γ activated bone marrow macrophages and differential susceptibility among strains of *Mycobacterium tuberculosis. J. Immunol. 138:*4408, 1987.

Gross, W. M., and Hawkins, J. E. Radiometric selective inhibition tests for differentiation of *Mycobacterium tuberculosis, Mycobacterium bovis,* and other mycobacteria. *J. Clin. Microbiol. 21:*565, 1985.

Lurie, M. B. Studies on the mechanism of immunity in tuberculosis. The fate of tubercle bacilli ingested by mononuclear phagocytes derived from normal and immunized animals. *J. Exp. Med. 75:*247, 1942.

Mackaness, G. B. The influence of immunologically committed lymphoid cells on macrophage activity *in vivo. J. Exp. Med. 129:*973, 1969.

Musial, C. E., Tice, L. S., Stockman, L., et al. Identification of mycobacteria from culture by using the Gen-Probe rapid diagnostic system for *Mycobacterium avium* complex and *Mycobacterium tuberculosis* complex. *J. Clin. Microbiol. 26:*2120, 1988.

Suter, E. Multiplication of tubercle bacilli within mononuclear phagocytes in tissue cultures derived from normal animals and animals vaccinated with BCG. *J. Exp. Med. 97:*235, 1953.

Witebsky, F. G., Keiser, J. F., Conville, P. S., et al. Comparison of BACTEC 13A medium and DuPont Isolator for detection of mycobacteremia. *J. Clin. Microbiol. 26:*1501, 1988.

16 *JOHN P. PHAIR, M.D.*

Fungal Infections of the Respiratory Tract

INTRODUCTION

Infections due to fungi are common. Most are superficial and caused by the dermatophytes, which involve the skin of the feet, groin, axillae, and other intertriginous areas. In contrast, the deep mycoses produce pulmonary infection and can disseminate in healthy individuals, and opportunistic fungi cause disease in immunocompromised patients (see Chapter 27). This chapter will review the epidemiology, microbiology, pathology, and clinical manifestations of the most common deep mycoses, as well as the opportunistic fungal infections. This separation is for convenience of presentation, but it should be realized that some fungi, such as *Cryptococcus neoformans,* infect healthy individuals as well as immunocompromised patients.

The pathogenic fungi can be classified as yeasts, which are spherical organisms that reproduce by budding, or molds, which have hyphae that branch, elongate, and release infective spores or conidia. Many of the deep mycoses are infections caused by dimorphic fungi, which exist as yeast forms in tissue and mold forms in the environment.

Diagnosis of fungal infections can be difficult and usually is best established by biopsy of involved tissue to demonstrate invasion by fungal elements. Fungal cultures can be slow to yield results, and laboratory isolation of an organism often does not distinguish between colonization and infection. Serologic tests can be useful in the differential diagnosis of histoplasmosis, coccidioidomycosis, and cryptococcal infections, but are not helpful in diagnosis of blastomycosis or the opportunistic infections due to *Candida* or *Aspergillus* species.

In general, the host defense mechanisms which control these infections involve the phagocytic cells, polymorphonuclear leukocytes, monocytes, and macrophages. In some instances, serum opsonins appear to augment phagocytosis, but for organisms such as *Histoplasma capsulatum* and *Coccidioides immitis*, cell-mediated responses involving lymphocytes and macrophages appear to be the primary host defense mechanism.

Mycotic infections generally result from exposure to environmental sources of the infecting organisms or activation of endogenous fungal flora secondary to other diseases or therapy for these illnesses. Except for candidal infections and superficial mycoses, there is no evidence of person-to-person spread. Culture of *C. immitis* and *H. capsulatum* should be attempted only in laboratories especially equipped to perform these isolation techniques, as laboratory personnel can be infected by the mold form of these organisms.

HISTOPLASMOSIS

H. capsulatum is an organism ubiquitous in the Ohio and Mississippi river valleys of the United States (Fig. 16–1). It has also been noted in tropical, subtropical, and temperate zones throughout the world. In 1905, Samuel Darling first noted and named the organism in autopsy tissue obtained in Panama. It was not until World War II that the widespread nature of this infection in endemic areas was appreciated. Culture of soil in endemic areas contaminated by bat excrement is usually positive, and localized outbreaks have occurred when such sites have been disturbed by construction. Bats, although carriers of the fungus, do not become infected or ill.

Pathology

Infection occurs following the inhalation of spores released from hyphae, which then germinate within tissue. Within days the yeast form of the fungus can be demonstrated in pulmonary macrophages. In the previously uninfected host, intracellular proliferation occurs. The mononuclear phagocytes containing the yeast can be found in regional nodes, and throughout the reticuloendothelial system within 2 weeks. This primary infection leads to an immune response,

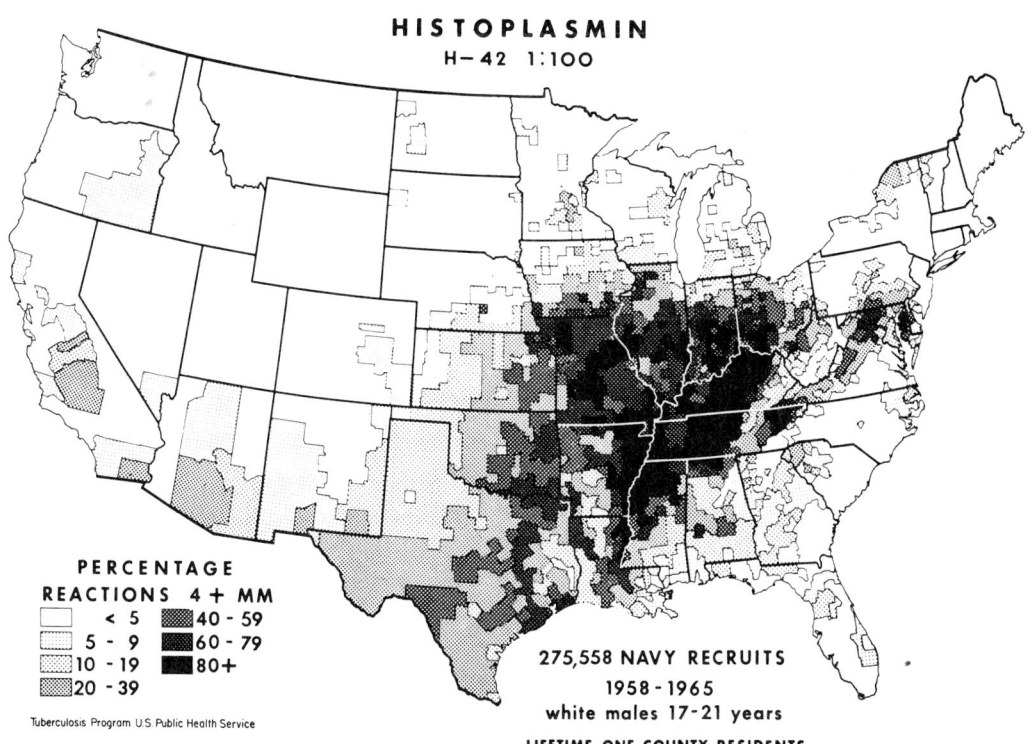

HISTOPLASMIN
H–42 1:100

PERCENTAGE
REACTIONS 4 + MM
< 5   40 - 59
5 - 9   60 - 79
10 - 19   80+
20 - 39

Tuberculosis Program U.S Public Health Service

275,558 NAVY RECRUITS
1958 - 1965
white males 17-21 years
LIFETIME ONE COUNTY RESIDENTS

Figure 16–1. Map shows incidence of skin reactivity to histoplasmin among naval recruits. In southern Kentucky, middle Tennessee, and other areas, the incidence of skin reactivity is as high as 90–95%. (From Edwards, L. B., Acquaviva, F. A., Livesay, V. T., et al. An atlas of sensitivity of tuberculin, PPD-B, and histoplasmosis in the United States. Am. Rev. Respir. Dis. 99:1, 1969.)

inflammation, and necrosis at the site of mononuclear cell accumulation. With the onset of the immune response, the macrophages are activated and kill the intracellular yeast. Ultimately the areas of caseous necrosis calcify; however, viable organisms can be recovered from such lesions long after the initial infection.

Symptoms related to the initial infection are uncommon, but constitutional and nonspecific symptoms can occur. When present, cough and chest discomfort point to the primary site of infection. Infection is extremely common in endemic areas, with 80% of persons growing up in the Ohio Valley having evidence of prior infection by age 18 years. If a large number of spores are inhaled, clinically apparent pneumonitis can occur. Rarely, the acute infection can be severe enough to produce life-threatening illness. In young children, the primary infection can be associated with evidence of dissemination including hepatic and splenic involvement. In normal adults, hepatosplenomegaly is uncommon, but histologic evidence of dissemination can be documented. In association with the immune response to infection with *H. capsulatum,* rashes such as erythema nodosum and erythema multiforme have been documented. In some outbreaks these cutaneous findings are extremely common.

Involvement of the pericardium, pleura, or mediastinal nodes or development of mediastinal fibrosis can complicate acute infection. The most serious complication, however, is uncontrolled dissemination. This is thought to occur almost exclusively in individuals with a defect in the host response to infection and has been well documented in patients with acquired immunodeficiency syndrome (AIDS). Disseminated histoplasmosis resembles miliary tuberculosis and can involve all organs; the diagnosis can most easily be made by examination and culture of the bone marrow. Hepatosplenomegaly, destruction of the adrenals, endocarditis, meningitis, and cerebral infection all have been reported. In children, dissemination is commonly accompanied by severe pulmonary involvement and pancytopenia due to infection of the marrow. In adults with chronic lung disease, *H. capsulatum* occasionally produces chronic cavitary disease of the upper lobes. Often these infected cavities represent superinfection of preexistent bullae.

Diagnosis

The diagnosis of histoplasmosis must be suspected clinically in order to be established. A fourfold or greater rise in the titer of complement-fixing antibody to *H. capsulatum* is generally considered diagnostic. Biopsy and culture of bone marrow or liver also can yield a diagnosis. Culture of blood using a technique that results in lysis of white cells, centrifugation of the cell lysate, and culture of the sediment on Saboraud's agar is often positive in cases of dissemination. Newer immunoprecipitation assays for antibody to *H. capsulatum* show promise, but are not widely available. Infection with this fungus stimulates a marked cell-mediated (T-cell) immune response, and skin testing with histoplasmin elicits a positive delayed hypersensitivity reaction beginning several weeks after initiation of infection. The skin test has been extremely useful in establishing the epidemiology of the infection in the United States. However, a positive skin test induces a rise in the serum complement-fixing antibody titer in previously infected individuals. Thus, individuals from an endemic area who have pulmonary disease, fever of unknown origin, or hepatosplenomegaly should not be skin tested. If they are tested, the resultant positive skin test will stimulate an antibody rise and provide misleading information.

Treatment

Treatment of acute histoplasmosis in the normal host is generally not necessary, being reserved for patients with evidence of disseminated disease or chronic cavitary pulmonary disease. The usual total adult dose of amphotericin B for such patients is 2.0 gm administered at 0.5–0.7 mg/kg every other day, or three times per week. Ketoconazole, an oral antifungal agent, can be substituted in treatment of disseminated disease in the absence of meningitis (the agent does not penetrate the blood–brain barrier) or endocarditis. This antibiotic is generally administered in a dose of 400 mg/day for 6–12 months. Ketoconazole should be reserved for individuals who are not immunocompromised. Treatment of meningitis and endocarditis requires amphotericin therapy.

BLASTOMYCOSIS

Blastomyces dermatitides also is endemic in the central United States; however, this disease extends further into the northern Midwest than does histoplasmosis (Fig. 16–2). Thus, in Chi-

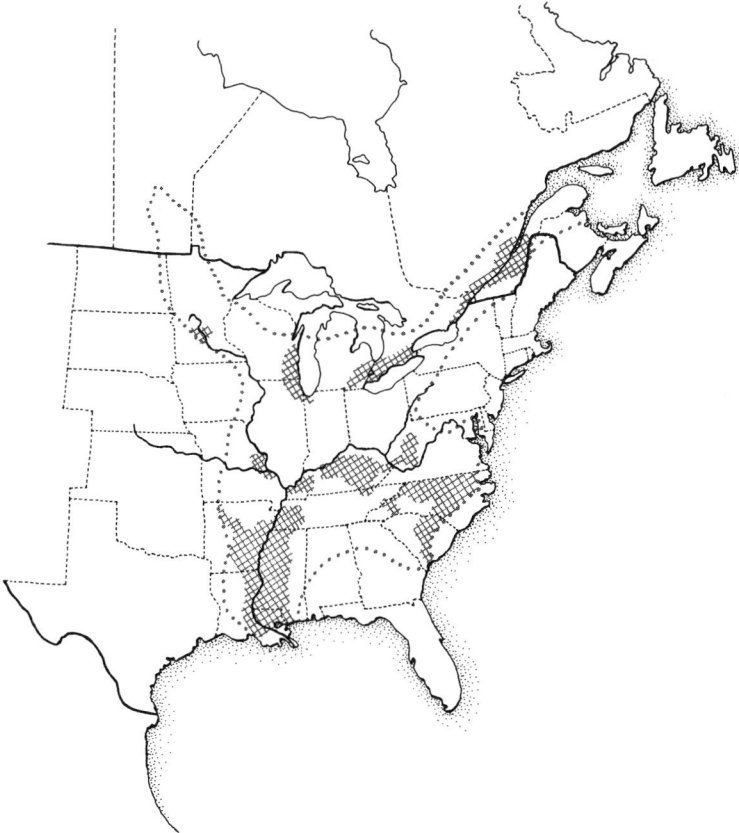

Figure 16–2. Blastomycosis. Incidence and prevalence of blastomycosis in North America. The dotted line indicates the known endemic region. The hatched areas are those with the highest incidence. (From Rippon, J. W. Medical Mycology. Philadelphia: W. B. Saunders Co., 1974.)

cago and Wisconsin, blastomycosis is more commonly diagnosed than histoplasmosis. The disease was originally described in Chicago by Thomas C. Gilchrist, who ultimately isolated the organism and proved that it was a fungus. At room temperature it grows as a mold with conidiospores which bud from the hyphae with terminal conidia—the infectious form of the fungus. At 37°C, however, the fungus grows as a yeast and in tissue is seen to bud with a characteristic broad base ("broad-based buds = blastomycosis"). Cases of blastomycosis are most common among individuals who work outdoors or who participate in activities such as hunting. The organism has not been isolated consistently from soil samples but there are recent reports of association of the mold with decaying vegetation.

Pathology

As with histoplasmosis, the primary site of infection by blastomycosis is the lung subsequent to inhalation of the conidia. At body temperature these convert to yeast forms which induce an inflammatory reaction with polymorphonu-

clear leukocytes and monocytes, and noncaseating granulomas result. The organism may disseminate.

The immune response has not been clearly defined in blastomycosis. As indicated, the inflammatory response involves polymorphonuclear leukocytes as well as mononuclear phagocytes. These phagocytic cells are capable of inhibiting replication of ingested organisms. In animal models, intracellular inhibition of proliferation is associated with previously induced cell-mediated immune responses. Cytokines, such as interferon and other lymphokines, have been shown to augment this cellular activity. Specific antibody can be detected, but because of difficulties in obtaining purified antigens, assays are difficult to interpret. Cross-reactivity with other fungal antigens is common.

It is assumed that the majority of acute pulmonary cases of blastomycosis are self-limited, as has been documented in small outbreaks. Individuals who seek medical attention generally have chronic disseminated disease. With a careful history, a long period of illness often can be documented. The organism can produce multisystem involvement, although skin ulcers are the most common manifestation. Bone, joint, genitourinary, and meningeal as well as chronic pulmonary involvement can occur. The pulmonary disease may resemble a chronic pneumonia but can also present as a dense mass, which is commonly misdiagnosed as carcinoma. The classic clinical triad of blastomycosis is pulmonary, skin, and bone lesions.

Diagnosis

The diagnosis of blastomycosis is established by demonstrating in tissue the characteristic budding yeast or by isolating the organism from secretions or tissue. Cytologic examination of sputum bronchial lavage fluid, pleura fluid, or pus can reveal these yeast forms and suggest the diagnosis.

Serologic tests to determine rises in specific antibody have been of only limited usefulness as noted above. Complement-fixing antibody to *B. dermatitidis* cross-reacts with other fungal antigens. Immunodiffusion has been used to detect antibody to the A antigen of *B. dermatitidis* in up to 70% of cases and appears to be the most useful serologic assay. Enzyme-linked and radioimmune assays to detect anti-*Blastomyces* antibody are under investigation and are not readily available.

Treatment

Treatment of blastomycosis is limited to those patients with disseminated disease. Intravenous amphotericin B has become the "gold standard" and is successful in 90% of the cases. Ketoconazole, however, is now clearly an alternative form of therapy which is more convenient (oral versus intravenous) and less toxic. Amphotericin B must be used for patients with central nervous system infection and for severely ill patients. A total adult dose of 2.0 gm is recommended.

SPOROTRICHOSIS

Pathology

Sporothrix schenckii produces primarily cutaneous infections in normal hosts. This organism is dimorphic, growing as a mold at room temperature and as a yeast at 37°C. The fungus is found in the soil, on plants, and on decaying vegetation. Infection occurs most commonly fol-

lowing puncture by thorns, which results in inoculation of the subcutaneous tissue. Therefore, sporotrichosis occurs most commonly in agricultural workers or gardeners.

Diagnosis

The cutaneous form of the disease begins as a red papule, which commonly ulcerates. Nodular lesions then are noted along the lymphatics draining the inoculation site. Nodal involvement and hematogenous spread of the fungus are rare. Histologic sections of the skin lesions reveal granulomas. Extracutaneous infection most commonly involves bone and joints. Pulmonary involvement is uncommon as is disease of other organs. Rarely, spread of infection to the meninges has been reported in immunocompromised patients.

Treatment

Therapy of extracutaneous disease requires amphotericin B, although the newer azoles (e.g., ketoconazole, fluconazole) are being tested as therapeutic agents. Cure of the cutaneous infection is generally accomplished by oral administration of a saturated solution of potassium iodide plus application of local heat. The mechanism of action of iodide is poorly understood.

COCCIDIOIDOMYCOSIS

Coccidioides immitis, the etiologic agent of coccidioidomycosis, is found in soil as a mold. Arthroconidia, barrel-shaped hyphae of the mold, form, break up, become airborne, and are inhaled. In pulmonary tissue they swell and develop a thick-walled structure termed a *spherule.* The spherule contains endospores which are released to form new spherules. *C. immitis* is found in the soil of the southwestern United States in a geographic area known as the Lower Sonoran life zone (Fig. 16–3). This area has high temperatures in the summer and mild winters. The spores can be blown for many miles by high winds. For example, following a storm, infection of immunocompromised patients in Sacramento, far from the classic endemic area in the lower San Joaquin Valley of California, was documented. As with histoplasmosis and blastomycosis, inhalation and pulmonary infection account for the majority of cases of coccid-

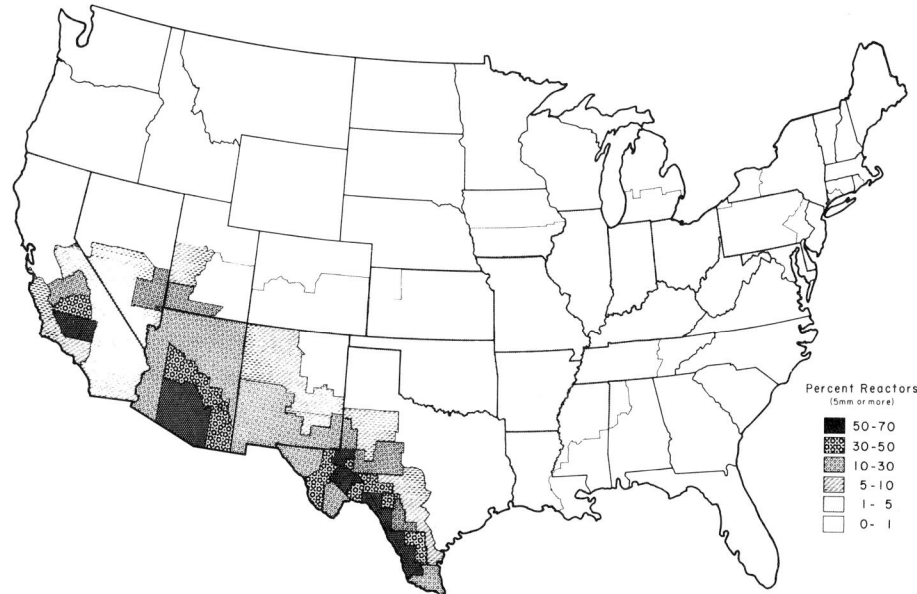

Figure 16–3. Geographic distribution of frequency of coccidioidin reactors among 48,676 young adults. Coccidioides immitis *is known to exist in areas of high incidence. A low incidence of positive reactions occurs in areas in which histoplasmosis is endemic. A low incidence of positive cutaneous reactions to coccidioidin also may be observed in certain other geographic areas, such as the Mississippi River and Ohio River regions, in which histoplasmosis is endemic, because of antigenic cross-reactivity between coccidioidin and histoplasmin skin-test reagents. (From Edwards, P. Q., and Palmer, C. E. Prevalence of sensitivity to coccidioidin, with special reference to specific and nonspecific reactions to coccidioidin and to histoplasmin.* Dis. Chest 31:*35, 1957.)*

ioidomycosis or San Joaquin fever. Person-to-person spread of these organisms does not occur except in extremely unusual circumstances.

Pathology

In tissue the spherules induce a granulomatous reaction and caseous necrosis. Yeast cells, macrophages, and neutrophils can be demonstrated at loci of infection. In the presence of ruptured spherules, neutrophils predominate but the spherules and endospores are resistant to both phagocytosis and killing by these cells. Activated macrophages are capable of killing the organisms following ingestion, and thus the lymphocyte-macrophage–mediated response is central to the control of this infection.

Diagnosis

The majority of coccidioidal infections are asymptomatic. Infected individuals who become symptomatic develop a productive cough, chest pain, and constitutional complaints of fever, night sweats, and fatigue. As with other fungal infections, erythema nodosum and erythema

multiforme occur. A chest radiograph may be normal or demonstrate pneumonia with or without pleural involvement. The hilar nodes are often enlarged. Five percent or fewer of infected normal individuals develop a cavity or a residual nodule, and very few progress to severe pneumonia or chronic pulmonary disease. Fewer than 1% of infections disseminate, this being a more common finding in men, persons of non-European ancestry, and pregnant women. Immunocompromised individuals are also vulnerable to disseminated disease. Chronic pulmonary coccidioidomycosis can resemble chronic cavitary histoplasmosis, tuberculosis, or bronchiectasis, and occasionally leads to development of a bronchopleural fistula.

Primary pulmonary infection with dissemination can lead to involvement of joints, bones, skin, and meninges. Meningitis is the most lethal complication if unrecognized or untreated. Early diagnosis is the essential element in successful treatment of this complication. Analysis of the cerebrospinal fluid (CSF) shows typical findings of low glucose, elevated protein, and a moderate mononuclear cell pleocytosis. Culture and tests for antibody in CSF, which is positive in 70% of cases, establish the diagnosis, which should be suspected in an individual with meningitis of unknown etiology who has been in an endemic area in the recent past (6–9 months).

The organism can be recovered from pus, sputum, bronchial washings, or joint fluid, but is rarely visualized in CSF or cultured from blood. Serum IgM antibody to *C. immitis* can be detected usually within 21 days of infection by precipitin or latex agglutination reactions. Complement-fixing IgG antibody develops later and persists for a longer time. Elevated serum levels of this antibody persist in disseminated disease, and serum titers continue to rise in the absence of effective treatment.

Positive delayed hypersensitivity skin-test reactions develop within 3 weeks of infection. Failure to become skin-test-positive suggests that the patient may have disseminated infection. Anergy to multiple T-cell-dependent antigens is very common in such individuals. The antigen utilized most frequently for skin testing is *coccidioidin,* which is derived from the mycelial phase. *Spherulin,* a newer skin-test reagent, is more reactive. Unlike in histoplasmosis, skin testing does not interfere with serologic assays by stimulating antibody responses.

Treatment

The basis of treatment of coccidioidomycosis is amphotericin B, which should be reserved for patients with severe primary disease or disseminated infection. Most patients require no therapy. Indications for treatment include persistent symptoms, rising complement-fixing antibody titers, and anergy. Chronic cavitary disease often requires surgical intervention. As well as requiring systemic amphotericin B, meningeal involvement may require intrathecal or intraventricular injection. As with cryptococcal meningitis, placement of a reservoir beneath the scalp connected via a cannula to the ventricular system is the most convenient way to deliver this drug to the central nervous system.

The orally administered azoles (miconazole, ketoconazole, fluconazole, and itraconazole) represent promising new therapy for this infection, except for coccidioidal meningitis. Fluconazole, however, penetrates the blood–brain barrier and may prove useful in the treatment of central nervous system infection.

CRYPTOCOCCOSIS

In contrast to the mycoses previously discussed, cryptococcosis is not associated with a specific

geographic locality. *Cryptococcus neoformans,* the causative organism, is distributed worldwide, occurs naturally in a wide variety of animal hosts, and has been isolated from soil contaminated with pigeon or other bird feces. Skin testing indicates that exposure followed by an immune response to the fungus is common.

Pathology

C. neoformans is a yeast surrounded by a polysaccharide capsule that effectively interferes with phagocytosis by neutrophils or macrophages. The organism is killed efficiently by neutrophils and macrophages that have been activated by T-cell-derived cytokines, and many patients who develop cryptococcosis have demonstrable defects in cell-mediated immunity. In addition, specific antibody is induced by infection and, in combination with complement, aids the cellular response to infection. The polysaccharide capsule and the cell wall of the fungus directly activate the alternative complement pathway.

Presumably, cryptococci are inhaled, and the lungs are the primary site of infection. The primary infection is generally asymptomatic; however, an occasional patient presents with a primary respiratory illness. This presentation has been more common in patients with AIDS than in other patient groups. Skin involvement, bone lesions, chorioretinitis, and myocarditis all have been reported to result from hematogenous dissemination of the fungus. The most common site of infection, however, is the central nervous system. Localization of the organism may be the result of the low level of complement in the CSF and the failure of the fungus to elicit cellular responses in brain tissue.

Diagnosis

Individuals predisposed to develop cryptococcal meningoencephalitis include diabetics, patients receiving corticosteroids, those with lymphoreticular malignancies, or severe immunodepletion secondary to human immunodeficiency virus (HIV) infection. However, approximately half of the diagnosed cases occur in individuals with no known defect in immunity or predisposing condition. The onset of the central nervous system infection can be acute but more commonly is subtle. In retrospect, patients may have had such symptoms as headache or change in mental status or vision for some time. The major site of infection is the meninges at the base of the brain. The cranial nerves are commonly involved, and diplopia due to involvement of the sixth cranial nerve may be the only sign of central nervous system disease. Patients may have a low-grade fever but often are afebrile. The neck is usually not stiff. Occasionally a cryptococcoma, or large granuloma in the brain, produces focal neurologic findings, but physical examination usually is not helpful except for the presence of cranial nerve abnormalities.

To establish the diagnosis requires a high degree of suspicion and a lumbar puncture. The CSF classically demonstrates low glucose and high protein concentrations plus a mononuclear cellular response, but it may be normal. Characteristically, cryptococcal organisms can be demonstrated by an India ink preparation. CSF is mixed with India ink, which is excluded by the polysaccharide capsule of the fungus, and examined microscopically. Thus, the yeast appears to be surrounded by a halo in the background of the dark ink. Cultures of CSF obtained by lumbar puncture are sometimes negative; CSF obtained from the cisterna magna by cisternal tap produces a higher yield of fungus. Meningitis is associated with antigenemia and free antigen in the CSF. Detection of cryptococcal antigen using latex beads coated with anticryptococcal antibody has been found to be a more sensitive diagnostic assay than either the India ink preparation or culture. Serum titers of free cryptococcal antigen can be quite high. False-positive reactions occur in the presence of serum antiglobulins (rheumatoid factors), and the cryptococcal antigen detection assay must be accompanied by controls to prevent misinterpretation on this basis.

Treatment

Treatment of cryptococcal infection is also based upon amphotericin B, but the addition of 5-flucytosine, 150 mg/kg/day in four divided doses, provides a synergistic antifungal effect. The combination enables a reduction of the daily dose of amphotericin B to 0.3 mg/kg/day and the completion of therapy within 6 weeks. Even this lowered dose of amphotericin can result in some renal insufficiency and accumulation of flucytosine (which is excreted by the kidneys). Excessive serum concentrations of flucytosine (>100 μg/mL) are associated with bone marrow depression. Therefore, renal function and flu-

cytosine levels, if available, should be monitored. The 6-week treatment course is reserved for patients whose CSF cultures become sterile within the first several weeks of therapy. With responses that are less satisfactory and in patients who are immunocompromised, therapy should be prolonged.

If single-drug therapy is chosen, amphotericin B, 0.4–0.6 mg/kg, is administered daily. Alternatively, up to 1.0 mg/kg can be given every other day. Flucytosine is not used alone because of the rapid development of resistance by the fungus. A newer azole, fluconazole, which can be administered orally, penetrates the blood–brain barrier and represents a useful alternative form of treatment for some cases of cryptococcal meningitis.

Relapses following therapy frequently occur and are especially common in immunocompromised patients. Patients must be monitored for at least 1 year following completion of apparently successful therapy. Cures can be effected in some difficult recurrent cases by use of local amphotericin B instilled through an Ommaya reservoir, which allows delivery of the antibiotic into a ventricle. Prolonged maintenance therapy with fluconazole may provide an especially useful means of preventing recurrences and of managing meningitis in immunocompromised patients.

CANDIDIASIS

Candida is a yeast, which reproduces by budding and has been isolated from soil, inanimate objects, the normal gastrointestinal tract, and the female genital tract. In disease states the yeast can be isolated from skin, sputum, urine, blood, and CSF. Presumably, most individuals are colonized during passage through the vagina at birth. Up to 80% of healthy individuals over 1 year of age exhibit cell-mediated delayed hypersensitivity skin-test reactions to candidal antigens. It follows then that the majority of clinically apparent candidal infections are the result of the failure or suppression of normal defense mechanisms.

Pathology

Candida species number in the hundreds, although only *C. albicans, C. guilliermondii, C. krusei, C. parapsilosis, C. tropicalis, C. pseudotropicalis, C. lusitaniae, C. rugosa,* and *C.*

glabrata (formerly *Torulopsis glabrata*) are common human pathogens. The host defenses against infection with these organisms are altered by diseases such as diabetes mellitus, infection with HIV-1 or -2, neoplasia, or therapy with antibiotics, corticosteroids, or neutropenia-inducing cytotoxic agents. The most common cause of candidal infection is the use of antibiotics which suppress the normal bacterial flora of the oropharynx, lower gastrointestinal tract, and vagina and result in proliferation of the yeast. Oropharyngeal (thrush) or vaginal overgrowth is the most common form of infection; however, fungemia may occur after lower gastrointestinal tract overgrowth of the fungus. The combination of gastrointestinal surgery or trauma and broad-spectrum antibiotic therapy is associated with an increased incidence of fungemia. Other conditions that predispose to candidemia include illicit use of intravenous drugs and parenteral hyperalimentation. The latter modality of therapy is associated commonly with prolonged use of a central venous cannula and hyperglycemia or hyperlipidemia, which provides a favorable growth medium, a means of entry, and a foreign body to enhance growth of candida.

Use of drugs which reduce the number of polymorphonuclear neutrophils or alter the function of these cells, such as corticosteroids, also favors infection with *Candida* species. Breaks in the skin due to maceration or burns predispose to colonization, tissue invasion, and fungemia in some cases. Finally, alteration in the lymphocyte-macrophage–mediated immune function leads to mucosal or skin infection with candida.

Diagnosis

The most common clinical manifestation of candidal overgrowth is oropharyngeal infection, or thrush. This is usually recognizable by creamy white patches that can be scraped from the mucosal surface, leaving raw bleeding surfaces. Potassium hydroxide smears of the scraped material can positively identify candida. Thrush can also present as atrophic lesions of the tongue and buccal membranes, and under dentures. Patients receiving antibiotics or inhaled corticosteroids, those with neoplastic disease or HIV-1 infections, and normal young infants or those with congenital T-cell defects all have an increased incidence of thrush. Since candida are part of the normal flora of the oropharynx, the isolation of candida from sputum, especially in

patients with pneumonia who are receiving antibiotics, presents a diagnostic challenge. To establish the diagnosis of candidal pneumonitis, documentation of pulmonary tissue invasion is required. This usually requires transbronchial or open lung biopsy. Other extremely common infections that occur with the use of antibiotics are candidal vaginitis and infection or colonization of the bladder in association with use of a Foley catheter. *Candida glabrata* urinary tract infection complicates diabetes mellitus, and in these patients can lead to pyelonephritis and, occasionally, to development of cortical and perinephritic abscesses.

Candidal involvement of the esophagus results in painful swallowing and the feeling of food "sticking" substernally. Candidal esophagitis occurs in neutropenic or immunodeficient patients and establishes the diagnosis of AIDS in an HIV-1 antibody–positive patient. In the neutropenic patient, involvement of the upper or lower gastrointestinal tract is well recognized as leading to fungemia and metastatic infection in bones and joints, cardiac valves, renal parenchyma, eye, and meninges, and to multiple small spleen and liver abscesses. This latter complication represents an increasingly prevalent problem in patients receiving intensive chemotherapy who have prolonged periods of neutropenia and have received antibiotic therapy for febrile illnesses.

Candidal endocarditis occurs in intravenous drug users, patients with prosthetic cardiac valves, and those with prolonged placement of central venous catheters (see Chapters 28 and 35). It represents the most common form of fungal endocarditis and presents a major problem of therapy. Surgical resection of the infected valve or other lesion is generally required for cure.

One of the more recently recognized manifestations of candidemia is endophthalmitis. Examination of the fundi reveals cotton-ball-like lesions in the choroid and retina. This may be the first indication that fungemia has occurred and can be sight-threatening. The funduscopic appearance is generally classic and establishes the diagnosis.

A very poorly understood syndrome is chronic mucocutaneous candidiasis. This term is used to describe several conditions manifested by chronic candidal infection of scalp, skin, mucous membranes, and nails that persists despite appropriate therapy. At least half of such patients are anergic in that they fail to respond to intradermal *Candida* antigen with a delayed cutaneous reaction. Exposure of thymus-derived lymphocytes to *Candida* antigen *in vitro* generally fails to result in the usual production of lymphokines or cellular proliferation in these patients (see Chapter 8). However, there are many variations of the defect. Thus, patients can be anergic but have lymphocytes that respond *in vitro* or vice versa. Some patients are anergic to multiple skin-test antigens and others have lymphocytes which fail to respond not only to *Candida* antigens but also to nonspecific mitogens. Approximately 50% of patients with this syndrome have a polyhypoendocrinopathy, most commonly hypoparathyroidism or hypoadrenalism. Chronic active hepatitis also is common in these patients.

Treatment

Management of candidal infections involves use of nonabsorbable antifungal agents, such as nystatin or clotrimazole for mucous membrane infection, nystatin ointment for infection of skin and nails, ketoconazole for refractory cases of thrush or esophagitis or urinary tract infection, and intravenous amphotericin B for patients with fungemia or visceral involvement. The role of fluconazole remains to be established in the management of severe infection. Approximately 50% of candida are susceptible to 5-flucytosine; however, when used alone, resistance develops rapidly. Therefore, use of 5-flucytosine is limited to the role of adjunct to therapy with amphotericin B.

ASPERGILLOSIS

Infection with *Aspergillus* species occurs primarily in patients with altered immunity, absent or dysfunctional polymorphonuclear neutrophils, or anatomic defects favoring growth of this fungus. The two species most commonly associated with human disease are *Aspergillus fumigatus* and *A. flavus*. *Aspergillus* species are ubiquitous and are found in decaying vegetation, but they can be isolated from room air. Most individuals have been exposed to aspergilli through inhalation of spores.

Pathology

Complement enhances the ingestion or killing of *Aspergillus* conidia by neutrophils and mono-cytes. Antibody is induced upon exposure, but whether or not the humoral response contributes to protection is unclear. In the neutropenic patient, hyphal forms of the fungus invade tissue and blood vessels. The hyphae are recognizable in histologic sections because they are wide and branching.

Diagnosis

Two common forms of human aspergillosis include sinusitis, which in the neutropenic patient is invasive but in noncompromised individuals usually is chronic; and allergic bronchopulmonary aspergillosis (ABPA), which is associated with elevated levels of specific IgG and IgE and with eosinophilia, recurrent wheezing, bronchial plugging, and ultimately bronchiectasis, but rarely with invasion of pulmonary parenchyma. The immune response to the fungus or to products produced by the organism is apparently central to the pathogenesis of ABPA. A third form of aspergillosis involves fungus balls or aspergillomas that develop in lung cavities associated with diseases such as tuberculosis, histoplasmosis, or sarcoidosis. The aspergilloma is usually asymptomatic; signs and symptoms are generally those of the underlying disease. Hemoptysis can occur but is usually not due to tissue or vascular invasion by the fungus.

The most serious form of aspergillosis is invasive disease of the lung, occurring in neutropenic patients. This illness is progressive and is associated with fever, a rapidly enlarging lesion on chest film, invasion of blood vessels, and spread to the pleura with chest pain. With involvement of the pulmonary vasculature, hemoptysis and hematogenous spread to other organs are common. However, it is uncommon to isolate the fungus from blood cultures even when it has colonized a heart valve or an intravascular prosthesis. Children with chronic granulomatous disease (see Chapter 8) also are highly susceptible to invasive aspergillosis. In this setting the disease is more indolent, but contiguous spread to pleura and vertebral bodies and hematogenous dissemination can occur.

Treatment

The treatment of invasive aspergillus is administration of amphotericin B. Surgical excision of a cardiac valve is essential for cure of endocarditis, and surgery has been successful in treating sinus infection. When massive hemoptysis occurs, surgery is required for treatment of pulmonary aspergilloma, but without hemorrhage antifungal treatment is generally all that is required. Amphotericin B is ineffective in treating a fungus ball. ABPA is treated with corticosteroids, which reduce the level of specific IgE, induce improvement in asthmatic symptoms, and possibly prevent the development of the central bronchiectasis.

MUCORMYCOSIS

Fungi of the order Mucorales are opportunistic pathogens that produce invasive sinusitis or pulmonary infection—infections referred to as mucormycoses. These organisms include *Rhizopus, Mucor,* and *Absidia* species, molds which grow ubiquitously in the environment and in tissue as hyphae. The various species of this order grow on decaying organic material, such as moldy bread. The high prevalence of these organisms in the environment results in universal exposure, but disease caused by these fungi occurs only in the presence of specific underlying host defects.

Pathology

The spores of these fungi are inhaled and colonize the nasal passages and respiratory tract. In individuals with normal immunity the spores are quickly ingested by neutrophils and alveolar macrophages.

Particularly in the presence of diabetic ketoacidosis, the spores can germinate in the sinuses, and tissue invasion by hyphae occurs, producing rhinocerebral mucormycosis. This is an extremely serious, life-threatening illness with invasion posteriorly into cerebral tissues. This clinical form of mucormycosis also occurs in patients who are neutropenic and who are also susceptible to pulmonary mucormycosis.

Diagnosis and Treatment

These ubiquitous organisms can cause cutaneous infection due to contamination of adhesive bandages. The primary manifestation is cellulitis secondary to inoculation of the fungus into skin under the adhesive. As with aspergillosis, Mucorales fungi invade blood vessels, resulting in tissue necrosis and hemorrhage. Rhinocerebral mucormycosis is recognized by the presence of

a black eschar in the nasal passages of a patient with ketoacidosis or neutropenia. There can be progression to involvement of the orbit with protrusion of the eye. Diagnosis requires a prompt biopsy demonstrating tissue invasion so that aggressive debridement and systemic therapy with amphotericin B can be instituted. In addition ketoacidosis should be corrected as rapidly as possible to eliminate this as a factor contributing to dysfunction of polymorphonuclears or macrophages. Amphotericin B is the only treatment of pulmonary infection.

SUMMARY

Fungi can produce disease in previously healthy individuals following inhalation of the infectious form of the endemic organisms such as *Histoplasma capsulatum, Blastomyces dermatitidis,* or *Coccidioides immitis.* In general, infection is asymptomatic or self-limited. In a minority of patients, chronic pulmonary disease or dissemination results. In compromised patients dissemination of these fungi and infection with fungi such as *Candida* or *Aspergillus* species or *Cryptococcus neoformans* is seen. Amphotericin B has been the therapy for serious fungal infections for many years. Recently, newer azole derivatives have been developed which offer alternative forms of treatment.

CASE HISTORY **1**

A 50-year-old professional gardener was admitted for evaluation of fever and weight loss noted over the past 6 months. In addition, he had developed a nonhealing skin ulcer on the left forearm. Physical examination revealed a moderately ill middle-aged man in no distress. His vital signs were within normal limits and, except for the ulcer, the examination did not reveal significant abnormalities. The hemoglobin was 11 gm/dL, and the white count 9000/mm³ with a normal differential. The platelets appeared to be moderately increased on smear, and the erythrocyte sedimentation rate was 60 mm/h. A chest x-ray revealed a fibronodular infiltrate in the right lower lung field. Serum was sent for antibody assay for fungal antibodies, and a punch biopsy of the ulcer showed histologic evidence of chronic inflammation with polymorphonuclear leukocytes and monocytes infiltrating the tissue. In addition, stains for

acid-fast bacilli were negative, but fungal stains revealed yeast which had broad-based budding. On the basis of the histologic features, treatment for blastomycosis was begun with amphotericin B. In association with the daily infusions of the drug, the patient complained of severe nausea, vomiting, rigors, and fever, despite pretreatment with salicylates and antiemetics. The patient was judged to be reliable, had normal liver function, and therapy was discontinued. Ketoconazole, 200 mg by mouth twice a day, was substituted for intravenous amphotericin B. The patient was discharged and followed biweekly in the infectious disease clinic. Within 2 months the ulcer was healed and a repeat chest x-ray demonstrated only residual scarring in the right lower lobe. Therapy was continued for 12 months with no alteration in liver enzymes.

CASE 1 DISCUSSION

This is a typical history for a patient with blastomycosis. The portal of entry is the respiratory system, and the fungus commonly disseminates. Skin is the most common site of metastatic infection. Amphotericin B produces both acute toxicity and, with chronic administration, anemia, hypokalemia, and renal insufficiency. Ketoconazole has been shown to be an effective alternative mode of therapy if there is no evidence of central nervous system infection. It is associated with hepatotoxicity in some patients.

CASE HISTORY 2

A 25-year-old diabetic man presented with bifrontal headache which had increased in intensity over the past 6 weeks. He had no other complaints except for double vision for the past 2 days, but he had noted glucosuria, despite continuing his usual insulin dose and diet. Physical examination recorded a temperature of 100°F rectally, pulse of 90/min, normal respirations, and a blood pressure of 120/80 mm Hg. No abnormalities except for minimal disconjugate gaze were noted. The neck was not stiff. Computed tomography of the head revealed no masses, and a lumbar puncture was performed. The fluid was clear, but there were 55 white cells/mm³ and 90% lymphocytes. The CSF glucose was 20 mg/dL (blood sugar was 350 mg/dL), and the CSF

protein 110 mg/dL. An India ink preparation was negative, but the latex agglutination assay for cryptococcal antigen was positive at a titer of 1:512. The bacterial cultures were sterile at 24 and 48 h. The fungal culture grew *Cryptococcus neoformans*.

After the result of the latex agglutination assay for cryptococcal antigen was known, therapy was initiated with amphotericin B and 5-flucytosine (5FC). The dose of amphotericin was increased to 0.3 mg/kg/day, and 5FC was administered orally at 37.5 mg/kg in four equal doses per day. Monitoring of the complete blood count, platelets, and serum creatinine was performed twice weekly. After 2 weeks of therapy, headache was gone, vision was normal, and diabetes was controlled with the usual insulin dose. Repeat CSF examination revealed the latex agglutination titer for cryptococcal antigen to be 1:64; however, the protein remained elevated and the glucose was less than 40% of the blood glucose. The hemoglobulin, platelet count, and creatinine remained within normal limits. The combined therapy was discontinued after 6 weeks. At discharge, the CSF was negative for cryptococcal antigen and the CSF chemistries were normal. The culture of CSF obtained at 2 weeks and at discharge remained negative. The patient was seen monthly as an outpatient for 3 months and then every 3 months for a year. He had no recurrence of headache or fever, and his diabetes remained under good control.

CASE 2 DISCUSSION

This is a typical presentation of cryptococcal meningitis in a diabetic patient. This indolent infection had produced headache, diplopia, and poor diabetic control. The combination of amphotericin B with 5FC allowed administration of a lower dose of the former drug, and the usual toxicities were avoided. The response was rapid and no relapse occurred during the year of follow-up.

REFERENCES

Books

Emmons, C., Binford, C., and Utz, J. *Medical Mycology.* 3rd ed. Philadelphia: Lea and Febiger, 1977.

Holmberg, K., and Meyer, R., eds. *Diagnosis and Therapy of Systemic Fungal Infection.* New York: Raven Press, 1989.

Rippon, J. W. *Medical Mycology.* 3rd ed. Philadelphia: W. B. Saunders, 1988.

Articles

Brown, J., Mucormycosis. *Semin. Respir. Med. 9:*191–175, 1987.

Drutz, D., and Catanzaro, A. Coccidioidomycosis. Parts 1 and 2. *Am. Rev. Respir. Dis. 117:*559–585, 727–771, 1978.

Edwards, J. Candida endophthalmitis. In: Bodey C. P., and Fainstein, V., eds. *Candidiasis.* New York: Raven Press, 1985: 211–225.

Fromthing, R., and Shadomy, H. An overview of macrophage-fungal interactions. *Mycopathogen 93:*77–93, 1986.

Gerson, S. L., Talbot, G. H., and Lusk, E. Invasive pulmonary aspergillosis in adult acute leukemia. *J. Clin. Oncol. 3:*1109–1115, 1985.

Glimp, R., and Bayer, A. Pulmonary aspergilloma diagnostic and therapeutic considerations. *Arch. Intern. Med. 143:*303–308, 1983.

Goodwin, R., Loyd, J., and DesPrez, R. Histoplasmosis in normal hosts. *Medicine 60:*231–266, 1981.

Klein, B. S., Vergeront, J. M., Weeks, R. J., et al. Isolation of *B. dermatitidis* in soil associated with a large outbreak of blastomycosis in Wisconsin. *N. Engl. J. Med. 314:*529–540, 1986.

Morduchowicz, G., Shmneli, D., and Shapira, Z. Rhinocerebral mucormycosis in renal transplant recipients. *Rev. Infect. Dis. 8:*441–453, 1986.

Patterson, R., Greenberger, P., Radin, B., et al. Allergic broncho-pulmonary aspergillosis: Staging as an aid to management. *Ann. Intern. Med. 96:*286–291, 1982.

Rinaldi, M. Invasive aspergillosis. *Rev. Infect. Dis. 5:*1061–1077, 1983.

Sarosi, G. A., and Davies, S. F. Blastomycosis. *Am. Rev. Respir. Dis. 120:*911–938, 1979.

Schaffner, A., Danis, C., Schaffner, T., et al. In vitro susceptibility of fungi to killing by neutrophil granulocytes discriminates between primary pathogenicity and opportunism. *J. Clin. Invest. 78:*511–524, 1986.

Thales, M., Tastakia B., Shawker, T., et al. Hepatic candidiasis in cancer patients: The evolving picture of the syndrome. *Ann. Intern. Med. 108:*88–100, 1988.

Williams, D. M., Krick, J. A., and Remington, J. Pulmonary infection in the compromised host. *Am. Rev. Respir. Dis. 114:*359–394, 1976.

Winegard, J., Merz, W., and Saral, R. *Candida tropicalis:* A major pathogen in immunocompromised patients. *Ann. Intern. Med. 91:*539–543, 1979.

V

Genitourinary Tract Infection

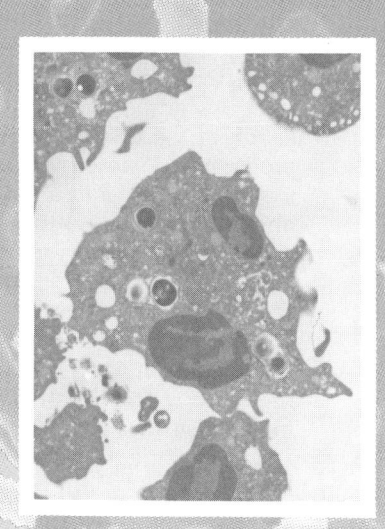

17 *ANTHONY J. SCHAEFFER, M.D.*

Urinary Tract Infections: Cystitis and Pyelonephritis

INTRODUCTION AND TERMINOLOGY

It is well established that the urine within the normal urinary tract is sterile, and consequently it appears likely that bacteria rarely colonize the mucosa lining the urinary tract. Recognition of the resistance of the normal urinary tract to infection is essential. Conversely, identification of bacteria in urine collected from the urinary tract is a probable indicator of bacterial colonization of the urinary tract mucosa and is highly predictive of subsequent infection, although the absence of associated pyuria occasionally leads observers to question this concept. Unresolved or recurrent bacteriuria must be assumed to reflect a predisposition resulting from a local or systemic abnormality.

Bacteriuria may result in a wide variety of clinical presentations. Asymptomatic bacteriuria probably reflects restriction of bacteria to the mucosal surface of the bladder or bladder urine. Asymptomatic bacteriuria is associated most frequently with a foreign body such as a urethral catheter and usually remits spontaneously once the foreign body is removed.

At the other end of the spectrum, bacteria may penetrate the deeper layers of the bladder and cause low-grade fever, frequent and urgent urination, and painful micturition, known as *dysuria*. These are the expected clinical manifestations of cystitis. In a very small proportion of patients, the bacteria in the bladder may gain access to the upper urinary tract, invade the mucosa of the renal pelvis, extend into the interstitial tissue of one or both kidneys, and cause acute pyelonephritis. Patients with acute pyelonephritis usually are very ill, with shaking chills, temperature spikes to approximately 40°C (104–105°F), paralytic ileus of a degree simulating an acute surgical abdomen, and excruciating pain in one or both flanks. The urine contains innumerable bacteria and leukocytes, a condition termed *pyuria.*

Acute pyelonephritis often follows interference with normal urine flow secondary to mechanical obstruction caused by a renal or ureteral stone, tumor, congenital abnormality, or an enlarged prostate gland. Altered urine flow also may result from neurophysiologic dysfunction with impaired ureteral contractions and imperfect emptying of the bladder (e.g., diabetic neuropathy). If the flow of urine through a ureter becomes totally obstructed, a grave emergency can arise, since the obstruction must be relieved within at least 36 h if function of the affected kidney is to be preserved.

The histopathologic changes of acute pyelonephritis are relatively well defined. There is an accumulation of inflammatory cells consisting predominantly of segmented neutrophils that encroach upon and invade the renal tubules, giving rise to "white blood cell casts." The inflammatory cells also infiltrate the interstitial tissue of the renal medulla and extend into the cortex. The glomeruli usually are not involved and often stand out conspicuously against a background of interstitial fibrosis, tubular dilatation, and degeneration. In most instances, bacteria are demonstrable in the urine or in cultures of affected renal tissue.

In chronic pyelonephritis, the identifying histopathologic changes are far less distinct and are thus difficult to define. There is a striking paucity of inflammatory cells. Obstructed and dilated tubules are often filled with hyaline material resembling colloid. Obstruction and loss of collecting ducts and inevitable fibrosis eventually result in an irregularly scarred and lobulated kidney of ever-decreasing size, which for decades was considered to be prototypic of end-stage chronic renal infection. One of the enigmas of chronic pyelonephritis is the frequent lack of any direct evidence of infection. The urine may contain neither formed elements nor bacteria and may be considered abnormal only because of persistent traces of proteinuria. Furthermore, bacteria almost invariably cannot be demonstrated in grossly abnormal areas of affected kidneys. Indeed, the absence of direct evidence supporting a role for bacteria in active chronic pyelonephritis has led several laboratories to search for noninfectious mechanisms that would account for relentless progression of the disease. Results of these studies are of considerable interest and are briefly summarized in a later section of this chapter.

From a large number of studies involving experimental animals and patients, it is clear that all the foregoing histopathologic changes, once accepted as characteristic of chronic pyelonephritis, may occur in other diseases of the kidney that do not have an infectious origin. Ischemia secondary to progressive nephrosclerosis, persistent obstruction of the urine outflow tract due to an intrarenal or extrarenal lesion, and analgesic nephropathy all may result in peritubular mononuclear cell infiltration, dilation of tubules, fibrosis, and microscopically or grossly evident scarring unaccompanied at any time by evidence of bacterial infection. The fact that a multiplicity of pathogenic mechanisms can cause renal injury indistinguishable from that of chronic pyelonephritis explains why the incidence of chronic renal infection, based on autopsy surveys, has been exaggerated over the years. This new perspective also means that chronic pyelonephritis is probably less important than formerly believed as a determinant of elevated blood pressure and such complications of pregnancy as prematurity and increased morbidity and mortality of newborns.

PREVALENCE, INCIDENCE, AND ECONOMIC IMPACT OF GENITOURINARY TRACT INFECTION

The prevalence of urinary tract infections appears to be influenced by many factors, including the age, sex, and personal habits of the patient. Asymptomatic bacteriuria is 10 times more common in male neonates than in females (incidences of 1.5% and 0.137%, respectively). Thereafter, the incidence of bacteriuria among children between the ages of 4 and 18 years is 1–2%. Noteworthy is the female-to-male ratio of 30:1, indicative of the predisposition of females to urinary tract infections. Recurrent urinary tract infections in girls usually become less frequent with onset of puberty, suggesting that hormonally induced alterations in the mucosal lining of the urogenital tract may be important. The prevalence of bacteriuria increases progressively among adult females and especially married women, presumably reflecting urethral trauma associated with sexual activity and pregnancy. It has been estimated that about 25% of women experience a urinary tract infection by their 30th year. In contrast, urinary tract infections are rare in young men. Structural or functional abnormalities in the urinary tract are much more common in men than women with recurrent bacteriuria. The approximately 10% prevalence of infection in elderly women and men is frequently associated with anatomic or physiologic changes in the urinary tract that cause urinary stasis and calculi. The incidence of urinary tract infection is even higher among hospitalized men and women, particularly those with serious illnesses. Urinary tract infections account for 30–40% of all nosocomial (i.e., hospital-acquired) infections. The majority of these episodes are associated with urinary catheterization (see Chap. 28).

The potential sequelae of bacteremia due to gram-negative microorganisms are more frequently preceded by bacteriuria than by any other infection (see Chapter 34). It has been estimated that at least 25% of the 70,000–150,000 documented bacteremic episodes each year prove to be fatal. Other potential sequelae of urinary tract infections include pyelonephritis, chronic renal disease, and stones that are formed in alkaline urine caused by urea-splitting bacteria. The estimated economic impact of urinary tract infection is great. The cost of treatment for a single urinary tract infection ranges from $100 to $175 for an outpatient. Patients who suffer a postoperative urinary tract infection spend several additional days in the hospital, and the hospital costs increase by over $1000 compared with those of closely matched controls. Clearly, urinary tract infections pose a major health problem in terms of the proportion of the population affected and the sequelae and cost of bacteriuric episodes. Fortunately, there is evidence that early detection and eradication of bacteriuria and prevention of recurrence reduce the incidence of subsequent life-threatening consequences of urinary tract infection.

MICROBE–HOST RELATIONSHIPS

Reservoir of Infection

Most urinary tract infections are caused by microorganisms that originate from the fecal flora of the lower bowel (see Chapter 2). Nearly 80% of infections occurring in nonhospitalized patients in the absence of obstruction are caused by *Escherichia coli*. Other gram-negative bacteria (e.g., *Klebsiella pneumoniae* and *Proteus* species) as well as gram-positive cocci (e.g., *Enterococcus faecalis* and *Staphylococcus epidermidis*) are also potential uropathogens. There is no convincing evidence that the numerically superior anaerobic bacteria in the intestinal microflora play a significant etiologic role in urinary tract infections.

When identification of specific strains of bacteria is possible, the same strain can be found in most instances simultaneously in the patient's urinary and intestinal tracts. It is also well established that relatively few strains account for most urinary tract infections. The basic question of whether the common strains that cause urinary tract infections are uropathogenic or whether they are simply the prevalent *E. coli* in the bowel at the time of a bacteriuric episode remains controversial.

Nosocomial urinary tract infections are caused by a wider spectrum of microorganisms, including *Pseudomonas aeruginosa*. Hospital-acquired strains are usually resistant to multiple antimicrobial drugs and probably possess virulence factors that facilitate their entry into the urinary tract and make the nosocomial urinary tract infection more difficult to treat.

Epidemiologic studies indicate that surprisingly rapid shifts occur in the intestinal microbial flora following hospitalization. Within 1–2 days, specific strains of *E. coli* demonstrable in the intestinal flora at the time of admission to the hospital begin to be replaced by increasing numbers of "hospital strains." Similar changes have been observed in the urethral meatal flora of hospitalized patients with indwelling urethral catheters. The urethral meatus appears to be an important reservoir of infection, since the density of bacteria at the urethral meatus is significantly greater in hospitalized patients who acquire catheter-associated bacteriuria than in those who remain abacteriuric.

Pathogens from extraintestinal reservoirs may also cause urinary tract infections. These include parasites (see Chapter 20) such as *Echinococcus*, primarily in the kidney; *Schistosoma haematobium* and *S. mansoni*, primarily in the bladder; protozoa such as *Trichomonas*, primarily in the urethra; yeast, usually occurring in debilitated patients treated with antibiotics (see Chapter 28); and *Mycobacterium tuberculosis*. Subcellular forms of bacteria such as protoplasts may play a role in the persistence of urinary tract infections, and their presence and importance are currently the focus of investigation.

Routes of Infection

Bacteria do not enter the urinary tract by filtration. Experiments in dogs, for example, have shown that during intravenous infusion of bacteria, the urine remains sterile. Recognized routes of entry allowing bacteria to gain access to the urinary tract include the following: (1) ascending, as in the presumed entrance of fecal bacteria into the bladder via the female urethra or into the kidney via the ureter; (2) hematogenous, as in staphylococcal infection of the renal cortex; and (3) direct extension, as in cystitis associated with an enterovesical fistula.

Ascending Infection

Most urinary tract infections are caused by bacteria from the fecal reservoir that colonize the perineum, the vaginal introitus (the area inside the labia minora at the entrance of the vaginal canal) in the female, and the urethra prior to the occurrence of bacteriuria. Sexual activity, poor toilet habits, and fecal incontinence are thought to promote retrograde spread of bacteria and contribute to the higher prevalence of infection seen in married women, among infants and children who are not toilet trained, and in elderly individuals with poor sphincter control. Both the proximity of the urethral and anal orifices and the short urethral conduit in women are believed to contribute to the strikingly higher susceptibility of women to urinary tract infection throughout most of their lives.

What scientific evidence is there to support the ascending infection theory? Stamey and his associates performed frequent cultures of the vaginal vestibule and urethra in women with recurrent bacteriuria and observed that colonization of the vaginal introitus by specific serotypes of *Escherichia coli* occurred prior to development of bacteriuria with identical serotypes. Vaginal carriage of the same strain frequently persisted between episodes of bacteriuria. These data not only show the importance of persistence of the pathogenic strain on the vaginal mucosa in the pathogenesis of recurrent urinary tract infection but also illustrate that recurrent infections caused by the same serotype may be separate events due to reentrance of bacteria into the urinary tract rather than "relapse" from a persistent renal bacterial focus. Thus, most recurrent urinary tract infections in women are probably due to persistence *outside* the urinary tract rather than relapse from a persistent focus *within* the kidney.

If vaginal colonization with uropathogenic bacteria plays a role in the pathogenesis of urinary tract infection, the vaginal mucosal flora in healthy women should differ significantly from that of patients with recurrent bacteriuria. Stamey and associates and Winberg and associates have shown that uropathogenic microorganisms rarely colonize the vaginal mucosa of women and girls. In contrast, between episodes of bacteriuria, the vaginal mucosa of women who have recurrent urinary tract infections frequently shows large numbers of these bacteria. Additional studies suggest that urethral colonization is in turn determined by the vaginal bacteria, presumably in part because the two mucosal surfaces are both derived embryologically from the urogenital sinus and are lined by squamous epithelial cells under the same hormonal control. Thus, susceptibility of the vaginal and urethral mucosa to colonization by urinary pathogens from the fecal flora clearly represents a major biologic alteration instrumental in the pathogenesis of urinary tract infections in females. There is considerably less evidence of retrograde spread of bacteria into the male urinary tract. Epidemiologic studies have demonstrated frequent colonization with *Proteus mirabilis* and other uropathogenic microorganisms of the anterior urethra in young uncircumcised boys with recurrent symptomatic bacteriuria. However, colonization of the adult male urethral mucosa with uropathogenic bacteria is infrequent in the absence of an anatomic abnormality such as a urethral stricture and rarely has been implicated as the source of recurrent bacteriuria. Most episodes of recurrent bacteriuria in men appear to be associated with bacterial prostatitis or urinary stasis caused by benign or malignant prostate growth, which impedes the natural bladder-emptying mechanism.

Very little is known about the specific events by which bacteria migrate into the bladder, colonize the mucosa, and establish infection. Normal voiding mechanisms have been shown to eliminate over 99% of experimental organisms inoculated intravesically. However, urinary obstruction severe enough to cause residual urine clearly represents a major impairment to the bladder defense mechanism and frequently is associated with bacteriuria. Adherence of bacteria to the uroepithelial mucosa (as discussed later) also appears to be an important step in the development of urinary tract infection. Adherence appears to involve a specific interaction that is influenced by bacterial and epithelial cell-surface characteristics. Endogenous surface mucopolysaccharides of the bladder wall, which in animal models appear to reduce bacterial adherence to the vesical mucosa, and hormonal and cell-mediated immune responses are probably also important urinary tract defense mechanisms. Once the bladder mucosa is infected, microorganisms begin to multiply in bladder urine. Urine can support limited bacterial growth above pH 5.5. At that pH, the stage is set for extension of the infection to the upper tract, that is, the ureter, renal pelvis, and kidney. Bacteriologic localization techniques involving ureteral catheters have shown that renal pelvic bacteriuria of either or both kidneys occurs in approximately 50% of men and women who have bladder bacteriuria and essentially normal intravenous urograms. Evidence of pyelonephritis, such as fever, chills, or flank pain, and destruction of renal tissue occurs rarely in these patients. In sharp contrast, upper tract bacteriuria in the presence of functional or anatomic obstruction of the urinary tract is frequently associated with symptoms of pyelonephritis, renal functional impairment, renal cortical scarring, and life-threatening urosepsis.

Hematogenous Infection

Bacteria as well as fungi and mycobacteria may invade the kidneys, bladder, or prostate gland by hematogenous spread from a distant focus of infection. In fact, fungal and mycobacterial infections of the urinary tract usually occur by this mechanism. Similarly, renal cortical and perirenal abscesses due to staphylococci or group A streptococci are usually secondary to bacteremia associated with extensive infection of other organ sites.

Direct Extension

Direct extension of bacteria from the enteric flora into the bladder, as in a colovesical fistula associated with diverticulitis of the colon, is an infrequent but important cause of recurrent bacteriuria. The infections are usually recurrent, caused by several different species of enteric bacteria, and accompanied by pneumaturia (air within the urinary tract).

HOST SUSCEPTIBILITY AND BACTERIAL VIRULENCE FACTORS

Clearly, contamination by fecal bacteria cannot be the sole determinant of urinary tract infec-

tions. As Chapters 2 and 3 emphasize, both host and bacterial factors must be instrumental in the pathogenesis of urinary tract infection. With regard to the host, both systemic and local factors may affect susceptibility to urinary tract infection. Any systemic abnormality decreasing host resistance (e.g., malnutrition, diabetes mellitus, or impairment of the immune system) may contribute significantly to the development and persistence of infection. Various studies discussed later also indicate that systemic changes in the adhesive characteristics of epithelial cells are associated with female susceptibility to urinary tract infections. The local factors usually considered of prime importance are urinary stasis and the presence of a calculus, essentially a foreign body. Urinary stasis may result from obstruction, such as with benign prostatic hypertrophy, external pressure, such as from a tumor, neuromuscular dysfunction, or a congenital or acquired abnormality, such as vesicoureteral reflux. It is essential to recognize that the presence of any foreign body such as an indwelling catheter or calculus can act as a nidus for microorganisms and make eradication of infection extremely difficult, if not impossible. Trauma is an additional local factor that experimentally permits development of infection and that has probable clinical significance in urinary tract infections developing after instrumentation and in the common occurrence of so-called honeymoon cystitis.

Certain species of microorganisms have a far greater capacity than others to initiate urinary tract infection, irrespective of how they gain access to this organ system. For example, *E. coli* represents a clear minority of the intestinal microflora, yet it is the most frequent and important pathogen in humans, presumably because of virulence factors that enhance its propensity to cause infection.

Bacterial Adherence

Numerous studies have demonstrated that bacteria may selectively adhere to mucosal surfaces and that the extent to which they adhere can influence the degree of colonization (see discussion in Chapter 2). Adhesion allows the microorganisms to resist being washed away by the fluids and secretions that bathe mucosal surfaces. There is now evidence to suggest that specificity is involved in the adherence process and that adhesion is an important virulence factor for a number of pathogenic bacteria.

The ability of bacteria to adhere to specific

epithelial cell surfaces is probably influenced by the characteristics both of cell types and of the secretions bathing them. Most studies of gram-negative bacteria have focused on hairlike surface proteins (pili). The first to be characterized were found in late stationary-phase cultures, commonly numbered between 100 and 400 per bacillus, and were over 7.0 nm in diameter and 1.5 μm long (type 1). They conferred on the organism the ability to adhere to a wide variety of cells, including guinea pig erythrocytes and squamous epithelial cells. Agglutination and adhesion by type 1 pili were inhibited by the monosaccharide D-mannose. These and other studies suggested that binding of some bacterial strains could occur via pili that act like lectins and presumably bind to mannose-containing receptors on the epithelial cell surface. Other types of pili, such as the P pilus of pyelonephritogenic *E. coli,* specifically agglutinate human erythrocytes, and such hemagglutination cannot be inhibited by D-mannose. The receptor sites frequently are sugar residues of glycolipids or glycoproteins in the cell membrane that may be genetically determined.

Nonspecific bacterial adhesion factors have also been identified, and they include (1) short-range attractive forces that act to overcome the repulsive forces between the negatively charged epithelial cells and bacteria, and (2) hydrophobicity. Studies have shown that adherence of nonfimbriated gonococci can be increased to the level of fimbriated organisms by chemical modification of the surface charges of the nonfimbriated bacteria. It has been suggested that fimbriae increase adherence by simply counteracting repulsive electrostatic forces. In other experiments, Smyth and associates found that *E. coli* strains possessing the K88 antigen were hydrophobic because they adsorbed to hydrophobic gels in interaction chromatography, whereas K88-negative strains did not adsorb to the gels.

Bacterial Adherence in Urinary Tract Infections

The role of bacterial adherence in urinary tract infections has been studied by *in vitro* assays in which the number of bacteria adhering to vaginal and uroepithelial cells is determined directly by light microscopy or indirectly by radiometric labeling techniques. Several groups of investigators observed that *Escherichia coli* strains isolated from urine adhere significantly better to uroepithelial and vaginal cells from women and children with recurrent urinary tract infec-

tions than to similar cells from healthy women who have never had an infection. This increased adherence in patients persisted despite temporary remission of infection, a finding that is consistent with the clinical observation that urinary tract infections in women usually recur despite spontaneous or pharmacologically induced remissions. Day-to-day variation was observed in all individuals studied, but the degree of variation was significantly greater in patients than in healthy controls. Similar results were obtained when buccal epithelial cells obtained from the same women were tested. Thus, susceptibility to recurrent urinary tract infection is associated with a widespread alteration in the surface characteristics of mucosal epithelial cells. Furthermore, the direct association between vaginal cell and buccal cell receptivity suggests that the adhesive characteristics of epithelial cells may be controlled in part by the same factor(s), such as genetic traits.

Scandinavian investigators have suggested that bacterial adhesive capacity is a factor both for selecting *E. coli* from the fecal flora that are capable of causing urinary tract infections and for determining the level of infection within the urinary tract. For example, strains of *E. coli* that cause pyelonephritis adhered better *in vitro* to uroepithelial cells from healthy women than did either strains causing cystitis or asymptomatic bacteriuria or fecal isolates from healthy individuals. The ability of the pyelonephritogenic *E. coli* strains to adhere to uroepithelial cells correlated with their ability to agglutinate human erythrocytes in the presence of mannose and their inability to agglutinate guinea pig erythrocytes. Thus, it was suspected that the uroepithelial cells and human erythrocytes had a common structural receptor site in their membrane. Subsequent studies showed that at least one of these receptors is a disaccharide that is a part of the antigenic determinants of the human P blood group system. Ninety-one percent of *E. coli* strains isolated from children with acute pyelonephritis had surface pili that reacted specifically with the P blood group–specific receptor (P pili). P-specific recognition was found in only 19% of the strains causing cystitis, 14% of the strains associated with asymptomatic bacteriuria, and 7% of fecal *E. coli* isolates from healthy controls. These studies suggest that P pili are markers of bacterial virulence in early episodes of acute pyelonephritis in children, but whether they contribute to pathogenicity in the kidney by promoting tissue invasion or by mediating adherence to vaginal cells remains to be established. Studies comparing the density of renal pelvis receptor mucosa with that of urethral or vaginal receptor density have not been reported. No similar studies have been reported in adults.

In contrast, other studies have failed to show an association between *E. coli* adherence to vaginal cells from normal women and clinical pathogenicity. Fecal strains that never caused infection in women with recurrent urinary tract infections adhered as well as strains isolated from urine. Over 90% of the fecal and urinary isolates adhered. Unfortunately, fecal isolates from healthy women were not tested. Controlled studies of the fecal isolates from healthy women and patients with urinary tract infections are needed to determine whether there is a relationship between adherence and pathogenicity. Various studies have shown a strong association between adherence and pathogenicity for vaginal isolates. *E. coli* strains that had the same O serotype as those later isolated from bladder urine adhered avidly to vaginal epithelial cells, whereas strains not associated with urinary tract infection adhered poorly or not at all. The possibility that bacteria exposed to the vaginal environment may undergo modulation that alters their ability to adhere to and multiply on the vaginal mucosa and subsequently invade the urinary tract warrants further investigation.

These data must be interpreted with consideration of the potential differences between *in vitro* assays and *in vivo* infections. Over 80% of the epithelial cells used in these assays are nonviable and may not be representative of the vaginal or uroepithelial cell lining that bacteria encounter in the patient. Furthermore, substances associated with the surfaces of transitional epithelial cells *in vivo* and Tamm-Horsfall mucoprotein, also called uromucoid, which is formed by and excreted from the ascending loop of Henle into the urine, may enhance or diminish adherence *in vivo*. *In vitro* growth conditions and duration of storage of bacteria can appreciably affect the number and type of bacterial adhesins as well as their ability to attach to epithelial cells. To avoid artifacts induced by laboratory culture techniques, investigators have assessed adherence of fresh bacteria from urine of patients with acute cystitis. The fresh isolates adhered to uroepithelial cells and expressed type 1 and/or P pili.

The bacterial population was frequently heterogeneous, in that both piliated and nonpiliated cells were seen. The ability of bacteria to express or not express (phase vary) pili and

other factors *in vivo* may enhance their virulence. For example, pili aid binding to epithelial cells, but also enhance phagocytosis. Therefore, pili would be beneficial in the initial phases of infection, and later their absence would be useful to protect against host defense mechanisms.

Bacterial K Antigens

Strains of *Escherichia coli* elaborate envelope or capsular acidic polysaccharide antigens called *K antigens*. Specific K antigens are associated with *E. coli* strains implicated in infections of many different tissues, including those of the urinary tract, particularly pyelonephritis. In several experimental studies of urinary tract infection in mice, it is quite clear that *E. coli* strains elaborating specific K antigens have a striking propensity to cause pyelonephritis, in contrast to other strains that elaborate either no K antigens or K antigens of other serotypes. These observations collectively suggest that certain K antigens endow strains of *E. coli* with enhanced pathogenic potential; that is, either they are themselves virulence factors or they serve as reliable markers for the presence of other determinants intimately associated with virulence of the specific bacterial strains.

Studies from several laboratories indicate that it is not merely the presence of certain K antigens but the quantity of K antigen synthesized by a given strain of *E. coli* that determines the degree of virulence of that strain. Production of K antigens appears to correlate with relative resistance of such microbial strains to the bactericidal activity of normal serum mediated by immunoglobulins in concert with complement.

Host Immune Response

Gram-negative microorganisms undergo dissolution when coated with specific antibody and exposed to serum complement. This antibody-complement–dependent bacteriolytic effect, observed with most normal sera, is the result of activation of the complement cascade, with C8 and C9 producing breaks in the integrity of the bacterial cell wall and membrane that lead to loss of internal contents, swift shifts in oncotic pressure, and bacterial lysis. From experimental studies in animals, deposits of bacterial antigen are known to persist in the kidney for long periods. Among infiltrating cells participating in the inflammatory response to infection are plasma cells that produce antibody specifically reactive with the bacterial antigen. An antibody response against the infecting organism occurs within the first week in patients with urinary tract infections. IgG and IgA are both synthesized by the bladder. IgM is synthesized only by kidney tissue.

Bacteria infecting the kidney are often coated by IgG as they pass down the ureter and into the bladder urine. Immunity induced by vaccination has been shown to protect against experimental hematogenous pyelonephritis in laboratory animals. The successful vaccines were boiled or formalin-killed whole bacteria and common pili. A protective effect in humans has not been demonstrated. Furthermore, the severity of infection has been shown to be unrelated to the rise in serum antibody during infection, and reinfections occur despite high serum antibody levels. Conspicuously lacking in most studies of urinary tract infection is attention to the role of cell-mediated immune responses. Delayed hypersensitivity reactions reaching peak intensity at 24 or 48 h can be demonstrated in bladder mucosa in the same manner in which one ordinarily performs a skin test. A transient, sparse T-cell infiltration occurs in the bladder, whereas in the kidney, T cells (mainly helper T cells) are persistent and abundant. Thus, it seems likely that cell-mediated immune responses play a role in host defense.

Unique Susceptibility of Renal Medullary Tissues

E. coli and other gram-negative enteric microorganisms have an extraordinary propensity for infecting renal peritubular and interstitial tissues. There is a very high solute concentration in the medulla, with values of sodium reaching 425 mmol/L and those of urea reaching 850 mmol/L. Tubular fluid osmolality ranges from less than 50 to more than 1300 mOsm/L, i.e., from approximately one sixth to four times the osmolality of plasma. Leukocytes show decreased migration and phagocytic activity in fluids of such hypo- or hypertonicity, and the high solute concentrations as well as the hypertonicity of the medullary environment lead to partial inactivation of complement. Furthermore, the production of ammonia specifically inactivates C4, a critical component in the classic complement pathway. These factors may explain why the otherwise potent antibody–complement bacteriolytic system appears relatively ineffective in the milieu of the renal medulla. Survival of gram-negative microorganisms in the form of protoplasts or spheroplasts (devoid of their rigid cell walls) has been demonstrated to occur in bladder urine with an osmolality of at least 100 mOsm/L. Presumably such defective bacteria would readily survive in the even more hypertonic milieu of the renal medulla. It has been postulated that bacteria injured by antimicrobial agents or by the host antibody–complement bacteriolytic system might survive as cell-wall-injured or cell-wall-deficient bacteria and account for the persistence and remittency of infection. However, most studies attempting to demonstrate a capacity of bacterial protoplasts to invade and infect host tissues in animals have been unsuccessful. Furthermore, most protoplasts, even though devoid of most of their cell-wall material, still possess critical antigenic constituents, including K antigens capable of binding specific antibody. Thus, the host should be able to react with and dispose of bacteria irrespective of whether they are in their conventional or a defective form.

Alternative Mechanisms of Renal Injury

Progression of pyelonephritis in the absence of bacteria in the urine or in biopsy specimens has led to the notion that mechanisms other than infection may be implicated in the production of renal damage. Experimental studies in mice and rats have revealed that microorganisms elaborating large amounts of urease, namely, strains of *Proteus mirabilis* and occasional *Klebsiella* species, may leave residual large deposits of this enzyme following their elimination from host tissues. The deposited enzyme may continue to create a high concentration of ammonia and a very high pH, approaching 8.0 to 8.5 or even greater, in extracellular fluids. Indeed, the presence of urine that contains bacteria and has a pH of 6.5 to 7.0 usually indicates infection due to *P. mirabilis* or another urea-splitting microorganism. An alkaline extracellular environment is well known to lead to cellular injury. Continued action of bacterial ureases may in this way lead to ongoing renal injury in the absence of any viable bacteria.

Mention has already been made of deposits of bacterial antigen within the kidney of animals with experimentally induced pyelonephritis. Using indirect immunofluorescence methods, some (but not all) groups of investigators have also demonstrated variable amounts of the so-called common antigen elaborated by most of the members of the family Enterobacteriaceae in human kidney biopsies or autopsy sections. Among the inflammatory cells in infected renal tissue are immunologically competent cells that actively elaborate antibodies specifically reactive with the bacterial antigenic constituents in question. In this manner, the stage could be set for renal cell injury caused by *in situ* antigen–antibody interactions (with or without complement) contributing to the injurious process.

Certain strains of *E. coli* have been found to elaborate antigenic constituents that cross-react with antigens of renal medullary cells of certain experimental animal species. Immune responses of the host to such bacterial antigens might well be expected to result in autoimmune renal damage. As yet, specific antibodies directed against kidney cells have not been found in the sera or renal tissue of animals with experimental pyelonephritis.

Pyelonephritis of rats induced by *Enterococcus faecalis* has reportedly been transferred to normal syngeneic Fisher rats by means of parabiosis. In this work, the prospective donors were infected with *E. faecalis* by a method previously established that regularly induces acute and chronic pyelonephritis in a high proportion of rats. The animals were subsequently treated with an antimicrobial regimen known to eradicate *E. faecalis* from renal tissues. The infected and treated rats were then placed in parabiotic union (cross-circulation) with normal Fisher recipients. Kidneys of the recipient parabionts were examined histologically at varying times during the 16-week period of parabiosis. Between 40% and 50% of the recipient Fisher rats developed histopathologic changes of pyelonephritis, including interstitial infiltration of mononuclear inflammatory cells, tubular and papillary distortion and degeneration, and fibrosis leading to significant scarring. Since antibodies reactive with normal rat kidney could be demonstrated in the sera of neither the donor rats nor the recipient parabionts, it was assumed that a cell-mediated immune mechanism was responsible for the pyelonephritis that was transferred.

DIAGNOSIS OF URINARY TRACT INFECTION

Patients with urinary tract infections can be asymptomatic but generally have symptoms related to the site and severity of the infection. Symptoms may include the following, alone or in combination: (1) chills, fever, flank pain, and often nausea and vomiting (usually associated with acute pyelonephritis); and (2) dysuria, frequency or urgency of urination, suprapubic pain, and hematuria (usually associated with cystitis). Patients with chronic urinary tract infection may experience the symptoms associated with acute urinary tract infection chronically or periodically or, alternatively, may be virtually asymptomatic until renal failure develops. Most patients with asymptomatic bacteriuria can recall having had urinary tract symptoms in the past, and many develop acute symptomatic infection. There is general agreement that asymptomatic bacteriuria associated with pregnancy or due to urease-producing organisms capable of forming urinary calculi should be treated. In other instances, therapy is optional and, in the presence of a foreign body such as a urethral catheter, ineffective. Physical findings such as flank mass and tenderness are characteristic of acute pyelonephritis, and prostatic or epididymal tenderness, swelling, and induration suggest acute prostatitis or epididymitis, respectively. However, the signs of urinary tract infection are usually ill defined.

Analysis and culture of the urine are essential to diagnosing urinary tract infection. Procurement of a urine sample that satisfactorily reflects the status of the bladder urine rather than urethral, vaginal, or skin contaminants is a challenging problem. Urine may be obtained by voiding, catheterization, or suprapubic aspiration. A voided urine sample should be obtained after satisfactory cleansing of the genitalia with a cotton swab and water. An antiseptic should not be utilized by women because it may contaminate the urine and produce a false-negative culture. Uncircumcised men should retract the foreskin, cleanse the glans with an antiseptic, and then remove the antiseptic with water before collection of the urine. No such preparation is necessary for circumcised men. In males, the first few milliliters of voided urine (first glass or urethral specimen) and a late midstream specimen (second glass or bladder specimen) should be obtained routinely. When prostatitis is suspected, secretions expressed by digital massage of the prostate and a subsequent few milliliters of voided urine should be collected. In women and children, the first specimen is frequently contaminated by bacteria from the vaginal or preputial mucosa. Therefore, only a late midstream urine specimen should be obtained.

Catheterization of the urinary bladder produces more accurate specimens, but occasionally this technique yields contaminated urine, and it may induce bacteriuria but rarely bacteremia and septic shock. Urine obtained by direct suprapubic percutaneous needle aspiration reflects the bacteriologic status of the urine most accurately, since contamination from urethral organisms is eliminated. This method is suited particularly to infants and other individuals who cannot void voluntarily and carries minimal risk when performed by a physician who is skilled in this technique.

Bacteriuria and pyuria, as determined by microscopic examination, are characteristic of infection. Unfortunately, these findings are nonspecific. "Clean" voided urine specimens frequently are contaminated by periurethral bacteria and white blood cells. Conversely, about 50,000 bacteria per milliliter of urine (uncentrifuged) produce 1 microorganism per high-power field microscopically. Thus, failure to identify bacteria by light microscopy never excludes a urinary tract infection. A *quantitative urine culture* is the definitive laboratory test for establishing the presence of bacteria in the urine and for diagnosing urinary tract infections. Since urine frequently can support bacterial growth and because the bladder is a reservoir usually emptying at 3–4-h intervals, urine from patients with urinary tract infection generally shows more than 100,000 colonies per milliliter. Increased fluid intake with resultant diuresis and frequent emptying of the bladder can easily reduce the number of microorganisms per milliliter to fewer than 10,000 and sometimes to 1000. The presence of antimicrobial agents in the urine or infection by fastidious microorganisms also may lower the colony count. Rarely, in patients with unilateral renal infection, complete obstruction of the ureter on the same side prevents bacteria and white blood cells from entering the bladder. Occasionally, a localized infection such as perinephric or renal abscess may be present despite a sterile urine culture.

False-positive urine cultures are not uncommon, particularly when voided urine specimens are obtained from women with heavy bacterial colonization of the vaginal mucosa. If a urine specimen that contains even a few contaminating bacteria is allowed to stand at room temperature prior to culture, bacterial multiplication soon produces high bacterial counts. For this reason, urine should be plated out on appropriate culture media within 1 h of collection or stored in a refrigerator at 4°C for no longer than 24 h before plating.

The vast majority of urinary tract infections are produced by a single microbial species. In the absence of a foreign body such as a urethral catheter, growth of two or three types of bacteria usually represents improper collection or handling of the specimen. If the clinical situation permits, a repeat urine culture should be obtained to confirm the growth of the same microorganisms before definitive antimicrobial therapy is initiated.

EVALUATION OF PATIENTS WITH BACTERIURIA

Appropriate evaluation of all patients with bacteriuria includes a complete history, physical examination, urinalysis, and urine culture. After the first infection in males and after the second or third infection in females, assessment of renal function by determination of serum creatinine and a search for congenital or acquired abnormalities by excretory urography or renal ultrasonography and cystoscopy are indicated. Excretory urography is not indicated in the vast majority of females with single or uncomplicated reinfections. Excretory urograms or sonograms are warranted, however, in high-risk patients with pyelonephritis, gross hematuria, obstruction, calculi, neurogenic bladder dysfunction, or renal damage associated with analgesic abuse or diabetes mellitus. Cystoscopy and urethral calibration should be performed on all women with recurrent infections.

All the aforementioned radiographic studies are performed to find a surgically correctable lesion. Excretory urography is the most useful study for demonstrating potential foci of bacterial persistence such as a calculus or diverticulum, causes of urinary stasis such as a ureteropelvic junction obstruction or ureterocele, and evidence of chronic pyelonephritis or tuberculosis. Ultrasonography is less specific but safer than excretory urography because intravenous contrast is not required. Renal tomograms should be obtained when recurrent infections are caused by urea-splitting microorganisms because the associated alkalinization of the urine can rapidly lead to formation of calculi, which are relatively radiolucent and easily missed on routine plain film radiographs. In children, voiding cystourethrography is a useful procedure for identifying those patients who, because of abnormalities such as urethral valves, have vesicoureteral reflux or bladder outlet obstruction or both. Most ureteral reflux secondary to urinary tract infection responds to eradication of infection; however, severe reflux requires surgical reimplantation of the ureters.

LOCALIZATION OF INFECTION SITE

Bacteriuria only confirms the presence of bacteria in bladder urine. The renal urine may be sterile. To determine the site of infection more accurately, investigators have devised various techniques and laboratory studies.

Ureteral Catheterization

This procedure is the "gold standard" for evaluating other techniques that may indicate renal involvement and is the only way to localize a unilateral renal infection accurately. In this procedure a cystoscope is introduced into the bladder, the bladder is washed with sterile irrigating solution, catheters are passed to each midureter, and urine is collected from both kidneys for culture and urinalysis. Comparison of the washed bladder and kidney specimens permits accurate determination of the site of infection.

Bladder Washout

In this procedure, a multilumen catheter is introduced into the bladder, and a baseline urine culture is obtained. The bladder is then filled for 30–45 min with a saline solution containing an aminoglycoside antibiotic, the solution is then washed out with saline, and serial urine cultures are obtained at 10-min intervals. In most cases of infection confined to the bladder, the postwashout cultures are sterile. If bacteria are detected, and especially if their numbers increase in the serial postwashout cultures, they are most likely emanating from the kidneys.

Detection of Antibody-Coated Bacteria in Urine

Detection of bacteria coated with specific immunoglobulins by indirect immunofluorescence has gained popularity as a noninvasive technique for differentiating renal from bladder infections. In most bacteriuric specimens, bacteria either are all fluorescent (antibody-coated) and thus presumably associated with pyelonephritis or are all nonfluorescent (non–antibody-coated). However, a number of specimens from patients with pyelonephritis yield equivocal results, and excretion of antibody-coated bacteria occurs in a high proportion of patients with prostatitis or hemorrhagic cystitis.

Other techniques, such as renal biopsy, determination of maximum renal concentrating ability, and serologic titers, all fail as adequate criteria for detecting chronic pyelonephritis.

MANAGEMENT OF URINARY TRACT INFECTIONS

Classification

The following classification devised by Stamey is based mainly on therapeutic and, to some extent, etiologic alternatives to management of the patient with urinary tract infection. This classification facilitates identification of high-risk and surgically curable patients and provides a rational framework for treating patients with recurrent urinary tract infection. All urinary tract infections are divided into the following three categories:

1. First infections
2. Unresolved bacteriuria
3. Recurrent bacteriuria
    a. Bacterial persistence
    b. Reinfections

First Infections

Approximately 80% of first infections are caused by *Escherichia coli,* are highly sensitive to many antimicrobial agents, and are eradicated by several days of empiric, inexpensive oral therapy. If the patient is hospitalized or has recently received oral antimicrobial agents, the bacteria may be more resistant and require specific therapy based on antimicrobial sensitivity patterns.

Unresolved Bacteriuria

Unresolved bacteriuria indicates failure to sterilize the urine despite antimicrobial therapy. Unless bacteriuria is resolved, a urinary tract infection cannot be considered cured, and an infection cannot be classified as recurrent. The most common cause of unresolved bacteriuria during treatment is the presence of organisms that were initially resistant or that became resistant to the antimicrobial agent selected to treat the infection. Approximately 10% of first infections are unresolved for this reason. During therapy, rapid reinfection with a new, resistant microorganism rarely occurs. Adjustment of therapy, based on antimicrobial sensitivity testing, usually eradicates the infection. Another cause of unresolved bacteriuria is failure to achieve an adequate concentration of an appropriate antimicrobial agent in the urine of a patient with renal failure, analgesic nephritis, or an excessive mass of bacteria (such as with a giant staghorn calculus). These patients remain bacteriuric despite taking an antimicrobial agent to which the microorganism is sensitive.

Recurrent Bacteriuria

Once bacteriuria has been resolved for several days and the antimicrobial drug stopped, the type of recurrent bacteriuria can be determined. Bacterial persistence *within* the urinary tract (e.g., in a renal calculus or in bacterial prostatitis) leads to recurrent infections with the same species. Surgery is usually required to eradicate the site of bacterial persistence and to cure the recurrent infections. Reinfections are caused by reintroduction of different bacteria from a reservoir *outside* the urinary tract. Most recurrent infections in females are reinfections and require antimicrobial prophylaxis rather than surgery. Vesicointestinal and vesicovaginal fistulae are uncommon causes of reinfection.

Acute Symptomatic Infection

Initial evaluation should determine whether a patient can be treated as an outpatient or whether hospitalization is necessary. Patients who have lower urinary tract infections, who are voiding adequately, and who are afebrile can be treated as outpatients. Patients with high fever and chills who are suspected of having bacteremia, as well as those with symptoms (e.g., colicky flank pain) or signs (e.g., palpable urinary bladder) of urinary tract obstruction, should be admitted to the hospital. Prompt evaluation by excretory urography or ultrasonography is frequently required, and drainage of obstruction (e.g., by passage of a urethral or ureteral catheter or ureterolithotomy) is mandatory. In addition to urinary tract obstruction, other major categories of increased risk of serious renal damage or poor response to therapy of urinary tract infection are (1) vesicoureteral reflux in children; (2) spinal cord injuries and other causes of neurogenic bladder; (3) pregnancy; (4) diabetes; (5) analgesic abuse; (6)

congenital anomalies that become secondarily infected; (7) urea-splitting organisms that cause struvite "infection" renal stones; and (8) renal failure. Inappropriate response to antimicrobial therapy should alert the managing physician to the possibility that one or more of these conditions are associated with an episode of bacteriuria and should lead to further diagnostic studies.

Eradication of bacteria from the urine by antimicrobial agents depends on the concentration of active antimicrobial drug in the urine. Most antimicrobial agents excreted by the kidneys are concentrated in the urine at levels 10–100 times greater than their peak serum levels. When selecting an antimicrobial agent, first consider whether an agent is capable of achieving urinary levels that exceed the minimum inhibitory concentration for the infecting bacterial strain by a great margin. In urinary tract infections, it seems to make little difference whether the mode of action of the agent is bacteriostatic or bactericidal as long as the microorganism is sensitive to the agent chosen.

Both an increase in antimicrobial-resistant strains of Enterobacteriaceae and a proliferation of *Candida albicans* in the fecal flora that accompanies even short-term, oral administration of tetracycline, ampicillin, sulfonamides, and cephalosporins are well documented. A wide range of microorganisms that are resistant to antimicrobial agents is also encountered in hospitalized patients. Antimicrobial drugs such as nitrofurantoin and trimethoprim-sulfamethoxazole, which are less likely to produce resistant microorganisms in the fecal flora, are particularly useful for antimicrobial prophylaxis in patients with increased susceptibility to recurrent urinary tract infections.

For most patients with an uncomplicated symptomatic infection, 3–5-day therapy with an inexpensive oral antimicrobial drug is effective. Several studies have advocated single-dose therapy for uncomplicated infections. Patients with evidence of systemic infection frequently require hospitalization for high-dose parenteral therapy. This is to assure the attainment of therapeutic serum levels, should coexisting bacteremia be present. Therapy is generally begun with ampicillin or a cephalosporin unless the patient acquired the infection while receiving antimicrobial agents or has some other underlying risk factor, in which case gentamicin or a third-generation cephalosporin drug is usually given. Outpatient therapy with a fluoroquinolone such as norfloxacin or ciprofloxacin may be used for less ill adult patients or when the results of bacterial antimicrobial sensitivity testing are available. Therapy is usually continued for 7–10 days. There is no convincing evidence that extension of therapy is necessary or that it improves the cure rate.

Asymptomatic Bacteriuria

Although controversy exists about whether all patients with asymptomatic bacteriuria should be treated with antimicrobial drugs, there is agreement that children, young adults, and pregnant women should be so treated. Patients with asymptomatic bacteriuria associated with indwelling catheters should generally *not* be treated with antimicrobial drugs unless they become symptomatic or the catheter is to be removed within 24 h. Although the incidence of catheter-associated bacteriuria is reduced for the first 2 or 3 days of catheterization, the incidence of infection is the same thereafter, and the infecting microorganisms are usually highly resistant to antimicrobial drugs. Any patient with bacteriuria due to a urea-splitting organism such as *Proteus mirabilis* should be treated to prevent formation of a struvite "infection stone."

Perinephric Abscess

Perinephric abscess formation is an uncommon but particularly serious problem. A mortality rate of over 50% has been reported; moreover, one third of the cases were undiagnosed before autopsy. The distinction between perinephric abscess and acute pyelonephritis is often difficult to make. Thorley, Jones, and Sanford, however, identified several distinctive features that aid differentiation between these two entities. Most patients with perinephric abscess, initially admitted with the diagnosis of acute pyelonephritis, were symptomatic and febrile for longer than 5 days. However, it should be noted that some patients with perinephric abscess have no urinary tract symptoms and are admitted to the hospital with a diagnosis of fever of unknown origin. A flank mass and an abdominal mass were noted in 27% and 35% of the patients, respectively.

The initiating event almost always is the rupture of an abscess within the renal parenchyma into the perinephric space. About two thirds of renal abscesses are believed to arise by direct extension from pyelonephritis and about one third by hematogenous spread. The etiologic bacteria reflect the pathogenesis. Perinephric abscesses associated with ascending infection are usually caused by Enterobacteriaceae; an abscess secondary to bacteremic spread is usually produced by *Staphylococcus aureus*. Occasionally, urine cultures are sterile. Any patient with presumed acute pyelonephritis who fails to improve as expected should be evaluated by ultrasound. On rare occasions, a computed tomographic scan may be required for diagnosis. The treatment of perinephric abscess is surgical drainage and antibiotics. Antimicrobial therapy alone is of little value and frequently results in death.

Recurrent Urinary Tract Infection

Recurrent urinary tract infections in men are usually associated with urinary stasis or bacterial prostatitis. Acute exacerbations of bacterial prostatitis are easy to recognize. Early symptoms include malaise, myalgia, and fever, often as high as 104°F (40°C). On rectal examination, the prostate is usually tense and exquisitely tender. Prostatic massage should be avoided to prevent bacteremia. Patients often respond dramatically to appropriate antimicrobial therapy, such as with an aminoglycoside or norfloxacin. Prostatic abscess is a rare complication that should be suspected if the prostate is fluctuant on rectal examination. Transurethral or perineal surgical drainage should be performed. A more common and more subtle sequela is chronic bacterial prostatitis. Between episodes of recurrent bacteriuria, the patients are asymptomatic, and the prostate is usually unremarkable by either rectal or cystoscopic examination. Comparison of quantitative cultures of urethral, bladder, and expressed prostatic fluid specimens is essential for documenting bacteria in the prostatic specimens that could not be accounted for by the urethral flora. Treatment is hampered by the inability of most antimicrobial drugs to diffuse from the plasma into prostatic fluid. Three-month therapy with trimethoprim-sulfamethoxazole or carbenicillin is effective in approximately 40% of patients. One-month therapy with a fluoroquinolone is effective in over 60% of patients. Those patients not cured may have prostatic calculi that act as a nidus for infection. Radical transurethral resection of the prostate and removal of prostatic calculi may be curative.

Recurrent urinary tract infections in women are due to reinfections in well over 95% of patients. Nevertheless, bacterial persistence associated with a structural or functional abnormality within the urinary tract should always be considered, particularly when the recurrent episodes are at close intervals, are caused by the same species of bacteria, or occur in young girls or elderly women. If bacterial persistence is suspected, evaluation by excretory urography, cystourography, and cystoscopy is indicated. Identification of a bacterial focus of infection is important because surgical removal and cure of recurrent bacteriuria can be accomplished in most cases.

Reinfection can be prevented by nightly low-dose antimicrobial therapy with agents such as nitrofurantoin or trimethoprim-sulfamethoxazole, usually continued for 6 months. In some patients, the infection rate can be reduced by postcoital antimicrobial prophylaxis. Antimicrobial therapy does not correct the basic underlying biologic abnormality; infections usually recur when the drug is discontinued.

Suppressive therapy should not be confused with preventive therapy. Suppressive therapy is given in the presence of bacterial persistence within the urinary tract, whereas preventive therapy is given after the urinary tract infection and focus of bacterial persistence has been eradicated. Suppressive therapy should be used when a focus of bacterial persistence such as a large calculus or bacterial prostatitis cannot be eradicated.

CASE HISTORY 1

A 58-year-old man presented with a 2-day history of malaise, dysuria, urgency, and suprapubic pressure. He had his first urinary tract infection (UTI) 12 years earlier with urinary frequency, dysuria, nocturia, and fever. Acute prostatitis was diagnosed, and he responded to a few days of sulfonamide therapy. He was well for 7 years and had another UTI that responded to a short course of sulfonamide. A third UTI occurred 1 year prior to admission, initially responding to sulfonamide, but recurring within 3 weeks of stopping the medication. Several other antimicrobial agents failed to cure the infection permanently. With each episode, symptoms were severe and quite similar to those of the first UTI. Previous urologic evaluation included excretory urography and cystoscopy demonstrating bilateral ureteral reflux with dilatation and 100 mL of residual urine.

On examination, the patient was acutely ill. His temperature was 99°F (37.2°C). The abdomen was soft, without a mass, and the bladder was not palpable. The genitalia were unremarkable. The prostate was slightly enlarged with minimal diffuse induration. Urinalysis revealed 10 white blood cells per high-power field and numerous bacilli. Urine culture was obtained and oral ampicillin, 250 mg four times per day, was started. Urine culture subsequently showed >100,000 *Escherichia coli* per milliliter. The patient became asymptomatic within 24 h. Ampicillin was continued for 30 days. Cultures of the first and second voided urine specimens yielded no bacterial growth. Cultures of both expressed prostatic secretions and postmassage urine revealed 4000 and 40 colonies of *E. coli* per milliliter, respectively. Both urine and prostate fluid *E. coli* isolates were sensitive to ampicillin (<1 μg/mL). Six months after discontinuation of therapy, another episode of dysuria, urgency, and frequency occurred. *E. coli* was again cultured in the midstream urine specimen. Sensitivities of the *E. coli* strain were ampicillin at 1 μg/mL and norfloxacin at <1 μg/mL. Norfloxacin was started at one 400-mg tablet twice daily for 30 days. He promptly became asymptomatic. Cultures of the urine and prostatic fluid showed no growth during therapy and for up to 6 months following therapy.

CASE 1 DISCUSSION

Case 1 illustrates the value of segmented culture techniques in the adult male for localizing urinary infections to the prostate. Although the infecting strain of E. coli *was sensitive to ampicillin, this drug was unable to eradicate* E. coli *from the prostate gland. The quinolone norfloxacin, however, appears to possess favorable diffusion characteristics that achieved a cure of recurrent prostatitis in this patient for up to 6 months. The presence of residual urine and bilateral ureteral reflux, however, place this patient at high risk for subsequent episodes of urinary tract infection.*

CASE HISTORY 2

A 34-year-old woman was admitted with history of recurrent left pyelonephritis characterized by fever, chills, nausea, and vomiting. She had her first UTI 12 years earlier, with one or two infections per year over the next 10 years. The patient had her first episode of pyelonephritis 1 year prior to admission. Intravenous excretory urography at that time demonstrated bilateral nephrocalcinosis. Metabolic evaluation for causes of stone disease was negative. Six months prior to admission, she had an *Escherichia coli* UTI treated with empiric antimicrobial therapy for 10 days. Follow-up cultures were not obtained. She remained asymptomatic until 3 days prior to admission, when she developed left flank pain, fever, chills, nausea, and vomiting. Examination showed an acutely ill woman with blood pressure 120/75 mm Hg; pulse 105/min; respirations 20/min; and temperature 104°F (40°C). The rest of the examination was normal except for left costovertebral angle tenderness on palpation. Laboratory studies showed a white blood count of 15,000/mm³ with a predominance of segmented neutrophils. Hemoglobin and hematocrit were normal. Urinalysis demonstrated pH of 7.0 and 30–40 leukocytes per high-power field in the centrifuged sediment. Midstream urine specimen was sent for culture.

Gentamicin, 60 mg every 8 h by intravenous infusion, was begun. Admission urine culture results reported on the second hospital day revealed *Proteus mirabilis* (100,000 colonies per milliliter), sensitive to gentamicin. The patient became afebrile, and subsequent cultures showed no growth. Repeat intravenous urogram demonstrated a 1 × 2 cm left renal pelvic calculus. Plain film tomograms showed another small calculus in the left renal pelvis. The patient underwent left extracorporeal shock wave lithotripsy. Stone analysis showed 82% struvite and 18% carbonate-apatite. The patient was treated with prophylactic antimicrobial therapy for 6 months postoperatively. Twenty-four-hour urine collections revealed idiopathic hypercalciuria, and diuretic therapy was started. Two episodes of *E. coli* lower UTI have occurred in the 3 years since discontinuation of prophylactic antibiotics. Repeat intravenous urograms demonstrated extensive bilateral nephrocalcinosis without evidence of struvite infection stones.

CASE 2 DISCUSSION

This case illustrates how subtle an early struvite infection stone can be. Clearly, the easiest way to make the diagnosis is to recognize that repeated cultures that show P. mirabilis *must be associated with an infection stone. This case also illustrates the value of plain film tomography in demonstrating the relatively radiolucent struvite stone. Despite recurrent urinary tract infections and evidence of increasing nephrocalcinosis, careful follow-up therapy has prevented recurrent formation of infection stones.*

REFERENCES

Book

Stamey, T. A. *Urinary Infections*. Baltimore: Williams & Wilkins Co., 1980.

Review Articles

Smith, H. Microbial surfaces in relation to pathogenicity. *Bacteriol. Rev. 41:*475–500, 1977.

Souney, P., and Polk, B. F. Single-dose antimicrobial therapy for urinary tract infections in women. *Rev. Infect. Dis. 4:*29–34, 1982.

Svanborg-Eden, C., and deMan, P. Bacterial virulence in urinary tract infection. *Infect. Dis. Clin. North Am. 1:*731–750, 1987.

Articles

Hacker, J., Hughes, C., Hof, H., et al. Cloned hemolysin genes from *Escherichia coli* that cause urinary tract infections determine different levels of toxicity in mice. *Infect. Immunol. 42:*57–63, 1983.

Hagberg, L., Engberg, I., Freter, R., et al. Ascending unobstructed urinary tract infection in mice caused by pyelonephritogenic *Escherichia coli* of human origin. *Infect. Immunol. 40:*273–283, 1983.

Hughes, C., Hacker, J., Roberts, A., et al. Hemolysin production as a virulence marker in symptomatic and asymptomatic urinary tract infections caused by *Escherichia coli. Infect. Immunol. 39:*546–551, 1983.

Johnson, J. R., Stamm, W. E. Diagnosis and treatment of acute urinary tract infections. *Infect. Dis. Clin. North Am. 1:*(no. 4) 773–791, 1987.

Komaroff, A. L. Urinalysis and urine culture in women with dysuria. *Ann. Intern. Med. 104:*212–218, 1986.

Korhonen, T. K., Vaisanen, V., Saxen, H., et al. P-antigen-recognizing fimbriae from human uropathic *E. coli* strains. *Infect. Immunol. 37:*286–291, 1982.

McKerrow, W., Davidson-Lamb, N., and Jones, P. F. Urinary tract infection in children. *Br. Med. J. 289:*299–303, 1984.

Mattsby-Baltzer, I., Hanson, L. A., Kaijser, B., et al. Experimental *Escherichia coli* ascending pyelonephritis in rats: Changes in bacterial properties and the immune response to surface antigens. *Infect. Immunol. 35:*634–646, 1982.

Orskov, I., Orskov, F., Birch-Andersen, A., et al. O, K, H, and fimbrial antigens in *Escherichia coli* serotypes associated with pyelonephritis and cystitis. *Scand. J. Infect. Dis. 33:*18–26, 1982.

Pitchon, H., Glassock, R., Kalmanson, G. M., et al. Experimental pyelonephritis. Effect of T-cell deficiency on the course of hematogenous enterococcal pyelonephritis in the mouse. *Am. J. Pathol. 115:*25–30, 1984.

Rene, P., Dinolfo, M., Silverblatt, F. J. Serum and urogenital antibody response to *Escherichia coli* pili in cystitis. *Infect. Immunol. 38:*542–547, 1982.

Schaeffer, J. K., Jones, J. M., Dunn, J. K. Association of in vitro *E. coli* adherence to vaginal and buccal epithelial cells with susceptibility of women to recurrent urinary tract infections. *N. Engl. J. Med. 304:*1062–1066, 1981.

Smyth, C. J. Differences in hydrophobic surface characteristics. *Infect. Immunol. 22:*462, 1978.

Stamm, W. E., Wagner, K. F., Amsel, R., et al. Causes of the acute urethral syndrome in women. *N. Engl. J. Med. 303:*409–415, 1980.

Svanborg-Eden, C., Freter, R., Hagberg, L., et al. Inhibition of experimental ascending urinary tract infection by an epithelial cell-surface receptor analogue. *Nature 298:*560–562, 1982.

Thorley, J. D., Jones, S. R., and Sanford, J. P. Perinephric abscess. *Medicine 53:*441, 1974.

Vaisanen-Rhen, V., Elo, J., Vaisanen, E., et al. P-fimbriated clones among uropathogenic *Escherichia coli* strains. *Infect. Immunol. 43:*149–155, 1984.

Winberg, J., Bollgren, I., Kallenius, G., et al. Clinical pyelonephritis and focal renal scarring. A selected review of pathogenesis, prevention and prognosis. *Pediatr. Clin. North Am. 29:*801–814, 1982.

18 *ROBERT L. MURPHY, M.D.*

Sexually Transmitted Diseases

INTRODUCTION

The clinical specialty in sexually transmitted diseases has evolved over the past two decades from a narrow field historically confined to the "classic venereal diseases" of gonorrhea, syphilis, chancroid, lymphogranuloma venereum and granuloma inguinale to a much expanded group encompassing illness produced by multiple bacteria, fungi, ectoparasites, protozoans, and viruses. This broader definition of sexually transmitted diseases essentially includes all pathogens that are capable of being transmitted human-to-human during intimate sexual activity.

Although sexually transmitted diseases are certainly not new (early references date back as far as the Old Testament), the evolution of sexually transmitted diseases as a distinct medical specialty has been fueled by three powerful social forces. First, the morbidity associated with these diseases has been more clearly elucidated. Not only do millions of patients experience acute sexually transmitted infections, but many more are diagnosed or suffer from the associated morbid complications such as infertility, pelvic inflammatory disease, ectopic pregnancy, cancer, congenital infections, and even death.

Second, it has become obvious that patients with sexually transmitted diseases differ from other patients with communicable diseases, in that most of them do not have specified notifiable diseases and many of them are completely asymptomatic. Multiple infections are common. The major issue which differentiates these patients from those with other communicable diseases is the sexual behavior that led to the disease. The intimate nature of acquiring these infections complicates or interferes with the necessary history taking and counseling, if not performed in an objective, nonjudgmental fashion. Lastly, the appearance of the human immunodeficiency virus type 1 (HIV-1) and the acquired immunodeficiency syndrome (AIDS) have jolted society and forced us to examine sexual behavior in terms that include potentially lethal complications. Not only is HIV-1 predominately a sexually transmitted infection and the cause of AIDS, but it appears to have a very significant impact on other sexually transmitted diseases, particularly syphilis, that has forced clinicians and public health authorities alike, to carefully reexamine old problems (see Chapter 26).

The trends in sexually transmitted diseases in the 1990s involve several significant changes in both the older "classic" venereal diseases as well as the more recently identified entities:

1. Although syphilis and chancroid had been declining in incidence during the early 1980s,

the latter half of the decade witnessed a disturbing rise that most likely will continue for the near future. This problem is complicated by the apparent association of these two infections with concomitant use of intravenous drugs and exposure to HIV-1.

2. Gonorrhea, although declining in incidence during the 1980s, has been associated with an increase in plasmid-mediated as well as chromosomally mediated resistance. As a result the Centers for Disease Control changed their treatment recommendations in 1989 from the inexpensive, convenient oral ampicillin/probenecid preparations to the more expensive, parenteral cephalosporin, ceftriaxone.

3. *Chlamydia trachomatis* infection is the most common of the sexually transmitted diseases in Western countries and remains an unreportable and difficult infection to confirm in most areas within the United States. Less than half of Americans aged 15–45 can even associate the name as being the cause of a sexually transmitted disease.

4. Human papillomavirus continues to be identified more and more frequently and is clearly associated with genital malignancies in both women and men.

5. HIV-1 is now behaving more like other sexually transmitted diseases as fewer homosexual and bisexual men and more heterosexual individuals contract the infection through intimate sexual activity.

ULCERATIVE GENITAL DISEASES

Syphilis

Introduction

Syphilis is an infectious disease of humans caused by the spirochete *Treponema pallidum* (Fig. 18–1). Although nonvenereal transmission may occur, most cases of syphilis are spread by sexual contact of one form or another. *T. pallidum* is indistinguishable by morphological or laboratory methods from the treponemes which cause yaws (*T. pallidum* subsp. *pertenue*) and pinta (*T. carateum*). Other multiple members of the genus *Treponema* are widely distributed in the environment and are not known to cause disease in humans. *T. pallidum* cannot be grown *in vitro*, a fact that has always severely limited the study of this organism and associated clinical syndromes. The organism can be cultivated in rabbit testes and rabbits can develop secondary

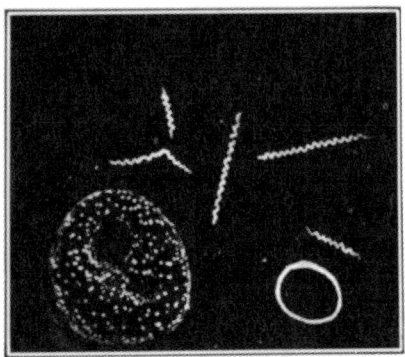

Figure 18–1. Treponema pallidum. *Diagrammatic sketch of the appearance of this spirochete under dark-field illumination, drawn to scale in comparison with a red corpuscle and a leukocyte. (From Joklik, W. K., and Smith, D. T., eds. Zinsser Microbiology, 15th ed. New York, Appleton-Century-Crofts, Publishing Division of Prentice-Hall, Inc., 1972.)*

but not tertiary lesions. All information concerning tertiary syphilis has been based on human data.

Epidemiology

Approximately one third of those who have sexual intercourse with an infected person themselves become infected. The incubation period ranges from 3 days to 3 months, averaging 3 weeks and is probably related to the inoculum size. The natural history of untreated syphilis was studied in two large clinical trials, the Oslo study of 1890–1910 and the Tuskegee study of 1932–1972; more recently the latter has been criticized as racist and unethical. In that study, initiated in rural Alabama in 1932, 412 black men with a history of untreated but inactive syphilis at the time of enrollment were followed until 1972. During that time they were not offered potentially curative therapy with penicillin and in fact actually were discouraged from such therapy. One of the original intentions of the study was to examine whether syphilis had a course different in blacks from that observed in whites. This objective was achieved, and the additional information gathered only helped to confirm the findings of the Oslo study of the latter half of the preceding century.

Following World War II the incidence of syphilis in the United States had generally declined until the late 1970s. After a brief period of increasing rates, the incidence again began to decline after 1982, primarily because of urban homosexuals and bisexuals, owing to their fear of contracting AIDS, altered their lifestyles to adopt significantly less risky sexual practices. However, this reduction in syphilis rates among homosexual and bisexual men stands in contrast to rates among urban heterosexuals, in whom the incidence has risen considerably from 1987 to 1990. Much of this increase has been associated with concomitant intravenous drug use, particularly of crack cocaine, and frequent ex-

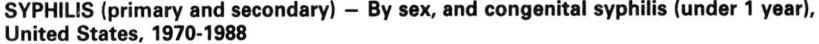

SYPHILIS (primary and secondary) — By sex, and congenital syphilis (under 1 year), United States, 1970-1988

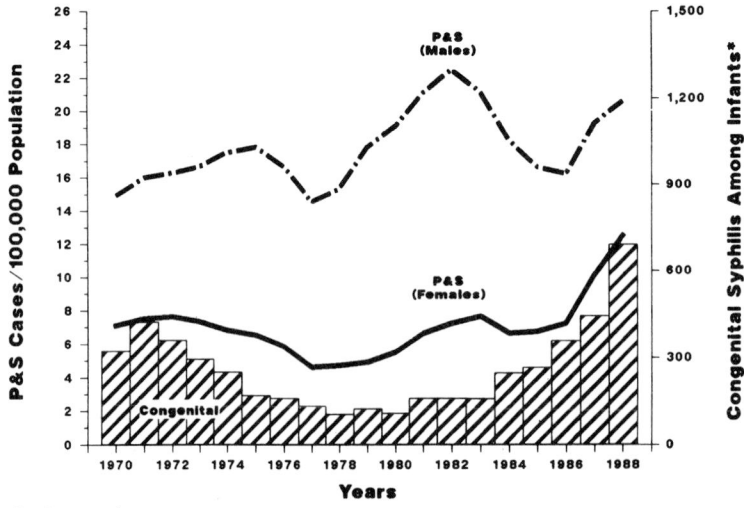

*Under 1 year of age.

*Figure 18–2. Occurrence of congenital syphilis (under 1 year) and primary and secondary (P&S) in the United States 1970–1989, by sex. *Under 1 year of age. (From Morbidity and Mortality Weekly Report, Summary of Notifiable Disease, United States 1988; MMWR, 38(54):40, 1989.)*

change of sexual services for drugs, a practice common among drug users. This rise in heterosexual infection has been followed by an alarming increase in congenital syphilis in many urban areas as shown in Figure 18–2.

Clinical Manifestations

Syphilis has three stages, which are related to the time of infection and may or may not be correlated with the appearance of cutaneous or visceral lesions.

Primary Syphilis. *Primary syphilis* is the term applied to the disease during the first 2–4 weeks following infection and is characterized by the appearance of a firm, usually nontender, cutaneous ulcer with a well-defined margin and indurated base at the site of inoculation of the spirochete. The classic ulcer is referred to as a *chancre*. Nontender, regional lymphadenopathy is common and may be unilateral or bilateral. Because atypical ulcers have become more common, any genital or oral lesion in sexually active patients should be suspected to be primary syphilis. Untreated chancres last for 10–14 days before healing spontaneously without leaving a scar.

Secondary Syphilis. The *secondary stage of syphilis* results from wide dissemination of the spirochete throughout the body and is characterized by a variety of mucocutaneous eruptions. This stage occurs 3–6 weeks following inoculation and may develop while the chancre is still present.

DERMATOLOGIC CONDITIONS. The most common manifestation of this phase is the skin rash, occurring in 75–100% of patients (Fig. 18–3). The rash is characterized as erythematous and papular and may spread to involve the entire body including the palms and soles. Rashes may be atypical and resemble folliculitis, annular lesions, or viral warts (condylomata acuminata). Essentially any clinical skin manifestations should be regarded as possibly syphilitic. Other manifestations of secondary syphilis include sore throat, fevers, hepatitis, diffuse lymphadenopathy, mucosal ulcerations, malaise, patchy alopecia, and thinning of the lateral one third of eye brows.

LATENT SYPHILIS. *Latent syphilis* is defined as that occurring in those patients with a positive serologic test for syphilis but without signs or symptoms of the disease. Latent syphilis is further defined as *early latent* if infection is thought to have been present for less than 1 year, and *late latent* if present for more than 1 year. *Early latency* is considered potentially infectious, with approximately one quarter of patients eventually developing signs of secondary syphilis, usually within the first year. Mothers giving birth during this time may deliver infants with congenital syphilis. *Late latent* syphilis is characterized by the development of immunity to relapse and acquired resistance to reinfection. Because of the difficulty in differentiating late latent from asymptomatic neurosyphilis, examination of the cerebrospinal fluid is essential to ensure that adequate therapy is prescribed.

Tertiary Syphilis. *Tertiary syphilis* is usually not clinically apparent until many years after the spontaneous clearing of the secondary stage. The lesions typical of tertiary syphilis are called *gummas*. They are granulomatous lesions that may affect skin or bones anywhere and, if left untreated, can permanently destroy the affected tissue: the cardiovascular, central nervous, or musculoskeletal system.

CARDIOVASCULAR SYPHILIS. Cardiovascular manifestations occur in up to 80% of untreated patients, although clinically apparent disease is seen in only 10% after a latent period of 15 or more years. The three major clinical cardiac conditions attributable to syphilis include thoracic aortic aneurysm formation, aortic valve incompetence, and coronary ostial stenosis.

Aortic Aneurysm. The aortic aneurysm is the most common clinical cardiac manifestation of tertiary syphilis. Over 60% of syphilitic aneurysms involve the ascending arch and 25% the transverse arch. Dissection does not occur. In general, patients are asymptomatic until the aneurysm has encroached on surrounding structures or has ruptured. Often, the earliest finding is an abnormal chest radiograph demonstrating a mediastinal mass with a typical, but nonspecific, eggshell calcification outlining the aneurysm. Surgical intervention may be required if symptoms are present.

Aortic Valve Incompetence. Aortic regurgitation occurs in 30% of patients with tertiary syphilis and appears to be due to aortic root dilation accompanied by stretching of the aortic valve, resulting in aortic valve incompetence. Patients are typically over 50 years of age and do not have other valvular conditions such as aortic stenosis. Aortic insufficiency is managed similarly to valvular disorders from other causes. Surgical repair can usually be accomplished well above the sinuses of Valsalva and appears no

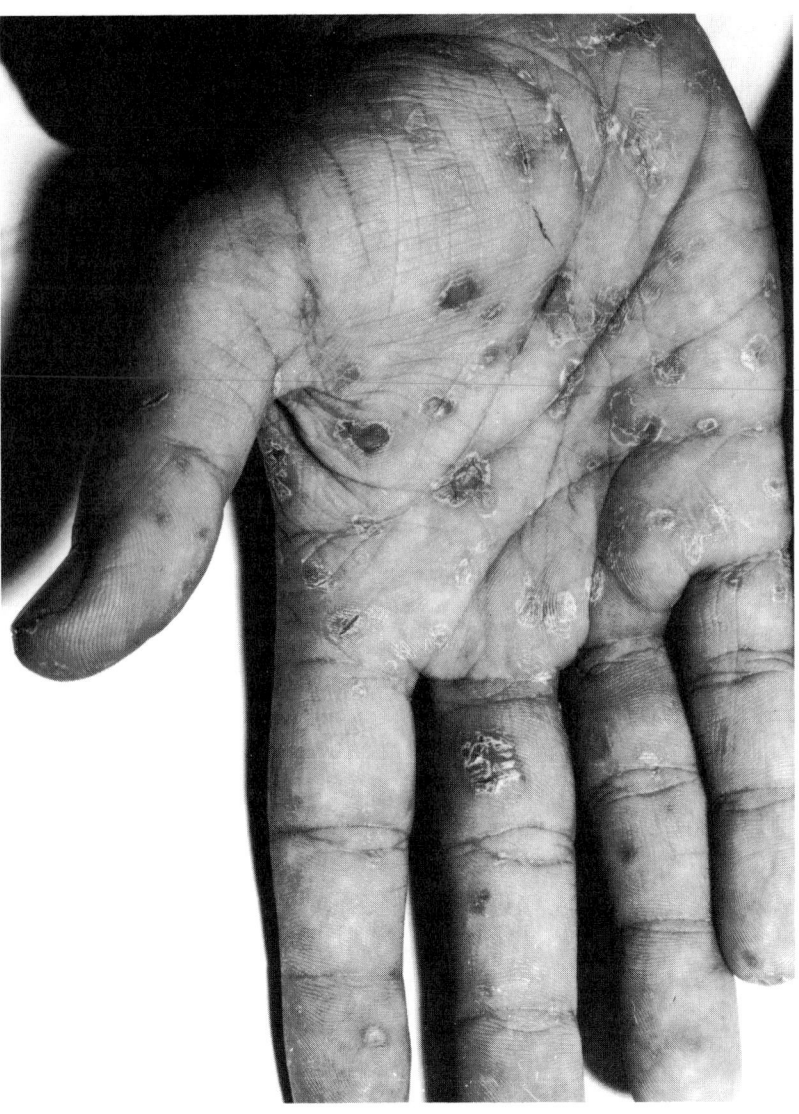

Figure 18–3. Secondary syphilis. For the past 6 weeks this 22-year-old student has had a scaling papular eruption of the palms and soles, an annular scaling plaque of the scrotum, and a mucous patch on the hard palate. Dark-field examination of the palmar lesions was negative. VDRL serologic test for syphilis was reactive. (From Shelley, W. B. Consultations in Dermatology II. Philadelphia, W. B. Saunders Co., 1974. Photo by Edward F. Gilfort.)

more technically difficult than for rheumatic valvular disease.

Coronary Ostial Stenosis. The proximal portion of the coronary arteries may also be involved in tertiary syphilis owing to an obliterative endarteritis. Symptoms are the same as for other causes of ischemic coronary artery disease. Typically, only proximal involvement is seen. Surgical management may be more difficult when the aorta is also involved because cross-clamping of severely calcified sections may be riskier and grafting of the vascular graft into the aorta more difficult.

NEUROSYPHILIS. Clinically apparent central nervous system syphilis occurs in 3–7% of untreated patients. It has become clear however, that subclinical central nervous system involvement is quite common even in the earlier stages of the disease. Recoverable spirochetes have been obtained from 15–40% of spinal fluids in early syphilis. Abnormal cerebrospinal fluid is just as likely, being noted in 13% of patients with untreated primary and 25–50% with untreated secondary syphilis. Neurosyphilis can be considered to be a form of chronic central nervous system infection capable of producing vascular and parenchymal lesions. The most common forms of neurosyphilis are the asymptomatic variety and tabes dorsalis. After these, the next most common forms are paresis and vascular neurosyphilis (Table 18–1).

Asymptomatic Neurosyphilis. Asymptomatic neurosyphilis is characterized by the absence of neurologic symptoms and the presence of cerebrospinal fluid abnormalities. It can be categorized into early (≤ 5 years) or late (≥ 5 years).

TABLE 18–1. *Relative Frequencies of Different Types of Neurosyphilis in 676 Patients Examined at Boston City Hospital 1932–1942**

	Percentage
Asymptomatic neurosyphilis	31
Tabes dorsalis	30
Paresis	12
Vascular neurosyphilis	10
Syphilitic meningitis	6
Taboparesis	3
Optic neuritis	3
Meningomyelitis (and other spinal cord involvement)	3
Deafness	1
Other	1

*From Merritt, H. H., et al. Neurosyphilis. New York: Oxford, 1946.

The frequency of asymptomatic neurosyphilis peaks at 12–18 months after initial infection and decreases with time. Progression to clinical neurosyphilis in the untreated patient has been observed in 23–87% of patients.

Blood serology for syphilis is almost always positive in asymptomatic neurosyphilis. The cerebrospinal fluid is characterized by a modest (<100 cells/mm³) lymphocytosis, a normal or slightly elevated protein, and a positive nontreponemal test.

Meningeal and Cerebrovascular Syphilis. Meningeal syphilis is quite rare and may mimic aseptic meningitis. The incubation period is usually less than 1 year and patients are generally younger. The cerebrospinal fluid nontreponemal tests are usually positive. Treatment with penicillin results in a prompt clinical response.

Cerebrovascular syphilis may involve any area of the central nervous system including the meninges as a result of infarction secondary to syphilitic endarteritis. Most cases occur in the younger adult population, 5–12 years after the initial infection. Common clinical manifestations include hemiparesis or hemiplegia, psychologic or behavioral changes, aphasia, and seizures. The diagnosis should be suspected in a young adult presenting with a stroke syndrome without obvious risk factors, with a positive syphilis serologic test and abnormal cerebrospinal fluid exam, as is seen with asymptomatic infection.

Paresis refers to a meningoencephalitis associated with direct invasion of the cerebrum by *T. pallidum*. The clinical presentation is that of chronic, progressive combined psychiatric and neurologic deterioration. The most common neurologic findings are pupillary abnormalities such as Argyll Robertson pupil, slurred speech, expressionless face, tremors, and deep-tendon reflex dysfunction. The blood nontreponemal

serology is usually positive. In the instances where it may be negative, there is often a history of treated syphilis. Cerebrospinal fluid abnormalities are found in nearly all instances. The spinal fluid nontreponemal test is very specific for neurosyphilis, but is less than 100% sensitive. In contrast, the spinal fluid fluorescent treponemal antibody (FTA) test may be more sensitive but false-positive reactions occur in 0.5–4.5% of cases.

Tabes Dorsalis. Tabes dorsalis had accounted for about one third of all cases of neurosyphilis in the prepenicillin era but now is quite rare in the United States. A clinical diagnosis is likely in a patient with lightening pains, ataxia, absent deep-tendon reflexes, Argyll Robertson pupil, and a positive Romberg sign. Cerebrospinal fluid abnormalities are common, but blood and spinal fluid serologies may revert to normal in treated and inactive cases with continuing symptoms.

CONGENITAL SYPHILIS. Congenital syphilis had been described in early medical writings as the "the French disease." The risks of developing congenital syphilis were well described in the Oslo study, in which it was shown that 26% of babies born to infected mothers were disease-free or recovered spontaneously, 25% remained seropositive but clinically unaffected, and 49% were symptomatic. Typical symptoms include hepatomegaly, splenomegaly, anemia, jaundice, rash, petechiae, "snuffles," abnormal bone radiograph, lymphadenopathy, and pseudoparalysis.

Diagnosis of congenital syphilis can be categorized as definite, compatible, or unlikely. A definite diagnosis requires confirmation of *T. pallidum* by darkfield examination, immunofluorescence, or histologic examination. A compatible diagnosis can be made by serologic testing although sensitivity and specificity issues abound because of the passive transplacental transfer of maternal antibody by the mother to the baby. Serial observation of the child's clinical condition, serologic and cerebrospinal fluid status, and bone findings are often the most effective ways to identify congenital syphilis.

The typical mother who delivers a baby with congenital syphilis is likely to have a history of other sexually transmitted diseases as well. The leading factor, however, appears to be lack of prenatal care, which has been associated with being single, young, poor, from a rural area, and with a lack of formal education. Total cases of congenital syphilis in U.S. children less than 1 year of age dropped below 200 cases in 1980,

TABLE 18–2. *Syphilis—Treatment Guidelines*

Early Syphilis

Primary and Secondary Syphilis and Early Latent Syphilis of Less Than 1 Year's Duration

Recommended Regimen

Benzathine penicillin G, 2.4 million U IM, in one dose.

Alternative Regimen for Penicillin-Allergic Patients (Nonpregnant)

Doxycycline, 100 mg orally two times a day for 2 weeks

or

Tetracycline, 500 mg orally four times a day for 2 weeks.

Doxycycline and **tetracycline** are equivalent therapies. There is less clinical experience with doxycycline, but compliance is better. In patients who cannot tolerate doxycycline or tetracycline, three options exist:

1. If follow-up or compliance cannot be ensured, the patient should have skin testing for penicillin allergy and be desensitized if necessary (see Appendix).
2. If compliance and follow-up are ensured, **erythromycin,** 500 mg orally four times a day for 2 weeks, can be used.
3. Patients who are allergic to penicillin may also be allergic to cephalosporins; therefore, caution must be used in treating a penicilin-allergic patient with a cephalosporin. However, preliminary data suggest that **ceftriaxone,** 250 mg IM once a day for 10 days, is curative—but careful follow-up is mandatory.

Follow-Up

Treatment failures can occur with any regimen. Patients should be reexamined clinically and serologically at 3 months and 6 months. If nontreponemal antibody titers have not declined fourfold by 3 months with primary or secondary syphilis, or by 6 months in early latent syphilis, or if signs or symptoms persist and reinfection has been ruled out, patients should have a CSF examination and be retreated appropriately.

HIV-infected patients should have more frequent follow-up, including serologic testing at 1, 2, 3, 6, 9, and 12 months. In addition to the above guidelines for 3 and 6 months, any patient with a fourfold increase in titer at any time should have a CSF examination and be treated with the neurosyphilis regimen unless reinfection can be established as the cause of the increased titer.

Lumbar Puncture in Early Syphilis

CSF abnormalities are common in adults with early syphilis. Despite the frequency of these CSF findings, very few patients develop neurosyphilis when the treatment regimens described above are used. Therefore, unless clinical signs and symptoms of neurologic involvement exist, such as optic, auditory, cranial nerve, or meningeal symptoms, lumbar puncture is not recommended for routine evaluation of early syphilis. This recommendation also applies to immunocompromised and HIV-infected patients, since no clear data currently show that these patients need increased therapy.

HIV Testing

All syphilis patients should be counseled concerning the risks of HIV and be encouraged to be tested for HIV.

Late Latent Syphilis of More Than 1 Year's Duration, Gummas, and Cardiovascular Syphilis

All patients should have a thorough clinical examination. Ideally, all patients with syphilis of more than 1 year's duration should have a CSF examination; however, performance of lumbar puncture can be individualized. In older asymptomatic individuals, the yield of lumbar puncture is likely to be low; however, CSF examination is clearly indicated in the following specific situations:

1. Neurologic signs or symptoms
2. Treatment failure
3. Serum nontreponemal antibody titer ⩾1:32
4. Other evidence of active syphilis (aortitis, gumma, iritis)
5. Nonpenicillin therapy planned
6. Positive HIV antibody test

Note: If CSF examination is performed and reveals findings consistent with neurosyphilis, patients should be treated for neurosyphilis (see next section).

Some experts also treat cardiovascular syphilis patients with a neurosyphilis regimen.

Recommended Regimen

Benzathine penicillin G, 7.2 million U total, administered as three doses of 2.4 million U IM.

Alternative Regimen for Penicillin-Allergic Patients (Nonpregnant)

Doxycycline, 100 mg orally twice a day for 4 weeks

or

Tetracycline, 500 mg orally four times a day for 4 weeks.

If patients are allergic to penicillin, alternative drugs should be used only after CSF examination has excluded neurosyphilis. Penicillin allergy is best determined by careful history taking, but skin testing may be used if the major and minor determinants are available (see Appendix).

TABLE 18–2. *Syphilis—Treatment Guidelines* Continued

Follow-Up

Quantitative nontreponemal serologic tests should be repeated at 6 months and 12 months. If titers increase fourfold, if an initially high titer (≥1:32) fails to decrease, or if the patient has signs or symptoms attributable to syphilis, the patient should be evaluated for neurosyphilis and retreated appropriately.

HIV Testing

All syphilis patients should be counseled concerning the risks of HIV and be encouraged to be tested for HIV antibody.

Neurosyphilis

Central nervous system disease may occur during any stage of syphilis. Clinical evidence of neurologic involvement (e.g., optic and auditory symptoms, cranial nerve palsies) warrants CSF examination.

Recommended Regimen

Aqueous crystalline penicillin G, 12–24 million U administered 2–4 million U every 4 h IV, for 10–14 days.

Alternative Regimen (if Outpatient Compliance Can Be Ensured)

Procaine penicillin, 2.4 million U IM daily

and

Probenecid, 500 mg orally four times a day for 10–14 days.

Many authorities recommend addition of **benzathine penicillin G,** 2.4 million U IM weekly for three doses after completion of these neurosyphilis treatment regimens. No systematically collected data have evaluated therapeutic alternatives to penicillin. Patients who cannot tolerate penicillin should be skin tested and desensitized, if necessary, or treated in consultation with an expert.

Follow-Up

If an initial CSF pleocytosis was present, CSF examination should be repeated every 6 months until the cell count is normal, If it has not decreased at 6 months, or is not normal by 2 years, retreatment should be strongly considered.

HIV Testing

All syphilis patients should be counseled concerning the risks of HIV and be encouraged to be tested for HIV antibody.

Syphilis in Pregnancy

Screening

Pregnant women should be screened early in pregnancy. Seropositive pregnant women should be considered infected unless treatment history and sequential serologic antibody titers are showing an appropriate response. In populations in which prenatal care utilization is not optimal, patients should be screened, and if necessary, treatment provided at the time pregnancy is detected. In areas of high syphilis prevalence, or in patients at high risk, screening should be repeated in the third trimester and again at delivery.

Treatment

Patients should be treated with the penicillin regimen appropriate for the woman's stage of syphilis. Tetracycline and doxycycline are contraindicated in pregnancy. Erythromycin should not be used because of the high risk of failure to cure infection in the fetus. Pregnant women with histories of penicillin allergy should first be carefully questioned regarding the validity of the history. If necessary, they should then be skin tested and either treated with penicillin or referred for desensitization (see Appendix). Women who are treated in the second half of pregnancy are at risk for premature labor and/or fetal distress if their treatment precipitates a Jarisch-Herxheimer reaction. They should be advised to seek medical attention following treatment if they notice any change in fetal movements or have any contractions. Stillbirth is a rare complication of treatment; however, since therapy is necessary to prevent further fetal damage, this concern should not delay treatment.

Follow-Up

Monthly follow-up is mandatory so that retreatment can be given if needed. The antibody response should be the same as for nonpregnant patients.

HIV Testing

All syphilis patients should be counseled concerning the risks of HIV and be encouraged to be tested for HIV antibody.

Table continued on following page

TABLE 18–2. *Syphilis—Treatment Guidelines* Continued

Congenital Syphilis

Who Should Be Evaluated

Infants should be evaluated if they were born to seropositive (nontreponemal test confirmed by treponemal test) women who:

Have untreated syphilis; *or*
Were treated for syphilis less than 1 month before delivery; *or*
Were treated for syphilis during pregnancy with a nonpenicillin regimen; *or*
Did not have the expected decrease in nontreponemal antibody titers after treatment for syphilis; *or*
Do not have a well-documented history of treatment for syphilis; *or*
Were treated but had insufficient serologic follow-up during pregnancy to assess disease activity.

An infant should not be released from the hospital until the serologic status of its mother is known.

Evaluation of the Infant

The clinical and laboratory evaluation of infants born to women described above should include:

A thorough physical examination for evidence of congenital syphilis
Nontreponemal antibody titer
CSF analysis for cells, protein, and VDRL
Long bone x-rays
Other tests as clinically indicated (e.g., chest x-ray)
If possible, FTA-ABS on the purified 19S-IgM fraction of serum (e.g. separation by Isolab columns)

Therapy Decisions

Infants should be treated if they have:

Any evidence of active disease (physical examination or x-ray); *or*
A reactive CSF-VDRL; *or*
An abnormal CSF finding (white blood cell count >5/mm^3 or protein >50 mg/dL)* regardless of CSF serology; *or*
Quantitative nontreponemal serologic titers that are fourfold (or greater) higher than their mother's; *or*
Positive FTA-ABS-19S-IgM antibody, if performed.

Even if the evaluation is normal, infants should be treated if their mothers have untreated syphilis or evidence of relapse or reinfection after treatment. Infants, who meet the criteria listed in "Who Should Be Evaluated" but are not fully evaluated, should be assumed to be infected and treated.

Treatment

Treatment should consist of: 100,000–150,000 U/kg of **aqueous crystalline penicillin G** daily (administered as 50,000 U/kg IV every 8–12 h) *or* 50,000 U/kg of **procaine penicillin** daily (administered once IM) for 10–14 days. If more than 1 day of therapy is missed, the entire course should be restarted. All symptomatic neonates should also have an ophthalmologic examination.

Infants who meet the criteria listed in "Who Should Be Evaluated," but who after evaluation do not meet the criteria lised in "Therapy Decisions," are at **low** risk for congenital syphilis. If their mothers were treated with **erythromycin** during pregnancy, or if close follow-up cannot be assured, they should be treated with **benzathine penicillin G,** 50,000 U/kg IM as a one-time dose.

Follow-Up

Seropositive untreated infants must be closely followed at 1, 2, 3, 6, and 12 months of age. In the absence of infection, nontreponemal antibody titers should be decreasing by 3 months of age and should have disappeared by 6 months of age. If these titers are found to be stable or increasing, the child should be reevaluated and fully treated. Additionally, in the absence of infection, treponemal antibodies may be present up to 1 year. If they are present beyond 1 year, the infant should be treated for congenital syphilis.

Treated infants should also be observed to ensure decreasing nontreponemal antibody titers; these should have disappeared by 6 months of age. Treponemal tests should not be used, since they may remain positive despite effective therapy if the child was infected. Infants with documented CSF pleocytosis should be reexamined every 6 months or until the cell count is normal. If the cell count is still abnormal after 2 years, or if a downward trend is not present at each examination, the infant should be retreated. The CSF-VDRL should also be checked at 6 months; if it is still reactive, the infant should be retreated.

Therapy of Older Infants and Children

After the newborn period, children discovered to have syphilis should have a CSF examination to rule out congenital syphilis. Any child who is thought to have congenital syphilis or who has neurologic involvement should be treated with 200,000–300,000 U/kg/day of **aqueous crystalline penicillin G** (administered as 50,000 U/kg every 4–6 h) for 10–14 days. Older children with definite acquired syphilis and a normal neurologic examination may be treated with **benzathine penicillin G,** 50,000 U/kg IM, up to the adult dose of 2.4 million U. Children with a history of penicillin allergy should be skin tested and, if necessary, desensitized. (see Appendix). Follow-up should be performed as described previously.

---

*In the immediate newborn period, interpretation of these tests may be difficult; normal values vary with gestational age and are higher in preterm infants. Other causes of elevated values should also be considered. However, when an infant is being evaluated for congenital syphilis, the infant should be treated *if test results cannot exclude infection.*

TABLE 18–2. *Syphilis—Treatment Guidelines* Continued

HIV Testing

In cases of congenital syphilis, the mother should be counseled concerning the risks of HIV and be encouraged to be tested for HIV; if her test is positive, the infant should be referred for follow-up.

Syphilis in HIV-Infected Patients

Diagnosis

All sexually active patients with syphilis should be encouraged to be counseled and tested for HIV because of the frequency of association of the two diseases and the implications for clinical assessment and management.

Neurosyphilis should be considered in the differential diagnosis of neurologic disease in HIV-infected persons.

When clinical findings suggest that syphilis is present but serologic tests are negative or confusing, alternative tests, such as biopsy of lesions, darkfield examination, and direct fluorescent antibody staining of lesion material, should be used.

In cases of congenital syphilis, the mother should be encouraged to be counseled and tested for HIV; if her test is positive, the infant should be referred for follow-up.

Treatment and Follow-Up

Penicillin regimens should be used whenever possible for all stages of syphilis in HIV-infected patients. Skin testing to confirm penicillin allergy may be used if minor and major determinants are available (see Appendix). However, data on its use in HIV-infected individuals are inadequate. Patients may be desensitized and treated with penicillin.

No change in therapy for early syphilis for HIV-coinfected patients is recommended. However, some authorities advise CSF examination and/or treatment with a regimen appropriate for neurosyphilis for all patients coinfected with syphilis and HIV, regardless of the clinical stage of syphilis. In all cases, careful follow-up is necessary to ensure adequacy of treatment.

HIV-infected patients treated for syphilis should be followed clinically and with quantitative nontreponemal serologic tests (VDRL, RPR) at 1, 2, 3, 6, 9, and 12 months after treatment. Patients with early syphilis whose titers increase or fail to decrease (see section on "Follow-Up, Early Syphilis") fourfold within 6 months should undergo CSF examinaion and be retreated. In such patients, CSF abnormalities could be due to HIV-related infection, neurosyphilis, or both. STD clinics and other providers of STD treatment should ensure adequate follow-up.

Appendix

Management of Patients with Histories of Penicillin Allergy

Currently, no proven alternative therapies to penicillin are available for treating patients with neurosyphilis, congenital syphilis or syphilis in pregnancy. Therefore, skin testing—with desensitization, if indicated—is recommended for these patients.

Skin Testing

Skin testing is a rapid, safe, and accurate procedure (see below). It is also productive; 90% of patients with histories of "penicillin allergy" have negative skin tests and can be given penicillin safely. The other 10% with positive skin tests have an increased risk of being truly penicillin-allergic and should undergo desensitization. Clinics involved in STD management should be equipped and prepared to do skin testing or should establish referral mechanisms to have skin tests performed.

Skin testing is quick; four determinants, along with positive and negative controls, can be placed and read in an hour. Skin testing is also safe, if properly performed. Patients who have had a severe, life-threatening reaction in the past year should be tested in a controlled environment, such as a hospital setting, and the determinant antigens diluted 100-fold. Other patients can be skin tested safely in a physician-staffed clinic. Patients with a history of penicillin allergy but with no reaction to penicillin skin tests, who are not on antihistamines, and who had a positive histamine control on skin testing, should be given **penicillin**, 250 mg orally, and observed for 1 h. Patients who tolerate this dose well may be treated with penicillin as needed.

Adapted from Centers for Disease Control. Sexually transmitted diseases treatment guidelines. *MMWR.* 38(S-8):6–12, 1989.

but this number had risen to over 600 by 1989. The reason for this increase is most likely related to the increase in syphilis seen in men and women who are also using intravenous drugs.

Syphilis and Human Immunodeficiency Virus Infection

The interaction between syphilis and HIV infection is not clearly defined; however, three important questions deserve attention: (1) Does syphilis, or other genital ulcer disease, enhance the risk of HIV transmission or acquisition? (2) Does coexistent HIV infection influence the natural clinical history of syphilis or its blood or cerebrospinal fluid manifestations? and (3) Are the current recommended therapies for syphilis adequate when HIV is also present?

Studies in Africa, as well as in North America, have demonstrated a strong association between evidence of past syphilis and risk of HIV infection. For men attending clinics treating sexually transmitted disease, other factors independently associated with HIV infection have included prostitute contact, foreign travel, prior *Herpes simplex* virus infection, history of genital ulcer disease and intravenous drug abuse.

The mechanism for the observed risk of HIV infection and prior genital ulcer disease is unknown. Disruption of the epithelial or mucosal surfaces may provide a more efficient portal of entry. Also, as Hook has postulated, the base of the syphilitic ulcerations are likely to contain large numbers of activated lymphocytes and macrophages, the potential target for HIV; thus, syphilis may enhance transmission as well as acquisition of HIV. Based on retrospective observations and theoretical concerns, the Centers for Disease Control has recommended serologic testing for HIV in all patients with newly diagnosed syphilis.

A large number of case reports have suggested that the clinical spectrum of syphilis and the rapidity of disease progression may be adversely modified by concomitant HIV infection. The frequency of such unusual clinical responses remains unknown. The reasons why the clinical course may be modified also remain obscure but most likely are due to the depressed cellular immunity and altered humoral immunity ascribed to HIV infection.

There have also been reports of increased treatment failure rates in HIV-infected patients with syphilis who have received the currently recommended therapy using benzathine penicillin. Although *T. pallidum* is quite sensitive to penicillin, the cerebrospinal fluid levels achieved after intramuscular benzathine penicillin administration do not reach spirocheticidal levels. This therapy may be enough to control syphilis in the otherwise normal host but not in those with the immunologic deficiencies associated with HIV infection. The Centers for Disease Control has recommended that serologic follow-up be performed monthly for at least 6 months after treatment in HIV-infected patients.

Treatment

The treatment of syphilis varies according to the stage of disease and allergic history of the patient. Table 18–2 outlines the current Centers for Disease Control recommendations.

Diagnosis

Microscopy. Since *T. pallidum* is very difficult to culture *in vitro,* the diagnosis of syphilis in the primary stage consists of demonstrating motile treponemes from the chancre. Treponemes can usually be found in a chancre from the early to late stages, but they are very sensitive to penicillin and cannot be found within 4 h after the drug is given. Demonstration of treponemes by darkfield examination may be the only way to establish the diagnosis in the initial stage of the disease, because diagnostic serologic changes usually do not begin to appear until 14–21 days after contact. Darkfield examinations are simple and easily done. The surface of the chancre is cleaned with a saline-moistened swab to clear away exudate and excessive bacterial contamination. Another swab is then applied to the chancre to irritate the surface and cause an outpouring of serous fluid containing treponemes. Using saline, serous fluid is then removed from the surface of the chancre by a small pipette or cover slip and placed on a microscope slide, protected by the coverslip, and examined with darkfield illumination. *T. pallidum* has an unforgettably rapid and purposeful corkscrewlike motion across the microscopic field. Darkfield preparations for motile treponemes should be examined within 10–15 min, as the treponemes are susceptible to a decrease in temperature and soon stop moving. The characteristic shape of the microorganism in darkfield illumination is not apparent when it is motionless. Motile treponemes can also be found in both skin lesions and enlarged lymph nodes in patients with secondary syphilis but not in the same numbers as in the primary chancre. Both primary and secondary lesions are contagious. Nonpathogenic treponemes are commonly isolated from the oral cavity and cannot be distinguished morphologically from *T. pallidum.*

Serology. Unfortunately, the cutaneous manifestations of primary and secondary syphilis are inconsistent. In many patients, the first symptom of the disease is the appearance of the tertiary form. Since the lesions of tertiary syphilis may be irreversible, it becomes increasingly important to recognize the disease and to give adequate therapy before tertiary lesions appear. This can be done with a high level of accuracy by using a variety of serologic tests for syphilis (STS).

In the discussion of any serologic test for syphilis, two terms, sensitivity and specificity, should be defined and the distinction between the two kept clearly in mind. *Sensitivity* is the ability of the test to be reactive in the presence of all cases of syphilis in all stages. As long as the test can detect all syphilis, it need not be expected to differentiate between syphilis and similar but nonsyphilitic diseases also reacting with the test. Highly sensitive tests are useful for preliminary screening. *Specificity* refers to the ability of a test to reject all cases that are not syphilis. This test may be applied to reactive cases selected by the high-sensitivity (screening) test and can discard all cases reactive on some basis other than syphilis. Until such time as a single test is both sensitive and selective, there is clearly a need for both kinds of tests. The ideal approach to the serologic diagnosis of syphilis is to use a highly sensitive test for screening purposes and a highly specific test for discrimination between syphilis and nonsyphilis among those reactive on the screening test.

Serologic tests for syphilis are divided into two broad categories: (1) tests to detect the presence of antibody to a cardiolipin antigen, the so-called Wassermann antibody; and (2) tests to detect antibody against treponemal antigens. In general, tests reactive for Wassermann antibody (see below) are useful as screening tests, and those based on detecting treponemal antibody are of help in establishing a specific diagnosis of syphilis.

WASSERMANN'S TEST. In 1906, one year after the treponeme causing syphilis had been identified, August Paul von Wassermann employed an aqueous extract of liver from an infant who died of congenital syphilis as an antigen for a complement fixation test. The liver contained large numbers of motile treponemes which Wassermann theorized would act as an antigen to combine with antibody in the serum of infected persons. Although the liver extract showed reactivity with sera of patients with syphilis, it was many years until it was recognized that the observed reactivity was not with treponemes but with intracellular, nontreponemal hepatocyte components. A similar substance could be isolated from other mammalian and plant sources. This substance is thought to be a component of mitochondrial membranes and has been called *cardiolipin.* Antibody to this antigen is known as *Wassermann antibody,* or reaginic antibody (not to be confused with IgE reaginic antibody).

VDRL Test. In 1922, R. L. Kahn developed the first precipitating test for syphilis, using an alcoholic extract of beef heart (cardiolipin). In 1941, lecithin and cholesterol were combined with cardiolipin, improving both the sensitivity and specificity of the test. This improved antigen led to the development of a slide microflocculation test by the Venereal Disease Research Laboratory of the United States Public Health Service (abbreviated as the VDRL test). The VDRL test is simple, inexpensive, and easy to perform on large numbers of sera in a short time. For these reasons, the VDRL has been the mainstay for screening sera for syphilis in many hospitals and public health laboratories for almost four decades.

Quantitation of Wassermann antibody can be determined by making twofold dilutions of the serum until the reaction disappears. Quantitative results of the VDRL test are reported as the reciprocal of the highest dilution of serum that precipitated with antigen, that is, the titer. The results of the quantitative test are then reported in terms of "dils," which is short for the Latin word *dilue,* meaning to dilute or dissolve.

Although these cardiolipin antigen tests have the advantages of ease, speed, and simplicity in the laboratory, it is necessary to inactivate complement and other inhibitors by heating the serum to be tested to 58°C for 30 min. This restriction, although not a problem in a well-equipped laboratory, limits application of the test in the field, where controlled test conditions may not be possible. More recently, the cardiolipin–lecithin–cholesterol complex has been stabilized with the addition of ethylenediamine tetraacetic acid (EDTA) and choline chloride to inactivate the inhibiting substances in unheated sera. This modification permits screening of large quantities of sera run under field conditions with minimal laboratory facilities. Several commercial variants of this test are available, e.g., the Plasmacrit and RPR (rapid plasma reagin) card test. The RPR test is performed by mixing the serum and reagent with an applicator stick on a hard piece of white cardboard. Experience has shown the RPR test to have equal and possibly better sensitivity and specificity than the VDRL test. One advantage of these tests is their ability to screen patients for Wassermann antibody at the time they visit a clinic or physician's office. This can facilitate the initiation of therapy when indicated.

Tests for Wassermann antibody are useful in screening large numbers of individuals for evidence of active syphilis, for example, tests performed for marriage license applications or prenatal blood tests for the prevention of congenital syphilis. Positive tests are considered to be diagnostic for syphilis when there is a high or increasing titer or when careful history taking and physical diagnosis reveal lesions consistent with primary or secondary syphilis. Tests for

Wassermann antibody are also useful in epidemiologic surveys for the investigation of patient contacts to find otherwise unrecognized active syphilis. In addition, Wassermann antibody tests may be of prognostic aid in following the response to therapy, since the VDRL titer falls over a 6–8-month period following adequate therapy.

Nonsyphilitic Antibodies to Wassermann Antigen. The cardiolipin Wassermann antigen is found in the mitochondrial membranes of many mammalian tissues. Similar antigenic material is present in other microorganisms, including mycoplasma, bacteria, and some yeasts. Thus, it is not surprising that antibodies to the Wassermann antigen appear in other diseases, such as infectious mononucleosis, hepatitis, and leprosy. These reactions have been called *biologic false-positive* (BFP) serologic tests for syphilis.

Antibodies to the Wassermann antigen may also occur in patients with collagen diseases or autoimmune disorders, such as systemic lupus erythematosus, rheumatoid arthritis, and Hashimoto's thyroiditis. The delayed onset of the tertiary stage of syphilis and the similarity of this condition to small-vessel disease with evidence of ischemic tissue damage have raised the possibility that the tertiary lesions of syphilis may be a manifestation of autoimmune disease. Further work to test this hypothesis is needed.

TREPONEMAL ANTIBODY TEST. The second type of serologic test is based on the use of whole treponeme or extracts of treponeme as antigen. The treponeme employed for this purpose may be either the virulent *T. pallidum*, grown only in rabbit testes, or a nonvirulent treponeme that can be cultivated in a special medium, for example, the Reiter's strain of *T. pallidum.*

TPI Test. The first successful treponemal antibody test was developed in 1949. During experiments to define growth characteristics of *T. pallidum* it was noted that serum from patients with active syphilis with guinea pig complement caused motile treponemes grown in rabbit testes to slow their active, corkscrewlike motion and to become immobilized (*T. pallidum* immobilization, or TPI, test). The antibody responsible for treponemal immobilization was found to differ from Wassermann antibody, in that Wassermann antibody was present in high concentration only during the early phase of infection, whereas immobilizing antibody persisted in high titer for many years. For many years this TPI test remained as a standard against which all other STS were measured and was considered

the ultimate criterion for presence or absence of antibody to *T. pallidum*. The TPI test is both sensitive and quite specific, but it is difficult to perform and requires closely supervised animal colonies and highly trained personnel. Sera tested for TPI are anticomplementary in 25–33% of patients, and if penicillin was given within the preceding month, traces present in the serum may immobilize the treponeme. The exacting conditions necessary to carry out the TPI test have limited it to only a few research laboratories.

The FTA and FTA-ABS Tests. In 1957, workers at the Venereal Disease Research Laboratory developed a test for antitreponemal antibody based on the principle of indirect immunofluorescence. This test essentially replaced the more cumbersome TPI test developed a decade earlier. A suspension of virulent *T. pallidum* from an infected rabbit testes is placed on a glass microscope slide and when overlaid with serum from a patient with antibody reactive with treponeme an antigen–antibody reaction occurs, with the antibody binding firmly to the surface of the treponeme. If the treponeme–antibody mixture is then exposed to antibody against human gamma globulin tagged with fluorescein and viewed under a strong ultraviolet light, the human antitreponemal antibody bound to the spirochete will be tagged with fluorescein dye and will outline the treponemal antigen. This test is called the fluorescent treponemal antibody test (FTA). It was then found that small amounts of antibody to endogenous treponemes normally present in humans could give a false-positive test unless absorbed with extracts of Reiter's treponemes. This test is called the fluorescent treponemal antibody absorption test (FTA-ABS).

The FTA-ABS can be performed in most clinical laboratories, and results are available within a day. Although the test is not difficult, the number of controls necessary and the experience and time required for reading the individual slides prevent the test from being used as a screening test as well as a test for specificity.

Microhemagglutination Tests. Within recent years, three microhemagglutination tests have been developed to test for treponemal antibodies. These tests are based on the principle of indirect hemagglutination using antigens of *T. pallidum* adsorbed onto erythrocytes. Two of the tests, the hemagglutination treponemal test for syphilis (HATTS) and the *T. pallidum* hemagglutination assay (TPHA) use glutaraldehyde-fixed turkey red blood cells. The third test, the microhemagglutination assay for antibodies to *T. pallidum* (MHA-TP) uses sheep red blood cells exposed to tannic acid and then fixed in formalin. Comparison of the three tests shows similar reactivity to each stage of syphilis with no evidence of one test being more sensitive than another. These tests are referred to collectively as the microhemagglutination (MHA) tests. Ease of performance, cost, and lack of need for expensive equipment are major factors in the popularity of the MHA tests when compared with the FTA-ABS. The MHA tests are more easily performed than are the other treponemal tests.

REACTIVITY OF SEROLOGIC TESTS. Comparison of the reactivity of various serologic tests to sera collected from well-documented cases of clinical syphilis can be helpful in determining the reliability of the tests for syphilis at varying stages of the disease. Table 18–3 lists the results of various serologic tests of sera from patients with well-documented primary or secondary syphilis. This table shows the FTA-ABS test to be reactive in a significantly higher number of patients with primary syphilis than are any other serologic tests, including the MHA and RPR. The FTA-ABS test is reactive in more than 90% of cases of darkfield-positive primary syphilis. If the FTA-ABS test is negative in a patient thought to have primary syphilis, it should be repeated on a second serum collected 7–10 days after the first. The FTA-ABS test is clearly the most reactive in all stages of syphilis. The MHA tests are likewise quite reactive, except in primary syphilis.

By the time secondary syphilis is well established, all tests give an acceptable result. If specific therapy for syphilis is instituted during the primary stage, and a Wassermann antibody test is positive, the test can be expected to become negative within 6–8 months. If therapy is delayed until the onset of the secondary stage of syphilis, 90–95% of adequately treated patients can be expected to be seronegative within 12 months. This characteristic is useful in monitoring the patient's response to therapy. If therapy is not begun until at least 2 years after the onset of disease, treatment will not significantly affect the serologic test, although it can be expected that about half the cases with active syphilis will become Wassermann antibody-negative over a 15–25-year period.

These findings are in contrast to those observed for tests for treponemal antibody. Of these, the TPI and FTA-ABS tests remain positive in a much higher percentage of cases (depending upon the stage at which therapy was started) and presumably reflect the total time and intensity of antigenic stimulation. Other than lower sensitivity in primary syphilis, the MHA tests compare favorably with the FTA-ABS. The MHA fails to detect antibodies in a few sera from persons with late syphilis, so it is wise to perform FTA-ABS tests on serum from suspected late syphilis if the MHA test is negative.

Although for many years nontreponemal STS have been required by many states on hospitalization or on application for marriage licenses, review of the results of these tests indicates a very low return of finding cases of active syphilis, with the prevalence of untreated syphilis approaching the rate of false-positive tests. The predictive value of a positive test when the prevalence of disease is reduced to the false-positive rate approaches 50% (i.e., as predictive as a coin toss). It is more efficient from a cost and detection standpoint to test only persons whose history places them in a high-prevalence group, such as persons with multiple sexual partners.

Both the FTA and MHA procedures have been applied to the detection of antibody against *T. pallidum* in cerebrospinal fluid, since treponemal tests are considered to be more specific than nontreponemal tests. Evaluation of these tests has shown both to be oversensitive, in that many persons without symptoms or other CSF findings have positive tests. No satisfactory explanation for the false-positive tests has been given. Currently, the best approach in diagnosing central nervous system syphilis is to use the

TABLE 18–3. *Reactivity of Nontreponemal and Treponemal Tests for Syphilis**

Stage of Syphilis	Percentage Reactive (Number Tested)				
	VDRL	*RPR*	*TPI*	*MHA*	*FTA-ABS*
Primary	70.5 (542)	80.6 (283)	57.3 (119)	77.3 (485)	91.5 (695)
Secondary	100 (182)	100 (74)	99.4 (156)	100 (166)	100 (309)
Latent	90.4 (521)	89.7 (195)	96.7 (60)	97.5 (836)	97.1 (681)
Late	68.2 (44)	75.0 (12)	91.7 (12)	94.7 (75)	100 (56)
Congenital	87.5 (7)	100 (10)		100 (17)	100 (25)

*From Huber, T. W. Syphilis serology. *Clin. Microbiol. Newsletter* 6:47, 1984.

VDRL test on CSF. This test is rarely positive in the absence of neurosyphilis, but it may lack sensitivity.

Recently, it has been recognized that serum from some patients with systemic lupus erythematosus may give an atypical, beaded appearance of fluorescence on treponemes with the FTA-ABS test (Fig. 18–4). In one study, 11 of 150 patients with lupus showed irregular, beaded fluorescence patterns. If the morphologic pattern of the test is not carefully differentiated, it can be confused with a positive test for syphilis.

Chancroid

Introduction

Chancroid is an acute, ulcerative disease caused by the gram-negative, facultative anaerobic bacillus, *Haemophilus ducreyi*. Chancroid is transmitted from person to person (usually during intercourse) and is more common in lower socioeconomic groups and uncircumcised men (particularly those who frequent prostitutes). Men are as much as 10 times more likely to develop clinical disease than women. In contrast to syphilis, there appears to be no latent or tertiary stages of disease. *H. ducreyi* can be cultured from approximately 50% of lesions.

Epidemiology

In the United States, the annual incidence of chancroid had decreased to fewer than 1000 reported cases in the early 1980s, but this figure had climbed to over 5000 cases by 1990. Chancroid remains a major public health problem in many Third World countries. The risk of enhanced transmission of HIV-1 in the presence of an active lesion has been suspected but not definitively proved.

Clinical Manifestations

H. ducreyi is a small, nonmotile, non–spore-forming organism that requires hemin for growth. The Gram's stain reveals typical streptobacillary chaining. The organism grows well on enriched media, such as chocolatized blood agar.

The incubation period for chancroid is usually between 4–7 days. There is no prodromal period. The presentation usually begins with a tender genital papule surrounded by erythema which evolves into a pustular, eroded ulceration, or chancre. The ulcer is well demarcated, has ragged undermined edges, and is without induration. There is little inflammation of the surrounding skin. Painful inguinal lymphadenitis is seen in up to one half of the cases and is usually unilateral. Buboes can progress and may spontaneously rupture. *H. ducreyi* does not disseminate further and is not known to be an opportunistic pathogen. Untreated infections may persist for several months.

Diagnosis

The diagnosis of chancroid is made by isolating *H. ducreyi* from a genital ulcer or bubo. A

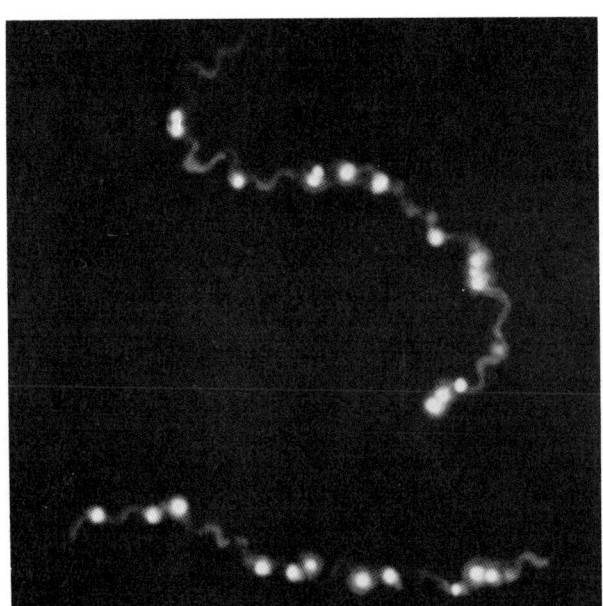

Figure 18–4. Atypical "beaded" spirochete fluorescence in FTA-ABS test with serum from patients with lupus erythematosus. (From Kraus, S. J., Haserick, J. R., and Lantz, M. A. Atypical FTA-ABS test fluorescence in lupus erythematosus patients. JAMA 211:2140, 1970. Copyright © 1970, American Medical Association.)

presumptive diagnosis can be made if the Gram's stain shows the characteristic features. A clinical diagnosis can be entertained in the presence of a compatible history and a painful genital ulcer and exclusion of other genital ulcer diseases, such as syphilis, herpes, lymphogranuloma venereum, and donovanosis.

Treatment

Treatment of chancroid is relatively easy. The sulfonamides, macrolides, cephalosporins, and quinolones have all been shown to be effective cures. The current Centers for Disease Control recommendation is for erythromycin, 500 mg orally 4 times daily for 7 days, or ceftriaxone, 250 mg intramuscularly as a single dose.

Granuloma Inguinale

Clinical Manifestations and Epidemiology

Granuloma inguinale (donovanosis) is a chronic, progressively destructive genital ulcer disease caused by *Calymmatobacterium granulomatis*, a gram-negative bacterium of uncertain affiliation. The primary lesion begins as an indurated nodule that slowly evolves into a granulomatous heaped ulcer. The pathognomonic feature of granuloma inguinale is the large infected mononuclear cell containing many intracytoplasmic cysts filled with deeply staining Donovan bodies. Hematogenous dissemination may occur.

Granuloma inguinale is rare in developed countries but is highly endemic in certain parts of the developing world. The role of sexual transmission is controversial, and the disease is only mildly contagious.

The incubation period may be as long as 80 days. Lesions are usually sharply defined, painless, and bleed readily on contact. Surrounding cellulitis is rare. Inguinal involvement is usually due to primary infection rather than to lymphangitic spread.

Diagnosis and Treatment

The diagnosis is usually made by clinical means. This can be confirmed by preparing a crush preparation from the lesion and observing clusters of blue- or black-staining organisms, referred to as Donovan bodies. No multinucleated giant cells and few lymphocytes are usually seen. The differential diagnosis of suspected granuloma inguinale includes carcinoma, chancroid, condylomata lata, and amebiasis.

The current treatment recommendation is for doxycycline, 100 mg twice daily for 10 days.

Herpes

Introduction

Genital herpes infection is caused by herpes simplex virus type 2. Genital herpes was originally thought to be due to the same herpesvirus that was responsible for herpes labialis, but studies in the 1960s revealed that there were two distinct antigenic types, each associated with a specific site of viral recovery. Newer type-specific serologic assays have been developed recently that avoid the cross-reactivity observed with older methods of testing. Seroepidemiologic surveys using these newer assays reveal that there is a wide disparity between antibody prevalence and history of clinical infection, indicating that many persons with infection are asymptomatic, have unrecognizable disease, or do not seek clinical care.

Epidemiology

The prevalence of genital herpes has increased over the past three decades. Although exact figures are not available, and vary according to the population studied, the observed increase of neonatal infection suggests that herpes prevalence has risen. Antibody to herpes simplex virus type 1 (HSV-1) is present in about 50% of the general U.S. population, but prevalence may be as high as 80% in lower socioeconomic groups. Antibody to herpes simplex virus type 2 (HSV-2) is usually not detected before puberty but rises to 50% in men and women attending clinics for sexually transmitted disease, nearly twice what is observed in the population at large. Higher rates have been reported in females, female prostitutes, homosexual men, and persons in lower socioeconomic groups.

Clinical Manifestations

Infection occurs after inoculation into small cracks in mucosal or skin surfaces. Initial infection is characterized by focal necrosis and inflammation with ballooning degeneration of cells. Concomitantly, HSV ascends peripheral sensory nerves and enters the nerve root ganglia where latency is established (regardless of whether the infection is symptomatic or asymptomatic). Reinfection with new strains can occur but is thought to be rare. Recrudescence may or may not be symptomatic and remains incompletely understood although recurrent skin lesions can be precipitated by local skin trauma such as sunburn or surgery.

Symptoms and Signs

The symptoms and signs of genital herpes vary greatly. First episodes of genital herpes can be classified as primary or nonprimary. Primary herpes is most often associated with systemic symptoms, more severe local involvement, and prolonged shedding of virus and duration of lesions. Patients with first episodes of genital herpes but who have clinical or serologic evidence of prior herpes infection, have a much milder clinical course. About one half of a group of patients presenting to an STD clinic in Seattle with herpes had primary infection. Most patients with nonprimary herpes have detectable antibody to HSV-1. Herpes simplex virus type 1 has been reported in 5–15% of all first episode herpes infections. There is no clinical difference in presentations of primary genital HSV-1 or HSV-2 infection.

Primary infections present after an incubation period of 5–14 days with pain, itching, dysuria, vaginal discharge, and tender inguinal adenopathy. The lesions usually start as erythematous papules or vesicles which spread rapidly to the surrounding area. Frequently, the vesicles coalesce and become pustular. Eventually, the lesions break, leaving tender, shallow ulcers that heal spontaneously without scarring. The mean time for viral shedding is 12 days and that to reepithelialization of the affected skin is 16–20 days. Ninety percent of women with primary HSV-2 infection have concomitant HSV cervicitis as well. In recurrent attacks, this rate drops to 12–29%. The clinical course of primary genital herpes infection is illustrated in Figure 18–5.

Recurrent genital herpes is a much milder disease and the duration of the episode ranges from 8 to 12 days or even less. Approximately 50% of patients experience a prodromal phase of the illness characterized by a tingling or shooting pain in the region of the outbreak that begins 1–48 h prior to eruption of the vesicular lesions. Lesions tend to occur unilaterally or on the buttocks or thigh, far removed from the inoculum site.

Asymptomatic shedding of virus is one of the least understood aspects of HSV infection. The source of the viral shedding in women is divided between the cervix and vulva and occurs in as many as 4% in the first year following a primary outbreak but drops to 0.5–2.0% in the following years. In men, the anatomical site is less well understood but is most likely due to small unrecognizable or atypical genital lesions rather than from semen.

Another aspect of HSV infection that is not well understood is the genital recurrence rate. Recurrence rates vary greatly among individuals. Following primary HSV-2 infection, 90% of persons have a recurrence within 12 months. The median rate of recurrence is five episodes in the 2 years following primary infection. Rates are lower following HSV-1 infection. Presence of serum HSV-1 antibody results in lower rates for new HSV-2 infections. Rates are also higher in persons with high titers of complement-independent neutralizing antibody, possibly indicating higher degrees of antigenic exposure.

Pharyngitis may be present in a significant number of patients with genital herpes and is usually accompanied by fever, headache, mucosal ulcerations, and cervical lymphadenopathy. Dysuria, urethritis, and a urethral discharge related to primary genital herpes may also be present and are more likely to be found in women. Women may also have evidence of lower urinary tract infection with HSV consistent with the signs and symptoms of the acute urethral syndrome.

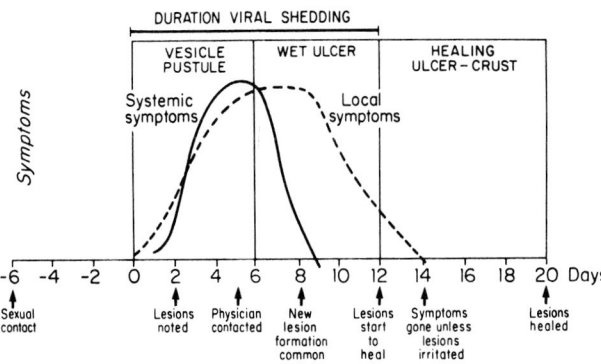

Figure 18–5. The clinical course of infection by primary genital herpes simplex virus. (From Corey, L., Adams, H. G., Brown, Z. A., et al. Genital herpes simplex virus infections: Clinical manifestations, course, and complications. Ann. Intern. Med. 98:958, 1983. Reproduced with permission.)

Aseptic meningitis is seen in more than one third of women and in approximately 10% of men with primary genital HSV-2 infection. Patients with aseptic meningitis may show increased CSF pressure and pleocytosis ranging as high as 300–400 cells/mm^3. There are usually no residual effects. In contrast to HSV-1, encephalitis from HSV-2 is rare.

Recently a syndrome of anorectal pain, discharge, constipation, and tenesmus was found in a group of sexually active homosexual males. These symptoms and findings are characteristic of herpes simplex virus proctitis. Serologic evidence indicated that 85% of the men with herpes proctitis were experiencing a primary HSV-2 infection. Other symptoms of herpes proctitis include sacral paresthesias, difficulty in urinating, and perianal skin and mucous membrane ulceration extending into the distal rectum.

Diagnosis

The diagnosis of herpesvirus infection is best established by recovery of the virus in cell culture. The virus grows in a wide range of diploid fibroblasts, including human embryonic tonsil, MCR-5, and WI-38. Growth is prompt, with early HSV cytopathic effect appearing in some cells by 24 h, in more than half by 48 h, and in almost all by 96 h.

Direct, Giemsa-stained smears from the base of ulcerated skin or mucous membrane lesions often show multinucleated giant cells, many with intranuclear inclusion bodies. Such large multinucleated cells are demonstrated in about 50% of patients who ultimately are found to have positive cultures. The use of fluorescein-tagged herpesvirus antibodies on smears from ulcerated lesions detects about 70% of patients who have positive cultures. The more recent application of fluorescein-tagged monoclonal antibodies to distinguish between HSV-1 and HSV-2 has shown this technique to produce the same results as the more time-consuming procedure of restriction endonuclease analysis. In addition, studies to establish DNA homology between culture specimens and herpesviruses as well as newly developed immunologic procedures are under way in the hope that they will provide rapid and specific identification of herpesvirus types 1 and 2.

Despite seroprevalence rates of between 30–70% in women attending prenatal clinics, clinical evidence of HSV is much less frequent. Although neonatal herpes is not a reportable disease, the estimated frequency of infection in the United States is approximately 1 in 7500 births, or about 700 cases annually. Recent studies indicate that most clinical manifestations of recurrent genital herpes are similar in pregnant and nonpregnant women. Visceral dissemination of herpes during primary infection in pregnant women has been reported, but fortunately appears to be rare. Pregnancy morbidity has been observed principally in primary cases.

The major identifiable source of HSV infection of the newborn is through contact with an infected birth canal. Approximately 70% of babies with neonatal HSV are born to mothers who were asymptomatic at delivery. The relative risk is much higher in primary cases. The risk of transmission by a mother with recurrent herpes ranges from 0 to 8%. In a remarkably large percentage of patients with neonatal herpes, the source is unknown.

Treating pregnant women who have a history of genital herpes remains problematic. Women should be advised to come to the delivery room early and to undergo a thorough examination of the vulvar area and cervix. A viral culture of the cervix and vulvar area should be taken. If no obvious lesions are present, the baby should be delivered vaginally. If any suspicious abnormality is present, a Caesarian section should be performed. Only 1–6% of infants exposed to HSV-infected maternal secretions develop neonatal herpes. Infants born to mothers with suspected active herpes should be placed in isolation and observed closely for signs of herpes infection. The benefit of early empiric antiviral therapy with acyclovir has not yet been determined.

Herpes and Human Immunodeficiency Virus Infection

Human immunodeficiency virus infection alters the course of HSV disease in many infected patients. Recurrences have been reported to be more frequent and more severe as the HIV-related disease progresses. In many cases, the genital, rectal, or oral HSV lesions become quite large, painful, and chronic. Patients with HSV ulcerations in which activated lymphocytes are present may be at the same higher risk of acquiring HIV as are patients with chancres. Many HIV-infected patients with active HSV may benefit from chronic suppressive therapy with acyclovir.

Treatment

Acyclovir is the only antiviral agent that has demonstrated a positive therapeutic effect in the

TABLE 18–4. *Genital Herpes Simplex Virus Infections—Treatment Guidelines*

Genital herpes is a viral disease that may be chronic and recurring and for which no known cure exists. Systemic acyclovir treatment provides partial control of the symptoms and signs of herpes episodes; it accelerates healing but does not eradicate the infection nor affect the subsequent risk, frequency, or severity of recurrences after the drug is discontinued. Topical therapy with acyclovir is substantially less effective than therapy with the oral drug.

First Clinical Episode of Genital Herpes

Recommended Regimen

Acyclovir, 200 mg orally five times a day for 7–10 days or until clinical resolution occurs.

First Clinical Episode of Herpes Proctitis

Recommended Regimen

Acyclovir, 400 mg orally five times a day for 10 days or until clinical resolution occurs.

Inpatient Therapy

For patients with severe disease or complications necessitating hospitalization.

Recommended Regimen

Acyclovir, 5 mg/kg body weight IV every 8 hours for 5–7 days or until clinical resolution occurs.

Recurrent Episodes

Most episodes of recurrent herpes do not benefit from therapy with acyclovir. In severe recurrent disease, some patients who start therapy at the begining of the prodrome or within 2 days after onset of lesions may benefit from therapy, although this has not been proven.

Recommended Regimen

Acyclovir, 200 mg orally five times a day for 5 days

or

Acyclovir, 800 mg orally twice a day for 5 days.

Daily Suppressive Therapy

Daily treatment reduces frequency of recurrences by at least 75% among patients with frequent (more than six per year) recurrences. Safety and efficacy have been clearly documented among persons receiving daily therapy for up to 3 years. Acyclovir-resistant strains of HSV have been isolated from persons receiving suppressive therapy, but they have not been associated with treatment failure among immunocompetent patients. After 1 year of continuous daily suppressive theapy, acyclovir should be discontinued so that the patient's recurrence rate may be reassessed.

Recommended Regimen

Acyclovir, 200 mg orally two to five times a day*

or

Acyclovir, 400 mg orally twice a day.*

Genital Herpes among HIV-Infected Patients

The need for higher than standard doses of oral acyclovir among HIV-infected but immunocompetent patients has not been established. Immune status, not HIV infection alone, is the likely predictor of disease severity and response to therapy. Case reports strongly suggest that patients with clinical immunodeficiency have a more severe clinical course of anogenital herpes than do immunocompetent patients, and some health care providers are using increased doses of acyclovir for patients with immunodeficiency. However, neither the need for nor the proper increased dosage of acyclovir has been conclusively established. Immunocompromised as well as immunocompetent hosts who fail initial therapy may benefit from an increased dosage of acyclovir. The indications for suppressive therapy among immunocompromised patients, and the dose required, are controversial. Clinical benefits to the patient must be weighed against the potential for selecting HSV strains that are resistant to acyclovir. Patients whose therapy for a recurrence fails because of resisant strains of HSV should be managed in consultation with an expert.

*Dosage must be individualized for each patient.
Adapted from Centers for Disease Control. Sexually transmitted disease treatment guidelines. *MMWR* 38(S-8):14–15, 1989.

treatment of genital herpesvirus infection. Acyclovir is selectively phosphorylated by cells infected with herpes simplex virus. Virus-specified thymidine kinase converts acyclovir to acyclovir monophosphate, which is then phosphorylated to acyclovir triphosphate, the form of the drug that ultimately acts as an inhibitor of herpes simplex virus DNA polymerase. Mutants of HSV that lack thymidine kinase are resistant to acyclovir.

Use of acyclovir as a topical cream after the appearance of skin lesions significantly shortens the time of viral shedding but has little effect upon the time to crusting and healing, to relief from pain, or upon the subsequent number of new skin lesions. The lack of significant symptomatic response to local therapy stands in contrast to the use of intravenous acyclovir in the treatment of first-episode genital herpes. When acyclovir is given every 8 h for 5 days, the clearance of shedding of herpes simplex virus from genital lesions, pharynx, cervix, and urethra, and in urine is greatly accelerated. In addition, the duration of local and systemic symptoms is shortened, and complications such as extragenital lesions and urinary retention are avoided. Thus, the use of intravenous acyclovir significantly decreases the symptoms, duration of lesions, and complications of primary genital herpes. However, as a parenteral agent its use remains impractical.

Oral acyclovir remains the mainstay of primary therapy and is nearly as effective as the intravenous preparation and much more convenient. Treatment of recurrent herpes outbreaks with shorter courses of acyclovir may benefit some patients. Long-term suppressive therapy for up to 1 year in patients with frequent recurrences can significantly reduce the number of outbreaks and appears to be well tolerated (Table 18–4).

GENITAL MUCOSAL DISEASES

Gonorrhea

Introduction

Gonorrhea is one of the oldest infectious diseases known that primarily involves the genitourinary tract, although the pharynx, rectum, eye, joints, and other organs may become involved as well. Hippocrates may have been the first to write extensively on the subject in the fourth and fifth centuries B.C. He referred to gonorrhea as "strangury" and associated it with "the pleasures of Venus." The term *clap,* which is still commonly used, first appeared in print in 1378 A.D. and most probably referred to the *Les Clappier* district of Paris, an area where prostitutes commonly worked at the time. Early on, it was thought that gonorrhea and syphilis were actually different manifestations of the same disease. It was not until Neisser's description of *Neisseria gonorrhoeae* in 1879 that scientists really began to understand the disease.

Clinical Manifestations

Neisseria gonorrhoeae is a small, gram-negative diplococcus whose only natural host is humans. Gonococci survive for only a very brief time outside the human body and despite the fact that these organisms can be cultured from an artificially inoculated toilet seat for up to 24 h, there are no documented cases of transmission except through intimate physical contact, specifically during sex. *N. gonorrhoeae* initially infects the mucosal surfaces of the genitourinary tract, primarily the urethra in males and the cervical endothelium in females. The rectum, pharynx, and conjunctivae can also become primarily infected. Ascending genital infection, salpingitis in females and epididymitis in males, as well as bacteremic dissemination, are relatively common and account for most of the serious morbidity due to gonorrhea.

More than 70 different strain types of *N. gonorrhoeae* exist. They can be differentiated by auxotyping, serotyping, or by antimicrobial sensitivities. The most useful and widely available method is by serotyping with monoclonal antibodies specific for various epitopes expressed on the outer membrane protein I. For epidemiologic purposes, typing of strains can be quite useful; to date, however, there appears to be no clinical need for such testing.

For infection to occur, gonococci must be able to adhere effectively to mucosal surfaces and to survive the usual mechanical forces present in the genitourinary system (Fig. 18–6). They are also capable of invading the mucosa and entering the bloodstream while evading the normal host defense mechanisms. Repeated reinfections in the same person by one strain strongly suggests that gonococci are able to evade local immune mechanisms or change surface antigens frequently. The considerable tissue damage that occurs following gonococcal salpingitis suggests that gonococci may produce a tissue toxin or evoke an immune response that results in damage to host tissues.

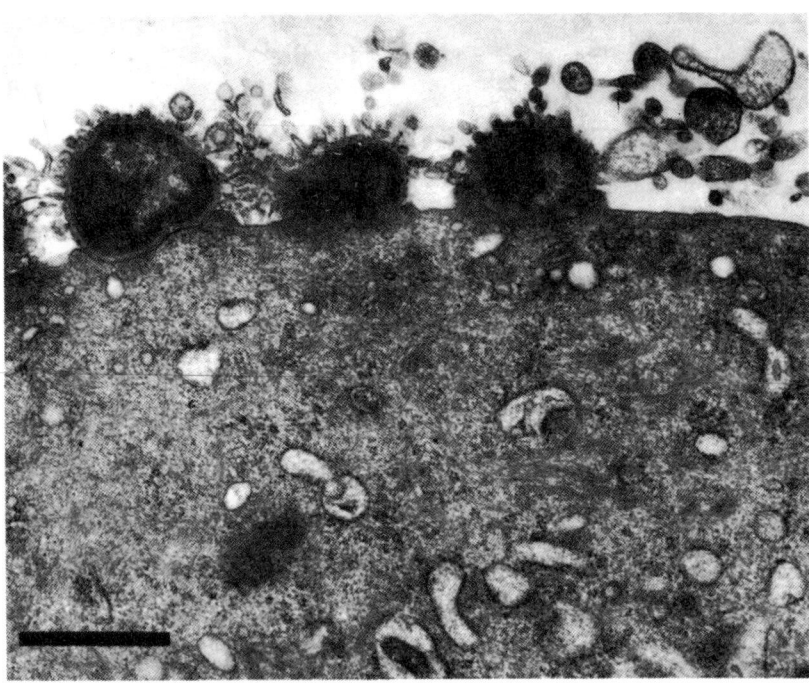

Figure 18–6. Electron micrograph showing gonococci closely attached to the surface of a urethral epithelial cell. The membrane of the host cell appears pushed up around the gonococcus to form cushionlike structures. The bar represents 500 nm (× 46,000). (From Ward, M. E., and Watt, P. J. Adherence of Neisseria gonorrhoeae *to urethral mucosal cells: An electron-microscopic study of human gonorrhea. J. Infect. Dis. 126:601, 1972. The University of Chicago Press, © 1972 by the* Journal of Infectious Diseases.)

Epidemiology

The incidence of gonorrhea varies considerably with age, sex, and race. Lower socioeconomic status, urban residence, unmarried marital status, and a past history of gonorrhea are also risk factors. Over 80% of reported cases in the United States in 1987 occurred in patients 15–29 years of age. The highest reported incidence of gonorrhea occurs among sexually active adolescent females, who have nearly twice the rate seen in sexually active women aged 20–24. Hook and Handsfield's published data revealed that in some census tracts in Seattle, the rate of gonococcal infection in sexually active African-American females aged 16–18 years was as high as 25%. In the 1980s, prostitution and illicit drug use appeared as new risk factors for gonorrhea. At the same time, male homosexuality and bisexuality are declining as risk factors because of the changing sexual practices in this group as a consequence of concerns regarding AIDS.

The number of reported cases of gonorrhea in the United States has been declining since 1975, 3 years after the initiation of a national gonorrhea control program. A significant portion of this decline relates to behavioral changes resulting from attempts to limit risk for HIV-1 infection. Not all groups have changed uniformly. For example, among white teenagers in the United States, rates may have actually increased.

The efficiency of transmission depends on the site of inoculation and the number of exposures. The best data are for men exposed to infected women: the attack rate after one such unprotected exposure during intercourse is 20% and rises to 60–80% following four such exposures. The attack rate among women may be as high as 50–90% following one such exposure to an infected man. The rates of infection following other types of sexual contact are less well defined. Anal intercourse appears to be a more efficient mode of transmission, and oral intercourse is less so. Barrier contraception with condoms, diaphragms, and spermicides clearly has a protective influence. Oral contraceptives may enhance transmission in women, but data in this regard are conflicting.

The acute clinical disease in men is associated with anterior urethritis that appears 1–8 days (mean 3–4 days) following exposure. The typical symptoms are dysuria and discharge, often purulent and profuse. A minority, 2–10%, never develop symptoms, partly as a result of the infecting strain type. The natural history of untreated gonorrhea is for spontaneous resolution of signs and symptoms over a period of weeks. Ninety-five percent of untreated patients become asymptomatic within 6 months. Complications of urethritis include epididymitis, acute or chronic prostatitis, and infections of Cowper's and Tyson's glands.

The acute clinical disease in women involves infection of the endocervical canal. Colonization of the urethra is common but rarely without concomitant endocervical involvement. Skene's and Bartholin's glands may also be infected. When present, symptoms include increased vaginal discharge, dysuria, abnormal uterine bleeding, and menorrhagia. The cervix may have obvious purulent discharge, erythema, or have areas of easily induced bleeding. Coexisting infection with other sexually transmitted diseases is common. Extension to the rectum frequently occurs in 20–50% of women with genital gonorrhea. Acute salpingitis, or pelvic inflammatory disease, is the most severe complication of gonorrhea, occurring in 10–20% of infected women. Salpingitis is the most important complication of gonorrhea both because of the potential severity of the acute disease and the secondary complications of infertility and ectopic pregnancy. Clinical findings of acute salpingitis include any combination of abdomenal pain, dyspareunia, abnormal menses, adnexal or cervical tenderness, abnormal cervical discharge, and fever.

Acute dissemination of gonorrhea occurs in 1–3% of untreated patients. Arthritis, tenosynovitis, and dermatitis are the most common findings, although any organ can become involved following hematogenous spread. Disseminated infection occurs more commonly in women than in men. Patients who are pregnant and those with pharyngeal infection or terminal complement component deficiency have higher rates of dissemination as well.

Diagnosis

Microbic Culture. The diagnosis of gonorrhea (in contrast to that of syphilis, in which the microorganism cannot be grown in artificial culture) depends on the culture and identification of the microorganism. A significant aid in improving gonococcal isolation has been the development of a selective culture medium that suppresses the growth of contaminating microorganisms that might otherwise overgrow and

mask the appearance of *N. gonorrhoeae*. This culture medium, named after the two men who developed it—James D. Thayer and John E. Martin—is known as Thayer-Martin (TM) medium. It is composed of chocolate agar containing a long, carefully compounded list of vitamins and cofactors and was originally prepared using the antibiotics ristocetin and polymyxin. When ristocetin was withdrawn from the market because of toxicity to humans, the antibiotics were changed to vancomycin, colistin, and nystatin (VCN). Currently, the terms Thayer-Martin (TM) and VCN refer to the same culture medium for the isolation of both *N. gonorrhoeae* and *N. meningitidis*.

The Venereal Disease Research Laboratory at the Centers for Disease Control has introduced a modification of the VCN medium, adding trimethoprim, a sulfonamidelike compound found to inhibit certain strains of *Proteus* that are resistant to vancomycin, colistin, and nystatin. The modified medium is poured into a small prescription bottle and capped under an atmosphere of 10% carbon dioxide. Cultures may be placed directly on this medium for transport to central processing laboratories. Recovery of *N. gonorrhoeae* is improved if the culture medium is incubated overnight at 37°C before forwarding to the microbiology laboratory. This latest modification of selective culture media for *N. gonorrhoeae* is called Transgrow and is available commercially for use in clinics and physicians' offices. The medium may be stored at 4°C until it is used, but it is important that it be warmed to either room temperature or preferably to 35 or 37°C before inoculation. *N. gonorrhoeae* is very sensitive to cold temperatures and can be killed if inoculated to medium just removed from a refrigerator. Many types of selective culture media have been introduced in recent years in an effort to materially increase the likelihood of the clinical laboratory's isolating *N. gonorrhoeae* from specimens collected from patients in physicians' offices or from individuals attending outpatient clinics.

Enzyme-Linked Immunosorbent Assay. Recently, the application of an enzyme-linked immunosorbent assay (ELISA) to test for specific gonococcal antigens has resulted in a sensitive method for identifying patients with gonorrhea. Since the results do not depend on recovery of the organisms by culture, the test can be completed within 3–4 h. In men, comparison of ELISA and culture results yielded a sensitivity of 94% and a specificity of 98%, which is essentially equivalent to the urethral Gram's stain. Subsequent studies in clinical settings have not been as encouraging, with sensitivity in the 70–80% range. In women, the immunoassay yielded a sensitivity of 78% and a specificity of 98% as compared with cervical culture. The ELISA test is significantly more sensitive than the cervical Gram's stain (78 vs. 48%). Neither prolonged transport nor refrigeration up to 30 days affects ELISA results. Thus, immunologic antigen detection for gonorrhea has certain advantages over cultures in early reporting of results or when there may be prolonged transportation periods that might affect organism viability.

Serology. For many years there has been a need for a serologic test to detect infection with *N. gonorrhoeae* that would serve the same purpose as the serologic tests for syphilis. The two infections are not comparable, however, since in gonorrhea the organism can be recovered and identified with moderate ease, a situation that does not exist with syphilis. In part because of a wide variety of potential antigens, including pili, polysaccharide capsules, and membrane and somatic proteins, as well as what appears to be considerable variation in strain specificity among isolates, the single best gonococcal antigen for screening purposes has not yet been determined. Similarly, increasing knowledge of the rather considerable antigenic heterogeneity of *N. gonorrhoeae* has led to a reconsideration of which antibody should be sought to establish specificity of infection. In contrast to the considerable variations in sensitivity and specificity that characterize serologic methods to identify gonococcal infection, culture of the infected site has an approximately 80% sensitivity and an almost 100% specificity for both symptomatic and asymptomatic infections. Although culture is considerably more expensive than most serologic procedures, the sensitivity and specificity of the culture ultimately make it a more economical screening procedure than most serologic tests.

Treatment

Sulfanilamide was the first antimicrobial agent of choice for the treatment of gonorrhea in the mid-1930s. However, this was replaced by penicillin in 1946, as many gonococcal strains had become resistant. Shortly after penicillin became available for treatment of gonorrhea, total dosage of as little as 100,000 U cured the infection. By the early 1970s, "low-level" chromosomally mediated penicillin resistance was observed in many parts of the world, particularly in Southeast Asia. Effective therapy with penicillin was maintained by increasing the total amount of penicillin or by giving probenecid or both. Probenecid blocks renal tubular secretion of penicillin and results in higher and more prolonged serum levels, thereby increasing the time the microorganism is exposed to effective levels of the drug. In 1983, "high-level" chromosomally mediated penicillin- and tetracycline-resistant strains were identified in North Carolina, resulting in penicillin treatment failure. By 1989, penicillin therapy was no longer effective at maximal doses in many parts of the United States, and the Centers for Disease Control recommended switching from penicillin or amoxicillin to intramuscular ceftriaxone therapy.

In 1976, the first two cases of infection with penicillinase-producing *Neisseria gonorrhoeae* (PPNG) were detected, in Maryland and in California. Over the next 15 months, 191 cases of PPNG infections were confirmed. In 177 patients for whom histories were available, 69 were traced to the Far East or West Africa. Prior to 1980, most infected patients with PPNG strains or their sex partners had traveled overseas. However, by 1980, PPNG had become endemic in many areas of the United States, and the prevalence of such isolates began to increase significantly. By 1988, PPNG accounted for more than 4% of all reported cases, over 40,000 cases per year. In South Florida, PPNG prevalence exceeded 33%.

By 1985, concomitant tetracycline was prescribed routinely for patients with gonorrhea as therapy for coexistent chlamydial infection. Tetracycline itself had been an effective agent for the treatment of gonorrhea and had been the treatment regimen of choice in penicillin-allergic patients. By 1985, high-level, plasmid-mediated resistance to tetracycline had become widespread, and tetracycline could no longer be recommended for therapy.

Spectinomycin, an aminoglycoside used exclusively for the treatment of gonorrhea, has been found to be very effective against uncomplicated infections with penicillinase-producing gonococci. In 1987, high-level, chromosomally mediated resistance to spectinomycin was reported in U.S. military personnel in Korea. At present, spectinomycin resistance remains rare in the United States. One disadvantage of spectinomycin is its failure in the therapy of gonorrheal pharyngitis. Patients with suspected or proven gonorrheal pharyngitis or their sexual partners who engage in oral sex should not be treated with spectinomycin.

In 1989, ceftriaxone became the recommended treatment of choice. Ceftriaxone eradicates gonorrhea from all potentially infected sites. A single intramuscular injection is highly effective (Table 18–5).

Chlamydia

Introduction

The most common sexually transmitted disease in developed countries is caused by *Chlamydia trachomatis,* an obligate, intracellular parasite that cannot be cultured on artificial media. Chlamydiae are distinct from all other microorganisms and have been placed in their own order, Chlamydiales, and family, Chlamydiaceae. Chlamydiae are responsible for several recognized forms of disease in humans: potentially blinding trachoma, infantile pneumonitis, sexually transmitted lymphogranuloma venereum, and genital mucosal disease (Table 18–6). Another species, *C. psittaci,* is a common pathogen in birds and domestic animals and only rarely affects humans.

Epidemiology

The prevalence of *C. trachomatis* ranges from 3–5% of asymptomatic men and women in general medical settings to over 20% in STD clinics. During pregnancy, 5–7% of women have been reported to be culture-positive for chlamydia. Neonates may acquire infection after passing through an infected birth canal. Teenage females have been shown to have the highest seroprevalence rates.

Clinical Manifestations

Clinical infection closely parallels that seen with gonorrhea. Chlamydial infection tends to have a longer incubation period (7–21 days), less frank purulence from inflamed sites, and is more likely to be asymptomatic than gonorrhea. Although both infections can become systemic, the manifestations associated with systemic chlamydial infection are more likely result from antigen–antibody complex formation rather than direct hematogenous spread of the organism as is seen with gonorrhea.

In men, the most common clinical condition associated with chlamydia is urethritis. Although symptoms are generally milder than with gonorrhea, there is enough overlap so that there is no clinical way to determine which agent is responsible for the urethritis. Chlamydia is the most common cause of nongonococcal urethritis. Sixty–75% of female partners of culture-positive men have proven infection.

Epididymitis may result from ascending chlamydial infection. In sexually active men under 35 years of age, chlamydia is the most common pathogen, in contrast to men over 35 in whom coliforms are the usual cause. Clinically, chlamydial epididymitis presents as unilateral scrotal pain, swelling, and tenderness of the epididymis. Therapy with tetracycline is usually rapidly effective. It is unlikely that chlamydia causes other forms of local infection, such as prostatitis.

The D, K, and LGV strains of chlamydia can produce proctitis which may be asymptomatic or appear as a purulent form indistinguishable from that caused by gonorrhea. Stamm and Holmes have reported that in their patient population, up to 15% of homosexual men presenting with proctitis were found to have chlamydia. Treatment with tetracycline is quite effective.

The most severe consequence of chlamydial infection is Reiter's syndrome (urethritis, conjunctivitis, and arthritis), a form of reactive tenosynovitis, or arthritis without other symptoms. Like postenteric Reiter's syndrome, patients are more at risk if they have the HLA-B27 haplotype (see Chapter 5). Reiter's syndrome is unlikely to occur if therapy with tetracycline is initiated promptly.

The most common chlamydial manifestation in women is cervicitis. Only one third of women are symptomatic. The most common finding is that of mucopurulent discharge, found in 37%. The presence of more than 30 polymorphonuclear leukocytes per high-power field is strongly suggestive of chlamydial or gonococcal cervicitis. The presence of cervical ectopy, common in teenagers, is a risk factor for infection. Oral contraceptives are also associated with increased risk of infection. Nearly all women with endocervical chlamydial infection develop antibody to *C. trachomatis*. Infection with chlamydia may persist for many months or resolve spontaneously.

Local extension or infection of the female urethra, Bartholin's glands, or endometrium is common and responds to the usual treatment regimen of tetracycline. The most severe form of chlamydial infection in women is salpingitis. The sequelae of salpingitis may include evolution to a tuboovarian abscess or severe inflam-

TABLE 18–5. *Gonococcal Infections—Treatment Guidelines*

Treatment of gonococcal infections in the United States is influenced by the following trends: (1) the spread of infections due to antibiotic-resistant *N. gonorrhoeae*, including penicillinase-producing *N. gonorrhoeae* (PPNG), tetracycline-resistant *N. gonorrhoeae* (TRNG), and strains with chromosomally mediated resistance to multiple antibiotics; (2) the high frequency of chlamydial infections in persons with gonorrhea; (3) recognition of the serious complications of chlamydial and gonococcal infections; and (4) the absence of a fast, inexpensive, and highly accurate test for chlamydial infection.

All gonorrhea cases should be diagnosed or confirmed by culture to facilitate antimicrobial susceptibility testing. The susceptibility of *N. gonorrhoeae* to antibiotics is likely to change over time in any locality. Therefore, gonorrhea control programs should include a system of regular antibiotic sensitivity testing of a surveillance sample of *N. gonorrhoeae* isolates as well as all isolates associated with treatment failure.

Because of the wide spectrum of antimicrobial therapies effective against *N. gonorrhoeae*, these guidelines are *not* intended to be a comprehensive list of all possible treatment regimens.

Treatment of Adults

Uncomplicated Urethral, Endocervical, or Rectal Infections

Single-dose efficacy is a major consideration in choosing an antibiotic regimen to treat persons infected with *N. gonorrhoeae*. Another important concern is coexisting chlamydial infection, documented in up to 45% of gonorrhea cases in some populations. Until universal testing for chlamydia with quick, inexpensive, and highly accurate tests becomes available, persons with gonorrhea should also be treated for presumptive chlamydial infections. Generally, patients with gonorrhea infections should be treated simultaneously with antibiotics effective against both *C. trachomatis* and *N. gonorrhoeae*. Simultaneous treatment may lessen the possibility of treatment failure due to antibiotic resistance.

Recommended Regimen

Ceftriaxone, 250 mg IM once

plus

Doxycycline, 100 mg orally twice a day for 7 days.

Some authorities prefer a dose of 125 mg ceftriaxone IM because it is less expensive and can be given in a volume of only 0.5 mL, which is more easily administered in the deltoid muscle. However, the 250-mg dose is recommended because it may delay the emergence of ceftriaxone-resistant strains. At this time, both doses appear highly effective for mucosal gonorrhea at all sites.

Alternative Regimens

For patients who cannot take ceftriaxone, the preferred alternative is **Spectinomycin,** 2 g IM, in a single dose (followed by **doxycycline**).

Other alternatives, for which experience is less extensive, include **ciprofloxacin***, 500 mg orally once; **norfloxacin***, 800 mg orally once; **cefuroxime axetil,** 1 g orally once with **probenecid,** 1 g; **cefotaxime,** 1g IM once; and **ceftizoxime,** 500 mg IM once. All of these regimens are followed by **doxycycline**, 100 mg orally, twice daily for 7 days. If infection was acquired from a source proven *not* to have penicillin-resistant gonorrhea, a penicillin such as **amoxicillin,** 3 g orally with 1 g **probenecid** followed by **doxycycline** may be used for treatment.

Doxycycline or tetracycline alone is no longer considered adequate therapy for gonococcal infections but is added for treatment of coexisting chlamydial infections. Tetracycline may be substituted for doxycycline; however, compliance may be worse since **tetracycline** must be taken at a dose of 500 mg four times a day between meals, whereas **doxycycline** is taken at a dose of 100 mg twice a day without regard to meals. Moreover, at current prices, tetracycline costs only a little less than generic doxycycline.

For patients who cannot take a tetracycline (e.g., pregnant women), **erythromycin** may be substituted (**erythromycin** base or stearate at 500 mg orally four times a day for 7 days *or* **erythromycin ethylsuccinate,** 800 mg orally four times a day for 7 days).

Special Considerations

All patients with gonorrhea should have a serologic test for syphilis and should be offered confidential counseling and testing for HIV infection. Most patients with incubating syphilis (those who are seronegative and have no clinical signs of syphilis) may be cured by any of the regimens containing beta-lactams (e.g., ceftriazone) or tetracyclines.

Spectinomycin and the quinolones (ciprofloxacin, norfloxacin) have not been shown to be active against incubating syphilis. Patients treated with these drugs should have a serologic test for syphilis in 1 month.

Patients with gonorrhea and documented syphilis and gonorrhea patients who are sex partners of syphilis patients should be treated for syphilis (see Table 18–2) as well as for gonorrhea.

Some practitioners report that mixing 1% lidocaine (without epinephrine) with ceftriaxone reduces the discomfort associated with the injection (see package insert). No adverse reactions have been associated with use of lidocaine diluent.

Treatment of Sex Partners

Persons exposed to gonorrhea within the preceding 30 days should be examined, cultured, and treated presumptively.

---

*Quinolones, such as ciprofloxacin and norfloxacin, are contraindicated during pregnancy and in children 16 years of age or younger. Adapted from Centers for Disease Control. Sexually transmitted disease treatment guidelines. *MMWR* 38(S-8):19–20, 1989.

Reprinted, by permission, from Schachter, J. Chlamydial infections. *N. Engl. J. Med. 298*:428, 1978.

TABLE 18–6. *Human Diseases Caused by Chlamydia (Exclusive of* C. pneumoniae*)*

Species	Serotype*	Disease
C. psittaci	Many unidentified serotypes	Psittacosis
C. trachomatis	L-1, L-2, L-3	Lymphogranuloma venereum
C. trachomatis	A, B, Ba, C	Hyperendemic blinding trachoma
C. trachomatis	D, E, F, G, H, I, J, K	Inclusion conjunctivitis (adult & newborn), nongonococcal urethritis, cervicitis, salpingitis, proctitis, epididymitis & pneumonia of newborns

*Predominant, but not exclusive, association of serotype with disease.

matory response leading to tubular scarring with subsequent infertility and risk for ectopic pregnancy. Another serious consequence of chlamydial infection is perihepatitis, or Fitz-Hugh–Curtis syndrome, also seen in gonococcal infections.

Diagnosis

The diagnosis of chlamydial infection can be made by inoculation of infected secretions onto McCoy or Hela cell-tissue culture. Tissue culture is relatively expensive and may require as long as 5–10 days for results. Rapid, nonculture methods for detection include direct immunofluorescence staining of smears with monoclonal antibodies, detection of chlamydial antigen by enzyme-linked immunoassay with polyclonal or monoclonal antibodies, and DNA probes, which have also been used with similar success. However, the nonculture methods have less than 100% sensitivity and specificity, resulting in unacceptably low predictive values in many lower risk groups. Fortunately, clinical diagnosis is relatively easy if pyuria (greater than 4 PMNs per high-power field) is present in men, or more than 30 PMNs are seen on endocervical Gram's stains.

Treatment

Tetracycline or doxycycline administered for 1 week is the therapy of choice. To date, no tetracycline resistance has been documented anywhere in the world. Other agents effective in treating chlamydia are the macrolides, sulfonamides, rifampin, and the quinolones.

Mycoplasmas

Introduction

Mycoplasmas are small gram-negative organisms that do not take up counter stain effectively and are therefore not seen on routine Gram-stained clinical specimens. They can be grown in beef heart infusion broth supplemented with yeast extract, and although commercially available, it is relatively expensive, and most clinicians do not have ready access to this culture media. Three mycoplasmas have been demonstrated to cause clinical disease in the genitourinary tract of sexually active patients: *Mycoplasma hominis*, *M. genitalium*, and *Ureaplasma urealyticum*.

Epidemiology

Ureaplasma urealyticum appears to cause a significant portion of the gonorrhea-negative, chlamydia-negative urethritis in men. Precise numbers do not exist because the recovery of *U. urealyticum* from the male urethra does not necessarily implicate ureaplasmas as the cause of urethritis because ureaplasmas also colonize the genital tract. The most convincing evidence that ureaplasmas may be pathogenic comes from a study in which two investigators inoculated themselves with a strain from a patient with apparent ureaplasma-induced disease. Both investigators developed urethritis associated with a transient antibody response.

The role of *Mycoplasma genitalium* as a pathogen causing urethritis is not as clear. Limited studies have suggested that it may be isolated more frequently from the urethra of men with urethritis when other pathogens are not present or have been specifically treated. Further studies are necessary to establish the role of *M. genitalium* in human urethritis. The possible role of the mycoplasmas in epididymitis, prostatitis, and Reiter's syndrome is unknown.

Data suggest that *M. hominis*, *M. genitalium*, and *U. urealyticum* can cause pelvic inflammatory disease. The data concerning local abscess formation, vaginitis, and cervicitis are not convincing.

Treatment

The usual treatment for *M. genitalium* or *U. urealyticum* infection is the same as that for chlamydial infection, that is, the tetracyclines. However, 10% of ureaplasmas are resistant to tetracycline and about 40% of the tetracycline-resistant strains are also resistant to erythromycin. Alternative therapy in this situation is limited. The quinolones, particularly ofloxacin, and spectinomycin have been shown to be the most active alternative agents to date.

EPIDERMAL DISEASES

Human Papillomavirus

Introduction

Anogenital warts are caused by specific types of human papillomaviruses (HPV)—small, naked viruses with an icosahedral symmetry and double-stranded circular DNA. Warts are benign, self-limiting tumors of the epithelium. Genital infection is caused primarily by HPV types 6, 11, and 16. Although caused by different strains of the same virus, there is no clinical or virologic evidence of any close association between genital warts and the common skin wart. Some human and animal papillomaviruses are associated with cancer, specifically types 16 and 18 which have been strongly linked with the development of cervical and vulvar carcinoma 5–30 years after infection.

Epidemiology and Clinical Manifestations

Anogenital warts are the most common sexually transmitted viral disease. They are three times more common than genital herpes and are exceeded in incidence only by gonorrhea and chlamydial infection. Human papillomavirus is transmitted during direct sexual contact, and the incubation period is 2–3 months. Infection may occur anywhere there is direct physical contact including the anus and oral cavity. Behaviors associated with increased risk for genital warts include having sex with a person with symptomatic or asymptomatic infection, smoking, and the long term use of oral contraceptives.

Genital warts in men can occur anywhere on the external genitalia, urethra, rectum, or bladder. When they are exophytic, the warts are referred to as condylomata acuminata. Warts are usually multiple and vary in size from 1 to 5 mm in diameter. They may be flat and are often inconspicuous, making diagnosis and treatment difficult.

In women, condylomata usually appear first on the vulva and in 20% of cases then rapidly spread to the perineum and perianal area. Subclinical infection of the cervix is common but is difficult to recognize without the aid of a colposcope. Studies with colposcopy, cytology, and histology have shown a 25–100% association between HPV infection and cervical intraepithelial neoplasia.

Diagnosis

Diagnosis of anogenital warts can be difficult. Warts must be distinguished from normal anatomical variants, tumors, and other infectious agents. The most similarly appearing such lesion is that of condylomata lata, a manifestation of secondary syphilis. Diagnosis is usually made on clinical, cytologic, or histologic grounds. The potential for the use of specific DNA probes appears promising but availability is limited at present.

Treatment

Treatment of anogenital warts is limited to chemical ablation with such agents as podophyllin, 5-fluorouracil, and trichloracetic acid. More complicated cases and treatment failures may require cryotherapy, surgery, electrocautery, or CO_2 laser treatment. Systemic interferon therapy has shown some benefit, particularly in patients with recalcitrant warts; however, the side effects are troublesome. Intralesional interferon injections have shown some promise although administration problems exist.

Molluscum Contagiosum

Epidemiology and Clinical Manifestations

Molluscum contagiosum is a benign papular lesion of the skin caused by the molluscum contagiosum virus, a member of the poxvirus family. Molluscum contagiosum can be spread by sexual as well as nonsexual routes. The incubation period ranges from 1 week to 6 months. The lesions are very characteristic: 3–5 mm in diameter, smooth, firm, dome-shaped, and grayish white in color with an umbilicated center.

Diagnosis and Treatment

Diagnosis is usually made on clinical grounds. Biopsy reveals characteristic large round intracytoplasmic molluscum bodies. Treatment is generally simple and easily accomplished by excisional curettage. In severely immunosuppressed patients such as those with AIDS, treatment is quite difficult and no therapy is very effective. New lesions appear faster than the existing lesions can be removed safely.

Ectoparasitic Diseases

Lice

Phthirus pubis, the crab louse, is transmitted from one person to another primarily during intimate contact but also, less frequently, after sharing bedding or toilet seats. It is more difficult to transmit than the other species of lice that infect man, *Pediculus humanus corporis,* the body louse, and *Pediculus humanus capitis,* the head louse. Lice must have human blood in order to survive. Once off the body, they die within a day.

The clinical manifestations of infection with the crab louse includes itching, which leads to scratching, erythema, and inflammation. Superinfection may occur. The diagnosis is made by careful visual inspection and identification of adult lice and their eggs (nits), which are firmly attached to the pubic hair.

The treatment for lice is permethrin 1% or lindane 1%. However, ridding the patient's clothing of nits and adult lice is also an important part of the treatment program.

Scabies

Sarcoptes scabiei is the mite responsible for scabies. Mites actually move quite rapidly and are quick to burrow into the horny layer of the skin and to begin laying eggs. Scabies is transmitted by any close personal contact. Household outbreaks are common. Scabies may also be transmitted by animals, particularly dogs. Animal mites are very similar to human mites but they differ biologically: their incubation period is shorter, typical burrows are absent, and household contacts need not be treated since the condition is not transmissible between humans.

The hallmark of scabies is pruritus, usually worse at night or after a hot shower or bath. The lesions associated with scabies may appear papular or eczematous. The hands are often the first place of involvement, particularly the finger webs. Skin folds are a common site of infection.

Lesions on the penis may mimic a chancre or superficial fungal infection. The pathognomonic burrow is a short, wavy, dirty-appearing line.

Diagnosis is often made on clinical grounds but can be confirmed by examination of a skin scraping or by prying a mite from its burrow with a needle. Treatment is relatively easy, with lindane being the most common preparation used in the United States.

ENTERITIS/DIARRHEAL SYNDROMES

Infections with pathogens that commonly cause enteritis or diarrhea traditionally have been associated with food or water-borne acquisition. Many are now known also to occur following sexual transmission, specifically anogenital or oroanal contact. Most of these infections occur in men who have had sex with other men. Although primary enteric infection with many of the sexually transmitted agents is possible (e.g., HSV, HPV, gonorrhea, and chlamydia), enteritis is generally associated with *Shigella* sp., *Salmonella* sp., and *Campylobacter* sp. The protozoans, *Entamoeba histolytica* and *Giardia lamblia,* are also known to cause diarrhea and be sexually transmitted.

Shigellosis

Shigellosis presents with an abrupt onset of diarrhea (sometimes bloody), fever, nausea, and cramps. The colonic mucosa is inflamed and friable. Diagnosis is made by culturing the organism, usually *Shigella sonnei* or *S. flexneri,* on selective media. Treatment consists of support and an antibiotic chosen based on local sensitivity patterns.

Salmonellosis

Less frequently, *Salmonella* sp. have been associated with sexual transmission. Findings are similar to other enteritides, and diagnosis is made by culture. Treatment is usually supportive. Since asymptomatic carriers are common, tracing sexual partners is extremely important. In the presence of concomitant HIV infection, long-term chronic therapy with one of the quinolone antibiotics may be warranted.

Campylobacteriosis

Campylobacter jejuni may actually be the most common bacterial cause of enteritis in homosexual men. Infection usually involves the upper abdomen, and abdominal pain is a common clinical feature. Diagnosis is made by culturing the organism on selective media in a microaerophilic atmosphere. Treatment consists of erythromycin or a quinolone.

Amebiasis

The etiologic agent of amebiasis is *Entamoeba histolytica.* It is not certain that *E. histolytica* actually causes illness in homosexual men since equal numbers of such patients with and without symptoms have organisms in their stool on wet mount exam. Most of these organisms appear to be nonpathogenic. When indicated, treatment is with metronidazole, with or without diiodohydroxyquin.

VAGINAL DISEASES

Vulvovaginal Candidiasis

Vulvovaginal candidiasis or candida vaginitis is most likely not a sexually transmitted disease of women. However, 20% of women with vulvovaginitis have a male partner who exhibits penile colonization with *Candida* but who may or may not be symptomatic. *Candida* sp. are found in up to 55% of asymptomatic women of childbearing age. Generally women with symptomatic vaginitis have some predisposing factor such as pregnancy, recent antibiotic use, diabetes, immunosuppression, or oral contraceptive use. Women in warmer climates or those who wear tight-fitting, ill-ventilated clothing are also at higher risk for clinical infection.

Diagnosis is made by examination of vaginal secretions by wet saline or 10% potassium hydroxide preparation or by culture. Treatment is uncomplicated with a variety of locally administered antifungal agents such as miconazole and clotrimazole.

Trichomoniasis

Trichomoniasis is a common sexually transmitted infection caused by the flagellated protozoan, *Trichomonas vaginalis.* The clinical syndrome in women ranges from asymptomatic carriage to frank vaginitis. Men tend to have more asymptomatic disease but may develop urethritis.

The prevalence of trichomoniasis in women attending sexually transmitted disease clinics ranges from 7 to 32%. Its presence is associated with nonuse of barrier or oral contraceptives. The organism is identified in up to 40% of male partners and 85% of female partners of infected index cases. Approximately 5% of girls born to infected mothers may acquire infection manifested as vaginitis.

Clinically, women present with a malodorous, frothy vaginal discharge and may have diffuse vaginal erythema. A wet preparation of the vaginal fluid reveals the typical motile trichomonads and an excessive number of polymorphonuclear leukocytes. Treatment of the patient and sexual partners with one 2.0-gm dose of metronidazole is effective.

Bacterial Vaginosis

Bacterial vaginosis is the most common vaginal disease in women of child-bearing age. Formerly referred to as nonspecific vaginitis, *Gardnerella* vaginitis, and *Haemophilus* vaginitis, this condition has been viewed as an inconsequential disease by many primary care providers. More recent evidence, however, has suggested an association between bacterial vaginosis and prematurity, chorioamnionitis, and pelvic inflammatory disease.

Bacterial vaginosis is present in up to one third of women visiting sexually transmitted disease clinics and in approximately 5% of women being seen for general medical reasons. Although originally thought to be caused by the anaerobic *Gardnerella vaginalis,* bacterial vaginosis is now thought to be due to the interaction of *G. vaginalis* with anaerobic bacteria and genital mycoplasmas which have replaced *Lactobacillus,* the normal vaginal flora. Male partners may or may not be colonized with *G. vaginalis.*

Vaginal discharge exhibiting an aminelike odor when treated with potassium hydroxide and having a pH greater than 4.7 is common, as are the presence of "clue cells" on a wet preparation. Clue cells are epithelial cells whose margins are obscured by adherent bacteria. Treatment recommendations are for metronidazole administered for 1 week. Routine treatment of male partners is not beneficial nor recommended.

CASE HISTORY

A 15-year-old African-American woman from Chicago was referred to the City of Chicago Social Hygiene Center (STD Clinic) by a disease intervention specialist who had phoned her. The reason for referral was that a recent sexual partner had been diagnosed with trichomonas urethritis and had listed her as a sexual partner.

The patient had no significant prior medical or STD history. She denied intravenous drug use at any time. No sexual partners were known to be bisexual, drug users, or hemophiliac. She had been sexually active for 3 years with fewer than 5 different partners, including a new partner (index case) during the prior 3 months. She had never undergone a pelvic examination. She had no known medicine allergies.

The patient admitted to no signs or symptoms, specifically, no vaginal discharge, dyspareunia, dysuria, abdominal pain, rash, or pruritus. Menstrual periods were regular; she had not missed a cycle. She was not using any form of contraception.

Physical examination revealed a thin female in no acute distress who appeared healthy. She was afebrile. The oral cavity, lymph nodes, skin, and abdomen were normal. The external genitalia were normal. The vagina was remarkable for the presence of a frothy, grayish white, malodorous discharge. The vaginal mucosa appeared beefy red. The cervix was erythematous and bleeding was easily induced. There was cervical motion tenderness and an endocervical whitish yellow discharge. Palpation of the adnexa was remarkable for left-sided tenderness, but no specific mass was appreciated. Rectovaginal exam also revealed some tenderness with abdominal palpation, but no discharge or intrarectal lesions were noted.

Laboratory evaluation was remarkable for the following: the wet preparation demonstrated trichomonas and "clue cells" but no yeast or hyphal elements; the Gram's stain of the endocervical secretions had greater than 50 PMNs per high-power field, but no predominant microorganisms and specifically no gram-negative intra- or extracellular diplococci; an RPR and urine pregnancy test were negative. An HIV antibody test was advised, but the patient declined.

Gonorrhea cultures of the throat, cervix, and rectum were obtained. An ELISA test for chlamydia was obtained from an endocervical specimen. A herpesvirus culture was taken from cervical secretion.

The patient was treated with empiric ceftriaxone (250 mg intramuscularly) and started on doxycycline (100 mg orally twice daily for 14 days), as well as metronidazole (500 mg twice daily for 7 days). She was instructed to return to the clinic within 48 h and to refer her sexual partners from the prior 3 months for evaluation and therapy.

After 48 h, she returned to clinic for evaluation. She still had no signs or symptoms. Examination revealed less cervical motion and adnexal tenderness but was otherwise unchanged. The gonorrhea cultures from the cervix and rectum were positive for *Neisseria gonorrhoeae*. The chlamydia and herpes assays were negative. A follow-up visit in 1 week was remarkable only for the presence of greater than 50 cells per high-power field and no other laboratory or clinical abnormalities. A repeat gonorrhea culture was negative as well.

CASE DISCUSSION

This case highlights many of the features seen in a variety of STD patients. The patient was initially referred for therapy by public health authorities as part of their routine contact tracing of a male with an atypical form of urethritis due to trichomonas. Although the patient admitted to no signs or symptoms of disease, her examination was quite abnormal. She was ultimately diagnosed with three separate infections: trichomonas vaginitis, bacterial vaginosis, and gonococcal cervicitis with salpingitis and rectal colonization. Infections such as these are common, particularly in patients with multiple sexual partners, who do not use barrier contraceptive methods, who become sexually active at a very early age and are from lower socioeconomic groups. Asymptomatic and multiple infections are likely, especially in this high-risk patient. Bacterial vaginosis, the most common infection in women attending STD clinics, may predispose patients to salpingitis. Fortunately for this woman, her infection was easily treated as an outpatient. Many patients with salpingitis require hospitalization and even surgery if a tuboovarian abscess forms. She is still at risk for potential infertility and ectopic pregnancy even though she received adequate therapy before becoming symptomatic.

REFERENCES

Books

Holmes, K. K., Mardh, P. A., Sparling, P. F., et al. *Sexually Transmitted Diseases.* New York: McGraw-Hill, 1990.
Jones, J. H. *Badblood.* New York: Free Press, 1981.
Merritt, H. H., et al. *Neurosyphilis.* New York: Oxford, 1946.

Review Articles

Centers for Disease Control. Sexually transmitted diseases treatment guidelines. September 1989. *MMWR 38:*(S-8):1, 1989.
Chapel, T. A. The signs and symptoms of secondary syphilis. *Sex. Transm. Dis.* 7:161, 1980.
Corey, L. Genital herpes. In: Holmes, K. K., Mardh, P. A., Sparling, P.F., et al., eds. *Sexually Transmitted Diseases.* New York: McGraw-Hill, 1990:391.
Fieldsteel, A. H., and Miao, R. H. Genetics of treponema. In: Schell, R. F., and Musher, D. M., eds. *Pathogenesis and Immunology of Treponemal Infection.* New York: Dekker, 1982:209.
Healy, B. P. Cardiovascular syphilis. In: Holmes, K. K., Mardh, P. A., Sparling, P. F., et al., eds. *Sexually Transmitted Diseases.* New York: McGraw-Hill, 1990.
Hook, E. Syphilis and HIV infection. *J. Infect. Dis.* 160(3):530, 1989.
Hook, E. W., and Handsfield, H. H. Gonococcal infections in the adult. In: Holmes, K. K., Mardh, P. A., Sparling, P. F., et al., eds. *Sexually Transmitted Diseases.* New York: McGraw-Hill, 1990:150.
Merritt, H. H. Early clinical and laboratory manifestations of syphilis of the central nervous system. *N. Engl. J. Med. 223:*446, 1940.
Musher, P. M. Biology of *Treponema pallidum.* In: Holmes, K. K., Mardh, P. A., Sparling, P. F., et al., eds. *Sexually Transmitted Diseases.* New York: McGraw-Hill, 1990:205.
Sparling, P. F. Biology of *Neisseria gonorrhoeae.* In: Holmes, K. K., Mardh, P. A., Sparling, P. F., et al., eds. *Sexually Transmitted Diseases.* New York: McGraw-Hill, 1990:131.
Stamm, W. E., and Holmes, K. K. *Chlamydia trachomatis* infection of the adult. In: Holmes, K. K., Mardh, P.A., Sparling, P. F., et al., eds. *Sexually Transmitted Diseases.* New York: McGraw-Hill, 1990:184.
Swartz, M. N. Neurosyphilis. In: Holmes, K. K., Mardh, P. A., Sparling, P. F., et al., eds. *Sexually Transmitted Diseases.* New York: McGraw-Hill, 1990:150.

Original Articles

Centers for Disease Control. Recommendations for diagnosing and treating syphilis in HIV-infected patients. *MMWR 37:*601, 1988.
Daling, J., et al. Sexual practices, sexually transmitted diseases, and the incidence of anal cancer. *N. Engl. J. Med. 317:*973, 1987.
Darrow, W. W., Echenberg, D. F., Jaffe, H. W., et al. Risk factors for human immunodeficiency virus (HIV) infection in homosexual men. *Am. J. Public Health 77:*479, 1987.
Dowdle, W. R., et al. Association of antigenic type of herpesvirus hominis with site of viral recovery. *J. Immunol.* 99:974, 1967.
Greenblatt, R. M., Lukehart, S. A., Plummer, F. A., et al. Genital ulceration as a risk factor for human immunodeficiency virus infection. *AIDS 2:*47, 1988.
Guinan, M. E., et al. Genital herpes simplex virus infection. *Epidemiol. Rev.* 7:127, 1988.
Madiedo, G., et al. False positive VDRL and FTA in cerebrospinal fluid. *JAMA 244:*688, 1980.
Olansky, S., et al. Untreated Syphilis in the male Negro. X: Twenty years of clinical observation of untreated syphilitic and presumably nonsyphilitic groups. *J. Chronic Dis.* 4:177, 1956.
Quinn, T. C., Glasser, D., Cannon, R. O., et al. Human immunodeficiency virus infection among patients attending clinics for sexually transmitted diseases. *N. Engl. J. Med. 318:*197, 1988.
Rockwell, D. H., et al. The Tuskegee study of untreated syphilis. *Arch. Intern. Med. 114:*792, 1964.
Stamm, W. E., Handsfield, H. H., Rompalo, A. M., et al. The association between genital ulcer disease and acquisition of HIV infection in homosexual men. *JAMA 260:*1429, 1988.
Taylor-Robinson, D., et al. Human intra-urethral inoculation of ureaplasmas. *Q. J. Med. 46:*309, 1977.

VI

Gastrointestinal Tract Infection

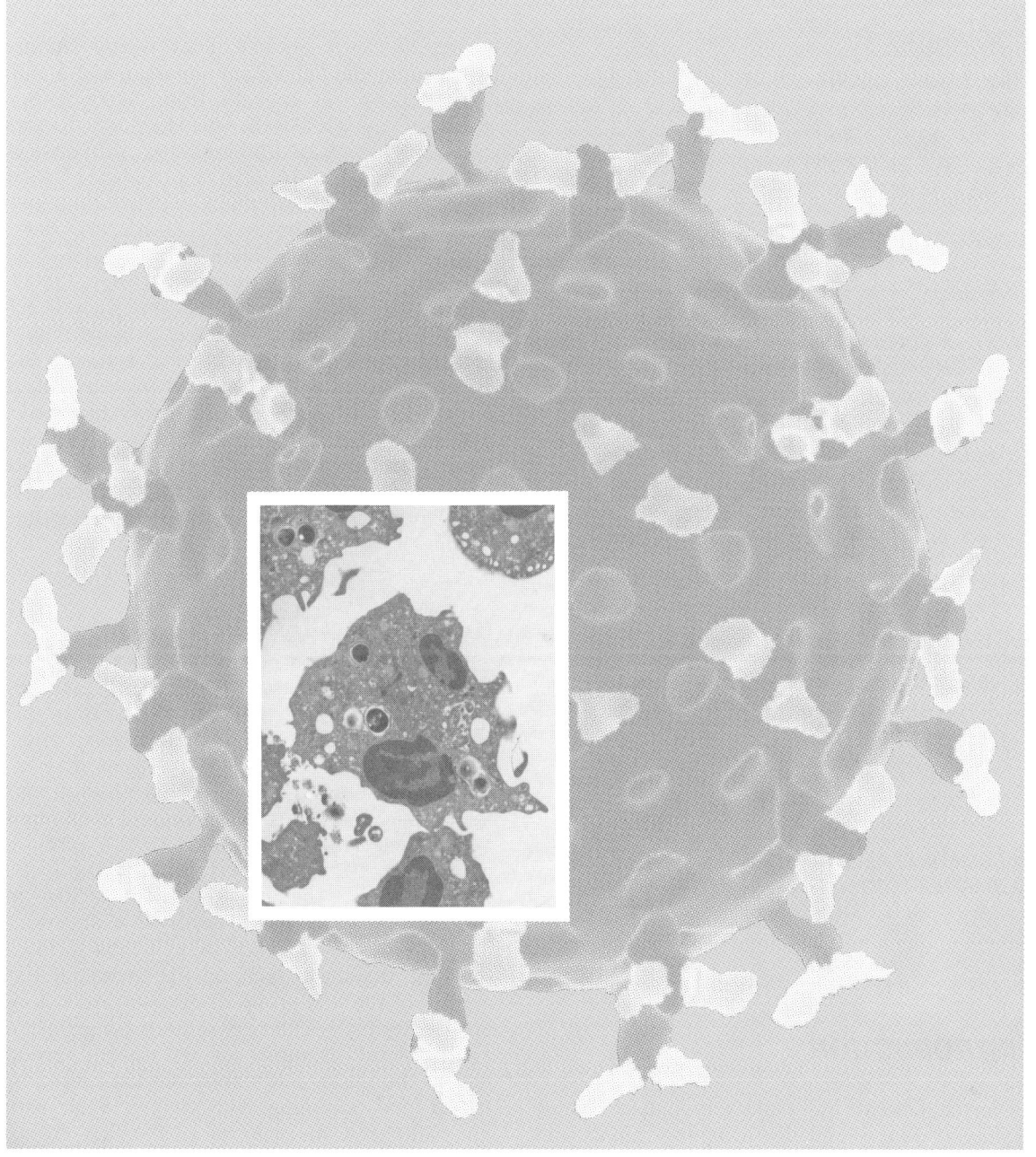

19

HERBERT M. SOMMERS, M.D. • STANFORD T. SHULMAN, M.D.

Infectious Diarrhea

INTRODUCTION

Diarrheal disease still ranks very high as a major cause of illness and death among infants and young children, especially in developing nations. Approximately 750 million illnesses and 5 million deaths result annually from diarrhea, primarily in young children. Socioeconomic factors manifested by clean drinking water, proper sewage disposal, and availability of balanced food supplies are most important in preventing gastrointestinal infections.

In 1900, the annual death rate from diarrheal disease in New York City was 5603 per 100,000 infants. In 1980, in the United States it was 3.5 per 100,000 infants, a decrease of more than 3 log. Although there has been a dramatic decrease in the number of deaths from diarrheal disease in the past 90 years, many outbreaks with substantial morbidity still occur. This chapter describes the more common infectious agents associated with gastrointestinal infection and compares the pathogenesis of the diseases they produce.

BACTERIAL DIARRHEA

Bacteria usually cause disease in the gastrointestinal tract by one of two mechanisms: (1) colonization and growth within the gastrointestinal tract, where the microorganisms may invade the tissues of the host or secrete exotoxins (a mechanism requiring the presence of replicating bacteria in the intestine) or (2) secretion of an exotoxin that is performed in food and then ingested by the host. This latter mechanism is more properly called *intoxication* and does not require the presence of living bacteria of the type that have secreted the exotoxin. Examples of the first group of diseases are salmonella enteritis, bacillary dysentery (shigellosis), and cholera; examples of the second group include botulism and staphylococcal and clostridial food poisoning. This chapter deals with the pathogenic mechanisms of the first group,

TABLE 19–1. *Characteristics of Enteropathogenic Bacterial Infections*

Organism	Diarrhea*	Dysentery†	Enterotoxin	Site	Pathogenesis	Extraintestinal Manifestations
Salmonella typhi	0	±	0	Small bowel	Penetrates mucosal cells, carried through body by macrophages	Fever, bacteremia
S. enteritidis	±	+	+	Small bowel	Penetrates mucosal cells	Fever, focal infection
var. typhimurium	±	+	+	Large bowel	Septicemia	Fever, focal infection
Shigella dysenteriae	+	+	+	Small bowel	Penetrates mucosal cells, multiplies within and kills epithelial cells.	Seizures, meningismus
S. flexneri	±	+	+	Large bowel	Cytotoxin contributes to ulceration and acute inflammatory reaction.	Focal infection rare
S. sonnei	±	+	?	Large bowel		
Vibrio cholerae	+	0	+	Small bowel	Attaches to mucosa, rarely penetrates but multiplies on cell surface. Toxin induces secretory diarrhea.	Dehydration, shock Hypokalemic nephropathy
Escherichia coli						
Enterotoxigenic	+	0	+	Small or large bowel		
Enteroinvasive	0	+	0	Small or large bowel	Various mechanisms	Shock, dehydration
Enteropathogenic	+	±	0	?		
Enteroadherent	?	?	0			
Enterohemorrhagic	+	+	+	Small or large bowel		

*Diarrhea: profuse, watery stool with no inflammatory cells.
†Dysentery: cramps, tenesmus, pus, blood in stools.

in which the replicating microorganism interacts with the host to cause disease. Infections caused by the protozoal parasites *Entamoeba histolytica* and *Giardia lamblia,* as well as the acute enteritis syndrome termed *cryptosporidiosis* (most frequently observed in the clinical setting of AIDS), are described in Chapters 20 and 27.

In the following discussion, the terms *dysentery* and *diarrhea* are used to distinguish between two distinct clinical syndromes. *Dysentery* refers to abdominal cramping, tenesmus, and pus and blood in the stool. These are symptoms associated with bacterial invasion of the intestinal wall, usually the colon, with epithelial necrosis, focal mucosal ulceration, and an acute inflammatory response as manifested by red blood cells and large numbers of neutrophils in the stool. Bacillary dysentery is produced by gram-negative bacteria of the genus *Shigella.* In contrast, the more common *diarrhea* syndrome refers to a profuse watery discharge usually from the small intestine. This syndrome does not produce histopathologic changes in the mucosa or submucosa of the intestine, and inflammatory cells are not present in the diarrheal stool. In the diarrhea syndrome, there is rapid, profuse secretion of fluid across the mucosal surface of the small intestine in response to a specific toxin (enterotoxin) secreted by the infecting microorganism. Examples of agents causing the diarrhea syndrome are *Vibrio cholerae* and toxin-producing enteropathogenic *Escherichia coli.*

In this discussion, the term *enterotoxin* refers to specific exotoxins secreted by several different bacteria that act at a specific site in the intestine. Enterotoxin is to be distinguished from *endotoxin,* the lipopolysaccharide found in the cell walls of many gram-negative bacteria. A brief summary of the characteristic distinguishing features of the most common causes of bacterial enteric disease is given in Table 19–1.

Salmonellosis

The salmonellae compose the most ubiquitous group of microorganisms that cause bacterial diarrhea. The widespread dissemination of these microorganisms reflects, in part, a vicious circle in the food-processing industry, particularly in egg and poultry production. Poultry growers use high-protein additives as food supplements. These additives are obtained from slaughterhouse by-products and mixed with feed grains. Many of the by-products are derived from animals with a high incidence of infection with salmonellae. Once ingested, the salmonellae proliferate within the bird's gastrointestinal tract. Varying numbers of salmonellae remain in the region of the cloaca, contaminating the surface of eggs and remaining in the bird after evisceration and dressing. For example, the incidence of salmonella contaminating 50-lb cans of pooled, frozen eggs has been found on occasion to be greater than 50%. Thus, the high availability of salmonellae in our food supply suggests that although more than 40,000 isolates of salmonella were recorded from humans in recent years, the actual incidence of salmonellosis is considerably greater. The possibility that most of the population in the United States has had mild clinical or subclinical disease, and therefore has been actively immunized by salmonella early in life, is suggested by Figure 19–1, in which the rate of isolation of salmonellae from humans is plotted against age. The large number of isolates from children under 10 years of age with a uniformly low incidence after age 10 may indicate a high proportion of immune persons, particularly in view of the potentially widespread exposure. As seen in Figure 19–2, the reported number of cases of salmonella infection in the United States has been rising steadily.

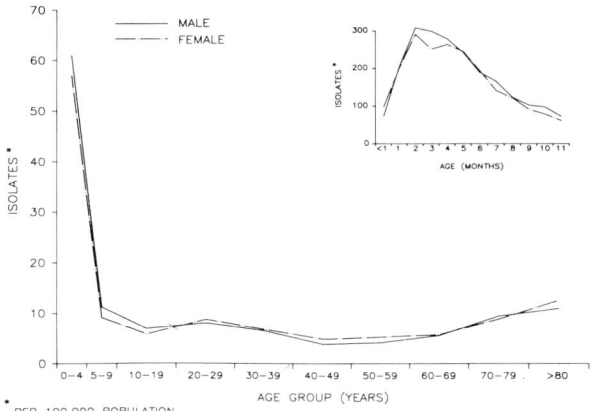

Figure 19–1. Rate of reported isolates of Salmonella, *by age in the United States in 1980. (From Centers for Disease Control.* Salmonella Surveillance, Annual Summary 1980, *U. S. Department of Health and Human Services, Public Health Service, December 1982, p. 3.)*

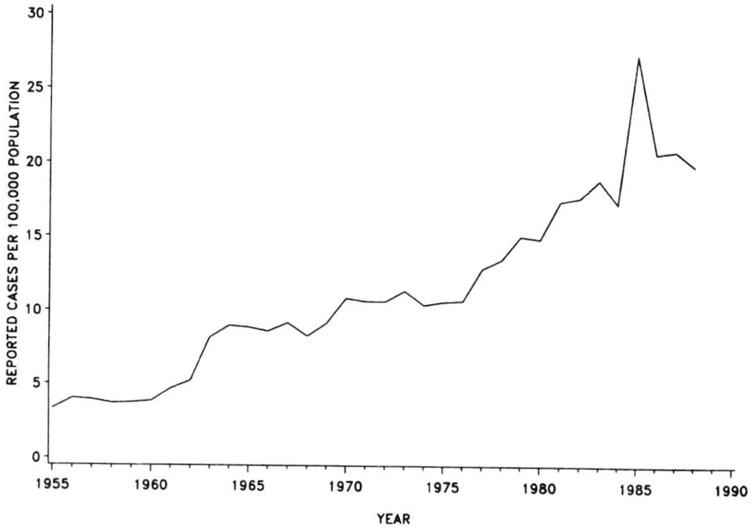

Figure 19–2. Salmonellosis (excluding typhoid fever): data for 1955–1988 (by year) for the United States. (From Morbidity and Mortality Weekly Report, Summary of notifiable disease, United States 1988. October 6, 1988, p. 36.)

Classification of the *Salmonella* species has only recently been simplified, a situation made necessary following the description of more than 1800 different serotypes. When the different *Salmonella* species are grouped according to host preference (e.g., those whose natural host is humans, those adapted primarily to animals, and those capable of inducing disease in both), three prototype species arise—*Salmonella typhi, Salmonella choleraesuis,* and *Salmonella enteritidis.* The first two species consist of a single serotype each, whereas more than 1800 different serotypes of *S. enteritidis* have been described, based upon the somatic cell-wall lipopolysaccharide (O) antigens and flagellar protein (H) antigens. Each of the individual serotypes listed under *S. enteritidis* is designated by a name following the abbreviation *var.* (variety) after the proper name *Salmonella enteritidis*—for example, *Salmonella enteritidis* var. *typhimurium, Salmonella enteritidis* var. *derby,* and so forth.

It is comforting to learn that the 10 most frequently reported serotypes generally account for about 70% of clinical isolates (Table 19–2). The similarity of serotypes between human and animal isolates illustrates the pattern of spread between humans and their food supply. In addition to serogrouping different *Salmonella* strains to identify specific organisms in epidemiologic studies, the finding of similar plasmids or antibiotic resistance patterns in epidemic strains has been useful in tracing outbreaks of salmonellosis, such as described in the next section.

Types of Infection from Salmonella

In humans, salmonella infection occurs in one of three forms: (1) enteric fever, such as typhoid or paratyphoid fever, (2) acute gastroenteritis, the most common form, and (3) extraintestinal focal infections, such as osteomyelitis, abscess,

TABLE 19–2. *Ten Most Common* Salmonella *Serotypes from Humans, U.S. 1986**

Rank	Serotype	No.	Percentage
1	S. typhimurium	10,888	26
2	S. enteritidis	5,967	14
3	S. heidelberg	5,595	13
4	S. newport	2,431	6
5	S. hadar	1,552	4
6	S. infantis	1,104	3
7	S. angona	912	2
8	S. montevideo	775	2
9	S. muenchen	694	2
10	S. braenderup	616	1
	Total	30,534	73
	Total (all serotypes)	42,028	

*From Centers for Disease Control, MMWR, Vol. 37, No. SS-2, 1988.

empyema, and concomitant with widespread reconstructive vascular surgery, local infection at the site of peripheral vascular prostheses.

Enteric Fever. Typhoid fever represents the classic enteric infection, spread by contaminated food or polluted water supplies. In contrast to simple salmonella gastroenteritis, *Salmonella typhi* causes gastrointestinal symptoms only late in the course of the disease, usually after prolonged fever, bacteremia, and finally localization of infection in the submucosal lymphoid tissue (Peyer's patches) of the small intestine. *S. typhi* is an example of a facultative intracellular parasite, surviving well within macrophages and requiring cell-mediated immunity for control. Establishment of chronic infection in the biliary tree may be related in part to intracellular persistence of the microorganism in macrophages, and is the mechanism by which chronic asymptomatic carriage ("Typhoid Mary") persists. In addition to protection of the bacteria from humoral defense mechanisms, intracellular residence within macrophages makes eradication by antibiotics difficult. Several serotypes of *S. enteritidis,* for example, var. *paratyphi A* and var. *schottmuelleri,* may also cause a clinical syndrome of enteric fever similar to that of *S. typhi,* with bacteremia. *S. choleraesuis* also is associated with enteric fever. Unlike salmonella gastroenteritis, enteric fever is a prolonged, generalized, usually serious infection that requires specific therapy. Fortunately, the incidence of typhoid fever in the United States has been falling since 1900, although the incidence has plateaued since the late 1960s. Approximately 500 cases occur annually in the United States, but it is estimated that 33 million cases with 500,000 deaths occur annually worldwide.

Gastroenteritis. Acute gastroenteritis related to the various serotypes of *S. enteritidis* varies from very mild to severe infection and may occasionally be associated with bacteremia or bacteriuria. In mild or moderate cases, prudent withholding of antibiotics does not slow the clinical recovery and results in more rapid clearing of the microorganism from the stool. The decision to withhold antibiotics depends on the severity of the illness in the individual patient and the presence of underlying disease, such as cancer, immunologic defects including AIDS, very young or very old age, or occlusive vascular disease (e.g., sickle cell disease), which could impair host defense mechanisms. Salmonella

gastroenteritis has its highest incidence in the first year of life.

Signs and symptoms of salmonella gastroenteritis vary widely, but usually include nausea, abdominal cramps, and diarrhea, which sometimes becomes bloody. The microorganisms may invade focal areas of the small and large intestine, where they are ingested by neutrophils and macrophages in the lamina propria (Fig. 19–3). Sigmoidoscopic and biopsy studies of humans with salmonellosis may show active colitis, with focal ulceration and submucosal microabscesses. The mechanism of diarrhea appears to involve both mucosal invasion and enterotoxin production.

Extraintestinal Infection. Extraintestinal infections with salmonella are frequently associated with other chronic disease or with a defect in host defenses. Patients with sickle cell disease are more susceptible to infection (particularly osteomyelitis) with salmonella, and patients with metastatic cancer are more prone to develop extraintestinal infections than the normal population. The increased incidence of salmonella disease in cancer and in sickle cell patients may be in part related to localization of microorganisms in foci of ischemia.

A variety of serotypes of *S. enteritidis* have been found to produce infections of peripheral vascular grafts. Grafts of abdominal aortic and femoral arterial bypasses frequently yield salmonella if individuals with these prostheses become infected. This may reflect continuing intake of the microorganisms from various food sources, with a resulting low-level intestinal colonization and periodic subclinical bacteremia. Intravascular salmonellae tend to localize at sites of atheromatous ulceration and set up foci of proliferation and infection. Two serotypes, *S. choleraesuis* and *S. enteritidis* var. *typhimurium,* are most commonly involved. The presence of foreign bodies in the vascular system, as elsewhere, predisposes to colonization by smaller numbers of microorganisms than otherwise are needed to initiate infection.

In choosing an antibiotic for salmonellosis, there is limited correlation of *in vitro* antibiotic susceptibility testing with therapeutic response. Despite *in vitro* sensitivity, the aminoglycosides are not clinically useful, presumably because of the acid pH in the phagolysosomes that usually contain the intracellular salmonellae. Ampicillin, amoxicillin, chloramphenicol, ceftriaxone, and trimethoprim-sulfamethoxazole are the agents least likely to be associated with clinical failure. However, antibiotic resistance has been

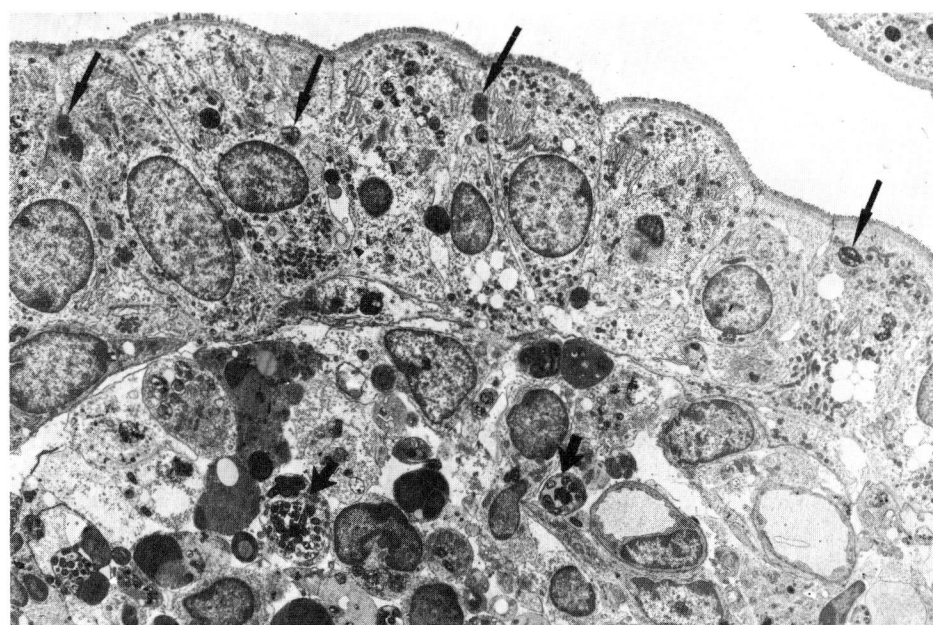

Figure 19–3. Salmonella *gastroenteritis. Cytoplasmic dense bodies (thin arrows) are readily identified. Bacteria are absent from epithelium. In contrast, many phagocytosed bacteria (thick arrows) are present in neutrophils and macrophages in the lamina propria (× 2500.) (From Takeuchi, A., and Sprinz, H. Electron-microscope studies of experimental* Salmonella *infection in the preconditioned guinea pig. Am. J. Pathol. 51:137, 1967.)*

increasing worldwide. Patients with a disseminated form of salmonellosis or enteric fever should be treated for 2–6 weeks. The dose and duration of treatment depends on the specific site of infection and its clinical manifestations.

Epidemiologic Notes*

Between March and May, 17 infections of *Salmonella agona* were detected in residents of a northeast Arkansas town. Four were hospitalized with symptoms of severe gastroenteritis, including nausea, diarrhea, fever, and abdominal cramps. The 13 remaining persons were asymptomatic. Five infected persons were detected through the routine salmonellosis screening program required by Arkansas state law for food handlers, and the remainder during routine follow-up of contacts of infected persons. Epidemiologic investigation revealed that the only common association of all infected persons was that they had all patronized a local drive-in restaurant (A). None of 23 individuals who had not patronized restaurant A became infected ($p = 0.004$). Analysis of food-specific attack rates for infected persons and 50 noninfected patrons and employees of restaurant A showed that the infection rate was significantly higher

*Adapted from report by Centers for Disease Control.

in persons eating cole slaw and onions (Table 19–3). Investigation of restaurant A revealed marginal sanitary conditions and numerous errors in food-handling procedures. The only work table was used to cut up chicken and catfish as well as cabbage, onions, and lettuce. Employees also ate at this table during lunch breaks. *Salmonella agona* was isolated from the table top, knives, meat slicer, sink, fresh-frozen catfish, fresh chicken parts, and lettuce. From the food-specific attack rates and the culture results, it was apparent that cross-contamination occurred from either raw chicken or catfish to other food items that were eaten raw.

Further investigation revealed that the chicken was the source of infection for restaurant A and came from a large Mississippi poultry operation. *Salmonella agona* was recovered from the slaughterhouse and from offal at the rendering plant but not from the hatchery, breeder, or broiler flocks nor from the complete feed or various feed ingredients. However, one or two deliveries of feed ingredients were made weekly, and samples were collected more than 2 months after the clinical cases occurred. Peruvian fishmeal made up 8% of the complete feed ration for the broiler flocks. The Food and Drug Administration, which is responsible for monitoring imported fishmeal for salmonella contamination, isolated *Salmonella agona* from

TABLE 19–3. *Food-Specific Attack Rates, Restaurant A, Arkansas**

Food Item	Ate			Did Not Eat		
	Infected	Noninfected	Attack Rate (%)	Infected	Noninfected	Attack Rate (%)
Slaw	15	29	34†	2	21	9†
Hamburgers	14	42	25	3	8	27
Hot Dogs	7	18	28	10	32	24
Chili Dogs	9	17	35	8	33	20
Coney Dogs	9	16	36	8	19	30
Chicken	11	24	32	6	27	18
Onions‡	10	16	39	2	20	9
French Fries	17	45	28	0	5	0

*From Centers for Disease Control, MMWR, Vol. 22, No. 4, 1973.
†$p < 0.05$
‡Interviewees were asked to add this item to the questionnaire, but not everyone did so.

Peruvian fishmeal and from Puerto Rican fishmeal on a number of occasions. Domestically produced fishmeal, which is also monitored for salmonella contamination, has never been found positive for this serotype. Investigation of this outbreak was facilitated by the fact that, at this time, *S. agona* was only rarely encountered. Frequently, plasmid profiles and antibiotic sensitivity pattern analysis are necessary to track a salmonella strain for epidemiologic purposes.

Shigellosis

Species of the genus *Shigella,* in contrast to those of *Salmonella,* are essentially restricted to humans as both a natural reservoir and as the major mode of dissemination. Shigellosis, or bacillary dysentery, is transmitted by the fecal–oral route, primarily by hand-to-mouth contact, but also by food handlers and insect vectors (e.g., flies) in areas of food preparation. Where outdoor latrines are prevalent, the incidence of the disease is sometimes directly related to the large number of flies attracted to the latrines. The availability of water for frequent washing of hands is of importance in controlling outbreaks. As few as 10 bacilli are said to be capable of causing bacillary dysentery, in contrast to the 10^5 organisms necessary to induce salmonella enteric fever. Because of inadequate sanitary precautions, both shigellosis and hepatitis are endemic in institutions for the care of mentally retarded children. Reflecting both the mode of fecal–oral transmission and perhaps some element of local immunization, the highest isolation rates for shigella are in children younger than 5 years old. Fatality rates are highest in young malnourished children. The incidence of bacillary dysentery in older age groups is similar to that for salmonellosis. In

contrast to salmonellosis, the reported incidence of shigella has been stable in the United States, after an earlier decline (Fig. 19–4).

Four species of *Shigella* are described: *S. dysenteriae,* with 10 subtypes, and *S. boydii,* both rarely seen; *S. flexneri,* with eight subtypes; and *S. sonnei,* having a single type. For reasons that are not apparent, the incidence of various species has varied in different parts of the world over cycles of several years. For many years, *S. flexneri* was the most common species isolated in the United States, but for the past 15 years, *S. sonnei* has been dominant. Several years ago, the appearance of the very virulent *S. dysenteriae* type I (Shiga's bacillus) from an endemic focus in Central America produced several outbreaks of severe disease in the southwestern United States.

Infections with shigella differ from those of salmonella in that tissue invasion in the former is usually limited to the lining of epithelial cells and possibly the submucosa of the colon. Rarely do the microorganisms penetrate beyond the submucosa, and extraintestinal infections with shigella seldom occur. Following invasion of the epithelial cell, a potent cytotoxin, which is a multimer of one A subunit and five B subunits with binding specificity for a microvillus membrane glycolipid receptor, is released (see below). Severe cases of dysentery may be associated with focal mucosal destruction and ulceration but do not extend beyond the intestinal tract. Shigellae are rarely found in blood cultures. The limited exposure of shigellae to deep structures in the body may account for the minimal amounts of circulating antibody found in convalescent patients.

Episomal Drug Resistance

In 1955, a woman returned to Japan from Hong Kong, ill with a strain of *Shigella* resistant

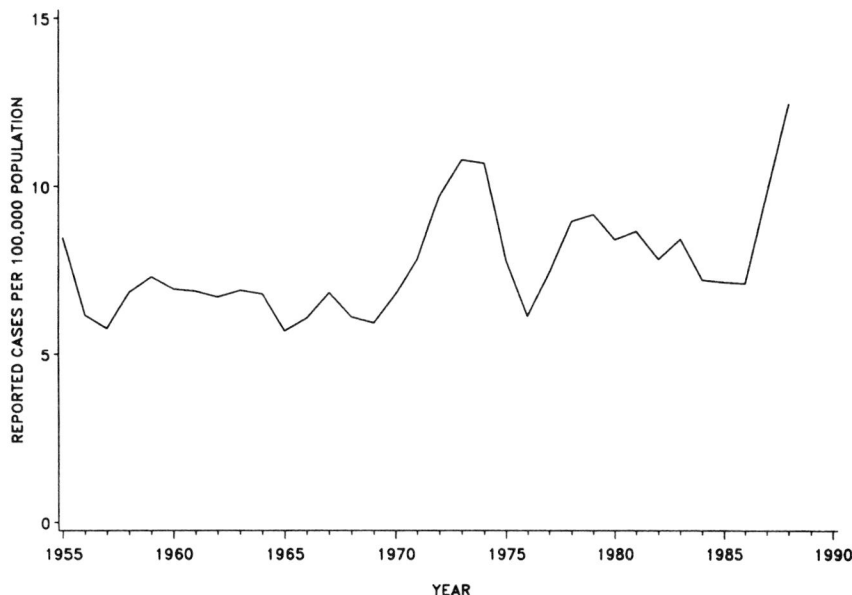

Figure 19–4. Shigellosis: data for 1955–1988 (by year) for the United States. Reported cases per 100,000 population. Data is from the National Shigella Surveillance System. (From Morbidity and Mortality Weekly Report, Summary of notifiable disease, United States 1988. October 6, 1989, p. 36.)

to several previously effective antimicrobial agents. Over the next few years, outbreaks of shigella dysentery appeared that were resistant to multiple antimicrobial agents. A combination of findings suggested that the multiple antibiotic resistance patterns could not be explained only by spontaneous mutation of the microorganisms with development of resistance to individual drugs. Both drug-sensitive and drug-resistant strains of *Shigella* could be isolated from a single outbreak and even from the same patient. It was also found that the administration of a single antimicrobial agent (e.g., sulfonamide) to a patient harboring drug-sensitive *Shigella* could promptly induce the appearance of strains resistant to four different antimicrobial agents, including drugs not previously used on that patient or in that outbreak. It was then noted that patients harboring drug-resistant mutants of *Shigella* also harbored *Escherichia coli* or other bacteria resistant to the same drugs. In contrast to these clinical findings, the development of multiple drug resistance from mutation by bacteria *in vitro* occurred very slowly by repeated subcultures to graded concentrations of single drugs. Taken together, these findings suggested that resistance to multiple antibiotics was being transferred by a genetic mechanism.

Such a mechanism is now known to function by means of sexual conjugation (Fig. 19–5).

Sexual conjugation of bacteria may result in the transfer of *episomes*, also called *resistance transfer*, or *R factors*. Episomes are nonchromosomal packets of genetic material that may control resistance of organisms to one or more antibiotics, as well as controlling other characteristics of the organism, for example, enterotoxin secretion. The finding that the transfer of episomes was not restricted to bacteria of the same species or genus but could also occur between widely varying bacteria was sobering. The possibility existed that the development of antibiotic resistance by such transfer factors might rapidly make existing drugs obsolete and quickly outdate new antibiotics. Several prospective

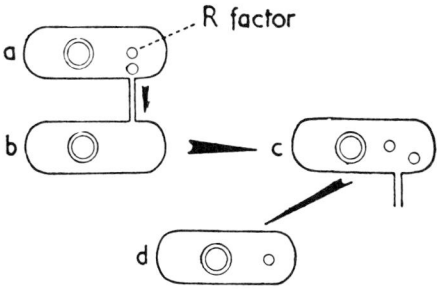

Figure 19–5. Transfer of drug resistance by conjugation (cytoplasmic R factor). (From Crofton, J. Some principles in the chemotherapy of bacterial infections. Br. Med. J. 2:209, 1969.)

studies have shown that a more significant factor in developing strains of bacteria resistant to antimicrobial agents has been the appearance of local "hospital" strains, not associated with transfer factors, that disseminate by interpersonal transfer. Although episomal transfer of antibacterial resistance remains a potential danger in clinical medicine, it has not developed into the serious problem that was initially feared, for reasons that are not completely clear. Episomal transfer is not frequent in the absence of an antimicrobial agent exerting selective pressure, and, once acquired, there is a tendency for the bacterium to lose the transfer factor after several generations.

Antibiotic resistance of *Shigella* to ampicillin has been increasing steadily, with more than 50% of recent U.S. isolates and up to 90% elsewhere resistant to ampicillin. In mild infections, the patient may clear the microorganism from the gastrointestinal tract more quickly if antibiotics are not used in therapy. An important exception is infection with *Shigella dysenteriae* type I. Disease from this microorganism is usually associated with significant morbidity and mortality, and it can produce devastating pandemics.

Shigella Enterotoxin

Previously it was thought that with the exception of *S. dysenteriae* type I (Shiga's bacillus), the shigellae did not secrete enterotoxin. It is now established that both *S. sonnei* and *S. flexneri* can produce a toxin quite similar to that of *S. dysenteriae*. These toxins can be neutralized by antibody to *S. dysenteriae* toxin. Conversely, *S. sonnei* and *S. flexneri* can stimulate production of an IgM antibody that neutralizes the Shiga toxin. Clinically, most patients with enteritis from *S. sonnei* and *S. flexneri* do not show the severity of illness associated with *S. dysenteriae* type I. It is now recognized that the shigellae secrete an enterotoxin that can bind to epithelial cells in the small intestine in a way that is somewhat analogous to the toxin of *Vibrio cholerae* (see below) and that has cytotoxic, neurotoxic, and enterotoxic (induces fluid secretion) properties.

Cholera

Cholera is a disease only of humans. People and their fecally contaminated water supplies are the major reservoirs of infection. Cholera is an ancient disease, having been known for thousands of years; epidemics consistent with cholera were described in Sanskrit writings. The disease has been endemic in Asia for centuries and is most prevalent along the great rivers of the Indian subcontinent. Since the 19th century, seven pandemics of cholera have appeared, each claiming large numbers of lives. In England in 1849, John Snow, a perceptive physician, became convinced that the disease was being spread by the drinking water in London. To stop the use of drinking water from one well in an area of high infection, Snow removed the handle of the Broad Street water pump, succeeding in reducing the number of new cases, and thereby helped establish the means of spread of the disease. This stands as one of the earliest examples of interventional epidemiology.

Although there has been very little cholera in most of the Western World since 1900, the reappearance of a pandemic in the Philippines in 1958 and its subsequent spread to Asia, Africa, Oceania, and the Middle East over the next 30 years are constant reminders of this disease. During the massive population shifts resulting from the Pakistani-Indian War in 1971, thousands of deaths from cholera occurred. An outbreak in Italy and an epidemic in Portugal occurred in 1973. A single case occurred along the Texas Gulf Coast in August, 1973, in a man who had not traveled out of the United States and had no known contact with foreign travelers.

In August and September of 1978, 11 cases of cholera occurred in residents living along the Louisiana coast. Most cases were associated with the ingestion of steamed crabs and were due to *Vibrio cholerae*, biotype *El Tor*, serotype *Inaba*. During the epidemiologic investigation, the organism was cultured from leftover steamed crabs as well as from stool specimens from several asymptomatic persons who had eaten the crabs at the same time as those who developed cholera. *V. cholerae* could be recovered from crabs boiled or steamed for 8 min but not from those cooked for 10 min. The U.S. Public Health Service has recommended that all crabs be boiled or steamed a minimum of 15 min before serving. Crabs from this Gulf Coast region are distributed by air freight to many cities in the United States.

Since the 1978 outbreak of cholera in Louisiana, individual cases and several small epidemics have occurred along the Gulf Coast from Florida to Texas. One reason for the increased incidence of laboratory-confirmed cholera is a heightened awareness of the disease and the more frequent practice of inoculating stool specimens onto the necessary selective culture media. Failure to consider the disease and to culture appropriately may have obscured outbreaks in the past.

In 1991 a major outbreak of cholera occurred in Peru, Ecuador, and other South American countries, affecting many thousands of individuals.

Clinical Disease

Clinically, the patient developing cholera first notices a slight fullness in the abdomen and loss of appetite. His hands and feet become cold, and he may vomit. Shortly thereafter he begins to have large numbers of liquid stools, first brown and then almost clear, which contain small amounts of mucus and are classically described as "rice water" stools. If fluids are not restored by aggressive oral or intravenous therapy, death from severe dehydration and hypovolemic shock can occur within hours or a few days (Fig. 19–6). In severe cases, a stool volume of up to 24 L/day may occur. In the acute disease, 50% or more of patients die unless proper fluid therapy is given.

Pathophysiology of Cholera

In contrast to salmonellosis and shigellosis, *Vibrio cholerae* does *not* penetrate the epithelial surface of the gastrointestinal tract to incite an inflammatory response but rather elicits its effects through the secretion of a potent enterotoxin (choleragen). The microorganism first colonizes the small intestine, and then secretes choleragen, which results in a massive outpouring of isotonic fluid from the mucosal surface of the small intestine. Grossly, the bowel may be slightly edematous, but histologically it appears normal (Fig. 19–7). Although occasional inflammatory cells can be seen, there is no significant cellular response, either within the mucosa or in the intestinal lumen.

Recent studies have provided a great deal of information on the mode of action of the toxin (Table 19–4). Since the toxin is essentially "outside" the body, it first must bind to the mucosal cell surface. Choleragen is an oligomeric protein toxin with a molecular weight of 84,000 d and is made up of one A and five B subunits. The B subunits each have a molecular weight of 11,000 d and the A subunit has a molecular weight of 27,000 d with two fragments, A_1 and A_2, held together by a disulfide bond (Fig. 19–8). When choleragen is exposed to small-bowel epithelial cells, the B subunits bind to G_{M1} ganglioside on the cell membrane. The A subunit passes through the cell membrane, where the disulfide bond is hydrolyzed and A_1 subunit is separated from A_2. The A_1 subunit possesses ADP-ribosyl transferase activity and stimulates the transfer of ADP-ribose from NAD to a GTP-binding protein that controls adenylate cyclase activity. ADP ribosylation of the GTP-binding protein inhibits the GTP turn-off reac-

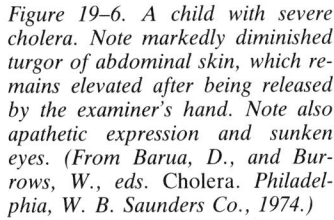

Figure 19–6. A child with severe cholera. Note markedly diminished turgor of abdominal skin, which remains elevated after being released by the examiner's hand. Note also apathetic expression and sunken eyes. (From Barua, D., and Burrows, W., eds. Cholera. Philadelphia, W. B. Saunders Co., 1974.)

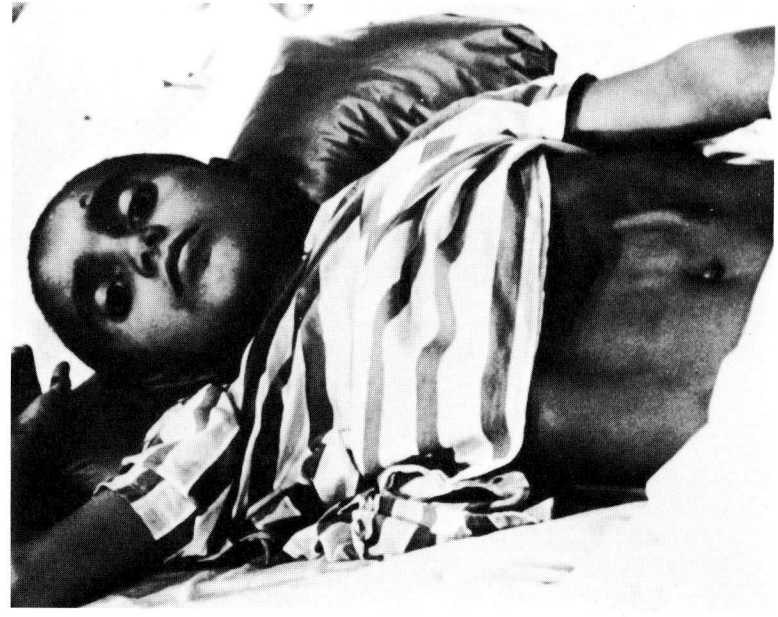

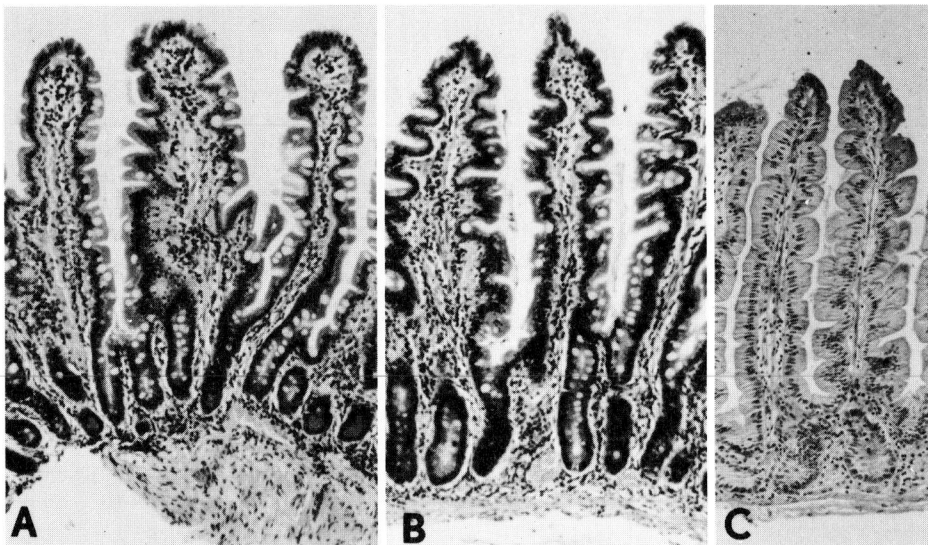

Figure 19–7. Three jejunal biopsies. All hemotoxylin and eosin (× 200). A. Small bowel biopsy from a 32-year-old Pakistani male with acute cholera of 38-hours' duration. Patient had received intravenous fluids for 24 hours. The epithelium is intact and the goblet cells, especially toward the tips of the villi, have discharged their mucus. A moderate inflammatory infiltrate composed of lymphocytes, monocytes, and plasma cells is present in the lamina propria. The subepithelial capillaries are hyperemic. B. Small bowel biopsy of a 28-year-old asymptomatic Pakistani male who served as a control. Biopsies A and B are almost identical. A similar degree of inflammatory infiltration is present in the lamina propria of both of these biopsies. (Pakistani biopsies courtesy of the Department of Experimental Pathology, Walter Reed Army Institute of Research.) C. Small bowel biopsy from a 30-year-old asymptomatic North American male. Very few inflammatory cells are present in the lamina propria of this biopsy. The villi are shorter in length, indicating that the biopsy was taken more distally than the biopsies in A and B. (From Barua, D., and Burrows, W., eds. Cholera. Philadelphia, W. B. Saunders Co., 1974.)

tion and causes a sustained increase in the adenylate cyclase activity. This results in increased intracellular cAMP, which through effects mediated by G proteins that interact with guanine nucleotides, causes secretion of isotonic fluid from the intestinal epithelial cell into the lumen of the small intestine.

The bound toxin does not block or prevent reabsorption of sodium and water by the small intestine or the colon. However, in acute cholera, the secretion of water and ions from the mucosal cells of the small intestine exceeds the capacity of the colon to absorb the loss. In mild to moderate cases, fluid balance can be achieved and water reabsorption facilitated by the use of oral rehydration solutions prepared from prepackaged envelopes containing 3.5 g NaCl, 2.5 g $NaHCO_3$, 1.5 g KCl, and 20 g glucose per liter of boiled water. Inclusion of 2–5% glucose or sucrose promotes sodium, electrolyte, and water reabsorption in both the small intestine and colon (Fig. 19–9). Inclusion of rice powder or other glucose polymers and amino acids has also proved effective. These solutions have been very successful in maintaining hydration in patients in parts of the world where intravenous fluids are not available. Widespread use of oral rehydration solutions, promoted by the World Health Organization, has substantially reduced mortality from gastrointestinal infections, particularly in young children.

Cholera is a self-limited disease, provided that the patient does not die from dehydration or shock before recovery. Although *Vibrio cholerae* is susceptible to tetracycline and other agents, the irreversible binding of the toxin to the epithelial surface of the mucosal cell results in little or no evidence of clinical effect from an antibiotic for at least the first 24–36 h. Twenty-four to forty-eight h is needed for new epithelial cells to extend from the mucosal crypts in the small intestine to the tips of the villi, replacing those cells that are bound by cholera toxin and thus are secreting large amounts of water and electrolytes. The resistance of *Vibrio cholerae* to tetracycline, chloramphenicol, and kanamycin has increased recently.

Immunity to Cholera

The issue of immunity to cholera is complex. Recurrent infections are rare, and highly effective immunity appears to develop. Humans produce both circulating vibriocidal immunoglobu-

TABLE 19–4. *Virulence Properties of* Vibrio Cholerae *and* Enterotoxigenic Escherichia Coli *(ETEC)**

| Property | V. cholerae O Group 1 | ETEC | |
		LT	ST
Enterotoxins			
Molecular weight	83,000	73,000	~ 1,500–5,000
Subunits	B and A	B and A	None identified
Mucosal receptors	G_{M1} ganglioside	G_{M1} ganglioside	None identified
Biochemical action	Activates adenylate cyclase	Activates adenylate cyclase	Activates guanylate cyclase
Physiologic action	Prolonged hypersecretion after lag	Prolonged hypersecretion after lag	Rapid-onset, short-lived hypersecretion
Immunologic properties	Closely related to LT	Closely related to cholera toxin and to other LT preparations	Not antigenic in natural state
Assay methods	Animal models, tissue culture, immunologic method, binding methods	Animal models, tissue culture, immunologic methods, binding methods	Animal models only
Genetic control in bacteria	Chromosomal	Plasmid	Plasmid
Colonization Factors	No structural proteins known; flagella may be important	CFA I and CFA II, plasmid-mediated; others have been identified as well	
Serotypes	*Ogawa, Inaba* (only two)	Most commonly O6:K15:H16, O8:K40:H9, O78:H11, O78:H12, O25:K7:H42, O15:H11, O115:H51, O128:H (variable), may be many others; geographically determined	
Antibiotic Sensitivities	Usually sensitive to tetracycline	In some parts of the world, unusually sensitive to antibiotics (Kenya, Morocco, United States, Bangladesh); in other parts of the world, antibiotic-resistance patterns similar to non-ETEC strains (Philippines, Thailand, Honduras)	

*Adapted from Sack, R. B. Enterotoxigenic *Escherichia coli:* Identification and characterization. *J. Infect. Dis.* 142:279, 1980. Reprinted with permission.
Note: LT = heat-labile toxin; ST = heat-stable toxin; B = binding; A = active; CFA = colonization factor antigen.

lins and local secretory IgA to the bacteria, as well as antibodies to the enterotoxin. Although circulating antibodies can readily cross the mucosa and enter the gastrointestinal tract, these antibodies may not survive enzymatic digestion. In the small intestine, secretory IgA develops soon after antigenic stimulus and is thought to function by preventing mucosal attachment of

toxin and to inhibit vibrio replication. Although secretory IgA is resistant to enzymatic digestion, it persists a relatively short time after antigenic stimulus.

Recently, vaccine preparations containing purified B subunits of choleragen have been developed. These preparations are effective toxoids and stimulate antibodies to prevent the

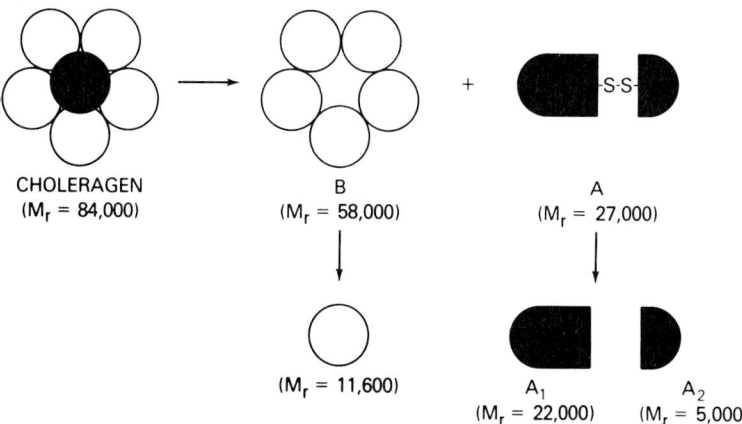

Figure 19–8. Subunit structure of choleragen. (From Fishman, P. H. Mechanism of action of cholera toxin: Events on the cell surface. In: Field, M., Fordtran, J. S., and Schultz, S. G., eds. Secretory Diarrhea. Clinical Physiology Series, American Physiological Society. Baltimore: Williams & Wilkins, 1981, p. 86.)

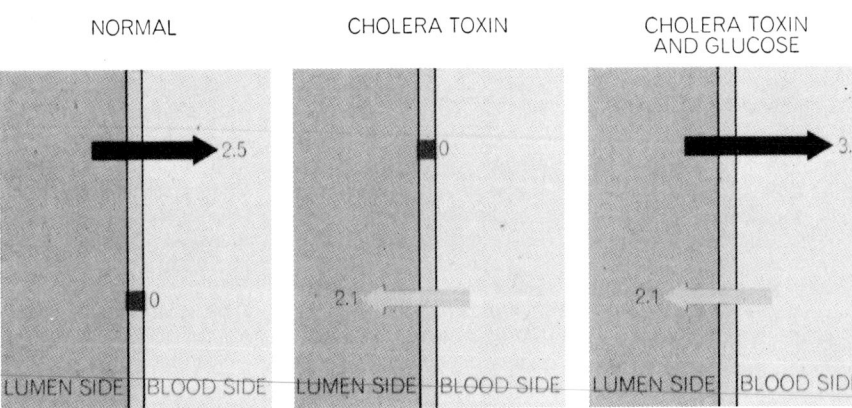

NORMAL   CHOLERA TOXIN   CHOLERA TOXIN
AND GLUCOSE

Figure 19–9. *Net ion flow across intestinal tissue is given in microequivalents per square centimeter per hour. The normal flow of sodium ion (top) and chloride ion (bottom) is reversed (center) if cholera toxin is added to fluid. Adding glucose on lumen side helps restore balance (right). (From Hirschhorn, N., and Greenough, W. B. III. Cholera.* Sci. Am. 225:15, 1971. Copyright © 1971 by Scientific American, Inc. All rights reserved.)

intact toxin from binding to intestinal cells. Oral immunization with the B subunit vaccine together with killed organisms stimulates secretory IgA responses and protection. Recombinant vaccines with B subunit are being developed and tested.

Infection with Vibrio parahaemolyticus

A related microorganism achieving increasing recognition as an agent of bacterial diarrhea is *Vibrio parahaemolyticus*. The disease caused by this microorganism may be sudden in onset with marked diarrhea. Usually, the symptoms and duration of the infection are not as severe as those of cholera. *V. parahaemolyticus* prefers salty environments and normally is found in seawater or tidal flats. For many years it has been the most common cause of food poisoning in Japan, usually transmitted by sashimi (raw fish). Although previously not recognized in the United States, within the last two decades *V. parahaemolyticus* has been found to be the cause of several outbreaks of food poisoning. Most recognized outbreaks have occurred along the Atlantic or Gulf Coasts and have involved steamed crabs. Other shellfish have also been found to contain the microorganism, and its survival in frozen shrimp has been described.

Non-O Group 1 (Non-O1) Vibrio cholerae

Non-O group 1 (non-O1) *V. cholerae* (previously known as nonagglutinating vibrios or non-

cholera vibrios) differs in the laboratory from the O group 1 strain, which causes clinical cholera, by its failure to agglutinate in vibrio O group 1 antiserum. The organism is not uncommon in the brackish water of bays and estuaries and has been isolated in both domestic animals and humans. Some human patients with infection give a history of foreign travel, whereas others report having recently ingested raw oysters. Symptoms include diarrhea, abdominal cramps, fever, and, in about one third of patients, bloody diarrhea. Vibrio species associated with non-O1 *V. cholerae* gastroenteritis include *V. alginolyticus, V. hollisae, V. mimicus, V. fluvialis,* and *V. vulnificus.* In addition to gastroenteritis, *V. mimicus* and *V. vulnificus* have been associated with infections of the external ear canal or with soft tissue wounds contaminated by either sea or brackish water. Although in the past most such isolates have been found in halophilic environments such as seawater, several patients in New Mexico and Oklahoma have developed wound infections following contamination with brackish water. Therefore, such infections are not limited to coastal communities. Species of *Vibrio* should be suspected in any serious wound or ear infection contaminated with brackish or seawater.

Enteropathogenic Escherichia coli

For many years, veterinarians have known that certain strains of *Escherichia coli* were associated with severe diarrhea in piglets and calves. Frequently, entire litters of piglets would die within a few hours to several days from a profuse, watery diarrhea.

In 1945 and 1947, a number of outbreaks of lethal diarrhea in human infants occurred in England, Mexico, and Scotland. Several of these outbreaks were associated with *E. coli* serotypes (O111:B4 and O55:B5) which caused diarrhea more readily in infants than other *E. coli* serotypes. In the years following these outbreaks, additional serotypes were described that were also isolated from babies with severe diarrhea. Most of the outbreaks of diarrhea in infants from enteropathogenic *E. coli* (EPEC) were found to be due to 12–15 specific serotypes. It is now clear that there are at least five different categories of diarrhea-producing *E. coli:* enterotoxigenic, enteroinvasive, enteropathogenic, enterohemorrhagic (or enterocytotoxic), and enteroadherent (or enteroaggregative). *E. coli* can produce disease resembling cholera or dysentery, depending on the strain involved.

Diarrhea Syndrome

Classically, this disease is seen in infants in hospital nurseries with a clinical picture of sudden onset of severe, watery diarrhea leading to dehydration and shock; a high mortality rate accompanies the disease. During 1960 and 1961 in Chicago, more than 1300 cases of gastroenteritis with 77 deaths occurred in infants and young children. The highest attack rate was in newborn infants, who also had the highest death rate (16%). Breast-fed infants were less likely to be involved, and the disease was thought to result from colonization of the small intestine by enteropathogenic strains of *Escherichia coli*. It has become clear that EPEC is among the most common causes of diarrhea worldwide, producing both epidemic and endemic disease in infants, as well as "traveler's diarrhea" (see below).

It was in the 1960s that enterotoxin-producing *E. coli* (ETEC) were first isolated from young domestic animals with severe diarrheal disease. The enterotoxic strains proved to be the same serotypes already known to cause diarrhea in these animals. Soon thereafter, strains of ETEC were described as the etiologic agents of severe choleralike illnesses in humans. These ETEC, however, did not belong to the EPEC serotypes previously known to cause diarrhea in babies.

ETEC produce one or both of two protein toxins, one heat-labile, which activates adenyl cyclase and is inactivated by heat (60°C), and the other heat-stable. The biochemical and physiologic characteristics of these two toxins are given in Table 19–5. Abbreviations commonly used for these two types of ETEC toxins are LT = heat-labile toxin; ST = heat-stable toxin. Additional virulence factors of ETEC include colonization factors CFA-I and CFA-II, necessary for the attachment of the organism to intestinal epithelial cells (see Table 19–4).

Both LT and ST, as well as CFA-I and CFA-II, are encoded by transferable plasmids. Of considerable importance is the fact that LT is immunologically similar to choleragen and has the same subunit structure. ST is a much smaller molecule than LT (molecular weight approximately 1500–5000 d) and is not antigenic. LT appears to be the same entity in all strains of ETEC, and the B subunit of LT binds to the G_{M1} ganglioside, as does the B subunit of choleragen. The mechanism of action of ST involves activation of guanylate cyclase.

Individual *E. coli* strains may produce one or both of the enterotoxins, depending on their plasmids. Organisms carrying both plasmids usually are associated with more severe diarrhea for a longer period than are those having plasmids producing only ST. There is some association between serotype and enterotoxin type.

The diagnosis of ETEC-mediated diarrhea requires demonstration of the presence of enterotoxins. This can be done by analysis of fluid accumulation in the ileal loop in various animal models (Table 19–5); by cell culture; by the immunologic demonstration of LT in the stool or culture fluid specimens; or by the identification of enterotoxin-producing genes by oligonucleotide probes. Culture of *E. coli* for unique biochemical or colonial characteristics is of little value.

E. coli strains associated with enterotoxin formation and watery diarrhea are only rarely found in infections of the urinary tract, wounds, meningitis, or other nonenteric sites.

Episomal Transmission of Toxin Production. The ability of EPEC to produce enterotoxin is determined by an episome that can be transmitted from one strain of *E. coli* to another by sexual conjugation. This may explain, in part, the finding of *E. coli* strains associated with diarrheal disease that do not belong to previously described enteropathogenic serotypes. Episomal coding of enterotoxin production is, therefore, similar to antimicrobial resistance transfer factor episomes. The loss of an enterotoxin-producing episome explains the previous paradox that certain isolates of *E. coli*, known to be the same serotypes as diarrhea-producing strains, could be isolated from patients lacking any symptoms of the diarrhea syndrome. The finding that transferable episomes mediate en-

TABLE 19–5. *Comparison of Heat-Labile (LT) and Heat-Stable (ST) Toxins of* Escherichia Coli

	Heat Resistance (100°C)	Immunologically Related to *Vibrio cholerae*	**Assay Model**			
			Y1 Hamster/Adrenal Tumor Cell Culture	Chinese Hamster Ovary Cell Culture	Rabbit Ileal Loop	Suckling Mouse
E. coli Labile toxin	−	+	+	+	+	−
E. coli Stable toxin	+	−	−	−	+	+

terotoxin production suggests that diarrhea-producing serotypes are particularly likely to accept the episome and to maintain it in order to produce enterotoxin. There is also the uncomfortable possibility that the episome might be passed to any strain of *E. coli* or a similar gram-negative bacterium, thus creating large numbers of enterotoxin-producing bacteria. Increased receptiveness to episomal transfer in enteropathogenic *E. coli* may explain the relatively high incidence of multiple antibiotic resistance in enteropathogenic *E. coli*. Multiple antibiotic resistance is a well-known therapeutic problem with this group of microorganisms and presumably results from episomes coding for antimicrobial inactivating enzymes.

Enteroinvasive Escherichia coli

A number of well-studied outbreaks of dysentery caused by *E. coli* have been described, particularly in adults. These outbreaks are similar to those caused by shigella, and the symptoms include severe abdominal cramping with bloody diarrhea. In these outbreaks, the isolated *E. coli* strains have the ability to penetrate and replicate within epithelial cells to cause focal epithelial necrosis, characteristics not possessed by enterotoxin-producing strains. The histologic differences between disease produced by ETEC and enteroinvasive *E. coli* are apparent in Figure 19–10. As in shigella, a large plasmid (120–140 Md) encodes for invasiveness.

Infection by Other Types of Escherichia coli

Enteropathogenic *E. coli* (EPEC). Currently the term *EPEC* is defined more narrowly than its original usage that encompassed all *E. coli* associated with diarrhea. Now EPEC refers to those strains of *E. coli* epidemiologically incriminated in diarrhea outbreaks, that are defined serologically, and that lack known virulence factors, such as invasiveness and enterotoxin production.

Enteroadherent *E. coli* (EAEC). These non-classic serotype strains are characterized by their ability to bind *in vitro* to Hep-2 cells. They possess no other marker of virulence. The importance of this group of organisms has yet to be defined.

Enterohemorrhagic *E. coli* (EHEC). In 1982, two outbreaks of acute hemorrhagic gastroenteritis occurred in Oregon and Michigan in association with hamburger patties served by a fast-food chain. At least 47 people were affected by an unusual syndrome characterized by severe crampy abdominal pains, grossly bloody copious diarrhea without fecal leukocytes, and little or no fever. No previously recognized pathogens were recovered from stool specimens. However, a rare *E. coli* serotype, O157:H7, was isolated from 9 of 20 cases (but not from controls) and from an implicated meat patty. The isolate was not toxigenic or invasive by standard tests. Plasmid profile analysis indicated that all outbreak-associated *E. coli* O157:H7 isolates were closely related. The pathogenic mechanism of *E. coli* O157:H7 probably relates to its production of a phage-encoded potent cytotoxin identical with Shiga toxin produced by *S. dysenteriae* type 1. An additional cytotoxin has also been discovered. *E. coli* O157:H7 appears to be responsible for outbreaks of hemorrhagic colitis and hemolytic-uremic syndrome.

Traveler's Diarrhea

"Traveler's diarrhea," well known to persons visiting Latin America, Asia, or Africa, can often be a serious medical problem. The chances of developing traveler's diarrhea depend on the traveler's country of origin, his destination, and what he does. A Latin American who travels to another Latin American country is at low risk.

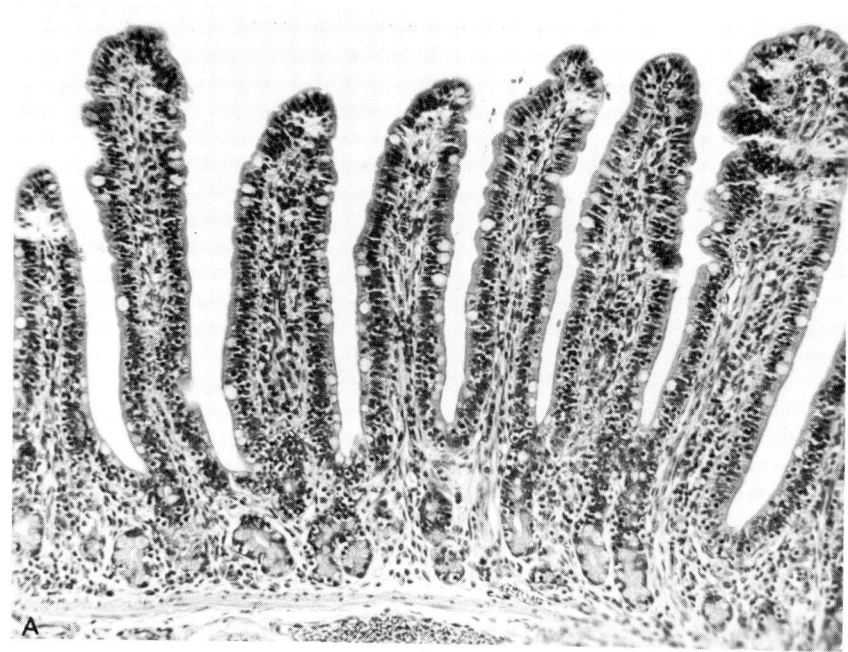

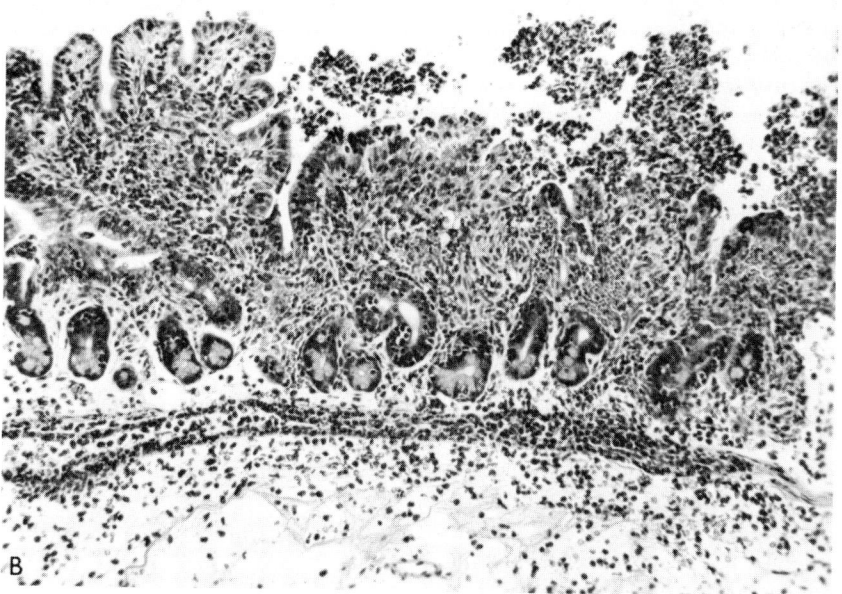

Figure 19–10. A. *Effects of enterotoxin-producing strains of* Escherichia coli *on rabbit ileum.* (× *170.) Section of ligated small bowel loop 7 h after inoculation with enterotoxin-producing organisms shows normal morphology.* B. *Effect of epithelium-penetrating strains of* E. coli *on rabbit ileum. Section of ligated loop 7 h after inoculation with penetrating organisms shows marked mucosal disarray, with necrosis, ulceration, and intense acute inflammatory reaction.* (*From DuPont, H. L., Formal, S. B., Hornick, R. B., et al. Pathogenesis of* Escherichia coli *diarrhea.* N. Engl. J. Med. 285:1, 1971. *Reprinted by permission from* The New England Journal of Medicine.)

Similarly, a North American who visits England is relatively safe, but the North American who visits a Latin American country is at high risk of developing diarrheal disease. The clinical illness is highly variable, reflecting the diverse causative agents. Typically patients experience watery diarrhea, cramps and nausea; vomiting, bloody diarrhea, and fever are less common. The diarrhea lasts a mean of 3 days. A study of a large group of American students on a 3-week visit to Mexico revealed that 30% developed diarrhea during the trip. Cultures of both sick and asymptomatic students yielded enterotoxin-producing strains of *Escherichia coli* in 72% of the sick and 15% of the nonsick students. In a study involving gastroenterologists traveling to a Latin American country for an International Congress, approximately 50% of the physicians and their family members developed traveler's diarrhea. An etiologic agent was identified in almost two thirds of those with diarrhea; the agents identified included enterotoxicogenic *E. coli*, salmonellae, shigellae, invasive *E. coli*, *Vibrio parahaemolyticus*, *Giardia lamblia,* and rotaviruses. Consumption of salads containing raw vegetables was significantly associated with enterotoxicogenic *E. coli* infection.

Several points should be made concerning prevention and therapy of traveler's diarrhea. The agents shown to prevent traveler's diarrhea include doxycycline, bismuth subsalicylate (Pepto-Bismol), trimethoprim-sulfamethoxazole (TMP-SMX), and bicozamycin. In general, however, prophylactic antibiotics are not recommended. Rather, avoidance of water and uncooked fruits and vegetables is prudent. Although TMP-SMX can be used as prophylaxis, it may well serve better as a therapeutic agent if acute diarrhea develops. In most areas of the world TMP-SMX is highly effective against ETEC and *Shigella,* the most common causes of traveler's diarrhea. Clinical improvement with TMP-SMX or with trimethoprim alone is usually seen within a day of the onset of symptoms, and the severity of the illness is reduced dramatically. It can be argued that early treatment is a reasonable alternative to prophylaxis with antimicrobial drugs.

The use of therapeutic agents such as paregoric, tincture of opium, or Lomotil (diphenoxylate and atropine sulfate) to reduce intestinal motility may block an important natural defense mechanism of the body for excreting disease-producing bacteria. Such agents should not be used frequently, nor should their use be prolonged for more than two to three doses.

Infection with Yersinia enterocolitica

Yersinia enterocolitica is a gram-negative bacillus that may cause severe enterocolitis and occasionally death. The disease has been reported more frequently in Scandinavia and other European countries than in the United States; in fact, it appears rather uncommon in the United States. Symptoms include fever, diarrhea, and severe abdominal pain. Occasionally, infection with *Y. enterocolitica* has been recognized only following surgery for suspected appendicitis or on culture of mesenteric lymph nodes. The organism has been found in wild and domestic animals and has been isolated from water, raw milk, and food. Recovery of *Yersinia enterocolitica* by culture is said to be greatly improved by "cold enrichment," for example, incubation of a rectal swab at 4°C for 2–3 weeks before inoculation to culture media. Unfortunately, this procedure, although providing valuable retrospective information, delays the prompt identification of this organism.

Yersinia enterocolitica causes a diffuse enterocolitis with focal mucosal ulcers and diffuse mesenteric lymphadenitis. The organism is invasive (encoded by a 42- to 44-Md plasmid) and elaborates a heat-stable toxin similar to the ST of *E. coli*. Strains isolated from human sources are much more likely to be enterotoxicogenic than are those recovered from water, milk, or food. Of particular interest is the association of erythema nodosum in 20–25% of cases and the appearance of reactive arthritis and occasionally Reiter's syndrome subsequent to infection. Salmonella, shigella, and helicobacter infection are also occasionally associated with reactive arthritis.

Epidemiologic Notes*

Multistate Outbreak of Yersiniosis. Between June 11 and July 29, 1982, a large interstate outbreak of enteritis caused by *Yersinia enterocolitica* occurred. Epidemiologic investigation implicated milk pasteurized at a plant in Memphis, Tennessee, as the vehicle of infection. One hundred seventy-two culture-positive *Y. enterocolitica* infections were identified in and around Little Rock, Arkansas; Memphis, Tennessee; and Greenwood, Mississippi. One hundred forty-eight patients (86%) had diarrhea and/or abdominal pain, usually accompanied by fever;

---

*Adapted from report by Centers for Disease Control.

24 patients had extraintestinal infections of the throat, blood, urinary tract, central nervous system, and wounds. Forty-one percent of cases occurred among children younger than 5 years of age. Most patients required hospitalization, and 17 underwent appendectomies. The epidemic strain was agglutinated most strongly by antisera to *Y. enterocolitica* O groups 13 and 18. Separate case-control studies in each city showed that drinking milk pasteurized by a plant in Memphis was associated with illness. Overall, 71% of patients and 39% of controls recalled drinking milk from the plant in the 2 weeks before the onset of symptoms.

In an effort to estimate the size of the outbreak, a survey was made by telephone of 100 randomly chosen households in Greenwood. Eleven cases of yersiniosis-like illness during the previous 6 weeks were identified among the 260 members of these households. All patients resided in households that used milk from the implicated plant, and 10 of the 11 (91%) recalled drinking its milk within the previous 2 months. Illness occurred in 6 of 50 households that used milk from the implicated plant and in none of 50 that did not use its milk ($p = 0.02$, Fisher's exact test). Of those individuals who drank milk from that plant, 8.7% had a yersiniosis-like illness. The total number of cases would appear to have been much higher than the 172 cases reported.

The outbreak appeared to end spontaneously. Milk from suspected lots was not available for culture, and *Y. enterocolitica* was not isolated from subsequent lots. Inspection of the plant identified neither a breach in pasteurizing technique nor an obvious source of contamination. In this investigation pasteurized milk was epidemiologically implicated as the vehicle of transmission of *Y. enterocolitica*. The temporal and geographic clustering of cases and the negative cultures of subsequent lots of milk are consistent with contamination of a single lot. The mechanism of contamination is unknown. *Y. enterocolitica* has been recovered from raw milk and has also been found in pasteurized milk. *Y. enterocolitica* generally does not survive standard pasteurization. However, if present in large enough numbers, viable *Yersinia* may persist after pasteurization. Once present in a pasteurized product, the organism grows well at refrigeration temperature. Therefore, pasteurization and proper handling of pasteurized milk may not ensure against enteric disease due to *Y. enterocolitica*. This 1982 yersiniosis outbreak was the largest ever reported in the United States.

Infection with Campylobacter jejuni

In recent years a distinctive syndrome of clinical enteritis, with campylobacter in the stool and the development of specific antibody against the organism, has drawn attention to *Campylobacter jejuni* as a cause of gastrointestinal infection. In many areas of the United States and Canada, this is now the most common bacterial cause of enteritis (Fig. 19–11). Several recent studies found the organism in the stool of 1% of asymptomatic children, but in 5–7% of those with diarrhea. In a recent collaborative study, *C. jejuni* was found twice as often as salmonellae. Isolation of the organism can be achieved by incubation at 43°C in a candle jar. A selective medium containing vancomycin, polymyxin B, trimethoprim, amphotericin B, and cephalothin facilitates the recovery of campylobacteria. The organism is fastidious and is unlikely to be recognized with the usual selective culture media for enteric bacteria, requiring the conditions noted above.

Enteric infection with *C. jejuni* is most common between the ages of 10 and 29 years, although it can occur at all ages. *C. jejuni* is widely available in the environment and has been isolated from the feces of 30–100% of chickens, turkeys, water fowl, and wild birds. It has also been isolated from healthy swine, cattle, sheep, and horses, and it may cause diarrheal disease in calves, lambs, dogs, cats, and monkeys. Household dogs and cats, especially young ones, are commonly infected. Feces from infected animals or persons may contain viable organisms for up to 4 weeks and may be a source for contamination of the environment.

Signs and symptoms of infection with *C. jejuni* include fever and malaise followed by diarrhea, often with severe, cramping abdominal pain. The stool contains many segmented neutrophils and frequently red blood cells. Both the jejunum and ileum appear to be involved, with fatal cases showing hemorrhagic necrosis of the small intestine and numerous hyperplastic mesenteric lymph nodes. The organism is resistant to the penicillin and cephalosporin antibiotics but susceptible to the tetracyclines and erythromycin. Like infection with salmonella or shigella, enteric infection with *C. jejuni* is frequently self-limiting, although relapses occur in up to 20% of untreated patients. In controlled trials, erythromycin did not alter the natural course of the disease in patients treated 4–6 days after the onset of symptoms. In selected patients with prolonged or severe symptoms or

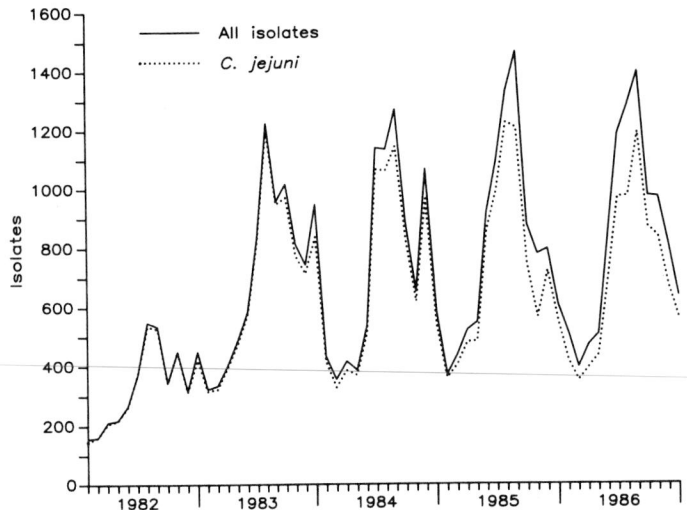

Figure 19–11. Reported Campylobacter isolates for 1982–1986 (by month and year) for the United States. (From Centers for Disease Control, MMWR, Vol. 37, No. SS-2, 1987.)

with high fever, treatment with erythromycin seems prudent.

ACUTE INFECTIOUS NONBACTERIAL GASTROENTERITIS

Acute infectious nonbacterial gastroenteritis is very common. It is one of the most frequent causes of illness in our society, second only to the common cold. This probably accounts for most of the nonspecific episodes of vomiting and diarrhea seen in the United States as well as in other parts of the world, particularly the tropics. It is surprising that so little information about the etiology and pathogenesis of nonbacterial gastroenteritis has been available until recently.

Two clinically distinct forms of nonbacterial gastroenteritis have been noted. One is associated with epidemic outbreaks of gastroenteritis and affects such groups as schoolchildren, members of families, or groups involved in a gathering at which a common meal is consumed. In this form of disease, patients have a rapid onset of gastroenteritis that lasts for 1–2 days. They usually develop diarrhea, vomiting, headache, fever, and muscle aches. Both children and adults may be involved. The second form of the disease is more often sporadic and only rarely epidemic. This occurs most frequently in children between 6 and 24 months of age. Symptoms include severe diarrhea lasting from 4 to 8 days, which may also be associated with vomiting and fever. Infants often suffer severe dehydration and may require hospitalization. Marked diarrhea can also occur in adults but is less common. The former epidemic form of

gastroenteritis is most often associated with the Norwalk group of viruses, whereas the latter endemic disease is associated with rotavirus or, less commonly, enteric adenoviruses.

Although until 1980 the recovery of viruses by tissue culture did not contribute significantly to the study of nonbacterial gastroenteritis, a variety of indirect techniques provided good evidence that viruses were responsible for many cases in children and for some in adults.

Much of the clinical and pathogenetic information about viral gastroenteritis has been gained through the use of human volunteers. Volunteers provide three important elements: (1) a source of infectious material, (2) an experimental host, and (3) the opportunity to study the clinical course and pathogenetic development of the disease under controlled conditions.

Norwalk Agent

The first intensively studied virus associated with acute infectious nonbacterial gastroenteritis was derived from an outbreak of "winter vomiting disease" in Norwalk, Ohio, in October, 1968. The "Norwalk agent" was recovered during an outbreak of illness at an elementary school where about half of the students became ill. Attempts to identify known bacterial or viral agents or filterable enterotoxins were unsuccessful. Three serial passages with stool filtrates from sick patients were made through human volunteers, with a resulting attack rate of 67%. The disease was characterized by an incubation period of 16–48 h, with symptoms lasting from 24 to 48 h, including low-grade fever and combinations of diarrhea, vomiting, abdominal cramps, malaise, and headache. Manifestations of the disease varied from one volunteer to another; vomiting was seen in some, and diarrhea in others (Fig. 19–12). Immunity to the agent, as shown by subsequent challenge of previously infected volunteers, showed two forms, one of short and the other of long duration. The organism has been visualized by immunoelectron microscopic studies of stool filtrates and found to measure 27 nm. The exact classification of the Norwalk virus will depend on its successful isolation and *in vitro* propagation so that an accurate determination of its nucleic acid type can be made. Preliminary studies using virus concentrated from stool suggest certain similarities to the RNA caliciviruses. Humans are probably the only natural host, as no animal models of the disease are known. The high rate of susceptibility to the disease in volunteers and the occurrence of community outbreaks suggest little widespread immunity.

Attempts have been made to isolate and grow the Norwalk agent in a culture system of human fetal intestinal organ. Although volunteers have become ill from ingestion of supernatants from such cultures, results have been inconsistent. The histopathologic changes of the mucosal architecture at the duodenal-jejunal junction have been studied by biopsy in a group of volunteers given the Norwalk agent. Abnormalities were found in all patients 12–48 h following challenge. The mucosal villi became shortened, the crypts hypertrophied, and the interstitial tissue of the villi became more cellular, containing both mononuclear cells and segmented neutrophils. Abnormal changes persisted for several days but cleared by 6–8 weeks after the acute illness (Fig. 19–13). In contrast to the abnormal findings in the small-intestine mucosa, biopsies of the rectosigmoid colon appeared normal, indicating a preferential localization to the small intestine.

Functional abnormalities of the small intestine during the acute and convalescent phases of this disease include abnormal D-xylose absorption, both in patients with acute clinical disease and in those who remain asymptomatic. Intestinal lactase deficiency also occurs transiently during the acute disease. Malabsorption of fat developed both in patients with clinical illness and in those without symptoms and cleared within 6 days after infection. No alteration of adenyl cyclase activity occurred.

Rotaviruses

In 1973, electron-microscopic studies of duodenal biopsies from nine children with acute

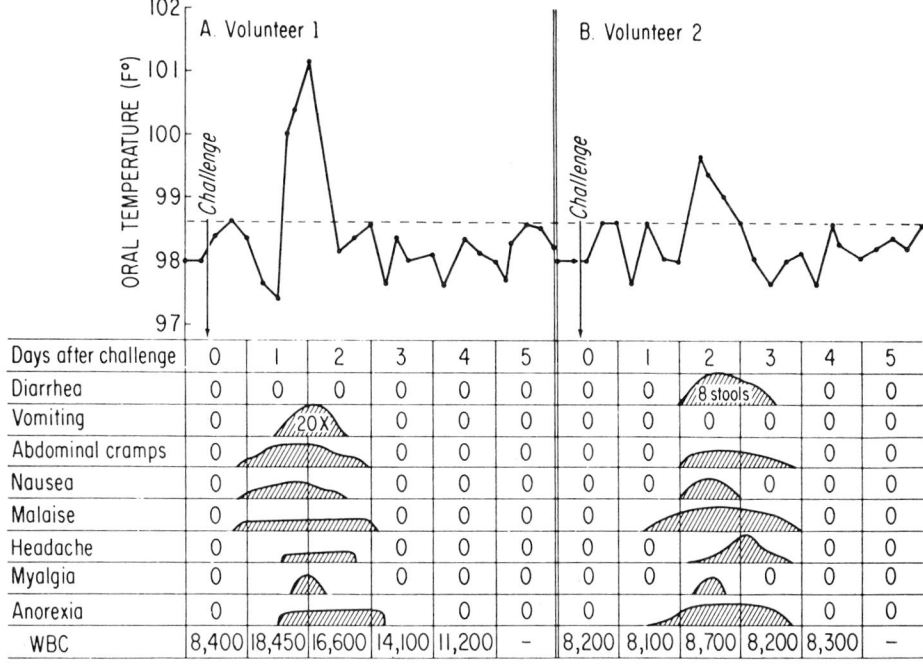

Figure 19–12. Response of two volunteers to oral administration of stool filtrate derived from a volunteer who received original Norwalk rectal-swab specimen. The height of the shaded curve is roughly proportional to the severity of the sign or symptom. (From Dolin, R., Blacklow, N. R., DuPont, H., et al. Transmission of acute infectious nonbacterial gastroenteritis to volunteers by oral administration of stool filtrates. J. Infect. Dis. 123:307, 1971.)

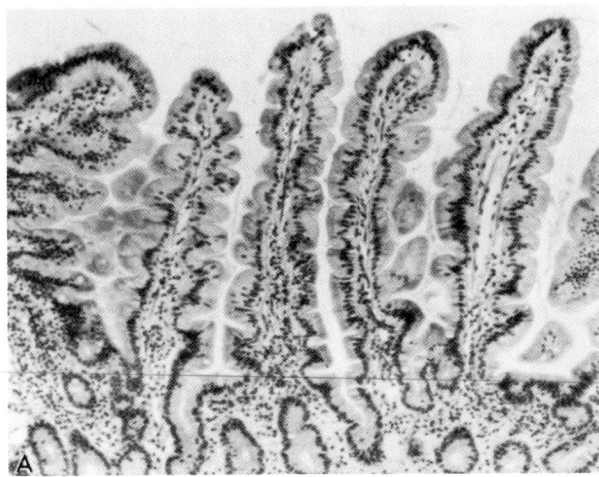

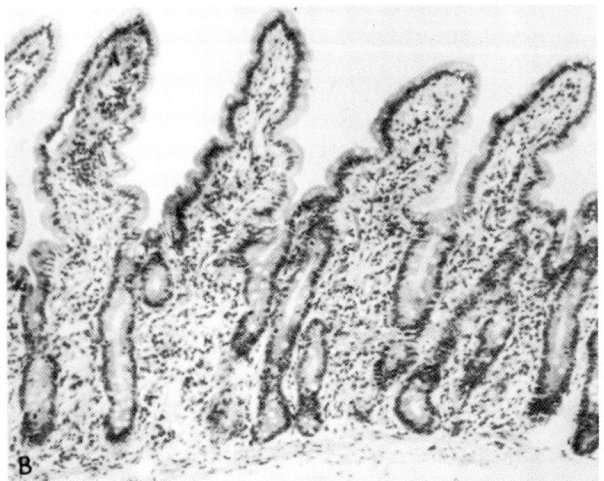

Figure 19–13. Biopsies of the small intestine before and after oral ingestion of Norwalk agent. Before ingestion (A), villi are tall, and the cellularity of the lamina propria is normal. Two days after ingestion (B), the villi are shortened, the crypts are hypertrophied and contain increased numbers of mitoses, and the cellularity of the lamina propria is increased. Six days after ingestion (C), shortened villi, hypertrophied crypts, and increased mitoses persist. (Hematoxylin and eosin stain, × 100.) (From Schreiber, D. S., Blacklow, N. L., and Trier, J. S. The mucosal lesion of the proximal small intestine in acute infectious nonbacterial gastroenteritis. N. Engl. J. Med. 288:1318, 1973. Reprinted by permission from The New England Journal of Medicine.*)*

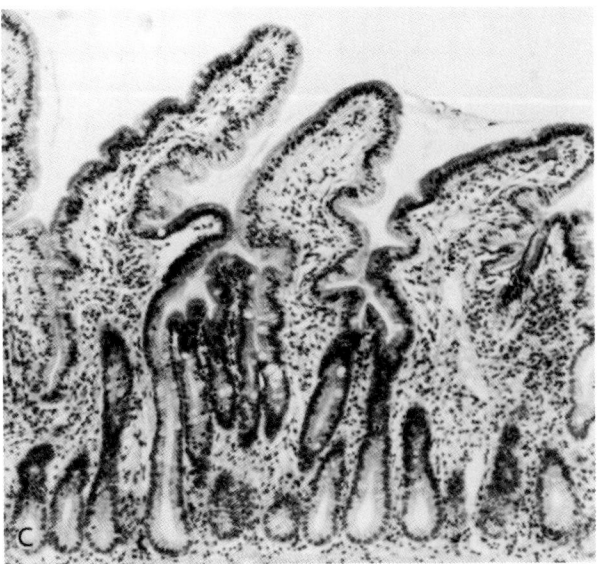

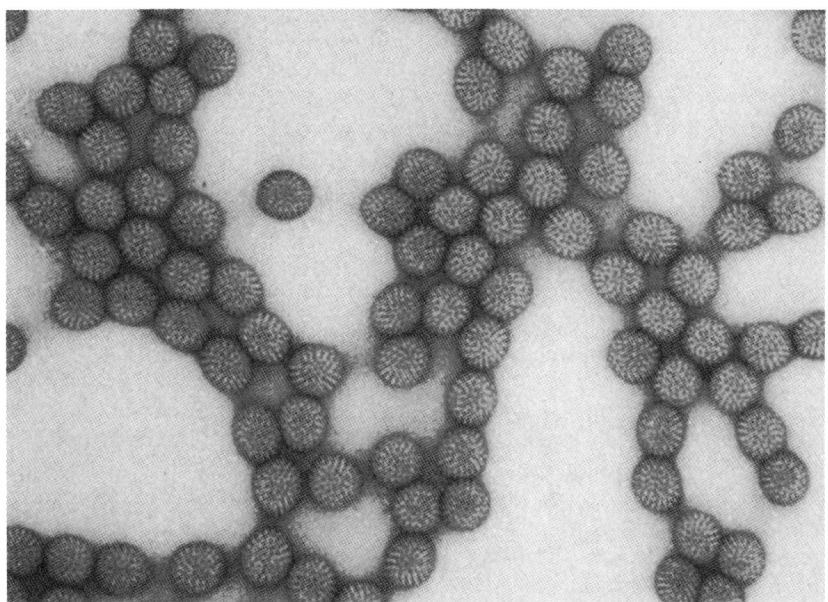

Figure 19–14. Purified rotavirus stained with 2% phosphotungstic acid (× 124,875). (From Gomez-Barreto, J., et al. Acute enteritis associated with reovirus-like agents. JAMA 235:1857, 1976. Copyright 1976, American Medical Association.)

infectious nonbacterial gastroenteritis revealed intracellular virus particles resembling human reoviruses. No viruses were found after clinical recovery. By electron microscopy, rotaviruses resemble a wheel with radiating spokes (Fig. 19–14). The name of the rotavirus group is derived from the Latin word *rota*, meaning wheel, because the circular outer capsid resembles the rim of a wheel connected to short spokes that radiate from a wide hub. Morphologically, rotaviruses resemble both reoviruses and orbiviruses, but each is serologically distinct. Rotavirus has many similarities to the Nebraska calf diarrhea virus (NCDV), an agent that causes a severe diarrheal disease in neonatal calves.

Rotavirus is unstable at pH less than 3.0 and may be destroyed by some proteolytic intestinal enzymes. After considerable difficulty getting rotavirus to grow *in vitro,* a human strain was recovered in cell culture after 10 serial passages in gnotobiotic (germ-free) piglets. Vaccine development has resulted, and several candidate vaccines are currently being tested. In addition, serologic tests for rotavirus antibody have been developed.

Epidemiologic studies of rotavirus infections have shown that gastroenteritis caused by this group of agents shows a distinct predilection for infants between 6 and 24 months of age. Infection is common in patients hospitalized for acute gastroenteritis, with up to 50% of infants and young children positive for rotavirus in stool.

Infection follows a characteristic seasonal pattern, with most infants hospitalized between November and April. Nearly 80% of infants in the hospital with acute gastroenteritis during December and January can be shown to shed the virus. Concurrent studies on the parents of clinically ill children show up to 40% to be infected, although most infections in adults are subclinical.

In addition to diarrhea, vomiting can be a serious problem contributing to dehydration. The disease is usually not fatal unless there has been severe dehydration or (in developing countries) is associated with preexisting malnutrition. Diarrhea begins somewhat later than vomiting and may reflect infection of the intestine at different levels. Mucosal abnormalities are similar to those seen in patients with Norwalk virus infections. Treatment is symptomatic, with fluid replacement being the most important factor.

Two serotypes of rotaviruses have been identified, types 1 and 2. Type 2 rotavirus constitutes nearly 80% of strains causing disease in humans, with the remainder being type 1. The distribution of the two serotypes is similar throughout the world. Most children have acquired antibody to rotaviruses by the time they are 2 years of age. In studies of children who develop reinfection, repeated illness is usually due to infection with a different serotype. Infection with one serotype does not appear to provide cross-protection from illness due to the other.

In general there are numerous virus particles

TABLE 19–6. *Diseases Associated with Fecal Leukocytes**

Disease	Number of Patients	Number with Fecal Leukocytes	Predominant Cell Type (Acute Illness)
Shigellosis	44	44	Polymorphonuclear (mean, 84%)
Salmonellosis	11	9	Polymorphonuclear (mean, 75%)
Typhoid fever†	8	8	Mononuclear (mean, 95%)
Invasive *Escherichia coli* colitis†	4	4	Polymorphonuclear (mean, 85%)
Ulcerative colitis	2	2	Polymorphonuclear (mean, 88%) and eosinophils (mean, 8%)
"Allergic" diarrhea	1	1	Mononuclear (mean, 95%)

*From Harris, J. C., DuPont, H. L., and Hornick, R. B. Fecal leukocytes in diarrheal illness. *Ann. Intern. Med.* 76:697, 1972.
†Experimentally induced.

in the stools of patients with rotavirus infections, making detection easy. Diagnosis of infection can be made by immunoelectron microscopy, counterimmunoelectrophoresis, radioimmunoassay, and most conveniently by enzyme-linked immunosorbent assay (ELISA). In some laboratories, rotavirus can be recovered by cell culture. A commercially available ELISA test has been most useful for the rapid and apparently specific identification of viral antigen in the stool.

Enteric Adenovirus

A subgroup of fastidious adenoviruses that are antigenically distinct and have specific tissue culture growth characteristics are associated with acute gastroenteritis. These viruses do not grow in the conventional cell lines used for other adenoviruses. Adenovirus diarrhea tends to be mild and self-limited, but can be very severe on occasion. Symptoms include low-grade fever, watery stools, emesis, and occasionally respiratory symptoms. Infants are particularly susceptible to these agents.

Gastrointestinal infection has also been described with caliciviruses and astroviruses, but the significance of infection, the number of patients infected, and the severity of illness have not yet been established.

FECAL INFLAMMATORY CELLS AND TYPE OF INFECTION

During the foregoing discussion, it has been stressed that infections in the gastrointestinal tract result either from the parasite invading the host, usually with an appropriate neutrophilic or mononuclear cell inflammatory reaction, or from the action of an enterotoxin causing fluid loss.

Understanding the pathogenesis of these infections has led to a simple, rapid, and reasonably specific test for the type of gastrointestinal infection. The test consists of making a stained smear of the stool or diarrhea contents and looking for inflammatory cells. If inflammatory cells are present, identification of the type (e.g., neutrophils or mononuclear cells) may be helpful in determining the kind of gastrointestinal infection. Typhoid fever is associated with a large number of mononuclear inflammatory cells. Shigella bacillary dysentery results in stool smears showing 80–90% neutrophils, reflecting the acute inflammatory reaction following mucosal penetration. Cholera and infection with enterotoxigenic *E. coli* or viral agents are characterized by the absence of inflammatory cells (Table 19–6). Exceptions to these generalizations, of course, can occur. Despite these exceptions, the relative number and type of inflammatory cells in the stool can be of help in determining the site of the infection and whether it is toxic or invasive.

REFERENCES

Books

Dupont, H. L., and Pickering, L. K. *Infections of the Gastrointestinal Tract*. New York: Plenum Press, 1980.
Field, M., Fordtran, J. S., and Shultz, S. G., eds. *Secretory Diarrhea*. Clinical Physiology Series—American Physiological Society. Baltimore, Williams & Wilkins Co., 1981.
Tzipori, S. *Infectious Diarrhea in the Young*. Amsterdam: Elsevier, 1985.

Review Articles

Blaser, M. J., Wells, J. G., Feldman, R. A., et al. Campylobacter enteritis in the United States. *Ann. Intern. Med.* 98:350, 1983.
Chalker, R. B., and Blaser, M. J. A review of human salmonellosis. *Rev. Infect. Dis.* 10:111, 1988.

Claeson, M., and Merson, M. Global progress in the control of diarrheal diseases. *Pediatr. Infect. Dis. J. 9:*345, 1990.

Cover, T. L., and Aber, R. C. *Yersinia enterocolitica. N. Engl. J. Med. 321:*16, 1989.

Keusch, G. T., and Bennish, M. L. Shigellosis: Recent progress, persisting problems and research issues. *Pediatr. Infect. Dis. J. 8:*713, 1989.

Levine, M. M. *Escherichia coli* that cause diarrhea: Enterotoxigenic, enteropathogenic, enteroinvasive, enterohemorrhagic, and enteroadherent. *J. Infect. Dis. 155:*377, 1987.

Robins-Browne, R. M. Traditional enteropathogenic *E. coli* of infantile diarrhea. *Rev. Infect. Dis. 9:*28, 1987.

Ryan, C. A., Hargrett-Bean, N. T., and Blake, P. A. *Salmonella typhi* infections in the United States, 1975–84: Increasing role of foreign travel. *Rev. Infect. Dis. 11:*1, 1989.

Original Articles

Bennish, M. L., Harris, J. R., Wojtyniak, B. J., et al. Death in shigellosis: Incidence and risk factors in hospitalized patients. *J. Infect. Dis. 161:*500, 1990.

Blaser, M. J., and Reller, L. B. Campylobacter enteritis. *N. Engl. J. Med. 305:*1444, 1981.

DuPont, H. L., Reves, R. R., Galindo, E., et al. Treatment of traveler's diarrhea with trimethoprim-sulfamethoxazole and with trimethoprim alone. *N. Engl. J. Med. 307:*841, 1982.

Gorbach, S. L. Traveler's diarrhea (editorial). *N. Engl. J. Med. 307:*881, 1982.

Ho, M. S., Glass, R. I., Pinsky, P. F., et al. Rotavirus as a cause of diarrheal morbidity and mortality in the United States. *J. Infect. Dis. 158:*1112, 1988.

Holmberg, S. D., Osterholm, M. T., Senger, K. A., et al. Drug-resistant salmonella from animals fed antimicrobials. *N. Engl. J. Med. 311:*617, 1984.

Johnston, J. M., Martin, D. L., Perdue, J., et al. Cholera on a Gulf Coast oil rig. *N. Engl. J. Med. 309:*523, 1983.

Kapikian, A. A., Kim, H. W., Wyatt, R. G., et al. Human reovirus-like agent as the major pathogen associated with "winter" gastroenteritis in hospitalized infants and young children. *N. Engl. J. Med. 294:*965, 1976.

Klipstein, F. A., Engert, R. F., Clements, J. D., et al. Vaccine for enterotoxigenic *Escherichia coli* based on synthetic heat-stable toxin crossed-linked to the B subunit of heat-labile toxin. *J. Infect. Dis. 147:*318, 1983.

Kuritsky, J. N., Osterholm, M. T., Greenberg, H. B., et al. Norwalk gastroenteritis: A community outbreak associated with bakery product consumption. *Ann. Intern. Med. 100:*519, 1984.

Lee, L. A., Gerber, A. R., Lonsway, D. R., et al. *Yersinia enterocolitica* 0:3 infections in infants and children associated with the household preparation of chitterlings. *N. Engl. J. Med. 322:*984, 1990.

Levine, M. M., Taylor, D. N., and Ferreccio, C. Typhoid vaccines come of age. *Pediatr. Infect. Dis. J. 8:*374, 1989.

Levy, S. B. Playing antibiotic pool: Time to tally the score (editorial). *N. Engl. J. Med. 311:*663, 1984.

Merson, M. H., Morris, G. K., Sack, D. A., et al. Traveler's diarrhea in Mexico: A prospective study of physicians and family members attending a congress. *N. Engl. J. Med. 294:*1299, 1976.

Morris, J. G., Jr., and Black, R. E. Cholera and other vibrioses in the United States. *N. Engl. J. Med. 312:*343, 1985.

Ormand, J. E., and Talley, N. J. *Helicobacter pylori:* Controversies and an approach to management. *Mayo Clin. Proc. 65:*414, 1990.

Pai, C. H., Gordon, R., Sims, H. V., et al. Sporadic cases of .hemorrhagic colitis associated with *Escherichia coli* O157:H7. *Ann. Intern. Med. 101:*738, 1984.

Palmer, D. L., Koster, F. T., Islam, A. F. M. R., et al. Comparison of sucrose and glucose in the oral electrolyte therapy of cholera and other severe diarrheas. *N. Engl. J. Med. 297:*1107, 1977.

Parsons, R., Gregory, J., and Palmer, D. L. Salmonella infections of the abdominal aorta. *Rev. Infect Dis. 5:*227, 1983.

Rubin, R. H. Human salmonellosis: Epidemiology, pathogenesis and clinical syndromes. *Infect. Dis. Pract. 6:*1, 1982.

Spika, J. S., Waterman, S. H., SooHoo, G. W., et al. Chloramphenicol-resistant *Salmonella newport* traced through hamburger to dairy farms. *N. Engl. Med. 316:*565, 1987.

Tacket, C. O., Barrett, T. J., Mann, J. M., et al. Wound infections caused by *Vibrio vulnificus*, a marine vibrio, in inland areas of the United States. *J. Clin. Microbiol. 19:*197, 1984.

Taylor, D. N., Wachsmuth, I. K., Shangkuan, Y. H., et al. Salmonellosis associated with marijuana. *N. Engl. J. Med. 306:*1249, 1982.

Wells, J. G., Davis, B. R., Wachsmuth, I. K., et al. Laboratory investigation of hemorrhagic colitis outbreaks associated with a rare *Escherichia coli* serotype. *J. Clin. Microbiol. 18:*512, 1983.

Yolken, R. H., Wyatt, R. G., Zissis, G., et al. Epidemiology of human rotavirus types 1 and 2 as studied by enzyme-linked immunosorbent assay. *N. Engl. J. Med. 299:*1156, 1978.

20 *BORIS REISBERG, M.D.*

Common Intestinal Parasitic Infections

INTRODUCTION

Parasitic infection of the human gastrointestinal tract is common, especially in those parts of the world where poor sanitation and an unprotected water supply exist. Although parasitic infection of the intestinal tract is rarely fatal, these infections contribute greatly to the global problem of diarrheal illness, malnutrition, and human suffering. Worse perhaps is the fact that infants and children bear the brunt of the morbidity and mortality associated with these infections. It is impossible to discuss all of the human intestinal parasitic infections in this chapter; therefore, the reader is referred to the references for texts devoted to parasitic infections. This chapter deals with common intestinal infections found in the United States.

The first part of this chapter deals with those parasites that are mainly responsible for diarrheal illness, namely *Entamoeba histolytica, Giardia lamblia, Isospara belli,* and *Cryptosporidium.* The second half of this chapter discusses common nematode infections.

ENTAMOEBA HISTOLYTICA INFECTION

Infection with the protozoan *Entamoeba histolytica* occurs throughout the civilized world, but is most commonly seen in countries with a warm climate where people live in poverty and sanitation is poor. In these tropical and semitropical areas of the world, there are an estimated 400 million infections and 30,000 deaths annually. On a global scale, death due to amebiasis is only exceeded by the parasitic infections malaria and schistosomiasis. Estimates of the incidence of *E. histolytica* infection in the United States have varied between 3 and 10%. With increasing international travel, amebiasis may occur in visitors to the United States from highly endemic areas, as well as in United States citizens who have traveled abroad.

Life Cycle of Entamoeba histolytica

Entamoeba histolytica, E. hartmanni, E. coli, and *E. gingivalis* are all capable of colonizing the mouth and intestinal tract of humans, but only *E. histolytica* is capable of producing disease. Man is the definitive host of *E. histolytica* and the only reservoir of infection.

Entamoeba histolytica exists in two distinct forms: as a cyst and as a motile, actively feeding trophozoite. Cysts are produced when the local conditions become unfavorable for trophozoite viability, which occurs when the stool is dehydrated in its passage from the colon to the rectum. In transforming into a cyst, the ameba discharges ingested food and rounds up to form

a precyst, containing a single nucleus. As the cyst matures, it forms a tough outer membrane and the nucleus divides. Immature cysts contain two nuclei; mature cysts, which measure 10–18 μm in diameter, have four nuclei. Cysts of *E. histolytica* are usually found in asymptomatic individuals whose stools are well formed. Infected individuals may excrete as many as 45 million cysts per day. The disease is spread by ingestion of food or water contaminated with *E. histolytica* cysts.

Once swallowed, the cysts, which are resistant to gastric juice, enter the small bowel. It is here that excystation occurs, liberating four trophozoites, which pass into the large intestine, their natural habitat. *Entamoeba histolytica* trophozoites are 12–50 μm in size and have a glassy green tinge when observed with a microscope. The nucleus is round, and on the inner surface of the thin nuclear membrane are minute deposits of chromatin (see Figs. 20–1, 20–2). In the center of the nucleus is a prominent karyosome (nucleolus). The structure of the nucleus is the most important morphologic feature in distinguishing *E. histolytica* from other intestinal amebae, with the exception of *E. hartmanni,* which has a similar appearing nucleus. Differentiation between these two amebae is made by size. Both the trophozoites and cysts of *E. hartmanni* are smaller than those of *E. histolytica.* The upper limit of the size of *E. hartmanni* cysts is 10 μm, and of the trophozoites, 12 μm.

E. histolytica trophozoites viewed in wet mount move rapidly and in one direction. This typical ameboid movement is accomplished utilizing pseudopodia. Multiplication is by binary division, as long as local conditions remain favorable. *Entamoeba histolytica* grow in and multiply best under anaerobic conditions. When they have invaded the bowel wall, the trophozoites reach sizes near the upper end of their size spectrum and are frequently observed to have ingested red blood cells. As metabolic conditions become unfavorable, precysts are formed, and the cycle begins again.

Pathogenesis of Infection

The initial step in the pathogenesis of amebiasis is the adhesion of *E. histolytica* trophozoites to the epithelium of the colon. Mechanically, this seems to be accomplished by formation of filopodia—long filamentous elements that extend outward from the amebic cell surface. Inhibition of this process by conditions known to prevent

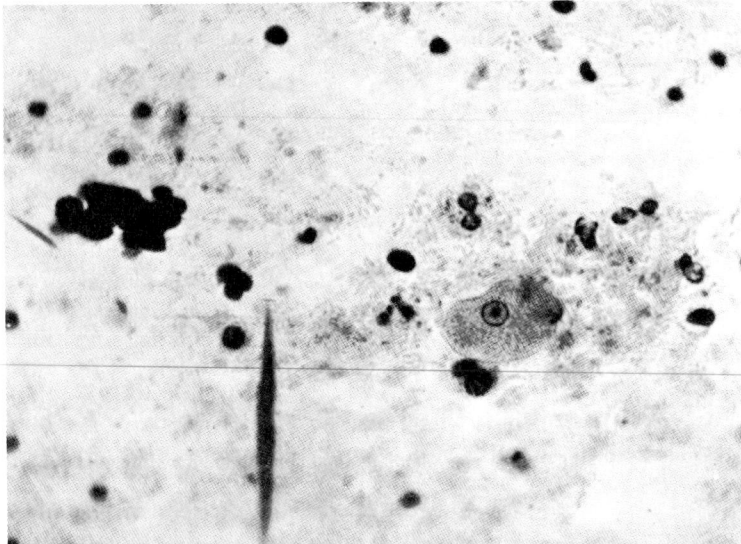

Figure 20–1. Trophozoite of Entamoeba histolytica *stained with iron hematoxylin. Note Charcot-Leyden crystals and clumped red blood cells. (Courtesy of Hunter, G. W., Shwartzwelder, J. C., and Clyde, D. F. Tropical Medicine. 4th ed. Philadelphia: W. B. Saunders Co., 1966.)*

microfilament formation causes a marked reduction in amebic adherence. Adherence of *E. histolytica* is also dependent on a specific carbohydrate-binding protein (lectin) on the amebic cell surface. The lectin of *E. histolytica* seems to bind preferentially to those polysaccharides and glycoconjugates that contain *N*-acetylgalactosamine. Attachment of *E. histolytica* to intestinal epithelial cells is also dependent on temperature, the amount of time elapsed since incubation, and pH. Experimentally, the optimal temperature has been found to be 35°–37°C; maximal adherence to a fixed epithelial cell monolayer is reached after 15 min of incubation and at a pH of 5.7–6.0.

Viable *E. histolytica* trophozoites are cytolethal to numerous tissue culture cell lines, and attachment is quickly followed by destruction of the intestinal epithelial monolayer. Although *E. histolytica* produces numerous proteases, hyaluronidase, and other hydrolytic enzymes, cell-free cytotoxicity has not been demonstrated *in vitro*. Contact between the target cell and the intact trophozoite is required for cytolytic effect. At the same time that cellular destruction is occurring, phagocytosis of viable or killed target cells also occurs. *E. histolytica* trophozoites are capable of destroying leukocytes on contact. Examination of tissue specimens obtained from patients reveals the presence of leukocytes only at the periphery of established lesions.

For many years, it has been recognized that

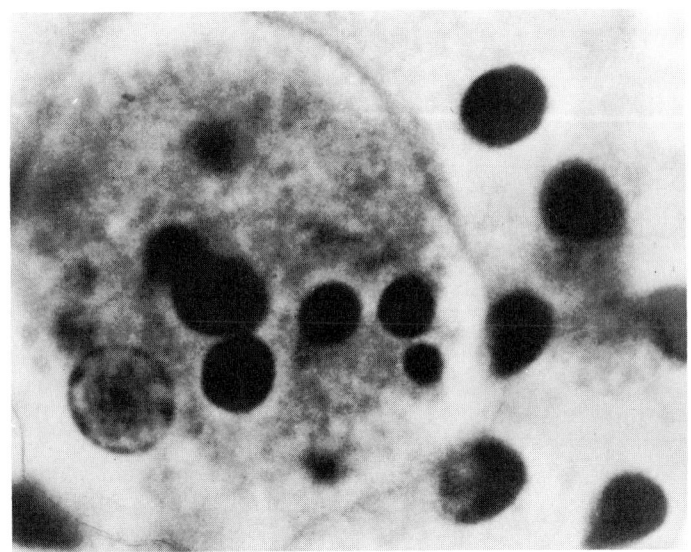

Figure 20–2. Entamoeba histolytica *trophozoite. Note ingested red cells (trichrome stain). (From Markell, E. K., and Voge, M. Medical Parasitology. 4th ed. Philadelphia: W. B. Saunders Co., 1976.)*

different strains of *E. histolytica* vary in pathogenicity. Amebae isolated from asymptomatic intestinal carriers do not produce lesions on intrahepatic inoculation of hamsters, whereas those strains isolated from symptomatic patients do produce liver abscesses. Pathogenic strains ingest greater quantities of human erythrocytes and have an isoenzyme electrophoretic pattern different from that of nonpathogenic strains. The intrinsic factors that determine the presence or absence of pathogenic activity are unknown, nor is it known if so-called nonpathogenic strains can revert under appropriate conditions and become invasive organisms.

Acute Intestinal Amebiasis

Disease is initiated by ingestion of food or water contaminated with fecal matter containing cysts of *E. histolytica.* Cysts are able to survive in moist soil for at least 1 week at temperatures of 28°–34°C, and even longer in colder temperatures. Cysts may also live for several days to weeks in water and are not killed by the concentration of chlorine usually present in municipal water. In many areas of the world, water used for drinking and washing may be contaminated by surface runoff into shallow wells, streams, or even by the discharge of untreated sewage into lakes and rivers. In the United States, several large epidemics of amebiasis have occurred in the past from the cross-contamination of fresh-water pipes by waste water. Cysts are killed by boiling water, desiccation, direct sunlight, heat, or by 200 ppm of iodine.

Contamination of food and water and direct person-to-person spread is usually accomplished by a totally asymptomatic cyst passer. In the majority of infected persons, *E. histolytica* lives as an asymptomatic commensal organism in the lumen in the large bowel. Trophozoites in these individuals are noninvasive and live on bacteria and debris. Invasion of the colonic epithelium and the production of symptomatic disease occur in less than 10% of infected individuals.

In patients who develop symptomatic disease, the onset of infection is usually gradual, with the patient complaining of abdominal pain and discomfort associated with frequent bowel movements. Rectal pain and urgency to defecate are also common. The stool is often noted to be loose and watery and to contain varying amounts of blood and mucus. Patients may have anywhere from a few bowel movements per day to several movements per hour. The combination of bloody diarrhea, abdominal pain, and

urgency is the classic presentation of amebic dysentery.

Fever and other constitutional symptoms are frequently absent, facts that are sometimes helpful in differentiating bacillary dysentery produced by *Shigella* from amebiasis. In approximately a third of patients with amebiasis, the onset of illness is acute, with profuse diarrhea containing blood and mucus, accompanied by high fever and signs of toxicity. These patients present in a manner identical to those with bacillary dysentery, and differentiation on clinical grounds is impossible. The abdominal pain is frequently most intense in the lower abdomen, and most commonly in the right lower quadrant. Abdominal tenderness is a frequent finding on physical examination. The combination of right lower quadrant pain and lower abdominal tenderness may be confused with acute appendicitis.

The characteristic colonic lesions produced by trophozoites of *E. histolytica* are discrete ulcers separated from each other by normal appearing intestinal mucosa. The ulcers vary in size from 2–3 mm to 1–2 cm. As trophozoites penetrate the submucosa, they spread out laterally, creating an ulcer shaped like an "inverted flask," the edges of which are thickened and shaggy and overhang the ulcer crater. The base of the ulcer is coated with a necrotic exudate (see Figs. 20–3, 20–4). Invasion of the bowel wall by trophozoites produces little in the way of an acute inflammatory reaction. Rarely, the ulcers may extend through the muscular layers of the intestine into the serosa. This is usually followed by frank intestinal perforation and amebic peritonitis.

A second local complication of amebic dysentery is massive lower intestinal hemorrhage, which occurs when the base of the ulcer crater erodes into an arteriole. Lower gastrointestinal hemorrhage usually responds to supportive care and specific antiamebic chemotherapy. Surgical exploration is not indicated. The majority of amebic ulcers are present in the cecum and rectosigmoid areas of the colon, but they may be found throughout the colon and even in the terminal ileum. Sigmoidoscopy is frequently helpful for diagnostic purposes. The presence of discrete ulcers with normal intervening mucosa makes ulcerative colitis and bacillary dysentery unlikely possibilities.

Although dysentery is the classic presentation of acute amebiasis, some patients may experience only mild diarrhea and abdominal pain, with no evidence of ulcerative lesions on sig-

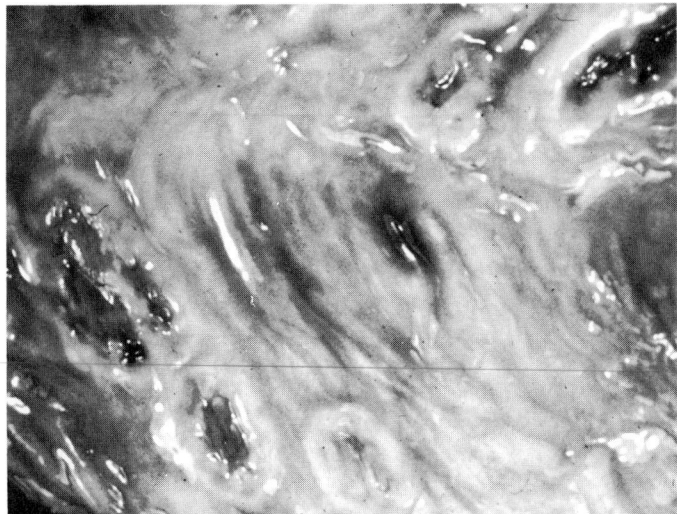

Figure 20–3. Amebic ulcers of the large intestine. Note raised margins of ulcers. (Courtesy of the Louisiana State University School of Medicine, New Orleans.)

moidoscopy. Stools may be watery or soft, but are free of blood and mucus. In these mild cases, the diagnosis is often overlooked because examination of the stool for amebic trophozoites and cysts is not requested by the physician.

Chronic Intestinal Amebiasis

Many patients with acute amebiasis, if left untreated, improve spontaneously, only to have a relapse within a short time. Such patients, especially if they reside in regions of low endemicity, such as the United States, may see several physicians before the possibility of amebiasis is considered. Physicians often neglect the possibility of amebiasis because in the United States intrinsic inflammatory bowel conditions, such as

ulcerative colitis and regional enteritis, are fairly common, and the signs and symptoms associated with these diseases may be indistinguishable from those of chronic amebiasis.

The patient with chronic amebiasis usually has frequent episodes of blood-tinged diarrhea, weight loss, and abdominal pain. These symptoms may be present for several months. Repeated examination of the stool may be negative for trophozoites, especially when they are sought following antibiotic therapy or barium contrast studies of the bowel. Barium roentgenograms of the colon in patients with chronic amebiasis may mimic those seen in patients with ulcerative colitis and regional enteritis, including the presence of skip lesions, thumbprinting, and loss of haustral markings. Rarely, toxic megacolon may develop in patients with acute or

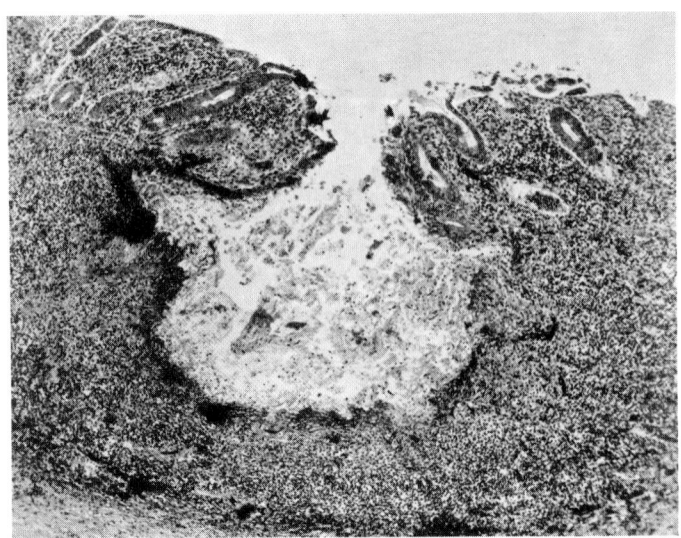

Figure 20–4. Section of colon showing flask-shaped chronic amebic ulcer involving the mucosa and submucosa. The neutrophilic infiltration of the border of the lesion suggests secondary bacterial invasion. (From Medical Museum Collection, Armed Forces Institute of Pathology.)

chronic amebiasis. This complication previously had been thought to occur almost exclusively in patients with ulcerative colitis. On sigmoidoscopy, characteristic ulcers may be seen. Biopsies and smears made of the ulcerative lesions may be positive for trophozoites at a time when stools have been negative on repeat examinations. Patients with chronic amebiasis almost always have a positive serologic test for amebiasis.

Other intestinal complications of amebiasis include intestinal stricture formation and amebomas. Strictures are usually asymptomatic but occasionally produce abdominal pain or difficulty with defecation. When present, they most frequently occur in the rectum, anus, and sigmoid colon. Strictures usually resolve following therapy with a tissue amebicide. Amebomas are tumors consisting of granulation tissue that arise from the colon; they are most commonly found in the cecum but may occur anywhere in the colon and rectum. Symptoms, if present, may include abdominal pain, alternating diarrhea and constipation, weight loss, and rarely, a mass that can be palpated on abdominal examination. On barium enema examination, an ameboma may appear as a polypoid lesion, a napkin ring deformity, or an area of bowel-wall infiltration, all of which may easily be mistaken for carcinoma of the colon, especially if the patient has no prior history of dysentery. Amebomas, like strictures, resolve with specific chemotherapy.

Extraintestinal Amebiasis

The most common extraintestinal site of *E. histolytica* infection is the liver, to which the trophozoites gain access via the portal circulation. Once infection is established in the liver, abscesses form. Almost all of the other extraintestinal sites of amebic infection follow the establishment of a liver abscess. Diagnosis of extraintestinal amebiasis is notoriously difficult, for most patients do not give a history of concomitant diarrhea or dysentery and may recall no gastrointestinal illness in the recent past. Stools are frequently negative on repeated examinations for trophozoites and cysts.

Liver Abscess

For reasons unknown, most patients who develop amebic liver abscess are male. The abscess is usually solitary and located in the right lobe of the liver. Pain and fever are the most common presenting symptoms. The pain is usually localized to the right upper quadrant, but may be present in the epigastrium or appear pleuritic in character over the right lower chest. Almost all patients are febrile. Those who present for medical attention with an abrupt onset of infection and symptoms for fewer than 10 days usually have high fever, whereas those with a more chronic presentation, with symptoms present for several weeks to several months, may have only a low-grade fever associated with night sweats. Occasionally, fever is the only presenting complaint, and the initial impression is that of fever of unknown origin.

On physical examination, the most frequent finding is tenderness in the right upper quadrant of the abdomen. The liver is usually palpable in those patients with a subacute or chronic presentation but is palpable in only one third or fewer of those patients with an acute illness.

Routine laboratory studies are not helpful. The white blood count is usually elevated but may be normal. There is no eosinophilia. Liver function tests are nonspecific; the most consistent abnormality is a rise in the serum alkaline phosphatase. High serum transaminase levels (SGPT, SGOT) correlate with more aggressive disease with multiple liver abscesses. Hyperbilirubinemia and jaundice are uncommon. Trophozoites or cysts are found in the stools of only 10% of patients. Most helpful in determining the extent and localization of amebic abscess has been the use of ultrasonography and computerized tomography (CT) of the liver and abdomen. Most patients are found to have a solitary abscess in the right lobe of the liver, but young patients with an abrupt onset of infection frequently are found to have multiple liver abscesses.

A definitive diagnosis may be made by performing needle aspiration of the abscess cavity and finding brown to brownish red, necrotic, non–foul-smelling material (the so-called anchovy paste) that is negative for bacterial growth. Trophozoites should be looked for in the aspirated material, especially in the final portions of the aspirate, although they are not commonly demonstrated. Fortunately, almost all patients with amebic liver abscess as well as other extraintestinal forms of amebiasis have a positive serum indirect hemagglutination test for amebiasis (see later discussion under Diagnosis).

Treatment consists of antiamebic chemotherapy, with or without needle aspiration of the abscess cavity. The major indications for therapeutic aspiration are the presence of an abscess cavity greater than 10 cm in diameter, an expanding abscess with rupture appearing imminent, or an abscess that has responded poorly to medical therapy. Small cavities respond well to medical therapy and do not need to be routinely aspirated.

Other Extraintestinal Sites of Infection

Less frequent complications of liver abscess are lung abscess and pericarditis. Lung abscess and empyema are almost always found in the right lower lobe and result from extension of an amebic liver abscess through the diaphragm. Amebic pericarditis is a rare complication of amebic liver abscess. Spread of infection to the pericardial sac is usually from an abscess in the left lobe of the liver, although pericarditis may be produced by contiguous spread from an adjacent lung abscess. Very rarely trophozoites reach the brain via the bloodstream to produce a brain abscess. Cutaneous amebiasis, usually of the perianal area, develops in a few individuals following prolonged contact of the perianal skin with *E. histolytica* trophozoites.

The vast majority of patients with invasive amebic infection develop circulating antibody within 1 week of infection. Specifically, antibody activity resides predominantly in the IgG fraction. Unfortunately, IgG plays little, if any, role in the intraluminal defense against invasive amebic disease. Population studies of individuals living in highly endemic areas also fail to provide evidence of protective immunity with advancing age. In fact, quite the contrary is found, with morbidity and mortality from *E. histolytica* infection increasing up to the age of 40–70 years.

Diagnosis

A definitive diagnosis of amebiasis is dependent on the demonstration of trophozoites or cysts in the stool or trophozoites in aspirated pus or tissue specimens. All patients suspected of amebiasis should have at least three stool specimens examined for trophozoites and cysts. The stool should be collected directly in a paper cup to prevent lysis of the trophozoites by water. Examination for motile trophozoites should be done within 1 h of obtaining the specimen. Specimens of stool that cannot be examined within 1 h should be kept in the refrigerator. If routine stool examinations are negative and the diagnosis of amebiasis is still strongly suspected,

a stool specimen should be obtained by saline purge if the patient can tolerate this procedure.

The initial examination of the stool should be a wet-mount preparation. A small sample of stool is placed on a microscope slide and emulsified with saline. A coverslip is added, and the slide is scanned under low power. The microscope should be equipped with an ocular micrometer so that the smaller trophozoites of *E. hartmanni* can be differentiated from *E. histolytica,* since, except for size, these organisms are morphologically identical. A second wet mount using a dilute iodine solution should also be used. Specimens that are negative on direct examination should be reexamined after concentration by the formol ether technique.

Identification of *E. histolytica* trophozoites requires an experienced technician. Trophozoites are usually only found in loose, watery, or dysenteric stools. White blood cells and macrophages with ingested red blood cells may be confused with trophozoites. *Entamoeba histolytica* trophozoites must also be differentiated from nonpathogenic amebae that may colonize the colon. Whenever possible, it is recommended that all parasitology laboratories preserve a portion of the stool with both 5% formalin and polyvinyl alcohol. Polyvinyl alcohol preserves the trophozoites, and the specimen preserved with 5% formalin can be examined for cysts. The preserved material can also be stained with either an iron hematoxylin or a Gomori-Wheatley trichrome stain, procedures which greatly aid in the differentiation of *E. histolytica* trophozoites from other protozoal trophozoites and white blood cells.

In patients with invasive intestinal amebiasis, the diagnosis may be strongly suspected by the finding of characteristic ulcers separated by normal appearing intestinal mucosa during sigmoidoscopy. Scraping of the exudate overlying the ulcer and material aspirated through the sigmoidoscope should also be submitted for parasitologic examination. At the time of sigmoidoscopy, a biopsy may also be obtained from an area of ulceration and serial sections of the biopsied tissue stained with PAS. Occasionally, the biopsy is positive when multiple stool examinations fail to demonstrate trophozoites.

If three stool specimens are examined, trophozoites will be demonstrable in 70–95% of patients with intestinal amebiasis. Unfortunately, many medications and roentgenographic contrast media interfere with the ability to find trophozoites and cysts in the stool. Among the substances that interfere with the diagnosis of amebiasis are antimicrobial, antiprotozoal, and antihelmintic drugs, bismuth, barium, kaolin, magnesium hydroxide, soap, and hypertonic salt enemas. These agents may cause the temporary disappearance of trophozoites and cysts from the stool for several weeks.

In recent years, serologic testing has played an important role in the diagnosis of amebiasis. The serologic diagnosis of amebiasis has been especially useful in cases of amebic liver abscess and other extraintestinal foci of infection in which the absence of trophozoites and cysts in the stool is quite common.

Of the several serologic tests currently available for diagnosis of amebiasis, indirect hemagglutination (IHA) seems to be the most sensitive. Of patients with amebic liver abscess, 90–100% have a titer of 1:128 or greater by IHA. Most patients (80–90%) with invasive intestinal amebiasis also have an elevated IHA titer. No serologic test is suitable for detecting asymptomatic cyst passers. Antibody titers measured by IHA usually revert to normal within 12 months of diagnosis and therapy. Complement fixation and gel diffusion titers usually return to the normal range within 6 months. Some individuals, however, continue to have elevated titers for several years without evidence of continued infection. Thus, a single serologic test is only suggestive of the diagnosis.

Treatment

Drugs used for the treatment of amebiasis can be divided into two major groups. The first encompasses those agents effective against the cyst form of the parasite, which are classified as intraluminal agents. The second group consists of those agents that are effective against the trophozoite, and which are classified as tissue amebicides. Of all the effective agents in use, only metronidazole (Flagyl) is effective against both cysts and trophozoites and is therefore listed as both an intraluminal agent and an amebicide. Outlined below is a therapeutic plan found clinically useful.

Intestinal Noninvasive Disease

Because of the potential for asymptomatic cyst passers to infect others, the consensus is that these individuals should be treated. The two major drugs effective against *E. histolytica* cysts are diloxanide furoate (Furamide),* which is

*Available only from the Parasitic Disease Division, Centers for Disease Control, Atlanta, Georgia.

given orally in doses of 500 mg three times a day for 10 days, and diiodohydroxyquin (Diquinol) in doses of 650 mg three times a day for 20 days. Of the two drugs, diloxanide furoate is better tolerated but more difficult to obtain. Diiodohydroxyquin has the potential to produce optic neuritis. Side effects of both drugs are mostly limited to gastrointestinal upset and hypersensitivity reactions.

Intestinal Invasive Disease

In recent years, metronidazole has been found to be a very effective agent in the therapy of amebiasis. It is effective against trophozoites present in tissue and relatively effective against cysts in the stool. Since the failure rate in treating asymptomatic cyst passers is between 12 and 19%, most clinicians combine metronidazole with either diiodohydroxyquin or diloxanide furoate, the dosages for which have already been outlined. Metronidazole is given orally in a dose of 750 mg three times a day for 5–10 days.

Extraintestinal Amebiasis: Liver Abscess

Although there have been some treatment failures, metronidazole administered as outlined above is the drug of choice. Some patients with extraintestinal amebiasis may be so ill that they are unable to take or cannot tolerate oral medication. For these patients, the same dose of metronidazole can be administered intravenously. If after 72 h the patient is still febrile and the response to metronidazole is perceived by the physician to be less than satisfactory, chloroquine phosphate and emetine hydrochloride should be added to the treatment regimen. Chloroquine phosphate is given at a dose of 1 gm orally each day for the first 2 days, then 0.5 gm daily for 2 weeks; emetine hydrochloride is given as well at a dose of 65 mg per day intramuscularly for 2 weeks.

Eradication of amebiasis can ultimately be accomplished only by governmental initiatives aimed at the elimination of poverty, poor sanitation, and the unsatisfactory living conditions of a vast portion of the world's population; unfortunately, these goals are unlikely to be achieved in the near future.

INFECTION WITH GIARDIA LAMBLIA

Giardia lamblia is a flagellated protozoan that inhabits the upper portion of the human small intestine. Both trophozoite and cyst stages of the parasite are found in humans. Trophozoites are usually found in duodenal aspirates and biopsy specimens of the duodenum and jejunum and are infrequently seen in stools. The trophozoite of *G. lamblia* has a characteristic pear shape and measures 10–18 μm in length and 5–15 μm in width. There are two anterior nuclei and two slender median rods (axostyles). Four pairs of flagella are attached to the ventral side, and attachment to the intestinal epithelium is accomplished by a large ventral sucking disc (see Fig. 20–5). Trophozoites are acid-intolerant and live optimally in the alkaline environment usually present in the upper small intestine.

Cysts of *G. lamblia* are thick-walled and oval in shape. Initially the cyst contains two nuclei that divide, forming four nuclei as the cyst passes down the intestinal tract and matures (Fig. 20–5). The cysts are the infective form of the parasite. Following ingestion, the cysts undergo excystation in the duodenum, forming two daughter trophozoites, completing the cycle.

Epidemiology

Giardia lamblia has a worldwide distribution; it has been reported in almost 100 different countries. There are, however, certain geographic areas where the incidence of infection is fairly high. In the United States, giardiasis is more common in residents of and travelers to the Rocky Mountain states than in the rest of the country. Giardiasis is the most commonly reported parasitic disease in the United States.

Giardia lamblia is the pathogen most frequently responsible for water-related outbreaks of diarrheal illness in the United States. Cysts are capable of remaining viable in cold or tepid water for 1–3 months and are able to survive in the concentrations of chlorine usually present in municipal water. Most community-acquired infections have occurred where surface water (streams, rivers, lakes) is the principal water source, and chlorination the principal method for disinfection. There is highly suggestive evidence that these surface waters may be contaminated by fecal material from infected beavers and perhaps other wild animals. Smaller outbreaks have been reported in campers and backpackers in the Rocky Mountains who drank from mountain streams or ponds. To eliminate the transmission of giardial infection from municipal water, filtration and coagulation–flocculation should be performed in addition to chlorination.

Infection may also occur by fecal-oral transmission. It does not take ingestion of many cysts to cause infection. When human volunteers were fed known numbers of giardial cysts in gelatin capsules, ingestion of 100 or more cysts produced infection in all volunteers, and as few as 10–25 cysts produced disease in 8 of 22 (36%) volunteers. Fecal-oral transmission occurs most commonly in sexually active male homosexuals but also occurs in children confined in institutions. Indirect modes of transmission include contamination of food by asymptomatic cyst passers.

Pathogenesis of Infection

The low pH of gastric secretions is probably somewhat protective against infection with *G. lamblia,* and it has been observed that individuals with achlorhydria and hypochlorhydria are at increased risk of developing infection. Genetic factors may also play a role in susceptibility to infection since giardiasis is seen more frequently in persons with type A blood and less frequently in persons with type O blood.

The mechanism by which *G. lamblia* produces diarrhea is not fully understood. From biopsy studies of the duodenum and jejunum, trophozoites of *G. lamblia* are most frequently found attached to the microvillus layer of the epithelium. In patients with severe disease, partial or subtotal villous atrophy is seen. Accompanying this change in villous architecture is a variable

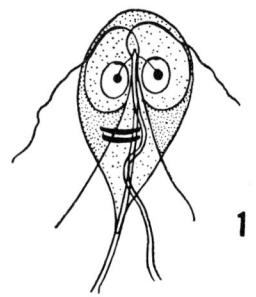 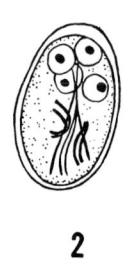 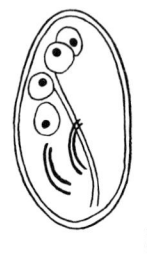

1   **2**   **3**

Figure 20–5. 1. Giardia lamblia *trophozoite;* 2, 3. G. lamblia *cysts. (From Markell, E. K., and Voge, M. Medical Parasitology, 4th ed. Philadelphia: W. B. Saunders Co., 1976.)*

inflammatory infiltrate in the lamina propria consisting of both lymphocytes and neutrophils. It is not known whether this inflammatory response is protective, pathogenic, or perhaps both. Rarely, trophozoites are found within the mucosa and lamina propria of the upper small intestine. Direct invasion of the mucosa is felt to be only coincidental and not responsible for the symptoms of infection.

There is good evidence for epithelial cell dysfunction of the upper small intestine. Quite commonly, the microvilli of the upper small intestine are found to be temporarily deficient in disaccharidase activity. Also, fat and vitamin B_{12} malabsorption are commonly observed, indicating that the absorptive dysfunction extends into the ileum. So far, no toxin has been found to explain the epithelial cell dysfunction, nor are there enough trophozoites present to mechanically block the enormous absorptive capacity of the small intestine. In many symptomatic patients with giardiasis, the biopsy of the upper small intestine is normal. This may be due in part to the patchy nature of the mucosal abnormalities, which can easily be missed when only a single biopsy is performed.

Host Response to Infection

Specific antibody to both cyst and trophozoite antigens can be found in the majority of patients recovering from *Giardia lamblia* infection. Even patients who are asymptomatic cyst passers have detectable circulating antibody. It has also been observed that residents of endemic areas are less commonly infected than are visitors. In the human intestine, it is quite possible that secretory anti-giardial IgA may interfere with adherence of this parasite to the gut epithelium and thus prevent the establishment of a new infection. There seems to be a definitely increased incidence of giardiasis in patients with common variable immunodeficiency. Not only is there an increased incidence of disease in such patients, but the illness is usually prolonged and more severe than in normal hosts.

Cellular immunity also appears to play a role in host defense against giardial infection. In the experimental mouse model, lymphocytes from an immune animal protect nonimmune mice from *G. muris* infection (a rodent strain of giardia). Athymic nude mice when infected with *G. muris* experience prolonged and severe infection suggesting that the host response to giardial infection involves cellular, as well as humoral, immunity. Patients with acquired immunodeficiency syndrome (AIDS), when infected with giardia, experience a severe and prolonged diarrheal illness.

Acute Symptomatic Infection

Following an incubation period of 1–3 weeks, an acute diarrheal illness lasting 5–7 days is the most common presentation of giardiasis. The acute illness is quite variable in severity. Some patients have an abrupt, explosive onset with frequent watery, foul-smelling stools, whereas others have only a few loose bowel movements. Most commonly, the patient also has abdominal cramps and complains of nausea, anorexia, and increased flatulence. Less often, fever, vomiting, and abdominal distention may be present. Blood or mucus is rarely present in the stool. In 86% of experimentally infected volunteers, cysts can no longer be found in the stool after 6 weeks. In some patients the acute illness may be prolonged, lasting 1–2 months. An even smaller percentage of infected individuals develop a subacute or chronic illness.

Chronic Giardiasis

In patients who have chronic giardiasis, diarrhea is often intermittent and less severe than in the acute illness. Stools are frequently foul-smelling, and foul-smelling gas may be passed from the rectum. Substernal burning, nausea, and anorexia may occur. Because of these symptoms, peptic ulcer disease, hiatal hernia, and gallbladder disease may be suspected.

Signs and symptoms of intestinal malabsorption are commonly present in patients with chronic giardiasis. As a result of chronic malabsorption, weight loss is frequently reported by the patient. These symptoms, in association with persistent or intermittent diarrhea, often lead first to a diagnosis of pancreatic insufficiency, celiac disease, regional enteritis, ulcerative colitis, or intestinal malignancy. In some patients frank steatorrhea develops, as evidenced by the passage of bulky, greasy, foul-smelling stools. In patients with steatorrhea, the absorption of vitamin A and folate are also frequently impaired. In some patients, absorption of vitamin B_{12} is abnormally low, implying that the absorption defect extends into the ileum. In addition to fat malabsorption, defects in the absorption of carbohydrates are found in up to 50% of patients with giardiasis, as indicated by decreased absorption of D-xylose. Intestinal biopsy also shows reduced activity of the disaccharidases, lactase, maltase, and sucrase, which may persist for some time even after completion of medical therapy.

Very rarely, there is extraintestinal extension of infection into the biliary tract. In patients so affected, the signs and symptoms of infection are identical to those seen in patients with classic, acute, or chronic cholangitis or cholecystitis.

Asymptomatic Carriers

Most people who become infected with *G. lamblia* do not recall experiencing a diarrheal illness. These individuals are usually discovered only when epidemiologic investigations are carried out. It has been found that in some regions of the United States, 5–10% of the population excrete cysts in their stools. The duration of asymptomatic carriage of *G. lamblia* is unknown.

Diagnosis

The diagnosis of giardiasis is most commonly made by finding cysts in the stool. Since the cysts passed in some patients may be intermittent or low in number and thus difficult to find, a stool specimen should be examined every other day for a total of three or four occasions. Stools should be examined directly and after concentration with formol ether or zinc sulfate and stained with Lugol's solution or iron hematoxylin. In the acute phase of the disease, when diarrhea is severe and transit time is short, trophozoites may also be found in the stool. In a small number of patients, cysts cannot be found in the stool, but a diagnosis can usually be made by duodenal intubation and aspiration, since trophozoites are frequently present in the fluid and mucus that is obtained. To increase the yield even further, biopsy of the duodenal and jejunal mucosa may be performed. A less invasive procedure is the "string test," in which the patient swallows a weighted capsule attached to a nylon line (Enterotest: available from Hedeco Co., Mountain View, California) long enough to pass into the upper small intestine. The capsule and line are removed after several hours, and the mucus adherent to the distal line is scraped onto a glass slide along with a few drops of saline and examined for trophozoites.

Recently, the detection of giardial antigen in the stool by the use of counterimmunoelectrophoresis and by enzyme-linked immunosorbent assay (ELISA) has been described. These techniques are able to detect very small numbers of organisms that are present in the stool or are seen only on duodenal aspiration and biopsy. In addition, these techniques require less skilled technician time and are more suitable to mass screening and epidemiologic studies than is routine stool examination.

Treatment

The drug of choice in the treatment of giardiasis is quinacrine (Atabrine). The usual dose for adults is 100 mg orally three times a day for 7 days. Children are given 7 mg/kg/day (maximum dosage, 300 mg/day). To decrease gastrointestinal upset, medication is given after meals. At this dose and duration of therapy, side effects are few and infrequent, but they include nausea, vomiting, abdominal cramps, toxic psychosis, exfoliative dermatitis, and rarely, yellowing of the skin and sclera. Ninety to ninety-five percent of the patients with giardiasis treated with quinacrine are cured. Treatment failures usually respond to a second course of therapy.

Metronidazole (Flagyl), 250 mg three times a day for 7 days, is also an effective agent in the treatment of giardiasis. Cure rates with metronidazole are in the range of 85–90%. A third agent now available for the treatment of giardiasis is furazolidone (Furoxone). This agent is not quite as effective in the elimination of infection as is quinacrine and metronidazole, but it is helpful in the treatment of children, since it is available as a pleasant-tasting liquid suspension. The usual oral dose for adults is 100 mg four times a day for 7 days, and for children 6 mg/kg/day divided into four equal doses. Side effects include nausea, vomiting, fever, and mild intravascular hemolysis with glucose-6-phosphate dehydrogenase deficiency. A disulfiram-like reaction may occur if alcohol is consumed during treatment.

INFECTION WITH ISOSPORA BELLI

Infection is initiated by swallowing food or water contaminated with sporocysts of *Isospora belli*. A higher incidence of *I. belli* infection has been observed in homosexual men, also suggesting that transmission of this parasitic infection may occur sexually. Excystation occurs in the upper small intestine with the release of four sporozoites from each sporocyst. Asexual development (schizogony) occurs within the cystoplasm of the epithelial cell with the development of trophozoites, schizonts, and finally, merozoites.

The merozoites are then released by the disintegrating schizont to invade other epithelial cells, and this cycle is repeated. At least 1 week later the sexual cycle (gametogony) begins with the production of micro- and macrogametocytes. Following fertilization of the macrogametocytes by the microgametocytes, the zygote, or oocyst, is formed. The oocyst, when shed into the bowel lumen, initially contains a single sporoblast. Following fecal passage of the oocyst, the sporoblast divides in two and secretes a cyst wall around itself (sporocyst). Within each sporoblast, four sporozoites develop. Ingestion of the sporocyst containing the sporozoites initiates the infection in the duodenum and upper jejunum.

Acute and Chronic Intestinal Infection

The most common symptom complex of *Isospora belli* infection is a self-limited diarrheal illness which lasts from 1–3 weeks. Watery diarrhea is frequently associated with cramping abdominal pain, fever, and weight loss. Some patients develop a chronic diarrheal illness frequently associated with malabsorption. *Isospora belli* infection in patients with AIDS is frequently a persistent protracted illness if left untreated.

On pathologic examination of the small bowel, villous shortening, hypertrophic crypts, and infiltration of the lamina propria with lymphocytes, plasma cells, and lymphocytes are frequently observed. Whether these mucosal changes alone are enough to account for the diarrheal illness is as yet unknown.

Diagnosis

Oocysts may be few in number or shed only intermittently in the stool. The cysts have an ovoid shape and measure 20–33 μm in length by 10–19 μm in width. Stools are best examined following a concentration technique. Identification of the cysts is also easier when the stool concentrate is stained with a modified Kinyoun stain. With this stain the oocysts of *Isospora*

belli stain bright red on a green background. If repeated stool examinations are negative, sometimes the only way to confirm the diagnosis of *I. belli* infection is by intestinal biopsy.

Treatment

Most infections with *Isospora belli* can be successfully treated with trimethoprim-sulfamethoxazole (Bactrim, Septra). In adults the usual dose is one double-strength tablet every 6 h by mouth for 10 days followed by one double-strength tablet every 12 h for an additional 3 weeks. An alternative regimen for the treatment of *I. belli* infection is pyrimethamine plus sulfadoxine (Fansidar) given orally. Patients with AIDS may require chronic suppression of this infection with weekly administration of trimethoprim-sulfamethoxazole.

INFECTION WITH CRYPTOSPORIDIUM

Cryptosporidium, like *Isospora belli,* is a coccidian protozoan capable of infecting the human intestinal tract, producing a diarrheal illness. Prior to 1976, infection with *Cryptosporidium* was felt to be confined to young farm animals (pigs, lambs, calves). In 1976, the first human case of cryptosporidiosis was described, and until 1982 there were only a handful of reported human cases. With the development of the AIDS epidemic, numerous cases of cryptosporidiosis have been described. This protozoan is now recognized as a major enteric pathogen of patients with AIDS, producing a severe, protracted diarrheal illness.

With the increased awareness of this protozoan as a cause of diarrheal illness and increased skill in routine identification of this parasite by parasitology laboratories, cryptosporidial infections have also been identified with increased frequency in normal hosts. The overall frequency of cryptosporidial infection in the United States has been estimated at 2.6%. A higher incidence of infection was found when selected day-care centers were sampled. Both human-to-human and animal-to-human transmission can occur. Nosocomial transmission between hospital staff and patients has been described, as well as an increased incidence of infection among household contacts of an infected patient. Individuals who work with animals, such as farm workers and veterinarians, also are at increased risk to develop infection.

Life Cycle

Infection is initiated by ingestion of small (2–5 μm) spherical oocysts. Excystation occurs in the upper intestinal tract with the liberation of four sporozoites. The entire asexual (schizogony) development of the parasite, with the production of trophozoites, schizonts, and merozoites, as well as the sexual cycle (gametogony), with the production of gametes, all occurs in a single host. This monoxenous life cycle lends itself to perpetuation of infection. The merozoites liberated from the schizonts within the intestinal tract are able to infect more enterocytes. Oocysts are excreted in the stool and are capable of infecting other humans or susceptible animals.

The life forms of *Cryptosporidium* are confined to the microvillous border of the intestinal epithelial cell. The parasite is enclosed in a vacuole, the membrane of which appears to be of host origin. Thus, the parasite is intracellular but extracytoplasmic. In patients with AIDS, cryptosporidia are found throughout the entire intestine and occasionally invade the gallbladder and biliary tree.

Acute and Chronic Intestinal Infection

In the normal host after an incubation period of 7–8 days, a self-limited watery diarrheal illness without blood or mucus ensues. Patients may also experience abdominal cramps and low-grade fever. The diarrheal illness usually resolves after 1 or 2 weeks, but excretion of oocysts may persist for 2–4 weeks after symptoms abate. In immunocompromised hosts, particularly in patients with AIDS, *Cryptosporidium* infection is severe and protracted. The diarrheal illness is often watery and voluminous, with fluid losses of up to 20 L/day described. This is often associated with malabsorption, significant weight loss, electrolyte imbalance, marked suffering, and poor quality of life for the patient.

Diagnosis

Oocysts can be easily demonstrated (after stool concentration) by a modified acid-fast stain, such as a cold Kinyoun stain. In the normal host, fewer oocysts are excreted during the diarrheal illness and several concentrated stools may need to be examined to establish a diagnosis.

Treatment

Presently there is no effective therapy for cryptosporidiosis. Although the macrolide antibiotic spiramycin initially was felt to be efficacious, subsequent studies have failed to confirm that benefit.

COMMON INTESTINAL NEMATODE INFECTIONS

Of the more than half million different species of roundworms, many of which infect animals and plants, only about 12 species are parasitic for humans. On a global scale infection with nematodes (roundworms) is more common than infection with any other group of pathogens. Enterobius and ascaris each account for a billion infections worldwide. Not far behind are infections with *Trichuris* and hookworm, which each produce a half billion infections annually. In the United States, it has been estimated that 54 million people, mostly children, are infected with nematodes. The intestinal nematodes are unsegmented roundworms with a cylindrical shape that is tapered at both ends. They are large parasites, all of which can be seen by the naked eye without magnification. The sexes of the roundworms are separate, with the male usually smaller than the female. Each roundworm has a complete digestive tract with an oral opening at one end and a distal anal opening.

Trichuris trichiura *Infection*

Trichuriasis, infection with *Trichuris trichiura* (or whipworm), is a common infection in the United States, especially in the southeastern portion of the country. It has been estimated that in the United States there are 2.2 million individuals infected with trichuris. Worldwide, the incidence of infection is even greater in tropical and subtropical areas of the world where there is overcrowding and poor sanitation.

Life Cycle

The life cycle of *Trichuris trichiura* is simple, and no intermediate host is required. Infection is initiated by the ingestion of the embryonated eggs present in soil that has been contaminated by human feces. The eggs are hardy and may remain viable in moist soil for years. In the small intestine the male and female larvae emerge and pass to the large intestine and cecum. Adult male and female worms develop in the large intestine. The adult worms have a characteristic appearance with a thin whiplike anterior portion and a stout hind portion, "the whip handle." The adults measure 30–50 mm in length. The slender anterior portion of the worm penetrates the mucosa of the large intestine anchoring the parasite while the posterior portion of the body protrudes into the bowel lumen facilitating copulation and oviposition. After the adult worms mature, the female is capable of laying 1000 eggs per day. The unsegmented eggs, passed into the feces, require about 2 weeks to embryonate in warm moist soil. Adult worms may live as long as a year in the intestinal tract.

Clinical Manifestations of Trichuriasis

Like all nematode infections, symptomatology is directly proportional to the extent of the infection (worm burden) and to the age and general health of the host. Most infections with trichuris are light to moderate. In these individuals symptoms of infection are uncommon. With heavy infections in children, complaints of abdominal pain, bloody or mucoid diarrhea, and weight loss may be experienced. Rarely, appendicitis secondary to appendiceal obstruction and prolapse of the rectum may occur.

Diagnosis

Diagnosis of *Trichuris trichiura* infection is made by finding the characteristic ovoid-shaped eggs with clear mucus plugs at each pole. Infections can be quantitated by counting the number of eggs found in a direct fecal smear. In light infections fewer than 10 eggs are present. In heavy infections 50 or more eggs are present in the fecal smear.

Treatment

Trichuris infections can be effectively treated with mebendazole 100 mg twice a day for 3 days. Mebendazole (Vermox) is poorly absorbed from the intestinal tract and has insignificant side effects.

Enterobius vermicularis *Infection*

Enterobiasis, infection with the pinworm *Enterobius vermicularis,* is the most common helminthic infection in the United States. An estimated 42 million individuals, mostly children, are infected with pinworms. Infections tend to spread within the family setting, especially if several children live in the same household or sleep in the same bed. Transmission of enterobius infection is by the fecal-oral route. This may be direct, from the unwashed hands of one child to the mouth of another, or indirect, by fecal contamination of sheets, linen, and night clothes.

Life Cycle

The life cycle of *Enterobius vermicularis* is very similar to that of *Trichuris trichiura* because it is direct, requiring no intermediate host.

Infection is initiated by swallowing the embryonated egg, which passes into the small intestine, releasing the enclosed larvae. The larvae migrate down the intestinal tract to the cecum and colon where the adult worms develop in about a month. The adult male is very small, measuring 2–5 mm in length, but the adult female is much larger, 8–13 mm long with a sharply pointed posterior end (pin). The fertilized females migrate at night to the perianal and perineal skin and deposit their eggs in this location. Each female pinworm is capable of laying 11,000 ovoid eggs which are surrounded by a thick wall and flattened on one side. The embryonated eggs, which develop within 6 h, are picked up by the child's hands or contaminate the bed clothes or linen and can initiate a new infection.

Clinical Manifestations of Enterobiasis

Most pinworm infections are asymptomatic. When symptoms are reported the most frequent complaints are perianal itching and restless sleep produced by the deposited eggs. Rarely in young girls a vaginitis or even salpingitis has been reported. Another rare complication of pinworm infection is appendicitis.

Diagnosis

Since eggs are rarely deposited into the stool, the most common method of confirming enterobius infection is the recovery of the characteristic eggs from the perianal skin. The most commonly employed method is the "Scotch-tape" swab. A piece of transparent adhesive tape backed by a tongue blade is pressed around the perianal skin early in the morning. The transparent tape is then transferred to a glass slide and examined under the microscope. A single Scotch-tape swab picks up eggs from at least 50% of those infected, and three swabs on consecutive days pick up eggs from 90%. In families with multiple children, all family members should be examined in this manner.

Treatment

Enterobius infection is effectively treated with a single 100 mg oral dose of mebendazole. Frequently physicians treat all children in the family if one child is discovered to have pinworms. Bed clothes and linen can be decontaminated by ordinary washing in hot water.

Ascaris lumbricoides *Infection*

Infection with *Ascaris lumbricoides* is the most common helmintic infection in the world, with over a billion humans infected. Infection is most common in tropical or subtropical areas of the world, where poor sanitation and overcrowding exist, but is not uncommon in temperate regions. In the United States an estimated 4 million people are infected with ascaris, mostly in the southeastern and Gulf states. Children bear the major brunt of this parasitic infection, with symptoms related to migration of the parasite through the lungs and to intestinal disease. Ascaris is the largest of the intestinal roundworms, with the female worm measuring 20–35 cm in length and the mature male 15–30 cm. The average life span for the adult worms is about 6 months.

Life Cycle

Infection is initiated by ingestion of embryonated eggs present in the soil. The larvae emerge in the small intestine and penetrate the bowel wall and into the portal circulation. They are carried via the bloodstream to the lungs, where they increase in size and molt twice. The larvae next break into the bronchial tree and travel up into the trachea and then into the esophagus. The swallowed larvae reach the small intestine where they develop into mature adults. From ingestion of the embryonated egg to the development of a gravid female takes about 8–12 weeks. Each female is capable of laying 200,000 eggs per day. Fertilized eggs require 2–3 weeks to develop in the soil before they are mature and are infective.

Clinical Manifestations of Ascariasis

In heavy infections, pulmonary infiltrates associated with peripheral eosinophilia may develop when the larvae migrate through the lungs. This self-limited pneumonia is associated with cough, dyspnea, fever, and scattered pulmonary infiltrates on chest x-ray. On repeated exposure to ascaris, allergic reactions may be responsible for bronchospasm (asthma) and cutaneous urticaria.

The symptoms of small-intestine infection are directly dependent on worm burden, with light infections being asymptomatic. In heavy infections with worm loads of several hundred to a thousand worms, abdominal pain, diarrhea, anorexia, and malnutrition may be experienced. Malnutrition is due to impaired absorption of carbohydrates and fat in the small intestine. In heavy infections symptoms may be secondary to a mass of tangled worms that can produce intestinal obstruction. Ascaris worms may also migrate into the common bile duct or pancreatic duct to produce obstructive cholecystitis and pancreatitis, or into the appendix with resulting appendicitis.

Diagnosis

Finding the characteristic ovoid eggs covered with an albuminoid shell in the feces is the most common method of confirming ascaris infection. On occasion adult worms may crawl out the nose, be vomited, or pass into the stool. In families with several children, all family members should have their stool examined for the presence of eggs.

Treatment

Mebendazole, 100 mg twice a day by mouth for 3 days, or pyrantel pamoate (Povan) as a single dose (11 mg/kg up to a maximum of 1 gm) are both equally effective agents in treating ascariasis.

Infection with Necator americanus *and* Ancylostoma duodenale

Infection with the hookworms *Necator americanus* and *Ancylostoma duodenale* dates to prehistoric times. These parasites are common in the tropical and subtropical areas of the world where there is overcrowding and poor sanitation. *Ancylostoma duodenale* (Old World hookworm) has been mostly found in southern Europe, the north coast of Africa, northern India, and China, and is not discussed at length in this section.

Necator americanus (New World hookworm) is present in the United States, mostly in the southeastern portion of the country, but is more frequently found in Central and South America, the Caribbean, Africa, and Asia. Together hookworm infection affects half a billion people throughout the world.

Hookworms derive their name from the teeth *(Ancylostoma)* or cutting plates *(Necator)* in the anterior buccal capsule, which allow the hookworm to attach to the intestinal mucosa and account for the significant blood loss experienced by heavily infected individuals.

Life Cycle

The life cycle of *Necator americanus* has been described as the skin-penetrating type. Infection is acquired by walking barefooted or in sandals in soil containing the filariform hookworm larva. The skin is penetrated by the larva, often producing a papular eruption and severe pruritus of the skin ("ground itch"). The filariform larva then enters the venous circulation and is carried to the pulmonary capillary bed. In the lungs *N. americanus* does not evoke an intense reaction as occurs in infection with ascaris or strongyloides (see description later in this chapter). The larva then breaks into the bronchial tree, migrates up into the trachea and then into the esophagus and is swallowed. In the small intestine the filariform larvae molt (third molt) and develop a temporary bacial capsule for attachment to the mucosa. Here the larvae grow and develop into adult male and female worms. After about a period of 5 weeks from initiation of infection, the female hookworms begin to oviposit. The hookworm eggs deposited with the feces into warm moist soil first develop into the rhabditiform larvae which are free-living and feed on bacteria and organic debris. By about a week the rhabdoid larvae develop into the nonfeeding filariform larvae capable of invading a new human host.

The life cycle of *Ancylostoma duodenale* is almost identical to that of *N. americanus* with the exception that infection can also be initiated by swallowing the filariform larva and that a developmental stage in the lungs is not required.

Clinical Manifestations of Hookworm Infection

As with most intestinal parasitic infections, symptoms are largely dependent on worm burden. In the United States most infections with *Necator americanus* are light and infections are usually asymptomatic. In heavy infections the major symptoms are secondary to anemia and hypoalbuminemia. Blood loss occurs secondary to ingestion of blood by the parasite, but to a much greater extent into the bowel lumen from the bleeding laceration created by the attachment of the cutting plates or teeth of the hookworm. It has been estimated that 0.03 mL of blood is lost per day for each adult *N. americanus* worm and 0.15 mL for each *A. duodenale* adult. In heavy infections, over a thousand adult worms may be present in the small intestine. The resulting anemia and hypoalbuminemia may be compounded in those individuals consuming diets poor in protein and iron. Occasionally a transient pulmonary infiltrate develops during the stage of pulmonary migration, associated with eosinophilia.

Humans may also develop a cutaneous eruption if they come in contact with the dog and cat hookworm larvae, *Ancylostoma braziliense* or *A. caninum*. These larvae penetrate the skin and migrate through the subcutaneous tissue, forming serpiginous tunnels associated with intense itching. Infection with these hookworms and this cutaneous eruption has been termed *cutaneous larva migrans*. The larva cannot complete the life cycle as human hookworms do and essentially remain trapped in the skin until they die, which may take several weeks.

Diagnosis

The diagnosis of hookworm infection rests on the demonstration of the characteristic eggs in the stool. The number of eggs can be quantitated, and egg counts greater than 2000 per gram of stool in children is considered clinically significant.

Treatment

Hookworms are very effectively treated with oral mebendazole, 100 mg twice a day for 3 days.

Strongyloides stercoralis *Infection*

Infection with *Strongyloides stercoralis* is most common in warm climates, but it is also present in temperate areas of the world. Strongyloides infection somewhat parallels hookworm infection. Infection in the United States has been reported mostly from the southeastern portion of the country. In addition to children being the most common target for infection, *S. stercoralis* may produce severe infection (hyperinfection) in the compromised host.

Life Cycle

The life cycle of *Stronglyloides stercoralis* is very similar to that of the hookworm in that infection is usually initiated when the infective filariform larvae penetrate the skin and make their way to the lung via the bloodstream. From the lungs the larvae migrate up the tracheobronchial tree and into the esophagus, and then into the upper small intestine. In the duodenum and upper jejunum the larvae mature into the adult worms, the female measuring about 2.5 mm in length. The gravid female lays her eggs, which usually hatch in the mucosal epithelium, producing rhabdoid larvae. The rhabdoid larvae are passed into the feces and in areas of poor sanitation are deposited in the soil. The rhabdoid larvae of strongyloides may exist in the soil as a free-living form or develop into nonfeeding, infective filariform larvae.

For reasons which are poorly understood, in some individuals, usually those who are immunologically compromised, the progression from rhabdoid to filariform larvae may occur in the lower intestine. The infectious filariform larvae thus produced are able to enter the host's circulation in the large intestine and rectum or through the perianal or perineal skin. This autoinfection (hyperinfection) leads to both persistence of infection and large numbers of worms infecting the host.

Clinical Manifestations of Strongyloidiasis

At the site of skin penetration a local pruritic inflammatory reaction may develop, but this occurs less frequently and is less symptomatic than with hookworm infection. When larvae penetrate the perianal skin, they may produce a serpiginous trail associated with urticaria. This creeping eruption has been termed *larva currens*. During the larva's migration through the lung, patchy infiltrates associated with peripheral blood eosinophilia may develop—Löffler's pneumonia.

With heavy intestinal infection, complaints of abdominal pain, weight loss, and diarrhea are common. The abdominal pain may be epigastric and burning in nature, similar to the pain produced by peptic ulcer disease.

Patients who are immunocompromised because of an underlying hematological malignancy, corticosteroid therapy, malnutrition, or AIDS are prone to develop hyperinfection. In these individuals infective filariform larvae develop from the rhabdoid larvae as the latter pass down the gastrointestinal tract. The filariform larvae penetrate the vascular system in the colon and rectum or through the perianal or perineal skin. Not infrequently after entering the host's circulation, these larvae follow an aberrant course and settle in various organs, producing local inflammatory disease. The lung is commonly involved in this process, but any organ may be affected. There may also be local ulcerations of the bowel, with the development of bacterial sepsis.

Diagnosis

The diagnosis of strongyloides infection rests on the demonstration of larvae in the stool, in bronchial secretions, or in duodenal fluid. Multiple stools should first be examined after concentration; if persistently negative, a duodenal aspirate obtained by intubation or material obtained by a "string test" (see diagnosis of giardiasis above) should be examined for the presence of larvae.

Treatment

Strongyloides infection can be effectively treated with thiabendazole (Mintezol), 25 mg/kg twice a day by mouth for 2 days. In patients with hyperinfection, treatment with thiabendazole should be extended for at least 1 week.

REFERENCES

Books

Bogitsh, B. J., and Cheng, T. C., eds. *Human Parasitology.* Philadelphia: Saunders College Publishing, 1990.

Cook, G. C. *Parasitic Disease in Clinical Practice.* New York: Springer-Verlag, 1990.

Leech, J. H., Sande, M. A., and Root, R. K., eds. *Parasitic Infections.* New York: Churchill Livingstone, 1988.

Original Articles

Adams, E. B., and MacLeod, I. N. Invasive amebiasis. I. Amebic dysentery and its complications. *Medicine* 56:315–323, 1977.

Adams, E. B., and MacLeod, I. N. Invasive amebiasis. II. Amebic liver abscess and its complications. *Medicine 56:*325–334, 1977.

DeHovitz, J. A. Management of *Isospora belli* infections in AIDS patients. *Infect. Med. 10:*437–440, 1988.

Guerrant, R. L. The global problem of amebiasis: Current status, research needs, and opportunities for progress. *Rev. Infect. Dis. 8:*218–226, 1986.

Healy, G. R. Immunologic tools in the diagnosis of amebiasis: Epidemiology in the United States. *Rev. Infect. Dis. 8:*239–246, 1986.

Katzenstein, D., Rickerson, V., and Braude, A. New concepts of amebic liver abscess derived from hepatic imaging, serodiagnosis, and hepatic enzymes in 67 consecutive cases in San Diego. *Medicine 61:*237–246, 1982.

Koch, K. L., Phillips, D. J., Aber, R. C., et al. Cryptosporidiosis in hospital personnel. *Ann. Intern. Med. 102:*593–596, 1985.

Nash, T. E., Herrington, D. A., and Levine, M. M. Usefulness of an enzyme-linked immunosorbent assay for detection of *Giardia* antigen in feces. *J. Clin. Microbiol. 25:*1169–1171, 1987.

Raizman, R. E. Giardiasis: An overview for the clinician. *Am. J. Dig. Dis. 21:*1070–1074, 1976.

Ravdin, J. I. Pathogenesis of disease caused by *Entamoeba histolytica:* Studies of adherence, secreted toxins, and contact-dependent cytolysis. *Rev. Infect. Dis. 8:*247–260, 1986.

Salata, R. A., Ravdin, J. I. Review of the human immune mechanisms directed against *Entamoeba histolytica*. *Rev. Infect. Dis. 8:*261–272, 1986.

Soave, R., and Armstrong, D. *Cryptosporidium* and cryptosporidiosis. *Rev. Infect. Dis. 8:*1012–1023, 1986.

Stevens, D. P. Giardiasis: Host-pathogen biology. *Rev. Infect. Dis. 4:*851–858, 1982.

Walsh, J. A. Problems in recognition and diagnosis of amebiasis: Estimation of the global magnitude of morbidity and mortality. *Rev. Infect. Dis. 8:*228–237, 1986.

Waterborne disease outbreaks 1986–1988. *MMWR 39:*1–13, 1990.

Viral Hepatitis

INTRODUCTION

Viral hepatitis is the term applied to those viral infections in which the liver is the dominant target organ. Other viral illnesses that may affect the liver but in which hepatic involvement does not usually dominate the clinical picture will not be discussed here. That jaundice could occur in an epidemic form was known to the Greeks and Romans of the 5th century B.C. During the 18th century, at least nine well-defined epidemics of jaundice were described in Central Europe, some including remarkably astute clinical observations. Subsequently, the infectious nature of hepatitis was clearly established by studies that strongly suggested fecal–oral transmission in some circumstances and transmission by blood or serum in other situations. An example of the latter was the early World War II outbreak of 50,000 cases of hepatitis among American soldiers who had received injections of yellow fever vaccine containing human serum. The fecal–oral form of hepatitis became known as *infectious hepatitis,* and the latter variety was termed *serum hepatitis.*

In the past two decades, there has been truly remarkable progress in identifying and characterizing the specific etiologic agents of viral hepatitis. This identification includes *hepatitis A virus* (HAV) as the etiology of infectious hepatitis; *hepatitis B virus* (HBV) as the etiology of serum hepatitis; the *delta hepatitis agent* as a novel defective viral pathogen; and most recently, *hepatitis C virus* (HCV) and hepatitis E virus (HEV). The latter two agents account for a large portion of the viral hepatitis not associated with HAV or HBV, which has become known as *non-A, non-B hepatitis.* This form of hepatitis includes infection by HCV and HEV and probably several additional agents. Diagnostic tests to measure specific well-characterized serologic markers now enable accurate identification of infection with HAV, HBV, the delta virus, and HCV. A highly effective HBV vaccine is available, and candidate HAV vac-

TABLE 21–1. *Characteristics of Viral Hepatitis*

	Hepatitis A	Hepatitis B	Delta Virus	Hepatitis C	Hepatitis E
Causative agent	27-nm RNA virus	42-nm DNA virus with surface and core components	36-nm RNA defective virus with HB$_S$Ag coat	RNA virus	32-nm RNA virus
Transmission	Fecal–oral	Parenteral	Parenteral	Parenteral; sporadic also (fecal–oral?)	Fecal–oral; contaminated water supply
Incubation	15–50 days	45–180 days	28–180 days	About 60–180 days	14–56 days
Period of infectivity	Late incubation to early clinical phase	When HB$_S$Ag positive	When anti-HDV seropositive	Unknown	Unknown
Fulminant hepatitis	Rare	Uncommon	Common	Uncommon	Common in third trimester; otherwise uncommon
Chronic hepatitis or carrier state	No	Common (5–10%)	Common	Common	No
Prophylaxis	Hygiene; ISG	Hygiene, HBIG; HBV vaccine	Hygiene; HBV vaccine	Screening blood; hygiene	Hygiene; safe water supply

cines are being developed and tested. Because similarity of the clinical manifestations of the several forms of viral hepatitis frequently makes differentiation on clinical grounds alone somewhat difficult, an accurate history of potential sources of infection together with serologic testing are required for accurate diagnosis of the specific type of viral hepatitis. Table 21–1 includes information about the five hepatitis virus–related illnesses.

HEPATITIS A: INFECTIOUS HEPATITIS

Virology

HAV was initially identified by electron-microscopic study of feces from patients with acute infectious hepatitis in 1973. By 1979, the virus was propagated in primate cell cultures, and by 1983 more than 99% of the viral genome had been cloned. HAV is classified as a picornavirus (genus Enterovirus) and morphologically is a nonenveloped spherical particle that is 27 nm in diameter with icosahedral symmetry; its genome is single-stranded RNA (Fig. 21–1 *A* and *B*). Marmosets, chimpanzees, and owl monkeys have been experimentally infected, and viral particles can be visualized in the resulting hepatocyte cytoplasm. HAV is a particularly hardy picornavirus: it is stable at 60°C for 1 h, withstands exposure to 10% ether at 4°C for 20 h, and can be stored at −20°C for at least 1½ years. It is destroyed by boiling for 15 min or

by autoclaving, and HAV can be inactivated but retain its antigenicity by boiling for 5 min, by exposure to ultraviolet light, or by exposure to 1:4000 formalin at 37°C for 3 days.

The HAV genome is 7478 nucleotides long with a poly(A) tail, and a viral protein is covalently linked to the 5′ terminus. The genome encodes four structural capsid proteins (VP1 to VP4) and seven nonstructural proteins (2A–2C, and 3A–3D). Only a single serotype of HAV is known, and the serologically recognized epitope of HAV is expressed on VP1 and probably on VP3. Vaccine development has included work with attenuated HAV strains containing a relatively small number of nucleotide changes in the genome.

Serology and Immunity

As with many other viral infections, the serologic response to HAV infection is characterized by a brief IgM–anti-HAV response, with subsequent prolonged synthesis of IgG–anti-HAV. The first available serologic test measured total serum anti-HAV, and thus reflected either recent or remote infection, but did not distinguish between them. The current assay is specific for IgM–anti-HAV and is very useful in clinical diagnosis of acute hepatitis A, because, unlike most other viral infections, IgM–anti-HAV is almost always detectable in serum at the time of clinical presentation of hepatitis A and persists for several months. In contrast, IgG–anti-HAV is present in convalescence and persists

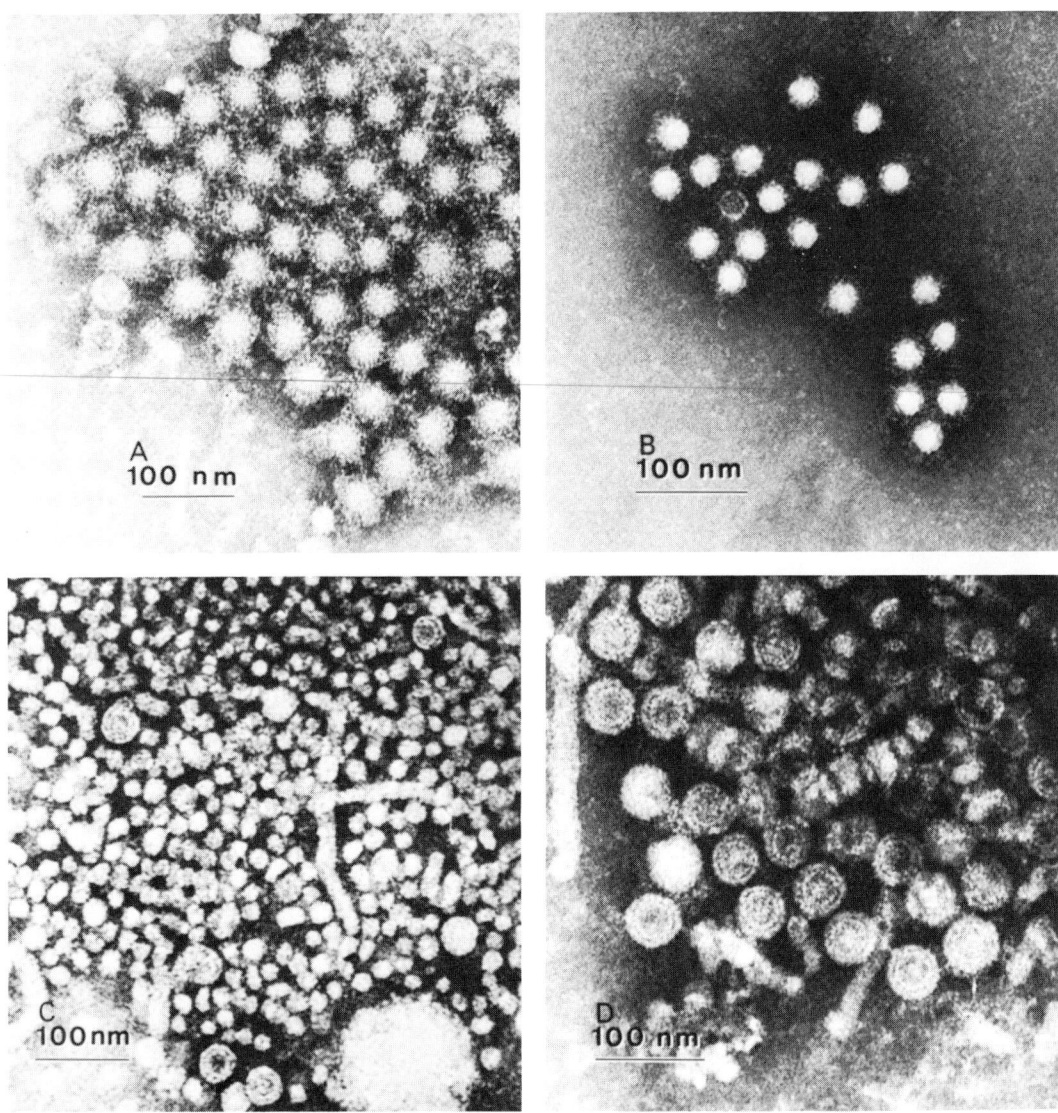

Figure 21–1. A. Hepatitis A viruses from human stool, aggregated by human antibody (4+). B. Hepatitis A viruses from chimpanzee stool, aggregated by human antibody (2+). C. Spherical and tubular forms of hepatitis B surface antigen and hepatitis B virus (Dane particle) aggregated by chimpanzee antibody. D. Aggregate of hepatitis B viruses concentrated by differential centrifugation. (From WHO Collaborating Centre for Reference and Research on Viral Hepatitis, Centers for Disease Control, Bureau of Epidemiology, Hepatitis Laboratories Division, Phoenix, Arizona. Photograph courtesy of Dr. Clifford Gravelle.)

for an extended time, perhaps for life (Fig. 21–2). Detectable serum IgG–anti-HAV confers immunity to HAV infection.

Pathogenesis and Infectivity

HAV replicates *in vitro* in human hepatoma cells and diploid fibroblasts without producing cytopathic changes; this also appears to be the case in hepatocytes *in vivo*. After oral inoculation, viral replication occurs in the liver accom-

panied by a brief viremic period during which virus is excreted into stool. In acute human and experimental infections, HAV is found in the hepatocyte cytoplasm and disappears coincident with recovery from hepatic injury. Extrahepatic sites of viral replication have not been found. HAV appears to enter hepatocytes after binding to a viral receptor on the cell membrane. Subsequently, uncoating occurs, viral RNA polymerase and viral protease are produced, viral RNA and proteins are synthesized, and new viral particles are assembled, which leave the

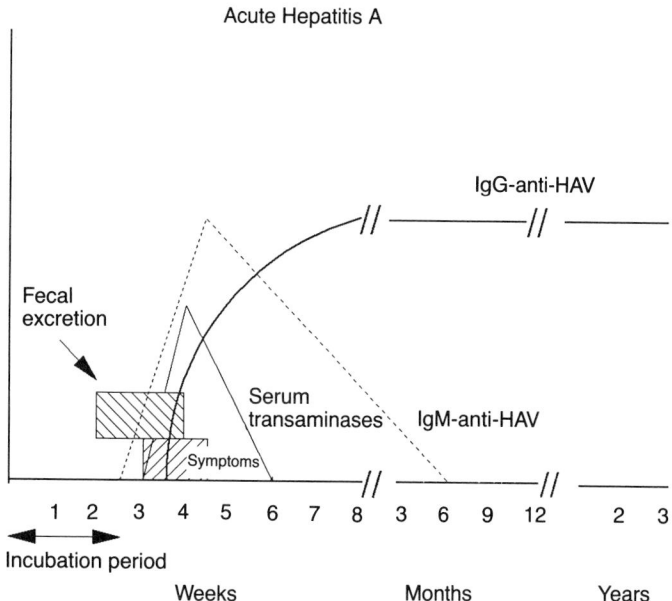

Figure 21–2. The course of acute hepatitis A. After a relatively brief incubation period, virus is excreted in feces, elevated serum transaminase levels develop, and symptoms may occur. IgM-anti-HAV is present in serum when symptomatic patients seek medical attention, and levels then wane. Serum IgG-anti-HAV is detectable relatively early and persists for decades, serving to protect against recurrent infection.

hepatocyte without producing cell lysis. The precise mechanisms of hepatocyte damage are unclear, although lymphocytic infiltration occurs and cytokines are released, suggesting that liver injury may be immunopathologically mediated. Vallbracht et al. recently showed that HAV-specific CD8$^+$ T lymphocytes isolated from liver in acute hepatitis A are specifically cytotoxic for HAV-infected cells. Hepatocyte injury is reflected by elevated serum levels of alanine aminotransferase (SGPT) and other hepatic enzymes and is apparent 15–50 days after infection. This becomes maximal within 3–7 days, and, except for the few patients who develop fulminant hepatitis A, patients typically recover completely. Fulminant hepatitis A has an approximately 50% mortality rate. Chronic infection with HAV does not develop.

Stool excretion of HAV occurs late in the incubation period and prior to onset of the clinical illness and, although somewhat variable, typically diminishes rapidly with the onset of clinical illness. It is most likely that fecal HAV is derived from hepatocytes via the bile ducts. Viral excretion is quite uncommon once serum transaminase levels have peaked. Therefore, patients are most infectious late in the incubation period, that is, before it is apparent that they are sick. This clearly complicates control of spread of HAV.

Clinical Disease

HAV infection in susceptible (anti-HAV–negative) individuals very frequently results in asymptomatic, subclinical infection. This is particularly true in children. Symptomatic infection occurs at all ages but is much more likely to occur in adults. The most common symptoms include the abrupt onset of nausea, vomiting, fever, and vague abdominal discomfort, developing 15–50 days (median is 30 days) after exposure. Smokers may lose their desire for tobacco. Headache and myalgias may occur, and some patients have shaking chills, high fever, and prostration, resembling acute bacteremia. On the other hand, symptomatic children frequently are only mildly ill, with symptoms that lead to the diagnosis of infectious hepatitis only if serum liver enzymes are measured. During the early preicteric phase of acute hepatitis A, few physical findings are apparent. Hepatomegaly with mild tenderness or right upper quadrant fullness may be noted. Laboratory studies show evidence of increasing hepatic dysfunction, with rising serum transaminase and other hepatic enzyme levels. Leukopenia is common, and atypical lymphocytes may be seen. IgM–anti-HAV is detectable, and total serum IgM levels are elevated (Fig. 21–2).

In many HAV-infected individuals, particularly children, symptoms subside after 3–7 days and recovery quickly ensues, with serum enzyme levels returning to normal. In others, however, particularly adults, an icteric phase occurs. The frequent absence of icterus in children contributes to their serving as efficient unsuspected transmitters of infection. Icterus is associated with increased serum bilirubin and enzyme levels, especially alanine aminotransferase (ALT, or SGPT) and aspartate aminotransferase (AST, or SGOT). Frequently, patients manifest improved appetite and decreased nausea and vomiting even as their icterus is worsening. Recovery ensues, and clinical and biochemical findings resolve within a few weeks. The exception to this pattern is the relatively infrequent patient with hepatitis A who develops fulminant hepatitis A, which has a very high fatality rate and which may require liver transplantation. Only a small fraction of all acute fulminant hepatitis is related to HAV, and a fatality rate of 0.14% for hospitalized patients with HAV has been reported. Unlike other forms of viral hepatitis, chronic hepatitis does not follow acute hepatitis A, even though occasional patients manifest elevated serum enzymes or intrahepatic cholestasis and icterus for several months, always with resolution. There is no known chronic carrier state, unlike hepatitis B and non-A, non-B hepatitis.

Epidemiology

HAV is present worldwide and is quite contagious. The dominant mode of transmission is the fecal–oral route, either through direct person-to-person spread or by ingestion of contaminated food or water. Thus, the epidemiology of hepatitis A is similar to that of other enteric infections, including poliomyelitis. As in the past with polio, seroepidemiologic studies in the United States show that prior HAV infection correlates with lower socioeconomic status. Although common source outbreaks are described, most cases are acquired through sporadic or endemic transmission, particularly from individuals in the preicteric phase of acute hepatitis A, when fecal excretion is maximal. In developing areas of the world where sanitation may be inadequate, transmission is widespread, with most infections occurring in the early years of life as subclinical or anicteric illnesses. Thus, immunity is acquired in childhood, and adults are protected. As sanitation improves, the risk of childhood infection decreases, and susceptibility more frequently extends to adulthood. Paradoxically, as sanitation improves, HAV can emerge as an increasing problem in developing nations.

In developed areas, such as the United States, hepatitis A is particularly endemic in day-care centers and institutions for the retarded, where fecal contamination is more common. Food-borne transmissions in these circumstances usually result from breaches in the usual sanitary safeguards. From 1983 to 1989, a 58% increase in the incidence of hepatitis A was recorded by the Centers for Disease Control in the United States. Specific identified risk factors associated with hepatitis A in the United States include contact with another person known to be infected with hepatitis, male homosexuality, foreign travel, and contact with a child attending a day-care center. Many community hepatitis A outbreaks can be traced to preschool day-care centers, particularly those large centers with long hours and a high proportion of children who are not toilet-trained. Transmission is common among these young children, who experience clinically inapparent infections and who efficiently transmit infection to older siblings, parents, and day-care center staff, who are much more likely to develop symptomatic, icteric hepatitis A. This form of transmission can account for a very substantial proportion of hepatitis A in a community, and intervention in day-care centers in which HAV transmission appears likely may reduce overall community rates of infection.

Sexual transmission of HAV is common among homosexual men, and viral hepatitis that occurs in such patients who have been immunized against hepatitis B virus is most often due to HAV. HAV is similar to other enteric pathogens that can be transmitted sexually. Parenteral HAV transmission is uncommon but can occur because there is a brief viremic phase early in the incubation period. Thus, posttransfusion hepatitis A has occurred, but only rarely. Nosocomial (hospital-acquired) HAV infections can occur if diarrhea or incontinence is accompanied by poor hygienic practices (i.e., insufficient handwashing).

Prevention

Sanitation

Careful disposal of excreta and avoidance of contamination of the water supply greatly reduce the risk of fecal–oral transmission of infectious agents like HAV. Handwashing is highly effective in preventing person-to-person spread. HAV transmission is particularly difficult to prevent completely because of both the high incidence of subclinical cases and the maximal viral excretion prior to onset of symptoms in those who do develop symptomatic disease.

Passive Immunization

Pooled human immune serum globulin (ISG) has been known since 1945 to provide protection against infectious hepatitis (hepatitis A), but its effectiveness depends on dosage and time of administration. When ISG is given in proper dosage (0.02 mL/kg) to household contacts within 2 weeks of exposure, prevention of symptomatic hepatitis A is documented to be up to 87% effective. ISG may prevent infection completely (particularly if given very soon after exposure) or may ameliorate symptoms, resulting in subclinical infection as well as in resultant long-term active immunity ("passive-active" immunity). ISG is recommended for all household contacts of individuals with hepatitis A and should be administered as soon as possible after exposure, since its prophylactic value decreases with time. ISG is generally *not* recommended for school exposures to HAV, but is valuable in limiting epidemics in institutions for the retarded and in day-care centers, as well as in preventing hepatitis A in travelers to foreign countries with high-risk for endemic HAV infection.

Active Immunization

An effective vaccine against hepatitis A is the goal of current research. The possibilities under study include an inactivated vaccine such as formalin-inactivated HAV, an attenuated live vaccine that lacks virulence but retains immunogenicity, and recombinant vaccines consisting of a viral surface polypeptide that possesses a critical neutralization epitope that could induce protection against HAV infection. Serum IgG antibody correlates with immunity to hepatitis A.

HEPATITIS B: SERUM HEPATITIS

Virology

The etiologic agent of hepatitis B is the hepatitis B virus (HBV), which was discovered serendipitously in 1965 during studies of genetic polymorphism, was associated with hepatitis in 1967, and led to the Nobel Prize in Medicine for Dr. Baruch Blumberg in 1976. In 1990, the World Health Organization estimated that a *billion* individuals then alive had been infected with HBV, that more than 200 million people worldwide were currently infected, and that 1–2 million deaths each year are attributed to HBV. Hepatitis B virus is the single most important cause of persistent viremia in humans. This agent is responsible for almost 80% of cases of primary hepatocellular carcinoma (hepatoma); it is second only to tobacco as a known human carcinogen. By electron microscopy there are three distinct kinds of particles in the serum of patients with HBV infection (Fig. 21–1 *C* and *D*). The intact virion, known as the Dane particle, is a 42-nm-diameter sphere made up of an outer shell 7-nm thick composed of hepatitis B surface antigen (HBsAg) and an inner core 28 nm in diameter possessing the hepatitis B core antigen (HBcAg), hepatitis B e antigen (HBeAg), DNA polymerase, and a small (3200 bases), circular, mostly double-stranded DNA genome. Smaller 22-nm spherical particles and tubular particles with a 22-nm cross-sectional diameter represent HBsAg produced in great excess. HBV has proved to be the prototype for a group of viral agents now termed the *hepadnaviruses* that include several animal viruses, such as the woodchuck hepatitis virus, duck hepatitis B virus, and ground-squirrel hepatitis virus, and agents that infect Taiwanese snakes, Himalayan marmots, and European herons; they all have similar structures and hepatotropism and are characterized by the unique presence of DNA polymerase and double-stranded DNA. HBV and several of the animal viruses are clearly oncogenic, leading to primary hepatic carcinoma (hepatoma), and all hepadnaviruses can produce either acute or chronic infections of the liver. HBV is resistant to many conditions that inactivate most viruses and bacteria, surviving storage at 60°C for 4 h, at room temperature for 6 months, or −10 to −20°C for 4½ years. It is inactivated by being kept at 60°C for 10 h or by boiling. HBV is phenol-resistant but is inactivated by chlorine (10,000 ppm for 10 min) or formalin and by heat or steam sterilization.

HBV Markers

The presence or absence of the various HBV antigens and the corresponding antibodies in patient serum specimens at different stages of HBV infection provides information regarding the stage of the infection, the presence of immunity, and the degree of infectivity.

Surface Antigen: HBsAg

This antigen was known previously as Australian antigen and hepatitis-associated antigen

(HAA), but it is now termed the HBsAg since it forms the outer coat of the intact HBV virus (Dane particle). HBsAg is composed of three large polypeptides (small protein, S; middle protein, M, which is made up of S plus 55 additional amino acids encoded by the pre-S2 region of the envelope gene; and large protein, containing the sequence of M and 108–109 additional amino acids encoded by the pre-S1 region of the envelope gene). The pre-S2 encoded sequence carries a receptor for polymerized human albumin that may be important in attachment of HBV to hepatocytes, and serum expression of pre-S1 antigen correlates with active HBV replication. The small spherical and the tubular particles seen by electron microscopy of serum represent HBsAg produced in great excess during HBV replication. This excessive envelope protein production is also characteristic of other hepadnaviruses. HBsAg expresses a single common group-specific antigen (a), either of two subtype antigens (d or y), and one of two allelic groups (r or w), resulting in four possible antigenic subtypes: adr, adw, ayr, and ayw. The subtype of the infecting strain of HBV does not appear to be a determinant of the severity or outcome of infection but is useful in epidemiologic studies. HBsAg is measured in blood and other body fluids by radioimmunoassay or ELISA; current assays detect 5–10 ng protein/mL, or 10^{10} particles per milliliter. HBsAg is widely distributed in body fluids including saliva, semen, and breast milk, but not feces, and its presence generally correlates with infectivity. HBsAg typically appears in serum late in the incubation period and persists through most or all of the clinical stages of acute hepatitis B (Fig. 21–3). Its disappearance almost always signals termination of hepatitis B infection and is shortly thereafter followed by detectable serum anti-HBsAg (Fig. 21–3). HBsAg in the liver is localized to the cytoplasm and to the nuclear membrane, cisternae, and endoplasmic reticulum. Individuals who fail to clear HBsAg from serum have chronic HBV infection, either associated with chronic liver disease or as a chronic HBsAg carrier without liver disease (Fig. 21–4). Chronic HBV infection is considered present if HBsAg-positivity persists longer than 6 months.

Core Antigen: HBcAg

This distinct antigen is associated with the core of the Dane particle in serum or in hepatocytes and with disrupted Dane particles. HBcAg is denser than HBsAg, having a buoyant density of 1.32 g/cm³ in $CeCl_2$, compared with 1.20 g/cm³ for HBsAg. In hepatocytes, exclusively nuclear localization of HBcAg is generally associated with viremia but rarely with active liver disease, whereas cytoplasmic HBcAg expression correlates with viremia and active liver disease. Unlike HBsAg, HBcAg is *not* found in serum. Anti-HBc, on the other hand, is readily demonstrable in serum by RIA and other techniques shortly after HBsAg is detectable and represents the earliest humoral immune response to HBV antigens (Fig. 21–3).

e Antigen: HBeAg

HBeAg is contained in a cryptic form within the Dane particle, revealed after proteolytic enzyme or detergent treatment, and in a soluble form in some HBsAg-positive sera. It is found in the nucleus of infected hepatocytes. Although it is known that there are two distinct HBeAg specificities, the biologic function of HBeAg remains obscure. However, it appears to have no role in viral replication. It has been suggested that HBeAg is the NH_2-terminal half of the HBcAg molecule and that it may be produced by proteolytic self-cleavage of HBcAg in infected hepatocytes. The clinical importance of HBeAg relates to its serving as a marker for significant chronic liver disease and for increased infectivity. HBeAg is correlated with DNA polymerase activity. Loss of HBeAg-positivity and appearance of anti-HBe in serum generally indicates lower infectivity and decreased severity of HBV-associated liver disease, but the absence of HBeAg does not negate potential infectivity.

DNA Polymerase and HBV DNA

Active HBV replication is reflected by the presence of serum DNA polymerase and HBV DNA (Fig. 21–3). The sustained disappearance of these markers of replication spontaneously or as a consequence of experimental therapeutic regimens (e.g., with alpha-interferon, acyclovir, or vidarabine) is evidence of terminated infection with HBV. Loss of viral replication is soon followed by evidence of sustained remission of chronic hepatitis B.

Antibodies against HBV Antigens

The earliest evidence of a humoral response to HBV is the presence of serum *anti-HBc* late in the incubation period, corresponding to the

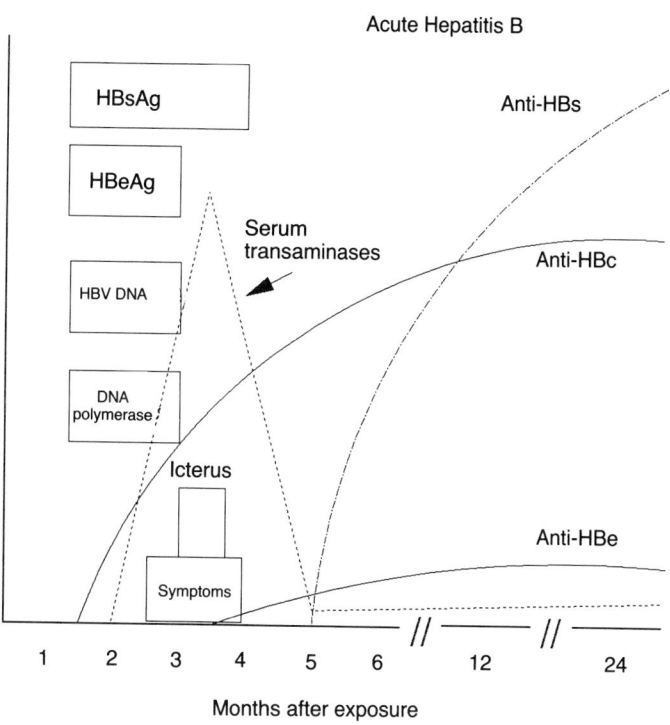

Figure 21–3. Time course of acute hepatitis B (HBV) infection. After an incubation period of several months, serum becomes positive for HBsAg, HBeAg, and markers of viral replication—HBV DNA and DNA polymerase. Shortly thereafter, serum transaminase levels rise, reflecting hepatocellular damage and then symptoms (often including icterus) develop. The earliest antibody response is anti-HBc, often preceding clinical manifestations. Serologic markers of active infection and viral replication disappear, and serum transaminases return to normal. Anti-HBc persists, whereas HBsAg and HBeAg are replaced by anti-HBs and anti-HBe, respectively. The appearance of anti-HBs generally confirms recovery from HBV infection and provides long-lived immunity against subsequent infection.

appearance of HBsAg (Fig. 21–3). Anti-HBc declines to low values with convalescence and can persist at low levels for many years. The presence of IgM–anti-HBc occurs early except in young infants and strongly suggests acute HBV infection. *Anti-HBs* is first detectable later in convalescence, often considerably after HBsAg has disappeared, and generally signifies termination of infection (Fig. 21–3). Anti-HBs lasts many years and is protective against reinfection. Anti-HBc may be the only marker of HBV infection in the interval between the de-

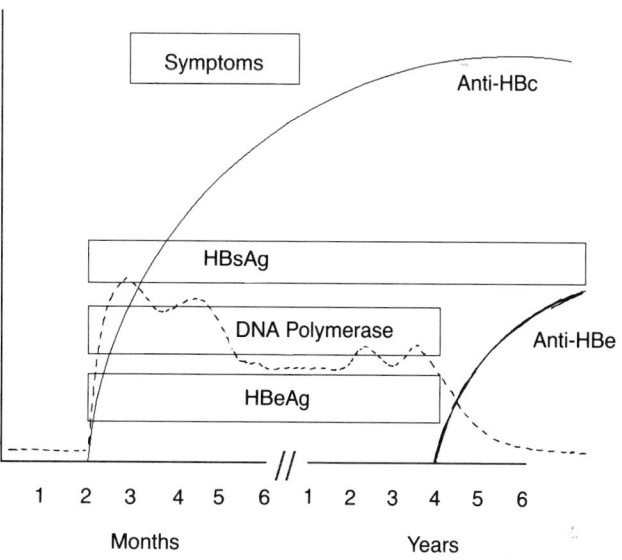

Figure 21–4. One of the patterns of chronic hepatitis B infection. After an incubation period of about 2 months, serum transaminase levels (dashed line) abruptly rise coincident with the appearance of several serologic markers (HBsAg, HBeAg, anti-HBc, and DNA polymerase) before the onset of symptoms. Serum transaminase levels fluctuate and eventually normalize, although serum HBsAg persists as a marker of chronic hepatitis B virus infection. DNA polymerase and HBeAg are no longer detectable in serum after 4 years, the latter replaced by anti-HBe. Anti-HBs never develops, since surface antigenemia never clears. Most such patients remain infected for many decades, and some develop chronic active hepatitis B, cirrhosis, and even hepatocellular carcinoma.

cline of HBsAg and the appearance of anti-HBs (the "core window"). Anti-HBe usually appears shortly after HBeAg declines in the early convalescent period. In individuals who develop chronic HBV infection, HBeAg usually persists and anti-HBe does not appear (Fig. 21–4).

Pathogenesis

The pathogenesis of hepatitis B infection is very complex. HBV is not hepatotoxic, as demonstrated by the fact that most chronic carriers of HBV, whose sera contain very high concentrations of viral particles, lack evidence of liver disease. Rather, it appears that the host response to HBV characterized by cytotoxic T cells and natural killer cells leads to hepatocyte necrosis, resulting in either *acute hepatitis* that subsides after a period of weeks to several months, or *chronic hepatitis* that may persist for many years. Apparently, HBV replication in the liver eventually ceases in some chronically infected individuals, even though viral DNA may remain integrated into the hepatocyte DNA and cells may continue to express HBsAg.

Late in the long (45–180 day) incubation period of HBV, at or shortly before the onset of hepatic inflammation and necrosis, some individuals develop hypersensitivity-like symptoms (arthralgia, skin rash, vasculitis) that are the result of circulating antigen–antibody complexes. A particularly severe form of HBV immune complex disease is adult periarteritis nodosa. In this disease a sizable portion of patients have evidence of HBsAg and immunoglobulin deposits within vessel walls.

Hepatocyte necrosis is probably a consequence of T-cell cytotoxicity directed against HBV or the hepatocyte membrane antigens expressed on the hepatocyte surface. The pre-S2 portion of HBsAg has been suggested to be the target of T cells infiltrating the liver in chronic hepatitis B. Individuals with some degree of impairment of T-cell function (such as those with Down syndrome, uremia, malignancy, HIV infection, neonates, etc.) are more likely to have a relatively mild degree of necrosis, incomplete elimination of HBV, and persistent smoldering chronic HBV infection. This situation is in contrast to individuals with normal T-cell function, who tend to have a more severe acute illness that includes termination of the infection, clearance of HBsAg from liver and serum, and development of anti-HBs. This host–virus relationship is further complicated by the fact that HBV DNA can be found integrated

into the genome of primary hepatocellular carcinoma (hepatoma) cells in HBsAg-positive individuals and into the genome of other nontumor host cells. This DNA integration is not associated with viral replication and suggests that, at least in some circumstances, integration inhibits replication and promotes malignant transformation. Individuals deficient in B-cell immunity are capable of developing acute or chronic hepatitis.

Chronic HBV infection in individuals also infected with HIV is associated with less severe histologic changes and lower serum transaminase levels. However, this milder hepatic involvement occurs in association with evidence of greater viral replication, including higher amounts of HBeAg, HBV DNA, and HBV DNA polymerase in serum and increased HBcAg and HBeAg expression on hepatocyte nuclei. These findings support the immune-mediated pathogenesis of hepatitis B and suggest that HBV in HIV-infected individuals will be more resistant to antiviral therapy.

Clinical Disease

The clinical picture of *acute hepatitis B* is similar in some respects to that of acute hepatitis A but tends to be a more serious illness, has a more insidious onset, has a propensity to linger or to become chronic, and typically affects somewhat older individuals. The incubation period between infection and onset of symptoms varies between 45 and 180 days, with HBsAg becoming detectable in serum several weeks before the clinical onset. Some patients develop hypersensitivity symptoms as noted above, whereas others manifest anorexia, fatigue, chills, and fever prior to the onset of jaundice. Coincident with the clinical onset, serum transaminases increase to reflect hepatocyte necrosis, and anti-HBc becomes detectable—initially of the IgM class and later of the IgG. Prior to the increase in serum transaminases, markers associated with the Dane particle (DNA polymerase, HBV DNA, HBeAg) are detectable in serum. The icteric phase of acute hepatitis B lasts 2–6 weeks, generally peaking in severity by 14 days and disappearing over a variable period. As jaundice worsens, fever, malaise, and weakness improve. Hepatomegaly frequently is present in the icteric phase, often with splenomegaly, and persists for some time after icterus clears. In children the illness is shorter and recovery generally faster. In approximately 90% of acutely infected individuals, Dane particle markers in the serum clear shortly after the serum transaminases peak and anti-HBe may become detectable, serum HBsAg disappears as transaminases reach near-normal values, and shortly thereafter, anti-HBs becomes detectable, signaling the successful termination of infection and establishment of long-term immunity against reinfection.

Hepatitis B infection is very different from hepatitis A in that a significant minority of HBV-infected individuals do not terminate their infection but become chronically infected, frequently for life. In these patients, HBsAg persists in serum, as does anti-HBc, HBeAg or anti-HBe, and Dane particle markers, such as DNA polymerase and HBV DNA. Chronic hepatitis B may take the histologic form of *chronic persistent hepatitis B,* which is associated with mild portal triaditis and mildly elevated serum transaminases. This form resolves within 1 year without development of cirrhosis. The more serious form of chronic hepatitis B is *chronic active (or aggressive) hepatitis B,* which is associated usually with more elevated transaminase levels and histologic evidence of T-cell inflammation that spills out of the portal triad, across the limiting plate, and into the lobules. This form has a tendency to produce bridging fibrosis and cirrhosis, leading in turn to portal obstruction and all of its complications. It is particularly these patients with cirrhotic chronic hepatitis B who are at dramatically increased risk for development of hepatoma. Treatment protocols that employ alpha-interferon, acyclovir, and/or corticosteroids for chronic hepatitis B infection are being evaluated.

Fulminant acute hepatitis B is relatively rare but is more common than other viral causes of fulminant acute liver failure, particularly in adults. These patients develop massive necrosis of virtually all hepatocytes, and 80% mortality is common. Fulminant hepatitis A is associated with a lower mortality rate, while fulminant non-A, non-B hepatitis has a higher mortality rate. Many such patients have been salvaged by hepatic transplantation in recent years, although HBV infection of the transplanted liver is common.

The *chronic HBsAg carrier,* in striking contrast, is classically an asymptomatic individual with minimal or no liver disease, who may or may not have had a symptomatic illness at the time of acquisition of HBV. Serum of such patients is chronically positive for HBsAg, anti-HBc, HBeAg or (more often) anti-HBe, HBV DNA, and DNA polymerase. Chronic HBsAg carrier rates as high as 20% or more are seen in some Asian populations. In the United States and Western Europe, chronic carrier rates are less than 1%.

Epidemiology

In a recent serologic survey representative of the entire U.S. urban (noninstitutionalized) population 6 months–74 years of age, serologic markers of HBV were found in 4.8% (3.2% of whites, 13.7% of blacks). No gender differences were noted but serologic markers increased in frequency with age. Overall, 0.3% were HBsAg-positive (0.19% in whites, 0.85% in blacks), indicating active infection.

HBV epidemiology resembles that of the human immunodeficiency virus (HIV) in many aspects. Transmission of HBV occurs primarily by parenteral, sexual, or vertical (maternal-infant) routes, and the fecal-oral route is relatively unimportant. This transmission pattern reflects the fact that HBV is present in virtually all body fluids of an infected individual, including blood, semen, saliva, and urine. Transmission generally requires either overt inoculation (transfusion of a blood product, injection with a contaminated needle, accidental needle-stick injury) or intimate personal contact (between sexual partners, or mother and neonate). Groups at particularly high risk for HBV infection include intravenous drug abusers who share needles, male homosexuals, the sexually promiscuous, health care workers, transfused patients, and hemophiliacs. In addition, certain geographic areas are known to be associated with relatively high rates of chronic HBsAg carriage and HBV-related liver disease with their concomitant risk of infectivity, including Southeast Asia (particularly China and Taiwan), sub-Saharan Africa, Oceania, and the Mediterranean region. In these regions, the role of vertical transmission from mother to neonate, resulting in long-term or even lifelong HBV infection, is thought to be crucial in maintaining high rates of HBsAg-positivity. This is particularly true in Southeast Asia. In the United States, the incidence of chronic HBsAg-positivity is approximately 0.1% but is higher in selected subgroups with specific ethnic or behavioral risk factors. HBV can contaminate all blood components except for preparations of gamma globulin, but the screening of blood products for HBsAg in order to exclude positive material has very substantially, but not completely, eliminated the problem of posttransfusion hepatitis B infection. Recent epidemiologic surveys suggest that homosexual activity has become a somewhat less important risk factor and that IV drug abuse and heterosexual activity have become relatively more important risk factors for acute hepatitis B infection. Even with extensive inquiry, however, the source of acute hepatitis B infection remains unknown in about 30% of instances.

Vertical transmission of HBV is an extremely important public health problem worldwide and contributes very substantially to the high rates of chronic HBV infection in many areas and to the resulting prevalence of chronic liver disease and hepatoma. For example, Beasley demonstrated that hepatoma was 223 times more common in middle-aged HBsAg-positive men in Taiwan than in HBsAg-negative controls, with hepatoma and cirrhosis accounting for 54% of deaths in HBsAg carriers but only 1.5% in noncarriers. Vertical transmission is possible from any HBsAg-positive mother to her off-spring but is particularly efficient when the mother is HBeAg-positive or when she experiences acute hepatitis B in the third trimester of pregnancy or in the early postpartum period. IgM–anti-HBc rarely develops after perinatal transmission of HBV and cannot be used for diagnosis in this situation. Prompt administration of anti-HBs (HBIG) and HBV vaccine to neonates is highly effective in preventing vertical transmission.

Hepatitis B is an occupational risk for medical personnel as well as a potential nosocomial risk. Staff and patients in dialysis, oncology, and transplantation units are at higher risk because exposure to blood products is common and HBV-infected patients are more likely to be asymptomatic chronic carriers.

Prevention

Highly significant advances have occurred in the past decade regarding prevention of HBV infection, including the development both of vaccines composed of purified HBsAg and an immune globulin containing high titer anti-HBs (HBIG).

General Measures

Even though HBV is much less commonly transmitted by the fecal-oral route than is HAV, the general hygienic measures noted above for hepatitis A are a necessary part of prophylaxis against HBV. In addition, used needles and other blood-contaminated materials should be properly discarded, and needle-recapping should be avoided. Barrier protection against splashes with blood-contaminated secretions by dentists, surgeons, and others is effective. Routine screening of blood donors to exclude HBV-infected individuals from the donor pool and utilizing volunteer blood donors rather than paid donors have been highly effective in reducing the incidence of posttransfusion hepatitis B. The risk of transmission of HBV by heterosexual and homosexual activity can be substantially reduced by the use of condoms.

Passive Immunization

Serum globulin preparations enriched in HBIG are used in certain circumstances to provide prompt passive immunity to HBV infection. These circumstances include (1) following an inadvertent needle-stick from a HBsAg-positive patient or accidental transfusion of HBsAg-positive blood products; (2) after an eye-splash or contamination of an open skin wound with HBsAg-positive material; (3) following accidental ingestion of HBsAg-positive material, for example, a pipetting accident; (4) for sexual partners of patients with acute hepatitis B within 14 days of contact; (5) household contacts under 1 year of age of patients with acute hepatitis B; and (6) infants born to HBsAg-positive mothers. In certain of these circumstances, active immunization with HBV vaccine is also indicated (see below). Ideally, it is best to be able to document that the "donor" is HBsAg-positive (and therefore infected) and that the "recipient" is anti–HBs-negative (and therefore susceptible) before administering this expensive reagent. This is not always possible or practical, however. In families of an acute hepatitis B patient, it is generally not indicated to give HBIG to children older than 1 year of age, since the risk of spread other than sexually is low; children younger than 1 year are given HBIG and HBV vaccine because their risk of severe or chronic HBV infection is greater.

Active Immunization

A safe and highly effective HBV vaccine consisting of HBsAg purified from chronic carrier donor plasma became available in 1983, and more recent HBsAg vaccines containing recombinant HBsAg synthesized by yeast (*Saccharomyces cerevisiae*) transfected with the gene for HBsAg subtype adw are now available. A regimen of three doses (at 0, 1, and 6 months) generally elicits anti-HBs in the recipient that serves to prevent HBV infection. Intramuscular injection is important, and sites with considerable adipose tissue (e.g., gluteus) should be avoided. The need for reimmunization has not been established. HBV vaccine is indicated for high-risk individuals, including health professionals (especially those at highest risk, such as dentists and their assistants, surgeons, dialysis staff), susceptible dialysis patients, hemophiliacs, certain residents and staff of chronic-care institutions, intravenous drug abusers, sexual and household contacts of a chronically HBsAg-positive individual, Alaskan Eskimos, Pacific Islanders, and other susceptible populations, and homosexual males. HBV vaccine should be combined with HBIG in the following circumstances: (1) after accidental needle-stick or splash exposures with HBsAg-positive or high-risk material, (2) for prevention of vertical transmission to neonates, and (3) for sexual contacts and for infant contacts younger than 1 year of patients with acute hepatitis B. Recently, it was shown that about half of HBV infections among children born in the United States to Southeast Asian refugees were not attributable to perinatal transmission. This indicates that child-to-child transmission may occur commonly, and it has been suggested that HBV vaccine should be given to all infants and young children of Southeast Asian ethnicity in the United States, regardless of whether there is HBV infection in family members.

Administration of HBV vaccine to individuals who are already immune is not harmful but represents an unnecessary expense. Approximately 90% of vaccine recipients develop anti-HBs, and about 10% appear to be unresponsive. Recombinant vaccine leads to early and high production of antibody to pre-S2 determinants of HBsAg and perhaps to earlier immunity. Interestingly, a primary antibody response is not detectable in about 70% of recipients, but secondary and tertiary responses are very common after the second and third vaccine doses. More than 20 countries, including China, Korea, and Taiwan, have initiated programs for universal newborn vaccination, and other large particularly high-risk ethnic groups are receiving widespread vaccine, including Aborigines in Australia, Maoris in New Zealand, and Eskimos in the United States.

HEPATITIS DELTA VIRUS

The hepatitis delta virus (HDV) is a defective spherical 36-nm virus composed of a core, con-

taining a circular, single-stranded, negative-polarity RNA genome of about 1750 bases, the delta antigen (a phosphoprotein that interacts with virion RNA and is possibly involved in viral replication), and a lipoprotein envelope made up of HBsAg. No viral polymerase activity or polymerase gene has been found in HDV particles. HDV appears to replicate through an RNA that is complementary to the viral genome. There is a strong analogy between HDV and certain pathogenic RNA agents of plants, including the viroids, virusoids, and satellite RNAs. Delta was first discovered as a novel antigen in hepatocyte nuclei of certain patients chronically infected with HBV, and viral replication appears to take place in hepatocyte nuclei. Replication of HDV is completely dependent upon the presence of HBV (or, experimentally, another hepadnavirus) and curiously is associated with suppression of HBV replication.

Thus, HDV causes infection only in individuals with coexistent active infection with HBV. Italian researchers have found evidence of HDV infection in some patients with inapparent HBV infection that is manifested only by IgM–anti-HBc, particularly in drug abusers. The presence of HDV infection is reflected by delta antigen and HDV RNA in liver and by serum antidelta antibody. In acute HDV infection IgM–anti-delta is demonstrable in serum. Newer techniques that demonstrate serum HDV antigen and HDV RNA appear to correlate with active replication. Transmission of HDV is by the identical routes that HBV is transmitted. Vertical transmission has been described from HBeAg-positive HDV-infected mothers but appears uncommon. The delta antigen comprises two major proteins of 24–27 kd and 27–29 kd, the functions of which are unknown. No other HDV-coded proteins are known.

HDV is important clinically in two circumstances. As a *coinfecting agent* with HBV in a previously non–HBV-infected individual, HDV is associated with more severe acute hepatitis as reflected, for example, by a higher rate of fulminant hepatitis and a higher fatality rate, as well as with a substantially increased risk for development and severity of chronic hepatitis B liver disease. As a coinfecting agent, the incubation period of HDV is the same as that of HBV. On the other hand, well-established HBV infection promotes efficient replication of HDV. Therefore, as a *superinfecting agent* in an already HBV-infected individual, HDV infection may produce an acute exacerbation of previously stable chronic hepatitis, increase the tendency for development of significant chronic active hepatitis B and cirrhosis, or accelerate the course of chronic liver disease. In this situation, the incubation period is about 4–8 weeks. The relationship of HDV to hepatoma is less clear. In both chronic active hepatitis B and chronic active delta hepatitis, T cells predominate in the liver inflammatory infiltrate, with helper T cells particularly in the portal tracts and suppressor/cytotoxic T cells particularly in the areas of piecemeal necrosis.

HDV is found worldwide but is uncommon in some HBV-infected populations, including male homosexuals and Southeast Asians. In the United States and Western Europe it is common only in intravenous drug abusers and hemophiliacs. Very high HDV rates are reported among HBV-infected individuals in the Amazon, the Middle East, Oceania, the Mediterranean area, the Balkans, and the European USSR. Screening of blood donors for HBsAg is highly effective in the prevention of transfusion-related HDV. Studies evaluating the efficacy of interferon in treatment of chronic HDV are proceeding.

NON-A, NON-B HEPATITIS

The term *non-A, non-B hepatitis* (NANB) has been used to connote viral hepatitis that is not due to infection with HAV, HBV, Epstein-Barr virus, or cytomegalovirus. Evidence that such illnesses are due to additional viral agent(s) includes experimental transmissibility to primates, epidemic occurrence, and an unequivocal relationship to transfusions. Very recently, many NANB hepatitis cases have been shown to represent HCV infection (see below).

Epidemiology and Clinical Features

The CDC estimates that almost 150,000 cases of NANB occur annually in the United States, of which 7,500–15,000 are transfusion-related. It is thought that about 75,000 individuals develop biochemical evidence of chronic liver disease and 15,000 progress to chronic active hepatitis or cirrhosis or both.

At least two distinct modes of transmission appear to exist for NANB, suggesting that at least two distinct viral agents exist: one transmitted parenterally, causing posttransfusion hepatitis and sporadic cases in developed coun-

tries, and a water-borne form with fecal–oral transmission that causes epidemics in developing countries. In the United States at present, at least 90% of posttransfusion hepatitis is classified as NANB hepatitis. Recent study of posttransfusion hepatitis demonstrates seroconversion to HCV in 85–90% of individuals. CDC surveillance studies have found that only 5–10% of NANB hepatitis cases are related to blood transfusions, whereas around 40% are associated with IV drug abuse, 5% to health care occupational exposure, and 10% to heterosexual activity with multiple partners or household or sexual contact with an individual with hepatitis. In about 40% there is no identifiable source of infection. This form of NANB hepatitis is characterized by long incubation periods (60–150 days), frequent subclinical or anicteric illnesses (25% become icteric), development of a chronic carrier state, and development of chronic liver disease, including chronic active hepatitis and/or cirrhosis in about 50% of patients. This illness resembles hepatitis B in many respects but is generally milder with lower serum transaminase and bilirubin levels. However, when NANB hepatitis manifests a fulminant course, 90% mortality has been reported.

Hepatitis E

A distinctive form of NANB hepatitis is characterized by fecal-oral transmission, and a shorter incubation period (usually 2–9 weeks, mean of 6 weeks), occurring either endemically for a number of months or in explosive waterborne epidemics related to fecal contamination of the water supply. This form particularly occurs shortly after the onset of the rainy season in developing countries. Clinical attack rates are highest among young adults. Fatality rates in epidemic water-borne NANB, which is reported primarily from India and Southeast Asia, are particularly high (10–20%) in pregnant women in the third trimester; in other individuals the disease has a fatality rate of 1–2%. Chronic liver disease has not been demonstrated following enterically transmitted NANB hepatitis. Viral particles 32–34 nm in diameter have been reported in feces of patients with this form of NANB hepatitis, and they react with convalescent sera from many geographic areas, as assessed by immune electron microscopy. The genome of this so-called E-NANB (epidemic, enteric NANB) hepatitis agent has been shown to be a single-stranded polyadenylated RNA of 7600 bases containing a sequence for an RNA-directed RNA polymerase. The agent has certain properties of some caliciviruses. The virus has been serially transmitted in cynomolgus monkeys, and viruslike particles were demonstrated in bile and feces. An antigen associated with E-NANB hepatitis (tentatively termed HEVAg, or E-NANB-Ag) has been identified in hepatocyte cytoplasm of experimentally infected primates. Reactivity with patient sera from many geographic areas indicates that one agent or class of similar agents is responsible for E-NANB hepatitis worldwide, and the term *hepatitis E virus* (HEV) has been proposed.

Hepatitis C

Recently, a positive-stranded RNA virus, probably related to the Flaviviridae or the Togaviridae, with a genome of about 10,000 nucleotides has been implicated as an extremely common cause of transfusion-transmitted NANB. This has been tentatively termed HCV. Seroconversion to HCV may not occur for as long as 6 months after infection and 4 months after onset of hepatitis. Half the individuals who acquire posttransfusion hepatitis C develop chronic hepatitis with the potential for cirrhosis. Seroepidemiologic studies have indicated that this is a major cause of blood-borne NANB hepatitis throughout the world and a common cause of sporadic or community-acquired NANB hepatitis among patients with no identifiable parenteral exposure. About 50% of the latter group are positive for HCV antibody within 6 weeks of illness onset and 90% by 6 months. Apparently, NANB patients without history of transfusion are just as likely as posttransfusion NANB patients to become seropositive for HCV and to develop chronic liver disease.

Interferon-alfa treatment of chronic hepatitis C has been shown to be effective in suppressing the activity of hepatitis and in improving hepatic histologic features.

Prevention

Efforts to prevent posttransfusion NANB have focused upon exclusion of paid blood donors, and until a serologic screening assay is widely available, exclusion of blood units that contain elevated serum transaminase levels or that show the presence of anti-HBc. Anti-HBc has been shown to be a nonspecific marker associated with transmission of NANB by blood transfusion. Studies recently have shown that institu-

tion of routine anti-HCV screening of blood donors can further reduce the small proportion of all HCV that results from transfusions. The possible value of immune serum globulin administered concomitantly with blood products in prevention of posttransfusion NANB has been suggested but not proved. Prevention of fecal-oral transmission of NANB is best achieved by making the water supply safe.

CASE HISTORY

A 19-year-old man presented with a lifelong history of factor VIII deficiency and a 5-day history of jaundice, malaise, anorexia, and low-grade fever. He had recently visited India, returning 4 weeks prior to examination. Examination demonstrated low-grade fever of 101°F (38.5°C), mild scleral icterus, a tender liver palpable 4 cm below the right costal margin, and evidence of previous intraarticular hemorrhages. The remainder of the examination was normal. Laboratory tests showed alanine aminotransferase and aspartate aminotransferase each of 1000 U/L (normal <40), total bilirubin of 9.3 mg/dL, with direct bilirubin of 4.0 mg/dL. Serologic studies were IgG–HAV-positive, IgM–HAV-negative, HABsAg-negative, anti–HBs-positive, anti-HBc-positive, and anti-HBe-negative.

CASE DISCUSSION

This patient falls into the category of multitransfused subjects, some of whom develop chronic hepatitis B infection that is evidenced most often as HBsAg-positive, anti–HBs-negative, and anti–HBc-positive. The last marker also correlates with increased risk for chronic NANB hepatitis. His HBV serologic studies are most consistent with resolved HBV infection. Similarly, his hepatitis A serologic studies indicate past infection with hepatitis A virus with resolution. This patient's clinical illness is highly suggestive of enterically transmitted acute E-NANB hepatitis acquired in India, although parenterally or nonparenterally transmitted hepatitis C is not ruled out by the information provided.

REFERENCES

Books

Gitnick, G., ed. *Modern Concepts of Acute and Chronic Hepatitis.* New York: Plenum, 1989.

Gust, I. D., and Feinstone, S. M., eds. *Hepatitis A*. Boca Raton, FL: CRC Press, 1989.

Nishioka, K., Blumberg, B. S., Ishida, N., et al., eds. *Hepatitis Viruses and Hepatocellular Carcinoma*. Tokyo: Academic Press, 1985.

Verme, G., Bonino, F., and Rizzetto, M., eds. *Viral Hepatitis and Delta Infection*. New York: Alan R. Liss, 1983.

Zuckerman, A., ed. *Viral Hepatitis and Liver Disease*. New York: Alan R. Liss, 1988.

Articles

Alter, H. J., Purcell, R. H., Shih, J. W., et al. Detection of antibody to hepatitis C virus in prospectively followed transfusion recipients with acute and chronic non-A, non-B hepatitis. *N. Engl. J. Med. 321:*1494–1500, 1989.

American Academy of Pediatrics. *Report of the Committee on Infectious Diseases*. 21st ed. pp. 214–220. 1988.

Beasley, R. P. Hepatitis B virus, the major etiology of hepatocellular carcinoma. *Cancer 10:*1942–1956, 1988.

Beasley, R. P., Hwang, L-Y., Lee, G. C., et al. Prevention of perinatally transmitted hepatitis B virus infections with hepatitis B immune globulin and hepatitis B vaccine. *Lancet II:*1100–1102, 1983.

Beasley, R. P., Hwang, L-Y., Lin, C. C., et al. Hepatocellular carcinoma and hepatitis B virus: A prospective study of 22,707 men in Taiwan. *Lancet II:*1129–1133, 1981.

Beasley, R. P., Hwang, L-Y., Stevens, C. E., et al. Efficacy of hepatitis B immune globulin for prevention of perinatal transmissions of the hepatitis B virus carrier state. *Hepatology 3:*135–141, 1983.

Bergmann, K. F., Cote, P. J., Moriarity, A., et al. Hepatitis delta antigen. *J. Immunol. 143:*3714–3721, 1989.

Brunetto, M. R., Oliveri, F., Rocca, G., et al. Natural course and response to interferon of chronic hepatitis B accompanied by antibody to hepatitis Be antigen. *Hepatology 10:*198–202, 1989.

DiBisceglie, A. M., and Negro, F. Diagnosis of hepatitis delta virus infection. *Hepatology 10:*1014–1016, 1989.

Fattovich, G., Boscaro, S., Noventa, F., et al. Influence of hepatitis delta virus infection on progression to cirrhosis in chronic hepatitis type B. *J. Infect. Dis. 155:*931–935, 1987.

Ganem, D., and Varmus, H. E. The molecular biology of the hepatitis B viruses. *Ann. Rev. Biochem. 56:*651–693, 1987.

Hadler, S. C., Francis, D. P., Maynard, J. E., et al. Long-term immunogenicity and efficacy of hepatitis B vaccine in homosexual men. *New Engl. J. Med. 315:*209–214, 1986.

Kao, H. W., Ashcavi, M., and Redeker, A. G. The persistence of hepatitis A–IgM antibody after acute clinical hepatitis A. *Hepatology 4:*933–936, 1984.

Kuo, G., Choo, Q-L., Alter, H. J., et al. An assay for circulating antibodies to a major etiologic virus of human non-A, non-B hepatitis. *Science 244:*362–364, 1989.

Mason, W. S., and Taylor, J. M. Experimental systems for the study of hepadnavirus and hepatitis delta virus infections. *Hepatology 9:*635–645, 1989.

Matsuda, K., and Ohori, H. Immunochemical characteristics of hepatitis B e antigen subspecificities, HBeAg/1 and HBeAg/2. *J. Immunol. 141:*1709–1713, 1988.

Maynard, J. E., Kane, M. A., and Hadler, S. C. Global control of hepatitis B through vaccination. *Rev. Infect. Dis. 11:*S574–578, 1989.

Miller, R. H. Proteolytic self-cleavage of hepatitis B virus core protein may generate serum e antigen. *Science 236:*722–725, 1987.

O'Grady, J. G., Alexander, G. J. M., Hayller, K. M., et al. Early indications of prognosis in fulminant hepatic failure. *Gastroenterology 97:*439–445, 1989.

Provost, P. J., Bishop, R. P., Gerety, R. J., et al. New findings in live, attenuated hepatitis A vaccine development. *J. Med. Virol. 20:*165–175, 1986.

Ramalingaswami, V., and Purcell, R. H. Waterborne non-A, non-B hepatitis. *Lancet I:*571–573, 1988.

Reyes, G. R., Purdy, M. A., Kim, J. P., et al. Isolation of a cDNA from the virus responsible for enterically transmitted non-A, non-B hepatitis. *Science 247:*1335–1339, 1990.

Scolnick, E. M., McLean, A. A., West, D. J., et al. Clinical evaluation in healthy adults of hepatitis B vaccine made by recombinant DNA. *JAMA 251:*2812–2815, 1984.

Szmuness, W., Dienstag, J. L., Purcell, R. H., et al. Distribution of antibody to hepatitis A antigen in urban adult populations. *New Engl. J. Med. 295:*755–759, 1976.

Vallbracht, A., Maier, K., Stierhof, Y-D., et al. Liver-derived cytotoxic T cells in hepatitis A virus infection. *J. Infect. Dis. 160:*209–217, 1989.

VII

Central Nervous System Infection

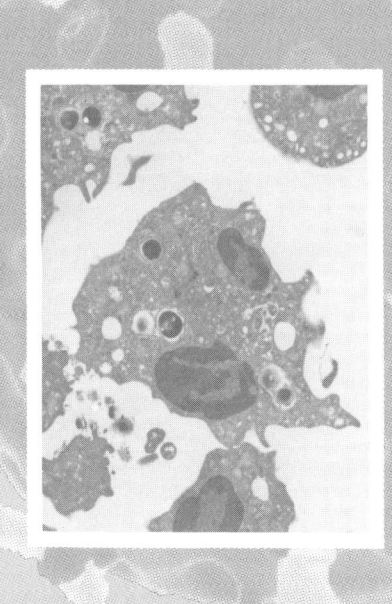

22

RAM YOGEV, M.D. • MOSHE ARDITI, M.D.

Introduction to Infections of the Central Nervous System

INTRODUCTION

The central nervous system (CNS) is unlike other organs in its closed confinement within rigid borders, its sequestration from the rest of the body by various barriers, and its relatively immunocompromised status. The brain is surrounded by the leptomeninges and bathed in the cerebrospinal fluid (CSF), which, in the case of infection, provides both a culture medium for the infecting organisms and a rapid means of disseminating the infection throughout the CNS.

The CNS is susceptible to a large number of infectious agents, and many viruses, bacteria, parasites, and fungi are implicated as the cause of CNS infections. CNS infections can be broadly divided into (1) *meningitis,* infection of the leptomeninges and the CSF, and (2) *encephalitis,* infection of the brain parenchyma. However, although these two conditions can be distinguished in many cases on clinical grounds, they frequently coexist and are referred to as *meningoencephalitis.* Three of the reasons for this phenomenon are:

1. During bacterial meningitis, the inflammatory mediators and toxins produced in the subarachnoid space diffuse into the brain parenchyma and cause an inflammatory response of the brain tissue.
2. In encephalitis, the inflammatory reaction reaches the CSF and produces symptoms of meningeal irritation in addition to those related to encephalitis.
3. Some etiologic agents may attack both the meninges and the brain.

Infections of the CNS, especially those that are bacterial, are often life-threatening situations that represent medical emergencies. There are very few other infections that demand such urgent medical attention and skill in differential diagnosis and antibiotic selection to effect a favorable outcome.

CLASSIFICATION AND PATHOGENESIS

Acute Bacterial Infections

Acute bacterial infections of the CNS can be divided into focal infection of the brain parenchyma (abscess) or diffuse inflammatory processes mainly involving the leptomeninges (meningitis) (Table 22–1). Brain abscesses usually develop from contiguous or adjacent anatomic tissues. Acute mastoiditis and sinusitis are examples of infections which, if not promptly treated, may serve as the source for direct bacterial invasion of the brain, causing focal cerebritis and later an abscess. Traumatic head injury or wound infections following neurosurgical or orthopedic procedures involving the calvarium or the spine may also lead to the formation of a brain abscess.

"Metastatic" infections (e.g., bacteria from other areas of the body seeding to the brain via the bloodstream) may lead to a brain abscess. Usually these bacteria originate from the mouth flora, and microaerophilic bacteria (such as *Haemophilus aphrophilus*) or anaerobic bacteria

(such as *Peptostreptococcus*) are the most common etiologic agents. Although bacteremia with *Streptococcus pneumoniae* or *Haemophilus influenzae* is common, especially in children (and in certain cases leads to meningitis), these bacteria very rarely cause brain abscesses. This observation suggests that specific receptors (yet unidentified) exist in the target tissue that allow the bacteria to adhere, multiply, and cause infection. These receptors apparently play a major role in the pathogenesis of infection by determining what type of bacteria produces infection in the brain or in the meninges.

Acute bacterial meningitis most commonly occurs in the very young and the very old. Despite immunization and antimicrobial prophylaxis aimed at decreasing bacterial meningitis, approximately 10,000–20,000 cases still occur annually in the United States in children

TABLE 22–1. *Classification of Infections of the Central Nervous System*

Type of Infection	Example	Pathogenesis	Most Frequent Causative Microorganisms
Acute bacterial ("suppurative"*)	Abscesses: brain, epidural, subdural	Hematogenous (lung, intestinal tract) or Direct invasion (trauma, ENT, sinuses, neuroorthopedic surgery)	Peptostreptococci *Bacteroides* sp. Staphylococci Group A or D streptococci
	Meningitis: neonates and young infants†	Hematogenous	*Escherichia coli* Group B streptococci *Listeria monocytogenes*
	Infants and young children‡	Hematogenous (nasopharynx) or Direct invasion—rarely	*Haemophilus influenzae*, type b *Streptococcus pneumoniae* *Neisseria meningitidis*
	Adults	Hematogenous (nasopharynx) or Direct invasion—rarely	*Streptococcus pneumoniae* *Neisseria meningitidis* (*Haemophilus influenzae*, rare)
	All ages	Direct invasion (head trauma, congenital neuromalformations, neurodiagnostic procedures, neuroorthopedic surgery)	Staphylococci Group A streptococci *Streptococcus pneumoniae* *Pseudomonas aeruginosa* *Escherichia coli* Other Enterobacteriaceae
Granulomatous meningitis	Tuberculous Cryptococcal	Hematogenous (lung) Hematogenous (lung)	*Mycobacterium tuberculosis* *Cryptococcus neoformans*
Acute viral ("aseptic")	Meningitis	Hematogenous (intestinal tract, oropharynx)	Enteroviruses Mumps virus Arboviruses Adenoviruses
	Encephalitis	Hematogenous (intestinal tract, arthropod vector feeding, respiratory tract)	Herpesvirus Enteroviruses Mumps virus Arboviruses Epstein-Barr virus

*Refers to predominance of neutrophils in the CSF.
†Less than 2–3 months of age.
‡2–3 months to 5 years of age.

under 16 years of age. In the preantibiotic era, fatality rates from bacterial meningitis ranged from 70 to 100%. Some progress was achieved when antiserum treatment was used. However, the most dramatic decrease in mortality occurred with the introduction of penicillin, whereupon mortality was reduced to 6% in infants and children and to 25–30% in neonates and the elderly. These mortality rates are still too high, and bacterial meningitis remains a life-threatening illness in all age groups. The mortality and morbidity of bacterial meningitis have not changed significantly in the five decades since the introduction of penicillin. Even the use of recently developed and more potent antibiotics has not substantially improved the outcome. This unexpected fact, despite seemingly more effective antimicrobial therapy as judged by more rapid sterilization of the CSF, may result from the harmful interaction between host inflammatory cells and bacterial components released into the CSF by multiplying bacteria or by antibiotic-induced bacterial lysis. This interaction, which continues despite bacteriologic cure, is believed to be the reason for the high percentage of neurologic sequelae currently observed in patients who recover from meningitis. As many as 25–40% of those who survive the infection may develop long-term sequelae. The major sequelae of meningitis consist of cognitive defects, hearing loss, motor lesions (including seizures, spasticity, and paresis), cranial nerve lesions, and behavioral disturbances. Sensorineural hearing loss, which occurs in 5–10% of cases, is the most serious neurologic sequela because in the very young it is likely to impair speech acquisition and learning. It has been estimated that approximately 37% of all hearing defects acquired postnatally are due to bacterial meningitis.

A wide variety of microorganisms can cause acute bacterial infection of the meninges (Table 22–2). In adults *Streptococcus pneumoniae* and *Neisseria meningitidis* are the most common causes of bacterial meningitis (about 40%). In recent years the number of infections due to gram-negative bacilli has increased significantly. This trend is not surprising since gram-negative bacillary meningitis is usually hospital-acquired and remains a major problem. In elderly patients (older than 60 years of age), *S. pneumoniae* is the most common cause of meningitis followed by gram-negative bacilli. *H. influenzae*, the most common cause of meningitis in the United States, has an annual incidence of 32–71/100,000 in children younger than 5 years of

age. This incidence is much higher among Navajo Indian and Alaskan Eskimo children (173 and 409/100,000/year, respectively), suggesting that genetic factors (yet undefined) play an important role in susceptibility to the infection. Susceptibility to bacterial meningitis is affected not only by age and genetics but also by acquired or congenital deficiencies in host defense mechanisms. Individuals with IgG or complement deficiencies, patients who have undergone splenectomy, or those with congenital or functional asplenia have an increased incidence of septicemia and meningitis caused by *S. pneumoniae* and *H. influenzae* type b. Patients with sickle cell anemia and other hemoglobinopathies are also at increased risk for developing meningitis (usually with *S. pneumoniae*) because of poor splenic function and a defect in the alternative complement pathway. Meningococcal infections occur with increased frequency in individuals who have a deficiency of the terminal components of the complement system (i.e., C5–C9) (see Chapter 23).

Certain environmental situations can increase the probability of acquiring meningitis. A higher incidence of *N. meningitidis* and *H. influenzae* type b meningitis has been reported in crowded households, day-care centers, classrooms, and college and military dormitories. Because the bacteria are transmitted from person to person through the air, the proximity of susceptible individuals in these situations facilitates the spread of infection and the occurrence of secondary cases.

Recurrent bacterial meningitis often suggests the presence of a communication between the subarachnoid space and the paranasal sinuses, nasopharynx, or middle ear. This communication results from fractures or congenital fistulae which transverse through the paranasal sinuses, cribriform plate of the ethmoid bone, or petrous bone. Some individuals have experienced more than 10 episodes of meningitis as a result of such lesions, which can be difficult to identify precisely. The most common bacterium recovered in such instances is *S. pneumoniae*. Therefore, any individual with a history of head trauma who develops meningitis should be promptly examined for excessively watery nasal or otic discharge, which is the result of intermittent or continuous drainage of CSF into the nasal cavities or into the ear through the fracture line. These conditions are called CSF rhinorrhea or CSF otorrhea.

Communication of the subarachnoid space with the skin is usually associated with congen-

TABLE 22–2. *Total Number of Bacterial Meningitis Cases Reported to the Centers for Disease Control between 1978 and 1981**

Organism	Cases Reported	Percentage of Total
Haemophilus influenzae	6,756	50.9
Neisseria meningitidis	2,742	20.7
Streptococcus pneumoniae	1,865	14.1
Group B streptococcus	476	3.6
Listeria monocytogenes	265	2.0
Escherichia coli	115	0.9
Staphylococcus aureus	84	0.6
Klebsiella-Enterobacter Serratia species	61	0.45
Other *Streptococcus* species	43	0.3
Other *Staphylococcus* species	35	0.25
Unknown	827	6.2
Total	13,269	100

*Adapted from cases reported from twenty-seven states participating in National Bacterial Meningitis Surveillance System. JAMA 253:1750, 1985.

ital midline defects of the skull or dura, such as cranial or lumbosacral dermal sinus, dermoid cyst, and myelomeningocele. The meningitis resulting from these lesions is often caused by gram-negative bacilli or staphylococci.

Acute Viral Meningitis and Encephalitis

Acute viral infections of the CNS are usually designated as aseptic meningitis, myelitis, or encephalitis (the last being characterized by altered cerebral function). However, a single satisfactory localization on the basis of clinical findings alone is often difficult. Thus, compound terms such as meningoencephalitis or encephalomyelitis are used to describe the spectrum of the disease. The term *aseptic* was used initially to describe an illness characterized by an acute onset, fever, CSF pleocytosis, with sterile bacterial cultures. With the use of viral isolation methods and new culture techniques to define other microorganisms, it has become clear that *aseptic* is not synonymous with *viral,* and that additional multiple etiologic agents can produce such syndromes (see Chapter 24).

Many viral pathogens cause CNS infections in humans. Some of the most common viruses are listed in Table 22–1. With the exception of herpes simplex encephalitis, the specific viruses causing CNS syndromes are frequently difficult, and sometimes impossible, to identify. Until recently, this lack of specific identification was moot because no useful antiviral therapy was available. With the development of antiviral therapy, increased attention has been focused on the pathogenesis and prompt and specific

diagnosis of the various viral infections of the CNS (especially herpes simplex encephalitis) so that appropriate therapy can be initiated promptly.

Viral CNS infections are common. Although all ages are involved, more than 90% of the patients are under 30 years of age. The viral etiology varies with the season of the year, the age of the patient, and the geographic location. In the United States, about 70% of cases are due to enteroviruses. The most common pathogens from this family are echovirus types 4, 6, 9, 11, 16, and 30 and coxsackieviruses A7, A9, and B2–B5. Most cases occur in children and in the late summer and early fall. Arboviral meningoencephalitis occurs mostly during the summer months because virus transmission occurs by an arthropod such as a mosquito or a tick active during this time of the year. Mumps virus infections are more frequent in the late winter and early spring. Herpesvirus and human immunodeficiency virus infections occur sporadically during the year. In immunocompromised patients other viruses such as adenovirus and cytomegalovirus may cause meningoencephalitis. Poliovirus and lymphocytic choriomeningitis virus, which are important causes of meningoencephalitis worldwide, cause remarkably few cases in the United States.

Viruses gain access to the CNS by one of two routes, hematogenous or neuronal. Most viruses that cause CNS infection do so hematogenously. Following multiplication at the site of entry or in regional lymph nodes that drain the entry site, the virus enters the bloodstream and reaches the CNS. For example, in arthropod-borne viral disease, the virus is transmitted by an insect bite to the skin, where the virus undergoes local replication. Transient viremia occurs with seeding of the virus to the reticuloendothelial system, particularly the liver, spleen, and lymph nodes. Following multiplication in these organs, a secondary viremia occurs leading to further seeding of the virus to other sites, including the CNS. Alternatively, viruses reach the CNS by peripheral intraneuronal routes as occurs with herpes simplex virus. Studies in animals and in humans have suggested that the olfactory tract may be a common route to the brain in cases of herpes simplex encephalitis. Another example of intraneuronal transmission of virus to the CNS is rabies. In this case, the limbic system is involved. Once the rabies virus has reached the CNS, subsequent replication can remain within the neurons or result in cell-to-cell or extracellular transmission.

The precise mechanisms by which viruses reach the CSF and produce neurologic damage are still under investigation. The pathologic findings in acute viral encephalitis are striking. Inflammation of cortical capillary vessels occurs primarily in the gray matter or at the junction of the gray and the white matters, and lymphocytic infiltration is seen in the perivascular areas. As the disease progresses, astrocytosis and gliosis become prominent histopathologic findings.

Viral meningitis is usually an acute, self-limiting illness which, in many instances, mimics other treatable life-threatening CNS infections. Therefore, it is important to recognize the similarities among viral meningitis, partially treated bacterial meningitis, tuberculous meningitis, and fungal meningitis.

As indicated above, the term *encephalitis* is used when there is clinical or pathologic evidence of cerebral involvement. Approximately 20,000 cases of encephalitis occur in the United States each year, with herpes simplex encephalitis accounting for approximately 10% of these cases. The arthropod-borne viruses (arboviruses), such as St. Louis encephalitis, Eastern or Western equine encephalitis, and LaCrosse virus, cause sporadic and epidemic CNS infections in the U.S. Japanese B encephalitis is the most common epidemic CNS infection outside of North America. In China alone, for example, more than 10,000 cases occur annually.

In general, viral encephalitis can be divided into four pathogenic categories: (1) acute primary viral encephalitis, (2) postinfectious encephalomyelitis, (3) slow viral infections of the CNS, and (4) chronic degenerative diseases of the CNS of presumed viral origin.

The acute primary form occurs when the virus directly invades and replicates within the CNS causing encephalitis.

Postinfectious encephalomyelitis is thought to be an autoimmune phenomenon initiated by a viral pathogen. There is a latent phase between the acute viral illness and the onset of neurologic symptoms. Histopathologic studies demonstrate perivascular inflammation and demyelination, but the virus cannot be recovered from the CNS. Postinfectious encephalomyelitis is most commonly associated with varicella and influenza in the United States. However, measles is the most common cause of postinfectious encephalitis worldwide, accounting for as many as 100,000 cases per year. The exact mechanisms that determine why only certain patients develop postinfectious encephalomyelitis are as yet unknown.

Neurodiagnostic techniques, including electroencephalography (EEG), computerized tomography (CT), and magnetic resonance imaging (MRI), may be of diagnostic help in cases of suspected encephalitis. Brain scan and EEG are especially of value in patients with herpes encephalitis. In these patients characteristic periodic high-voltage spike activity, particularly emanating from the temporal regions, and a background of slow-wave complexes are highly suggestive of herpes simplex infection of the brain. Brain biopsy is the most sensitive and specific means of diagnosis for differentiating between herpes simplex encephalitis and other diseases that mimic it.

Granulomatous Meningitis

In granulomatous meningitis the term *granulomatous* refers to the histopathologic characteristic of this infection—formation of granulomata. The granuloma is a collection of lymphocytes and histiocytes derived from mononuclear cells, epithelioid cells, and multinucleated giant cells. Granulomatous meningitis is characterized by a subacute and progressive clinical course and may be remittent, with definite remissions and relapses.

Mycobacterium tuberculosis and *Cryptococcus neoformans* are the most common causes of granulomatous meningitis (see Table 22–1). Both organisms usually infect the CNS in the course of hematogenous dissemination of infection originating in the lungs. Meningitis may be the initial clinical manifestation of tuberculosis or cryptococcal disease when dissemination of the organisms to the CNS is intense. In such cases chest roentgenograms may show little or no evidence of underlying infection. (See Chapters 15 and 27.)

Tuberculous meningitis in adults frequently results from reactivation of an old tuberculous CNS focus that had developed many years earlier and then spread to the subarachnoid space. Tuberculous meningitis is typically associated with active, progressive systemic disease. Tuberculosis of the CNS may also present as a tuberculoma of the brain, which is a well-circumscribed intraparenchymal mass that may slowly enlarge (up to several centimeters in diameter) and may significantly increase intracranial pressure because of its mass. Biopsy of such a lesion usually shows a central core of caseous necrosis surrounded by a typical tuberculous granulomatous reaction. Organisms can often be seen with acid-fast stains, and calcification frequently occurs in inactive lesions. Although seen less frequently in the United States and Europe, tuberculomas still constitute up to 25% of intracranial masses in India and South America. In about 25% of the cases, multiple lesions are found. In children tuberculomas are usually found in the posterior fossa, whereas in adults they are predominantly supratentorial. History of exposure to a patient with tuberculosis may give an important clue to this treatable disease.

In contrast, exposure history for cryptococcus is of little value since this fungus is a widespread saprophyte. Evidence of underlying cellular immune dysfunction is more important because it predisposes the patient to this infection. The development of subacute or chronic meningitis in patients with Hodgkin's disease or lymphosarcoma, in those receiving high-dose daily corticosteroids, or in those at risk for AIDS should raise the possibility of cryptococcal meningitis. Initial manifestations of cryptococcal meningitis may be unexplained fevers and chronic headaches.

Chronic meningitis in the immunosuppressed patient with impaired cellular immunity requires special consideration because of the distinctive differential diagnosis. *Listeria monocytogenes, Mycobacterium avium-intracellulare, Toxoplasma gondii,* and *Nocardia, Histoplasma,* and *Coccidioides* sp. are some of the other etiologic agents of chronic meningitis in such patients which should be considered in the differential diagnosis. The list of opportunistic agents associated with chronic meningitis in individuals with AIDS is even longer, including papovavirus, cytomegalovirus, *Treponema pallidum, Candida* sp., and the human immunodeficiency virus itself.

CLINICAL ASPECTS

Manifestations of Meningitis

Fever, headache, vomiting, impairment of consciousness, and stiff neck and back are common manifestations of meningeal irritation in adults, irrespective of its etiology. The headache is usually generalized and persistent. Unfortunately it is a manifestation that children younger than 2 years of age cannot communicate; they are usually irritable, which is not as specific an indicator of a CNS process. Nuchal rigidity (the most pathognomonic sign of meningitis in adults) is resistance to flexion of the neck caused by cervical and upper thoracic paraspinal muscle spasm as a result of meningeal inflammation. True nuchal rigidity, which usually indicates meningeal inflammation, should be distinguished from meningismus (e.g., painful or difficult flexion or rotation of the head), which is caused by posterior cervical or shoulder girdle muscle spasm related to acute pharyngitis/tonsillitis, especially peritonsillar abscess, or acute posterior or anterior cervical lymphadenitis. Torticollis and other processes in the neck can cause symptoms that simulate nuchal rigidity.

Meningitis presents as two symptom patterns in infants and young children. The first is insidious and develops progressively over several days; it may be preceded by a nonspecific febrile illness or an upper respiratory-like infection. In this setting, it is usually difficult, if not impossible, to time the exact onset of meningitis, especially if another infection, such as otitis media, is diagnosed and oral antibiotics given. The second pattern is acute and fulminant, with the manifestations of sepsis and meningitis developing rapidly over a few hours. This rapidly progressive form may be associated with severe brain edema that can provoke herniation of the cerebellar tonsils, resulting in death.

In children, the presenting symptoms are often nonspecific. Fever, listlessness, sleepiness, irritability, and vomiting are commonly found, and there is a higher incidence of seizures. In neonates as well as in very old patients, the signs and symptoms of meningitis may be even more subtle, consisting of only fever, confusion, and poor feeding; unstable or low temperature is not rare. Stiff neck or fullness of the anterior fontanelle are relatively late signs of meningitis in infants and may not be present in all cases. It is important to consider the possibility of meningitis in any patient with fever and unexplained alteration in mentation or level of alertness and consciousness. Whereas judgment based upon clinical findings is certainly important, the adage "If you think about doing a spinal tap to verify the diagnosis, do it" still holds. The potential diagnostic value of a lumbar puncture far outweighs the very small risk of harm from the procedure.

Several features which may be found during the physical examination warrant specific mention. Petechiae, especially in association with fever, should always raise the possibility of bacteremia and meningitis. Although petechiae classically are associated with meningococcal infection, they can occur with *H. influenzae, S. pneumoniae,* and many viral infections. It is important to note that pediatric patients with meningitis may also have an extrameningeal focus of infection, such as buccal or periorbital cellulitis, otitis media, or pneumonia. Therefore, if such a focus is found, the patient's status (e.g., age, immune competence, severity of symptoms in relation to the identified focus, and symptoms unexplained by the known focus) should be carefully assessed before a decision is made not to do studies for determining the presence of meningitis. Focal neurologic signs, such as hemiparesis, quadriparesis, or cranial nerve palsy, occur in about 15% of patients with meningitis and reflect the possible presence of cortical venous or arterial thrombosis secondary to edema and inflammation. Papilledema is uncommon early in the course of acute meningitis and, when present, should prompt an evaluation for venous sinus thrombosis, subdural collection of fluid, or brain abscess.

Differential Diagnosis of CNS Infections

Because the signs and symptoms of CNS infection are very diverse and are not pathogno-monic, many other diseases should be considered in the differential diagnosis (Table 22–3). Even distinguishing among the various infectious processes that may occur in the CNS, such as viral meningitis, fungal meningitis, tuberculous meningitis, brain abscess, early bacterial meningitis, subdural empyema, and others, may be difficult. In some instances, the initial laboratory findings are nonspecific and serial cerebrospinal fluid evaluation is necessary to identify the etiologic agent or the response to therapy. Clues to the specific diagnosis may come from careful history of potential exposure (e.g., tuberculosis, or specific viral, bacterial, or fungal exposure), meticulous physical examination (e.g., lesions outside the CNS with potential to spread, systemic manifestations of noninfectious diseases), careful examination of cerebrospinal fluid, immunologic studies, and roentgeno-graphic studies.

Brain tumors and brain abscesses are frequently indistinguishable by their clinical presentation alone. Increased intracranial pressure may be the only presenting neurologic sign, and lumbar puncture may not be helpful in differentiating between these two entities because the CSF may be entirely normal, except for the fact that its pressure is increased. Epidural or subdural spinal abscesses usually present with spinal cord compression, symptomatology that can simulate noninfectious diseases such as Guillain-Barré syndrome, spinal cord tumor, meningioma, and herniated disc. Emergency myelography is often essential to differentiate spinal cord compression from other processes. The urgency of myelography cannot be overemphasized because, when abscess formation occurs within the spinal canal, the spinal cord must be decompressed promptly by appropriate neurosurgical means if return of normal neurologic function is to be expected.

Neoplastic metastases involving the meninges may produce the same clinical manifestations as granulomatous meningitis. The CSF abnormalities may also be identical to those that are typically seen in tuberculous or cryptococcal meningitis. Only special studies such as careful examination of the cells in the CSF, special staining procedures (e.g., acid-fast or India ink), and biopsy may be helpful in the diagnosis.

CEREBROSPINAL FLUID ABNORMALITIES

Lumbar puncture to obtain CSF is essential for the evaluation of a patient with CNS infection.

TABLE 22–3. *A Partial List of Differential Diagnoses of CNS Infections*

Noninfectious	Infectious
Brain tumors	Viral meningoencephalitis
Leukemia	Bacterial meningitis
Lymphoma	Tuberculosis
Subarachnoid hemorrhage	Brain abscess
Subdural hematoma	Parameningeal infections
Systemic lupus	Lyme disease
erythematosus	Syphilis
Malignant hypertension	Brucellosis
Multiple sclerosis	Toxoplasmosis
Sarcoidosis	Cysticercosis
Mollaret's (recurrent)	Cryptococcosis
meningitis	Fungal meningitis
Behçet's disease	Rickettsia
Ruptured dermoid cyst	
Ruptured spinal	
ependymoma	

There are very few conditions which contraindicate the prompt performance of a lumbar puncture. These conditions include (1) the presence of obvious signs of increased intracranial pressure (e.g., papilledema, altered pupillary responses, increased blood pressure with bradycardia), (2) significantly unstable cardiopulmonary status (e.g., with severe sepsis) that might be aggravated by the procedure, and (3) infection in the area that the needle must traverse to obtain CSF. If signs of increased intracranial pressure are present, removal of even small amounts of CSF (3–4 mL) may result in downward displacement of the brain into the foramen magnum, compressing the cerebellar peduncles against the lower medulla and leading to brain stem compression. Sudden removal of CSF under increased pressure may also cause shifting of the brain with transtentorial herniation of some portion of the cerebral hemispheres into the posterior fossa. Foraminal or transtentorial herniation of the brain is an extreme emergency situation which requires immediate neurosurgical decompression to save the patient. For the above reasons, if increased intracranial pressure is suspected, noninvasive neurodiagnostic procedures, such as a CT scan or MRI should be performed before lumbar puncture is performed.

The typical CSF abnormalities associated with types of CNS infections are shown in Table 22–4. When the CSF is obtained, it should be examined immediately. The total number of white blood cells should be counted in a counting chamber, and, following centrifugation, a differential cell count should be performed on a Wright-stained smear of the sediment. Normally the CSF has fewer than 5–10 mononuclear leukocytes/mm^3 and no polymorphonuclear neutrophils (PMNs). Therefore, the presence of a single PMN is abnormal and suggests the possibility of CNS infection. In addition, if the number of mononuclear cells is higher than 10, a CNS process (including infection) should be suspected. Although the differential count is more likely to disclose a predominance of PMNs in bacterial meningitis and a predominance of mononuclear cells in viral, tuberculous, or fungal meningitis, there is an overlap between these groups. Up to one third of cases with tuberculous or viral meningitis demonstrate a predominance of PMNs, and as many as 10% of cases of early or partially treated bacterial meningitis have a predominance of lymphocytes. The CSF protein concentration (normally less than 40 mg/dL) and the CSF glucose concentration (normally above 40 mg/dL) and its ratio to the simultaneous blood glucose concentration (normally above 0.4) may help in the diagnosis.

The CSF abnormalities associated with tuberculous, fungal, and viral meningitis overlap even more, and it may be impossible to separate one from the other (see Table 22–4). The CSF findings in tuberculous meningitis usually consist of a lymphocytic pleocytosis (25–500 cells/mm^3), increased protein concentration, and depressed

TABLE 22–4. *Cerebrospinal Fluid Abnormalities Often Associated with CNS Infections*

	Leukocytes		Cerebrospinal Fluid Findings			
Condition	*No per* mm^3	*Predominant Cell*	*Glucose*	*Protein*	*Stained Smear*	*Result of Culture*
Bacterial meningitis ("purulent")	0–60,000	Segmented neutrophils	Very low (<5–20 mg%)	Elevated	Usually positive*	Usually positive*
Partially treated meningitis	0–2,500	Neutrophils and mononuclear cells	Normal to slightly reduced	Elevated	Often negative	Often negative
Tuberculous meningitis	25–500	Mononuclear cells	Low (20–40 mg%)	Elevated	Usually negative	Usually negative
Fungal meningitis	0–1,000	Mononuclear cells	Low	Elevated	Often positive	Usually positive
Viral meningitis ("aseptic")	0–1,000	Mononuclear cells (neutrophils in early phase)	Normal (65–70 mg%)	Slightly elevated early in illness	Negative	Negative
Brain abscess	10–200	Lymphocytes or neutrophils	Normal	Elevated	Usually negative	Usually negative
Syphilis	30–500	Lymphocytes	Normal	Elevated	Usually negative	Usually negative
Sarcoidosis	50–200	Mononuclear cells	Normal	Elevated	Negative	Negative

*A major exception is bacterial meningitis caused by *Neisseria meningitidis*, in which the Gram's strain of cerebrospinal fluid sediment often fails to reveal microorganisms, and cultures may be negative for growth.

glucose level. CSF acid-fast smears are positive in 10–22% of the cases, and CSF cultures are positive in 38–88% of the cases.

Antituberculous therapy should be initiated promptly if the clinical setting suggests infection with *M. tuberculosis,* since delay in treatment may preclude full recovery. Typical CSF findings in cryptococcal meningitis include a mild lymphocytic pleocytosis (0–400 cells/mm^3) and a depressed glucose level in 55% of cases. It is important to note that in AIDS patients, currently the most common patients with this infection, the CSF often shows little evidence of an inflammatory reaction. India ink staining of CSF is positive in over half of the cases, demonstrating the cryptococcal cells with their large capsules. The yield is highest in patients with acute infection. More than 85% of patients have cryptococcal polysaccharide antigen in the CSF. Although the initial CSF culture is positive in only three quarters of the patients, additional CSF cultures increase the yield and are indicated.

Because it is not justified to exclude bacterial meningitis and to defer antimicrobial therapy solely on the basis of the CSF parameters, the sediment of centrifuged CSF should be Gram stained and examined thoroughly. A positive Gram's stain provides helpful information, but a negative stain does not rule out bacterial meningitis. The probability of visualizing bacteria on a Gram's stain is dependent upon the number of organisms present. The percentage of positive Gram-stained smears is less than 25% when there are fewer than 10^3 organisms/mL. The percentage is higher (up to 40–50%) when there are 10^4–10^5 organisms/mL. When more than 10^5 organisms/mL are present, 97% of Gram's stains are positive. Staining of the CSF with acridine orange and examination with fluorescence microscopy may increase the sensitivity of the method, and bacteria not observed by the usual Gram's stain may be found. Pretreatment with oral antibiotics may only slightly modify the results of Gram's stains and cultures with some bacteria (e.g., *H. influenzae*), but with others (e.g., *S. pneumoniae* and *N. meningitidis*) the changes are significant. Rapid tests (within 1 h) are available to detect bacterial antigens associated with *H. influenzae* type b, *S. pneumoniae, N. meningitidis,* and group B streptococcus in both CSF and urine. The most sensitive test is the latex agglutination test. Various latex agglutination tests typically demonstrate sensitivity of 90–100% as compared with 65–75% for counterimmunoelectrophoresis

(CIE). These tests are especially helpful for patients in whom pretreatment has rendered the interpretation of bacterial cultures difficult (partially treated meningitis). However, failure to detect antigen in the CSF using these tests does not rule out bacterial meningitis. Again, the sensitivity of the test is in direct correlation to the number of bacteria in the CSF; if they are below 10^2–10^3/mL, the test result is usually negative.

Detection of endotoxin in the CSF or measurement of CSF C-reactive protein, lactic acid concentration, and lactic dehydrogenase (LDH) activity have been reported to be helpful in differentiating bacterial from viral meningitis. The accuracy and usefulness of these tests are uncertain because they have not been extensively used and thus need further evaluation.

In addition to CSF cultures, blood cultures should be obtained for every patient with suspected bacterial meningitis. These cultures are positive in 80% of children with *H. influenzae* meningitis, in 50% with *S. pneumoniae* meningitis, and in a third of patients with *N. meningitidis* meningitis.

From the above discussion of the CSF findings in CNS infections, it should be obvious that, despite the availability of many sensitive tests for detecting various etiologic agents, the differential diagnosis relies heavily on the physician's ability to consider these tests in the context of the clinical setting of the individual patient. Only then can reasonable decisions concerning antimicrobial therapy be made.

THEORETICAL AND PRACTICAL CONSIDERATIONS OF ANTIBIOTIC THERAPY

General Approach to Antimicrobial Therapy

Prompt treatment of bacterial meningitis with an appropriate antibiotic is essential to minimize the occurrence of additional nervous system damage. The development of serious neurologic complications such as seizures, hemiplegia, hearing impairment, and personality dysfunction is correlated with the type of bacteria causing the meningitis, with its concentration in the CSF, and with very low CSF glucose concentrations (less than 20 mg/dL). The initial antimicrobial regimen chosen for treatment should be sufficiently broad to affect all likely pathogens that commonly cause meningitis in the patient's age group. Remember that the Gram's stain can be misinterpreted and that rapid antigen tests do not provide information regarding antimicrobial susceptibility. Therefore, the preferred initial antimicrobial regimen varies with the expected pathogens, their susceptibilities, and the age of the patient.

Entry of Beta-Lactam Antibiotics into the CSF

A number of new beta-lactam antibiotics have been evaluated recently for the treatment of meningitis, and several have been shown to be very effective in eradicating bacteria. Multiple factors influence the penetration of beta-lactam antibiotics into the CSF. The blood-brain barrier and the blood-CSF barrier restrict penetration of most antimicrobial drugs into the brain and CSF, respectively. Concentration of antibiotics in these two CNS areas in normal volunteers and in experimental animals are approximately 1/200–1/500 those achieved in the serum. Penetration of antibiotics into the CSF is by passive diffusion, and inflammation of the pia-arachnoid during infection enhances the permeability of the barrier, with subsequent increase in CSF antibiotic concentrations. The blood-brain barrier acts like a lipid layer. As a result, highly lipophilic substances (e.g., drugs such as chloramphenicol, rifampin, isoniazid) enter readily into the CSF, whereas certain cephalosporins and aminoglycosides do not.

Most antibiotics that diffuse into the CSF are removed from the subarachnoid space by "bulk-flow" mechanisms across the arachnoid villi. In addition, penicillins, cephalosporins, and aminoglycosides are transported out of the CSF to the intravascular region by an energy-requiring exit pump in the choroid plexus. This active exit pump of the choroid plexus rapidly moves antimicrobial agents back into the systemic circulation, making it even more difficult to achieve and maintain high concentrations of antibiotics in the CSF or brain tissues.

Two other considerations are relevant to the penetration of antibiotics into the CSF following the disruption of the blood-brain barrier:

1. The penetration of antibiotics declines as meningeal inflammation subsides during the course of treatment of meningitis. For example, on the first day of therapy for bacterial meningitis, ampicillin levels in CSF are about 40% of serum levels, but after 7 days of treatment the CSF level is less than 20% of the serum level; therefore, the dosage of the antimicrobial agents must not be reduced during therapy.

2. Experimental meningitis studies in animals show that antiinflammatory agents, such as corticosteroids, decrease meningeal inflammation and thus may reduce permeability of the blood-brain barrier.

Need for Bactericidal Activity in CSF

The blood-brain barrier and the blood-CSF barrier restrict delivery of antibodies and complement to the nervous system. Thus, host immune responses outside the CNS have a very limited effect on the invading pathogen after it enters the CNS. Some evidence exists that active production of IgM and IgG by antibody-secreting B lymphocytes that have entered the CNS as part of the inflammatory response may be important in combating invading bacteria. However, phagocytosis of encapsulated meningeal pathogens is inefficient in CSF *in vivo*, resulting in unhindered bacterial proliferation and ultimately in high bacterial concentrations within the CSF. These observations suggest that antibiotics are of paramount importance in treatment of bacterial CNS infections. Unfortunately, an antibiotic not only must reach the affected area of the CNS but also must achieve concentrations that exceed the minimum bactericidal concentration (MBC) of the antibiotic for the invading bacteria (as determined *in vitro*).

The need for high bactericidal activity in the CSF to effect a desirable outcome has been demonstrated in experimental models of meningitis. CSF concentrations of beta-lactam or an aminoglycoside agent that are at least 10 times higher than the MBC of the infecting pathogen were necessary to achieve optimal bacterial eradication.

An innovative approach to assist in the choice of an effective antibiotic is to combine *in vitro* data (e.g., the MBC) with *in vivo* data (e.g., CSF antibiotic levels) to produce an index which reflects the degree to which the achievable CSF antibiotic levels exceed the MBC of the bacteria. This ratio, called the Inhibitory Quotient, should exceed 10 if the desired bactericidal effect is to be achieved. For example, an *H. influenzae* isolated from a patient with meningitis was found to be killed *in vitro* (MBC) by drug A at a concentration of 0.5 µg/mL and by drug B at 0.05 µg/mL concentration. From data in the literature, it is known that drug A produces CSF levels of 4 µg/mL and drug B only 2 μg/mL. From the equation Inhibitory Quotient = CSF drug level ÷ MBC, the inhibitory quotient for drug A is 8 (4 ÷ 0.5), and for drug B it is 40 (2 ÷ 0.05). Although drug A achieves absolute CSF levels higher than drug B, drug B is predicted to be more efficient in eradicating the bacteria (e.g., Inhibitory Quotient > 10) and should be the preferred drug.

Antimicrobial Drug Resistance

In recent decades, some bacteria that cause meningitis have changed their susceptibility to antibiotics. A substantial proportion of strains of *H. influenzae* type b, the leading etiologic agent of childhood meningitis, have become resistant to ampicillin and, to a lesser extent, to chloramphenicol. Most of the resistant strains contain a plasmid that mediates production of a beta-lactamase that hydrolyzes penicillins and some cephalosporins. Although chloramphenicol is still highly effective against strains that produce beta-lactamase, on very rare occasions a strain of *H. influenzae* may be resistant to both ampicillin and chloramphenicol. It is predicted that the prevalence of these strains may increase in the next several years. Thus, the traditional combination of ampicillin and chloramphenicol as the initial therapy for *H. influenzae* meningitis may warrant modification. Newer cephalosporins, such as ceftriaxone or cefotaxime, are highly active against *H. influenzae,* including organisms that produce beta-lactamase or that are multiresistant, and should be considered strongly as the initial therapy.

The same scenario pertains to *S. pneumoniae.* Five–fifteen percent of *S. pneumoniae* strains in the United States are relatively resistant to penicillin. If this antibiotic is used for treatment of meningitis, it may be ineffective. Most of the relatively penicillin-resistant strains are susceptible to chloramphenicol, but an occasional strain may also be resistant to that agent. Antibiotics such as cefotaxime, ceftriaxone, or vancomycin appear to be effective against such strains. The newer cephalosporins are being used with increasing frequency as a single-drug regimen for the therapy of bacterial meningitis.

Need for Adjunctive Antiinflammatory Therapy

A major goal of antimicrobial therapy has been to achieve sterilization of the CSF as rapidly as possible. However, there have been concerns that rapid lysis, particularly of gram-negative bacteria, may result in a massive release of endotoxin that could be harmful to the host. Studies in animals and humans have shown that products of bacterial lysis, such as cell fragments and lipopolysaccharides (e.g., endotoxin) induced by cell wall–active antibiotics, can cause a transient increase of locally produced cytokines. These proinflammatory agents may amplify and augment tissue injury. In fact, although the newer antibiotics are much more efficient in sterilization of the CNS compared with older agents, there has been little improvement over earlier treatment trials. In animal experiments, use of the corticosteroid dexamethasone (given prior to or concomitant with the first dose of antibiotic) was found to be effective in preventing the antibiotic-induced burst of cytokines in the CSF, and thus augmentation of the inflammatory response was aborted. At present, the addition of dexamethasone to antimicrobial therapy for patients with bacterial meningitis is controversial, and further confirmatory studies are needed.

Duration of Therapy

Regimens used for the therapy of bacterial meningitis are largely empiric and are based upon antibiotic pharmacokinetic data and clinical experience. The duration of antibiotic therapy for meningitis continues to be somewhat controversial: the patient needs to be treated long enough to effect permanent cure but not any longer. For example, in neonates, the suggested duration of therapy for *Escherichia coli* meningitis is the longer time of (1) 14 days after the documentation of sterile CSF, or (2) 21 days total. In older infants, children, and adults, shorter courses of therapy are used. The clinical and bacteriologic responses of patients with meningococcal meningitis and *H. influenzae* type b meningitis suggest that a 7–10-day course of therapy is sufficient in the majority of cases.

VACCINE IMMUNOPROPHYLAXIS OF MENINGITIS

Capsular polysaccharides appear to be the major antigenic determinants of many of the major bacterial pathogens that play an important role in causing meningitis. Vaccines employing some of these bacterial polysaccharides have proved to be highly immunogenic and protective, especially in adults. Currently, vaccines for protection against selected strains of *S. pneumoniae, N. meningitidis,* and all *H. influenzae* type b are available.

The available meningococcal vaccines are monovalent serogroup A or C, bivalent A/C, and quadrivalent A/C/Y/W-135. The monovalent A or C vaccines are recommended for use in epidemics caused by these two serotypes. The immunogenicity of these vaccines differs in various age groups. For example, monovalent serogroup A polysaccharide vaccine is highly immunogenic in children 3 months of age and older and is effective in preventing meningitis. In contrast, the serogroup C polysaccharide vaccine is immunogenic only in adults and children 2 years of age or older. The use of this vaccine in army recruits decreased the incidence of meningococcal meningitis by 90%. To date, no immunogenic meningococcal serogroup B vaccine has been prepared.

Pneumococcal vaccine was first licensed in the United States in 1978 and was composed of 14 common capsular serotypes. It has now been reformulated to include 23 common serotypes. Despite this broader spectrum of serotypes, pneumococcal vaccine still does not prevent all pneumococcal infections, because many pneumococcal serotypes are not included and because insufficient responses to serotypes included in the vaccine occur, especially in very young and very old patients. The pneumococcal vaccine is recommended for individuals older than 2 years of age who are at increased risk of developing disseminated infection with *S. pneumoniae.* This targeted population includes those patients with functional asplenia (e.g., sickle cell disease) or traumatic asplenia, nephrotic syndrome, HIV infection, and other individuals with increased risk for serious pneumococcal infections.

The prevention of *H. influenzae* type b meningitis is another important target of vaccine immunoprophylaxis. Although immunization of adults and children older than 18 months of age with purified *H. influenzae* type b capsular polyribose phosphate (PRP) has shown it to be highly immunogenic and to provide protection, the response of infants younger than 18 months of age is poor because of an impaired ability of their immune system to respond to purified polysaccharide (T-independent) antigens. This poor response is due to the relative immaturity of the immune system. Similarly, most children who develop *H. influenzae* type b meningitis during the first 18 months of life do not produce anti-PRP antibody exceeding the minimum levels associated with protection. These data point to the need for more effective vaccines to improve the immune responses of children younger than 18 months of age, who are most susceptible to this serious infection. One approach to augment the immunogenic potential of polysaccharide antigens is to link the capsular polysaccharide to a protein molecule. In such conjugates, the polysaccharide is converted from being a T-cell–independent antigen to a T-cell–dependent antigen. This conversion not only increases the B-cell response to the polysaccharide moiety but also induces memory T cells, which enhance amnestic responses to the antigen. Conjugate vaccines of *H. influenzae* type b (such as PRP conjugated to diphtheria toxoid or PRP conjugated to an outer membrane protein of *N. meningitidis*) have recently been shown to be highly immunogenic even in children as young as 2 months of age. Since approximately 60% of all *H. influenzae* type b meningitis in the United States occurs in children younger than 15 months of age, the potential for these vaccines to prevent meningitis more effectively is obvious. (See Chapters 23 and 40.)

REFERENCES

Books

Johnson, R. T. *Viral Infections of the Nervous System.* New York: Raven Press, 1982.

Swosh, M., and Kennard, C., eds. *The Scientific Basis of Clinical Neurology.* London: Churchill Livingstone, 1985.

Review Articles

Balows, A., and Tilton, R. C. Body fluids and infectious diseases. *Am. J. Med.* 75(1B):98–138, 1983.

Connolly, K. D. Lumbar punctures, meningitis and persisting pleocytosis. *Arch. Dis. Child* 54:792–793, 1979.

Ellner, J. J., and Bennett, J. E. Chronic meningitis. *Medicine* 55:341–369, 1976.

Greenlee, J. E. Anatomic considerations in central nervous system infections. In: Mandell, G. L., Douglas, R. G., and Bennett, J. E., eds. *Principles and Practice of Infectious Diseases.* 3rd ed. New York: Churchill Livingstone, 1990:732–741.

Johnson, R. T. The pathogenesis of acute viral encephalitis and postinfectious encephalomyelitis. *J. Infect. Dis.* 155:359–364, 1987.

Meyers, B. R. Tuberculous meningitis. *Med. Clin. North Am.* 66:755–762, 1982.

Whitley, R. J. Herpes simplex virus infections. In: Remington, J. S., and Klein, J. O., eds. *Infectious Diseases of the Fetus and Newborn Infant.* Philadelphia: W. B. Saunders, 1990:282–305.

Whitley, R. J. Viral encephalitis. *N. Engl. J. Med.* 323:242–249, 1990.

Common Etiologic Agents of Bacterial Meningitis

Although bacterial meningitis can be caused by virtually any organism, *Streptococcus pneumoniae, Haemophilus influenzae* type b, and *Neisseria meningitidis* are by far the most common pathogens isolated. Various predisposing host factors, such as age, race, immunodeficiency, and specific environmental situations, are discussed in Chapter 22. In this chapter we discuss the common bacteria causing meningitis, their virulence factors, and the interactions between the host and the infecting organism.

HAEMOPHILUS INFLUENZAE

Morphology

Haemophilus influenzae is a small, nonmotile, non–spore-forming, gram-negative, pleomor-

phic bacterium (rod). When the cells are young and growing under optimal conditions, they appear more like a coccobacillus than a true bacillus. Short chains may be found which, with improper decolorization of the Gram's stain, may be mistakenly identified as *Streptococcus pneumoniae*. In older cultures or when growth occurs under unfavorable conditions, the rods become elongated and frequently appear filamentous (Fig. 23–1). Many other bacteria also have a gram-negative pleomorphic appearance on Gram's stain. A partial list of these bacteria is given in Table 23–1.

Growth

Haemophilus influenzae grows either in the presence (aerobe) or the absence (facultative anaerobe) of oxygen. This microorganism belongs to a group collectively referred to as the hemophilic bacteria, which require enriched media for growth, and most must have available either one or both of two growth factors, referred to as X and V. X factor has been identified as hemin (or related protoporphyrins), and V factor is found to be replaceable by NAD+ (nicotinamide adenine dinucleotide) or NADP (nicotinamide adenine dinucleotide phosphate).

H. influenzae is incapable of synthesizing hemin (or related protoporphyrins) from delta-aminolevulinic acid, and its NAD requirement for growth is absolute. By heating blood agar at 50°C for approximately 15 min until a brown color appears (hence the name chocolate agar), red blood cells are destroyed and hemin and NAD+ are released to the media. At the same time, enzymes that inactivate V factor are destroyed, but V factor, which is heat-labile, is

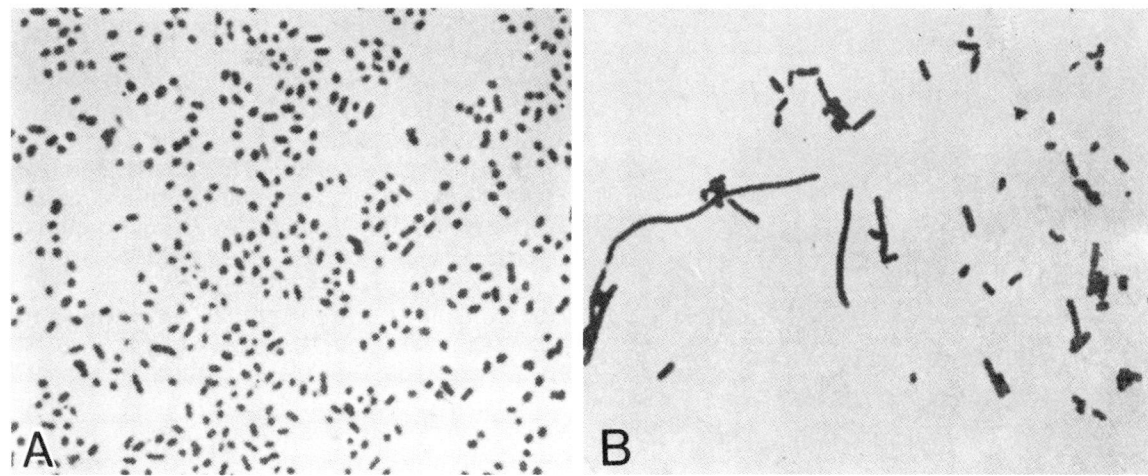

Figure 23–1. Gram's stain of Haemophilus influenzae. A. *Growing under optimal conditions.* B. *Growing under unfavorable conditions (e.g., older cultures, presence of antibiotics).*

not inactivated. *H. influenzae* does not grow on blood agar but grows profusely on chocolate agar. This preferential growth may serve as the first clue that an unknown pathogen might be *H. influenzae.*

Although *Haemophilus influenzae* requires both X and V factors for growth, not all the species of bacteria in the genus *Haemophilus* do; some require only one. Table 23–2 lists the members of this genus, their requirements for X and V factors, and their capacity to lyse red blood cells. The growth requirements outlined in the table are useful for differentiating members of this group.

V factor necessary for the growth of *Haemophilus influenzae* can also be furnished by other microorganisms. For example, colonies of staphylococci on blood agar may produce enough V factor to permit the growth of *H. influenzae* in the immediate vicinity of the staphylococcal colony. This is known as the satellite phenomenon (Fig. 23–2). It is not known whether the production of V factor by other microorganisms or by the host may contribute to the growth of *H. influenzae in vivo* and, therefore, to its pathogenicity.

One practical problem may arise from the fact that *Haemophilus haemolyticus* and staphylococci are components of the normal oropharyngeal microbial flora, especially in children. Because of production of V factor by the staphylococci, *H. haemolyticus* colonies surrounded by areas of complete (beta-type) hemolysis may be present on blood agar plates streaked with throat swabs. These colonies may be mistaken for group A streptococci. This problem can be avoided by using agar plates prepared from sheep blood rather than blood of other species, since the hemolysin produced by *H. haemolyticus* does not lyse sheep erythrocytes. When group A streptococci are suspected to be the hemolytic colonies in close proximity to other microorganisms on a plate streaked with a throat swab, a Gram's stain also prevents mistaken identity.

H. influenzae can use glucose, xylose, and galactose as carbon sources, but it cannot ferment sucrose or lactose. In addition many strains produce urease, ornithine decarboxylase, alkaline phosphatase, and indole. Using some

TABLE 23–1. *Partial List of Gram-Negative Coccobacilli*

Actinobacillus actinomycetem comitans
Bordetella pertussis
Brucella melitensis
Cardiobacterium hominis
Eikenella corrodens
Francisella tularensis (also called *Pasteurella tularensis*)
Haemophilus species
Campylobacter fetus
Streptobacillus moniliformis

TABLE 23–2. *Differential Growth Characteristics of the* Haemophilus *Group*

Species	Growth Factors		Hemolysis
	X	V	
Haemophilus influenzae	+	+	–
H. parainfluenzae	–	+	–
H. aegypticus	+	+	–
H. ducreyi	+	–	+
H. suis	+	+	–
H. haemolyticus	+	+	+
H. parahaemolyticus	–	+	+
H. aphrophilus	+	–	–

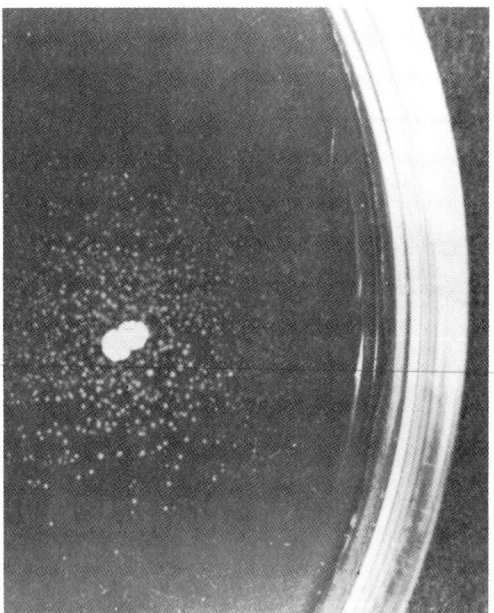

Figure 23–2. Satellite phenomenon. Colonies of Haemophilus influenzae *growing only in vicinity of staphylococcal colonies of agar medium lacking V factor. The agar, which contained blood autoclaved to destroy the V factor, was uniformly seeded with a heavy inoculum of* H. influenzae *and a very light inoculum of* Staphylococcus aureus. *(From Davis, B. D., et al.* Microbiology. *3rd ed. Hagerstown, MD: Harper & Row, 1980.)*

of these capabilities a biotyping system has been devised (Table 23–3). By use of the biotyping system it became clear that *H. aegyptius* is not a distinct species but rather *H. influenzae* biotype III. This observation is strengthened by examining the mean guanosine plus cytosine (G + C) base composition of *H. aegyptius*, which is exactly the same as *H. influenzae*. The biotyping system is also very helpful in epidemiologic studies. For example, Brazilian purpuric fever (BPF), a life-threatening infection which presents as an acute febrile illness in children 3 months to 10 years in age with abdominal pain or vomiting and hemorrhagic skin lesions, was recognized during 1984 in the state of São Paulo, Brazil. Epidemiologic investigations could not identify a pathogen, but a history of conjunctivitis in the 30 days preceding the fever was identified as a common denominator in all 10 children who died of BPF. When conjunctival cultures from children with acute febrile illnesses became positive for *H. influenzae* biotype III (*aegyptius*) this agent was identified as the cause of BPF. Further investigation confirmed that this "new" disease arose probably from a single clone of *H. influenzae* biogroup *aegyptius* with unique invasive potential. Other epidemiologic studies found that most cases of *H. influenzae* meningitis are caused by biotype I, which is rarely isolated from the respiratory system of well children. In addition, resistance to antibiotics may be related to the biotype. For example, ampicillin resistance is less frequent among biotype I isolates as compared with other biotypes.

Antigenic Structure

H. influenzae strains can be encapsulated or nonencapsulated. The major antigenic capsular component of encapsulated strains is a polysaccharide. Six distinct antigenic types have been identified and labeled a–f (Table 23–4). Serologic tests such as precipitation, agglutination, or quelling (capsular swelling) can be used to differentiate among the various serotypes. The most common test used clinically is latex agglutination. For this test, latex particles are coated with antibodies specific for a particular antigenic type. When aliquots of an unknown clinical sample (like CSF) are added to the various antibody-coated particles, agglutination occurs only between the specific antigen (for example, type b) and its specific antibody, producing visible precipitation within 10 min (Fig. 23–3). No precipitation is observed with the other antibodies. Thus, a specific definitive identification of *H. influenzae* type b is provided within minutes. Virulence appears to be related to the specific serotype. For example, the capsular polysaccharide of *H. influenzae* type b, by far the most frequent cause of serious infection in

TABLE 23–3. Haemophilus influenzae *Biotypes**

| | Reaction | | |
Type	Indole Production	Ornithine Decarboxylase	Urease Activity
I	+	+	+
II	+	−	+
III	−	−	+
IV	−	+	+
V	+	+	−

*Only the more common biotypes are presented.

TABLE 23–4. *The Carbohydrate Component of* Haemophilus influenzae *Capsules*

Serotype	Carbohydrate
a	Glucose
b	Ribose, ribitol
c	Galactose
d	Hexose
e	Hexosamine
f	Galactosamine

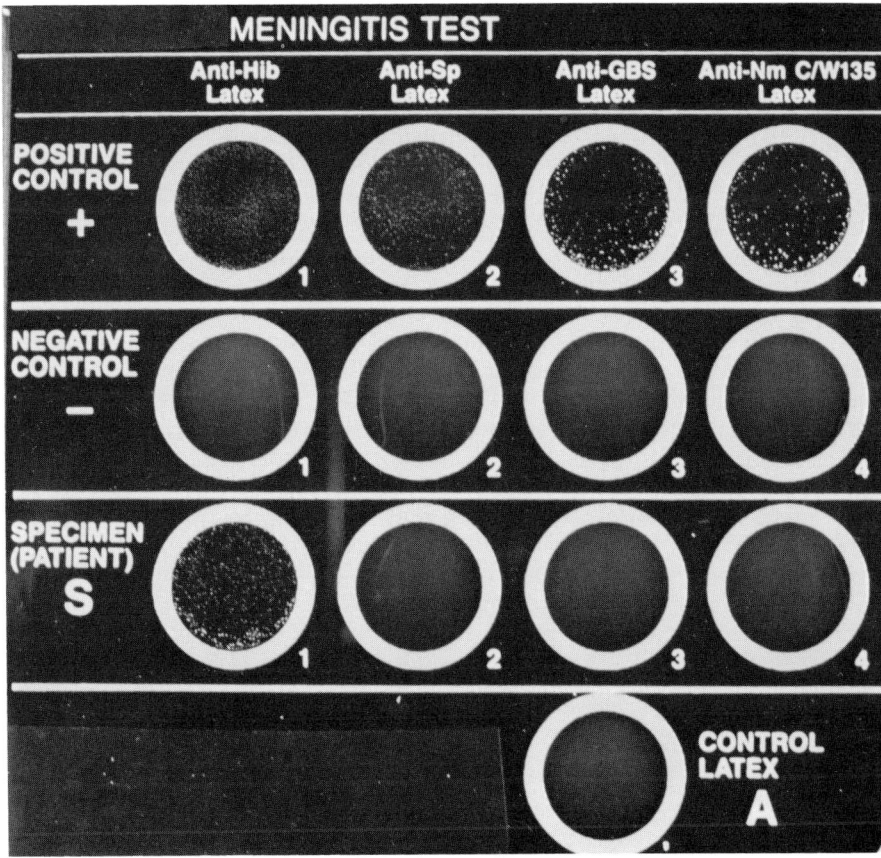

Figure 23–3. Results of latex agglutination test of CSF from a child with Haemophilus influenzae *type b meningitis. Note the positive agglutination in the left-hand well in the third (patient specimen) row.*

humans, contains ribose. The next (although much less common) virulent serotype is type a, in which ribose is replaced by glucose. The structures of the other four types are less closely related, and they are also less virulent even though they are more commonly found in the nasopharynx of children.

Protection (e.g., antibody formation) against *H. influenzae* type b develops slowly during infancy (see below). In most cases the formation of these natural antibodies is due to cross-reacting polysaccharides from other bacteria. For example, type b cross-reacts with *S. pneumoniae* types 6, 15, 29, and 35; type c cross-reacts with *S. pneumoniae* type 11; and type a cross-reacts with *S. pneumoniae* type 6. Other cross-reactions have been noticed as well. For example, type b cross-reacts with antigens found in *Staphylococcus aureus*, *Bacillus subtilis*, and some strains of *Escherichia coli*. The antigen in *E. coli* that cross-reacts with the *H. influenzae* polyribose phosphate capsule has been identified as a surface-stable, acidic capsular polysaccharide which is part of the *E. coli* K antigen.

Other antigenic structures of *H. influenzae* are part of the cell envelope and include the outer membrane proteins (OMPs) and lipopolysaccharide (LPS). Using gel electrophoresis, which separates the OMPs according to their molecular weight, 6 major and (at least) 20 minor OMPs differing in antigenic specificity are found. Infection with *H. influenzae* induces production of antibodies against certain OMPs, and in experimental animal infections these antibodies are protective. These observations suggest that OMPs may have an important role in the virulence of *H. influenzae*. Subtyping *H. influenzae* type b isolates from patients with invasive infections on the basis of the molecular weight of OMPs revealed that six subtypes caused 90% of all infections. In addition, OMP subtyping of nontypable (nonencapsulated) *H. influenzae* strains revealed that one subtype was more predictive of pathogenicity. This specific subtype was more commonly found in strains isolated from blood, a very rare occurrence of invasion for nontypable *H. influenzae*. OMP subtyping can be very useful in epidemiologic studies of, for example, an outbreak of *H. influenzae* infection in household contacts or day-care centers.

The lipopolysaccharide of *H. influenzae* is chemically distinct from that of Enterobacteriaceae. Although the lipid composition is the same, the saccharide component in *H. influenzae* LPS is smaller and less heterogenous. Nevertheless, the biologic activity (and toxicity) seem to be similar. Again the antigenic variability of LPS in various *H. influenzae* strains may serve as a tool for epidemiologic studies.

LPS (also referred to as endotoxin) is likely another virulence factor of *H. influenzae,* and following an infection, serum antibodies to LPS increase. Surprisingly, these anti-LPS antibodies did not prevent bacteremia in an animal model experiment. This failure of protection may be explained partially by changes in the bacteria which result in resistance to the complement-mediated bactericidal effect of anti-LPS antibodies. However, anti-LPS antibodies probably prevent some of the adverse effects of endotoxin released during invasive infections with *H. influenzae.*

Pathogenesis

H. influenzae infection in susceptible children probably starts with colonization of bacteria in the nasopharynx. Carrier rates in children may be as high as 90%, but these organisms are usually unencapsulated. Encapsulated strains, mostly type b, are encountered in only 5–10% of preschool children. To establish itself in the nasopharynx, the bacteria need to adhere to the epithelial cells. One mechanism of adherence used by *H. influenzae* is pili—filamentous projections from the surface of the bacteria that increase bacterial ability to adhere to human epithelial cells. Another potentially important virulence factor of invasive *H. influenzae* strains is IgA1 protease. This protease can cleave the principal defensive immunoglobulin of mucosal surfaces, paving the way for bacterial invasion through the mucosa. This enzyme appears not to be present in nonencapsulated *H. influenzae* strains. Although the potential mechanisms for pili and IgA1 protease described above are logical, their precise role in colonization and in producing disease remains to be defined.

The exact mechanism by which *H. influenzae* moves from the surface of the nasopharyngeal epithelial cells into the blood is unknown. One mode of transportation may be via the lymphatics following a nasopharyngeal inflammatory response. The inflammatory response needed to initiate the process is probably caused by a "trivial" coincident viral infection. Studies in infant rats showed that preinoculation of the nose with virus increased nasal colonization with *H. influenzae* and led to a higher rate of bacteremia. In addition to the increase in inflammatory cells in the nasopharynx following influenza virus infection, other host protective mechanisms are adversely affected. This includes reduced bacterial killing due to a defect in phagosome-lysosome fusion, reduced macrophage function, and decreased neutrophil chemotaxis. It is interesting that this synergy between influenza virus and haemophilus was erroneously interpreted during the influenza pandemic of 1918. Because the virus had not yet been isolated at that time (it was first isolated from humans in 1933) and "bacillus influenzae" was isolated from patients who died with influenzal pneumonia, the latter was thought to be the cause of the epidemic and was consequently called *H. influenzae.* In patients colonized with nontypable (nonencapsulated) *H. influenzae,* the bacteria may spread locally to the sinuses, middle ear, bronchi, or lung, probably following a viral infection or when other underlying conditions which modify the host defense mechanisms exist.

Although *H. influenzae* is one of the most common causes of suppurative otitis media in children (about 20% of all cases), most of the *H. influenzae* strains isolated from this condition are nontypable, whereas *H. influenzae* type b is responsible for only 5–10% of otitis media caused by *H. influenzae.*

It is probably safe to conclude that virtually all disease due to *H. influenzae* results from microorganisms originally harbored in the upper respiratory tract. Thus, sporadic cases are the common rule. However, in the case of *H. influenzae* type b, the organisms may be acquired from other carriers and lead to bacteremic infections, causing small epidemics in household contacts or day-care centers.

Bloodstream invasion by encapsulated *H. influenzae* type b is associated with more serious diseases. The bacteria multiply in the blood rapidly, reaching levels of 10^2–10^6 organisms/mL of blood within 12–48 h. The rate of bacterial growth is dampened by the host defenses, which clear it from the blood. In young children and nonimmune adults, serum bactericidal activity for *H. influenzae* is diminished because of the lack of antibodies against the polyriboseribitol phosphate (PRP) of the capsule and against the outer membrane proteins. In addition, animal experiments have shown that the reticuloendothelial system and the alternative complement pathway (opsonic antibodies) are very important components in the host defenses against *H. influenzae*. If these components are nonfunctional (e.g., because of splenectomy, sickle-cell anemia, or C3 deficiency), both the incidence and the magnitude of bacteremia increase. If the primary bacteremia is of low magnitude (10^1–10^3 organisms/mL of blood), it is clinically represented only as low-grade fever with a relative paucity of symptoms. This type of low-grade bacteremia is relatively common in children with otitis media or acute epiglottitis. However, if the magnitude of bacteremia reaches $>10^3$–10^4 organisms/mL of blood, spread of infection to serous surfaces (e.g., meninges, pericardium, joints) or other tissues (e.g., skin and bone) frequently occurs.

Meningitis

One of the most frequently seen manifestations of bacteremic spread of *H. influenzae* is meningitis. The organisms reach the CSF compartment via the choroid plexus of the lateral ventricles and then spread to the extracerebral CSF space. The bacteria are usually confined to the subarachnoid space which is continuous around the brain and the spinal cord. However, it is important to note that the subarachnoid space is in direct contact with the extracellular space of the brain parenchyma through the perivascular spaces. It is probable that through this intimate connection, bacteria and the inflammatory response produce the brain damage which is observed as a frequent sequela of meningitis.

The factors which lead to meningeal localization of *H. influenzae* are not completely clear. One possibility is that the polysaccharide capsule of *H. influenzae* type b possesses unique neurotropism. This possible role of the polysaccharide is suggested by the observation that only certain capsular types of *S. pneumoniae*, *N. meningitidis*, *H. influenzae*, and *E. coli* cause meningitis. These observations also suggest the presence of specialized receptors on endothelial cells lining the blood vessels supplying the brain. Additional factors may include initial viral infection of the meninges or facilitated entry of bacteria into the subarachnoid space due to disruption of the blood-CSF barrier by circulating endotoxin or other mediators.

Once bacteria reach the CSF, they multiply rapidly because the subarachnoid space and CSF are devoid of complement, opsonic antibodies, and phagocytic cells. It has been shown in experimental *H. influenzae* meningitis that only a single viable bacterium is needed to initiate infection in the CSF. The ingress of antibody, complement, and phagocytic cells that occurs later during the course of meningitis is too late to abort the progression of the infection.

The specific pathophysiologic changes leading to cerebral dysfunction and damage during bacterial meningitis are probably induced by both bacterial products and by the host inflammatory response and are generally well underway by the time a clinical diagnosis of meningitis can be made. *H. influenzae* LPS is probably the first molecule to be recognized by the host. This recognition triggers an intense inflammatory reaction, which includes the induction and release of several inflammatory mediators (cytokines, such as tumor necrosis factor [TNF], interleukin 1 [IL-1], platelet-activating factor [PAF]) (Fig. 23–4). The receptor(s) in the CNS that recognizes the bacterial products and initiates the cytokine release has not yet been identified. The cytokines induce an influx of polymorphonuclear leukocytes and serum proteins into the CSF. In addition, the breakdown of the blood-brain barrier (BBB) increases brain water content, leading to increased intracranial pressure and to decreased cerebral perfusion. The degree of increased permeability of the BBB correlates directly with the number of bacteria in the subarachnoid space. The influx of serum albumin into the CSF is accompanied by other low-molecular-weight proteins of the complement cascade which produce intense chemotactic activity within 10–12 h after the infection began. The major mediator of this chemotactic activity is C5a. Several hours later, an intense PMN leukocyte influx occurs. The role of PMNs in eliminating the bacteria from the CSF is limited. This was illustrated in a study of normal and neutropenic rabbits who were inoculated with intracisternal (cisterna magna) organisms. There was no significant difference in bacterial growth rate or peak bacterial concentration at 24 h after inoculation between the normal rabbits and the neutropenic rabbits. The role of "activated neutrophils" (and the highly reactive oxygen radicals and lytic enzymes they release) in potentiating brain damage is not completely clear. However, some investigators suggest that limiting the number of white blood cells in the CSF during meningitis may be beneficial to the patient with respect to neurologic sequelae.

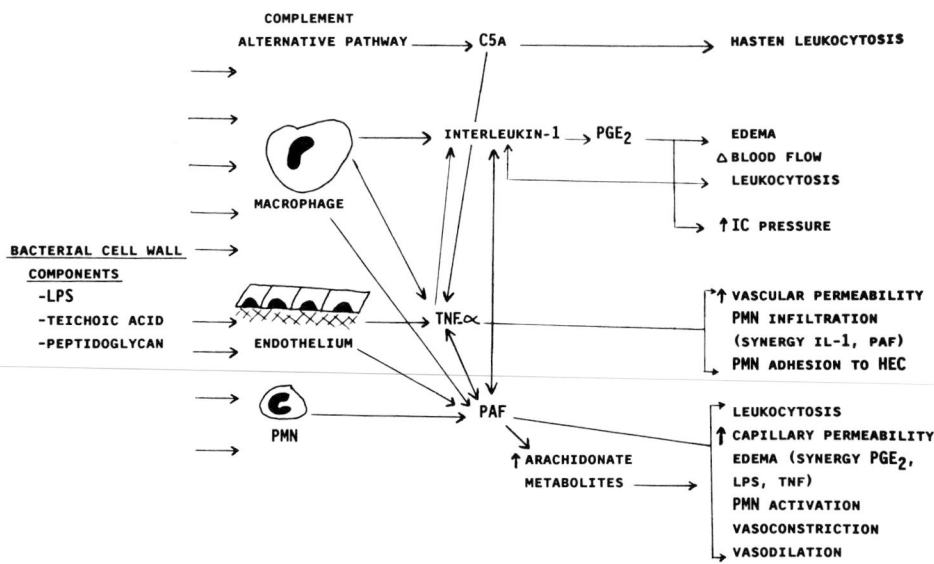

Figure 23–4. Hypothetical scheme for the generation of inflammation in bacterial meningitis. (HEC) human endothelial cell, (PGE₂) prostaglandin E₂, (IC) intracranial, (PMN) polymorphonuclear cells, (LPS) lipopolysaccharide, (TNF) tumor necrosis factor, (PAF) platelet activating factor.

Recent experimental studies showed that purified endotoxin or cytokines, such as TNF or IL-1, induce intense meningeal inflammation when injected intracisternally, similar to that induced by live organisms. Blockage of TNF or IL-1 by specific antibodies downregulates the subarachnoid inflammation. In addition, intravenous dexamethasone reduced the release of these cytokines into the CSF, followed by an attenuated inflammatory response. Thus, antiendotoxin or anticytokine therapies will play a major role in future attempts to improve the outcome of bacterial meningitis.

During meningitis, the subarachnoid space, which normally absorbs CSF, contains purulent material that may interfere with the normal flow of CSF, resulting in obstructive hydrocephalus. Since the subarachnoid space is transversed by vascular structures which bring blood to and from the brain, these vessels are frequently involved in the inflammatory process and areas of focal vasculitis can develop. Cortical venous thrombosis causes areas of hemorrhagic cortical infarction, and arteritis of major vessels leads to foci of ischemic cerebral infarction. In addition, venous obstruction resulting from purulent material in the veins can contribute to cerebral swelling. A vicious cycle then develops in which cerebral edema contributes to further venous obstruction and stasis, and phlebitis further accelerates cerebral swelling. Focal ischemia of the cerebral tissues may constitute a principal source of permanent neurologic impairment.

The reduction in cerebral blood flow is also associated with regional hypoxemia and lactate production due to a shift to anaerobic glycolysis.

Increased intracranial pressure (ICP) is a common acute phenomenon in *H. influenzae* meningitis. Increased ICP manifests itself as headache in adults, but the fontanelle bulges in about 60% of cases in infants with an open anterior fontanelle. Papilledema, a common finding of increased ICP in adults, is rarely found in children, but when present in an infant, other complications of meningitis, such as venous sinus thrombosis, brain abscess, or subdural empyema, should first be ruled out. Several mechanisms may contribute to increased ICP: (1) the increased fluid leakage through the BBB affected by the cytokines, (2) abnormal patterns of cerebral blood flow due to loss of autoregulation, (3) hypoventilation (which occurs in some patients with meningitis) causing hypercarbia, which increases cerebral blood flow through its effect on cerebral vascular tone, (4) abnormal collection of subdural fluid or development of hydrocephalus, and (5) interstitial cerebral edema as a result of metabolic abnormalities developing in the brain cells. Severely increased ICP can cause trans-tentorial herniation of the brain. This complication is relatively frequent in adult patients with meningitis, but is found in less than 5% of pediatric patients. When trans-tentorial herniation occurs, the patient's respiration and hemodynamic patterns worsen, pupillary reaction to light becomes sluggish, and the patient responds only to noxious stimuli. The presence of these symptoms defines patients with serious morbidity and higher mortality rate. It has been suggested that diagnostic lumbar puncture in patients whose cardiorespiratory system is unstable or who suffer from advanced symptoms of increased ICP can cause a sudden decrease in CSF pressure. In addition, the neck flexion required for performing a lumbar puncture decreases cerebral venous return and increases cerebral blood flow. These effects may shift brain substance through the tentorium or the foramen magnum, causing herniation.

No specific clinical signs and symptoms differentiate *H. influenzae* meningitis from that caused by other organisms. Usually the symptoms of meningitis develop relatively slowly (2–3 days). However, in some cases, a fulminant course with a mean of less than 24 h from the onset of symptoms to death is observed. The CSF findings (WBC and differential, protein, glucose, and lactate) in patients with *H. influenzae* meningitis are similar to those seen with other bacterial meningitis (see Chapter 22). Gram's stain is positive in more than 80% of cases, and the latex agglutination test is positive in more than 90% of cases.

About 50% of patients with *H. influenzae* meningitis do well in all respects. An additional quarter to a third of the surviving patients have a significant handicap, the most common being hearing loss, followed by language disorders and mental retardation. The mortality rate is less than 5%.

Other Systemic Infections

Other systemic diseases caused by *H. influenzae* type b include pneumonia, epiglottitis, septic arthritis, and cellulitis. Rarely, *H. influenzae* type b causes osteomyelitis, abscess, endocarditis, peritonitis, pericarditis, or neonatal sepsis.

About one quarter to one third of documented bacterial pneumonia in children is caused by *H. influenzae* type b. The age distribution is similar to that of meningitis, with most cases occurring in infants younger than 2 years of age. In older children and adults, *H. influenzae* type b is rarely the cause of pneumonia, except in patients with chronic obstructive pulmonary disease. About 50% of patients with *H. influenzae* pneumonia also have clinical or radiologic evidence of pleural involvement. Pneumonia is confined to one lobe in the majority of the cases, and fewer than 15% of the patients present with bronchopneumonia. Pneumatocele

and interstitial pneumonia are very rare. The peripheral WBC is usually elevated with a shift to the left. The best diagnostic test is blood culture, which is positive for *H. influenzae* in almost 80% of the cases. Gram's stain of the pleural fluid may be helpful in diagnosis but is prone to possible misinterpretation. Detection of capsular polysaccharide (PRP) from urine or pleural fluid by the latex agglutination test is rapid and reliable and, thus, should always be performed. Usually the outcome is excellent, with a negligible mortality rate.

A less common but even more serious disease caused by *H. influenzae* type b is epiglottitis. Epiglottitis is a rapidly progressive cellulitis of the epiglottis. The typical patient is a child between 2 and 5 years old who develops a sore throat with the abrupt onset of fever and toxicity. The disease progresses rapidly over the first 12–24 h and includes respiratory distress, dysphagia, and drooling. To keep the airway open the patient insists on sitting and breathes with an open mouth. In most cases bacteremia is documented, although it is unclear if infection of the epiglottis occurs directly from the colonized nasopharynx or follows bacteremia. The diagnosis is based on the clinical presentation. Direct observation of the epiglottis should be avoided because it may trigger acute respiratory obstruction. In adults, examination of the epiglottis is safer than in children. Lateral neck x-ray emphasizing the soft tissues is very useful in confirming the diagnosis. Early nasotracheal intubation for 2–3 days is probably the most important treatment. Antibiotics should be added but they are secondary to respiratory support. Rarely, other manifestations of *H. influenzae* infection present concomitantly with epiglottitis, including pneumonia, cervical adenitis, and, very rarely, meningitis.

Although *Staphylococcus aureus* is a very common cause of septic arthritis in children, in infants younger than 2 years of age *H. influenzae* is more common. There are no clinical or laboratory features which can distinguish between the two pathogens except Gram's stain and culture of joint fluid or the latex agglutination test of urine and joint fluid. The larger joints are usually involved, and if the hip joint is involved, emergency surgical drainage is required to save the intracapsular blood supply to the head of the femur.

Cellulitis (an acute infection of the skin) is usually caused by *S. aureus* and group A streptococcus. In infants 6 months to 3 years of age, cellulitis of the face, head, or neck is more likely to be due to *H. influenzae*. An acute cellulitis of the cheeks with violet discoloration is highly suggestive of *H. influenzae* infection, but *S. pneumoniae* can also present in this way. Because a high percentage of patients with *H. influenzae* cellulitis are also bacteremic, initial antibiotic therapy should be given intravenously to prevent spread of bacteria to other organs (especially the meninges).

Epidemiology

It has already been noted that *Haemophilus influenzae* is a normal inhabitant of the upper respiratory tract. Sixty to ninety percent of children of various ages carry unencapsulated *H. influenzae* in the nose or throat, but only 5% of them are colonized with type b. As with meningitis caused by *N. meningitidis*, *H. influenzae* type b meningitis is primarily a disease of pharyngeal carriers. The incidence of *H. influenzae* type b meningitis in the United States has been relatively constant in recent years, and the current estimate is that 10,000–15,000 cases occur each year, with 500–800 deaths. *H. influenzae* type b meningitis usually occurs in the very young. The peak incidence is below 1 year of age, and 85% of cases occur in infants younger than 2 years of age. Most cases of *H. influenzae* septic arthritis, cellulitis, and pneumonia also occur in infants younger than 2 years old. In contrast, epiglottitis typically occurs in children older than 2. The reasons for this age difference are not clear.

Certain racial differences in susceptibility to infection with *H. influenzae* have been noted. The incidence of *H. influenzae* meningitis is four times greater in blacks than in whites. Navajos and Alaskan Eskimos have an even higher incidence than blacks. These findings suggest a genetic role in susceptibility to *H. influenzae* type b meningitis. However, the higher incidence in these populations may also reflect lower socioeconomic status, which in some unknown way could reduce resistance to this microorganism.

As with other respiratory pathogens, family size and living conditions may also affect risk. Secondary cases of meningitis are more common in household contacts of primary meningitis cases than in the general population.

Immunity

Immunity to infection with *Haemophilus influenzae* is related directly both to age and to the amount of serum bactericidal antibody. Figure 23–5 shows the relationships among age, incidence of *H. influenzae* type b meningitis, and the presence of circulating bactericidal antibody. Subsequent studies demonstrated that most of the bactericidal activity was due to antibodies directed against capsular PRP. *In vitro* experiments showed that purified IgG antibodies against PRP were opsonic and bactericidal to *H. influenzae* type b. Since the major effect of this protective antibody is to promote phagocytosis through opsonization, opsonization and phagocytosis are probably the major immune factors that account for the protection of humans against infection.

The increased immunity to *H. influenzae* infections that occurs with age is accompanied by an increase in antibody to PRP capsular polysaccharide. It has been assumed that the development of antibody with increasing age is due to subclinical exposure to *H. influenzae* types residing in the nasopharynx. This assumption is partially supported by the observation that the contacts of a child with *H. influenzae* type b meningitis in a day-care center had higher anti-PRP antibody titers than controls. Because they also had a higher carrier rate of *H. influenzae* type b in their nasopharynx, it was concluded that "natural" antibody may result from colonization with the virulent bacteria. But this type of antigenic exposure is only partly responsible for the development of immunity, and a variety of other bacteria which normally colonize the gut also contribute. Although anticapsular antibodies play a major role in protection against *H. influenzae* invasive disease, other noncapsular antibodies contribute to this protection, as discussed above.

The fact that the most serious disease caused by *H. influenzae* occurs in infants and young children should particularly recommend these individuals for vaccination with PRP. However, investigators have found that particularly children younger than 18 months of age do not respond well immunologically to PRP capsular material, or to other polysaccharide antigens. In addition, lower anti-PRP titers were found in children recovering from *H. influenzae* type b meningitis compared with those from siblings and controls. Thus, the possibility that covalent coupling of PRP to immunogenic *H. influenzae* OMPs results in an augmented response of protective antibodies in infants as young as 2 months of age has been assessed. Recently, coupling of PRP to OMP from *N. meningitidis* (PRP-OMP) or to nontoxic diphtheria toxoid

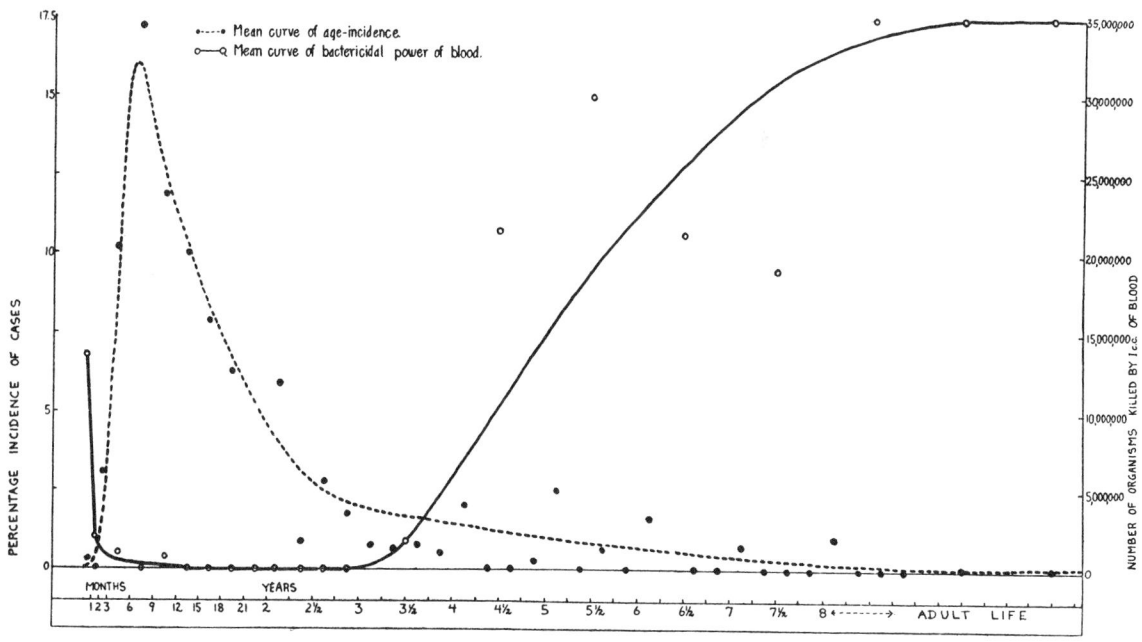

Figure 23–5. Relation of the age incidence of Haemophilus influenzae *meningitis to bactericidal antibody titers in the blood. (From Fothergill, D., and Wright, J. Influenzal meningitis: The relation of age incidence to the bactericidal power of blood against the causative organism.* J. Immunol. *24:281, 1933. © 1933 The Williams & Wilkins Co., Baltimore.)*

(PRP-CRM) was shown to be immunogenic in infants when given at 2, 4, and 6 months of age. PRP-OMP also proved to be protective in Navajo infants in whom 22 episodes of *H. influenzae* type b meningitis occurred in 2500 infants who received placebo as compared with only one episode in 2500 infants who received the vaccine. These effective vaccines are now available to prevent this common form of bacterial meningitis.

STREPTOCOCCUS PNEUMONIAE

The characteristics of this organism are described in Chapter 13.

Streptococcus pneumoniae, the second most common cause of bacterial meningitis, commonly colonizes the upper respiratory tract. Of the 86 known serotypes defined by the capsular polysaccharide, only 10 are commonly associated with meningitis. In contrast to *H. influenzae, S. pneumoniae* causes meningitis in all age groups, and in patients older than 40 years of age it is the most common etiologic agent. Like *H. influenzae, S. pneumoniae* meningitis is the result of hematogenous spread. *S. pneumoniae* also reaches the meninges by spread from contiguous infections such as mastoiditis or sinusitis, or by direct invasion through communication between the upper respiratory tract and the

meninges. This communication may be congenital (e.g., Mondini defect, or a sinus tract) or the result of a skull fracture, especially if the fracture reaches the paranasal sinuses. If the communication persists, recurrent episodes of meningitis may result. *S. pneumoniae* meningitis occurs more frequently in blacks. An increased incidence has been noted especially in children with sickle cell disease. From available data, it was estimated that 4% of children with sickle cell disease may develop *S. pneumoniae* meningitis by 4 years of age.

The clinical manifestations of *S. pneumoniae* meningitis are indistinguishable from those of meningitis due to other bacteria. A definitive diagnosis can be made by examining the CSF. Gram's stain shows the typical gram-positive diplococci, and the latex agglutination test is positive for *S. pneumoniae.* However, it is important to note that, in contrast to *H. influenzae* in which pretreatment with antibiotics rarely affects the Gram's stain and culture results, such therapy may cause the Gram's stain to be negative and the culture to be sterile in pneumococcal meningitis. In addition, certain strains of *S. pneumoniae* (types 6, 15, 29, and 35) have some immunologic cross-reactivity with *H. influenzae* type b, which may produce a positive result for *H. influenzae* type b in the latex agglutination test. With the effective antimicrobial therapy currently available, most patients with *S. pneumoniae* meningitis survive, but they frequently have complications. Almost 50% have some hearing loss. Visual problems, paralysis, and mental or neurodevelopmental impairments occur. Even severe neurologic defects present at the time of discharge may resolve or improve with time. Patients with *S. pneumoniae* meningitis have the highest overall rate of sequelae of bacterial meningitis in non-neonates.

Although there is a vaccine for the clinically most important serotypes of *S. pneumoniae*, its efficacy in preventing *S. pneumoniae* meningitis is unknown.

NEISSERIA MENINGITIDIS

Epidemic cerebrospinal meningitis was first described in 1805, and since then meningococcal meningitis has continued to be a cause of endemic and epidemic disease worldwide, with a propensity for afflicting young children and military recruits. *Neisseria meningitidis* also may produce fulminating sepsis and death within a very short time. The rapid onset of the disease, its often fulminant course, and its high mortality evoke anxiety among both laymen and physicians.

Morphology

Neisseria meningitidis is a nonmotile, non–spore-forming, gram-negative coccus that typically appears in pairs with the opposing sides flattened or indented, giving them the appearance of "kidney bean" diplococci. Other gram-negative cocci include bacteria from the genera *Branhamella* and *Veillonella*. On suitable solid media, *N. meningitidis* isolates from blood or cerebrospinal fluid form transparent or semilucent, nonpigmented, nonhemolytic colonies approximately 1–5 mm in diameter. In contrast, organisms isolated from the nasopharynx of healthy individuals often grow as opaque colonies. Colonies are convex and, if large amounts of polysaccharide are present, appear mucoid rather than smooth.

Growth

Many *Neisseria* strains are considered fastidious and require the use of appropriate media and conditions. The *Neisseria* are aerobic and prefer a humid environment at a temperature of 37°C

TABLE 23–5. *Sugar Fermentation by* Neisseria *species*

Species	Sugar		
	Glucose	**Maltose**	**Sucrose**
Neisseria gonorrhoeae	+	−	−
N. meningitidis	+	+	−
N. sicca	+	+	+
N. flavescens	−	−	−
N. mucosa	+	+	+
N. subflava	+	+	±

for optimal growth; isolation and growth are enhanced by a concentration of 5–10% CO_2. Some *Neisseria* species such as *N. meningitidis* and *N. gonorrhoeae* require a specially treated medium to improve their growth. Heavy metals, fatty acids, and other heat-labile components are some of the growth inhibitors that should be eliminated. Therefore, most clinical laboratories prepare chocolate agar plates by heating sheep blood in molten agar at 80°–90°C for the isolation and propagation of the sensitive *Neisseria* strains. Another medium (devised by Mueller and Hinton) is particularly good as a basic culture medium for cultivating *N. meningitidis*. The genus *Neisseria* includes six important species: *N. gonorrhoeae*, *N. meningitidis*, *N. flavescens*, *N. subflava*, *N. mucosa*, and *N. sicca*. They are distinguished by a series of biochemical tests. *N. meningitidis* ferments glucose and maltose, whereas *N. gonorrhoeae* ferments only glucose (Table 23–5). *N. meningitidis* also produces catalase and indophenol oxidase. To perform the oxidase test, colonies are flooded with a solution of dimethyl- or tetramethylparaphenylenediamine, and if they turn pink or dark blue (depending on which reagent is employed), the test is positive. A positive oxidase test is often cited as useful for identifying *N. meningitidis;* however, nonpathogenic *Neisseria* may give a positive test result too. Thus, the identification of *N. meningitidis* from nasopharyngeal cultures should not rely on the results of the catalase test alone.

Antigenic Structure

The cell wall of *N. meningitidis* is typical of gram-negative bacteria; it contains a peptidoglycan backbone and lipopolysaccharide (endotoxin) complexed with protein in the outer membrane (Fig. 23–6). The organism produces a polysaccharide capsule which is the basis of the serogroup typing system. There are 16 different polysaccharide groups, 9 of which are listed in Table 23–6. Capsules of *N. meningitidis*

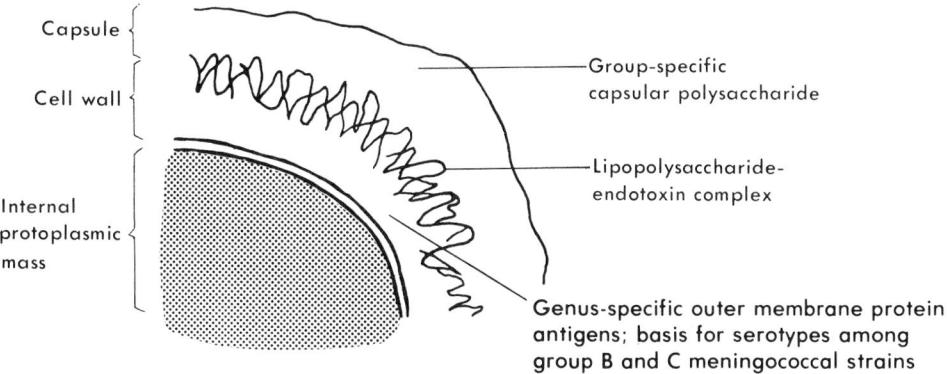

Figure 23–6. Major antigenic and virulence determinants of Neisseria meningitidis.

strains can be identified by the quelling reaction in the presence of appropriate serogroup antibody. Almost all isolates from invasive disease can be grouped based on the capsular polysaccharide, with the most important groups being A, B, C, W-135, and Y. Group A strains historically have been responsible for worldwide epidemic outbreaks involving large numbers of individuals and occurring cyclically. Therefore, group A *N. meningitidis* has traditionally been considered to be the epidemic type. In contrast, groups B and C *N. meningitidis* tended to cause sporadic cases or limited outbreaks of meningococcal disease. Thus, group B and C strains were considered to be the endemic serotypes. However, a progressive shift in the relative importance of these serotypes and other serotypes occurred since the early 1960s. Group B strains increasingly have been the cause of the majority of community-acquired cases of meningococcal disease, and new groups have been reported more often. Since 1980, group W-135 has been the second most frequent strain causing invasive disease. In addition, the spectrum of

N. meningitidis infections has changed. The W-135 strains appear to have a propensity for causing bacteremia, whereas serogroup Y frequently induces pulmonary disease. In addition to the group-specific polysaccharide antigens, subgrouping is possible within groups B and C meningococci based on differences in outer membrane proteins. Group B can be subgrouped to at least 12 different serotypes on this basis. Interestingly, serotype 2 is the most frequently isolated (more than 50% of serogroup B) and is also an antigenic determinant in group C strains. The importance of the subgrouping based on OMP pattern relates to epidemiologic studies and vaccine development.

Another principal outer membrane antigen is the lipooligosaccharide (LOS), which is analogous to the lipopolysaccharide (LPS) of enteric gram-negative bacilli. The LOS is serologically diverse, with at least 12 different serotypes. Again, this diversity of LOS can be used as an epidemiologic tool to show that various isolates are related or nonrelated.

TABLE 23–6. *Capsular Polysaccharides of* Neisseria meningitidis *Groups**

Group	Capsular Polysaccharide
A	O-Acetylated 2-acetamido-deoxy-D-mannose-6-phosphate
B	α2,8, N-Acetylneuraminic acid
C	α2,9, O-Acetylneuraminic acid
D	Composition not known
X	Alternating sequence of D-glucose-4-phosphate
Y	O-Acetylated alternating sequence of D-glucose and N-acetylneuraminic acid
Z	Composition not known
29E	3-Deoxy-D-manno octulosonic acid
W-135	Alternating sequence of D-galactose and N-acetylneuraminic acid

*Partial list.

Pathogenesis and Immunity

The meningococcus is an exclusively human parasite. It can exist as an apparently harmless member of the normal flora of the nasopharynx or produce acute disease. Carrier rates of *N. meningitidis* in the upper respiratory tract are usually from 5–15% in healthy adults and children. Higher colonization rates can be found in closed populations such as in military recruit camps or boarding schools. A close relationship has been noted between the carrier rate in a population and the onset and decline of an epidemic. It has been suggested that when the carrier rate exceeds 20% in the community, the danger of an epidemic (due to the predominant serotype) increases. Recent studies have indicated that *N. meningitidis* pili, which have been demonstrated on the surface of many meningococci, provide a means for meningococci to attach selectively to nonciliated human pharyngeal mucosal cells. Although the organisms appear to attach selectively to the nonciliated columnar epithelium, they also cause damage to the ciliated cells, possibly by direct action of meningococcal lipooligosaccharide. *N. meningitidis* preferentially colonizes the nasopharyngeal region of the upper respiratory tract, rather than the oropharynx. Although the nasopharynx provides a significantly more humid environment with a higher carbon dioxide content than the oropharynx, a more likely explanation for this preferential colonization seems to be the presence of a higher density of specific receptors for *N. meningitidis* pili on nasopharyngeal epithelial cells. The preference of *N. meningitidis* to attach to the nasopharynx has a practical diagnostic application; cultures of the nasopharynx are the best way to determine if a person is a carrier of *N. meningitidis*. Carriers can be divided into three groups: chronic (constantly colonized for up to 2 years), intermittent, and transient. Coincidental viral infection may affect acquisition of meningococcal nasopharyngeal carriage. Household contacts of a patient with *N. meningitidis* infection who have a recent history or symptoms of upper respiratory infection have significantly higher carriage rates compared with household members without such symptoms. Many studies suggest that the vast majority of people exposed to a pathogenic strain of *N. meningitidis* become carriers rather than develop active infection.

It is possible that viral infection may initiate invasive meningococcal disease. This was suggested because both diseases have peak incidence in the winter, and statistically patients with invasive meningococcal disease are often found to have serologic evidence of viral infection (such as influenza). Once the attached bacteria start to invade, the organisms penetrate the epithelial cells and enter the subepithelial spaces and adjacent lymphoid tissue, subsequently reaching the systemic circulation. A possible mechanism for the survival of *N. meningitidis* is induction of secretory IgA production. Group C polysaccharide was found to induce secretory IgA antibody, which blocks the bacteriolytic effect of IgG or IgM antibodies plus complement. Such a mechanism enables the bacteria to reside in the nasopharynx or to initiate penetration without being eradicated. In addition, many meningococcal strains produce IgA1 protease which can degrade mucosal IgA and facilitate access of the bacteria to the vascular system. Although the circumstances that determine whether an individual remains a carrier or progresses to invasive disease are not known, it is believed that the capsular polysaccharide of *N. meningitidis* is an important virulence factor. This capsular polysaccharide helps the bacteria to invade the blood and survive by inhibiting complement activation, thus making the bacteria more resistant to opsonization and phagocytosis.

Protective antibodies are usually acquired as a result of carriage, subclinical, or overt infections. However, natural immunization may not require infection or colonization with each serogroup or even with *N. meningitidis*. Antibodies may be produced in response to cross-reacting antigens of other *Neisseria* species and even of other nonrelated bacteria that carry cross-reactive antigens. Susceptibility or resistance to clinical meningococcal disease is determined by the absence or presence of serum bactericidal activity, that is, bacteriolysis. This killing effect is mediated by specific IgG or IgM antibodies in concert with the terminal components (C5–C9) of the complement system. These circulating bactericidal antibodies appear to prevent multiplication and dissemination to other tissues (particularly the central nervous system) of *N. meningitidis* that have invaded the bloodstream. The importance of the complement system in protection against *N. meningitidis* is evident from the striking association of recurrent meningococcemia in patients with deficiency of one of the terminal complement components. Circulating group-specific opsonic and bactericidal antibody are present in the serum of many adults. This antibody explains why the peak incidence of serious *N. meningitidis* infections (like that of *H. influenzae* infections) is between 6 months and 2 years of age, which corresponds to the time between loss of transplacental antibodies and the appearance of naturally acquired antibodies. Infections later in life appear in populations where many people carry a virulent strain and are in close contact with susceptible individuals lacking specific antibodies.

Group C and group A capsular polysaccharides induce specific antibodies of either IgG or IgM class. These antibodies have a bactericidal effect in two ways. First, IgG and perhaps IgM act as opsonic antibody to augment phagocytosis and subsequent killing by polymorphonuclear neutrophils. Second, following binding of IgG or IgM antibodies to *N. meningitidis* capsular antigen, activation of the complement cascade via the classic pathway causes a point injury of the bacterial cell-wall membrane.

Group B capsular polysaccharide is relatively nonimmunogenic. Data suggest that humans are immunologically unresponsive, or "tolerant," to group B meningococcal polysaccharide because of its extraordinary similarity to host autologous tissue constituents (e.g., neuraminic acid residues of mammalian cell membranes and polysialosyl glycoproteins of nervous tissue). Even after full recovery from group B *N. meningitidis* infection, only low titers of IgM antibodies can be found. These antibodies had low binding affinity and only modest bacteriolytic activity against the offending bacteria.

A significant portion of the meningococcal cell wall consists of lipopolysaccharide-endotoxin complex (see Fig. 23–6). During the growth phase of *N. meningitidis* or with its death, endotoxin is released into the extracellular environment. Group C meningococci, more than other serotypes, releases capsular polysaccharide and endotoxin into the extracellular environment during growth. Therefore, detection and quantitation of capsular polysaccharide or endotoxin in blood or cerebrospinal fluid can be useful in assessing the severity of infection in an individual patient. Such information can be of considerable diagnostic and prognostic importance. Multiple *in vitro* and *in vivo* studies show that endotoxin is directly responsible for the fulminant course of *N. meningitidis* sepsis and its high mortality rate. Endotoxin derived from *N. meningitidis* has been used extensively in studies of tissue injury caused by gram-negative bacillary endotoxins. Many of the pathophysiologic and immunohistopathologic changes observed in patients developing meningococcal sepsis and shock are elicited by endotoxin, which in turn induces the host's inflammatory mediators. These events include: (1) activation of the clotting system with extensive deposits of fibrin in glomerular arterioles and small vessels of other tissues, (2) hemorrhage of the adrenal glands (Waterhouse-Friderichsen syndrome) and hemorrhagic necrosis of other organ systems, and (3) altered peripheral vascular resistance, circulatory failure, and death.

Epidemiology

Infection due to *N. meningitidis* remains an important worldwide health problem. It has been estimated that during the period 1939–1962 there were almost 600,000 cases of meningococcal disease in the world and that more than 100,000 were fatal. Most cases occurred in children. The case rate in endemic situations varies widely, and in the United States it has almost doubled over the 6-year period 1975–1981 (from 1 to 2 per 100,000 population). In 1981, 3525 cases were reported to the Centers for Disease Control, compared with 1478 cases reported in 1978. Infants and children between 1 and 4 years of age accounted for 51% of the 1981 patients. Relatively more cases are reported in children and adolescents (ages 5–19) during an epidemic than during nonepidemic circumstances. Therefore, careful surveillance of age distribution patterns may be valuable in recognizing an epidemic during its inception. Currently, about 50% of all cases are caused by serogroup B and another 20% by serogroup C. The remainder are primarily serogroup Y and serogroup W-135. All meningococcal infections occur primarily as isolated cases, sporadic small epidemics, or closed-population outbreaks (such as recruits). However, group A strains have the potential to cause widespread epidemics, which have appeared in 8–12-year cycles. Between the peaks of the cycle, group A meningococci almost disappear and cause only 1–2% of reported cases. It has been more than 40 years since an epidemic due to group A *N. meningitidis* occurred in the United States, but serious epidemics with this serogroup have occurred in Brazil and South Africa in recent years.

The fatality rate varies depending upon the prevalence of disease, the nature of the infection, and socioeconomic conditions. In industrialized countries during endemic periods, the fatality rate can be as low as 7% for meningitis and as high as 19% for meningococcemia without meningeal involvement. However, during epidemics, mortality from meningitis varies from 2 to 10% and death rates from meningococcemia can be as high as 70%, particularly in developing countries.

As discussed above, colonization of the upper respiratory tract of a new host is an immunizing process, and circulating bactericidal and hemagglutinating antibodies are generally detectable within 7–10 days. From a variety of studies it is clear that only a brief period of colonization by *N. meningitidis* is needed before invasive disease occurs. This period is usually 10 days or less, and in a small proportion of patients, even less than 1 day.

Clinical Aspects of Meningococcal Disease

The clinical manifestations of *N. meningitidis* infection range from transient fever and bacteremia to fulminant sepsis with death ensuing within hours. A few patients may present with an upper respiratory illness or viral-like exanthem and recover without specific antimicrobial therapy; only later are blood cultures reported positive for *N. meningitidis*. The most frequent disease due to *N. meningitidis* is meningococcemia, which may follow a fulminant course with rapid progression to septic shock (Waterhouse-Friderichsen syndrome) or a much slower course producing meningitis. Some patients present with features of both sepsis and meningitis. In most series, the peak incidence of invasive disease occurs in the late winter and early spring. The disease has been reported in all age groups, but the majority of cases occur in infants younger than 2 years of age.

The patient with sepsis usually presents with skin rash, malaise, weakness, headache, and hypotension developing on admission or shortly thereafter. The patient with meningitis presents with fever, headache, meningeal signs, and mental status varying from fully alert to comatose. Variations of these manifestations can occur, and patients can progress from one syndrome to the other during the course of the disease. Because of the wide range of clinical expressions of *N. meningitidis* infection, a high index of suspicion and a careful search for clues of disease are required for early diagnosis. Erroneous diagnosis and inappropriate therapy can have fatal consequences.

Meningococcal sepsis is commonly accompanied by cutaneous lesions of a petechial or purpuric nature (Figs. 23–7 and 23–8). Occasionally if the patient is not completely undressed when examined, these important lesions can be missed. Purpura, which is separate and distinct, is a feature of fulminating disease and does not arise from the petechiae which are seen in milder cases. The petechial rash is manifested as discrete lesions 1–2 mm in diameter on the extremities and trunk. The wrist and forearm are frequently involved as well as the lower leg and ankles. The petechiae may spare the palmar and plantar surfaces. They are commonly seen in clusters under areas where pressure has been applied to the skin by the elastic in underwear or stockings. These petechial lesions can coalesce to form larger lesions that appear ecchymotic. The petechiae correlate with the degree of thrombocytopenia present, and they are important as a clinical indicator of the severity of disease and of development of disseminated intravascular coagulation (DIC). It is important to follow the progression of petechial lesions, both to monitor the effectiveness of therapy and to assess whether additional therapies become necessary. A simple way of accomplishing this is to circle areas of petechiae and to document the number of petechial lesions

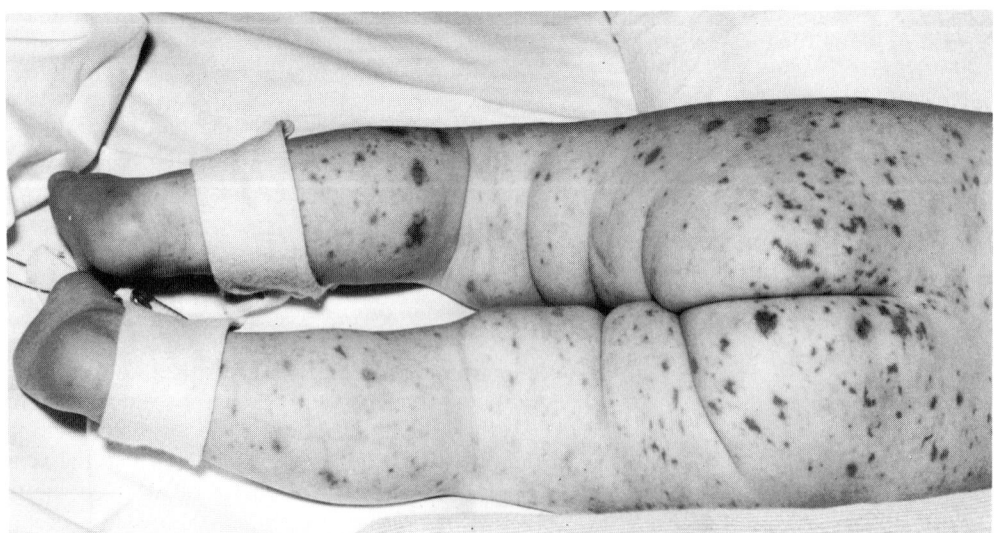

Figure 23–7. Representative cutaneous eruption of acute meningococcemia in a young child with meningococcal meningitis. (From Bell, W. E., and McCormick, W. F. Neurologic Infections in Children. 2nd ed. Philadelphia: W. B. Saunders Co., 1981.)

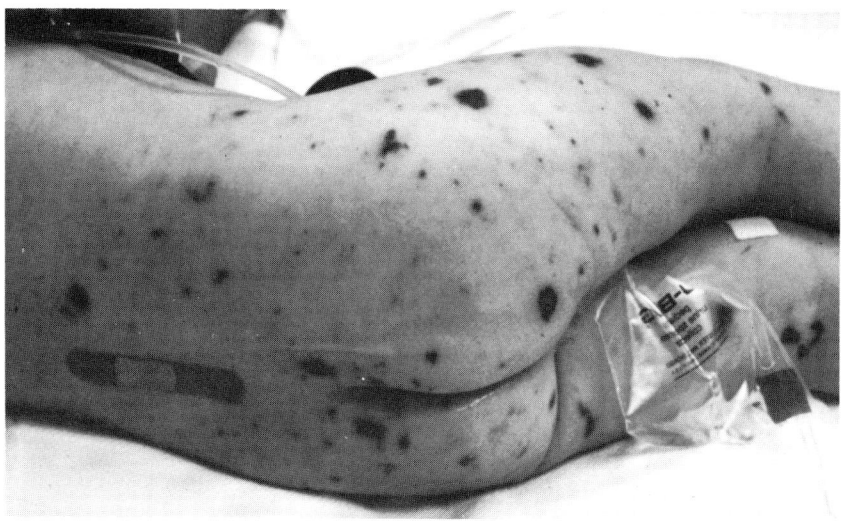

Figure 23–8. More extensive purpuric skin lesions characteristic of acute meningococcemia in a child with meningococcal meningitis and septic shock. Systemic hypotension is also present and there is laboratory evidence of disseminated intravascular coagulation. (From Bell, W. E., and McCormick, W. F. Neurologic Infections in Children. *2nd ed. Philadelphia, W. B. Saunders Co., 1981.)*

and time of the count on a flow sheet. Counts within each circle should be performed periodically until the patient's condition stabilizes. Several other diseases may produce skin lesions resembling the petechiae of *N. meningitidis* septicemia. These diseases include Rocky Mountain spotted fever, rubella, rubeola, secondary syphilis, bacterial endocarditis, and cutaneous eruptions associated with drug allergies. Moreover, in infants and children, *Haemophilus influenzae* type b or, very rarely, pneumococcal sepsis can also present with similar clinical manifestations of petechial or purpuric skin lesions, DIC, and shock. Therefore, the therapeutic approach to pediatric patients with this syndrome must include antimicrobial therapy effective against *N. meningitidis, H. influenzae,* and *S. pneumoniae.* To facilitate identification of the etiologic agent, a urine sample should be tested by the latex agglutination technique for specific antigens. In addition, a representative skin lesion can be incised under sterile conditions, and two or three drops of tissue fluid expressed for Gram's stain and culture. The presence of polymorphonuclear neutrophils with gram-negative cocci or diplococci within or outside of these phagocytic cells is highly suggestive (even pathognomonic) of *N. meningitidis* infection. Culture of the fluid from the incised lesion is best done by placing one or two drops directly onto chocolate agar at the bedside. Isolation of *N. meningitidis* from skin lesion or blood provides a definitive diagnosis of meningococcemia.

The shock state which frequently develops in patients with meningococcemic sepsis dominates the clinical picture and is an ominous prognostic sign. Such a patient is poorly responsive, showing both peripheral vasoconstriction and cyanotic, poorly perfused extremities. There is evidence of acidosis, hypoxia, and DIC. Clinical evidence of DIC includes increased numbers of petechiae within circumscribed areas, gastric or gingival bleeding, or oozing at the sites of venipuncture or intravenous infusions. Myocardial failure as evidenced by congestive heart failure and pulmonary edema may occur, and histologic evidence of myocarditis is present in more than 50% of patients who die from meningococcal disease.

The clinical manifestations of *N. meningitidis* meningitis overlap with those of meningitis due to *H. influenzae* type b or *S. pneumoniae.* These manifestations are discussed in Chapter 22.

Meningococcal pneumonia has been reported in as many as 10–20% of patients with meningococcemia or meningitis. However, primary meningococcal pneumonia, once considered a rare disease, is now recognized as one of the more common forms of meningococcal disease in military recruits, and it has been reported to cause 4.5% of all bacterial pneumonias in a general hospital population. Pulmonary infection is probably disseminated via airborne droplets. Thus, respiratory isolation of patients with pneumonia is indicated. Most primary meningococcal pneumonias are caused by serogroup

Y, whereas groups B and C are mostly involved in pneumonia associated with meningitis or septicemia. Usually the onset of primary *N. meningitidis* pneumonia is gradual and the clinical symptoms do not differ from those of other pneumonias. The chest x-ray examination generally shows lung consolidation with patchy alveolar infiltrates. Establishing the diagnosis is difficult. Because nasopharyngeal carriage of meningococci is common, isolation of the bacteria from the sputum does not establish the diagnosis. Transtracheal aspirate, pleural effusion culture, and blood culture yielding *N. meningitidis* are accepted confirmatory diagnostic tests.

Chronic meningococcemia is defined as persistent meningococcal bacteremia associated with low-grade fever, chills, rash, arthralgia, and headache, but without clinical evidence of sepsis. The reported mean duration of illness is 6–8 weeks. Symptoms tend to be intermittent; the rash often appears in association with fever and then disappears. Bacteremia and arthralgias also tend to be intermittent. The pathophysiology of chronic meningococcemia is not well understood, but a defect in host immunity which allows the bacteria to survive, rather than a change in bacterial virulence, seems to be a reasonable explanation. Interestingly, the skin changes suggest a hypersensitive reaction secondary to antigen-antibody complexes.

Other Diseases and Complications

Infections of the genitourinary tract with *N. meningitidis* have been reported. These infections include: proctitis, urethritis, vaginitis, and cervicitis. That some infected patients have pharyngeal colonization with the same strain suggests that sexual habits may be related to the genitourinary infections.

Approximately 50 cases of primary meningococcal conjunctivitis have been reported, most in children. Meningitis, corneal ulceration, and corneal opacity are the most frequent complications.

Serous membranes are sometimes involved in *N. meningitidis* disease, presenting as pleuritis, pericarditis, peritonitis, or arthritis. Aspiration of the affected area often reveals predominance of mononuclear cells, and Gram's stain and culture are negative. These findings suggest an immune-complex–mediated hypersensitivity phenomenon which usually occurs when the patient with invasive meningococcal disease is otherwise improving.

REFERENCES

Book

Sande, M. A., Smith, A. L., and Root, R. K., eds. *Bacterial Meningitis.* New York: Churchill Livingstone, 1985.

Articles

Arditi, M., and Yogev, R. Convalescent therapy for selected children with acute bacterial meningitis. *Semin. Pediatr. Infect. Dis. 1*:404–410, 1990.

Beutler, B., and Cerami, A. Cachectin: More than a tumor necrosis factor. *N. Engl. J. Med. 316*:379–385, 1987.

Haven, P. L., Garland, J. S., Brook, M. M., et al. Trends in mortality in children hospitalized with meningococcal infection, 1975 to 1987. *Pediatr. Infect. Dis. J. 8*:8–11, 1989.

Kaplan, S. L. Recent advances in bacterial meningitis. In: Aronoff, S., Hughes, W., Kohl, S., et al., eds. *Advances in Pediatric Infectious Disease.* Chicago, Year Book Publishers, Vol. 4, 1988: 83–101.

Klein, J. O., Feigen, R. D., and McCracken, G. H., Jr. Report of the task force on diagnosis and management of meningitis. *Pediatrics 78*(suppl):959–982, 1986.

Lebel, M. H., Freij, B. J., Syrogiannopoulos, G. A., et al. Dexamethasone therapy for bacterial meningitis. Results of two double-blind, placebo-controlled trials. *N. Engl. J. Med. 319*:964–971, 1988.

McGee, A. Z., Stephens, D. S., Hoffman, L. H., et al. Mechanisms of mucosal invasion by pathogenic *Neisseria. Rev. Infect. Dis. 5*:708S, 1983.

Sande, M. A., Tauber, M. G., Scheld, W. M., et al. Report of a second workshop: Pathophysiology of bacterial meningitis. *Pediatr. Infect. Dis. J. 8*:901–933, 1989.

Scheld, W. Theoretical and practical consideration of antibiotic therapy for bacterial meningitis. *Pediatr. Infect. Dis. J. 4*:74–83, 1985.

Scheld, W. M., and Wispelwez, B. Meningitis. *Infect. Dis. Clin. N. Am. 4*(4):555–584, 1990.

Smith, A. L. Neurologic sequelae of meningitis. *N. Engl. J. Med. 319*:1012–1014, 1988.

Yogev, R. Advances in diagnosis and treatment of childhood meningitis. *Pediatr. Infect. Dis. J. 4*:321–325, 1985.

24

STEVEN M. WOLINSKY, M.D. • *MICHELE TILL, M.D.*

Viral Infections of the Central Nervous System

INTRODUCTION

Viral meningitis is generally a benign illness of limited duration characterized by signs and symptoms of fever, headache, and meningeal irritation. The term *aseptic meningitis* also includes a variety of nonviral clinical syndromes indistinguishable from viral meningitis. These conditions include partially treated bacterial meningitis; suppurative parameningeal infections; infective endocarditis; mycoplasma, treponemal, rickettsial, and parasitic infections; meningeal metastases; intracranial tumors; vasculitides; sarcoidosis; and Mollaret's, Behçet's, and Vogt-Koyanagi-Harada recurrent meningitides. Therefore, the term *aseptic meningitis* is not synonymous with viral meningitis but encompasses other entities as well.

Viral encephalitis, unlike viral meningitis, is generally a very serious disease with significant morbidity and mortality. The characteristic features of viral encephalitis are the prominent clinical findings of cerebral dysfunction. Signs and symptoms include confusion, stupor, coma, and seizures, in addition to fever, headache, and meningeal irritation. The term *meningoencephalitis* is used to connote a syndrome, usually viral in etiology, that combines encephalitic features with clinical or laboratory evidence of meningeal involvement.

Subacute sclerosing panencephalitis (SSPE), progressive multifocal leukoencephalopathy (PML), and the transmissible spongiform encephalopathies are a group of clinical syndromes characterized by a prolonged incubation period followed by progressive deterioration of neurologic function. The diverse clinical signs and symptoms of these slow infections of the central nervous system reflect the regional foci of myelin destruction and neuronal loss. SSPE and PML each have a defined viral etiology, whereas the transmissible spongiform encephalopathy (Creutzfeld-Jacob disease) is caused by an undefined transmissible agent. These clinical entities are considered separately from viral meningitis and encephalitis.

VIRAL MENINGITIS AND ENCEPHALITIS

Etiology

Table 24–1 lists the pathogenic viruses associated with meningitis and meningoencephalitis in

TABLE 24–1. *Viral Causes of Meningitis and Meningoencephalitis*

Togaviridae
alphaviruses
  Eastern equine encephalitis virus
  Western equine encephalitis virus
  Venezuelan equine encephalitis virus
Flaviviridae
  St. Louis encephalitis virus
  Powassan virus
Bunyaviridae
California encephalitis viruses
  LaCrosse virus
  Jamestown Canyon virus
  other bunyaviruses
Paramyxoviridae
paramyxoviruses
  mumps virus
  parainfluenza virus
morbillivirus
  measles virus
Orthomyxoviridae
influenza A
influenza B
Arenaviridae
lymphocytic choriomeningitis virus
Picornaviridae
enteroviruses
  polioviruses
  coxsackievirus A
  coxsackievirus B
  echoviruses
Reoviridae
orbivirus
  Colorado tick fever virus
Rhabdoviridae
rabies virus
vesiculoviruses (?)
Retroviridae
lentiviruses
  human immunodeficiency virus type 1 and type 2
oncornaviruses
  human T-lymphotropic virus type 1
  human T-lymphotropic virus type 2
Herpesviridae
herpesvirus
  herpes simplex virus type 1
  herpes simplex virus type 2
  varicella-zoster virus
  Epstein-Barr virus
cytomegaloviruses
  human cytomegalovirus
Adenoviridae
adenoviruses

the United States. The most common of these agents are the enteroviruses, mumps, herpes simplex virus (HSV), Epstein-Barr virus (EBV), and the arthropod-borne agents. These viruses differ in their primary tropism and modes of transmission. The enteroviruses are usually acquired by fecal-oral transmission and generally remain localized to the gastrointestinal tract. Respiratory viruses are usually acquired by respiratory, hand-to-nose, or hand-to-eye transmission. These viruses generally remain confined to the respiratory tract (see Chapter 14). The arthropod-borne viruses, or arboviruses, are acquired by a bite from an infected blood-feeding insect. Following viremia in the inoculated host, other blood-feeding insects can become infected and subsequently perpetuate the infectious cycle. Viruses can also be transmitted congenitally; by inoculation, including by animal bites and intravenous drug abuse; and by sexual contact.

Enteroviruses

Enteroviruses are small, nonenveloped RNA viruses which belong to the Picornaviridae family. The enteroviruses have been divided into polioviruses, coxsackievirus groups A and B, and echoviruses on the basis of antigenic relationships. The echovirus serotypes 4, 6, 9, 11, 16, and 30 and the coxsackievirus serotypes A7, A9, B2, B3, B4, and B5 are most frequently implicated in sporadic and community outbreaks of viral meningitis. Enteroviral infections occur primarily in late summer and early fall.

Respiratory Viruses

Adenoviruses. The viruses which belong to the Adenoviridae family have a double-stranded, linear DNA genome in an icosahedral virion. Subgroup A, hemagglutination group IV (serotype 12, among others) and subgroup B, hemagglutination group I (serotypes 3 and 7, among others) have been most closely associated with sporadic meningoencephalitis. Serotypes 1, 6, 7, and 12 have been associated with meningoencephalitis complicating respiratory epidemics. Adenovirus serotypes 7, 12, and 32 can cause a chronic meningoencephalitis in patients with hypogammaglobulinemia.

Paramyxoviruses. The Paramyxoviridae family includes the paromyxoviruses (mumps, parainfluenza), the morbillivirus (measles), and the pneumovirus. These viruses have a linear RNA genome encapsidated in a cylindrical nucleocapsid which is surrounded by an envelope. These viruses vary greatly in size. The viral envelope, which is partially derived from the cytoplasmic membrane of the host, contains both neuraminidase and hemagglutinin activity (paramyxoviruses) or hemagglutinin activity alone (measles). After the enteroviruses, mumps is the second most common cause of viral meningitis and encephalitis in the United States. Measles commonly infects the central nervous system. Most infections are asymptomatic; however, 0.1–0.2% of patients develop clinical signs and symptoms ranging from mild to severe. A large number of patients who recover from measles encephalitis have neurologic sequelae. Subacute sclerosing panencephalitis (SSPE) is now a rare, chronic, fatal, and progressive encephalitis associated with natural measles infection early in life (see below).

Orthomyxoviruses. The Orthomyxoviridae family includes influenza virus type A and influenza virus type B. These viruses have a segmented single-stranded RNA genome encapsidated in a nucleoprotein capsid which is surrounded by a lipid bilayer containing neuraminidase and hemagglutinin glycoproteins. The orthomyxoviruses have been associated with Reye syndrome, which is a postinfectious noninflammatory encephalopathy, and with some cases of viral encephalitis.

Arboviruses

Arboviruses were originally named for their *ar*thropod-*bo*rne mode of transmission. The arthropod vector, including mosquitos, ticks, and flies, becomes infected by ingesting the blood of a vertebrate host during the viremic phase of infection. The infected arthropod then transmits the disease by biting a new susceptible host. Arbovirus infections occur particularly in the summer and fall months.

Viruses transmitted by arthropod vectors are chiefly members of the Togaviridae, Flaviviridae, Reoviridae, and Bunyaviridae families. These viruses, with the exception of members of the Reoviridae family, have a single-stranded RNA genome in an enveloped nucleocapsid. Reoviruses are nonenveloped particles which have a double-stranded RNA genome encapsidated in an icosahedral capsule.

The Togaviridae family contains the alphavirus genus which is transmitted by arthropod vectors. The alphaviruses include the Eastern, Western, and Venezuelan equine encephalitis species. Encephalitis caused by the Eastern equine encephalitis virus generally has a more severe course and a higher fatality rate than encephalitis caused by the other viruses. Neurologic sequelae including mental retardation, behavior changes, and seizure disorders are common following encephalitis caused by alphaviruses. Vertebrate reservoirs include horses and birds.

The Flaviviridae family includes St. Louis encephalitis virus and Powassan virus, among others. Japanese B encephalitis virus is a major mosquito-transmitted cause of encephalitis in the Far East. St. Louis encephalitis virus has been associated with major epidemics of viral meningitis and encephalitis. In general, neurologic sequelae from St. Louis encephalitis are rare. St. Louis encephalitis has a predominantly avian reservoir, whereas Powassan's reservoir is small mammals, particularly groundhogs.

The Reoviridae family contains the orbivirus genus. Colorado tick fever is the only known human disease caused by an orbivirus in the United States. Generally, Colorado tick fever is a self-limited disease. However, central nervous system infection in children may produce serious neurologic sequelae.

The Bunyaviridae family contains the California encephalitis viruses, including the LaCrosse, Jamestown Canyon, and several other unnamed bunyaviruses. After St. Louis encephalitis, these agents, particularly the LaCrosse virus, are the major cause of mosquito-borne encephalitis in the United States. Encephalitis primarily occurs in children. Seizures are a common clinical manifestation, with epilepsy a frequent neurologic sequela. Overall, bunyavirus infections are relatively mild, although fatalities have occurred.

The arthropod-borne viruses of the Rhabdoviridae family include the vesiculoviruses. Vesicular stomatitis virus (VSV) commonly infects domesticated animals and is occasionally transmitted to humans as an incidental host. Infected hosts may be asymptomatic or have a self-limited flulike syndrome. Although neurologic involvement has not been reported with VSV, a related virus has been isolated from a child thought to have Reye syndrome. The significance of this is unclear.

Sexually Transmitted Viruses

Retroviruses. The Retroviridae family includes the Oncovirinae, Spumavirinae, and Lentivirinae subfamilies. The retrovirus virion consists of a lipid-containing envelope surrounding an icosahedral capsid that contains two copies of a single-stranded RNA genome. The Onco-virinae [human T-lymphotropic virus types I (HTLV-I) and II (HTLV-II)] and Lentivirinae, [human immunodeficiency virus types 1 (HIV-1) and 2 (HIV-2)] infect the central nervous system and are transmitted by sexual contact, transfusion, and use of contaminated needles (see Chapter 26).

Herpesviruses. The Herpesviridae family includes the herpesvirus and cytomegalovirus genera. The herpesvirus genus contains herpes simplex virus types 1 and 2, varicella-zoster virus, and Epstein-Barr virus. The human cytomegalovirus belongs to the cytomegalovirus genera. Viruses in the Herpesviridae family have a double-stranded DNA genome encapsidated in an icosahedral capsid and surrounded by a lipid-containing envelope. A characteristic of viruses in this family is their ability to establish a latent state in the host cell they infect. Each of these viruses has been implicated in central nervous system infection, specifically meningitis (herpes simplex virus type 2) and meningoencephalitis (herpes simplex virus type 1, varicella-zoster virus, Epstein-Barr virus, and the human cytomegalovirus). Herpesviruses are transmitted sexually or by exposure to infected body fluids.

Viruses with Other Modes of Transmission

The Rhabdoviridae family contains rabies and the rabies-related viruses. The surface glycoprotein is capable of inducing virus-neutralizing antibody. Immunization with this glycoprotein has been shown to be protective in animals against a subsequent rabies virus challenge. Antinucleocapsid antibodies are useful for detecting the intracytoplasmic eosinophilic inclusions, or Negri bodies, which are characteristic of rabies infection in tissues. Transmission occurs mainly by animal bite with salivary inoculation into the wound.

The Arenaviridae family contains the lymphocytic choriomeningitis (LCM) virus. The arenavirus genome consists of two single-stranded RNA molecules joined in a circle. The genome is encapsidated in a circular nucleocapsid which is surrounded by a lipid envelope. LCM virus primarily infects mice and hamsters, with humans being an incidental host. Transmission modes appear to include aerosols, direct rodent contact, and rodent bites.

Epidemiology

The etiology of the viral meningitides and encephalitides differs with the geographic location, season, and age of the patient. Encephalitides transmitted by mosquitos, ticks, flies, and other insect vectors are limited to the location and time of year that these insects are feeding, particularly the late summer and autumn months. Mumps infections peak in the late winter and early spring, but occur year-round. Enterovirus spread is facilitated by close family and school contacts. Enteroviral meningitis, as well as the other viral meningitides, is usually a disease of the young, rarely occurring in adults older than 40.

The rabies virus is primarily transmitted by domestic animal bites (approximately 80%), with wild animal bites, particularly those of bats, skunks, raccoons, and foxes accounting for the remainder of the cases. Small rodents, reptiles, and birds have not been found to be reservoirs of the virus in nature.

Lymphocytic choriomeningitis virus and poliovirus are very infrequent causes of meningitis in the United States, but are significant etiologic agents in other geographic locations. LCM virus infection is more prevalent in the winter months and is spread among persons living in rodent-infested regions. Mice, laboratory animals, and some household pets, such as hamsters, excrete the virus in their stool and urine. Poliovirus infection essentially occurs almost exclusively in immunocompromised recipients of live polio vaccine, since paralytic polio has been virtually eradicated from the Western hemisphere.

Geographic location and travel history facilitate the diagnosis of encephalitis transmitted by an arthropod-borne vector. For example, St. Louis and California encephalitides are most common in the midwestern United States, whereas Eastern equine encephalitis is found primarily in the regions bordering the Atlantic and Gulf coasts. Colorado tick fever is confined to the western United States.

Viral meningitis caused by herpesvirus and the human immunodeficiency virus occurs sporadically throughout the year without seasonality. Immunocompromised patients may also have viral meningitis caused by cytomegalovirus, echoviruses, or adenoviruses.

Pathogenesis

Clinical manifestations of central nervous system infection can be produced by either direct infection of the neural parenchyma or infection of contiguous tissues. In addition, some manifestations reflect the effect of host immune responses upon infected neural elements. Neurotropic viruses most commonly enter the central nervous system by hematogenous spread from an extraneural site of viral replication. The primary site of replication is usually the respiratory tract for measles, mumps, and influenza viruses; the gastrointestinal tract for enteroviruses; and the subcutaneous tissues for the arboviruses. Thus, respiratory droplets, fecal-oral contamination, and direct inoculation of the host either by an animal bite or an insect bite are the major routes of infection. Transplacental infection also occurs in the case of rubella or cytomegaloviruses and involves the fetal central nervous system and other tissues as well.

During the course of many viral infections, initial virus replication at an extraneural site is followed by hematogenous dissemination. Viral particles are then cleared by the reticuloendothelial system. This mechanism of viral clearance may be detrimental to the host if a population of these reticuloendothelial cells is susceptible to viral infection. Virus may then replicate in these cells and further disseminate. Viruses in the Orthomxyoviridae and Paramyxoviridae families escape clearance by the reticuloendothelial system by adsorption to red blood cells. The paramyxoviruses and morbilliviruses propagate within leukocytes where they remain in an immunologically privileged site.

Viruses enter the central nervous system by one of several mechanisms. Most commonly, viruses cross the cerebral capillary endothelial cells of the blood-brain barrier. Some viruses can directly infect the endothelial cells of the cerebral microvasculature and then infect contiguous neural tissue. Infected leukocytes can also transport viruses into the central nervous system. In addition, the epithelium of the choroid plexus may represent another portal of entry.

Alternatively, viruses can enter the central nervous system by retrograde migration within sensory or motor axons. Rabies and poliovirus infections reach the central nervous system by this route. Herpes simplex virus and varicella-zoster virus invade sensory axons from the skin or mucous membranes at the time of the primary infection and ascend to ganglia. During the typical exacerbations, the infection is reactivated at the primary site after antegrade transport from the ganglia to the periphery. Reactivated virus also reaches the central nervous system by retrograde transport. Retrograde transport of herpes simplex virus from the trigeminal ganglia to the brain appears to account for the preferential localization of infection with this virus to the temporal lobe.

The olfactory pathway received early attention as a possibly important route of spread of viruses to the central nervous system. Fibers of the olfactory nerve extend through the nasal submucosa and epithelial cells and thus make direct contact with the environment. Togaviruses and herpesviruses have been shown to infect the olfactory and frontal lobes of experimental animals after inoculation into the nasal mucosa. However, spread of infectious organisms via the olfactory route has been found to be of clinical significance only in the entry of free-living amoebas, such as *Naegleria*.

Following entry of virus into the central nervous system, selected cells may become infected. Infection of specific cells (neuronal or oligodendrial) is contingent upon the presence of suitable cell-surface receptors for virus attachment and the ability of the virus to replicate within the infected cell. The virus may then disseminate by spread to contiguous cells, either through extracellular gaps, or along the extensive network of neural axons and dendrocytes.

The immune response of the central nervous system to viral infection is not fully understood. Inflammation is immunologically mediated predominantly by lymphocytes sensitized by the infecting agent and predominately distributed perivascularly. The sensitized lymphocytes are activated by locally released cytokines. Some polymorphonuclear cells are evident in the inflammatory infiltrate. As the inflammatory response develops, the blood-brain barrier is altered to allow immunoglobulins and other serum proteins to enter the cerebrospinal fluid. B lymphocytes, which also enter the cerebrospinal fluid, differentiate into plasma cells which synthesize immunoglobulins locally. Locally synthesized immunoglobulins have been found for the mumps virus, varicella-zoster virus, and the human immunodeficiency virus when they infect the central nervous system.

In general, T-lymphocyte–mediated responses are more important than B-lymphocyte responses for viral clearance. Failure to clear the infecting virus often occurs in patients with depressed cell-mediated immunity who may develop a chronic, active encephalitis.

Neuropathology

Viral meningitis is an inflammatory process involving the leptomeninges. Since this is usually a benign, self-limiting illness, its pathologic correlates are not as well characterized as those of viral encephalitis. The usual histologic appearance of viral meningitis when it is associated with fatal encephalitis consists of an inflammatory infiltrate that is generally confined to the leptomeninges. The inflammatory infiltrate consists primarily of mononuclear cells with some PMNs.

Encephalitis is a diffuse inflammatory process involving the brain parenchyma and usually, although not invariably, the leptomeninges as well. Hematogenous dissemination of a virus to the brain results in a predominantly perivascular inflammatory reaction within the brain parenchyma. The inflammatory reaction is primarily composed of mononuclear cells, although a few polymorphonuclear cells may be present. Polymorphonuclear cells may also predominate early in the course of infection. Neurons may show changes ranging from minimal swelling and hyalinization to complete destruction. Neuronal engulfment and phagocytosis by macrophages may be observed. In severe cases, destruction of nerve and supporting cells may be so complete that cystic areas of necrosis and hemorrhage may develop in the brain, a condition termed *porencephaly*. Edema may occur as a direct consequence of infection or as a result of inappropriate antidiuretic hormone (ADH) secretion.

The viruses associated with encephalitis generally do not produce characteristic pathologic changes that enable precise histologic diagnosis. Herpes simplex virus, poliovirus, and rabies are commonly localized to certain parenchymal regions. Herpesvirus, adenovirus, rabies virus, and some forms of measles virus infections have characteristic intranuclear inclusion bodies that can be diagnostic. Brains of patients with acquired immunodeficiency syndrome (AIDS)–related dementia demonstrate glial nodules and myelin pallor. Meningeal involvement may also occur.

Rabies and LCM virus produce disease without pathologic evidence of an acute cytolytic effect on cells of the central nervous system. In the case of LCM virus, relatively few cells are infected, and they usually do not lyse or die as a result of infection. Rather, they survive in an antigenically altered state that reflects virus-induced changes in the outer cell membrane. Because these cells have been modified by viral antigen(s) present within or on their surfaces, they are recognized as "non-self" by the immune system of the infected host. A vigorous immune-mediated attack may ensue against virus-infected host cells, including those within the central nervous system. This immune response may induce injury or death of virus-infected host cells, which in turn may result in tissue injury and inflammation extending to nearby noninfected cells. Therefore, the host immune response in fact contributes to tissue injury and disease. The virus-host reaction to LCM virus serves as an example of a form of viral central nervous system disease that is immunopathologically mediated.

Postinfectious encephalomyelitis as a complication of viral respiratory or exanthemous infections and postvaccinal encephalomyelitis may occur without direct infection of the central nervous system. The pathogenesis of Guillain-Barré syndrome and postinfectious myelitis or encephalomyelitis appears to involve the immune response induced by sensitization of the patient to peripheral or central myelin, respectively. Demyelination results from this response. A similar demyelinating syndrome was seen with the early rabies vaccines originally formulated from virus cultivated in neural tissue. These vaccines could sensitize the recipient to neural antigens and lead to tissue damage. An animal model of immune-mediated demyelination, termed *experimental autoimmune encephalitis*, has clarified a number of issues related to these disorders. Perivascular infiltration by mononuclear cells and perivenous demyelination are the characteristic pathologic changes of postinfectious and postvaccinal encephalomyelitis. The fibrinoid necrosis, hemorrhage, and perivenous demyelination seen in acute hemorrhagic leukoencephalitis probably represent a more severe form of postinfectious encephalomyelitis.

Reye syndrome is characterized by acute noninflammatory cerebral edema and fatty liver and usually follows a respiratory, cutaneous, or enteric viral infection in children. The pathogenesis of Reye syndrome is not known, but it appears to be a postinfectious encephalopathy rather than an encephalitis. Influenza A and B and varicella virus infections are most commonly associated with Reye syndrome. This syndrome is associated with salicylate ingestion during the preceding viral infection. In recent years, Reye syndrome incidence has declined sharply, paralleling the sharp decline in administration of aspirin to children.

Clinical Manifestations

Viral meningitis is usually a benign disease of limited duration. Common prodromal symptoms of viral meningitis include fever, malaise, anorexia, myalgia, and sore throat. After a period of 3–14 days, signs of meningeal irritation including headache and stiff neck become apparent. Other symptoms of meningitis may include fever, severe frontal or retroorbital headache, photophobia, lethargy, nausea, and vomiting. Mucocutaneous manifestations of infection include a nonpruritic, maculopapular rash associated with enterovirus infections, herpangina associated with group A coxsackievirus infection, and vesicular eruptions associated with herpesvirus type 2 infection.

The characteristic clinical presentation for encephalitis is evidence of cerebral dysfunction. The signs and symptoms of encephalitis include altered state of consciousness, abnormal behavior, seizures, and deterioration in cognitive function accompanied by prominent memory deficit. Signs of temporal lobe dysfunction, including bizarre behavior and visual or auditory hallucinations, are commonly associated with herpes encephalitis. In addition, signs and symptoms of meningeal irritation as well as fever, headache, malaise, nausea, vomiting, and anorexia are also frequently present in acute encephalitis. A much more insidious onset is characteristic of the chronic encephalitis of Creutzfeldt-Jakob disease, AIDS-related dementia, tropical spastic paraparesis, and progressive multifocal leukoencephalopathy. Depending on the region of the brain affected, neuronal involvement may result in focal or generalized seizures. Coma or respiratory failure can occur if there is brain stem involvement.

Physical findings may include frank neurologic defects such as pathologic reflexes, cranial nerve weakness, seizures, tremors, altered consciousness, and obvious meningeal signs with nuchal rigidity. Papilledema and third- and sixth-nerve cranial palsies can result from an increase in the intracranial pressure. Involvement of the hypothalamic region can contribute to disturbances of temperature, water, and electrolyte regulation.

Laboratory Findings

Laboratory studies of the peripheral blood are of limited value in diagnosing viral meningitis or encephalitis. The peripheral white blood cell count is normal or somewhat elevated. Other routine hematologic and chemical tests are usually normal. The serum amylase may be elevated if mumps virus is the cause of meningitis. Serum transaminases may be elevated in illnesses due to HSV, EBV, and adenovirus.

Examination of the cerebrospinal fluid (CSF) obtained by lumbar puncture is the single most useful procedure for the diagnosis of viral meningitis. The CSF opening pressure is usually elevated, and there is a lymphocytic pleocytosis in the range of 50–500 cells/mm^3. As a general rule, cell counts exceeding 250 cells/mm^3 give the CSF a slightly hazy appearance to the naked eye. CSF counts seldom exceed 1000 cells/mm^3. Usually, the differential cell count reveals a predominance of mononuclear cells. However, early in the course of infection (within the first 24–48 h), the CSF may have a predominance of segmented neutrophils. Repeat examination of the CSF shows that lymphocytes have become the dominant inflammatory cell. Other CSF abnormalities may include a moderately elevated protein, usually 65–150 mg/dL. Normal CSF glucose concentration is common. However, in about 10% of patients with mumps meningitis and occasionally in other viral meningitides (especially due to HSV type 1 and LCM virus), a low glucose concentration may be seen. Histochemical staining and microscopic examination of the centrifuged CSF sediment reveals neither bacteria nor fungi. However, cultures of the blood and CSF should be obtained. Virus can occasionally be isolated from the CSF early in the course of infection with enteroviruses and with the human immunodeficiency virus, but CSF viral culture overall is of low yield. Throat washings and stool should be obtained for viral culture, and acute and convalescent sera should be tested for antibody titers. Computerized axial tomography and magnetic resonance imaging studies are useful for ruling out other clinical situations which can mimic viral meningitis, including parameningeal, brain, subdural, and epidural abscesses; neoplasia; and viral encephalitis.

Diagnosis

It is important to emphasize that the frequency with which a specific virus can be identified as responsible for meningitis depends on the thoroughness with which virologic studies have been pursued and the time after onset of illness when CSF or other specimens for culture are collected. The success rates for isolating an enterovirus from the cerebrospinal fluid of patients of various ages vary as follows: <1 year (60%); 1–19 years (26%); >19 years (close to 0%). Although some series report as high as a 75%

recovery rate for a virologic agent using standard virologic techniques, most consider the usual recovery rate to be 25–33% of those infected. Even these percentage figures are rather high, since they reflect the results of virologic studies initiated in carefully selected patient populations. For example, results of viral studies by the Centers for Disease Control on CSF specimens from a more general population group indicate that, overall, the etiology of aseptic meningitis is established in only 20% of cases.

In general, it is important to obtain both acute and convalescent serum specimens for antibody titer changes. Both serum specimens should be obtained so that a diagnostic fourfold or greater increase in titer can be sought. The timing of specimen acquisition is critical. The first serum specimen should be obtained as soon as the suspicion of viral meningitis arises, and the convalescent serum specimen should then be obtained 2–3 weeks later. In addition to serum, CSF should be obtained for attempted virus isolation, although as noted above this procedure often fails to yield a specific agent. Inability to recover a specific virus in viral meningitis results in part from the rapid elimination of virus from the central nervous system. Finally, throat washings and especially stool specimens should also be obtained for virus isolation in the acute stage, irrespective of whether there have been symptoms or signs implicating the gastrointestinal tract as the organ system primarily infected. Since enteroviruses are the leading cause of viral meningitis, and stool specimens contain relatively large amounts of enterovirus for at least several days after the onset of clinical signs of disease, there is a reasonable probability of recovering the etiologic agent from the stool.

If an enterovirus is isolated by either of these procedures, serum can then be tested for antibody against the specific enterovirus, and, if a fourfold rise in antibody titer is demonstrated, a reasonably certain diagnosis of enteroviral meningitis can be made. Without an enteroviral isolate from throat washings or stool specimens, attempts at serologic tests are usually not practical because of the large number of serotypes represented by the enteroviruses.

Mumps virus and arboviruses are the agents most frequently recovered from proven cases of viral encephalitis. When epidemics of viral encephalitis occur, arboviruses are the agents most frequently recovered from proved cases. During nonepidemic periods, sporadic cases of viral encephalitis are most often caused by herpes simplex virus. Unfortunately, figures for prevalence of specific viruses are imprecise because a specific viral agent is identified in only about 30% or fewer of reported cases of encephalitis in the United States.

Examination of the CSF is critical also for establishing the diagnosis of viral encephalitis. The total white blood cell count in the CSF ranges from 10 to 2000 cells/mm^3. Although mononuclear cells predominate late, polymorphonuclear cells may be the primary cell type early in the course of the infection. Therefore, repeat lumbar puncture in 12–24 h can be useful. Red blood cells may be found in the CSF of patients with herpes encephalitis.

The CSF protein level is usually elevated, reflecting nonspecific protein exudation as part of the acute inflammatory reaction. However, plasma cells, which infiltrate the central nervous system later in the infection, may lead to elevation of specific antibody to the certain inciting agents. Antibody to herpes simplex, varicella-zoster, and mumps virus have been detected at levels equal to or greater than simultaneously assayed serum levels, suggesting local production. The CSF glucose level and the microscopic examination of the centrifuged sediment are generally unremarkable for the viral encephalitides.

HSV antigen has been detected in CSF late in the course of the infection but not reliably enough to be very useful. Detection of viral DNA or RNA by molecular hybridization techniques or by polymerase chain reaction holds considerable promise for the early diagnosis of several forms of viral encephalitis.

The electroencephalogram may be useful for localizing cerebral lesions. Characteristic periodic epileptiform foci that localize to the temporal lobe can be found in some patients with herpes encephalitis.

Definitive diagnosis of herpes encephalitis depends on prompt brain biopsy (usually of the frontal lobe) and demonstration of the virus or viral antigens within biopsied brain tissue. The most reliable method of demonstrating HSV is to isolate the etiologic agent in suitable tissue culture lines. Alternatively, one may detect HSV antigen by immunofluorescence, using highly specific antibody probes. Detection of antigen is more rapid but is not as sensitive or specific a diagnostic procedure as virus isolation. Opinions vary widely regarding the advisability of brain biopsy in patients suspected to have herpetic encephalitis.

Differential Diagnosis

Since meningitis and encephalitis may be life-threatening diseases, it is important to establish as early as possible the specific etiologic agent producing the infection. It is particularly important to differentiate among bacterial meningitis, nonviral causes of aseptic meningitis, and viral meningitis. Once it is clear that bacterial meningitis is not the diagnosis, meningitis resulting from infection with other potentially treatable microorganisms needs to be ruled out. Tuberculous and fungal meningitis should be considered, as well as parameningeal infections, such as epidural or subdural abscesses.

Leptospirosis, an uncommon disease, may manifest clinically as an aseptic meningitis syndrome. Usually, the initial symptoms of fever, chills, meningismus, and nausea and vomiting are followed by signs of renal and hepatic injury. The diagnosis can be substantiated by a history of exposure to water that also has been in contact with rodents. The diagnosis can be established by serologic tests documenting a four-fold rise in agglutinin titers.

An aseptic meningitis-like syndrome can be associated with infective endocarditis. Meningeal inflammation occurs either because of emboli or as a result of immune-complex-mediated vasculitis in the vicinity of the leptomeninges. Clinical findings resembling aseptic meningitis may divert attention from subtle cardiac abnormalities, allowing the underlying endocardial infection to be overlooked. In all instances of so-called aseptic meningitis in adults, blood cultures are advisable.

Neoplasms and dermoid or epidermoid cysts adjacent to the subarachnoid space can present clinically as aseptic meningitis. Certain drugs, such as trimethoprim-sulfamethoxazole, azathioprine, and nonsteroidal antiinflammatory agents have been associated with a clinical syndrome resembling aseptic meningitis. Recurrent meningitides (including Mollaret's and Behçet's) and meningitis associated with systemic lupus erythematosus and other vasculitides (including Kawasaki disease, sarcoidosis, tumor necrosis, and Lyme borreliosis) have laboratory findings consistent with an aseptic meningitis syndrome.

Encephalitis must be differentiated from tumor, intracranial abscesses, hemorrhage, and other intracranial processes.

Course and Treatment

Treatment of viral meningitis is symptomatic. When appropriate supportive care is administered, the prognosis is excellent, with full clinical recovery and low mortality the rule. Complications such as weakness of a specific motor group

may occur, but they are usually mild and generally resolve. Since antibody is known to restrict or inhibit cell-to-cell spread of echoviruses, intravenous administration of large amounts of high-titer antibody has been used to treat chronic echovirus meningoencephalitis in children with hypogammaglobulinemia. The results have been disappointing because of the inability of antibody to penetrate the blood-brain barrier and gain access to the central nervous system compartment in significant amounts. The benefit of periodic intraventricular infusions of echovirus antibody-containing immunoglobulin was reported for a boy with sex-linked hypogammaglobulinemia who had persistent, progressive type 5 echovirus encephalitis. These data provide support for the suggestion that intraventricular antibody infusions might be of benefit in the treatment of other viral encephalitides such as rabies.

In general, when the diagnosis of viral meningitis is unequivocal, hospitalization is not necessarily required unless the illness is severe. However, because it is very difficult to be certain that a patient has viral meningitis at the outset, hospitalization is often recommended to permit adequate evaluation of other diagnostic possibilities and sometimes to permit repeat lumbar puncture. Initially, segmented neutrophils may represent the majority of the white blood cells in CSF obtained early after the onset of viral meningitis. Such a high proportion of neutrophils may lead to diagnostic uncertainty and to empiric antibiotic treatment until the diagnosis of viral meningitis is established. Since the change from neutrophils to lymphocytes occurs within 12–24 h in most cases of aseptic meningitis, repeat lumbar puncture and reexamination of CSF after an appropriate interval is often advocated to gain additional support for the diagnosis of viral meningitis.

Supportive treatment is indicated for comatose patients with encephalitis since recovery can occur after a prolonged period of unconsciousness. Supportive measures include monitoring and correction of electrolyte imbalances, control of seizure activity, and thermal regulation. Corticosteroids and/or mannitol may be useful to reduce cerebral edema and increased intracranial pressure.

Vidarabine and acyclovir have proved efficacious in treating HSV encephalitis. However, intravenous acyclovir is more effective and less toxic than vidarabine and has become the drug of choice. For rabies, preexposure or postexposure prophylaxis (rabies vaccine, hyperimmune serum) prior to the onset of signs and symptoms has been shown effective. It is possible that the antiretroviral agent zidovudine (AZT) may benefit HIV-1 infected patients who have neurologic involvement.

SLOW VIRUS INFECTIONS

Etiology

Measles-like Virus

Subacute sclerosing panencephalitis is caused by a measles-like virus which has been isolated from cultures of brain cells from SSPE patients. The SSPE paramyxovirus differs from measles in its genomic RNA, structural proteins, morphologic appearance under electron microscopy, and growth properties in tissue culture. In addition, the SSPE virus has reduced synthesis of the major M matrix structural protein. Serum and cerebrospinal fluid antibodies to M protein are absent in patients with SSPE, despite high-titered antibodies to the other paramyxovirus structural proteins.

Papovaviruses

The JC polyomavirus is a member of the Papovaviridae family which includes the papillomaviruses and polyomaviruses. These viruses have a double-stranded DNA genome encapsidated in a nonenveloped icosahedral particle. The majority of viruses isolated from pathologic specimens from patients with progressive multifocal leukoencephalopathy (PML) have been strains of the JC virus.

Transmissible Spongiform Encephalopathy

Kuru and Creutzfeldt-Jakob disease (CJD) are the two subacute spongiform encephalopathies that occur in humans. They are related to scrapie and transmissible mink encephalopathy in animals. Both kuru and CJD are caused by transmissible agents which are not conventional viruses. These agents do not have a demonstrable nucleic acid genome. A major component of the scrapie agent is a 27–30 kd hydrophobic protein. Infectivity of the scrapie agent can be reduced by proteolytic enzymes and protein-denaturing agents. Both the kuru and CJD agents are characterized by their small size (filterable to 100-nm pore size) and resistance to inactivation by physical (heat to 80°C, and

gamma and ultraviolet irradiation) and chemical (formaldehyde) means. The kuru and CJD agents can persist *in vitro* and can be transmitted to primates. No humoral or cellular immune response to these agents has been identified.

Epidemiology

SSPE is a very rare disease with fewer than 40 new U.S. cases reported annually. The majority of cases occur in the first and second decades of life. The decreasing incidence rate has been associated with the increasing use of measles vaccination and the resulting decreasing prevalence of wild measles. One epidemiologic study indicated that the majority of SSPE patients had a history of measles much earlier in life (mean of 15 months) than a matched control group (mean of 48 months).

PML is a rare disease associated with the immunocompromised host. PML has been reported in patients with collagen vascular diseases, AIDS, and in renal transplant recipients. PML has a worldwide distribution, with the age of first clinical manifestation between the fifth and seventh decades of life in non-AIDS patients and between the third and fourth decades for adult AIDS patients.

Kuru is confined to the Fore people of eastern New Guinea. Transmission has been associated with ritualistic cannabalism of dead relatives, which was practiced as a rite of mourning. Consumption of brain tissues was limited to children and adult women, thus accounting for the unusual age and sex distribution of the disease. The incidence of kuru has experienced a steady decline since the cessation of this ritualistic cannabalism.

CJD has a worldwide distribution, with an estimated prevalence of 1 per million persons. Transmission has been associated with ingestion of the scrapie agent from hogs or sheep, and there is an autosomal dominant familial form. Transmission by corneal transplants and by human pituitary extract has been documented. The majority of cases occur in the fifth to seventh decades of life.

Pathogenesis

The pathogenesis of SSPE is not known. Recent data, however, indicate that the host immune response may play an important role in the causation of this disease.

The pathogenesis of PML is clearly associated with the underlying immunoincompetence of the host. Antibodies to the JC virus are common in the general population. The development of PML may be related to activation of latent virus in the brain parenchyma.

Kuru and CJD are caused by transmissible agents. Cases of CJD have been documented following direct inoculation through corneal transplantation and contaminated stereotactic brain electrodes. There is no increased prevalence of CJD in medical personnel.

Neuropathology

SSPE is characterized by a diffuse infiltrate of lymphocytes and plasma cells and neuronal destruction in the white and grey matter of the brain and brain stem. Gliosis and myelin degeneration are seen in more chronic cases. Cowdry type A intranuclear inclusion bodies composed of paramyxoviruslike nucleocapsids are seen in neurons, oligodendrocytes, and astrocytes. Therefore, SSPE is a fatal, progressive subacute encephalitis which causes a nonselective loss of all cells in the brain parenchyma.

PML is characterized by discrete foci of demyelination which become confluent and form large plaques. Within the plaques, oligodendrocytes show characteristic nuclear enlargement and giant astrocytes that are morphologically similar to the predominant cell type seen in glioblastoma. Viral particles and antigens can be detected in the lesions by electron microscopy and immunofluorescence, respectively.

Spongiform encephalopathy is characterized by diffuse neuronal loss, proliferation of astrocytes, and vacuolization of astroglial and neuronal processes. This last symptom corresponds to the spongy histopathologic state. Demyelination and inflammation are conspicuously absent.

Clinical Manifestations

SSPE generally has two stages of neurologic decline. The first is characterized by the insidious decline of intellectual performance and the onset of behavioral abnormalities. Following a period of several weeks to months, the patient has the sudden onset of severe intellectual deterioration, seizures, myoclonus, and visual disturbances which rapidly progress to multifocal myoclonus, depression of consciousness, and development of a decorticate state.

Patients with PML deteriorate rapidly; death occurs 2–4 months after the presenting neurologic symptoms. Signs and symptoms are diverse, reflecting the random distribution of lesions in the central nervous system. Personality changes, paresis, and cortical blindness progress to quadriparesis, dementia, and coma.

Spongiform encephalopathy is characterized by rapidly progressing dementia with myoclonus following a prolonged incubation period. Patients present with alterations in behavior and memory, emotional lability, and visual distortions. Patients rapidly progress to dementia within 6 months. Myoclonus can be induced by sudden physical stimuli. Signs and symptoms also include dysarthria, ataxia, and delirium. Kuru is additionally characterized by pyramidal and extrapyramidal signs. Death results from inanition, usually within 1 year after the onset of symptoms.

Laboratory Findings

Patients with SSPE have elevated IgG concentrations and very elevated measles antibody levels in both serum and CSF. Antibody levels are substantially higher in SSPE patients than in patients who have had measles or have been vaccinated. Patients have characteristic electroencephalographic and computed cranial tomographic abnormalities.

Patients with PML usually have normal cerebrospinal fluid. The electroencephalogram shows diffuse nonspecific slowing. Computed cranial tomography can detect the large demyelinated foci. Since antibodies to JC virus are prevalent in the general population, serologic studies are not useful.

The CSF is also usually normal in patients with CJD. A distinctive electroencephalogram pattern is found in the late stages of the disease. The rapid progression of cerebral atrophy can be appreciated using serial computed cranial tomography.

Course and Treatment

There is no current treatment for SSPE, PML, kuru, or CJD. SSPE can be prevented by measles virus vaccination and prevention of wild measles. There is no known prevention for PML. Since CJD is transmissible from human to human, precautions are necessary for handling potentially infectious material and caring for patients. CJD patients can not be permitted to donate organs or blood. Accidental exposure to infected material should be treated by washing with soap or detergent. Percutaneous exposure should be treated by cleansing the site with 0.5% hypochlorite or iodine. Surgical instruments and electrodes should be autoclave sterilized.

CASE HISTORY 1

A 36-year-old white male with a 10-year history of intravenous drug abuse was hospitalized with a 3-day history of malaise, myalgia, anorexia, and nausea. On the day of admission he had developed a severe headache and photophobia. He had been previously well except for a history of acute hepatitis B several years earlier. He was taking no medications and had last used intravenous cocaine 2 weeks prior to admission. There was no history of recent travel.

The patient was alert and responded appropriately to questions. Temperature was 39°C, pulse was 118/min, and respirations were 20/min. Physical examination was significant for mild nuchal rigidity and pain with neck flexion and a fine maculopapular exanthem distributed over the trunk. There were no other physical or neurologic abnormalities.

Laboratory studies included a peripheral leukocyte count of 4800/mm^3, with 68% segmented neutrophils, 25% lymphocytes, 5% monocytes, and 2% atypical lymphocytes. Heterophil antibody and VDRL were negative. Lumbar puncture revealed an opening pressure of 120 mm of water (normal <180 mm of water) and clear, colorless fluid. Microscopic examination revealed 188 leukocytes/mm^3, of which 86% were mononuclear cells. Protein was 60 mg/dL (normal <45 mg/dL), and the glucose was normal. Gram's stain and India ink analysis failed to demonstrate any microorganisms. Blood cultures and cerebrospinal fluid cultures were negative. An EIA for HIV-1 antibody was negative. However, serum was positive for HIV-1 p24 core antigen.

The patient's fever slowly disappeared over a 5-day period. His symptoms also resolved, and he was discharged and followed as an outpatient. Six weeks later, a repeat EIA was positive for antibodies to HIV-1.

CASE DISCUSSION

No specific antimicrobial therapy was given to this patient since his clinical presentation and laboratory findings were consistent with an acute viral syndrome. In addition, the patient's history of intravenous drug abuse placed an HIV-1–related acute retroviral syndrome in the differential diagnosis. Symptoms of this syndrome include fever, night sweats, meningismus, myalgias, anorexia, nausea, vomiting, diarrhea, and a nonexudative pharyngitis. Signs include a maculopapular or urticarial exanthem generally localized to the trunk in 25–50% of patients.

The acute retroviral syndrome usually occurs 1–6 weeks after exposure to the virus. The incidence is unknown since symptoms can be mild and resemble a minor flulike illness. Although this syndrome occurs prior to antibody production, the p24 core antigen of HIV can often be detected in the serum or cerebrospinal fluid. Occasionally, the virus can be cultured from the spinal fluid. HIV-1 antibody is usually detected 2–3 months later, by which time antigenemia has usually cleared.

The differential diagnosis of an acute retroviral syndrome includes influenza, infectious mononucleosis, measles, mumps, cytomegalovirus infection, secondary syphilis, and, rarely, acute viral hepatitis.

CASE HISTORY 2

A 21-year-old college student was hospitalized in January after a few days of malaise, headache, and low-grade fever. The patient was brought to the hospital after friends found him behaving strangely. He was also having difficulty speaking. On examination in the emergency room, the patient was confused, oriented to person only, and complaining of a severe headache. His speech was moderately impaired. His temperature was 40°C. The remainder of the physical and neurologic examinations were unremarkable.

Routine laboratory studies and computerized cranial tomography were normal. Lumbar puncture revealed an opening pressure of 280 mm^3 water and slightly cloudy fluid. There were 300 white cells/mm^3 and 53 red cells/mm^3. Ninety-eight percent of the white cells were lymphocytes. The glucose was 65 mg/dL (serum glucose was 88 mg/dL) and protein was 95 mg/dL. No organisms were visible on

Gram's stain or by India ink. An EEG showed a spike and slow wave pattern localized to the left temporal lobe.

The patient was treated with intravenous acyclovir at 10 mg/kg every 8 h. After 2 days, the patient was less confused, but still had spiking fevers and difficulty speaking. After the fifth day of therapy, fever had disappeared. Although his speech improved, he complained of difficulty with his memory. The patient completed a 14-day course of intravenous acyclovir and was discharged in good condition. Some memory problems persisted.

CASE DISCUSSION

This patient's clinical course is typical of herpes encephalitis. His illness was heralded by malaise, headache, and low-grade fevers, which progressed to spiking fevers with behavioral changes. The virologic diagnosis is presumptive because a brain biopsy was not performed. However, the clinical and laboratory findings, EEG results, and apparent good clinical response to acyclovir are consistent with HSV infection of the central nervous system. Magnetic resonance imaging would have been more sensitive than computerized cranial tomography for demonstrating an early abnormality. Magnetic resonance imaging can also be used to localize a lesion if a biopsy is to be done.

This patient responded to antiviral therapy. Early treatment with acyclovir, which is well tolerated with few side effects, has significantly reduced mortality in herpes encephalitis. However, residual neurologic deficits are still common. Therefore, patients with a clinical presentation consistent with viral encephalitis are often treated empirically with acyclovir. Recently, several viral isolates have been found to be resistant to acyclovir. This emerging resistance may complicate treatment in the future.

A brain biopsy remains the only definitive means for diagnosing herpes encephalitis and excluding other treatable diseases. This differentiation is particularly important when dealing with the immunocompromised host, such as AIDS patients who may be coinfected with other pathogens.

REFERENCES

Review Articles

Berger, J. R., Kaszovitz, B., Post, M. J., et al. Progressive multifocal leukoencephalopathy associated with human immunodeficiency virus infection. A review of the literature with a report of sixteen cases. *Ann. Intern. Med. 107*:78, 1987.

Choppin, P. W. Measles virus and chronic neurological diseases. *Ann. Neurol. 9*:17, 1981.

Dupont, J. R., and Earle, K. M. Human rabies encephalitis: A study of forty-nine fatal cases with a review of the literature. *Neurology 15*:1023, 1965.

Gabuzda, D. H., and Hirsch, M. S. Neurologic manifestations of infection with human immunodeficiency virus. *Ann. Intern. Med. 107*:383, 1987.

Ho, D. D., moderator. The acquired immunodeficiency syndrome (AIDS) dementia complex. *Ann. Intern. Med. 111*:400, 1989.

Hollander, H., and Stringari, S. Human immunodeficiency virus-associated meningitis. *Am. J. Med. 83*:813, 1987.

Joffe, A. M., Farley, J. D., Linden, D. L., et al. Trimethoprim-sulfamethoxazole-associated aseptic meningitis: Case reports and review of the literature. *Am. J. Med. 87*:332, 1989.

Johnson, K. P., Lepow, M. I., and Johnson, R. T. California encephalitis I. Clinical and epidemiologic studies. *Neurology (NY) 89*:250, 1968.

Johnson, R. T., and Mims, C. A. Pathogenesis of viral infections of the nervous system. *N. Engl. J. Med. 278*:23, 84, 1968.

Johnson, R. T., and Ter Meulen, V. Slow infection of the nervous system. *Adv. Intern. Med. 23*:353, 1978.

Pachner, A. R. Neurologic manifestations of Lyme disease, the new "great imitator." *Rev. Infect. Dis. 11* (suppl 6):S1482, 1989.

Ratzan, K. R. Viral meningitis. *Med. Clin. North Am. 69*:399, 1985.

Reik, L. Disorders that mimic CNS infections. *Neurol. Clin. 4*:223, 1986.

Shimizu, T., Ehrlich, G., Inaba, G., et al. Behçet's disease (Behçet's syndrome). *Semin. Arthritis Rheum. 8*:223, 1979.

Sperber, S. J., and Schleupner, C. J. Leptospirosis: A forgotton cause of aseptic meningitis and multisystem febrile illness. *South. Med. J. 82*:1285, 1989.

Stern, B. J., Krumholz, A., Jons, C., et al. Sarcoidosis and its neurologic manifestations. *Arch. Neurol. 42*:909, 1985.

Tenser, R. B. Herpes simplex and herpes zoster nervous system involvement. *Neurol. Clin. 2*:215, 1984.

Articles

Carne, C. A., Tedder, R. S., Smith, A., et al. Acute encephalopathy coincident with seroconversion for anti-HTLV-III. *Lancet 2*:1206, 1985.

Chonmaitree, T., Menegus, M. A., and Powell, K. R. The clinical relevance of 'CSF viral culture.' *JAMA 247*:1843, 1982.

Cizman, M., Mozetic, M., Radescek-Rakar, R., et al. Aseptic meningitis after vaccination against measles and mumps. *Pediatr. Infect. Dis. J. 8*:302, 1989.

Dagan, R., Jenista, J. A., and Menegus, M. A. Association of clinical presentation, laboratory findings, and virus serotypes with the presence of meningitis in hospitalized infants with enterovirus infection. *J. Pediatr. 113:*975, 1988.

Dwyer, J. M., and Erlendsson, K. Intraventricular gamma-globulin for the management of enterovirus encephalitis. *Pediatr. Infect. Dis. J.* 7:S30, 1988.

Erlich, K. S., Mills, J., Chatis, P., et al. Acyclovir-resistant herpes simplex virus infections in patients with the acquired immunodeficiency syndrome. *N. Engl. J. Med. 320:*293, 1989.

Gajdusek, D. C., Gibbs, C. J., Asher, D. M., et al. Precautions in medical care of, and in handling materials from, patients with transmissible virus dementia (Creutzfeldt-Jakob disease). *N. Engl. J. Med.* 297:1253, 1977.

Grinnell, B. W., Padgett, B. L., and Walker, D. L. Distribution of nonintegrated DNA from JC papovirus in organs of patients with progressive multifocal leukoencephalopathy. *J. Infect. Dis. 147:*669, 1983.

Hall, W. W., and Choppin, P. W. Measles-virus proteins in the brain tissue of patients with subacute sclerosing panencephalitis. Absence of the M proteins. *N. Engl. J. Med. 304:*1152, 1981.

Hemachudha, T., Griffin, D. E., Giffels, J. J., et al. Myelin basic protein as an encephalitogen in encephalomyelitis and polyneuritis following rabies vaccination. *N. Engl. J. Med. 316:*369, 1987.

Johnson, R. T., Griffin, D. E., Giffels, J. J., et al. Measles encephalomyelitis—Clinical and immunologic studies. *N. Engl. J. Med. 310:*137, 1984.

Johnstone, J. A., Ross, C. A. C., and Dunn, M. Meningitis and encephalitis associated with mumps infection: A 10-year study. *Arch. Dis. Child. 47:*647, 1972.

Kelsey, D. S. Adenovirus meningoencephalitis. *Pediatrics 61:*291, 1978.

Kessler, H. A., Blaauw, B., Spear, J., et al. Diagnosis of human immunodeficiency virus infection in seronegative homosexuals presenting with an acute viral syndrome. *JAMA 258:*1196, 1987.

Lin, F. H., and Thormar, H. Absence of M protein in a cell-associated subacute sclerosing panencephalitis virus. *Nature 285:*490, 1980.

Masters, C. L., and Richardson, E. P., Jr. Subacute spongiform encephalopathy (Creutzfeldt-Jakob disease): The nature and progression of spongiform change. *Brain 101:*333, 1978.

McDonald, J. C., Moore, D. L., and Quennec, P. Clinical and epidemiologic features of mumps meningoencephalitis and possible vaccine related disease. *Pediatr. Infect. Dis. J.* 8:751, 1989.

McKinney, R. E., Katz, S. L., and Wilfert, C. M. Chronic enteroviral meningoencephalitis in agammaglobulinemic patients. *Rev. Infect. Dis.* 9:334, 1987.

Nahmias, A. J., Whitley, R. J., Visintine, A. M., et al. Herpes simplex virus encephalitis: Laboratory evaluations and their diagnostic significance. *J. Infect. Dis. 145:*829, 1982.

Prusiner, S. B., Groth, D. F., Bolton, D. C., et al. Purification and structural studies of a major scrapie prion protein. *Cell 38:*127, 1984.

Rennels, M. B. Arthropod-borne virus infections of the central nervous system. *Neurol. Clin.* 2:241, 1984.

Rowley, A. H., Whitley, R. J., Lakeman, F. D., et al. Rapid detection of herpes-simplex-virus DNA in cerebrospinal fluid of patients with herpes simplex encephalitis. *Lancet 335:*440, 1990.

Soong, S-J., Watson, N. E., Caddell, G. R., et al. Use of brain biopsy for diagnostic evaluation of patients with suspected herpes simplex encephalitis: A statistical model and its clinical implications. *J. Infect. Dis. 163:*17, 1991.

Whitley, R. J., Cobbs, C. G., Alford, C. A., et al. Diseases which mimic herpes simplex encephalitis: Diagnosis, presentation, and outcome. *JAMA 262:*234, 1989.

Whitley, R. J., Soong, S-J., Linneman, C., et al. Herpes simplex encephalitis. Clinical assessment. *JAMA 247:*317, 1982.

VIII

Infection in the Immunocompromised Host

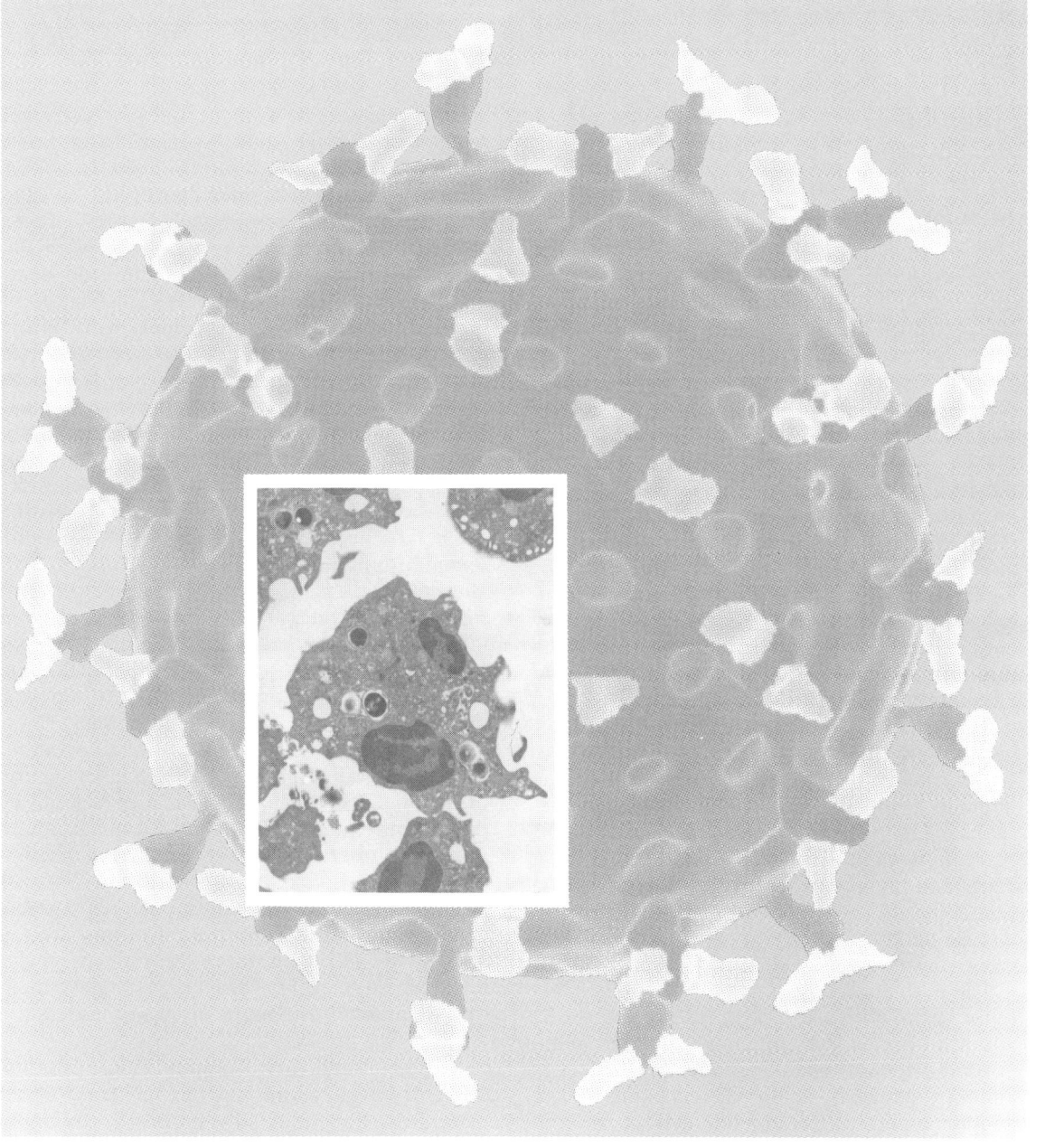

25

JOHN P. PHAIR, M.D.

Syndromes of Host Immunoincompetence

INTRODUCTION

Advancing knowledge of the interrelationship of infection and host defenses has provided much of the impetus for the development of modern immunology. The observation of Major Ogden Burton in 1952 that hypogammaglobulinemia was associated with repeated infection by encapsulated pyogenic organisms represented the first recognition of a defined failure of immunocompetence. Later studies of children with a variety of deficiencies provided further insight into the relationship of immunity to specific infections, and the interaction of the immune response with the inflammatory response. The need to delineate the mechanisms of graft rejection, the study of the effects of drugs and radiation therapy, and the investigation of the effects of infectious and noninfectious disease upon the ability to control invasive microorganisms have yielded more information.

The evaluation of a patient's immunocompetence begins with a thorough history. Thus, the absence of recurrent childhood infection is important evidence against a congenital defect in antibody synthesis, cell-mediated immunity, or another aspect of the immune system. In con-

trast, the history of a splenectomy or sickle cell anemia should alert the physician to the possibility of overwhelming infection due to *Streptococcus pneumoniae*, meningococcus, or *Haemophilus influenzae*. Postsplenectomy sepsis due to these organisms is associated with disseminated intravascular coagulation and death in as many as 50% of patients. This syndrome occurs most commonly in patients with serious underlying disease but has also been reported in patients with congenital absence of the spleen and in individuals who have undergone splenectomy secondary to trauma. This susceptibility is most apparent within the first 2 years following splenectomy, but sepsis has been reported more than 15 years after loss of the spleen. A history of chemotherapy for neoplastic disease, homosexual orientation, or illicit intravenous drug abuse should also alert the physician to a possible defect in the patient's ability to respond to infectious agents.

Recurrent infections or a single "deep-seated" infection, especially due to unusual pathogens, such as *Aspergillus, Candida, Cryptococcus, Toxoplasma gondii*, or *Pneumocystis carinii*, should prompt systematic investigation of host defense mechanisms. If a defect can be defined, the patient is categorized as an immunocompromised host and should be managed as outlined in this chapter.

The physical examination should be complete and specifically note the presence, absence, or hyperplasia of lymph nodes, tonsillar tissue, or hepatosplenomegaly. The laboratory assessment of the immune response is discussed in detail in Chapter 8.

A difficult and very common clinical problem is recurrent infections, such as recurrent upper respiratory tract infections, bronchitis, or staphylococcal skin infections in either an adult or a child. In the great majority of these patients, the most careful and detailed examination of the immune system fails to detect a deficit. Alternatively, a number of disorders are non-immunologic but are associated with recurrent infections, for example, the inherited ciliary dysfunction associated with sinopulmonary infections such as occurs in half of patients with situs inversus viscerum, the so-called Kartagener's syndrome, in which an anatomic abnormality exists in the structure of the dynein arms of the cilia of the respiratory epithelium.

The wide range of potentially pathogenic microorganisms is mirrored by the multiple mechanisms which have evolved to provide resistance by the host. It should be noted that many organisms which rarely cause disease in an individual with a normal immune or inflammatory response can produce severe, or even lethal, infection in the compromised host. Thus, the fungus (once thought to be a protozoan) *P. carinii* is known to infect 80% of children within the first several years of life and may account for some pneumonitis in the infant. In the overwhelming majority of infants and young children, the clinical infection is self-limited or asymptomatic. The organism, however, is not eradicated by the immune response and persists. If the immune status of the individual is impaired at a later time, either by infection with an immunosuppressive agent, such as the human immunodeficiency virus (HIV), or by immunosuppressive therapy, the organism replicates and produces a severe form of pneumonia. A similar phenomenon occurs with reactivation of tuberculosis in elderly individuals in association with loss of their previously fully effective cell-mediated immunity.

This chapter reviews the various deficiency states by grouping them with the cells responsible for the specific defense mechanism. Table 25–1 lists common defects and the diseases associated with specific deficiencies. Table 25–2 lists the infections associated with defective function of specific cells. Although these listings provide a useful framework, it must be understood that there is often overlap and that patients frequently manifest multiple defects.

THE SEGMENTED NEUTROPHIL

Neutrophils, to accomplish their task of killing microorganisms, must be produced in appropriate numbers and arrive at the site of invasion. The most prevalent immune system defect is a

TABLE 25–1. *Common Disorders and Therapies Associated with Secondary Host Defense Abnormalities*

Neutropenia
Leukemia
Rheumatoid arthritis and Felty's syndrome
Cytotoxic therapy
Neutrophil Dysfunction
Solid tumors
Hodgkin's disease
Cirrhosis
Diabetes
Uremia
Rheumatoid arthritis
Systemic lupus erythematosus
Corticosteroid therapy
Acute alcoholism
Hypogammaglobulinemia/Defective Opsonins
Chronic lymphocytic leukemia
Paraproteinemias
Multiple myeloma
Sickle cell anemia
Thermal injury
Depressed Cell-Mediated Immunity
Leukemia
Hodgkin's disease
Non-Hodgkin's lymphoma
Solid tumors
Sarcoid
Aging
Major surgery
Protein-calorie malnutrition
Systemic lupus erythematosus
Acquired immunodeficiency syndrome
Acute viral infections

deficiency in the number of these cells (neutropenia) due to diseases such as leukemia, congenital or cyclic neutropenia, or cytotoxic therapy. Infections which occur in patients with neutropenia include those due to aerobic gram-negative bacilli and *Staphylococcus aureus* and to specific fungal infections, such as candidiasis and aspergillosis. It is uncommon for patients with low neutrophil counts to develop infections until the absolute neutrophil count (ANC) falls below 1000/mm³, and the great majority of individuals do not become infected until the neutrophil count decreases to less than 500/mm³. Fever in neutropenic patients must be considered to be due possibly to infection even if other potential causes of temperature elevation, such as recent transfusions, are present. It should not be assumed that the fever is the consequence of the underlying disease, as up to 60% of temperature elevations in neutropenic adults are the consequence of infection. This percentage is lower in children. Bacterial or fungal infections in the neutropenic patient may progress rapidly and may result in sepsis and death within hours. Therefore, evaluation, including appro-

TABLE 25–2. Infections Associated with Specific Defects

Defect	Typical Infection
Polymorphonuclear neutrophils	Staphylococci, *Corynebacterium,* enteric gram-negative bacilli
	Fungi (candida or aspergillus)
B cell (hypogammaglobulinemia)	*Streptococcus pneumoniae*
	Haemophilus influenzae
	Neisseria meningitidis
T-cell and macrophage deficiencies	Herpes simplex
	Herpes zoster
	Cytomegalovirus
	Epstein-Barr virus
	Mycobacteria
	Listeria monocytogenes
	Salmonella
	Legionella infection
	Disseminated fungal infections
	Coccidioidomycosis
	Cryptococcosis
	Blastomycosis
	Histoplasmosis
C3 deficiency	Staphylococci
	Aerobic enteric organisms
	Encapsulated organisms
Terminal complement component deficiencies	*Neisseria*

priate cultures, should be completed rapidly and empiric broad-spectrum antibiotic therapy initiated without waiting for the results of cultures. Once antimicrobial therapy is begun, the patient should be monitored closely. Approximately 20% of febrile neutropenic adult patients (and a lower percentage of children) prove to be bacteremic or fungemic. Another fifth of the patients have a bacteriologically documented nonbacteremic infection, such as pneumonia, urinary tract, or soft tissue infection. A further 20% have clinical evidence of an infection, but cultures are negative. If a positive culture is obtained, the empiric antibiotics should be altered according to the susceptibility test results.

There is evidence that administration of synergistic combinations of antibiotics, empirically or rationally chosen, results in a better outcome for neutropenic patients. Thus, the choice of empiric antibiotics should be based upon the pathogens commonly isolated in the specific hospital or service treating these patients. The most widely used therapy combines a broad-spectrum penicillin, such as piperacillin, mezlocillin, or azlocillin, with an aminoglycoside. Equally good results are seen with the combination of a broad-spectrum cephalosporin with an aminoglycoside (see Chapter 39). The avail-

ability of the third-generation cephalosporins and imipenem has led to the suggestion that monotherapy with one of these agents is as effective as combinations of a beta-lactam plus an aminoglycoside. However, such therapy often is not as effective as a combination of antibiotics against such gram-positive organisms as *S. aureus*. Infection with this organism is increasingly a problem with the prevalent use of long-term intravenous catheterization.

Several outcomes are possible following initiation of empiric antibiotic treatment. If effective antibiotics had been chosen and an organism isolated, appropriate therapy should continue until the bone marrow recovers and the absolute neutrophil count exceeds 500 or 1000/mm³. If culture results are negative but the patient responds, the empiric antibiotics also should be continued until the bone marrow recovers. If fever persists despite 5–7 days of antibiotics and the cultures are not definitive, antibiotic treatment must be altered. Some authorities have suggested that in the presence of an indwelling intravenous catheter, therapy should be initiated for methicillin-resistant *S. aureus* or *S. epidermidis*. Most, however, feel that the empiric use of vancomycin, the agent of choice for such infections, is not justified because blood cultures are only rarely negative in the presence of intravascular infection with these organisms. A second strategy is to alter the aminoglycoside, substituting amikacin for either gentamicin or tobramycin, because few aerobic gram-negative bacilli are resistant to this agent.

A third approach is to add an antifungal agent to the combination of antibiotics being administered. Data from National Institutes of Health studies indicate that continued use of broad-spectrum antibacterial agents in nonresponsive febrile neutropenic patients is associated with the frequent finding of deep fungal infections at autopsy. Therefore, amphotericin B is given in rapidly increasing doses over a 24-h period and then administered at doses of 0.5 mg/kg/day in adults (1.0 mg/kg/day in children) until the marrow recovers. The new azole, fluconazole, a promising antifungal agent, may prove useful in this situation (see Chapter 39).

In febrile neutropenic patients with pneumonia, aggressive steps should be taken to establish an etiology. If induction of sputum is not diagnostic, it should be followed by bronchial lavage. Transbronchial biopsy is usually precluded because of thrombocytopenia accompanying the neutropenia. In the neutropenic patient pneumonia due to gram-negative bacilli is highly lethal, and the combination of multiple antibiotics to cover all possible causes of infection can be highly toxic.

The prototypic congenital qualitative defect in neutrophils is *chronic granulomatous disease,* a genetic defect in intracellular killing of phagocytosed catalase-positive bacteria. This defect is described in detail in Chapter 3.

Certain disease states are associated with an increased concentration of serum inhibitors of neutrophil chemotaxis which block the response of neutrophils to chemotactic factors. Included in this group of diseases are common problems, such as hepatic cirrhosis. In addition, some children with eczema and extremely high serum levels of IgE have impaired leukotactic responses thought to be due to effects of histamine on neutrophils. In contrast to humoral modulation of neutrophil mobility, intrinsic abnormalities of neutrophil chemotaxis have been described in children with the "lazy leukocyte syndrome," patients with diabetes mellitus, and first-degree relatives of diabetic patients.

For neutrophils to be effective, serum opsonins (activated complement or antibody) must be available and functional. Absence of the third component of complement is associated with the same bacterial spectrum of infections noted in neutropenic patients. Other congenital defects in the complement cascade also have been described. Terminal component deficiency, C5–C9, is associated with recurrent meningococcal and disseminated gonococcal infections. These organisms are sensitive to the bactericidal (lytic) action of fresh serum which is mediated by these complement components (see Chapter 3).

B LYMPHOCYTES (B CELLS)

Lymphocytes derived from bone marrow (B cells) are the antibody-producing precursors of plasma cells. Absent B-cell progenitors, defects in B-cell maturation, B-cell dysfunction, or lack of helper T-cell activity can all lead to agammaglobulinemia, hypogammaglobulinemia, inability to produce a specific antibody class or subclass (dysgammaglobulinemia), or failure to respond to specific antigens. Thus, there are a variety of clinical syndromes associated with B-cell defects which will be briefly reviewed.

X-linked (Bruton's) agammaglobulinemia is due to absent B-cell precursors or the failure of B cells to mature. No B cells, therefore, can be found in the peripheral blood or lymphoid tissue. There is a virtual absence of the immuno-globulins IgG, IgA, and IgM in serum and body secretions. As the defect is X-linked, boys are affected and mothers (who are healthy) are carriers.

Common variable hypogammaglobulinemia occurs in both children and adults but is more frequently diagnosed in adults. The cellular changes that have been cited as underlying this heterogeneous form of hypogammaglobulinemia include increased suppressor T-cell activity, failure of helper T-cell function, deficient B-cell activation, and lack of B cells. These patients have variable patterns of low but not absent serum levels of immunoglobulins.

A delay in the onset of production of IgG in infants has been termed transient hypogammaglobulinemia of infancy. IgM and IgA are present in normal concentrations in serum, and usually there is recovery within the first several years of life. Prior to recovery, otitis and upper respiratory infections are prevalent; severe infections, such as pneumonia, are uncommon.

In addition to these forms of agammaglobulinemia and hypogammaglobulinemia, children have been described with selective IgG2 subclass deficiency. Such children fail to respond to immunization with polysaccharide vaccines. These children have recurrent otitis, sinusitis, and pneumonia caused by organisms with polysaccharide capsules (*S. pneumoniae, H. influenzae* type b, etc). Another group of children have been described who have normal IgG subclass concentrations but manifest recurrent infections, such as those seen with IgG2 subclass deficiency. These children fail to respond to *H. influenzae* vaccines but usually do produce antibody to pneumococcal vaccine and to protein antigens, such as diphtheria and tetanus toxoids. IgG subclass deficiency has been noted in a sizable minority of patients with food allergy, asthma, diabetes mellitus, Henoch-Schönlein purpura, intractable epilepsy of childhood, Friedreich's ataxia, and autoimmune cytopenias. Relatives of persons with IgA deficiency and of patients with common variable immunodeficiency also can have subclass deficiencies. These patients may be asymptomatic but some have sinopulmonary infections, recurrent *Herpes simplex* infections, bone infections, group B streptococcal sepsis, and urinary tract infections. As discussed below, primary T-cell deficiencies also can result in hypogammaglobulinemia.

A number of other distinct diseases have been associated with deficiencies of immunoglobulin and/or specific antibody responses. Some clearly benefit from replacement therapy and in others the relevance of the immunoglobulin deficiencies to infection has not been established. As an example, group B streptococcal sepsis and meningitis of the newborn have been shown to be associated with low maternal levels of anti-group B streptococcal type-specific opsonic antibodies. Some preliminary studies indicated that human immune globulin therapy may be effective in preventing neonatal sepsis due to this organism, but larger trials have not confirmed this.

In general, however, it should be noted that it is not clear what lower limits of IgG subclass levels are compatible with freedom from infection. Although IgG2 deficiency has been definitely associated with poor responses to bacterial polysaccharide, no correlation of deficiencies of other IgG subclasses has been so well defined. It has been suggested that frequent viral upper respiratory infections are associated with IgG3 deficiency, but this is not firmly established.

Following trauma or major surgery, changes in the immune status, including depressed serum immunoglobulin levels, serum subclass concentrations, serum concentrations of complement components and T-cell phenotypes, have been noted. The direct relevance of these changes to infection in these patients has not been defined. Many hematologic malignancies of adults are complicated by hypogammaglobulinemia. Included in this group are multiple myeloma, the paraproteinemias, and chronic lymphocytic leukemia. Infections with the encapsulated organisms occur in these patients; however, the chemotherapy these patients receive also leads to neutropenia and to the typical infections associated with that defect.

It has been recognized for years that replacement therapy with immunoglobulin preparations benefits some hypogammaglobulinemic patients. The relatively recent availability of preparations that safely can be administered intravenously has led to renewed interest in exploring the benefits of this therapy in a wide variety of immunodeficiencies.

T LYMPHOCYTES

The contribution of thymic-dependent lymphocytes to host defense is complex (see Chapter 8). Cooperation between T and B cells is required for maturation of antibody production by B lymphocytes, for example, switching of secretion from IgM to IgG. IgA and IgE pro-

duction also requires interaction between helper T cells and B lymphocytes. The expansion of the B-cell response involves well-characterized soluble factors produced by T lymphocytes and by macrophages. T-cell factors include interferon and interleukin-2 (formerly known as lymphocyte activating factor, or T-lymphocyte growth factor). However, the number of T-cell interleukins identified which have important functional activities continues to increase. The macrophage, in addition to "processing" antigen necessary for induction of an immune response, produces interleukin-1 (endogenous pyrogen) which stimulates B cells directly, upregulates T-cell "helper" function, and serves to augment delivery of phagocytic cells to sites of inflammation. Suppressor T cells, alone or in combination with monocytes, dampen antibody production and T-helper activity, thus serving as modulators of hormonal and cellular immune responses.

Other cytokines, such as migration inhibitory factor (MIF), produced by T cells and B cells under specific conditions, act to amplify the *host response* by interacting with macrophages and neutrophils. (See Chapters 3 and 6 for additional discussion of activated lymphocyte and macrophage products.) Interferons are antiviral factors released following exposure to virus-specific antigen, or nonspecifically after exposure of lymphocytes to mitogens. In addition to the alfa and gamma interferons produced by lymphocytes, fibroblasts produce beta interferon. An example of the importance of the role of interferon in viral infection is found with disseminated herpes zoster infection occurring in patients with malignant disease. In such patients, there is impaired production of local interferon at the time of dissemination. Early systemic administration of interferon to patients with disseminated cutaneous zoster is successful in limiting further spread of the infection, suggesting that interferon therapy corrects a host deficiency. Clinical investigation also has demonstrated the potential efficacy of interferon treatment of cytomegalovirus (CMV), chronic hepatitis B, chronic hepatitis C, chronic granulomatous disease, and possibly HIV-1 infection. Recombinant DNA technology now enables large-scale production of pure interferons and further evaluation of potential therapeutic benefits. Synergistic effects between interferon and other antiviral compounds, such as zidovudine, are being evaluated. Finally, transfer factor, a polypeptide of approximately 10,000 mol wt is another cytokine which has been extensively studied. It can convert nonsensitized lymphocytes to an antigen-responsive state and thus acts to amplify the immune response.

Defects in thymic-dependent responses are due to multiple causes. Congenital thymic aplasia (DiGeorge's syndrome) represents an embryologic failure of development of the thymus and parathyroid glands from the third and fourth pharyngeal clefts. In this disorder the immunologic defect improves somewhat with time. The prototypic T- and B-lymphocyte disorder, severe combined immunodeficiency (SCID), is due to failure of hematopoietic stem cells to differentiate normally. SCID can be X-linked or inherited as an autosomal recessive deficit; deficiency of the cellular enzyme adenosine deaminase is responsible in some patients for this defect. A small number of cases of pure T-cell defects also are due to nucleoside phosphorylase deficiency. Depressed cellular immune responses are also found in a number of neoplastic diseases. Hodgkin's disease represents an example of such an acquired T-lymphocyte dysfunction. Depression of T-cell function due to enhanced suppressor-cell activity and alteration of lymphocyte traffic to lymph nodes has been noted also in certain intracellular infections, such as lepromatous leprosy, disseminated tuberculosis, coccidioidomycosis, and histoplasmosis. Measles is the classic example of a viral illness which transiently depresses cell-mediated immunity. Long before the mechanisms of cellular immunity were delineated it was recognized that a measles epidemic among children with quiescent tuberculosis led to exacerbations of the mycobacterial disease. Depression of cell-mediated immune responses (skin tests, *in vitro* lymphocyte responses, and change in T-cell numbers) has been noted following influenza, rubella, infectious mononucleosis, cytomegalovirus infection, severe bacterial pneumonia, bacteremia, and immunization with live viral vaccines. Depressed *in vitro* lymphocyte responsiveness and skin-test reactivity are also found in aged individuals and in patients with protein-calorie malnutrition.

In the late 1970s and early 1980s, infections due to *Pneumocystis carinii*, fungi, cytomegalovirus, and atypical mycobacteria were noted in male homosexuals, users of illicit intravenous drugs, patients with hemophilia, and others. Profound defects in cell-mediated immunity, and increased occurrence of the rare vascular neoplasm, Kaposi's sarcoma, as well as lymphoproliferative tumors, were reported. The cause of the alteration in immune regulation is a depletion of helper T cells as a consequence of infection with HIV. Chapter 26 discusses this important infectious cause of immunodeficiency in detail.

THE MONONUCLEAR PHAGOCYTE

The third cell involved in host defenses against microorganisms is the phagocytic monocyte, or macrophage (see Chapter 3 for overview). These cells, which are derived from bone marrow, are located in the peripheral blood (monocytes) or in specific organs, including liver, spleen, and pulmonary alveoli (histiocytes, or macrophages). Monocytes can leave the vascular compartment, enter tissues and organs, and participate in cell-mediated reactions. With appropriate stimulation, the number of mononuclear phagocytic cells in the liver (Kupffer's cells) can greatly increase due to both local proliferation and recruitment from blood.

Macrophages have receptors for IgG and complement that enhance their adherence to and facilitate their ingestion of opsonized particles. They also are capable of non–immune-mediated phagocytosis. Phagocytosis and digestion of antigen by macrophages play an important role in processing and presentation of antigen to lymphocytes—a precondition for T- and B-cell immune responses. In addition, macrophage factors, such as interleukin-1, or cell-to-cell contact between macrophages and lymphocytes facilitates lymphocyte responses to antigens and to mitogens.

Mononuclear phagocytes demonstrate a metabolic burst that is keyed to activation of the hexose monophosphate shunt following ingestion of bacteria. Killing bacteria requires the production of H_2O_2 and the fixation of halide, as happens in neutrophils. Enzymes within macrophages aid in the digestion of macromolecules. However, cationic proteins, necessary for bacterial killing by neutrophils, are lacking in these cells. Some microorganisms have evolved the ability to survive within macrophages. The tubercle bacillus (*Mycobacterium tuberculosis*), for example, survives and replicates within non-activated macrophages. Other organisms such as *Toxoplasma gondii* also resist killing unless coated with antibody.

Dysfunction of macrophages has been demonstrated in chronic granulomatous disease, in certain hematologic neoplasms, in malacoplakia (an uncommon acquired granulomatous disease associated with chronic infection), in systemic lupus erythematosus, HIV infection, and during corticosteroid therapy. Disseminated infections due to intracellular pathogens may represent examples of intrinsic dysfunction of these phagocytes. However, a failure of macrophage-lymphocyte interaction or an inherent lymphocyte defect may be at fault.

MULTIPLE DEFICIENCIES

It should be clear that patients can have multiple defects in their immune or inflammatory responses. As suggested in the discussion of B-cell deficiencies, a disease such as multiple myeloma typically leads to infection with pneumococci. However, treatment of this hematologic neoplasm often leads to neutropenia secondary to cytotoxic agents and to subsequent infection with gram-negative bacteria, *S. aureus*, or fungi.

An instructive example of a single patient with multiple defects that occur sequentially is a recipient of an allogenic bone marrow graft for the treatment of aplastic anemia or leukemia. The cytotoxic treatment and/or radiotherapy administered to produce the ablation necessary for transplantation is associated with the usual infections associated with neutropenia. Viral infections are uncommon. With production of leukocytes by the transplanted marrow, infections markedly diminish. However, with a partial mismatch, graft-versus-host disease leads to disruption of the integrity of skin and intestinal mucosa and to infections involving skin and enteric organisms. Cytomegalovirus infections follow as a consequence of the defects in cell-mediated and humoral immunity associated with graft-versus-host reactions. If immune function is restored by the graft, the patient is often left with deficiencies of IgG subclasses 2 and 4 and with resultant susceptibility to infection by pyogenic encapsulated bacteria. Use of protective isolation and antibiotic prophylaxis reduces the risk of the early infections. A good match for histocompatibility antigens and use of CMV-free blood products decreases the risk of both graft-versus-host disease and cytomegalovirus infection. Finally, administration of immunoglobulin preparations and antibiotics can ameliorate the effect of selective deficiency of IgG subclasses.

CASE HISTORY

A 12-year-old girl was referred to the hospital for fever of 8 weeks' duration associated with weight loss and night sweats. A thorough history revealed that the child's pet monkey had died 12 weeks earlier while the girl was convalescing from measles. When the fever began, the physician, recognizing the known risk of tuberculosis in monkeys, placed an intradermal purified protein derivative (PPD) skin test on the child. The test was negative. The physical examination was unrevealing except for a temperature of 38.5°C. The initial laboratory studies, including a chest x-ray, were not helpful. A consultant noted several exudative lesions upon careful examination of the retina. A presumptive diagnosis of miliary tuberculosis was made and therapy initiated. A repeat skin test using intermediate strength PPD (5 TU) caused an area of erythematous induration 22 mm in diameter. A repeat chest x-ray demonstrated multiple nodular densities 7 days after admission. The child's fever resolved 14 days after initiation of antituberculosis therapy, which was continued for 1 year.

CASE DISCUSSION

This case illustrates the effects of viral infection (measles) upon cellular resistance to tuberculosis and the ability to react to skin-test reagents. The physician correctly thought of tuberculosis in this clinical setting, but skin-tested the child only once and did not determine whether or not she was anergic. Testing with several antigens such as candida extract would have demonstrated anergy and should have prompted a continued search for tuberculosis. The recognition of the eye lesions after referral led to the correct diagnosis and initiation of appropriate therapy. In addition it should be recognized that for up to 6 weeks after initial infection with Mycobacterium tuberculosis, *PPD skin tests can remain negative and that miliary disease itself can result in anergy (see Chapter 15).*

REFERENCES

Books and Symposia

Allen, J., ed. *Infections and the Compromised Host. Clinical Collaborations and Therapeutic Approaches.* 2nd ed. Baltimore: Williams and Wilkins, 1987.

Berger, M., and Kliegman, R., eds. Neonatal sepsis and the role of immunotherapy: A symposium. *Rev. Infect. Dis.* 12(Suppl. 4):S393, 1990.

Verhoef, J., Peterson, P., and Quie, P., eds. *Infections in the Immunocompromised Host: Pathogeneses, Prevention and Therapy.* Amsterdam: Elsevier, 1980.

Articles

Bagdade, J., Root, R., and Bulger, R. Impaired leukocyte function in patients with poorly controlled diabetes. *Diabetes 23:9,* 1974.

Bodey, G., Buckley, M., Sathe, Y., et al. Quantitative relationships between circulating leukocytes and infection in patients with acute leukemia. *Ann. Intern. Med. 64:328,* 1966.

Brayton, R., Stokes, P., Schwartz, M., et al. Effect of alcohol and various diseases on leukocyte mobilization, phagocytosis and intracellular killing. *N. Engl. J. Med. 282:123,* 1970.

DeMeo, A., and Anderson, B. Defective chemotaxis associated with a serum inhibitor in cirrhotic patients. *N. Engl. J. Med. 286:735,* 1972.

Good, R., and Pahwa, R., eds. The recognition and management of immunodeficient disorders. *Pediatr. Infect. Dis. J. 7:S2,* 1988.

Phair, J., Kauffman, C., Bjornson, A., et al. Host defenses in the aged: Evaluation of components of the inflammatory and immune response. *J. Infect. Dis. 138:67,* 1978.

Phair, J., Riesing, M., and Metzger, E. Bacteremic infection and malnutrition in patients with solid tumors: Investigation of host defense mechanisms. *Cancer 45:2702,* 1980.

26

JOHN P. PHAIR, M.D. • ELLEN G. CHADWICK, M.D.

Human Immunodeficiency Virus Infection and AIDS

INTRODUCTION

In 1981, several investigators reported the occurrence of opportunistic infections due to intracellular microbial pathogens and a rare cancer, Kaposi's sarcoma, in epidemiologically restricted populations. This illness, first noted in mid-1979 and characterized by profound immune defects, was termed acquired immune deficiency syndrome (AIDS). Initially cases were reported in homosexually active males and intravenous drug abusers. Individuals who received blood transfusions or blood component therapy, children born to mothers who were intravenous drug abusers or prostitutes, and sexual contacts of bisexual males and drug users later were identified as having similar defects and clinical manifestations. Many persons with AIDS have had a prodromal illness of varying duration characterized by fever, generalized lymphadenopathy, malaise, weight loss, oral thrush, and diarrhea. This prodromal syndrome was termed the AIDS-related complex (ARC). Investigation of symptomatic and asymptomatic individuals in the high-risk groups documented that an altered immunoregulatory state precedes the development of AIDS. The diagnosis of AIDS is based upon the clinical findings of an opportunistic infection, Kaposi's sarcoma, or central nervous system non-Hodgkin's lymphoma (usually of the B-cell type), or severe wasting—conditions suggestive of a defect in cell-mediated immunity.

The most common presentation of AIDS has been pneumonia due to *Pneumocystis carinii* (PCP), which has accounted for 55% of cases. Another 15–20% of AIDS patients have Kaposi's sarcoma (KS) alone, and 5–10% have both KS and PCP. An additional subgroup present with other opportunistic infections including central nervous system toxoplasmosis, mycobacteriosis (especially infections due to *M. avium*-complex), and disseminated fungal or herpes virus infection. Finally, a small group of patients present with encephalopathy or wasting.

This chapter reviews the etiology, epidemiology, immunopathogenesis, diagnosis, natural history, and treatment of patients with HIV infection and AIDS. Specific issues relevant to maternal–fetal transmission and manifestations of human immunodeficiency virus infection in children are also addressed.

ETIOLOGY

The cause of the immune dysfunction that leads to AIDS is infection with a retrovirus, the human immunodeficiency virus type 1 or 2 (HIV-1, HIV-2). These retroviruses are related to a number of primate retroviruses which cause a similar syndrome in specific species of Old World monkeys. HIV-1 was the first to be recognized and was isolated in three laboratories in 1983–1984. Initially, it was termed lymphadenopathy associated virus, human T-cell lymphotropic virus type III (HTLV-III), or AIDS-related-virus (ARV). Genetic analysis indicated that HIV-1 and HIV-2 are closely related to the lentivirus group of retroviruses and by consensus the name human immunodeficiency virus was assigned to these new human viruses.

HIV-1 is epidemic in Central and East Africa, and is associated with cases of AIDS in Europe, North America, Oceania, and Asia. HIV-2 is found in West Africa and is the cause of imported cases of AIDS in Western Europe and in North America.

HIV are RNA viruses. The genetic material is contained within a protein core of 24,000 mol wt, termed p24. Closely associated with the RNA is an enzyme, reverse transcriptase, which transcribes DNA from RNA after the virus core enters a human cell. Surrounding the core is a multilayered outer envelope composed of an inner protein coat of 18,000 mol wt, termed p18. This protein lines a lipid layer into which is inserted a glycosylated protein of 41,000 mol wt (gp41). Attached to gp41 is a larger molecular weight glycosylated protein, gp120, of 120,000 mol wt. This gp120 protein contains a sequence of amino acids which recognize and adhere to surface CD4 molecules of a number of human cells, most prominently the helper T (CD4+) lymphocytes. A subset of monocyte/macrophages and B lymphocytes also bears small numbers of CD4 molecules and can be

infected with HIV-1 or HIV-2. There is suggestive evidence that endothelial cells, rectal mucosal cells, and possibly lymphocyte progenitor cells can be infected although CD4 surface molecules have not been identified on the surface of these cells.

Once the virus attaches to the surface of CD4+ lymphocytes, its core is internalized, the RNA uncoated, and, through the action of reverse transcriptase, viral DNA is transcribed. The DNA is circularized and inserted into the DNA of the infected lymphocyte. This proviral DNA can remain in a latent state in the cell for months to years. *In vitro* stimulation of the infected cell by mitogens or antigen induces a replicative infection. The proviral DNA transcribes viral mRNA which encodes the specific viral components. Specifically, there is a region which transcribes the precursor protein of the internal structural proteins (gag), the viral enzymes (pol), and the outer envelope components (env). The virion is assembled in the cytoplasm of the infected cell and buds from the cell surface.

EPIDEMIOLOGY

Infection with HIV-1 and AIDS were first recognized in homosexual men and intravenous drug users in New York, San Francisco, and Los Angeles in 1979–1980. Since the initial recognition of the syndrome, persons with AIDS have been diagnosed in all 50 states and all inhabited continents. In the United States the proportion of AIDS cases occurring in homosexual or bisexual men during the 1980s has slowly decreased, whereas the number of cases among illicit drug users, their sexual contacts, and children born to infected women has increased. Cases continue to be reported among recipients of contaminated blood and blood component therapy. For the most part such individuals were infected with HIV before donors of blood were screened for high-risk behavior, symptoms related to HIV, and antibody to the virus (before March 1985).

The majority of persons with AIDS are male and between the ages of 20 and 50. Infection in older adults generally has been associated with receipt of HIV-infected blood. In the latter half of the 1980s, an increasing number of women have been diagnosed with AIDS as a result of drug use or sexual contact with men who are bisexual or drug users. All racial groups are represented among cases reported to the Centers for Disease Control as part of the national surveillance program.

As of April 1991, more than 170,000 cases have been reported, and it is estimated that approximately 1 million residents of the United States are infected. The coincident epidemic of intravenous drug use in this country has resulted in an increasing number of economically disadvantaged people from the inner cities being infected and developing AIDS. Thus, African-Americans and Hispanics, especially women and children, are disproportionately represented among those persons with AIDS.

IMMUNOLOGY AND IMMUNOPATHOGENESIS

The primary targets of HIV are the CD4-bearing lymphocytes (helper T cells), macrophages/monocytes, and B cells. The CD4+ lymphocytes play a central role in the regulation of the immune system, releasing a number of cytokines necessary for normal function of this response. Through a variety of mechanisms, HIV infection results in depletion and dysfunction of the CD4+ lymphocytes. The infection of the mononuclear phagocytes does not apparently produce cell death, but the depletion of the CD4+ lymphocytes results in decreased serum concentrations of lymphokines, such as IL-2 and gamma interferon, and consequent macrophage/monocyte dysfunction. Infection of B lymphocytes induces autonomous production of immunoglobulins and hypergammaglobulinemia. Paradoxically, however, the loss of CD4+ cells and B-cell infection induce a state in which the infected individual cannot respond to new antigens with specific antibody production.

The mechanism underlying the depletion of the CD4+ lymphocytes remains obscure to some extent. Replication and budding of the virus does result in cell death, but relatively few lymphocytes have been shown to be productively infected in the first period of infection, 1 in 10,000–50,000 cells. Infection with HIV *in vitro* induces cell fusion and giant-cell formation, but this is not a consistent or prevalent finding upon histologic examination of tissues from infected individuals. Antibody-mediated cell cytotoxicity or lymphocytoxic antibody possibly mediates destruction of HIV-infected lymphocytes, and both forms of antibody have been associated with decreasing CD4+ cell numbers as infection advances.

The result of the immunologic perturbation is a defect in both cell- and antibody-mediated responses. In adults, the first defect predominates, and infection with intracellular pathogens, such as fungi, protozoa, mycobacteria, and herpesvirus, is characteristic of advanced HIV infection. The failure to produce specific antibody is associated with bacteremic infections due to encapsulated pyogenic organisms, such as *Streptococcus pneumoniae* and *Haemophilus influenzae*.

DIAGNOSIS OF HIV INFECTION

Following the isolation of HIV-1, an immunoassay was developed to detect serum antibodies to virus. This enzyme-linked immunoassay (EIA) was developed to screen blood donors and is highly sensitive, being able to detect 99% of infected individuals. It is highly specific, with a false-positive rate of 1% or less. However, the estimated infection rate in low-risk populations in the United States is 0.2% or less. Widespread testing in low-risk populations results in 5–10 falsely identified infected persons for every truly infected individual. Therefore, a confirmatory assay is required before a definitive diagnosis of HIV-1 infection can be established. The most commonly used confirmatory test is the Western blot assay. The EIA tests primarily detect antibody to the core protein, p24, and to the glycosylated envelope protein, gp41. The EIA is relatively inexpensive and is semiautomated. In contrast, the Western blot can detect antibody to all viral proteins but is more expensive and labor intensive and relies upon a subjective interpretation by a technician. The Western blot, by consensus, is not interpreted as positive unless there is evidence of antibody to products of two of the three major gene regions, gag, pol, or env. Blots which have no bands are negative, whereas those that have bands but are not diagnostic are termed indeterminate.

Alternative confirmatory tests include a radioimmune precipitation assay (RIPA) and an immunofluorescent assay. At present neither is as widely used as the Western blot and neither offers an improvement in terms of convenience or expense.

A major limitation of the assays for antibody is the fact that following infection there is a period of variable length in which antibody cannot be detected in serum. This period is analogous to the "window" seen in persons recently infected with hepatitis B. There have been documented instances of individuals in the window donating blood which produced HIV-1 infection in recipients. It is presumed that sexual contact with a person in the window also could result in transmission of HIV-1.

Other techniques can detect infection before antibody can be measured. However, they either are of limited usefulness or are available only in research laboratories. Following infection and during the window, the core protein, p24, circulates in blood for a period of 2 weeks or less and can be detected with an enzyme-linked assay using antibody for p24. Once antibody to this antigen is produced by the infected patient, p24 is usually cleared from the blood. Studies of this assay's potential usefulness in blood donors and retrospective testing of stored serum obtained from high-risk individuals who later developed antibody indicate that this technique has limited usefulness as a means of detecting infected individuals who are antibody-negative.

Virus has been isolated from peripheral blood lymphocytes of seronegative individuals at high risk of infection. In addition, using the polymerase chain reaction (PCR), enzymatic amplification of proviral DNA has been documented from lymphocytes of antibody-negative individuals, months before seroconversion. These findings demonstrate the ability of HIV-1 to produce latent infection which induces an attenuated or absent immune response and which has little or no impact on the immunologic status of the infected individual. It is not known whether latently infected persons transmit the infection sexually, and the frequency of prolonged latency is unknown, but is presumed to be low.

NATURAL HISTORY OF HIV-1 INFECTION

Following infection with HIV-1 there is an immediate rise in the proportion and number of CD8+ lymphocytes and a decrease in the proportion and number of CD4+ lymphocytes. Approximately 50% of individuals experience a self-limited mononucleosis-like syndrome manifested by fever, malaise, sore throat, and generalized lymphadenopathy. A few individuals develop aseptic meningitis, which is symptomatic for 2 weeks or less. A large number of HIV-1-infected individuals, however, are asymptomatic immediately after infection and remain asymptomatic for a prolonged period. A subset of individuals develop asymptomatic generalized lymphadenopathy.

With time, the majority of infected individuals demonstrate a decrease in CD4+ lymphocytes, but in some the numbers of these cells plateau

at relatively normal values. Other infected persons have a progressively rapid fall in CD4+ cell counts. Infected persons who experience the acute syndrome described above are more likely to demonstrate rapid immunodepletion. The rapidity and degree of the decrease serves as the most accurate prognostic indicator for the development of the opportunistic diseases which define AIDS. The normal adult number of helper T cells approximates $1000 \pm 300/mm^3$ and represents 40–45% of T cells in the peripheral circulation. As infection progresses and CD4+ cell counts approach $200/mm^3$, symptoms such as unexplained fever, malaise, weight loss, diarrhea, oropharyngeal thrush, or hairy leukoplakia are noted in approximately one third of patients. At or below counts of $200/mm^3$ (or 20%) helper T cells, there is an increasing risk of developing *Pneumocystis carinii* pneumonia, or other AIDS-defining conditions.

In association with the fall in CD4+ cells, serum concentrations of beta$_2$-microglobulin and neopterin increase. Both are nonspecific markers of immune activation of lymphocytes and monocyte/macrophages. In addition, approximately 20–25% of HIV-infected persons with CD4+ cell counts between $200/mm^3$ and $400/mm^3$ demonstrate p24 antigen in serum in association with a decline in antibody to this core protein. Knowledge of the level of these markers adds prognostic information because increases in p24 concentrations are associated with an increased risk of developing AIDS.

Although it is not known whether all HIV-infected individuals will progress to AIDS, it has been estimated that 50% of those who do develop AIDS do so within 9–10 years. In adults, it is very uncommon to establish a diagnosis of AIDS within the first 12 months following seroconversion, and 90% of infected adults are AIDS-free 3 years after the appearance of specific antibody. Once an individual's CD4+ count approaches $200/mm^3$, the occurrence of fever and thrush adds significantly and independently to the risk of developing AIDS.

TREATMENT OF HIV INFECTION

Although in 1991 only one FDA-approved agent, zidovudine (formerly known as AZT), was generally available for therapy of HIV infection, a rapidly increasing number of potential agents are being developed and evaluated. To prevent adherence of the virus to cells with CD4 receptors on their surface, recombinant soluble CD4 is being tested. Other agents which potentially interfere with this initial step are sulfonated analogues of dextran sulfate and heparin, which prevent infection of cells by HIV-1 *in vitro* by altering surface characteristics of lymphocytes.

The substituted nucleosides, such as zidovudine (AZT), dideoxycytidine (ddC), and dideoxyinosine (ddI) inhibit reverse transcriptase and terminal chain transcription. These agents thus interfere with the transcription of proviral DNA by viral RNA, which occurs after cellular internalization of the virus. To attack later stages of viral replication, protease inhibitors are being developed which block enzymatic production of core proteins from precursor molecules. Interferons which have been evaluated as immunomodulators also interfere with the final steps of viral assembly and budding.

Zidovudine, the currently available therapeutic agent, has been documented in double-blind trials to extend survival of patients with AIDS, and those with severe immunosuppression and HIV-related signs and symptoms (AIDS-related complex). In recent trials this agent has also reduced the frequency of progression to AIDS when administered to asymptomatic persons and to those with mild AIDS-related complex. This agent is not curative; viral resistance develops over time, and there are toxicities. The most prominent adverse effect is bone marrow suppression. Both anemia and leukopenia commonly occur, especially in severely ill individuals. The other substituted nucleosides do not induce hematologic toxicity but do produce neurotoxicity.

A less frequent adverse reaction to zidovudine in persons who have received the agent for a year or more is myopathy. In most individuals this is manifest only as a rise in serum muscle enzymes. A minority of individuals also develop symptoms of pain, weakness, and wasting. Often the myopathy and hematologic toxicity can be managed by dose reduction. In many persons, however, therapy must be discontinued temporarily or permanently.

MANAGEMENT OF OPPORTUNISTIC INFECTIONS

The most common AIDS-defining complication of HIV-1 infection during the first 10 years of the epidemic has been pneumonia due to *Pneumocystis carinii*, accounting for up to 55% of AIDS diagnoses (see Chapter 27). It is estimated that approximately 70% of patients with AIDS ultimately develop this form of pneumonia during their HIV-1 infection. It is now possible to reduce the frequency of PCP, which represents a reactivation of infection originally established in early childhood. Eighty percent of children by age 6 have antibody to this organism. The alteration or failure of the immune system secondary to steroid therapy, hypogammaglobulinemia, or HIV infection allows replication of *P. carinii* and development of pneumonia. Prophylaxis in the form of (a) single monthly administration of pentamidine by aerosol; (b) daily oral administration of trimethoprim-sulfamethoxazole or dapsone; or (c) weekly administration of oral pyrimethamine-sulfadoxine has proved effective. Inhaled pentamidine produces mild to moderate respiratory symptoms and the oral prophylactic regimens are associated with allergic reactions. Prophylaxis should be initiated in adults when the CD4+ cell count falls to 200/mm^3.

Diagnosis of PCP requires a high degree of suspicion, for the pneumonitis can present as fever of unknown origin with or without respiratory symptoms or as a life-threatening pulmonary infection. Induction of sputum can be used to demonstrate the cysts of the organism, but up to 50% of cases require bronchoscopy with lavage to demonstrate the agent. The chest x-ray can be normal but more commonly demonstrates bilateral interstitial pneumonia. Therapy is generally initiated with intravenous trimethoprim-sulfamethoxazole. The high rate of adverse reactions (approximately two thirds of patients develop rash, fever, or neutropenia) requires that intravenous pentamidine frequently be substituted in order to complete the required 3 weeks of therapy. Adverse effects of intramuscularly injected pentamidine include hypoglycemia, pancreatitis, renal and hepatic toxicity, and sterile abscess formation. In patients who fail therapy with either of the two primary antibiotics, experimental agents such as trimetrexate, another antifolate, are available for treatment. Clindamycin plus primaquine, and daily aerosol pentamidine have been successfully used in mild cases of PCP. Adjunctive use of corticosteroids is associated with improved survival from an episode of acute PCP if begun within the first 2–3 days of antibiotic therapy. With early diagnosis and aggressive management, survival from the initial episode of PCP should approach 90%. Recurrent PCP has a higher mortality. All patients surviving PCP should receive maintenance aerosol pentamidine or oral prophylaxis to reduce the frequency of recurrences.

Cryptococcal meningitis and cerebral toxoplasmosis are treated with amphotericin B and sulfadiazine-pyrimethamine, respectively. These infections of the central nervous system should be suspected when an individual presents with headache or focal neurologic findings. Cerebral imaging techniques are utilized to rule out masses due to toxoplasma, Kaposi's sarcoma, or B-cell lymphoma. In the absence of such findings, a lumbar puncture should be performed to determine if cryptococcal antigen is present in the cerebrospinal fluid (CSF). This immunoassay is more sensitive than the India ink test used to demonstrate the fungus in CSF. Culture for cryptococci and mycobacteria, as well as the usual cell counts and assays for protein and sugar, are also necessary. If the diagnosis of cryptococcal meningitis is established and initial treatment is successful, maintenance amphotericin administered once weekly is required to prevent relapse. Fluconazole, an oral antifungal agent, is available both for initial and maintenance therapy for this infection.

Antibiotic therapy for presumptive cerebral toxoplasmosis should be administered for 2 weeks to individuals with multiple mass lesions identified by computerized tomography (CT) or magnetic resonance imaging (MRI). After completion of the initial therapy, the CT or MRI should be repeated. If the lesions have diminished in size, a full course of treatment should be completed and followed by maintenance therapy to prevent relapse. If the lesions are unchanged after 7–10 days or if there is a solitary lesion, a brain biopsy is necessary to rule out cerebral lymphoma or Kaposi's sarcoma.

Infections due to herpes simplex or herpes zoster can be managed successfully with acyclovir. Ganciclovir is now available for therapy of cytomegalovirus (CMV) retinitis. Although successful in reversing or slowing the progression of sight-threatening retinitis, discontinuation of the agent is associated with a progression of the infection. Unfortunately ganciclovir therapy is not effective treatment for CMV pneumonitis and induces neutropenia when given with zidovudine. Though disseminated fungal infections, such as histoplasmosis and blastomycosis, can be treated successfully with amphotericin B, sufficient experience has not accumulated to determine if maintenance therapy is required to prevent relapses. Disseminated mycobacterial infection due to the tubercle bacilli can be managed with the usual antituberculous agents. The most common mycobacterial infection in persons with AIDS is due to the *Mycobacterium*

avium complex and is resistant to isoniazid and rifampin. Combination therapy with experimental agents and second-line antituberculous drugs is generally unsuccessful in eradicating the organism but is often associated with clinical improvement.

Other infections which cannot be cured because of the lack of effective agents include cryptosporidiosis, a protozoal infection of the gastrointestinal tract, and progressive multifocal leukoencephalopathy due to papovavirus, the virus associated with plantar warts.

LATE MANIFESTATIONS OF HIV INFECTION AND AIDS

A problem unrelated to opportunistic infections is dementia due to HIV infection of the central nervous system. Studies indicate that neurologic manifestations are uncommon before the diagnosis of AIDS. However, up to 40% of persons with AIDS develop CNS disease, and a significant proportion is due to HIV encephalopathy. Ninety percent of autopsied cases show evidence of HIV effects upon the central nervous system, and cerebrospinal fluid pleocytosis is common even in asymptomatic HIV-infected individuals. The neurons are not infected, although virus can be demonstrated in glial cells of central nervous system. The pathogenesis of dementia has not been elucidated. The dementia presents with memory defects, and in untreated patients progresses to coma and death in weeks or months. There are reports of responses to zidovudine therapy.

A second apparently related condition is severe wasting. In Africa this is especially common and has been termed "slim disease." The pathogenesis of this manifestation of HIV infection is unknown but may be related to malabsorption due to viral effects upon the mucosal epithelial cells of the small intestine.

OTHER MANIFESTATIONS OF HIV INFECTION

Until the outbreak of AIDS, Kaposi's sarcoma was seen rarely in North America and Europe. It is a tumor of endothelial origin occurring in men over the age of 60 in Europe and North America. The lesions are found on the lower extremities, and the disease is indolent in nature. In Central Africa, in contrast, KS is most commonly seen in young men, is widely disseminated, and involves the viscera, including the bronchi and gastrointestinal tract. KS represents the second most common tumor of males in this region of Africa. The virulence of KS in persons with AIDS resembles that of the African type. In the decade before the recognition of AIDS, KS was increasingly reported in patients with renal allografts, emphasizing the role of an altered immune response in the pathogenesis of this tumor. Although KS has been used to establish the diagnosis of AIDS, there is recent evidence to indicate that it is due to infection with a second, as yet undefined, sexually transmitted agent.

B-cell lymphomas are becoming increasingly prevalent as a presenting, AIDS-defining condition as effective prophylaxis for opportunistic infections is developed. Similar neoplastic complications have been recorded in transplant patients. Epstein-Barr virus coinfection accounts for a subset of the lymphomas that occur as a result of the profound immunosuppression induced by HIV (see Chapter 10).

Thrombocytopenia mediated by immunologic mechanisms is also common in advanced HIV disease. Auto-antibodies directed at both platelet antigens or immune complexes adhering to the platelet surface have been demonstrated in thrombocytopenic HIV-infected patients. Anemia and neutropenia are common in patients with AIDS as well, independent of therapy. These cytopenias are the result of direct HIV infection of the bone marrow, presumably of the stem cells.

PEDIATRIC HIV INFECTION

Transmission

One of the major features differentiating HIV infection in children from that in adults is the mode of transmission. Among children younger than 13 years of age who have AIDS, approximately 80% have been perinatally infected during gestation or delivery from an HIV-seropositive mother, 13% have been infected via contaminated blood transfusions prior to 1985, and 5% received contaminated clotting factors in the treatment of hemophilia and other coagulation disorders. In adolescents, the routes of acquisition are more typical, that is, transfusion of blood or coagulation factors (39%), sexual transmission (41%), or intravenous drug use (11%).

There are three postulated routes by which perinatal HIV transmission occurs: (1) transpla-

cental infection *in utero,* (2) exposure to blood and cervical secretions during delivery, and (3) postpartum ingestion of breast milk containing the virus. *In utero* HIV infection has been demonstrated by isolating the virus from aborted 13–20-week fetuses. The virus has been isolated in cord blood, and the placenta has been shown to contain cell-surface CD4 that serves as receptor for HIV. Therefore, HIV may directly infect the placenta, facilitating transplacental spread of the virus. The ability to recover HIV from cervical secretions supports the possibility of intrapartum transmission, similar to the mechanism seen in infection by hepatitis B virus. Several infants have been reported to have acquired HIV infection postnatally via breast milk, because their mothers' only HIV risk factors were postpartum blood transfusions from donors subsequently found to have AIDS. Although this mode of transmission appears to be very rare, it is recommended in the United States that HIV-infected mothers refrain from breast-feeding. However, in developing countries, where it is the cornerstone of infant nutrition and prophylaxis against diarrheal disease, the advantages of breast-feeding appear to outweigh the risk.

The rate of HIV transmission from infected mother to infant has been studied in numerous centers throughout the world and appears to approximate 30%. However, factors associated with transmission are poorly understood. Clinical evidence of disease in the mother is not an important factor affecting transmission, as the majority of women giving birth to infants who are ultimately proved to have HIV infection are asymptomatic. Viremia during gestation is an attractive hypothesized mode of transmitting the infection. However, some infants remain uninfected despite repeated isolation of HIV from the mother's peripheral lymphocytes throughout pregnancy and from the placenta at delivery. The route of delivery does not appear to affect infectivity; both cesarean and vaginal deliveries have produced HIV-infected infants. Some studies have suggested that low maternal numbers of CD4+ lymphocytes may enhance the risk for fetal transmission, but this has not been well documented. Repeated pregnancies in the same woman may produce alternately infected and uninfected infants. Further complicating this picture are transmission data in twin pairs. In two reported sets of dizygotic twins, infections occurred in all four offspring; however, in two sets of monozygotic twins, only one member of each twin pair was HIV-infected. Thus, the factors that determine the relatively low perinatal transmission rate of 30% need further research to be fully understood.

Diagnosis

Serodiagnosis of HIV infection is more difficult in infants and young children than in adults. There is no consistent IgM response by the infected infant to enable diagnosis of prenatal infection. Furthermore, methods to detect IgM anti-HIV are neither sensitive nor specific. As a result of placental transfer of maternal IgG antibody to HIV, virtually all neonates born to seropositive women are HIV-antibody-positive at birth, and this maternally derived antibody may persist for up to 15 months of age. Serial testing by the Western blot technique in uninfected infants may reveal a decay of viral bands representing loss of maternal antibody, but this requires at least several months of observation. A small proportion of HIV-infected children are hypogammaglobulinemic, leading to false-negative antibody tests once they catabolize the maternally derived antibody. For other children who have a "window period" between their loss of maternal antibody and their onset of producing endogenous antibody, repeated testing is necessary. Others may never develop detectable levels of HIV antibody, despite having positive viral cultures from the blood or repeated HIV antigenemia. Finally, children recently transfused with large volumes of seronegative blood may demonstrate false-negative antibody tests. Children in whom clinical suspicion for HIV infection is high, but who become seronegative, should be further evaluated. Clearly, a single positive antibody test in an infant does not identify HIV infection and a negative result does not rule it out. Knowledge of the clinical status and longitudinal testing are necessary to accurately interpret HIV antibody determinations in young infants and children.

Although viral culture is capable of identifying more than 80% of infected infants, a negative culture does not exclude infection. Furthermore, because it is a cumbersome and costly technique, few laboratories are equipped to provide viral culture for routine clinical diagnostic purposes. Although p24 antigenemia is sometimes demonstrated in infants, it is generally not detectable in neonates, presumably because p24 antigen is bound by high levels of circulating maternal anti-p24.

Newer methods that may enable neonatal diagnosis include the polymerase chain reaction (PCR) technique and *in vitro* antibody production. PCR identifies the presence of HIV DNA in peripheral blood mononuclear cells using enzymatic amplification of highly conserved sequences of proviral DNA. The advantage of PCR over serologic testing is that it provides direct evidence of HIV infection regardless of the serologic status of the infant. To date, this molecular biology technology has appeared highly sensitive and specific for diagnosis of HIV in young infants, but more data are needed. The *in vitro* production of HIV-specific antibody by cultured peripheral lymphocytes appears to be a promising technique; however, sensitivity and specificity data are not yet available.

To simplify the difficulties of diagnosis in the pediatric population, the Centers for Disease Control (CDC) has set out guidelines for the definition of HIV infection in children (Table 26–1). Children younger than 15 months of age who were born to seropositive mothers are considered to be definitely infected only if (1) they have AIDS by clinical criteria (that is, manifest opportunistic infections), (2) HIV can be detected in blood or tissues, or (3) they are seropositive with evidence of both humoral and cellular immunodeficiency as well as characteristic symptomatology. In older children or in children infected by routes other than perinatally, evidence of a positive serologic test by EIA and by a confirmatory test, such as the Western blot, is definitive of HIV infection.

Clinical Manifestations

Pediatric AIDS is largely a disease of young children. Most infected infants have no manifestations of the disease at birth, but 50% of HIV-infected children are symptomatic in the first 12 months of life, and 78% by 2 years of age have clinical disease. The CDC has developed a classification system for pediatric HIV infection that describes the clinical presentation of the disease, including both asymptomatic (class P-1) and symptomatic HIV infection (class P-2) (Table 26–2). The P-0 classification is reserved for those HIV-seropositive asymptomatic infants younger than 15 months of age in whom it is unknown whether they are infected, until they can be reclassified later as either infected or uninfected.

Nonspecific Findings

Most children with symptomatic HIV infection have several of the following symptoms, which

TABLE 26–1. *CDC Definition of HIV Infection in Children Younger Than 13 Years of Age**

Children younger than 15 months of age with perinatal infection must have one of the following:
1. HIV in blood or tissues confirmed by culture or other laboratory detection method
2. Symptoms meeting CDC case definition for AIDS
3. Antibody to HIV (repeatedly reactive screening test plus positive confirmatory test result) and evidence of both cellular and humoral immunodeficiency (elevated immunoglobulin levels, decreased absolute helper T-cell count, absolute lymphopenia, decreased helper/suppressor T-cell ratio) and symptoms (class P-2 [Table 26–2])

Older perinatally infected children or children who acquired infection through another mode of transmission must have one of the following:
1. HIV in blood or tissues confirmed by culture or other laboratory detection method
2. Antibody to HIV (repeatedly reactive screening test plus positive confirmatory test result)
3. Symptoms meeting CDC case definition for AIDS

*Adapted from Centers for Disease Control: Classification system for human immunodeficiency virus (HIV) infection in children under 13 years of age. *MMWR* 36:225–236, 1987.

are present in descending order of frequency: lymphadenopathy, hepatomegaly, splenomegaly, poor growth, recurrent diarrhea, more than 10% weight loss, and more rarely, parotitis. The most debilitating of these is significant weight loss, or the wasting syndrome, which may be life-threatening.

TABLE 26–2. *Classification for HIV Infection in Children Younger Than 13 Years of Age**

Class or Subclass	Symptomatology
Pediatric HIV Infection	
Class P-0	Indeterminate infection
Class P-1	Asymptomatic infection
Class P-2	Symptomatic infection
Classification of Asymptomatic HIV Infection (Class P-1)	
Subclass A	Normal immune function
Subclass B	Abnormal immune function
Subclass C	Immune function not tested
Classification of Symptomatic HIV Infection (Class P-2)	
Subclass A	Nonspecific findings
Subclass B	Progressive neurologic disease
Subclass C	Lymphoid interstitial pneumonitis
Subclass D	Secondary infectious diseases
	D-1: opportunistic infections
	D-2: recurrent bacterial infections
	D-3: other infections
Subclass E	Secondary cancers
Subclass F	Other diseases possibly caused by HIV infection

*Adapted from Centers for Disease Control: Classification system for human immunodeficiency virus (HIV) infection in children under 13 years of age. *MMWR* 36:225–236, 1987.

Progressive Neurologic Disease

The majority of neurologic manifestations of pediatric AIDS are believed to be the result of direct infection of the brain by HIV. A characteristic encephalopathy occurs that consists of developmental delay or deterioration of motor milestones, intellectual ability, or behavior. Paresis, pyramidal tract signs, ataxia, abnormal muscle tone, or pseudobulbar palsy may also occur. Acquired microcephaly is the result of poor brain growth, and computerized tomography scans frequently reveal basal ganglia or frontal calcifications and cerebral atrophy. The progression of neurologic disease may be static, or slowly or rapidly progressive. The majority of symptomatic HIV-infected children have some degree of neurologic involvement, and encephalopathy may be the dominant manifestation of the disease in children.

Lymphocytic Interstitial Pneumonitis

Lymphocytic interstitial pneumonitis (LIP) is a chronic interstitial pneumonia that results from nodular peribronchiolar lymphoid aggregates or diffuse infiltration of the alveolar septa and peribronchiolar areas by lymphocytes and plasma cells. The exact role of Epstein-Barr virus (EBV) in LIP is not clear, but it is likely that an interaction between HIV and EBV-infected B cells in the lungs may account for the pathogenesis of this condition. Both EBV DNA and HIV RNA have been demonstrated by *in situ* hybridization in lung tissue from children with LIP, and patients with LIP usually have high anti-EBV IgG titers with atypical antibody responses to EBV. Clinically, the lungs are without such auscultatory symptoms as rales, especially early in the disease, but clubbing of the fingers and hypoxemia (with or without respiratory distress) are frequently present. The clinical presentation of LIP is usually subtle with gradual progression. Symptomatic hypoxemia is generally well controlled by treatment with oral corticosteroids. These drugs diminish the lymphocytic infiltrate sufficiently to allow more normal gas exchange in the lung. Approximately 50% of children with hypoxemia due to LIP become steroid-dependent (that is, attempts to decrease corticosteroids are associated with reappearance of hypoxemia); the remainder may be successfully weaned from corticosteroids within several weeks to months.

LIP occurs at some time in approximately 40% of children with AIDS, but is quite rare in adults. The mean survival time of children diagnosed with LIP is 91 months, and LIP predicts a better prognosis than for children who never develop LIP but who manifest opportunistic infections.

Opportunistic Infections

As in adults, *Pneumocystis carinii* pneumonia (PCP) is the most common opportunistic infection in children with AIDS, occurring in approximately half of the population. However, with the more widespread use of prophylactic agents, such as trimethoprim-sulfamethoxazole and pentamidine, PCP has become less prevalent. The children at greatest risk appear to be infants younger than 8 months of age who have not been recognized previously to be HIV-infected and who therefore have received no prophylaxis.

Other important opportunistic infections include disseminated *Mycobacterium avium* complex infection, *Candida* esophagitis or pneumonia, disseminated cytomegalovirus or herpes simplex infection, and intestinal cryptosporidiosis. Certain opportunistic infections which are common in adult AIDS patients, such as disseminated *M. tuberculosis* infection, toxoplasmosis, cryptococcal meningitis, and progressive multifocal leukoencephalopathy, have occurred in less than 1% of children with AIDS.

Recurrent Bacterial Infections

One of the more common problems associated with HIV infection in children is recurrent bacterial infections, such as sepsis, meningitis, pneumonia, and soft tissue abscesses. Encapsulated organisms, such as *Haemophilus influenzae* and *Streptococcus pneumoniae,* are most commonly observed—a pattern similar to that seen in primary antibody deficiency syndromes. Indeed, the laboratory hallmark of infection in pediatrics is polyclonal hypergammaglobulinemia, and paradoxically, many symptomatic patients fail to mount primary or secondary antibody responses to antigens they have not previously encountered. Recurrent bacterial infections occur in approximately 30% of children with AIDS, whereas these infections are considerably rarer in adults. Less severe bacterial infections, such as chronic otitis media and sinusitis, also occur very frequently.

Other Infections

Viral infections not categorized as opportunistic can also cause significant morbidity and mortal-

ity in pediatric AIDS patients. Primary varicella can result in disseminated infection involving the lungs, liver, coagulation system, and brain. In addition, chronic or recurrent herpes zoster frequently follows primary varicella. These lesions may be atypical and become necrotic and are usually quite painful. Severe rubeola may occur, with complications such as pneumonia and encephalitis, sometimes in the absence of the typical rash. Chronic oral candidiasis is exceedingly common, and herpetic gingivostomatitis may be recurrent.

Malignancies

Cancer accounts for only 2% of AIDS-defining illnesses in children. Kaposi's sarcoma, so typical of adult AIDS, has been reported in fewer than 20 children. B-cell lymphoma and primary lymphoma of the brain also occur in pediatric HIV-infected patients, but strikingly less often than in the adult population. Recently, very rare soft tissue sarcomas were reported with increased frequency in HIV-infected children. Other unusual malignancies may be associated with pediatric AIDS as a result of decreased immune surveillance.

Other Diseases Possibly Caused by HIV Infection

Abnormalities of virtually any organ system can occur with HIV infection. Hepatitis with fluctuating transaminase levels is frequently seen without an identifiable alternative infectious cause. On biopsy, a form of chronic active hepatitis is present with accompanying lymphoid aggregates in the portal and lobular regions. HIV-nephropathy generally presents with massive proteinuria and edema and may progress to frank renal failure. Histologically, focal and segmental glomerular sclerosis is the rule. Cardiomyopathy culminating in congestive heart failure has been described. The hematologic system is almost universally affected, and most children have anemia of chronic disease. More rarely, hemolytic anemia with positive direct and indirect Coombs's tests may be found. Autoimmune thrombocytopenia and neutropenia are frequently encountered. Many of the therapeutic agents used to treat children with HIV infection may exacerbate these problems, most notably zidovudine, which often causes anemia and neutropenia, and trimethoprim-sulfamethoxazole, which commonly causes neutropenia. A variety of routine dermatologic abnormalities often become extensive in HIV-infected children, such as seborrheic dermatitis, molluscum contagiosum, and common warts.

Prognosis

In children with perinatal infection, survival from the onset of clinical disease depends on multiple factors. In one series of 172 congenitally infected infants in Miami, 50% had died by 36 months of age. Factors associated with a poor prognosis include onset of symptoms before the first birthday, opportunistic infections (especially infantile PCP), and progressive encephalopathy. Laboratory findings suggesting disease progression are absolute CD4 lymphopenia, hypogammaglobulinemia, and progressively elevated p24 antigen levels in the blood.

Supportive and General Treatment

Children who are HIV-seropositive should be followed closely by a multidisciplinary team of specialists. Frequent checkups allow for early recognition of neurologic deterioration or failure to thrive. Aggressive nutritional support is very important, with calorie-enriched formulas, supplemental nasogastric feedings, and, in some cases, intravenous hyperalimentation. Diphtheria, pertussis, and tetanus immunizations should proceed normally, and the inactivated polio vaccine should be substituted for the live attenuated (oral) polio vaccine (Chapter 40). Because of the severe morbidity and mortality associated with measles in these children, it has been recommended that most HIV-infected children receive the measles-mumps-rubella vaccine, regardless of their degree of immune deficiency, even though it is a live virus vaccine. *Haemophilus influenzae* vaccine should be given on a routine schedule, and pneumococcal vaccine at 2 years in an effort to prevent some of the invasive infections common in pediatric AIDS. It is important to recognize, however, that the antibody response to many of these immunizations may be impaired.

Prophylaxis against Specific Infections

In contrast to adults, young children with HIV infection, especially those with onset of symptoms before the age of 2 years, are susceptible to PCP well before their absolute CD4 cell counts drop below 200/mm^3. Consequently, many physicians recommend the institution of anti-PCP prophylaxis in infants <12 months with CD4 counts below 1500/mm^3, and in children 1–2 years of age with CD4 counts <1000/mm^3. Monthly intravenous gammaglobulin therapy has been used in an attempt to prevent recurrent bacterial infections in children with AIDS by providing preformed passive antibody and has been shown to decrease serious bacterial infections in children whose CD4 counts exceed 200/mm^3.

Antiretroviral Therapy

The principles of controlling HIV replication in children are similar to those in adults. The more important differences revolve around when best to initiate therapy, especially in relation to efforts to prevent perinatal transmission. Studies are currently being designed to treat pregnant HIV-seropositive women with antiretroviral agents like zidovudine during the third trimester to prevent viral transfer across the placenta late in gestation. Other studies will address whether intrapartum therapy for the mother or immediate postpartum therapy for the neonate will prevent transmission. Finally, when reliable neonatal diagnosis becomes achievable through techniques such as PCR, *in vitro* antibody production, and viral culture, very early antiviral intervention will be possible.

Social Issues

The social complexities of treating a child with AIDS are frequently formidable. Many infected children have parents who are ill or dying, drug abusers, poor, homeless, or all of the above. The variety of medical specialties necessary to care for such a child may be overwhelming to the parent, and the financial burdens may be staggering. Finally, many families may feel isolated or discriminated against, and children may be excluded from school and church. For these reasons, the role of the social worker in coordinating the care of a child with AIDS may be equally important to that of the medical providers.

The issues that relate to infected adolescents are different. Although several hundred teenagers in the United States between the ages of 13 and 19 years have been recorded as having

AIDS, the 20,000 AIDS cases in adults aged 20–29 years suggests that many of these infections were acquired during adolescence. The risk-taking attitudes of teenagers and the growing number of teen runaways (many of whom engage in prostitution to support themselves) signal this as a target population for whom education on AIDS prevention is critical.

PREVENTION OF HIV INFECTION

Although an intensive effort is under way to develop a vaccine, to date none is available. Recombinant DNA technology has been utilized to produce purified components of the outer envelope of the virus for use in immunization. Trials in volunteers have been conducted that demonstrate immunogenicity of a number of candidate vaccines. None has been demonstrated to be protective in humans, but there are recent reports of successful immunization of monkeys to prevent infection with simian immunodeficiency virus, which is related to HIV. Therefore, prevention of infection can result now only from behavioral change. Education aimed at reducing the use of illicit intravenous drugs and unsafe sexual practices must be augmented in order to reduce transmission of the virus. Heat treatment of factors VIII and IX or use of factors derived from recombinant technology has reduced the frequency of infection following therapy for coagulation defects. Testing of donated blood and encouragement of voluntary testing and counseling of individuals at risk represent the foundation of efforts to reduce the risk from blood transfusion.

The risk of transmission of HIV-1 to medical personnel is low but does exist through exposure to infected blood or other body fluids. To reduce the risk, hospitals have adopted a policy of "universal precautions" which is designed to lower the chance of exposure to contaminated blood or secretions and accidents with sharp instruments, such as needles and scalpels. Personnel performing procedures in which there is a possibility of aerosolization or splashing should wear goggles and masks to reduce the risk of mucous membrane exposure. It is estimated from studies conducted by the CDC that there is a 0.35% risk of infection with each accidental parenteral exposure to contaminated blood.

CASE HISTORY 1

A 35-year-old homosexual man is seen for advice regarding possible exposure to HIV. He is asymptomatic, but has a history of repeated sexual contacts with individuals who are infected. Serologic studies reveal a positive enzyme-linked immunoassay for antibody to HIV that is confirmed by Western blot. T-cell phenotyping demonstrates that CD4 (helper T) cells account for 22% of his peripheral blood lymphocytes; the absolute CD4 count is 360/mm³. The proportion of CD8 (T-cytotoxic) cells is 33% with an absolute count of 540/mm³. A repeat study 1 month later reveals similar T-cell proportions and numbers. Although offered therapy with zidovudine (ZVD or AZT) he refuses because he is asymptomatic and worried about adverse effects. Repeat evaluation in 3 months reveals a decrease in the CD4 cell number to 300/mm³. Physical examination now reveals thrush. He again refuses AZT therapy. Prophylaxis to prevent *Pneumocystis carinii* pneumonia (PCP) is discussed, and he agrees to take trimethoprim-sulfamethoxazole daily. In addition, a course of ketoconazole is begun to treat the oropharyngeal candidal infection. Three months later he is asymptomatic, but the CD4 count is 270/mm³. With the evidence that the CD4 number is continuing to fall, he agrees to begin AZT at 500 mg/day. Two weeks later he reports mild nausea but otherwise no difficulties with the therapy, and his hemoglobin has remained stable. One month later, however, he reports development of a rash over his back and chest which is associated with itching and fever. He is diagnosed as hypersensitive to trimethoprim-sulfamethoxazole and monthly aerosolized pentamidine is substituted for the oral antibiotic. With AZT therapy the CD4 cell count has risen to 400/mm³, and with clearance of the drug rash he feels well. He is monitored by obtaining an interval history, physical examination, CD4 counts, and complete blood counts every 3 months for the next 15 months. At that point his CD4 count drops to 200/mm³. Serologic studies reveal the presence of p24 HIV antigen. The decision is made to discontinue AZT and begin therapy with dideoxycytidine. The patient is warned about the possible development of peripheral neuropathy with this inhibitor of viral reverse transcriptase. He tolerates the drug, p24

antigenemia clears, and the CD4 count rises to 280/mm³.

CASE 1 DISCUSSION

This case illustrates the prolonged course and need for close monitoring of HIV-infected patients. The psychologic problems of acceptance of potentially toxic therapy is an issue the physician will need to grapple with. In addition to anti-HIV therapy, treatment of intercurrent infections and institution of prophylaxis is indicated at specific times in the natural history of the infection. Generally, PCP prophylaxis is indicated in adult patients with fewer than 200/mm³ CD4 cells; however, the risk of PCP is great in individuals who have CD4 counts between 200 and 350/mm³ and who also have minor infections, such as thrush. Many physicians, therefore, begin PCP prophylaxis before the CD4 cell count reaches 200/mm³. AZT is effective in stabilizing the immunodepletion induced by HIV for 12–24 months. Resistance through mutation of the viral reverse transcriptase is associated with declining efficacy of the drug, as manifested by a decrease in CD4 cell number and development of antigenemia. Fortunately, the newer substituted nucleosides, such as dideoxycytidine and dideoxyinosine, continue to be effective inhibitors of reverse transcriptase and can be substituted for AZT. With time it is likely that this patient will develop a complication of HIV-induced immunosuppression, such as disseminated fungal infection, lymphoma, HIV-wasting syndrome, or encephalopathy, despite antiretroviral therapy.

CASE HISTORY 2

A 15-month-old boy is referred for evaluation of recurrent infections. He was the 7-pound, 8-ounce full-term product of an uncomplicated pregnancy and delivery, born to a 23-year-old single woman who had no known risk factors for HIV infection. In the first year of life, the baby experienced four episodes of diarrhea, recurrent otitis media, and one episode of bronchiolitis. His growth had been adequate, although his weight and height were never greater than the fifth percentile. At 14 months of age, he developed a fever of 104°F without localizing signs, and a blood culture revealed

S. pneumoniae. He recovered uneventfully with intravenous penicillin and was referred for evaluation.

On initial examination the child was small for his age, but appeared healthy. Remarkable physical findings included dull tympanic membranes, mild bilateral parotid enlargement, diffuse lymphadenopathy measuring 0.5–1 cm in the anterior and posterior cervical chains and in the axillary and inguinal regions. Pulmonary and cardiac examinations were normal, and the liver and spleen were enlarged (5 cm and 3 cm below the costal margins, respectively). The diaper area revealed an erythematous rash typical of *Candida* infection. Neurologic examination revealed decreased tone and inability to stand unsupported.

Laboratory examination revealed a WBC of 8600/mm³ with a normal differential, hemoglobin of 9.5 gm/dL, and positive HIV antibody by EIA and Western blot. Serum immunoglobulins revealed IgG of 1696 mg/dL (normal is 345–1213 mg/dL) and the total CD4 count was 1044/mm³. Chest x-ray revealed a diffuse bilateral reticulonodular pattern involving all lobes of the lung, but a pulse oximetry test demonstrated normal blood oxygen saturation.

AZT therapy was initiated, and the child was followed monthly. Three months later, he developed another bacteremic illness with *S. pneumoniae* and was again treated uneventfully with antibiotics. A screening chest x-ray at 20 months of age revealed an increase in the reticulonodular infiltrates, which was not associated with pulmonary symptoms.

When the parents of the child were tested for HIV antibody, the mother was found to be positive by EIA and Western blot; the father was negative. The mother then recalled that two of her previous sexual partners may have used recreational drugs and, therefore, may have been HIV-infected.

CASE 2 DISCUSSION

This case illustrates a variety of features of pediatric HIV infection. Many HIV-positive women, especially those who are asymptomatic, may not recognize that they have been exposed to HIV through sexual contact, and, therefore, do not report having risk factors. It is not

uncommon for the child to be the first family member recognized to be HIV-positive. Developmental delay and recurrent diarrhea accompanied by poor growth in the first year of life are common presentations of perinatally acquired HIV infection. One of the hallmarks of pediatric HIV infection is recurrent serious bacterial infections. Although AZT therapy appears to lessen the frequency of some opportunistic infections, experience to date does not suggest that it modifies the frequency of bacterial infections. Helper T-cell counts in normal children tend to be higher than those in adults, and may be correspondingly higher in HIV-infected children than in HIV-infected adults. Although a helper T-cell count of 1044/ mm³ is not normal for a child this age, it is not so low that he is at particularly high risk for an opportunistic infection. Children with lymphocytic interstitial pneumonitis (LIP) are more likely to have generalized enlargement of the salivary glands and lymph nodes and may remain asymptomatic for prolonged periods despite marked chest x-ray abnormalities. It is highly likely that this child will eventually develop poor oxygenation and respiratory distress as a result of progressive LIP, but this can be successfully reversed with administration of systemic corticosteroids, such as prednisone.

REFERENCES

Books

Leoung, G., and Mills, J., eds. *Opportunistic Infections in Patients with Acquired Immunodeficiency Syndrome.* New York and Basel: Marcel Dekker, Inc., 1989.

Levy, J. A. ed. *AIDS Pathogenesis and Treatment.* New York and Basel: Marcel Dekker, Inc., 1989.

Sande, M. A., and Volberding, P. A., eds. *The Medical Management of AIDS.* Philadelphia: W. B. Saunders Co., 1990.

Review Articles

Centers for Disease Control. Guidelines for prophylaxis against *Pneumocystis carinii* pneumonia for children infected with HIV. *MMWR 40* (RR-2): March 15, 1991.

Colgate, S. A., Stanley, E. A., Hymen, J. M., et al. AIDS and a risk-based model. *Los Alamos Science 18:*2–39, 1989.

Falloon, J., Eddy, J., Wiener, L., et al. Human immunodeficiency virus infection in children. *J. Pediatr. 114:*1–30, 1989.

Nara, P. AIDS virus of animals and man: Non-living para-

sites of the immune system. *Los Alamos Science 18:*54–89, 1989.

Original Articles

Blanche, S., Rouzioux, C., Moscato, M. L. G., et al. A prospective study of infants born to women seropositive for human immunodeficiency virus type-1. *N. Engl. J. Med. 320:*1643–1648, 1989.

Centers for Disease Control: Classification system for human immunodeficiency virus (HIV) infection in children under 13 years of age. *MMWR 36:*225–236, 1987.

Centers for Disease Control: Current trends. First 100,000 cases of acquired immunodeficiency syndrome—United States. *MMWR 38:*561–563, 1989.

Chadwick, E. G., Yogev, R., Kwok, S., et al. Enzymatic amplification of the human immunodeficiency virus in peripheral blood mononuclear cells from pediatric patients. *J. Infect. Dis. 160:*954–959, 1989.

Chadwick, E. G., Connor, E. J., Hanson, C. G., et al. Tumors of smooth-muscle origin in HIV-infected children. *JAMA 263:*3182–3184, 1990.

DeWolf, F., Lange, M., and Houweling, J. Appearance of predictors of disease progression in relation to the development of AIDS. *AIDS 3:*563–569, 1989.

Hesletine, W. Development of antiviral drugs for treatment of AIDS: Strategies and prospects. *J. AIDS 2:*311–334, 1989.

Masur, H., Ognibene, P., Yarchoan, R., et al. CD4 counts as predictors of opportunistic pneumonia in human immunodeficiency virus (HIV-1) infection. *Ann. Intern. Med. 111:*223–231, 1989.

The NICHD intravenous immunoglobulin study group. Efficacy of intravenous immunoglobulin for the prophylaxis of serious bacterial infections in symptomatic HIV-infected children. *N. Engl. J. Med.* 1991, in press.

Oxtoby, M. J. Human immunodeficiency virus and other viruses in human milk: Placing the issues in broader perspective. *Pediatr. Infect. Dis. J. 7:*325–335, 1988.

Peterlin, B., and Lucillo, P. Molecular biology of HIV. *AIDS 2:*529–540, 1988.

Phair, J., Munoz, A., Detels, R., et al. The risk of PCP among men infected with HIV-1. *N. Engl. J. Med. 322:*161–165, 1990.

Phair, J., and Wolinsky, S. Diagnosis of infection with the human immunodeficiency virus. *J. Infect. Dis. 159:*320–323, 1989.

Pizzo, P. Pediatric AIDS: Problems within problems. *J. Infect. Dis. 161:*316–325, 1990.

Rubenstein, A., Morecki, R., Silverman, B., et al. Pulmonary disease in children with acquired immune deficiency syndrome and AIDS-related complex. *J. Pediatrics 108:*498–504, 1986.

Schoenbaum, E., Hartel, D., Selwyn, P., et al. Risk factors for human immunodeficiency virus infection in intravenous drug users. *N. Engl. J. Med. 321:*874–879, 1989.

Scott, G. B., Hutto, C., Makuch, R. W., et al. Survival in children with perinatally acquired immunodeficiency virus type 1 infection. *N. Engl. J. Med. 321:*1791–1796, 1989.

Selwyn, P., Feingold, A., Hartel, D., et al. Increased risk of bacterial pneumonia in HIV-infected intravenous drug users without AIDS. *AIDS 2:*267–272, 1988.

Selwyn, P., Hartel, D., Lewis, N., et al. A prospective study of the risk of tuberculosis among intravenous drug users with human immunodeficiency virus infection. *N. Engl. J. Med. 320:*545–550, 1989.

Wolinsky, S., Rinaldo, C., Kwok, S., et al. Human immunodeficiency virus type 1 infection a median of 18 months before a diagnostic Western blot. *Ann. Intern. Med. 111:*961–972, 1989.

27 *ROBERT MURPHY, M.D.*

Infection in the Compromised Host

INTRODUCTION

Spectrum of Immunodeficiencies

The earlier chapters of this book emphasized the importance of host defense mechanisms. This chapter describes the various immunodeficiencies and defects that may occur in the host and correlates those specific deficiencies with the types of infection likely to result from them.

Clinical well-being is a relatively temporary condition. As discussed in earlier chapters, many microorganisms are capable of successfully evading the competent host's defense system to cause clinical or subclinical disease. When these defenses have been altered congen-

itally or by acquired conditions or invasive procedures, the *usual* clinical syndromes may occur more frequently or be more virulent, and the *unusual* clinical syndromes caused by what are referred to as opportunistic microorganisms begin to appear. This process can be illustrated by the following two examples.

In 1976, an outbreak of an unusual pneumonia occurred in guests of a hotel in Philadelphia, resulting in 34 deaths in 221 clinical cases of pneumonia. The etiology of this pneumonia was not known for several months until it was discovered ultimately to be due to a previously unidentified bacterium subsequently named *Legionella pneumophila*. Retrospective seroprevalence studies revealed that this was not a new infection at all. Prospective studies have indicated that this organism accounts for 1–15% of all community-acquired pneumonias occurring in presumably normal adult hosts and is associated with lower mortality. The reason for the increased mortality (15%) among the 221 people who developed Legionella pneumonia while visiting Philadelphia was that this group was not a *community* group. It was, in fact, a group with significant numbers of compromised members. Cigarette smoking, heavy alcohol use, underlying chronic lung disease, immunosuppression for a variety of reasons, recent surgery, and advanced age have all been implicated as enhancing the risk for developing Legionella pneumonia. The 1976 outbreak illustrates how a ubiquitous bacterium can cause disease in the normal host, but in the presence of altered host defenses infection occurs with much higher frequency and significantly greater mortality.

The other type of infection in the immunocompromised host is the opportunistic type that occurs *only* in the presence of altered host defenses. For example, in 1981, a cluster of *Pneumocystis carinii* pneumonia (PCP) infections was identified in a group of young, otherwise healthy men. Pneumocystis pneumonia previously had been observed exclusively in severely immunocompromised hosts such as those with underlying hematologic malignancies, tumors, and profound malnutrition. Ultimately, these men were found to be infected concomitantly with the human immunodeficiency virus, type 1 (HIV-1), which resulted in a cellular immune defect which uniquely predisposes to PCP infection.

Host Defenses

A compromised host is defined as an individual with an underlying abnormality or defect in any of the host defense mechanisms that predisposes to infection, whether due to an opportunistic or more common microorganism. The immunodeficiency is associated with specific host defense mechanisms that are either altered or deficient. These may be acquired or, in some cases, congenital and include the following:

1. Granulocytopenia related to underlying hematologic malignancies, cancer chemotherapies, alcohol, and specific bacterial and viral infections
2. Cellular immune dysfunction due to congenital disorders, diseases such as Hodgkin's disease and AIDS, and immunosuppressive therapies administered for leukemia or organ transplants
3. Humoral immune dysfunction due to agammaglobulinemia, diseases such as multiple myeloma and chronic lymphocytic leukemia, and splenectomized patients
4. Foreign body exposure during invasive procedures such as venipuncture, endoscopy, and surgery or by the placement of semipermanent devices such as central venous catheters, grafts, shunts, and artificial joints
5. Tumors and other medical conditions that may block the natural drainage of secretions in vital organs leading to obstruction, abscess formation, and infection

The spectrum of host immunodeficiencies and associated conditions is outlined in Table 27–1. Although primary immune abnormalities, such as sex-linked agammaglobulinemia, have attracted much attention, they occur infrequently. The focus of this chapter is on acquired deficiencies and defects. The subject of AIDS is discussed in considerably more detail in Chapter 26.

TABLE 27–1. *Host Immunodeficiencies and Associated Clinical Syndromes*

Immunodeficiency	Clinical Syndromes
Granulocytopenia	Bacteremia, sepsis, pneumonia, urinary tract infection, sinusitis caused by aerobic gram-negative bacilli, *Staphylococcus* sp., *Candida* sp., and *Aspergillus* sp.
Cellular immune disorders	*Pneumocystis carinii* pneumonia, *Toxoplasma gondii* infection, *Cryptosporidium* enteritis, herpesvirus stomatitis and proctitis, cytomegalovirus retinitis and enteritis, disseminated mycobacterial disease, invasive candidiasis
Humoral immune disorders	Bacteremia, sepsis, meningitis, and pneumonia due to *Streptococcus pneumoniae, Haemophilus influenzae*
Foreign bodies (indwelling central venous catheters)	*Staphylococcus aureus, Staphylococcus epidermidis,* JK group corynebacterium

COMPROMISED HOST DEFENSES

Granulocytopenia

The most thoroughly investigated and a very common immune defect is granulocytopenia, a condition most frequently associated with acute leukemia, aplastic anemia, and intensive myelosuppressive chemotherapy or other drug reactions. The lower the absolute number of circulating granulocytes, the higher the risk for serious bacterial and fungal infections. In acute leukemic patients, this risk becomes most evident when the absolute granulocyte count drops below 100 cells/mm^3 of whole blood. Other associated risks include the duration of granulocytopenia and the rate of granulocyte decline. The more rapidly the granulocyte count drops and the longer it stays suppressed at low levels, the higher the risk for serious infection.

Granulocytopenia associated with other immunodeficiencies, particularly altered mucosal membranes, leads to even higher infection rates. The typical leukemic patient who has recently undergone intensive chemotherapy is also likely to have damaged mucosal surfaces as a direct effect of the agents administered. These patients are also likely to have central venous catheters or similar devices in place. This combination of defects places these patients at extremely high risk for infections that originate from the gastrointestinal tract, oral cavity, lung, or skin. These infections result primarily from organisms that had colonized the host initially and that, under such altered conditions, are able to cause clinical infectious syndromes. Bacteremia (with or without sepsis), pneumonia, cellulitis, and urinary tract infections are quite common in this patient population.

If patients have been hospitalized prior to their development of infection, they are likely to be colonized with a different array of bacteria and fungi that are likely to have antimicrobial resistance patterns reflective of the institutional setting where they were acquired. The hospital-acquired bacteria are usually more resistant to the usual antimicrobial agents employed and vary widely from hospital to hospital. The recent emergence of methicillin-resistant *Staphylococcus aureus* is an example of a microorganism that is primarily hospital-acquired, whereas sensitive strains remain the rule in the community. Knowing the type of organism likely to be colonizing a patient is critical to providing prompt empiric antimicrobial therapy in these high-risk patients.

A lack of granulocytes diminishes the overall inflammatory response that a patient is able to generate. This makes diagnosing infections even more difficult and makes empiric therapeutic decisions even more critical. Table 27–2 outlines the common pathogens affecting granulocytopenic patients.

Cellular Immune Dysfunction

Cellular immune dysfunction refers to the immune defect resulting from the inability of the

TABLE 27–2. *Pathogens Common in Granulocytopenic Patients*

Gram-Negative Bacilli
  Escherichia coli
  Klebsiella sp.
  Pseudomonas aeruginosa
  Enterobacter cloacae
  Serratia sp.
  Proteus sp.
  Salmonella sp.

Gram-Positive Cocci and Bacilli
  Staphylococcus aureus
  S. epidermidis (and other coagulase-negative species)
  Streptococcus pneumoniae
  S. pyogenes
  E. faecalis

Anaerobes
  Bacteroides sp.
  Clostridium sp.
  Fusobacterium sp.

Fungal
  Candida sp.
  Aspergillus sp.

TABLE 27–3. *Most Common Pathogens Associated with Cellular Immune Dysfunction*

Bacteria
  Legionella pneumophila
  Listeria monocytogenes
  Mycobacterium sp.
  Nocardia sp.
  Salmonella sp.

Fungi
  Coccidioides immitis
  Cryptococcus neoformans
  Histoplasma capsulatum
  Pneumocystis carinii

Viruses
  Cytomegalovirus
  Herpes simplex
  Varicella–zoster

Protozoa
  Cryptosporidium
  Toxoplasmosis gondii

Helminths
  Strongyloides stercoralis

---

monocytes/macrophages to kill effectively intracellular pathogens. Common causes of impaired cellular immune function include certain diseases such as Hodgkin's disease and chronic granulomatous disease; drugs such as corticosteroids, cyclosporine, and cytotoxic agents; irradiation; and infection with viruses such as cytomegalovirus and human immunodeficiency virus type 1. The types of drugs commonly used following renal or bone marrow transplantation, acute lymphocytic leukemia, and some collagen vascular diseases are all likely to cause cellular immune dysfunction.

The type of pathogen able to cause clinical infection in the patient with a cellular immune defect is unlikely to be associated with significant disease in the normal host. *Pneumocystis carinii*, originally thought to be a protozoan but now thought to be a fungus, is ubiquitous in nature and infects nearly everyone; however, it produces clinical illness only in those with marked cellular immune deficiencies, such as AIDS or hematologic malignancies. *Toxoplasma gondii*, a protozoan, infects 10–40% of Americans and a substantially larger percentage of residents of developing countries as well as France, but again rarely causes disease unless the host's immune system is markedly impaired. Table 27–3 outlines the pathogens common to hosts with cellular immune dysfunction.

Humoral Immune Dysfunction

Humoral immune dysfunction can be described as the defect in host defenses that results from the impairment of specific antibody binding to respective antigens. This antigen–antibody binding plays an important role in opsonizing microorganisms for phagocytosis and for neutralizing toxins. Multiple myeloma, splenectomy, and other conditions associated with hypogammaglobulinemia, such as chronic lymphocytic leukemia, result in humoral immune dysfunction and a significantly high risk for the development of infections caused by encapsulated pyogenic bacteria. The most common of such infections are those due to *Streptococcus pneumoniae* and *Haemophilus influenzae.*

Multiple myeloma is a disease classically associated with humoral immune dysfunction. Normal immunoglobulin production is suppressed to varying degrees in these patients. As the disease progresses, the degree of suppression of antibody production increases as does the risk for infection with encapsulated organisms.

Splenectomy, whether it be due to trauma, staging in Hodgkin's disease, autosplenectomy as seen in patients with sickle cell anemia, or is congenital, is associated with a decrease in antibody production, particularly of the IgM class, and with a high incidence of infection with the encapsulated bacteria. The severity of infection is also increased (with overwhelming sepsis being a relatively common clinical manifestation), and this appears to be inversely associated with age. Immunization with vaccines directed against *Streptococcus pneumoniae* and *Haemophilus influenzae* is an important part of the treatment of patients who have undergone splenectomy.

Foreign Bodies

Peripheral and central indwelling vascular catheters, surgically implanted prosthetic devices, vascular grafts, and impregnated shunts and pacing devices have become increasingly common in the past two decades. They present a unique dilemma for the practicing clinician. On the one hand, they have become an integral part of the treatment of many patients: administering blood products, chemotherapy, and parenteral hyperalimentation; replacing obstructed veins and arteries; replacing various joints and valves; pacing irregularly beating hearts, among other functions. On the other hand, these foreign bodies serve as the sites that compromise host defenses.

Bacteria and fungi may attach to the foreign body and then, in selected cases, gain access to the bloodstream, causing clinical disease. Treatment is often difficult and requires prolonged intensive antibiotic therapy and/or removal of the infected device.

The type of infection likely to occur in a patient with an indwelling catheter or implanted medical device is likely to depend on the underlying disease and its associated immunodeficiencies, but there is a predilection for certain types of infection. Indwelling central venous catheters commonly used in cancer and AIDS patients are most likely to become infected with gram-positive organisms, usually the coagulase-negative staphylococci. These infections can usually be treated with such parenteral antibiotics as vancomycin and do not necessarily require removal of the infected catheter. Infections with gram-negative bacteria and candida more often necessitate catheter removal as well as aggressive systemic antimicrobial therapy.

Tumors and Other Medical Conditions

Most malignant processes lead to some degree of impaired host defenses. Depending on the nature of the malignancy, any of the major host defense mechanisms may become impaired. In addition to the primary immunodeficiencies associated with specific malignancies, tumors may also obstruct vital organ functions. In the case of bronchogenic carcinoma, obstruction of the bronchus may lead to postobstructive pneumonia. Colon carcinoma may lead to obstruction of the intestinal tract and an acute abdomen with accompanying abscess formation, phlegmon, perforation, or bacteremia. In these situations, the infecting organisms are usually the ones colonizing the site near the tumor. The normal flora found at the site of the tumors are likely to be affected by the hospitalization of the patient, prior antibiotic therapies, and medical and surgical procedures.

Any disease or condition that affects normal function of organ systems may significantly impair the host defenses. Loss of the normal gag reflex and of the ability to cough, as seen in neurologic conditions, usually results in some degree of aspiration of oropharyngeal microflora into the lung, resulting in aspiration pneumonia. Patients with chronic obstructive lung disease, cystic fibrosis, or asthma are all likely to have more frequent and more serious infections in the lung. In the case of cystic fibrosis, pseudomonas pneumonitis may be quite common and associated with frequent relapses. Diabetics are very prone to infection of the feet, partially due to their inability to feel pain and partially due to other alterations in their defense mechanisms.

OPPORTUNISTIC PATHOGENS AND CLINICAL INFECTION

Gram-Positive Bacteria

Both *Staphylococcus aureus* and the coagulase-negative *Staphylococcus epidermidis* have a characteristic propensity for invading skin and adjacent tissues at cutaneous puncture sites as well as at the sites of indwelling intravenous catheters (see Chapter 28). Within 48–72 h, staphylococci are demonstrable on these foreign bodies. Clinical infection occurs with increasing frequency the longer the catheters remain in place. During the last decade, the use of long-term central access devices, such as the external long-term central venous (Hickman) catheters and subcutaneous implantable ports (Port-a-Cath), have become commonplace, particularly in leukemic patients. Infections associated with these devices are relatively common and present as exit site infections of the surrounding skin structures or as intravascular infections with subsequent bacteremia. Although it is relatively easy to change peripheral intravascular catheters when infection is suspected or at least every 24–36 h, replacing the central devices is problematic in, for example, the pancytopenic, very ill leukemic patient. Fortunately, removing these catheters is not always necessary, and parenteral antibiotic therapy is frequently effective, particularly in gram-positive infections. When evaluating patients with unexplained fever, the astute clinician should inspect all intravascular catheter sites thoroughly for signs of infection and should culture the blood. While awaiting results, empiric therapy directed against the more likely pathogens, such as the staphylococci and group JK corynebacteria, is often indicated.

Streptococcus pneumoniae infection, as noted above, occurs at a higher frequency in patients with humoral immune deficiencies, particularly those who have undergone splenectomy (see Chapter 13). Patients with multiple myeloma, who are unable to produce adequate antibody to the streptococcus, are also at risk, and for unclear reasons are more likely to present with pneumococcal pneumonia than with bacteremia or meningitis.

Infections with the gram-positive bacillus, *Listeria monocytogenes,* occur in patients with hematoproliferative disorders, as well as in the elderly and in newborns. In the neonate, infection is usually first manifested as bacteremia, whereas in the leukemic patient, meningitis is more likely. A Gram's stain of the cerebrospinal fluid revealing gram-positive bacilli should alert clinicians to the possibility of listeria infection. In some instances, these organisms may be mistaken for diphtheroids and discarded as contaminants, with disastrous consequences.

Gram-Negative Bacteria

Granulocytopenia is the major risk factor associated with aerobic gram-negative infections. Septicemia is the most common clinical manifestation, and in about one third of such patients, no other source of infection is ever documented. The clinical presentation of this type of infection ranges from low-grade fever to overt septic shock, which is described in more detail in Chapter 34.

The most common pathogen identified in these patients is *Escherichia coli.* When the absolute granulocyte count drops below 500/mm^3 of blood, the risk of *Pseudomonas aeruginosa* bacteremia rises precipitously. *P. aeruginosa* is able to invade the endothelial cell lining of major blood vessels, which may serve as foci of infection. The mortality rate in these infections is considerably higher than that associated with other gram-negative organisms.

One of the complications of gram-negative septicemia is its dissemination to other sites, particularly the lung. When this occurs, mortality rates are generally twice as high as those for bacteremia alone. Early on, the clinical signs of pneumonia may be minimal and the chest radiograph normal. A lack of granulocytes reduces the initial inflammatory response and makes the clinical diagnosis more difficult.

Empiric therapy directed against gram-negative bacteria, including *P. aeruginosa,* is critical in the treatment of the granulocytopenic patient. Prompt initiation of broad-spectrum, usually synergistic combinations of antibiotics (an aminoglycoside plus a beta-lactam or two beta-lactams together), is associated with decreased mortality in this patient population. Interestingly, the relative proportion of gram-negative infections in these patients has declined over the past 10 years, with a corresponding increase in gram-positive infections. Early initiation of empiric antibiotic therapy in febrile patients, oral antibiotic prophylaxis, and the widespread use of indwelling central venous catheters all likely contribute to this shift in types of infections occurring in the granulocytopenic patient.

Acid-Fast Bacteria

Reactivated *Mycobacterium tuberculosis* infection occurs more frequently in patients receiving immunosuppressive therapy, in patients with AIDS, and in malnourished and alcoholic patients (see Chapter 15). Pulmonary disease and disseminated miliary tuberculosis are the most common clinical presentations.

Other mycobacteria are also likely to occur in the compromised patient. In patients with severe underlying chronic lung disease, *Mycobacterium avium* complex (MAC) is associated with an indolent pulmonary process that may persist for many years. It only rarely becomes aggressive and life-threatening. In patients with AIDS, the clinical syndrome caused by MAC is quite different, and the clinical presentation is one of dissemination. Blood and bone marrow cultures are usually positive. Any organ system may be heavily infected with the organism. Currently, MAC is responsible for the most common severe bacterial infection seen in patients with AIDS. As AIDS patients live longer because of improved antiviral and antimicrobial chemotherapy and prophylaxis, there will likely be an increase in incidence of infection related to the dissemination of MAC. This infection is very difficult to treat and requires three- to five-drug regimens that are not tolerated well by many patients.

Despite the fact that *Nocardia asteroides* is a true bacterium, its acid-fast staining characteristic and the morphologic shape of the organism had led to its erroneous classification as a fungus. At times, it may be confused with mycobacteria on stained smears; however, *N. asteroides* causes a very different type of disease, consisting of abscess formation, especially in the lung, which is the organ initially infected. Spread of the organism occurs via the bloodstream and commonly results in abscess formation in the brain, and less frequently, in skin, soft tissues, and other internal organs. The typical patient infected with nocardia is receiving long-term maintenance immunosuppressive therapy.

Protozoans

Defects in cell-mediated immunity are associated with infections with two protozoans, *Toxoplasma gondii* and *Cryptosporidium*. *Pneumocystis carinii,* originally considered a protozoan, is now thought to be a fungus, and is discussed separately.

Toxoplasma infects many animals worldwide. The definitive host is the cat, which appears to be responsible for the bulk of transmission to other animals as well as to humans. *Toxoplasma gondii* infection appears in four clinical settings: (1) an asymptomatic infection of older children and adults from ingestion of contaminated undercooked meat or vegetables; (2) an acute infection in pregnant women, in whom transmission to the fetus results in congenital infection of the fetus; (3) in persons receiving long-term immunosuppressive drugs, as in transplant recipients; and (4) in persons with the marked cell-mediated immunodeficiency associated with AIDS.

In the competent host, acute infection with toxoplasma is infrequently associated with any symptoms. When present, they usually consist of lymphadenopathy and mononucleosis-like symptoms. The clinical course is self-limited and benign. In the compromised host, the clinical picture is quite different. In this situation, *T. gondii* has a striking propensity to invade and establish persistent infection in the brain. Toxoplasmic encephalitis presents clinically with findings such as cranial nerve abnormalities, focal seizures, mental status changes, or localized headache. Computerized tomographic or magnetic resonance imaging of the brain usually reveals several space-occupying vascular lesions typical of *T. gondii*. The cerebrospinal fluid may be normal.

Ocular toxoplasmosis presents as chorioretinitis, mostly as a result of congenital infection. Patients are usually asymptomatic until reaching their 20s and 30s. Relapse of toxoplasmic chorioretinitis may occur during periods of immunosuppression associated with the chemotherapy given for various malignancies.

Cryptosporidium is a protozoan that may cause diarrhea in infected turkeys, cattle, sheep, and humans. In the competent host, disease is self-limited and requires no specific therapy. In the presence of severe cell-mediated immunodeficiency, such as AIDS, the diarrhea can be relentless and chronic, resulting in profound malnutrition, dehydration, electrolyte imbalances, and even death. The diagnosis of cryptosporidiosis is made by examining the stool. The cryptosporidial oocysts characteristically take up acid-fast stain. Unfortunately, there is no antimicrobial treatment effective against

Cryptosporidium. Limited experience with spiramycin and diclazuril has not been promising.

Fungi

Pneumocystis carinii, a fungus-like organism, formerly classified as a protozoan, is able to cause pneumonia and, rarely, other organ system infections in the host with compromised cell-mediated immunity. *P. carinii* pneumonia (PCP) is the most common, severe, life-threatening infection among AIDS patients in the United States (Fig. 27–1). The organism is ubiquitous in nature and infects three fourths of children by age 4. A small percentage of self-limited infantile pneumonitis is due to pneumocystis. However, severe clinical infection requires profound immunosuppression. Adults and children at risk for this infection include patients with hematologic malignancies, those with severe malnutrition, and patients with AIDS.

The typical clinical presentation of PCP in the compromised host includes fever, nonproductive cough, and shortness of breath or chest tightness. Symptoms may be present for days to months, particularly in AIDS patients. Chest radiographs classically reveal diffuse, interstitial processes. Arterial blood gases demonstrate hypoxia. In early cases, chest radiographs may be normal. In patients with suspected disease and a normal chest radiograph, aggressive evaluation should continue. When PCP is suspected, sputum should be obtained for cytologic examination. Appropriate specimens may be generated after 3% saline mist inhalation for 20–40 min. This is a so-called induced sputum. In the event this sample is negative, fiberoptic bronchoscopy with lavage and transbronchial biopsy usually results in the correct diagnosis. Rarely, an open lung biopsy may have to be considered if bronchoscopy is negative and the clinical diagnosis remains in question.

PCP is fatal if not treated, and when sus-

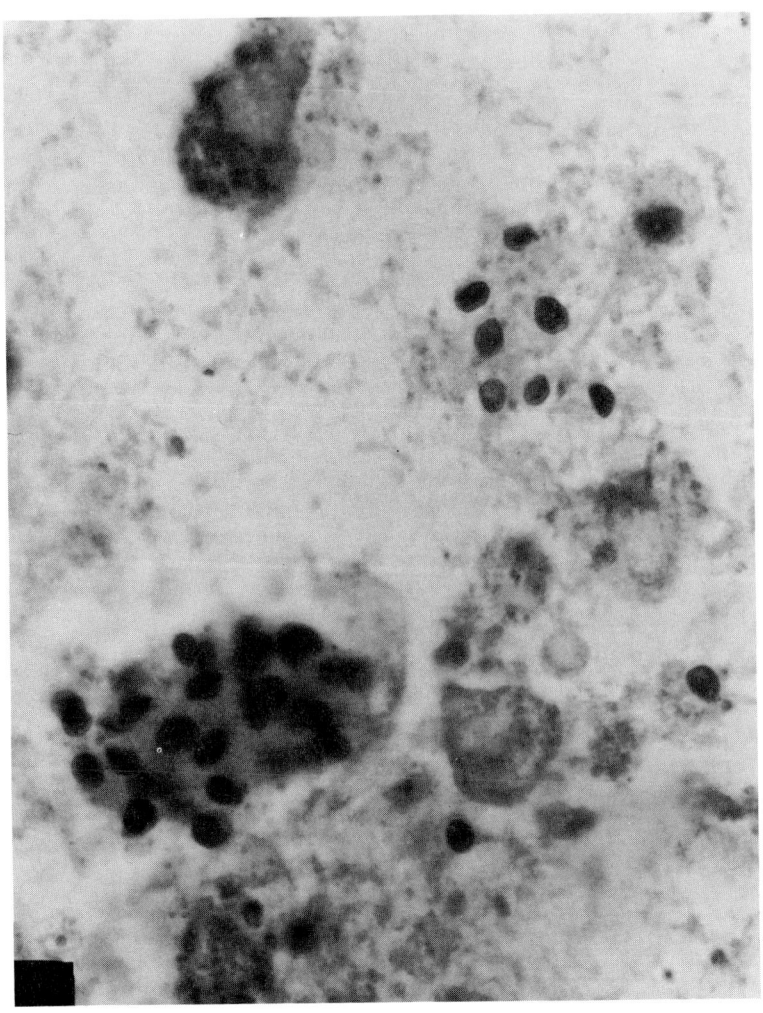

Figure 27–1. Section of autopsy lung specimen from an AIDS patient, stained with Gomori's and illustrating Pneumocystis carinii *microorganisms within an alveolus filled with a protein-rich intraalveolar menstruum. Note the stained, somewhat elliptical, cyst-like structures arranged in tight or loose aggregates. Cystic forms of* P. carinii *are thought to initially increase numerically within alveolar septa; maturing trophozoites eventually break out of the cysts, spilling into the alveolar spaces. Also note inconspicuous host inflammatory response, in terms of only slight infiltration by mononuclear cells/macrophages, even at this terminal phase of the pulmonary infection. (Photomicrograph × 800 provided through the kindness of Dr. M. D. Rowland and Dr. W. E. Farrar, Medical University of South Carolina, Charleston, South Carolina.)*

pected, empiric therapy with either pentamidine or trimethoprim-sulfamethoxazole is indicated until the diagnosis can be confirmed. Significant adverse reactions are associated with both of these regimens in the HIV-1 infected host. To date, trimetrexate, dapsone-trimethoprim, and clindamycin-primaquine have all been used with some success in limited studies in patients who are intolerant of the standard regimens.

Relapse of PCP is common in the face of persistent immunodeficiency; however, relapse rates can be significantly reduced if prophylactic doses of trimethoprim-sulfamethoxazole or monthly inhaled aerosol pentamidine is taken. In patients who are receiving aerosol pentamidine prophylaxis for PCP, the clinical presentation of pneumonitis may be atypical. Normal radiographs and upper lobe disease are more common. Induced sputum examinations and fiberoptic bronchoscopy are more likely to yield negative results even when clinical disease is present.

Infection with *Cryptococcus neoformans,* a true fungus, has long been associated with malignant lymphoma, especially Hodgkin's disease. Dissemination of cryptococcus occurs by the fecal droppings of pigeons, which harbor the organism, with subsequent inhalation of viable fungus by humans and development of symptomatic or asymptomatic pulmonary infection (Fig. 27–2). Hematogenous spread from the lungs leads to metastatic disease in a variety of organ systems. However, there is a propensity for infection of the central nervous system. The most common clinical manifestation of disseminated cryptococcal disease is that of relatively slowly evolving meningitis in a patient with underlying lymphoma or AIDS. Symptoms range from mild headache to obtundation with fever and coma. The cerebrospinal fluid is mostly remarkable for its rather bland characteristics; often there are no inflammatory cells whatsoever. There usually are viable organisms seen in the India ink preparation (Fig. 27–3), the cryptococcal capsular polysaccharide antigen, as measured by a relatively sensitive latex agglutination test, is uniformly present, and the fungal culture is positive. Management of cryptococcal disease is with the rather toxic antifungal agent amphotericin B. In 1990, oral fluconazole, an azole derivative, was approved for use in cryptococcal disease. Fluconazole appears considerably less toxic than amphotericin B and is effective in managing milder forms of acute disease as well as in maintenance therapy following initial treatment (see Chapter 16).

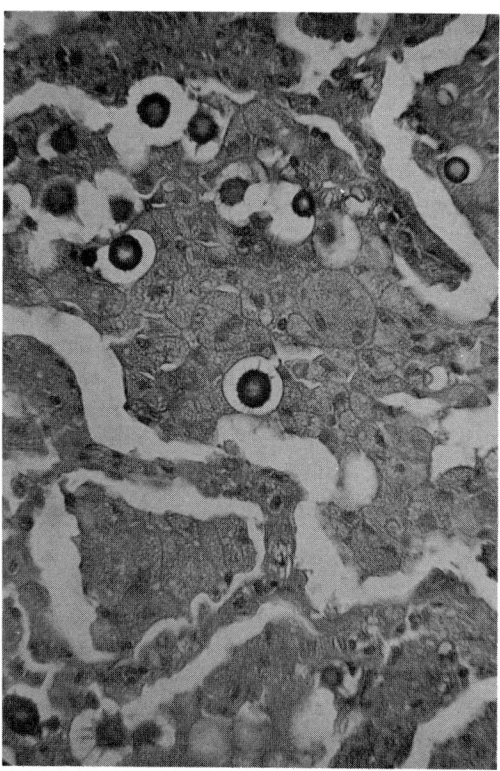

Figure 27–2. A section of a lobe of the lung removed at the time of surgical exploration for a presumed malignancy involving the lower right lung of a middle-aged male with a history of heavy cigarette smoking. Morphologic details of the cryptococcal yeast cells are seen especially well with the methenamine-silver stain used in this instance. The patient made a complete and uneventful recovery. Lack of demonstrable involvement of any other organ system led to a decision to withhold treatment with amphotericin B after the diagnosis of cryptococcal infection of the lung was established postoperatively. Fungi identified as Cryptococcus neoformans *were isolated from the surgically removed lung specimen. The only evidence of altered host defense in this patient was a persistently low serum concentration of gamma globulin.*

Candida albicans and *Aspergillus* sp. are common offending fungal pathogens associated with granulocytopenia and with cellular immunodeficiencies (see Chapter 25). In granulocytopenic patients, these infections are likely to be life-threatening. Factors predisposing to serious fungal infections include prolonged broad-spectrum antimicrobial therapy, indwelling intravascular catheters, prolonged hospitalization, corticosteroid therapy, and hyperalimentation—all factors common in the severely ill cancer patient.

One of the major practical problems with these fungal infections is that isolation of the organisms is not sufficient evidence to document clinical infection. These fungi commonly colonize mucosal surfaces throughout the body.

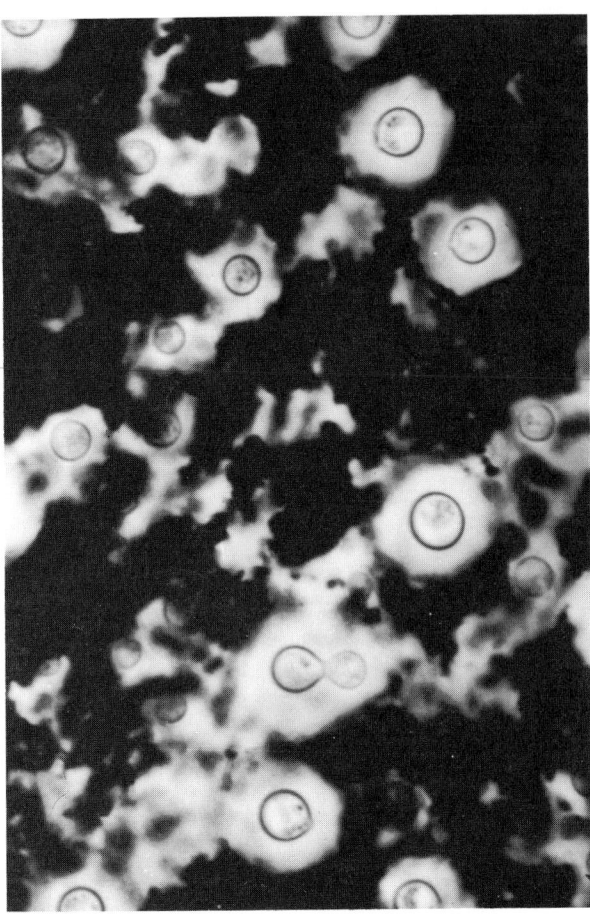

Figure 27–3. Cerebrospinal fluid sediment (from a 36-year-old male) mixed with India ink illustrates heavily encapsulated yeast cells, one of which is in the process of budding. Clinical signs of meningitis prompted hospitalization of this patient. Initial cerebrospinal fluid findings included a total cell count of 340 cells/mm³; glucose was 32 mg/100 mL and protein was 128 mg/100 mL. Culture of the cerebrospinal fluid yielded a yeast identified as Cryptococcus neoformans. *The history revealed that 8 months previously the patient had received a renal allograft for endstage chronic glomerulonephritis. Allograft function has been maintained by an immunosuppressive regimen consisting of azathioprine and prednisone.*

Documenting invasive disease is more difficult. A high index of suspicion is warranted in treating the granulocytopenic cancer patient. Empiric antifungal therapy with amphotericin B is indicated when no other source of fever or infection is documented in patients who are already receiving antibiotic therapy without apparent response. Superinfection with *Aspergillus* sp. may be more common in patients receiving oral ketoconazole or fluconazole, because neither of these agents is effective in treating or preventing aspergillosis.

Viruses

Three DNA viruses commonly cause infection in immunocompromised patients, particularly those receiving long-term immunosuppressive therapy for malignancies or as a result of organ transplantation and in patients with AIDS. These viruses are herpes simplex virus, the varicella–zoster virus, and the cytomegalovirus. All three are capable of producing disseminated disease.

Herpes simplex usually presents as an extensive, cutaneous infection that may spread locally to involve the gastrointestinal tract, particularly the esophagus and the rectum. These infections actually represent reactivation. In the presence of persistent immunosuppression, the infection may become chronic.

Varicella–zoster is also associated with extensive local dermatomal eruptions, and, in severe cases, involves multiple dermatomal areas. Reactivated disease may disseminate widely. Immunocompromised patients who have never experienced childhood varicella infection are highly susceptible to it and may experience widely disseminated disease involving the lungs as well. Exposure of the immunocompromised child or susceptible adult to varicella warrants therapy with concentrated varicella–zoster immunoglobulin (VZIG) because of the relatively high mortality associated with these infections.

Cytomegalovirus (CMV) infection may involve multiple organ systems. Acute infection may mimic infectious mononucleosis or hepatitis. In organ transplant patients receiving immunosuppressive agents, pneumonia and hepatitis are not uncommon clinical manifestations. In AIDS patients, retinitis and gastrointestinal involvement are the more common presentations.

The most common clinical presentation of CMV infection in the compromised host is that of a mononucleosis-like syndrome with fever, myalgias, and hepatosplenomegaly. The next most common syndrome is that of pneumonia. Typically the pneumonia due to CMV is an interstitial process associated with fever and nonproductive cough. Symptoms may be indistinguishable from PCP pneumonia. The onset of CMV pneumonitis is typically 6–8 weeks following organ transplant. The severity of disease is generally related to the severity of the immunosuppression. No effective therapy exists for the treatment of CMV pneumonitis; ganciclovir with intravenous gamma globulin is the best option. Other organ systems infected with CMV may respond to intravenous ganciclovir therapy. This is particularly true in regard to treating CMV retinitis in AIDS patients.

DIAGNOSTIC APPROACHES

The diagnosis of infection in the compromised host is often hindered because of the lack of inflammatory and other host responses. A lack of granulocytes often causes late-appearing or atypical clinical manifestations of disease. If this results in delayed initiation of appropriate antiinfective therapy, this can be catastrophic for the patient. This is a tragic outcome for patients who could be cured potentially with appropriate antimicrobial drugs. A persistent and aggressive diagnostic approach is warranted in immunosuppressed patients with signs of potential infection. Available serologic, microbiologic, and radiographic procedures should be employed, as well as invasive and noninvasive procedures, as necessary. It must be kept in mind that identification of certain pathogens, such as *Candida* sp., is in itself not confirmation of a significant fungal infection. This type of infection often requires histologic proof of tissue invasion prior to committing the patient to weeks or months of potentially toxic therapies.

One of the most common sites of infection in the compromised host is the lung. The clinical setting usually involves a granulocytopenic patient receiving chemotherapy who develops fever and an increasing respiratory rate. Early on, the patient may not even complain of shortness of breath and the chest radiograph may be normal; however, hypoxemia is usually present.

Routine sputum cultures are generally unhelpful and reveal only the presence of normal microflora. Induced sputum and blood cultures are often negative, particularly if empiric antibiotics have been started, as is often necessary. In this situation, the diagnostic and therapeutic possibilities are numerous. At a minimum, induced sputum cultures and smears should be obtained for bacteria, fungi, and acid-fast organisms. Cultures for *Legionella pneumophila* and direct smears for *Pneumocystis carinii* should be obtained as well. Serologic studies for Legionella, histoplasmosis, coccidioidomycosis, and blastomycosis are indicated. Broad-spectrum antimicrobial therapy with at least two agents is indicated initially. These agents should provide coverage for the usual pathogens associated with the underlying condition. In granulocytopenic cancer patients this therapeutic regimen means including agents effective against pseudomonas. If therapy is not successful and improvement is not observed in the first 2 days, further invasive procedures such as bronchoscopy and transbronchial biopsy should be considered. At this point, the antibiotic regimen should be expanded to include coverage for Legionella and pneumocystis. After 4 days, this coverage needs to be extended to include antifungal therapy as well. If a diagnosis is still not forthcoming and the patient is deteriorating, open lung biopsy is indicated. Procrastination and temporizing may result in a lost opportunity to diagnose a potentially reversible infectious process.

THERAPEUTIC APPROACHES

Broad-spectrum antimicrobial therapy is the key to treating the clinically ill compromised host. The mainstay of such treatment, especially in febrile, granulocytopenic patients, includes at least two bactericidal antibiotics effective against pseudomonas and other aerobic bacteria. An aminoglycoside plus an antipseudomonal beta-lactam antibiotic or two antipseudomonal beta-lactams are the usual initial choices. Indwelling central venous catheters can usually be left in place unless gram-negative, *Candida, Corynebacterium,* or *Bacillus* sp. are recovered from blood or line site. If a diagnosis cannot be confirmed because the patient is too ill to undergo the procedures required, expansion of the antimicrobial regimen may be required, the specific choices depending on the site of suspected infection. If lesions are present that may represent typical or atypical viral infection, antiviral therapy should be initiated as well. Empiric antiviral therapy without some clinical suspicion is not indicated.

Granulocyte transfusions can provide only short-term benefit to the critically ill granulocytopenic patient. Their use should be limited to controlling known bacterial infection in those patients receiving appropriate antibiotics who continue to fail to respond to therapy.

Specific monoclonal antibody therapy is currently being investigated in controlled trials and may add to the management of some of the infections seen in these compromised hosts.

CASE HISTORY

A 20-year-old male restaurant worker presented to his local emergency room complaining of shortness of breath and increasing edema of the lower extremities. His past medical history was remarkable for aplastic anemia at age 7 while living in St. Louis. He had a partial remission and was able to complete high school and to work. During the past 3 years, he required periodic blood and platelet transfusions. He also underwent several experimental therapies for anemia at various medical centers in the Chicago area as well as in Los Angeles. He was considering a bone marrow transplant at the time of his current hospitalization.

Physical examination revealed a grossly edematous 20-year-old male who appeared older than his stated age and who was in mild respiratory distress. His temperature was 102.1°F, pulse 120 and regular, respiratory rate 28/min, and blood pressure 100/60 mm Hg. Soft palatal and conjunctival petechiae were present. The lung examination was remarkable for bilateral rales halfway up both fields. The heart examination revealed sinus tachycardia and a grade III systolic murmur. There was 2 + pitting edema of both lower extremities and in the sacral area. There were two tender, swollen areas on the right lateral thigh measuring 4 × 6 cm. The overlying skin was normal. The remainder of the examination was normal.

The hemoglobin was 3.9 gm/dL; WBC was 1100/mm³ with a granulocyte count of 400/mm³. Platelets were 12,000/mm³. The serum transaminase levels were two times the upper limits of normal. Chest radiograph revealed bilateral alveolar and interstitial infiltrates,

predominantly of the lower lobes. The echocardiogram findings were negative.

Blood cultures on admission grew *Staphylococcus aureus*, methicillin-sensitive. A sputum culture grew normal flora as well as *S. aureus*. On the fifth hospital day, one of the tender nodules on his leg was aspirated by needle. The Gram's stain revealed gram-positive cocci in clusters; however, the culture was negative for growth.

The patient was initially treated with an aminoglycoside and an antipseudomonal beta-lactam antibiotic. He was transfused with packed red blood cells and platelets. Diuretics were given with gradual improvement of the respiratory complaints and pitting edema. When culture results became available, a primary antistaphylococcal agent was added to his regimen. Despite significant clinical improvement, he remained febrile and dependent on multiple blood product transfusions. He developed multiple additional nodules in other areas of the body similar to the ones on his leg. Several of the nodules developed into frank abscesses and required surgical drainage. He was treated with parenteral antibiotics for 2 months and was discharged home to receive an oral antistaphylococcal antibiotic. He was evaluated for a possible bone marrow transplant but was rejected because his infection was never completely controlled. One month after discharge from the hospital, he developed high spiking fevers with rigors and died as a consequence of septic shock.

CASE DISCUSSION

This young man had a chronic illness characterized by an inability to produce significant quantities of blood components. For the last 3 years of his life, he was able to function surprisingly well despite severe pancytopenia. On his final admission to the hospital, he had a widely disseminated staphylococcal infection and high-output cardiac failure. It was most likely that he did not have bacterial pneumonia, and his rather rapid clinical response to diuretics was more likely related to congestive heart failure.

He had a relentless bacterial infection that disseminated to his muscles. He was unable to form abscesses except in a few areas because of chronic granulocytopenia. It is somewhat surprising that he never developed a gram-negative infection; however, these infections are associated more often with rapid drops in granulocyte count and particularly with absolute granulocyte levels below 100/mm³. He ultimately died because his underlying disease never improved. His last hope for remission or cure with bone marrow transplantation was dashed by his incurable infection.

REFERENCES

Books

Grieco, M. H., ed. *Infections in the Immunocompromised Host.* New York: Yorke Medical Books, 1980.

Mandell, G. L., Douglas, R. G., Bennett, J. E., eds. *Principles and Practice of Infectious Diseases.* 3rd ed. New York: Churchill Livingstone, 1990.

Rubin, R. H., and Young, L. S., eds. *Clinical Approach to Infection in the Compromised Host.* 2nd ed. New York: Plenum Press, 1988.

Sherris, J. C., ed. *Medical Microbiology.* 2nd ed. New York: Elsevier, 1990.

Articles

Bennett, J. E. Rapid diagnosis of candidiasis and aspergillosis. *Rev. Infect. Dis. 9:*398–402, 1987.

Chaisson, R. E., and Slutkin, G. Tuberculosis and human immunodeficiency virus infection. *J. Infect. Dis. 159:*96–100, 1989.

Corey, L. C., and Spear, P. G. Infections with herpes simplex viruses. *N. Engl. J. Med. 314:*686–691, 749–757, 1986.

Hughes, W. T., Armstrong, D., Bodey, G. P., et al. Guidelines for the use of antimicrobial agents in neutropenic patients with unexplained fever. *J. Infect. Dis. 161:*381–396, 1990.

Mills, J. *Pneumocystis carinii* and *Toxoplasma gondii* infections in patients with AIDS. *Rev. Infect. Dis. 8:*1001–1011, 1986.

O'Hanley, P., Easaw, J., Rugo, H., et al. Infectious disease management of adult leukemic patients undergoing chemotherapy: 1982 to 1986 experience at Stanford University Hospital. *Am. J. Med. 87:*605–613, 1989.

Strauss, S. E. Varicella–zoster virus infection. *Ann. Intern. Med. 108:*221–237, 1988.

Winn, W. C., Jr. Legionnaires disease: Historical perspective. *Clin. Microbiol. Rev. 1:*60–81, 1988.

Woods, G. L., and Washington, J. A., II. Mycobacteria other than *Mycobacterium tuberculosis. Rev. Infect. Dis. 9:*275–294, 1987.

Nosocomial Infections

INTRODUCTION

Hospital-acquired, or nosocomial, infections represent an increasing problem in the United States. The composition of hospital populations has changed under pressure of policy and insurance requirements; patients admitted to hospital are more acutely ill, require more medical and surgical intervention, and are at increased risk of developing infection. It is estimated that approximately 5% of patients acquire infection while hospitalized (Table 28–1).

These infections involve all of the major organ systems, can result in bacteremia, and are commonly lethal, especially in elderly debilitated patients. Nosocomial urinary tract infections alone are thought to result in more than 50,000 deaths per year. This chapter reviews the epidemiology, etiology, management of, and techniques for preventing nosocomial infections.

EPIDEMIOLOGY

The most common nosocomial infection involves the urinary tract and generally follows urologic manipulation, including use of indwelling urinary catheters. Few nosocomial urinary tract infections result in bacteremia except in the presence of obstruction. Although women more frequently are infected, elderly men more commonly develop bacteremia.

Pneumonia represents an especially troublesome form of nosocomial infection, and elderly or very young patients are at high risk. Other determinants of predisposition to infection include depressed mental status leading to aspiration of pharyngeal flora, and endotracheal intubation. During the postoperative period patients are extremely vulnerable to pulmonary infection. The patient is often immobile (which favors aspiration); not ventilating fully; and receiving medication for pain that impairs coughing, the cough reflex, and swallowing. Thoracic or high abdominal incisions, antecedent respiratory infections, and obesity also add to the risk. Finally, therapeutic reduction of gastric acidity increases the risk of nosocomial pneumonia.

Skin and soft tissue infections occur in the hospital as a result of immobilization and development of pressure sores (decubitus ulcers) or invasive procedures that violate the integrity of the skin (wound infections). Few decubitus ulcers or wound infections are associated with bacteremia. At highest risk for this potentially

TABLE 28–1. *Nosocomial Infections*

Site	Risk
Urinary tract	Instrumentation
	Diabetes
Pulmonary	Intubation
	Depressed cough
	Congestive heart failure
Skin and soft tissue	Immobilization
	Pressure
	Invasive procedures
	Burns and wounds
	Diabetes
	Ischemia and/or necrosis
Primary bacteremia	Intravascular lines
	Vascular shunts

lethal complication are immobile elderly patients and patients who have just had bowel, rectal, or urologic surgery.

Primary bacteremia generally occurs in hospitalized patients with central indwelling intravenous or intraarterial lines. The prevalence of infection in association with use of intravascular catheters is increased with prolonged placement of the catheter. These infections account for one fifth of bacteremic nosocomial infections but represent only 3% of all nosocomial infections.

ETIOLOGY

Shortly after penicillin became widely available, penicillin-resistant *Staphylococcus aureus* was noted to be a cause of infection in hospitalized patients. By the mid 1950s, nosocomial *S. aureus* infection, due to the specific phage type 80/81, was a worldwide problem that resulted in the closure of some surgical and neonatal units and the development of infection control programs. Coincident with the introduction of penicillinase-resistant penicillins the frequency of these infections decreased and nosocomial infections due to aerobic gram-negative bacilli became a major problem. The past 10 years has seen the reemergence of *S. aureus* (now methicillin-resistant), enterococcal species, fungi, and, in specific situations, viruses as the cause of nosocomial infection problems. The majority of nosocomial infections continue to be caused by aerobic gram-negative bacilli; however, in specific situations, such as following colonic surgery, anaerobic organisms produce hospital-acquired infections (Table 28–2).

The aerobic gram-negative bacilli associated with nosocomial infection include enteric bacilli, such as *Escherichia coli, Proteus mirabilis, Klebsiella,* and *Enterobacter* species. *Serratia marcescens* and *Pseudomonas* species also are frequently isolated in specific clinical situations. Members of the *Bacteroides* genus are most often the anaerobic organisms causing nosocomial infection. Rarely, *Clostridium* species and group A streptococci cause serious infections of surgical wounds. *S. aureus* and *S. epidermidis* are associated with infection occurring with intravenous catheter use and intraarterial monitoring.

The etiology of a nosocomial infection often can be suspected from the location of the infection or the underlying clinical problem. Examples include the association of staphylococci with intravascular devices, *Pseudomonas aeruginosa*

TABLE 28–2. *Etiology of Nosocomial Infections*

Gram-positive bacteria
  Staphylococcus aureus (methicillin-resistant)
  Coagulase-negative staphylococci
  Enterococci

Gram-negative bacteria
  Escherichia coli
  Proteus mirabilis
  Klebsiella/Enterobacter/Serratia sp.
  Pseudomonas sp.
  Bacteroides sp.

Fungi
  Candida sp.
  Aspergillus sp.

Virus
  Hepatitis B
  Hepatitis C
  Human immunodeficiency virus
  Cytomegalovirus
  Respiratory viruses
  Herpes simplex

in patients with third-degree burns and in patients with neutropenia, and *Enterococcus faecalis,* which commonly infects patients receiving enhanced-spectrum cephalosporins. There is a well-recognized association of candida infection in patients with a disrupted gastrointestinal tract who are receiving multiple antibiotics or parenteral hyperalimentation. Up to 1% of babies in the intensive care unit at Children's Memorial Hospital in Chicago develop candidemia in association with gastrointestinal surgery, broad-spectrum antibiotics, indwelling lines, and hyperalimentation. Intraabdominal or pelvic infections are commonly caused by both aerobic and anaerobic organisms, such as *Bacteroides* species. Enteric infection with *Clostridium difficile,* an anaerobic spore-forming organism which produces an enterotoxin, occurs in hospitalized patients receiving antibiotics, especially clindamycin, penicillins, or cephalosporins, and chemotherapy for neoplastic disease. It is felt that the majority of cases are due to overgrowth of endogenous organisms, but there have been documented outbreaks that have occurred as a result of cross-infection in hospitals.

Viral infections, as well as bacterial and fungal infections, can occur during hospitalization. A major cause of such infections in adults is the transfusion of blood. The three agents of most concern are hepatitis C (see Chapter 21), the cause of many cases of non-A, non-B hepatitis; cytomegalovirus (see Chapter 10), which causes a mononucleosis-like syndrome in normal hosts and severe pneumonitis or hepatitis in immunocompromised patients; and human immunodeficiency virus (HIV) (see Chapter 26), the cause of the acquired immunodeficiency syndrome (AIDS). The vast majority of nosocomial viral infections, however, occur in pediatric populations and are primarily caused by the respiratory agents, including respiratory syncytial virus, influenza, parainfluenza, adenovirus, rhinovirus, as well as varicella and measles. Hospital outbreaks of these infections reflect their presence in the community and are the result of patient contact with infected hospital staff or visitors. Children at risk are those who lack specific immunity to these agents, rather than individuals predisposed to infection by therapy or underlying disease. Nosocomial varicella–zoster virus infection, however, may produce severe, often fatal, infection in immunocompromised nonimmune children or adults. It is highly contagious, producing infection in 80% of nonimmune individuals. Outbreaks can occur as a result of contact with patients or staff with unrecognized chicken pox or herpes zoster.

A major advance in determining whether a cluster of nosocomial infections is due to a single organism has resulted from the use of molecular techniques to identify the causative agents. In the past, epidemiologists used antibiotic susceptibility patterns, phage typing of *S. aureus,* and other phenotypic characteristics of the microbe to demonstrate that an outbreak was due to a single strain of the bacteria. However, molecular techniques identify genetic or enzymatic characteristics of isolates, enabling investigators to document that the outbreak in a unit or an institution is the result of the spread of a single organism from patient to patient or from staff to patients.

PATHOGENESIS

Nosocomial infections generally occur when natural barriers to microbial invasion are violated or when the patient is debilitated. The skin, mucous membranes of the gastrointestinal tract, urinary tract, and upper airway act as natural barriers to the establishment of infection. Much of modern therapy, including surgery and utilization of techniques to support life, such as nasotracheal intubation or intravascular catheters, violates these barriers. Nasogastric tubes, and reduction of gastric acidity through the use of H_2 blockers or antacids, also decrease the efficiency of important defense barriers. In addition, the normal flora of the oropharynx and lower intestinal tract is altered through elimination of oral intake or use of antibiotics, enhancing colonization of these locations by potential pathogens.

Control of the majority of bacterial infections depends upon an adequate number of normally functioning polymorphonuclear leukocytes (PMNs) and the effective interaction of these phagocytes with the serum opsonins, complement, and antibody. A number of diseases and therapies interfere with this primary systemic mechanism of host response to microbial invasion (see Chapter 3).

Advanced age is associated with an increased susceptibility to nosocomial infection. This has been well documented in a number of published series. A specific age-related defect in the inflammatory response, however, has been difficult to identify. A reasonable explanation for the association of age and nosocomial infection is the prevalence of such diseases as cancer, diabetes, and cerebrovascular disease in the elderly. All of these diseases require use of therapy that alters PMN number, are associated with altered PMN function, or result in the use of support systems which bypass natural barriers. For instance, hematologic malignancies are treated with cytotoxic agents that induce bone marrow suppression or are associated themselves with hypogammaglobulinemia. Solid tumors obstruct organs, resulting in undrained secretions that, when infected, result in abscess formation or bacteremia. Specific tumors, such as bronchogenic carcinoma and Hodgkin's lymphoma, are associated with serum inhibitors of PMN chemotaxis, an important component of the inflammatory response. Corticosteroid therapy used in therapy of a number of neoplastic conditions also interferes with PMN adherence to endothelial cells, resulting in poor delivery of the phagocytes to the locus of infection in tissue. Diabetes is associated with defective PMN chemotaxis and, in association with ketoacidosis, deficient intracellular killing of bacteria, such as *Staphylococcus aureus*. Although it is difficult to document that infections occur with greater frequency in diabetics, the infections that do occur result in an increased morbidity and mortality.

Nosocomial pneumonia with aerobic gram-negative bacilli is associated with tracheal intubation, use of antibiotics, reduction of gastric acidity, and augmented acuity of illness, all of which are associated with colonization of the upper airway or tracheal tube with these organisms. Decreased gag and cough reflexes enhance the possibility of aspiration of these organisms and ultimate development of pneumonia. A specific nosocomial pneumonia that occurs in normal as well as in individuals with an altered immune response is that due to *Legionella* species. Legionella pneumonia occurring in hospitals has been especially troublesome in oncology and transplant units. This organism is capable of surviving and replicating in any standing water and is aerosolized from water taps and shower heads.

MANAGEMENT

Nosocomial infections are defined as those developing after the patient has been hospitalized for longer than the incubation time of the agent. For bacterial infections this is usually 3 days after entry into the hospital. The classic signs of infection, tachycardia, fever, and toxicity, can be muted by therapy or attributed to the admitting illness. Therefore, the diagnosis requires that the physician have a high degree of suspicion for patients at greatest risk of acquiring nosocomial infection. All postoperative patients, those who are intubated, and those in whom an intravascular device or urinary catheter is placed should be considered as susceptible. Additions to this high-risk group of patients are those receiving cytotoxic therapy, intravenous infusions which can be contaminated in manufacture or preparation, antibiotics, or glucocorticosteroids.

As mentioned, clinical signs and symptoms can be incomplete. Unexplained fever or hypothermia, change in mental or respiratory status, and development of hypotension should stimulate a search for infection. Laboratory findings in association with these signs include either leukocytosis or leukopenia, thrombocytopenia, or evidence of disseminated intravascular coagulation. These clinical or laboratory alterations can occur together or alone in both bacteremic and nonbacteremic infections.

When a hospital infection is suspected, two blood cultures separated by at least 10–15-min intervals should be obtained. A thorough review of the hospital course, therapy, and invasive intervention, plus a complete physical examination, should be performed. If possible, Gram's stain and culture of urine, sputum, draining secretions, or pus should be performed. A chest x-ray can often be useful. Ultrasonography and computerized tomography (CT) can be extremely helpful in specific situations. If a focus of infection can be identified that can be removed or drained this should be done expeditiously. In patients about whom there is any

suspicion of central nervous system involvement, including those having undergone neurosurgery, examination of the cerebrospinal fluid is mandatory. It may be necessary to use imaging techniques, such as cerebral CT, to determine if there is an intracerebral mass producing increased intracranial pressure before performing a lumbar puncture. In the neutropenic patient, empiric antibiotics should be initiated immediately after obtaining blood cultures. Patients with evidence of septic shock should be treated immediately. In addition to antibiotics, reconstitution of the intravascular volume with fluid replacement is necessary. In less acutely ill patients, therapy can be delayed until the evaluation is completed.

The choice of empiric antibiotics can be based upon the organisms frequently isolated in a specific hospital or unit. For example, in some oncology units, gentamicin-resistant *Pseudomonas aeruginosa* are frequent causes of infection in neutropenic patients. Therefore therapy with another aminoglycoside (amikacin, tobramycin) plus an enhanced-spectrum penicillin or cephalosporin effective against this gram-negative bacilli would be the treatment of choice. In patients whose infection is intraabdominal, therapy should include antibiotics with activity against the anaerobe *Bacteroides fragilis* in addition to aerobic enteric bacilli. Methicillin-resistant *Staphylococcus aureus* should be suspected in patients with sepsis who have an indwelling intravenous catheter, as the prevalence of such resistant organisms is increasing in hospitals.

The dose and interval of antibiotic therapy is determined by the physiologic state of the patient. Thus, in patients with renal insufficiency, the interval between doses of aminoglycoside is prolonged. The same strategy is required for all agents that are excreted by the kidneys, such as vancomycin, penicillins, and cephalosporins. It is important to remember that some decrease in renal function is present in the majority of elderly patients even with a normal serum creatinine. If empiric antibiotic therapy is initiated, results of culture should be used to select later the safest and most effective antibiotic or combination of antibiotics to complete the treatment.

The duration of treatment is dependent upon the course of the nosocomial infection, the clinical condition of the patient, and the responses to therapy. Bacteremia due to *S. aureus* in association with the use of an intravenous catheter can be treated safely with 2 weeks of an effective parenteral antibiotic if the catheter is removed, the patient responds, has no defect in resistance to infection, and has normal cardiac valves. Four to six weeks of antistaphylococcal antibiotic therapy is necessary if the patient has cardiac valvular disease or is immunocompromised. Nonbacteremic urinary tract infection can be effectively treated with a week of orally administered antibiotics in the absence of obstruction to urine flow. Pseudomembranous enterocolitis due to *Clostridium difficile* is managed by discontinuation of antibiotics (if possible) and administration of vancomycin (250 mg by mouth every 12 h) or metronidazole (250 mg by mouth or intravenously every 6–8 h) (see Chapter 29). Parenteral vancomycin is ineffective for treatment of this infection.

PREVENTION

The prevention of infection in hospitalized patients requires a commitment by physicians and by the hospital to institute procedures and programs designed to reduce the prevalence of this major cause of morbidity and mortality (Table 28–3). The Joint Commission on Accreditation of Healthcare Organizations mandates that each institution establish a committee to supervise this effort. The major vectors of transmission of the majority of bacteria and viruses causing nosocomial infections are the hands of medical personnel. Washing of hands between caring for each patient is essential to reducing the spread of hospital infections. A second major technique, reduction of the use of therapy or support devices that enhance risk of infection, should be implemented wherever possible. Thus, the use of antibiotics should be limited to situations where these agents have been proved to be necessary and effective. Intravascular lines should be left in place only as long as absolutely necessary. There is documentation that phlebitis or arteritis and sepsis directly correlate with the duration of time such lines are left in place. The diagnosis of catheter-related sepsis can be estab-

TABLE 28–3. *Prevention of Nosocomial Infections*

HAND WASHING
Intelligent use of instrumentation
Limitation of use of antibiotics
Prophylactic antibiotics in specific situations and for short duration
Limitations of transfusions
Barrier precautions
Surveillance
Frequent change of intravenous lines

lished by use of quantitative cultures of blood obtained through the catheter and peripherally. If the number of organisms in the catheter blood is 5–10 times the number isolated from peripheral blood, the catheter is usually the source of the bacteremia. The prevalence of catheter infections can be reduced by use of an attachable subcutaneous cuff impregnated with antibacterial agents. Urinary catheters should be used as sparingly as possible. Blood transfusions must be justified by the clinical situation and should not be used "to promote healing" or for other nonspecific reasons. The risk of transmitting HIV infection is estimated to be 1 in every 42,000 units of blood transfused; the risk of transmitting non-A, non-B hepatitis is considerably greater. It has also been suggested that administration of nonabsorbable antibiotics by mouth to patients with nasogastric tubes or to those receiving H_2 blockers and antacids reduces the frequency of nosocomial pneumonia.

There is increasing evidence that in specific surgical situations the judicious use of prophylactic antibiotics reduces the prevalence of postoperative infection. Surgery conducted in contaminated sites, such as the head and neck or colorectal or pelvic areas, is associated with high rates of wound infection in the absence of prophylactic antibiotics. The antibiotics must be initiated shortly before or during surgery with the aim of providing effective blood and tissue levels during and immediately after the procedure. Prolonged preoperative antibiotic administration or continuation beyond 8–12 h postoperatively, however, does not enhance the efficacy of prophylaxis and is clearly associated with the subsequent carriage of antibiotic-resistant organisms and adverse reactions. Surgery, such as herniorrhaphy, uncomplicated cholecystectomy, or for peptic ulcer disease, performed at uninfected, clean sites does not require antibiotic prophylaxis. Placement of a prosthetic device, such as a cardiac valve or a prosthetic joint, however, has been demonstrated to require prophylaxis to prevent a devastating infection of the prosthesis.

There is increasing evidence that administration of oral prophylactic antibiotics reduces the infection rate in neutropenic patients. However, this form of prophylaxis is associated with increased colonic carriage of antibiotic-resistant bacteria and (in some series) an increased frequency of fungal infection and thus can have untoward effects.

If a patient is admitted to the hospital with a virulent, highly contagious infection, develops an infection with an antibiotic-resistant organism while in the hospital, or has a draining infected wound, appropriate isolation techniques should be instituted to prevent spread of the infection. Medical personnel must scrupulously utilize gowns and gloves. Hands, the major vector of infection, must be washed to avoid transferring organisms from one patient to another. Prevention of nosocomial viral and a few bacterial infections requires that hospital personnel be removed from patient care if they are infected or have been exposed and are known to be susceptible. Examples of such infections include measles, mumps, pertussis, rubella, and varicella. Personnel who are actively infected with hepatitis B or are chronically HBs-antigenemic should glove for patient interactions which involve invasive procedures. The same is true for HIV-infected personnel. Routine contact does not pose a risk to patients. Finally, susceptible hospital staff should receive available viral vaccines including hepatitis B to protect themselves and their patients.

During the early 1980s, when AIDS was recognized before its etiology was established, concern was raised regarding spread of the syndrome from patients to health care workers. It was quickly realized that AIDS was probably caused by an infectious agent, transmitted by sexual activity and exposure to blood, much as is the case for hepatitis B. With the identification of HIV, this etiology was confirmed and health care organizations instituted so-called universal precautions to limit the risk of nosocomial acquisition of the virus. Universal precautions are designed to limit exposure of personnel and patients to contaminated blood or body secretions by establishing physical barriers (gowns, masks, gloves).

If a nosocomial outbreak occurs in a specific unit (such as an intensive care area), frequently the unit must be closed to new admissions. Those patients in the unit are all assumed to be potentially infected and kept in the area until discharge. Investigation of the reason for spread of the infection in the unit should be undertaken, and only when secondary infections cease can the unit be allowed to admit new patients. The investigation of reasons for the outbreak can involve obtaining cultures from personnel, evaluation of patient care techniques used in the unit, and a search for possible vectors, such as infected disinfectant, intravenous solutions, or a break in sterilization techniques of critical care equipment.

A program of surveillance must be instituted by each hospital under the direction of its infection control committee. A staff physician, preferably someone with an interest or expertise in nosocomial infections, should chair the committee and take responsibility for the program. Sufficient numbers of nurse epidemiologists, at least one per 250 beds as recommended by the Centers for Disease Control, should be hired and trained to conduct surveillance of infections occurring in the hospital and to detect outbreaks of unusual infections. These personnel are responsible for in-service education of hospital personnel, and they must have authority to carry out policies designed to reduce the risk of infection. To accomplish infection control the team must have the active support of the medical staff and hospital administration.

CASE HISTORY

A 55-year-old man was admitted to the hospital with crushing chest pain and profound hypotension. A diagnosis of myocardial infarction was established. His hemodynamic status was rapidly stabilized after emergent placement of a subclavian catheter to administer intravenous fluids and an intraortic balloon pump. On the fourth hospital day, while making a good recovery in the intensive care unit, the patient developed a fever of 104°F following a rigor (chill). He did not complain of headache, sore throat, cough, shortness of breath, chest pain, pain on urination, abdominal discomfort, or diarrhea. Examination revealed a supple neck, a clear chest, no cardiac murmur, and a soft, nontender abdomen with good bowel sounds. There was minimal erythema surrounding the site of the intravenous catheter which had not been changed since arrival in the emergency room. Suspecting bacteremia due to an infected venous catheter, his physician obtained two blood cultures using blood obtained from each antecubital vein, a third blood culture drawn from the venous catheter, urine for analysis and culture, a complete blood count, and a portable chest x-ray. The subclavian venous catheter and aortic balloon were removed and cultured, and venous access was maintained with a peripheral intravenous line.

The white cell count was 15,500/mm³ with 40% segmented neutrophils and 35% band forms. The urine contained no leukocytes or

erythrocytes, and the chest x-ray was normal. Vancomycin, 1 g administered intravenously every 12 h, was begun for possible infection with methicillin-resistant *S. aureus* (MRSA).

The patient's temperature was normal within 24 h. All blood cultures and the venous catheter tip culture grew MRSA. Examination after 14 days of therapy revealed no evidence of metastatic infection or cardiac murmur. It was decided that it was safe to discontinue the antibiotic and to proceed with coronary angiography and possible angioplasty or coronary artery bypass if necessary.

CASE DISCUSSION

The emergent placement of an intravenous catheter and intraaortic balloon to treat shock due to myocardial infarction are common occurrences. However, the situation described above often prevents complete asepsis during the placement of the catheter. The intravenous catheter was left in place for 4 days rather than being replaced within 48 h, and bacteremia secondary to S. aureus *resulted. This oversight complicated the patient's recovery, delaying evaluation of the coronary arteries and prolonging hospitalization. In similar patients who do not have the complication of infection, angiography and angioplasty could have been carried out and the patient discharged much earlier.*

The use of empiric vancomycin for treatment of a suspected S. aureus *infection was appropriate because* S. aureus *or* S. epidermidis, *resistant to penicillinase-resistant penicillins, is a very common cause of "line sepsis." The discontinuation of therapy at 14 days in the absence of evidence of infection in* bones or joints, on a cardiac valve, or of the pericardium is justified.

REFERENCES

Books

Bennett, J., and Brachman, P., eds. *Hospital Infections.* 2nd ed. Boston: Little Brown & Co., 1986.

Van Saene, H., Stanetenbeck, C., Lowin, P., and Ledingham, I., eds. *Infection Control in Intensive Care Units by Selective Decontamination.* Berlin: Springer-Verlag, 1989.

Weber, J., and Rubula, W., eds. *Nosocomial Infections: New Issues and Short Strategies for Prevention.* Inf Dis Clinics of North America. Vol. 3. Philadelphia: W. B. Saunders Co., 1989.

Wenzel, R. P. *Prevention and Control of Nosocomial Infections.* Baltimore: Williams and Wilkins, 1987.

Articles

Cox, C. Nosocomial urinary tract infections. *Urology* 32:210–215, 1988.

du Moulin, G., Paterson, D. Hedley-White, J., et al. Aspiration of gastric bacteria in antacid-treated patients: A frequent cause of postoperative colonization of the airway. *Lancet 1:*242–245, 1982.

Haley, P., Hooton, T., Culter, D., et al. Nosocomial infections in U.S. hospitals 1975–1976: Estimated frequency by selected characteristics of patients. *Am. J. Med. 70:*947–959, 1981.

Johanson, W., Pierce, A., and Sanford, J. Changing pharyngeal bacterial flora of hospitalized patients. *N. Engl. J. Med. 281:*1137–1140, 1969.

Johanson, W., Pierce, A., Sanford, J., et al. Nosocomial respiratory infections with gram-negative bacilli: The significance of colonization of the respiratory tract: *Ann. Intern. Med. 77:*701–706, 1972.

Schaberg, D., Weinstein, R., and Stamm, W. Epidemics of nosocomial urinary tract infection caused by multiply resistant gram-negative bacilli: Epidemiology and control. *J. Infect. Dis. 133:*363–366, 1976.

Stamm, W. Infections related to medical devices. *Ann. Intern. Med. 8*(part 2):764–769, 1978.

IX

Additional Infections

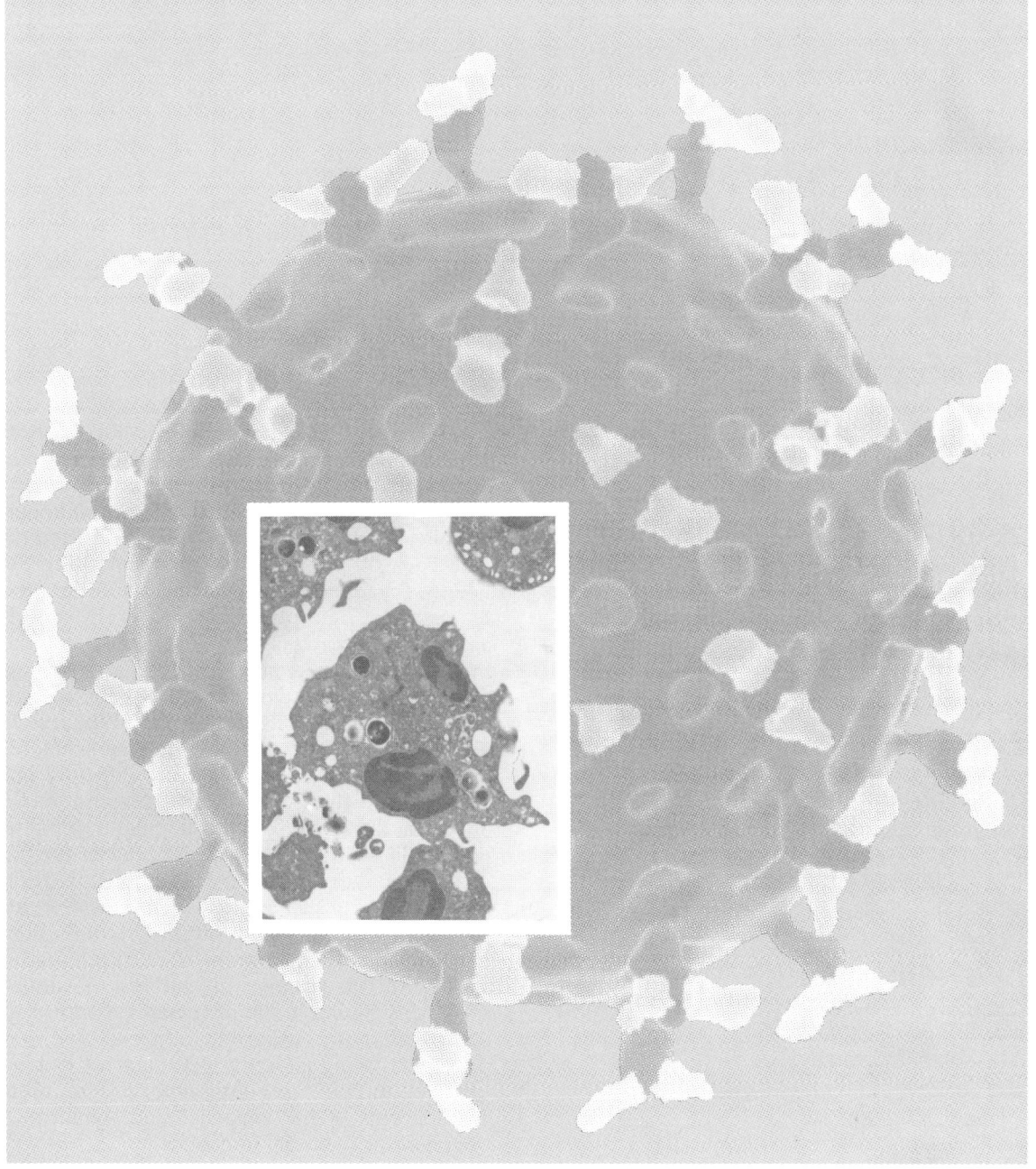

29 *HERBERT M. SOMMERS, M.D. • STANFORD T. SHULMAN, M.D.*

Infections Caused by Anaerobic Bacteria

INTRODUCTION

Anaerobic bacteria outnumber aerobic and facultative anaerobic bacteria in the colon by from 300:1 to 1000:1. They also outnumber aerobic and facultative anaerobic bacteria in the mouth, vagina, and other sites in the body, although not always at the same ratio. Facultative anaerobic bacteria are those bacteria that can grow in either the presence or the absence of oxygen, for example, Enterobacteriaceae, staphylococci, and streptococci. It is surprising that despite the predominance of anaerobic bacteria in the indigenous flora, relatively little had been written of anaerobic bacterial infections until the last 20 years. Perhaps one of the more significant restrictions has been the technical difficulty encountered in the isolation and identification of anaerobic bacteria. The development and general application of improved procedures for the recovery and classification of anaerobic bacteria have shown anaerobes to be more widely involved with disease at all sites in the body than had previously been recognized. Widespread application of sensitive procedures to culture specimens results in the increased isolation and identification of anaerobic bacteria, and improved recovery of anaerobic bacteria can be expected to result in a realignment of our present concepts of the incidence and significance of anaerobic bacterial infections.

FACTORS ASSOCIATED WITH ANAEROBIC INFECTION

Oxidation–Reduction Potential (E_h)

Disease caused by anaerobic bacteria may be defined in a broad sense as tissue disease or severe systemic intoxications due to microorganisms growing in an environment with low oxidation-reduction potential, or in the absence of oxygen. The oxidation–reduction potential (E_h), like the hydrogen ion concentration (pH), can be measured and expressed in terms of defined units. Oxidation is defined as a reaction in which electrons are lost, whereas a reaction in which electrons are gained is called reduction. Any compound with a tendency to be oxidized can be thought of as possessing a corresponding measure of electrons available for donation. If a solution of such a compound is arranged to form a half cell in a circuit with a different half cell of known potential, a potential difference is set up whose magnitude is related to the oxidizing (or reducing) power of the compound and can be expressed in volts. Oxidation–reduction potential is expressed by the positive or negative electric potential across a calomel half cell and can be measured in either *in vivo* or *in vitro* culture systems. The oxidation–reduction potential at any site in the body is usually but not necessarily related to the distance of that site from oxygen-carrying red blood cells and the integrity of the vascular capillary network. The E_h of the blood depends on the oxygen saturation of hemoglobin in red blood cells and, to a lesser but significant extent, on dissolved oxygen content in the serum. The E_h in most tissues in the body varies between $+0.126$ V and $+0.246$ V, depending on blood supply and whether the measurement is taken near sites of high (arterial) or low (venous) oxygen saturation. Anaerobic bacteria will not grow in tissues with these E_h values. For example, the highest E_h recorded for germination of *Clostridium tetani* is $+0.110$ V, whereas clostridial spores usually need an E_h less than -0.100 V for germination and growth. The majority of anaerobic bacteria require an E_h of -0.100 V to -0.250 V for growth *in vitro*. The oxidation–reduction potential of normal tissue therefore prevents growth of anaerobic bacteria unless blood flow is reduced and the E_h falls. The presence of oxygen can also very effectively prevent the growth of certain anaerobic bacteria, even with an E_h of -0.50 V. Both the presence or absence of oxygen and the proper oxidation–reduction potential of the tissue are important determinants of the growth of anaerobic bacteria.

Those parts of the body removed from active capillary perfusion, such as the lumen of the colon or the vagina, and the oral cavity, have large populations of anaerobic bacteria. Other regions where anaerobic bacteria are found in high concentration include the nasal sinuses, tonsillar crypts, and other parts of the body where the microorganisms are kept warm and moist and are protected from oxygen concentrations that would inhibit or prevent growth.

Effect of Tissue Injury on E_h

Inasmuch as anaerobic bacteria are normally present in well-defined sites throughout the body, conditions that predispose to disease can in part be predicted. This is particularly true at sites adjacent to mucous membranes where large numbers of anaerobic bacteria are part of the indigenous microbiota. Any injury that produces interruption of the capillary blood flow, with a resulting decrease in tissue E_h at that site, predisposes to anaerobic bacterial replication and, in the case of clostridia, toxin production. Injury may result from surgery, trauma, arteriosclerosis, or growth of a malignant tumor with ischemic necrosis. The importance of the reduction of blood flow and its subsequent effect on the decrease in the tissue E_h have been illustrated by experimental clostridial infections in animals. Production of vascular spasm and ischemia by injecting epinephrine and a suspension of *Clostridium perfringens* into the hind leg of a guinea pig reduces by 1000-fold the number of microorganisms required to initiate infection.

Variability of Anaerobic Bacterial Requirements

Some anaerobic bacteria are more fastidious than others in their need for a low oxidation–reduction potential. *C. perfringens,* the microorganism most frequently associated with gas gangrene, will grow with only a slight reduction of oxygen tension, 70–80 mm Hg (normal, ~150 mm Hg), whereas *C. tetani* has been reported to be intolerant of oxygen concentrations greater than 2 mm Hg. This variation of oxygen sensitivity suggests that the number and types of microorganisms isolated by the clinical laboratory depend on the method of collection of the specimen, protection of the specimen from exposure to air or oxygenated mediums, and the speed of delivery of the culture to the laboratory. Table 29–1 lists the oxygen tolerance of different strains of anaerobic bacteria found in association with dental plaque and shows that some microorganisms are much more tolerant of oxygen than others. The number of species of anaerobic bacteria isolated by the laboratory, therefore, reflects the effort expended to maintain anaerobiosis during the collection of the specimen, isolation of the organism, and the identification procedure.

Most species of anaerobic bacteria must have certain conditions necessary for growth before they can cause disease. Frequently, these conditions can be met more rapidly in company with other anaerobic or facultative anaerobic bacteria. *In vitro* experiments have shown that dilute suspensions of anaerobic bacteria, incapable of growth when widely dispersed in a fresh broth culture medium, demonstrate rapid growth when centrifuged to concentrate the microorganisms in a smaller volume of medium. The change from a stationary to a rapidly growing bacterial population is thought to be due to the ability of bacteria to reduce the immediate microenvironment by metabolism of residual oxygen, thus making rapid growth possible. This same principle of rapid utilization and depletion of available oxygen facilitates the development of anaerobic disease. Facultative anaerobic bacteria, such as *Escherichia coli* or *Klebsiella pneumoniae,* metabolize and use available oxygen, thereby reducing the E_h of the *in vivo* microenvironment to a level where strict anaerobic bacteria can grow. With reduction of the tissue E_h, the anaerobes start to grow, producing necrosis, toxins, or other virulence factors. The ability of microcolonies of mixed bacteria to reduce the E_h of their immediate environment helps explain the otherwise confusing finding that large numbers of anaerobic bacteria can be cultured from the mouth, nasal sinuses, and lower respiratory tract—areas that might usually be considered unlikely sites for colonization with anaerobic bacteria.

CULTIVATION AND IDENTIFICATION OF ANAEROBIC BACTERIA

Most anaerobic bacteria have two cardinal requirements for growth—a low oxidation–reduction potential and the absence of oxygen. The critical factors necessary for a low E_h are not clearly understood. Peroxides formed during aerobic metabolism may be toxic and are usually inactivated by catalase, an enzyme that many anaerobes lack. Exposure to oxygen may be fatal to a large number of anaerobes. However, exposure to oxygen is not the only factor involved, since it is known that oxygen can be bubbled through a culture medium containing growing anaerobes if a low oxidation–reduction potential is maintained by strong chemical reducing agents. In contrast, studies with *Bacteroides fragilis* have shown that chemical changes in E_h do not impair growth if no oxygen is introduced, but that growth stops abruptly when oxygen is provided; these results suggest a direct toxic effect of oxygen. The presence of the enzyme superoxide dismutase in aerobic and facultative anaerobic bacteria but not in many of the fastidious anaerobic bacteria also plays a role. Superoxide (O_2^-) is a highly reactive compound produced when oxygen is reduced by a single electron, and it is generated during the normal catalytic action of a number of enzymes. Superoxide dismutase catalyzes the conversion of two molecules of superoxide to one molecule of oxygen and one molecule of hydrogen peroxide. The absence of superoxide dismutase in obligate anaerobic bacteria creates obvious disadvantages to survival. The ability to produce

TABLE 29–1. *Oxygen Sensitivity of Various Anaerobic Bacteria** *

Species	Oxygen in Gas Atmosphere (Percentage)					
	0.1	*0.5*	*1.0*	*3.0*	*6.0*	*10*
Treponema macrodentium	+ +†	0				
T. denticola	+ +	0				
Butyrivibrio fibriosolvens	+ +	+	0			
Clostridium haemolyticum	+ +	+ +	0	0		
C. novyi type A	+ +	+ +	+ +	0		
Bacteroides oralis	+ +	+ +	+ +	+ +	+,V	0
B. melaninogenicus	+ +	+ +	+ +	+ +,V	+,V	0
Fusobacterium nucleatum	+ +	+ +	+ +	+ +	+ +	0
Bacteroides fragilis	+ +	+ +	+ +	+ +	+,V	0

*Adapted from Loesche, W. J. Oxygen sensitivity of various anaerobic bacteria. *Appl. Microbiol. 18*:723, 1969.
†Symbols: + +, growth; +, slight growth; V, growth varied with strain or length of incubation (or both); 0, no growth.

this enzyme may provide varying degrees of protection to individual bacteria upon exposure to different amounts of oxygen.

Many, but not all, anaerobic bacteria grow more slowly in culture than do facultative anaerobic bacteria and usually require 48 h for colony formation. This means that the isolation, separation, and complete characterization of individual species may take 3–10 days or longer.

Collection of Specimens

For the optimal recovery of anaerobic bacteria, cultures should be taken in a manner that minimizes exposure to air. When cultures for anaerobes are to be obtained, oxygen-free tubes and vials should be used (Fig. 29–1). A variety of methods for taking cultures are available, but most are based on the use of containers with an atmosphere free of oxygen and incorporation of a reducing agent to diminish the effect of residual air. Collection of quantities of aspirated fluid or pus is preferable to collection of specimens by swabs, even when transported in anaerobic containers. Precautions should be taken to reduce contamination of the indigenous microbiota from contiguous sites of infection, such as oropharyngeal or vaginal secretions. Prompt delivery to the laboratory and inoculation to prereduced culture media greatly improves recovery of fastidious anaerobic bacteria. Direct smears for Gram's stains should be made when the culture is taken to correlate the bacterial forms present with bacteria isolated by culture.

Methods for Culture

One of the earliest methods used to create an anaerobic environment was to place a handful of oat seeds in a dish of water, close the container tightly, and wait until the oat seeds germinated; the process of germination effectively used all available oxygen and produced small amounts of carbon dioxide. The period of time necessary to achieve anaerobiosis precluded the study of any microorganisms except the spore-forming clostridia, since non–spore-forming anaerobic bacteria would perish long before the oxygen was utilized by the seeds. Considerable progress has been made since the time when this method was used. Many of the more current useful techniques have been borrowed from veterinary microbiologists who developed sensitive methods for studying the complex anaerobic microbial flora of the cow's rumen.

The standard procedure for isolation of anaerobic bacteria in many clinical laboratories includes the use of a Brewer jar to obtain anaerobiosis. Culture plates are placed in a plastic or glass jar, and hydrogen is added by evacuation and replacement with a mixture of 80% N_2, 10% CO_2, and 10% H_2, or by a disposable H_2-CO_2 generating system. This latter system consists of a metal foil envelope activated by adding water to sodium borohydride to generate hydrogen and a tablet of citric acid and sodium bicarbonate to make CO_2 (Gas-Pak) (Fig. 29–2). Five–10% CO_2 is added to stimulate the growth of anaerobes. Hydrogen reacts in the presence of a catalyst with atmospheric oxygen to form H_2O. In the past, the catalyst was a coil of platinum that required heating by an electrical element for activation. Enthusiasm for the use of this chamber was dampened when breaks in the safety screen occasionally resulted in explosions. Currently, most anaerobic jars contain catalysts of palladinized alumina pellets that do not need to be heated and require less than 10% hydrogen to convert remaining atmospheric oxygen to water.

One of the more recent methods facilitating work with anaerobic bacteria utilizes small cannulas that carry a slowly moving stream of oxygen-free gas, usually carbon dioxide. When culture tubes containing anaerobic bacteria are opened for transfer or staining, the cannula is placed in the tube and prevents the entry of atmospheric oxygen (Fig. 29–3). This method is frequently called the "VPI System," referring to the Virginia Polytechnic Institute, where it was developed for clinical laboratories by Drs. Holdeman and Moore. Another technique for working with anaerobic bacteria in the absence of oxygen is the use of an anaerobic "glove box," a closed chamber of plastic film with transfer ports in which cultures can be handled in a completely controlled, oxygen-free atmosphere. These chambers may be heated and may serve as both an incubator and a work area.

Culture Media for Anaerobes

Most culture media for anaerobic bacteria require components not found in standard media. Reducing agents may be necessary to keep the E_h in the -0.010 V range or less. Anaerobic culture media contain an indicator showing when the E_h of the media is above a certain level. The most commonly used indicator is resazurin, colorless when reduced and pink when oxidized. Recovery of different bacterial

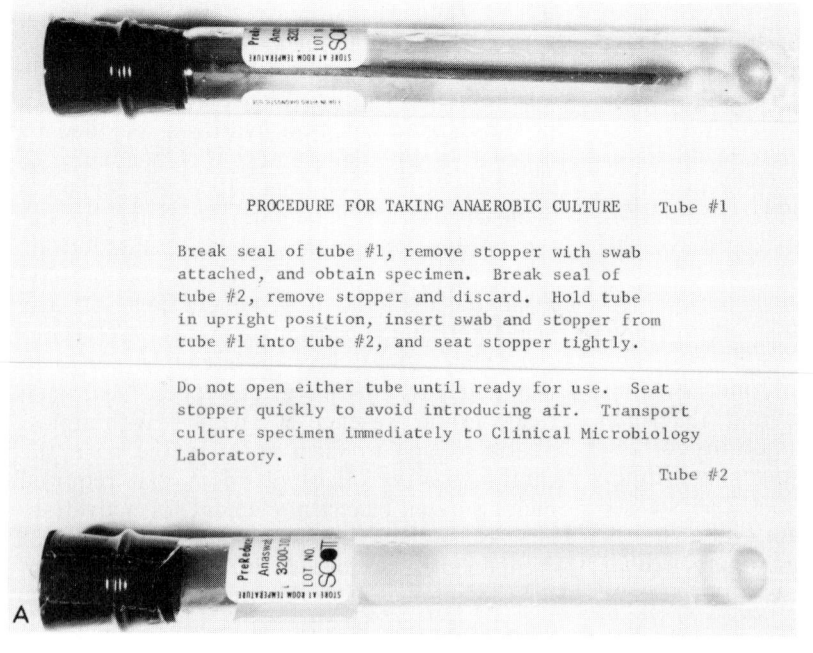

Break seal of tube #1, remove stopper with swab
attached, and obtain specimen. Break seal of
tube #2, remove stopper and discard. Hold tube
in upright position, insert swab and stopper from
tube #1 into tube #2, and seat stopper tightly.

Do not open either tube until ready for use. Seat
stopper quickly to avoid introducing air. Transport
culture specimen immediately to Clinical Microbiology
Laboratory.

Tube #2

Figure 29–1. A. *Collection kits for obtaining specimens for anaerobic culture. Directions are attached. Each tube contains an oxygen-free atmosphere and a small quantity of a reducing agent.* A. *Smear for a Gram stain should be made with a second swab to correlate the bacterial forms present with subsequent isolates.* B. *Oxygen-free transport vial for anaerobic culture of pleural, peritoneal, or other fluids.*

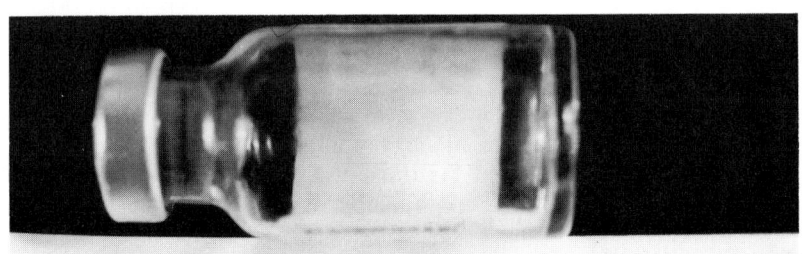

USE OF OXYGEN-FREE TRANSPORT VIALS FOR
ANAEROBIC BACTERIAL CULTURE

Use sterile needle and syringe to aspirate
specimen. Expel all air from needle and
syringe prior to inoculation into vial.
Inject specimen through rubber stopper.
Send immediately to Clinical Microbiology
Laboratory.

species may be enhanced if different additives are incorporated, such as bile for the stimulation of growth of *Bacteroides fragilis* or hemin and menadione (vitamin K) for the growth of *Bacteroides melaninogenicus.*

The best results for the isolation and identification of anaerobic bacteria are reportedly obtained by the use of prereduced, anaerobically sterilized culture media. These are prepared under an oxygen-free gas, usually nitrogen, reducing exposure to air or oxygen during preparation. Culture media exposed to air and oxygen during preparation may form "toxic peroxides," which will inhibit growth of fastidious microorganisms. One such microorganism, *Clostridium haemolyticum,* is said not to be able

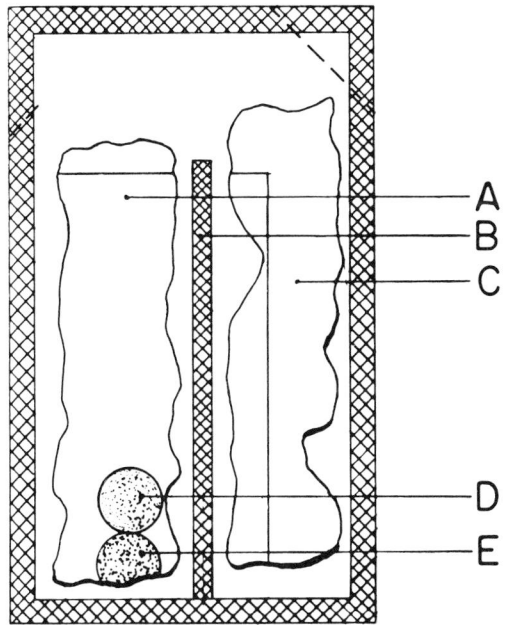

Figure 29–2. Cutout view of the hydrogen–carbon dioxide generator (Gas-Pak). (A) Filter; (B) heat seal; (C) water added to this side; (D) CO_2 tablet; (E) H_2 tablet. (From Brewer, J. H., and Allgeier, D. L. Safe self-contained carbon dioxide–hydrogen anaerobic system. Appl. Microbiol. *14:985, 1966.)*

to grow on a blood agar plate exposed to atmospheric air for longer than 3 h.

Identification of different species of anaerobic bacteria has been facilitated by the use of gas chromatography for the detection and semi-quantitation of volatile fatty acids produced by different bacterial species. Propionibacteria will produce propionic acid; lactobacilli, lactic acid; butyrobacteria, butyric acid; and so forth. Production of volatile acids by anaerobic bacteria in the intestine is one of the mechanisms that retards experimental colonization of *Salmonella typhimurium* in the colon of animals and presumably of humans as well. The strong and offensive odor often associated with anaerobic disease is in part related to the release of volatile fatty acids and the formation of strongly aliphatic amines, such as cadaverine and putrescine, by biosynthetic and biodegradative decarboxylases.

It is evident from the foregoing discussion that several points should be kept clearly in mind when taking cultures for the purpose of establishing disease due to anaerobic bacteria. First, the culture should be collected and promptly transported to the laboratory in a manner that excludes or minimizes exposure of the specimen to air. Second, special media needed for anaerobic bacteria and the unique

slow growth of these bacteria are frequently reflected in the prolonged time required for species identification and the reporting of results to the physician. Third, the extra effort necessary for identification of anaerobic bacteria results in an increased cost for processing the culture. The return for this effort is justified if specific microorganisms are isolated and identified, thereby permitting definitive therapy to be initiated in the patient under study and gaining valuable treatment time for the next patient the physician sees with a similar disease.

ANTIMICROBIAL THERAPY

Since the nature of anaerobic disease tends to predispose to abscesses and localized collections of pus in a closed space, the primary treatment is surgical. Even so, therapy with an appropriate antimicrobial agent may significantly affect patient survival. Higher mortality is associated with the use of an antimicrobial agent effective only against members of the family Enterobacteriaceae in patients with disease caused by both aerobic and anaerobic bacteria. When the agent selected is effective primarily against anaerobic bacteria, mortality is lower.

Penicillin is useful against many species of anaerobic bacteria, but it is almost totally ineffective against *Bacteroides fragilis*, a fact that obviously limits the use of penicillin against disease possibly caused by *B. fragilis*. One exception to this limitation is pulmonary infection. Infections in the lung from *B. fragilis* and other species of anaerobic bacteria frequently respond clinically to penicillin, although penicillinase-producing organisms are isolated in 15–20% of cases.

Both chloramphenicol and clindamycin are usually quite effective against the penicillin-resistant species of *Bacteroides*, but the threat of potentially toxic effects on the bone marrow by chloramphenicol and the development of pseudomembranous colitis from clindamycin restrict their use to serious infections. Recently, imipenem has been found to be effective against many anaerobic bacteria, and metronidazole (an antiparasitic agent useful against *Trichomonas vaginalis*) has been found to be very effective against *Bacteroides fragilis* and other penicillin-resistant *Bacteroides* species.

The beta-lactamase–resistant cephalosporin cefoxitin is useful in the antimicrobial therapy of anaerobic infections, being considerably active against the penicillin-resistant species of *Bacteroides in vitro*.

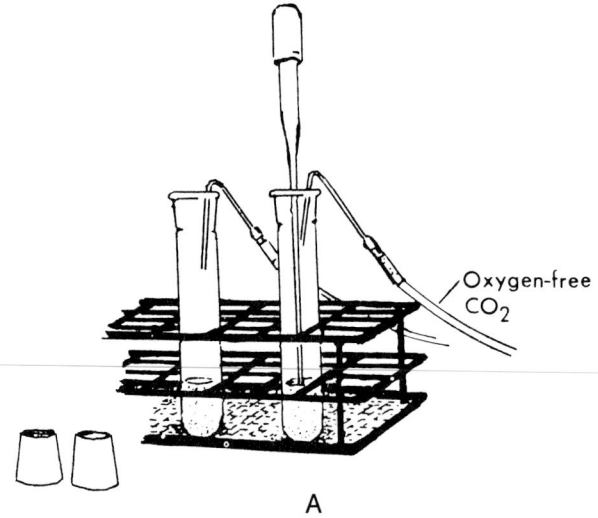

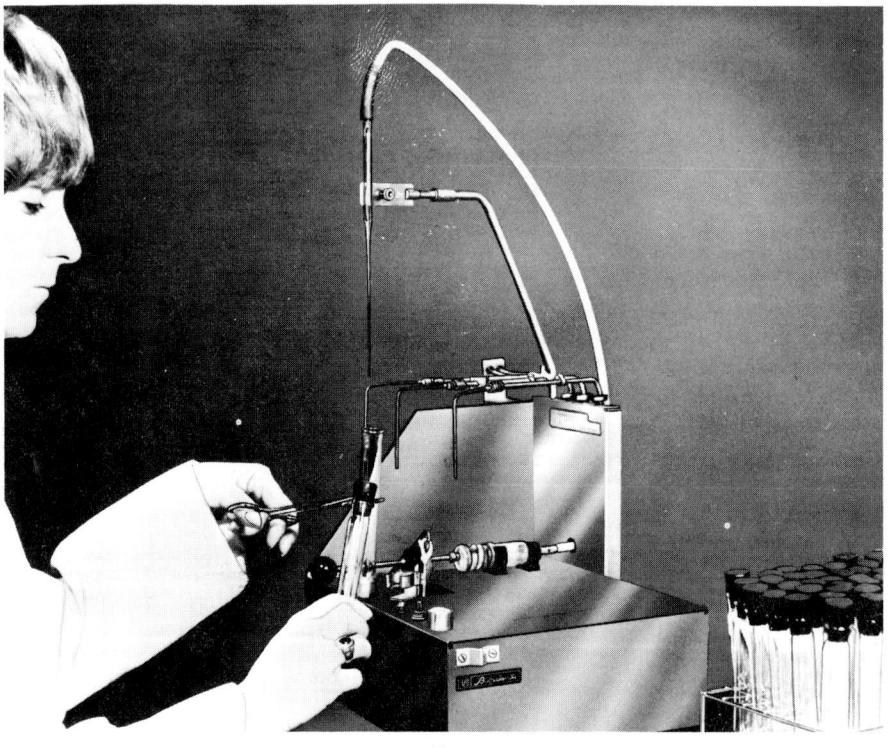

Figure 29–3. A. Simple transfer of anaerobic culture. (From Holdeman, L. V., and Moore, W. E. C., eds. Anaerobe Laboratory Manual. *3rd ed. Blacksburg, VA: Virginia Polytechnic Institute and State University Anaerobe Laboratory, 1975. Drawing by Dr. W. E. C. Moore.) B. Virginia Polytechnic Institute anaerobic culture system. (Courtesy of Bellco Glass, Inc., 340 Edrudo Rd., Vineland, NJ 08360.)*

ANTIMICROBIAL SUSCEPTIBILITY TESTING

Determining susceptibility of anaerobic bacteria to antimicrobial agents has posed a technical problem for a number of years. A frequently used procedure, that of measuring a zone of growth inhibition around a paper disc impregnated with a known amount of antibiotic, does not have the same validity for the slowly growing anaerobic bacteria that has been shown for rapidly growing bacteria. The composition, pH, and depth of the growth medium, and the number of microorganisms inoculated have not been standardized for the anaerobic bacteria in the same manner as for rapidly growing bacteria (see Chapter 38). Information derived from testing drug susceptibility of anaerobic bacteria by measuring zone diameters on agar plates tends to vary widely from one laboratory to another.

The use of an agar growth medium containing varying dilutions of antimicrobial drugs has given results more uniform than those produced by disc diffusion. This procedure has been used at several medical centers, and has proved to be reproducible and clinically useful. Under the auspices of the National Committee for Clinical Laboratory Standards, a single culture medium and a standardized procedure have been developed for determining the antimicrobial susceptibility of anaerobic bacteria. Adaptation of this medium and procedure to microtiter plates provides many small clinical laboratories with the means for identification and susceptibility testing previously possible only in larger or more specialized laboratories.

Certain anaerobic bacteria with a slow rate of growth and fastidious culture requirements have defied all methods of susceptibility testing. Such microorganisms include species of *Peptostreptococcus* isolated from patients with endocarditis. Treatment of disease due to these microorganisms is usually empirical.

POLYMICROBIC NATURE OF ANAEROBIC DISEASE

Disease due to non–spore-forming anaerobic bacteria is commonly associated with localized, necrotizing abscesses, each of which may yield 2–13 different strains of bacteria. Because of the multiple species that can be isolated, the term *polymicrobic disease* is sometimes used to refer to anaerobic bacterial abscesses. For this reason, diseases caused by anaerobic bacteria stand in sharp contrast to the "one microorganism—one disease" concept that characterizes many infections, such as typhoid fever, cholera, and diphtheria. Anaerobic disease commonly results from the contamination or extension of the indigenous microflora to adjacent, submucosal tissues. Improved isolation and identification techniques for anaerobic bacteria have reemphasized the need for a better understanding of the interaction of one microorganism with another.

The most clinically important anaerobic bacterial genera are listed in Table 29–2 organized on the basis of Gram's-stain reactivity and morphologic appearance. Although additional genera exist, they are only rarely associated with disease. Within genera, there may be a large number of different species; this is particularly true for clostridia and bacteroides.

Clinically, the significance of "polymicrobic" infection can be difficult to evaluate. The interaction between different species of bacteria may be antagonistic, synergistic, or indifferent. Several examples, which follow, serve to underline this point. A classic example of a synergistic infection involves a series of four organisms that can together cause a serious necrotizing infection of the oral mucous membranes. None of the four can cause the infection independently. One of the organisms, a diphtheroid, is known to contribute to the virulence of the infection by secreting vitamin K, a growth factor needed by *Bacteroides melaninogenicus*, another one of the four. *Bacteroides melaninogenicus* in turn secretes numerous proteolytic enzymes toxic to the host. The contributions of the other two organisms are not apparent. Another form of interaction between two bacterial species that can be detrimental to the host is the protection of one species by another from the action of an antibiotic. In experimental animals penicillinase-producing *Bacteroides fragilis* can prevent the successful treatment of infection by penicillin-susceptible *Fusobacterium necrophorum*. Protection can occur even with only small numbers of *B. fragilis* injected as long as 24 h after the infecting dose of *F. necrophorum*. A third example of "polymicrobic" interaction concerns the number and size of intrahepatic abscesses that can develop in experimental infections in mice. The combination of different strains of *B.*

TABLE 29–2. *Major Clinically Important Anaerobic Bacterial Genera*

Gram-Positive Cocci
Peptococcus
Peptostreptococcus
Gram-Negative Cocci
Veillonella
Gram-Positive Bacilli
Clostridium (spore-forming)
Actinomyces
Lactobacillus
Gram-Negative Bacilli
Bacteroides
Fusobacterium

fragilis with other gram-negative non–spore-forming anaerobic bacteria can result in widely varying numbers and sizes of hepatic abscesses, suggesting synergism of virulence factors between some bacterial strains but not others.

Most Enterobacteriaceae are susceptible to the aminoglycoside antibiotics and resistant to clindamycin. In contrast, disease-associated anaerobic bacteria are susceptible to clindamycin but resistant to the aminoglycosides. This fact provided an interesting experimental model to study the contribution of both types of organisms to peritoneal infection. Gelatin capsules containing rat colonic contents were placed in the peritoneal space of rats. The infection that developed had two stages. In untreated animals, acute peritonitis occurred first and was associated with a mortality rate of 37%. All control animals surviving the initial infection went on to develop chronic intraabdominal abscesses caused by strict anaerobic bacteria. When the rats were treated with gentamicin, the initial mortality rate decreased to 4%, but 98% of the survivors had anaerobic intraabdominal abscesses. When clindamycin was given alone, the early mortality rate became similar to control levels (35%) but the incidence of intraabdominal abscesses decreased to 5%. When both gentamicin and clindamycin were given, the early mortality rate was 7% and the incidence of intraabdominal abscess 6%. These findings suggest that the Enterobacteriaceae are the organisms most significantly associated with the early mortality from acute peritonitis, whereas obligately anaerobic bacteria are primarily responsible for chronic intraabdominal abscesses. For this reason, therapy for "polymicrobic" infections usually requires antimicrobial agents effective against both the Enterobacteriaceae and anaerobic bacteria.

ADVANTAGES OF ANAEROBIC BACTERIAL IDENTIFICATION

Progress toward understanding the host–parasite interaction first requires the accurate identification of all participating parasites. One example of why such identification is advantageous is illustrated by the clinical information provided by the identification of certain members of the genus *Bacteroides*. Of the many species that make up this genus, one, *Bacteroides fragilis*, is more frequently isolated than are other *Bacteroides* species from abscesses and other sites of clinical infection, even though it is present in the colon in considerably smaller numbers than

other species of *Bacteroides* (Chapter 2). In contrast to other species in this genus, *B. fragilis* has a polysaccharide capsule that appears to confer the ability to incite abscess formation either by live or by heat-killed bacteria, a finding not shared by unencapsulated strains. The capsular polysaccharide of *B. fragilis* has also been shown to stimulate circulating serum antibody and thereby appears to be one of the more important virulence factors associated with infection by this organism. For this reason the specific identification of *B. fragilis* indicates to the clinician that active therapeutic measures should be taken, in contrast, for example, to the isolation of *B. vulgatus,* an organism often associated with fecal contamination but uncommonly the cause of infection.

CLINICAL SETTINGS SUGGESTING INFECTION WITH ANAEROBIC BACTERIA

Certain clinical findings associated with infection suggest a strong possibility of anaerobic bacterial disease. These findings include a foul-smelling discharge, infection located in or adjacent to a mucous membrane, or the presence of gangrene, necrotic tissue, or a pseudomembrane. Gas in the tissues or in serous discharges may suggest infection by members of the genus *Clostridium.* Patients with clinical evidence of endocarditis but with no growth of bacteria in aerobically incubated blood cultures may have infection from anaerobic bacteria. Infections associated with malignancies or other conditions resulting in necrotic tissue or developing during therapy with aminoglycosides should be considered to be due to anaerobic bacteria until shown to be otherwise. Patients with septic thrombophlebitis or infected human or animal bites often have primary infections by anaerobic bacteria. Discharges from sinus tracts containing "sulfur granules" or bacteremia with jaundice may also signify serious underlying anaerobic infections.

In the section to follow we are unable to cover all aspects of infections caused by anaerobic bacteria, but the general principles and predisposing factors associated with anaerobic infections in several organ systems are described. The bizarre clinical symptoms associated with the very potent toxins secreted by certain clostridia are briefly reviewed.

PREDISPOSITION TO THROMBOPHLEBITIS

Disease produced by all types of bacteria commonly causes an associated local thrombophlebitis. This is particularly true in anaerobic bacterial pelvic disease in females, but it is also a feature accompanying anaerobic disease elsewhere. The reason for what appears to be a greater incidence of thrombophlebitis in anaerobic bacterial disease is not clear. It has been reported that certain strains of bacteroides and fusobacteria secrete a heparinase which may predispose to clotting.

One result of thrombosis and thrombophlebitis associated with anaerobic disease is an increased incidence of embolism to the portal or pulmonary venous systems. Such emboli predispose to infarcts in the liver, lung, brain, or other organs, resulting in a decreased E_h and conditions advantageous to growth of anaerobic bacteria. This is one way anaerobic disease can "metastasize" from a primary locus to elsewhere in the body.

Severe septicemia from gram-negative anaerobic bacteria may cause disseminated intravascular thrombosis. The mechanism is considered to be similar to that related to other gram-negative bacteria, such as meningococci, and is thought to be mediated through endotoxin release from the bacterial cell walls. Disseminated intravascular coagulation may also be seen in severe disease due to streptococci and is not solely restricted to infections with gram-negative bacteria.

DISEASES CAUSED BY NON–SPORE-FORMING ANAEROBES

Upper Respiratory Tract Infections

It is now well established that chronic infection of the paranasal sinuses or mastoids may be caused by anaerobic bacteria alone or in combination with facultative anaerobic bacteria. In one study, over half of 83 patients with chronic sinusitis were found to be harboring anaerobic bacteria either in pure culture or in combination with facultative anaerobic bacteria. Peptostreptococci, *Bacteroides fragilis*, *B. funduliformis*, and *B. melaninogenicus* are among the most commonly isolated bacteria. Acute sinusitis is, however, only rarely associated with anaerobes.

Anaerobic bacteria can be isolated from the mouth, particularly in the presence of dental caries and infection of the adjacent gingival tissues (see Chapter 11). Almost all dental infections are caused by anaerobic bacteria. It is probably significant that strains found in the oral cavity, including *B. melaninogenicus, B.*

oralis, Fusobacterium nucleatum, and numerous species of *Peptostreptococcus* and *Veillonella* are also among the most commonly isolated anaerobic bacteria associated with pulmonary disease (see Chapter 12).

Lower Respiratory Tract Infections

Anaerobic disease of the lung may occur in one of several forms. It may be an *abscess,* defined in this context as a solitary or dominant pulmonary cavity frequently measuring at least 2 cm in diameter. A diffuse pulmonary infiltrate without evidence of cavitation is called *anaerobic pneumonia,* and the term *necrotizing pneumonia* is applied to disease characterized by multiple areas of necrosis and cavitation within one or more pulmonary segments or lobes. Extension of intrapulmonary disease to the surface of the lung with involvement of the pleural space is called *empyema* and may or may not occur as a sequela to pulmonary abscess or anaerobic or necrotizing pneumonia (Fig. 29–4).

The pathogenesis of these different disease processes varies, but the similarity of the bacteria isolated from most patients with anaerobic pulmonary disease to the indigenous flora of the oropharynx supports the theory that aspiration of oropharyngeal secretions is an important contributing factor. Thromboemboli from abdominal or pelvic disease associated with thrombophlebitis may contribute significantly to the development of an anaerobic bacterial abscess. Staphylococci are commonly associated with anaerobic pulmonary abscess formation (particularly in nosocomial infections) and may contribute to this process by production of necrotizing toxins (see Chapter 36). The resulting ischemia provides a proper environment for growth of anaerobic bacteria, and they in turn bring about further tissue destruction.

The microorganisms found in anaerobic pulmonary disease include *Bacteroides melaninogenicus, Fusobacterium nucleatum,* peptostreptococci, *Veillonella,* and other anaerobic cocci. In contrast to anaerobic abscesses elsewhere in the body, surgical drainage of anaerobic abscesses in the lung is often not necessary, and treatment with clindamycin alone is adequate unless empyema is present. With empyema, drainage is usually necessary.

Intraabdominal Infections

In view of the large numbers of anaerobes indigenous to the gastrointestinal tract (see

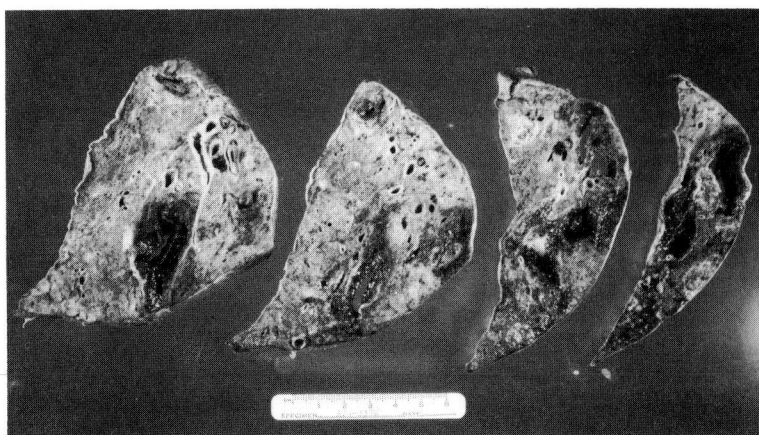

Figure 29–4. Serpiginous anaerobic bacterial abscess in the lower lobe of a lung. Extension to the pleural surface is seen in the section on the right and was associated with empyema. Culture revealed Staphylococcus aureus *and four separate anaerobic bacterial species.*

Chapter 2), it is not surprising that anaerobic infections within, adjacent to, or related to disease of the gastrointestinal tract account for a significant number of cases of clinical disease due to anaerobes. Ulceration of the gastrointestinal tract, by either inflammatory disease, ischemia, or malignant tumor, can provide a portal of entry, first to the regional lymphatics and later to the intravascular compartment. Septicemia with anaerobic bacteria should prompt a search for an overt or inapparent lesion of the gastrointestinal tract, such as an ulcerated tumor of the right colon, diverticulitis, or mucosal ulceration of the small intestine or colon from leukemia or lymphoma.

Anaerobic bacterial disease following intestinal surgery, ruptured appendicitis, or penetrating trauma to the intestinal tract is usually associated with multiple species of anaerobic bacteria. Contamination of the peritoneum with large numbers of obligate and facultative anaerobic bacteria results in the rapid lowering of the local oxidation–reduction potential and creates conditions advantageous for disease. Anaerobic disease, once established in the peritoneum, can be self-sustaining, with the E_h reaching a very low level and thereby permitting growth of even the most fastidious microorganisms. Abscesses within the peritoneal cavity or beneath the diaphragm are often very difficult to treat unless drained surgically.

Abscesses in the liver frequently yield anaerobic bacteria when properly cultured. Inflammatory disease of the intestine or partial or complete obstruction of the biliary tract are predisposing factors. The blood supply to the liver, predominantly venous from the intestine, results in a low oxidation–reduction potential compared with other tissues of the body with an intact blood supply. Thrombophlebitis in mesenteric or portal veins with embolism to the liver can initiate anaerobic disease and abscess formation. In addition, certain anaerobic bacteria, such as *Bacteroides fragilis* and *Clostridium perfringens,* have a potential advantage over other bacteria in causing infection in the liver or biliary tract in that they can grow in high concentrations of bile. They are also the most commonly isolated anaerobic bacteria from cultures of the gallbladder at the time of cholecystectomy. The ability to grow in high concentrations of bile is probably of importance in the association of *C. perfringens* with both primary and postsurgical biliary tract infection.

Female Genital Tract Infections

The large majority of female genital infections that are not caused by sexually transmitted pathogens are due to anaerobes. Anaerobic bacteremia and septicemia can be complications of pregnancy. Septicemia may also result from induced or spontaneous abortion. Presumably, the anaerobic and facultative aerobic flora of the vagina gain entrance to the endocervical canal when the embryo or fetus and fetal membranes are being expelled. The highly vascularized endometrial surface is particularly susceptible to bacterial invasion during pregnancy, and septicemia may result. Bacteremia associated with abortion is usually transitory and clears promptly following curettage of the uterus.

In the female pelvis, anaerobic infectious disease not associated with pregnancy may cause salpingitis or result from a complication of gynecologic surgery. Careful bacteriologic study of pelvic infections yields numerous microorganisms similar to those of the vagina and lower genitourinary tract of the female. The most commonly isolated bacteria are species of peptostreptococci, peptococci, and occasional species of *Bacteroides* and *Clostridium*.

Endocarditis

Endocarditis from anaerobic bacteria is probably more common than has been recognized in the past. Endocarditis due to true anaerobic bacteria differs from that due to facultative anaerobic streptococci and other common aerobic types of bacteria. Preexisting heart disease is less frequent in patients with anaerobic endocarditis, and embolic complications are more common. The oropharynx and inflammatory lesions of the gastrointestinal tract are the usual sources of infection. *Bacteroides fragilis, Fusobacterium nucleatum,* and *F. necorphorum,* as well as *Clostridium perfringens* and other clostridial species, rarely cause endocarditis. *Propionibacterium acnes,* a normal anaerobic inhabitant of the skin, has caused endocarditis in a number of patients following prosthetic valve replacement. Endocarditis complicating a prosthetic valve replacement may be resistant to treatment despite the use of large amounts of an appropriate antimicrobial agent (see Chapter 35) and may require removal of the infected prosthesis. In many instances, the presenting symptoms in patients with anaerobic bacterial endocarditis are related to embolic complications (Fig. 29–5).

Central Nervous System Infections

In the brain, disease due to anaerobes may be the result of direct extension from infections in the paranasal or mastoid sinuses, causing epidural abscess or meningitis. Anaerobic brain infection also may appear as a metastatic abscess from an embolus secondary to infection in the lungs or a vegetation on a heart valve. Patients with cyanotic congenital heart disease (with a right-to-left shunt), whose arterial blood supply has a lowered oxygen saturation that bypasses the normal pulmonary capillary filter, are at greater risk of developing cerebral abscesses from anaerobic bacteria than are normal persons. The association of recent cerebral infarction with anaerobic bacterial abscess has also been noted and is thought to reflect the decreased oxidation–reduction potential in the ischemic tissue. Brain abscesses are most often polymicrobic.

DISEASES CAUSED BY SPORE-FORMING ANAEROBES (CLOSTRIDIA)

General Characteristics

The clostridia are gram-positive, spore-forming, anaerobic bacilli. Most species form spores, but some sporulate only under special conditions. Although there are more than 50 species of clostridia described and classified, disease in humans is caused by fewer than 10–12 species. Wide variation exists in the ability of different species of clostridia to tolerate oxygen. Some are considered to be aerotolerant, whereas others germinate and grow only under strictly anaerobic conditions.

Different species of clostridia vary widely in

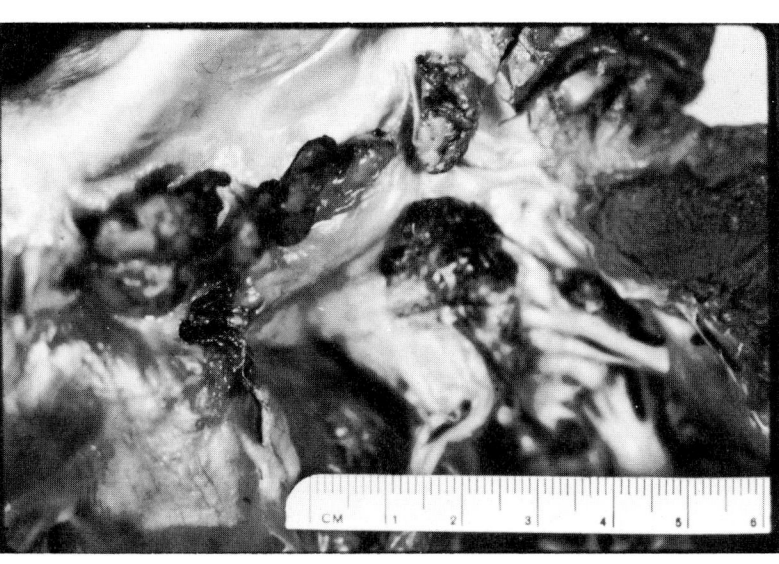

Figure 29–5. Anaerobic bacterial endocarditis with destruction of the aortic valve and colonization of the ventricular surface of the anterior mitral leaflet. Note the large friable verrucae. The patient had two metastatic anaerobic bacterial abscesses of the brain.

their ability to utilize carbohydrates and split proteins. Such characteristics are helpful in the laboratory for purposes of identification and classification, but they also aid in explaining clinical manifestations of diseases caused by individual species. For example, *Clostridium perfringens,* the microorganism most often associated with gas gangrene, produces strong proteolytic and saccharolytic enzymes, which contribute to the spread of infection. Glycogen, present in large amounts in skeletal muscle, is fermented with almost explosive formation of gas, and when coupled with collagenase and other proteolytic enzymes secreted by the microorganism, contributes to the rapid spread of disease. By contrast, *C. tetani,* the microorganism that causes tetanus, has few enzymes for carbohydrate fermentation or protein degradation. Therefore, growth of *C. tetani* with production of toxin can occur without evidence of an inflammatory reaction.

Exotoxins

A characteristic of the clostridia that are pathogenic for humans is the production of one or more potent exotoxins which usually contribute significantly to the ability of these microorganisms to cause disease. Tetanus and botulism are each due to a single toxin having a well-defined mode of action. Table 29–3 lists some of the exotoxins produced by important clostridia. *C. perfringens* produces at least 10 separate toxins

that facilitate production of disease. Secretion of toxins is a highly specialized function of microorganisms in general and, in clostridia, requires a suitably low E_h. As the E_h increases, toxin production ceases before death of the bacterium. This concept is important, since any mechanism (including use of hyperbaric oxygen) that increases the oxidation–reduction potential at the site of bacterial growth first interrupts toxin formation and then threatens the survival of the microorganism. *C. perfringens* is normally present in the gastrointestinal tract of 25–35% of humans and the urogenital tract of a significant number of adult females. Toxins of the clostridia are some of the most potent poisons known. Figure 29–6 lists representative toxins from animal and bacterial sources and highlights the very low human lethal doses for botulinus and tetanus toxins.

Gas Gangrene

The classic disease caused by *C. perfringens* is gas gangrene. The organism can be isolated from the skin of many noninfected hospitalized patients. These patients are at risk of developing gas gangrene postoperatively under appropriate conditions. In World War I, gas gangrene associated with traumatic wounds from shell fragments was responsible for a huge number of fatalities. In most cases, the wounds were contaminated with soil that had been fertilized with animal and human waste. The presence of mul-

TABLE 29–3. *Exotoxins Produced by Principal Toxigenic Bacteria Pathogenic for Humans**

Bacterial Species	Disease	Toxin	Action
Clostridium botulinum	Botulism	Six type-specific neurotoxins	Paralytic
C. tetani	Tetanus	Tetanospasmin	Spastic
		Tetanolysin	Hemolytic cardiotoxin
C. perfringens	Gas gangrene	Alpha-toxin†	Lecithinase: necrotizing hemolytic
		Beta-toxin	
		Gamma-toxin	
		Delta-toxin	
		Epsilon-toxin	Necrotizing
		Eta-toxin	
		Theta-toxin	Hemolytic cardiotoxin
		Iota-toxin	Necrotizing
		Kappa-toxin	Collagenase
		Lambda-toxin	Proteolytic
C. septicum	Gas gangrene	Alpha-toxin	Hemolytic
C. novyi	Gas gangrene	Alpha-toxin	Necrotizing
		Beta-toxin	Lecithinase: necrotizing, hemolytic
		Gamma-toxin	Lecithinase: necrotizing, hemolytic
		Delta-toxin	Hemolytic
		Epsilon-toxin	Lipase: hemolytic
		Zeta-toxin	Hemolytic

*Modified from van Heyningen, W. E. In Florey, H. W., ed. *General Pathology.* 3rd ed. Philadelphia, W. B. Saunders Co., 1962, p. 754.
†The designation of toxins by Greek letters is based on the order in which they were identified.

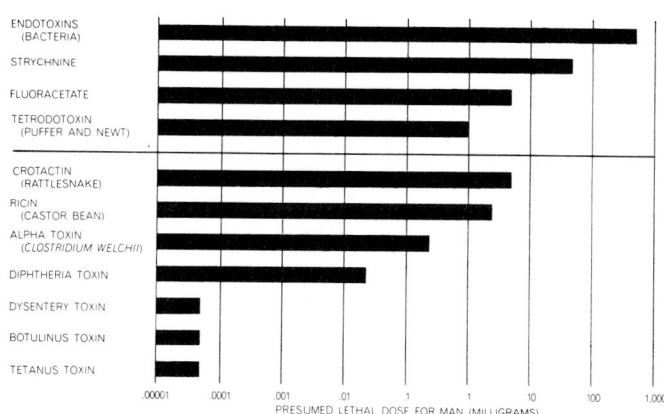

tiple species of clostridial spores in the soil frequently resulted in infections with more than one clostridial species, including *C. novyi* and *C. septicum,* as well as *C. perfringens.*

Clinical manifestations of gas gangrene are due to the vigorous utilization of glycogen and other fermentable carbohydrates, resulting in the rapid production of lactic acid and gas. Increased tissue tension from gas formation causes decreased blood flow, a lowered tissue oxidation–reduction potential, and more favorable conditions for growth of anaerobic bacteria and toxin formation. Absorption of the toxins has a profound effect on the patient and results in a marked but not well understood "toxicity." Adequate control of disease can usually be achieved by surgical excision of tissue from accessible sites and the prompt administration of antibiotics. In more severe or generalized infections, hyperbaric therapy should be used.

Hyperbaric therapy is the exposure of the patient to increased atmospheric pressure of air or oxygen for short periods. This exposure does not significantly change the oxygen-carrying capacity or saturation of the red blood cells, but does result in a small but significant increase in the oxygen tensions of the serum and of the interstitial tissues. The increase in interstitial oxygen tension resulting from 1–2 h in a hyperbaric chamber may be sufficient to interrupt toxin formation and microbial replication. Normal phagocytic and host defense mechanisms may then be able to control the infection. Hyperbaric chambers are not always necessary for the treatment of gas gangrene, but on occasion they can be lifesaving.

Although gas gangrene has classically been an infection associated with trauma and devitalized tissue, it is occasionally seen in hospitalized patients in situations in which necrosis, vascular insufficiency, and possible fecal contamination

occur. Invasion of the bloodstream by *C. perfringens* may result from ulcerating lesions of the gastrointestinal tract. Recovery of *C. septicum* by blood culture has a high correlation with malignant tumor in the gastrointestinal tract. As long as the clostridia remain in the blood and do not localize at a site where there is a low tissue oxidation–reduction potential, they will not replicate. Isolation of *C. perfringens* from skin wounds or cultures from the female genital tract in asymptomatic patients should be neither viewed with alarm nor dismissed as contaminants. Such patients should be observed carefully and given an appropriate antimicrobial agent if indicated.

Disease due to *C. perfringens* also occurs at several other sites in the body. As indicated above, *C. perfringens* is a not infrequent inhabitant of the gallbladder and may cause cholecystitis. The diagnosis should be considered when a roentgenogram of the abdomen taken when the patient is in an upright position shows a gas–fluid level in the region of the gallbladder. Care should be taken to distinguish air–fluid levels that may be present in the same area from ileus of the small intestine (which is frequently present in acute cholecystitis) or a gas bubble in the hepatic flexure of the colon. Figure 29–7 shows the appearance of a gas-filled gallbladder with gas outlining the thin wall and extending through small mucosal diverticula. Other gas-forming bacteria, such as species of *Klebsiella* and peptostreptococci, may also cause gas production. Gas gangrene may occur as a postoperative complication in patients, diabetics in particular, with amputations of extremities for peripheral arteriosclerosis. Disease under these circumstances results from decreased blood flow, decreased tissue oxidation–reduction potential, and necrosis from the surgical procedure. The microorganism presumably was

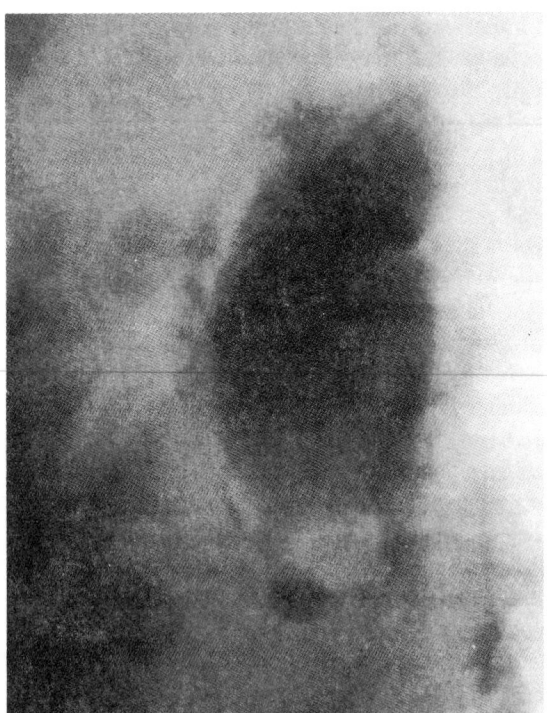

Figure 29–7. Gas-filled gallbladder. Note the extension of gas through the wall to small mucosal diverticula. Radio lucencies below the gallbladder represent accumulations of gas in the intestine.

present on the skin, possibly as a contaminant from the flora of the large bowel.

Infectious complications of spontaneous or induced abortion are well known to involve *C. perfringens*. Clostridial endometritis is due to a low tissue oxidation–reduction potential, endometrial necrosis, and bacterial contamination from the vagina. One of the toxins (alpha-toxin) produced by *C. perfringens* is lecithinase, which acts on the surface membrane of red blood cells. Under optimal conditions, large amounts of alpha-toxin can be secreted, which may result in massive intravascular hemolysis.

Tetanus

Tetanus is a disease caused by *C. tetani*, a spore-forming, gram-positive, anaerobic bacillus with a ubiquitous distribution in soil fecally contaminated by humans and animals. Although most cases of tetanus result from contamination of wounds by soil or objects that have been in contact with soil, tetanus may also be transmitted in drug addicts by dirty hypodermic needles or contaminated skin surfaces ("skin poppers"). As seen in Figure 29–8, the incidence of tetanus

in the United States has dropped dramatically in the past three decades, with most cases occurring in the elderly.

Clostridium tetani is considered to be part of the indigenous intestinal microbial flora of humans and domestic animals and is widely available in the soil. The spores are resistant to wide temperature changes and may remain viable for years in both soil and cicatrized wounds. In contrast to *C. perfringens*, *C. tetani* requires a very low oxidation–reduction potential (E_h) for toxin production. Wounds are usually the site of infection, owing to the interruption of blood flow in traumatized tissue, which results in a decreased tissue E_h. A further decrease in the E_h can occur if there are contamination and growth of facultative anaerobic bacteria. Clinical tetanus from spores, presumably introduced into wounds months or years previously, has been reported and may reflect either additional injury or continued cicatrization with a further decrease in blood supply and lowering of tissue E_h. The lack of significant numbers of proteolytic and saccharolytic enzymes in *C. tetani* tends to minimize any inflammatory reaction that may develop from germination of spores and toxin formation. This means that in occasional cases the site of infection and toxin production in patients with tetanus may not be apparent (cryptogenic tetanus).

Tetanus toxin blocks transmission of inhibiting impulses of the internuncial neurons, producing prolonged muscular spasms of both the flexor and extensor muscle groups. Studies have shown that the toxin moves by retrograde axonal transport from the site of infection to synapses in the central nervous system (Fig. 29–9). Inasmuch as the flexor muscles of the body are usually dominant, the patient with advanced tetanus shows generalized flexion contractures. Severe, prolonged spasm of the masseter muscle may restrict opening of the mouth and has led to the condition known as *lockjaw*. Progression of the disease to include the muscles of respiration may result in respiratory failure. In less severe cases, loss of control of pharyngeal musculature can lead to tracheobronchial aspiration and death from pneumonia.

Not well known in the United States is the considerable worldwide mortality rate from neonatal tetanus, which is one of the major causes of death from infectious disease. Although the incidence of neonatal tetanus is very low in the United States—only a few cases occurring each year—it follows the epidemiologic pattern seen elsewhere in the world and appears in areas

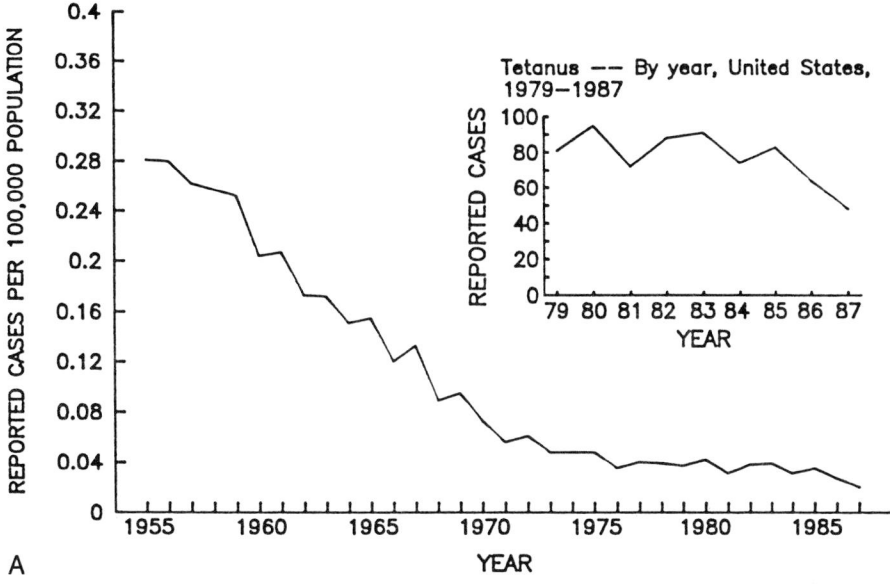

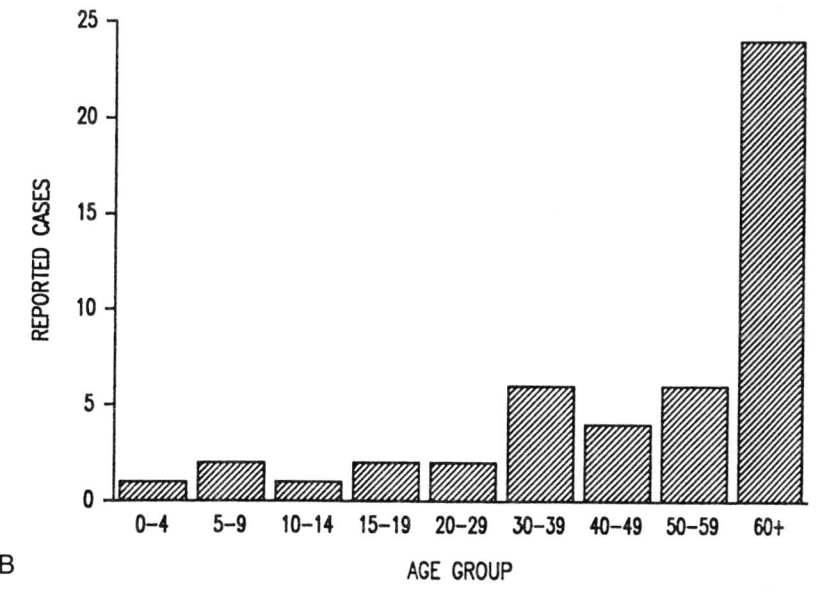

Figure 29–8. Incidence of tetanus in the United States. A. From 1955 to 1987 (by year). B. Incidence by age group for 1987. (From Morbidity and Mortality Weekly Report, Summary of notifiable disease, 1988. October 6, 1989, p. 39.)

where there are poverty, crowded living conditions, and lack of even minimal medical care. Neonatal tetanus usually results from contamination of the umbilical cord of newborns with tetanus spores. In India, it has been reported that in cases of severe dystocia, packing of the birth canal with cattle dung, a practice in those regions where religious significance is assigned to cows, can result in contamination with tetanus spores of both the umbilical cord and the endometrial surface.

Tetanus is a disease produced by an exotoxin that can be inactivated by an antitoxin. Therefore, tetanus is a *preventable* disease. Tetanus

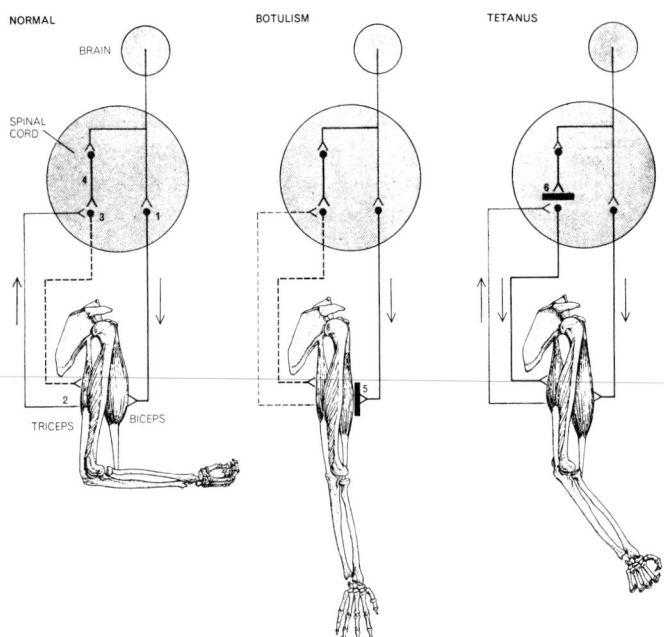

NORMAL   BOTULISM   TETANUS

Figure 29–9. Nervous control of muscles that raise and lower the forearm is diagrammed schematically. In a normal individual (left) impulses from the brain can excite a motorneuron (1) to cause the biceps to contract, stretching the triceps. A stretch-sensitive receptor (2) in the triceps would thereupon cause a triceps motorneuron (3) to fire and oppose the stretching—except that this firing is inhibited by impulses from an inhibitory nerve (4). In botulism (center) the neuromuscular junction is blocked (5), causing flaccid paralysis. In tetanus (right) the inhibitory impulses to the triceps motorneuron are blocked (6); both muscles contract, causing a spasm. (From van Heyningen, W. E. Tetanus. Sci. Am. 218:69, 1968. Copyright © 1968 by Scientific American, *Inc. All rights reserved.)*

toxin can be made nontoxic by the addition of small amounts of formalin, thereby forming a toxoid. This modification does not change the antigenicity of the toxin. Preparations of toxoid are made with alum to facilitate slow absorption and prolonged antigenic exposure (see Chapter 40). Current recommendations for primary immunization call for giving alum-precipitated toxoid at 2, 4, and 6 months of age, followed by a "booster" dose 12 months and 4 years later. Such a schedule will produce active immunity to the toxin; this immunity is reported to be protective for 12–20 years. Recent studies have shown that the routine practice of giving boosters or "recall" injections of fluid toxoid as a part of emergency room care following minor trauma to patients known to be adequately immunized is unnecessary. Administration of unneeded toxoid adds considerably to the incidence of allergic reactions.

Patients who develop and recover from clinical tetanus should undergo a primary immunization series with toxoid because, by getting tetanus once, these patients have demonstrated that they live and work in a manner that predisposes them to future exposure.

Passive protection in patients not previously actively immunized with toxoid can be temporarily provided by the use of antitoxin. Hyperimmune human gamma globulin is now used for this purpose. Experience with the human hyperimmune gamma globulin has shown it to be at least as effective as the previously used equine antiserum in treating and preventing tetanus,

but it has the important advantage of eliminating serum sickness and allergic reactions to the animal sera. Benzathine penicillin, released over a 28-day period, is recommended for inactivating vegetative bacteria.

Botulism

Botulism should more properly be called an intoxication than an infectious disease. In most cases of botulism, the toxin is formed outside the body in food and is then ingested with the tainted food.

In addition to classic botulism, cases of botulism that result from wounds contaminated with *Clostridium botulinum* have recently been recognized. In these patients there is usually a history of a traumatic injury with contamination by soil. Pathogenesis of the infection is presumed to be similar to that of tetanus, with growth of the organism in the depths of the wound and subsequent production of the toxin. Systemic absorption of the toxin occurs at the wound site.

The toxin of botulism acts at the neuromuscular junction of skeletal muscle, blocking neural transmission (Fig. 29–9). Symptoms of botulism are due to a progressive decrease of skeletal muscle function, which eventually results in paralysis. The first muscles to become affected are the small muscles of the eye, larynx, and pharynx; consequently, diplopia and dysphonia develop early. Later, weakness of the extremities may appear, and impairment of the muscles of respiration may occur. Death usually is caused by cardiac arrest due to inadequate respiratory exchange.

Six serotypes of *C. botulinum,* types A–F, are known, with types A, B, and E most often seen in humans. Types A and B are associated with the growth of the microorganism in home-prepared meats (the word *botulus* is Latin, meaning "sausage") and in vegetables. *C. botulinum* type C causes limberneck in fowl, and type D causes botulism in cattle but not in humans. Type E botulism is most frequently acquired from fish or marine animals, whereas type F has caused disease in several outbreaks, one from home-canned mushrooms and a second from home-prepared venison jerky. Type F *C. botulinum* has also been isolated from salmon and soil. Spores from all types of *C. botulinum* are in the soil and may be present on plants and vegetables. The spores can be washed by rains into rivers, lakes, or the sea. Spores of *C. botulinum* are resistant to heat, and if contaminated food is not thoroughly heated during preparation, anaerobic conditions resulting from the canning procedure may allow germination, growth, and production of toxin. This is particularly dangerous in home-canned or home-prepared foods, when canning temperatures are not always carefully controlled.

Although spores of *C. botulinum* are resistant to heating, the toxin is susceptible to increased temperatures and may be inactivated by heating at a temperature as low as 60°C for 30 min. Type A *C. botulinum* is apparently more lethal than type B, as the mortality rate in patients ingesting type A toxin is 60%; in those with type B toxin it is slightly less (48%).

Several outbreaks of botulism caused by *C. botulinum* type E involving smoked whitefish from the Great Lakes prompted investigation of the incidence of spores in fish taken from Lake Michigan. These studies showed that type E *C. botulinum* spores could be recovered from up to 13% of whitefish being transferred from brine vats to smoking rooms; the presence of the spores was the result of cross-contamination with infected fish. This would indicate that the potential for clinical botulism would be considerably greater than documented cases indicate.

One interesting characteristic differentiating types A and E *C. botulinum* is the minimal proteolytic activity of type E toxin compared with type A toxin. Patients who had ingested food contaminated with type A *C. botulinum* usually remember that the food tasted spoiled, but few patients complain of the bad taste or evidence of spoilage with type E *C. botulinum.* Type E *C. botulinum* has fewer proteolytic enzymes than type A organisms and presumably produces fewer offensive end products.

Clinically, botulism caused by type E *C. botulinum* presents with signs of acute gastrointestinal disease simulating intestinal obstruction. Neurologic signs may occur later and initially be overlooked because of the intensity of the patient's vomiting and acute distress.

The diagnosis of botulism is best established by demonstration of toxin in the serum of the sick patient and in the suspected food. Even minute quantities of toxin may be detected by injecting mice with serum from patients ill with the disease or with extracts of the suspected food. The presence of toxin is shown by the development of paralysis in the animal. The toxin type is then determined by pretreating a second set of mice with specific antisera.

The treatment of botulism should be directed toward removing unbound toxin from the circulation with either specific or polyvalent equine type A, B, and E antitoxin. Because progressive disease usually causes death by paralysis of the muscles of respiration, patients with botulism must be watched carefully for need of respiratory assistance. With the exception of wound-associated botulism, the toxin is not produced within the body and antibiotics are not helpful. Heat lability of the toxin suggests that the best therapy is prevention. Heating all food at 60°C for 30 min or boiling for 10 min inactivates the toxin.

Infant Botulism

In 1976, several pediatricians in central California became aware of a syndrome in infants suggesting botulism. They noticed several infants between 5 and 13 weeks of age who had constipation and muscle weakness as manifested by less vigorous sucking from breast or bottle, a weak cry, and loss of neck and limb strength, creating a "floppy" appearance. Although serum specimens were negative for toxin, the stools of all infants were positive for both *C. botulinum* organisms and toxin. In contrast to food-borne botulism, the disease appeared to result from the ingestion of *C. botulinum* spores with intracolonic growth and toxin formation. Presumably the colon is less permeable to the toxin than is the small intestine, and thus there is decreased absorption of toxin with low or undetectable levels in the serum of most affected infants. This is correlated with a less severe form of disease. In some infants the organism and toxin can be found in the stools for as long as 100 days following discharge from the hospital for the acute illness. Antitoxin has not been considered necessary in treatment. Therapy has been based on general supportive measures, although complete recovery may require several months.

Despite intense epidemiologic surveys, no common source of the organisms implicated in the syndrome described above has been determined. Approximately 60% of the infants studied have had type A organisms and 40% type B. No preformed toxin has been found in any food source, although *C. botulinum* spores have been isolated from honey obtained from several different states and from corn syrup, both used as formula additives. As pediatricians have become more aware of this syndrome, the number of known cases has increased. Approximately half of all known cases have been found in California, but confirmed cases have also been identified elsewhere.

Because of the paralytic effects of botulism toxin on skeletal muscles, there was a possibility that infant botulism might be a contributing factor to the sudden infant death syndrome (SIDS). This syndrome is characterized by the unexpected death of an infant, usually at less than 6 months of age. Most SIDS victims are found dead in their cribs without signs or symptoms of antecedent illness or an adequate explanation for their death on autopsy examination. The age similarity between SIDS and infant botulism cases is of interest, but no recent data have supported a relationship between these two conditions.

ANTIBIOTIC-ASSOCIATED DIARRHEA AND PSEUDOMEMBRANOUS COLITIS

For many years it has been known that antimicrobial agents can be associated with the development of diarrhea or colitis. Antimicrobial agents incriminated or known to have caused diarrhea in humans include penicillin G, ampicillin, cephalexin, tetracycline, chloramphenicol, co-trimoxazole, lincomycin, and clindamycin. The most serious of the gastrointestinal complications associated with antibiotics is pseudomembranous colitis. Pseudomembranous colitis is characterized clinically by abdominal pain, leukocytosis, fever, and profuse diarrhea.

Mortality rates as high as 60% were reported initially in untreated patients. The changes noted in the colon include the presence of yellow, plaquelike lesions on the mucosa with diffuse infiltration of neutrophils, disruption of the villous tips, and the presence of fibrin, bacteria, and inflammatory cells (pseudomembrane) on the surface of the intestinal epithelium. Sigmoidoscopic changes in patients with antibiotic-associated diarrhea that is not related to pseudomembranous colitis reveal only edema and hyperemia of the colonic mucosa.

Following the introduction and increasing use of clindamycin for anaerobic bacterial infections, pseudomembranous enterocolitis began to occur sporadically in treated patients. There appeared to be wide variation in the incidence of the disease following the use of clindamycin. In some hospitals the incidence was as high as 10%, whereas other large centers had no reported cases. Efforts to determine the cause of this disease had included extensive studies to isolate and to identify bacteria, viruses, and other infectious agents, all without success. Then it was found by several investigators working independently that when stools or aqueous extracts of stools from patients with pseudomembranous colitis were added to tissue cultures in an effort to isolate viruses, cytopathic effects developed very rapidly, often within hours, precluding the role of a more slowly growing virus. These studies suggested the presence of a bacterial toxin. About the same time, investigators studying an animal model of pseudomembranous enterocolitis noted that clindamycin given to hamsters resulted in the overgrowth of the colonic flora by several species of clostridia. Pseudomembranous colitis was consistently produced by intracecal injection of either the whole bacterial cells or cell-free broth filtrates of these clostridial strains. Identification of these organisms revealed two species, *C. difficile* and *C. sordellii*. Injection of hamsters intracecally with cultures or cell-free culture filtrates of *C. difficile* resulted in pseudomembranous colitis, whereas injection of *C. sordellii* or its culture filtrates did not. Further studies showed that *C. sordellii* antitoxin neutralized the toxin derived from *C. difficile*. In addition, passive immunization with antitoxin from *C. sordellii* was found to protect hamsters from clindamycin-associated colitis, suggesting that the disease is mediated by a toxin of *C. difficile*.

Studies on humans developing pseudomembranous colitis after taking clindamycin, ampicillin, or one of the cephalosporin drugs have shown the toxin of *C. difficile* to be present in stools in high titer in most patients. In contrast to pseudomembranous colitis, patients with simple antibiotic-associated diarrhea do not have colitis, and their stools contain little or no toxin. *Clostridium difficile* toxin is rarely found in the stools of normal controls or in stools of patients with other types of inflammatory bowel disease.

Clostridium difficile is considered to be a member of the normal flora of the colon, although it is present only in small numbers. The incidence of isolation in previous studies (2%) may represent a lack of sensitivity in the isolation procedure, since this species is a fastidious, and not easily identifiable, organism. Fewer than half of the isolates of *C. difficile* isolated from patients without colitis produce the toxin. *Clostridium difficile* toxin is a large immunogenic molecule that is both heat- and acid-labile. The toxin does not activate adenyl cyclase.

The diagnosis of antibiotic-associated colitis is made by the clinical and sigmoidoscopic picture of pseudomembranous colitis, the demonstration of toxin by cytopathic effect in tissue cell culture systems, and the neutralization of the toxin by antitoxin. The organism can be isolated and identified but may require special procedures and 3–7 days' time.

Clostridium difficile is susceptible to vancomycin, tetracycline, and metronidazole. Therapy with oral metronidazole or oral nonabsorbable vancomycin are approximately equally efficacious, but the former is much less expensive. Recurrence of pseudomembranous colitis is known to occur following cessation of vancomycin therapy.

In summary, the current findings in patients with pseudomembranous colitis indicate that toxin-producing clostridia are responsible for the disease. It is likely that the clostridia are selected by virtue of their resistance to antibiotics being administered to the patient and subsequently overgrow adjacent flora to produce varying amounts of toxin. The mechanism of action of the toxin is not yet known.

CASE HISTORY 1

A 62-year-old white woman was admitted to the hospital complaining of polydipsia, nocturia, fever, and increasing shortness of breath of 10 days' duration. She had noted a poor appetite for the preceding 8 months and had shown a 60-lb weight loss. The patient lived by herself but had moved to her daughter's apartment 8 days before she was hospitalized. While living with her daughter, the patient was found to have a temperature of 101°–102°F (38.3°–38.9°C), for which her physician prescribed cephalexin. During this period, the patient asked her daughter about the symptoms of hemorrhoids and complained of vague discomfort in the perineal region.

Physical examination at the time of hospitalization revealed an elderly white woman who appeared dehydrated and lethargic. The blood pressure was 146/90 mm Hg, and the pulse rate 126/min and regular. Examination of the optic fundi revealed venous congestion and hyperemia of the discs but no evidence of exudates, hemorrhages, or microaneurysms. The heart had a rapid but regular rate. No murmurs were heard. The right lung was resonant, and the left revealed coarse rales. The abdomen was soft and scaphoid, and no masses were palpable. The skin was rough and dry, although warm to the touch. Deep tendon reflexes were present and within normal limits.

At the time of hospitalization, the white blood count was 44,000/mm³, with 76% segmented neutrophils. The blood glucose was 900 mg/100 mL, and the urine was strongly positive for reducing substances. A chest roentgenogram showed patchy infiltrates in the left lower lung field. The patient was started on 6-h management for what was presumed to be diabetes mellitus. On the morning of the third hospital day, she was found in a coma and had a fever of 102°F (38.9°C). Four blood cultures taken at that time were subsequently reported to be negative for bacteria. Because of the fever, gentamicin was added to the cephalexin the patient had been receiving. Control of the diabetes proved difficult, and on the eleventh hospital day two decubitus ulcers were noted over the sacrococcygeal region. By the 13th hospital day, the decubiti were associated with a fluctuant mass. This mass was surgically incised, releasing a large amount of foul-smelling, clay-colored material. Culture of the material was reported to yield beta-hemolytic streptococci. Following the incision and drainage, the patient appeared to improve, although blood glucose levels continued to show wide fluctuation, reaching 465 mg/100 mL on one occasion. Because of a continued decline in her clinical course, the patient was transferred to a second hospital on the 16th hospital day.

At the time of admission to the second hospital, the patient was lethargic and responded poorly to questioning. Her temperature was 101°F (38.3°C); blood pressure, 85/50 mm Hg; pulse, 140/min, and respirations, 48/min. The chest was said to be clear to auscultation and percussion. The abdomen was distended, with voluntary guarding and diffuse tenderness to palpation. Examination of the gluteal region revealed a large fluctuant mass extending from the sacrococcygeal region laterally through the left gluteus maximus to the left femoral trochanter. The skin had a brownish discoloration over the mass. Arterial blood gases were pO_2, 108 mm Hg, pCO_2, 12 mm Hg, and pH, 7.05. The white blood count was 45,000/mm³; the blood glucose, 183 mg/100 mL; and the blood urea nitrogen, 141 mg/100 mL. The patient was started on 6-h management of diabetes, which included vigorous fluid replacement and intravenous sodium carbonate, plus clindamycin in preparation for surgery to drain the abscess. Cultures were obtained from the abscess. Attempts to probe the extent of the abscess cavity were only partially successful, and the patient was scheduled for a more complete incision and drainage of the gluteal region the following morning. Approximately 4 h after admission, the patient had a cardiac arrest. Resuscitation procedures were not successful.

Blood cultures taken shortly after death failed to grow bacteria, although a blood culture taken from the right ventricle at the time of autopsy grew *Clostridium perfringens*. At autopsy, a large, necrotic abscess cavity was found extending from the sacrococcyx laterally through the left gluteus maximus to the region of the left greater trochanter. The culture taken from the abscess shortly before death revealed the following:

Anaerobic Bacteria (large numbers of all strains)

1. *Clostridium perfringens*
2. *Bacteroides vulgatus*
3. *Bacteroides thetaiotaomicron*
4. *Bacteroides* species #1
5. *Bacteroides* species #2
6. *Bacteroides melaninogenicus*
7. *Bifidobacterium adolescentis* var. B
8. *Peptostreptococcus anaerobius*
9. *Peptococcus prevotii*

Facultative Anaerobic Bacteria

1. *Enterococcus faecalis*—moderate numbers
2. *Escherichia coli*—few
3. *Pseudomonas aeruginosa*—rare

Fungi

1. *Candida albicans*—few

The remainder of the autopsy showed multiple organizing thromboemboli with infarcts and cavity formation in the lower lobe of the right lung and the lingular portion of the upper lobe of the left lung. Focal thrombi in small vessels consistent with disseminated intravascular coagulation were found in the adrenals and kidneys.

CASE 1 DISCUSSION

The patient was initially hospitalized with symptoms of uncontrolled diabetes mellitus. This was evident by the history of polydipsia, nocturia, weight loss, and increasing shortness of breath. Whether she had an infection in the sacrococcygeal region at the time of admission to the first hospital is not clear, but the history of vague pain or discomfort mentioned to her daughter would suggest the possibility. It is likely that the infection in the sacrococcygeal region was the factor that precipitated diabetic coma on the third day. Severe infection in the diabetic may lead to uncontrolled hyperglycemia and coma. The presence of infarcts in both lungs, with organizing thrombi, would suggest embolization from a peripheral site. One such source could have been the gluteal abscess, although the autopsy did not provide for careful examination of veins draining from this region.

In reviewing the bacteria isolated from the sacral abscess, it is difficult to decide which of the 12 strains were responsible for the septic shock which probably caused the patient's death. Clostridium perfringens *is known to be associated with severe infection and septicemia, but there was no evidence either before or after death to support gas or lecithinase production in the patient. Each of the other*

TABLE 29–4. *Antimicrobial Susceptibility Studies**

Microorganism	Chloramphenicol†	Clindamycin†	Penicillin†	Tetracycline†	Gentamicin†
Clostridium perfringens	8	1	1	≤2	>8
Bacteroides vulgatus	8	1	>4	>16	>8
B. thetaiotaomicron	8	1	>4	>16	>8
Bacteroides species #1 and #2	≤2	≤0.12	≤0.03	≤2	8
Bifidobacterium adolescentis var. B	≤8	≤0.12	≤0.03	≤2	≤0.25
Peptostreptococcus anaerobius	8	≤0.12	≤0.03	≤2	4
Peptococcus prevotii	≤2	≤0.12	≤0.03	8	1

*Minimal inhibitory concentrations
†μg per mL.

microorganisms isolated can also be associated with severe infection, but what role each played or how they may have interacted cannot be determined in retrospect.

When the bacteria recovered from the abscess culture were tested for susceptibility to gentamicin, C. perfringens and the Bacteroides species were found to be resistant to achievable serum levels (see Table 29–4). All isolates were sensitive to clindamycin.

In retrospect, if cultures for anaerobic bacteria had been obtained in the first hospital, the difficulty in bringing the patient's diabetes under control should have alerted her physicians to the significance of the underlying infection. The recognition of a polymicrobic abscess from anaerobic bacteria should have prompted more careful attention to an appropriate antimicrobial agent. Gentamicin, although a very good agent against many gram-negative bacteria, is ineffective against anaerobic bacteria. In this instance, either clindamycin, chloramphenicol, or cefoxitin would have been a better selection.

Treatment of anaerobic bacterial infections with antimicrobial agents not effective against anaerobic bacteria results in a significantly decreased survival rate of seriously ill patients. When facultative anaerobic and strict anaerobic bacteria are present in the same infection, survival of the patient is significantly aided when agents are employed that are selected for use against the anaerobic bacteria.

This patient had an anaerobic bacterial infection of the skin and subcutaneous tissue called necrotizing fasciitis. *Diseases of this type are almost always due to mixed anaerobic bacterial species and are frequently associated with some underlying host defect, such as diabetes mellitus. Adequate control of infections of this type usually requires aggressive surgical*

incision and drainage as well as an effective antimicrobial agent.

CASE HISTORY 2*

Case A. **Four hours after a lunch that included home-canned gefilte fish that had been stored in a refrigerator for 7 weeks, a 57-year-old woman with mild hypertension complained of headache, epigastric distress, hoarseness, and mild dyspnea. The woman vomited repeatedly and experienced dryness of the mouth, weakness, constipation, and urinary retention. Examination that evening revealed an anxious, moderately obese woman with a respiratory rate of 26/min, blood pressure of 80/58 mm Hg, and a pulse rate of 110/min. Her pupils were equal in size and somewhat dilated; they were reactive to light. Extraocular movements were normal, and no facial weakness was noted. The patient's mouth and throat were dry, and her voice was hoarse. Bowel sounds were decreased, but her abdominal examination was otherwise normal. Examination of the chest and heart was normal. Because of hypotension and epigastric distress, the patient was hospitalized on the suspicion of myocardial infarction.**

On admission, hemoglobin, hematocrit, and white blood cell count and differential were normal, as was urinalysis. The next morning serum electrolytes, bilirubin, amylase, and serum protein were normal, as were chest and abdominal roentgenograms and electrocardiogram. The patient was treated symptomatically with antacids and with nasogastric and intravenous fluids. Thirty-six hours later the patient had a cardiopulmonary

*Adapted from Armstrong, R. W., Stenn, F., Dowell, V. R., Jr., et al. Type E botulism from home-canned gefilte fish. JAMA 210:303, 1969.

arrest and was resuscitated. Spontaneous respiration did not recur, and breathing was maintained on a mechanical respirator. The following day no apparent benefit resulted from the administration of 80,000 U of bivalent (types A and B) botulism antitoxin and 10,000 U of type E botulism antitoxin, which were given intravenously. One day later the patient died.

At autopsy the patient had generalized ischemic changes in the central nervous system, moderate arteriosclerosis of the coronary arteries, and mild hypertrophy of the left ventricle. The liver and spleen were enlarged and hyperemic. The lungs showed pulmonary edema and focal acute bronchopneumonia.

Case B. A 39-year-old man, an employee of the patient in case A who also consumed one portion of the gefilte fish that day, was anorectic and tired that evening. The next day, recurrent vomiting, periumbilical cramping, progressive abdominal distention, constipation, and a dry mouth developed. He was hospitalized 3 days later. Findings on physical examination were normal except for increased bowel sounds.

Results of laboratory studies were normal. An abdominal roentgenogram showed a distended small bowel with air–fluid levels. Findings from barium enema were consistent with those of small-bowel obstruction. Attempts to pass a nasogastric tube were unsuccessful.

The patient was treated with intravenous fluids and antiemetics. By 12 h after admission, abdominal distention had increased. For the next 2 days the patient complained of weakness, sore throat, dry mouth, and slightly blurred vision. No objective facial weakness, extraocular motion, disturbance of accommodation, or changes in the pharynx could be found on examination. Three days later the symptoms had disappeared and the patient was discharged from the hospital.

Case C. A 28-year-old woman who was 7 months pregnant, the daughter-in-law of the patient in case A, had a brief dizzy spell followed by nausea, profound weakness, and slight distortion of hearing. She had eaten half a portion of the gefilte fish. Recovery was spontaneous, and she had no further symptoms. Two months later she gave birth to healthy twins.

On the first, second, and third days after the patient in case A (who later died) ate the gefilte fish, type E botulinus toxin was detected in her serum. No toxin was detected in the serum samples from the other two patients. The fish contained 10 mouse intraperitoneal 50% lethal doses (IP LD_{50}) of type E botulinus toxin per gram of food. Trypsinization of the food extract increased the toxin activity to 780 mouse IP LD_{50}/gm. Cultures of the gefilte fish yielded *C. botulinum* type E. Extracts from the patient's myocardium, psoas muscle, kidney, brain, liver, and proximal jejunum taken at autopsy failed to show any toxin activity. Type E antitoxin had been given to the patient 10 h before her death, and serum obtained at autopsy neutralized type E toxin.

CASE 2 DISCUSSION

Type E botulism can present a confusing clinical picture in that neurologic signs may be less prominent than the acute, severe gastrointestinal symptoms. The clinical illnesses of the patients described in cases A, B, and C illustrate how the prominence of gastrointestinal symptoms in type E botulism can be confused with symptoms of bowel obstruction or myocardial infarction, thus delaying specific treatment of the intoxication.

In case A, hypotension, epigastric distress, and tachycardia suggested myocardial ischemia and possible myocardial infarction. In both cases A and B, severe gastrointestinal symptoms initially suggested intestinal obstruction, a characteristic of type E botulism. Another characteristic feature, urinary retention, was observed in case A.

These cases are noteworthy because of the lack of classic ocular and facial muscle manifestations, although transitory blurring of vision was reported in one patient, and dilated but not fixed pupils were seen in another.

Clostridium botulinum *type E is widely distributed. Its spores have been demonstrated in sediment and in fish from all northern oceans and from waterways and soils of all northern continents, including the Great Lakes and the Atlantic, Gulf, and Pacific coasts of North America. The greatest concentration of the spores is in the sediments of shallow offshore waters, especially near the mouths of rivers. All of the major commercial fishing areas are thus well seeded with the microorganism. The type E spores and microorganisms are mainly confined to the fish intestine and are present in low numbers. Type E spores are relatively more heat-labile than those of other* C. botulinum *types, but in processing, the whole fish may become contaminated. Smoking or light cooking may not be sufficient to inactivate all spores. Of freshly smoked fish examined at one processing plant, 1% contained detectable* C. botulinum. *In contrast to other varieties of* C. botulinum, *type E spores germinate and produce toxin at refrigerator temperatures. Therefore, in fresh or processed fish, lethal accumulations of botulinus toxin may develop when a lightly contaminated fish is held at low temperatures under anaerobic or nearly anaerobic conditions.*

Thus far, the majority of reported type E botulism cases have resulted from the consumption of home-preserved fish or fish products. Because of the wide distribution of the microorganism, the potential problem of future outbreaks from commercially processed fish products remains.

REFERENCES

Books and Symposia

Balows, A., DeHaan, R. M., Dowell, V. R., et al., eds. *Anaerobic Bacteria: Role in Disease.* Springfield, IL: Charles C Thomas, 1974.

Brook, I. *Pediatric Anaerobic Infection—Diagnosis and Management.* 2nd ed. St. Louis: C. V. Mosby Co., 1989.

Finegold, S. M. *Anaerobic Bacteria in Human Disease.* New York: Academic Press, 1977.

Finegold, S. M. International Symposium on Anaerobic Bacteria and Their Role in Disease. *Rev. Infect. Dis. 6* (suppl): S1–S299, 1984.

Laboratory Manuals

Dowell, V. R., and Hawkins, T. M. *Laboratory Methods in Anaerobic Bacteriology. CDC Laboratory Manual.* Atlanta, GA: Centers for Disease Control, 1974.

Holdeman, L. V., Cato, E. P., and Moore, W. E. C., eds. *Anaerobe Laboratory Manual.* 4th ed. Blacksburg, VA: Virginia Polytechnic Institute, 1977.

Sutter, V. L., Vargo, V. L., and Finegold, S. M. *Wadsworth Anaerobic Bacteriology Manual.* 5th ed. Belmont, CA: Star Publishing Co., 1985.

Review Articles

Bartlett, J. G. Recent developments in the management of anaerobic infection. *Rev. Infect. Dis. 5:*235, 1983.

Gorbach, S. L., and Bartlett, J. G. Anaerobic infections. *N. Engl. J. Med. 290:*1177, 1237, 1289, 1974.

Simon, G. L., and Gorbach, S. L. Intestinal microflora. *Med. Clin. North Am. 66:*557, 1982.

Styrt, B., and Gorbach, S. L. Recent developments in the understanding of the pathogenesis and treatment of anaerobic infections. *N. Engl. J. Med. 321:*240, 298, 1989.

Original Articles

Armstrong, R. W., Stenn, F., Dowell, V. R., et al. Type E botulism from home canned gefilte fish. *JAMA 210:*303, 1968.

Arnon, S. S., Midura, T. F., Clay, S. A., et al. Infant botulism. Epidemiological, clinical and laboratory aspects. *JAMA 237:*1946, 1977.

Bartlett, J. G., Chang, T. W., Gurwith, M., et al. Antibiotic-associated pseudomembranous colitis due to toxin-producing clostridia. *N. Engl. J. Med. 298:*531, 1978.

Bartlett, J. G., Gorbach, S. L., Tally, F. P., et al. Bacteriology and treatment of primary lung abscess. *Am. Rev. Respir. Dis. 109:*510, 1974.

Berthrong, M., Sabiston, D. C., Jr. Cerebral lesions in congenital heart disease. *Bull. Johns Hopkins Hosp. 89:*384, 1951.

Black, R. E., and Arnon, S. S. Botulism in the United States, 1976. *J. Infect. Dis. 136:*829, 1977.

Brook, I. Recovery of anaerobic bacteria from clinical specimens in 12 years at two military hospitals. *J. Clin. Microbiol. 26:*1181, 1988.

Carlson, J., Wrethen, J., and Beckman, G. Superoxide dismutase in *Bacteroides fragilis* and related *Bacteroides* species. *J. Clin. Microbiol. 6:*280, 1977.

Centers for Disease Control. Botulism in the United States. Review of cases 1899–1967. Public Health Services, Department of Health, Education and Welfare, 1967.

Chang, T. W., Gorbach, S. J., and Bartlett, J. G. Neutralization of *Clostridium difficile* toxin by *Clostridium sordellii* antitoxins. *Infect. Immunol. 22:*418, 1978.

Clabots, C. R., Peterson, L. R., and Gerding, D. N. Characterization of a nosocomial *Clostridium difficile* outbreak by using plasmid profile typing and clindamycin susceptibility testing. *J. Infect. Dis. 158:*731, 1988.

Dowell, V. R. Botulism and tetanus: Selected epidemiologic and microbiologic aspects. *Rev. Infect. Dis. 6*(suppl): S202, 1984.

Drewett, S. E., Payne, D. J. H., Tuke, W., et al. Skin distribution of *Clostridium welchii:* Use of iodophor as sporocidal agent. *Lancet 1:*1172, 1972.

Edsall, G., Elliott, M. W., Pebbles, T. C., et al. Excessive use of tetanus toxoid boosters. *JAMA 202:*17, 1967.

England, D. M., and Rosenblatt, J. E. Anaerobes in human biliary tracts. *J. Clin. Microbiol. 6:*494, 1977.

Felner, J. M., and Dowell, V. R. Anaerobic bacterial endocarditis. *N. Engl. J. Med. 283:*1188, 1970.

Frederick, J., and Braude, A. I. Anaerobic infection of the paranasal sinuses. *N. Engl. J. Med. 290:*135, 1974.

George, W. L., Sutter, V. L., and Finegold, S. M. Antimicrobial agent-induced diarrhea. A bacterial disease. *J. Infect. Dis. 136:*822, 1977.

Jousimies-Somer, H. R., and Finegold, S. M. Problems encountered in clinical anaerobic bacteriology. *Rev. Infect. Dis. 6*(suppl.):S45, 1984.

Kasper, D. L., Onderdonk, A. B., and Bartlett, J. G. Quantitative determination of the antibody response to the capsular polysaccharide of *Bacteroides fragilis* in an animal model of intraabdominal abscess formation. *J. Infect. Dis. 136:*789, 1977.

Levine, L., McComb, J. A., Dwyer, R. C., et al. Active–passive tetanus immunization. *N. Engl. J. Med. 274:*186, 1966.

Lusk, R. H., Fekety, R., Silver, J., et al. Clindamycin-induced enterocolitis in hamsters. *J. Infect. Dis. 137:*464, 1978.

Merson, M. H., and Dowell, V. R., Jr. Epidemiologic, clinical and laboratory aspects of wound botulism. *N. Engl. J. Med. 289:*1005, 1973.

Price, D. L., Griffin, J., Young, A., et al. Tetanus toxin: Direct evidence for retrograde intraaxonal transport. *Science 188:*945, 1975.

Rosenblatt, J. E., and Schoenknicht, F. Effect of several components of anaerobic incubation on antibiotic susceptibility tests results. *Antimicrobiol. Agents Chemother. 1:*433, 1972.

Thadepalli, H., Gorbach, S. L., Broido, P. W., et al. Abdominal trauma, anaerobes, and antibiotics. *Surg. Gynecol. Obstet. 137:*270, 1973.

Walden, W. C., and Hentges, D. J. Differential effects of oxygen and oxidation–reduction potential on the multiplication of three species of anaerobic intestinal bacteria. *Appl. Microbiol. 30:*781, 1975.

Weinstein, W. M., Onderdonk, A. B., Bartlett, J. G., et al. Antimicrobial therapy of experimental intraabdominal sepsis. *J. Infect. Dis. 132:*282, 1975.

30

STANFORD T. SHULMAN, M.D.

Rickettsial Diseases

INTRODUCTION

The rickettsioses are caused by a group of small coccobacilli (rickettsiae) that share certain features of viruses and bacteria, but more closely resemble bacteria. Although like viruses they grow only intracellularly, they resemble bacteria by multiplying by transverse binary fission; by containing both DNA and RNA; by possessing Krebs's cycle (tricarboxylic acid cycle), electron transport, and protein synthetic enzymes; and by being susceptible to several antibacterial agents. Rickettsiae were named to honor Dr. Howard Taylor Ricketts, who, in studies from 1906 to 1909, elucidated the etiology of Rocky Mountain spotted fever and who died of typhus in 1909 while working to determine the etiology of that disorder. Ricketts clearly established the importance of ticks and lice as vectors for these disorders.

For all major rickettsioses except louse-borne typhus, man is only an incidental and accidental host, with the reservoir of rickettsial infection existing in lower animals or in the vectors. The rickettsiae include four genera, *Rickettsia, Coxiella, Ehrlichia*, and *Rochalimaea*, that are grouped together because they share certain characteristics:

1. They are of similar size (0.3 μm × 1–2 μm) and shape, appearing as nonmotile, gram-negative, pleomorphic coccobacilli (Figs. 30–1 and 30–2).
2. They occur naturally in insects (lice and fleas) or in arachnids (ticks and mites) that, except for *C. burnetii*, serve as the major mode of transmission to humans.
3. They multiply within certain host cells, many particularly within endothelial cells.
4. They characteristically produce a widespread vasculitis of small blood vessels.
5. They all result in an acute infection characterized by fever, headache, and rash, with the exception of Q fever, which has no rash.
6. They are all inhibited by certain antibiotics, particularly chloramphenicol and tetracyclines.
7. Except for Q fever and rickettsialpox, rickettsial infections induce agglutinins to *Proteus vulgaris* OX-19, OX-2, or OX-K antigens (Weil-Felix reaction).

Clinical and epidemiologic features facilitate presumptive diagnosis of the rickettsioses, and laboratory confirmation is provided by Weil-Felix reaction and particularly by specific complement-fixing antibody responses (Table 30–1). Because antibiotic therapy must be instituted early in the course of rickettsial infection to be effective, clinical suspicion must be high to

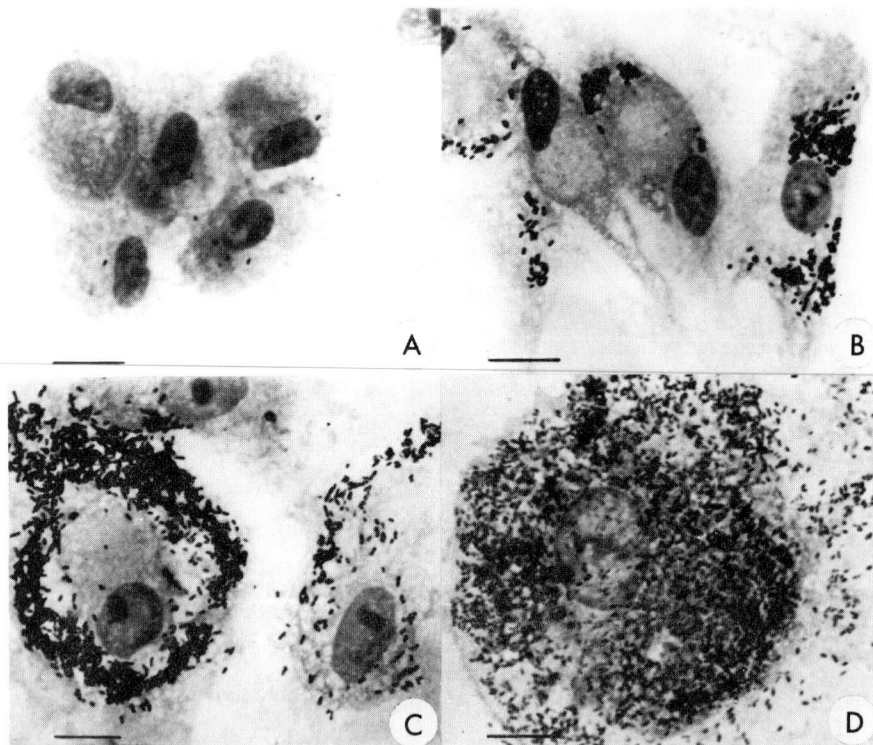

Figure 30–1. Photomicrographs of growth of Rickettsia mooseri *in macrophages in cell culture containing normal human serum (Giménez stain). (Solid bars, 10 µm.)* A. *After 2 h of exposure to* R. mooseri *suspension (× 1480).* B. *Day 3 after infection (× 1400).* C. *Day 6 after infection (× 1400).* D. *Day 6 after infection. Destruction of* R. mooseri *infected macrophage (day 6) with release of microorganisms (× 1560). (From Gambrill, M. R., and Wisseman, C. L., Jr. Mechanisms of immunity in typhus infections. I. Multiplication of typhus rickettsiae in human macrophage cultures in the nonimmune system: Influence of virulence of rickettsial strains and of chloramphenicol. Infect. Immun. 8:519, 1973.)*

achieve consideration of these diagnoses prior to serologic confirmation. Except for scrub typhus, long-lived immunity results from rickettsial infection.

The rickettsial genome is composed of a single circular chromosome of $1.0–1.5 \times 10^9$ d. Although physiologically similar to bacteria, with multiple enzymatic systems, including oxidative phosphorylation and glutamate oxidation for energy production, rickettsiae appear to require certain cofactors provided by the host cell. Except for *C. burnetii*, the rickettsiae quickly lose viability outside host cells. Polychromatic stains such as Giemsa stain are superior to Gram's stain for identification of intracellular rickettsiae.

PATHOGENESIS

After the bite of an infected vector, rickettsiae invade endothelial cells of small blood vessels and are demonstrable in both the nucleus and cytoplasm; they then multiply within those cells and are widely disseminated by the bloodstream. Focal areas of endothelial cell damage and proliferation with perivascular mononuclear cell infiltration result in local areas of hemorrhage and thrombosis. Postulated mechanisms of cell damage include: (1) toxic rickettsial metabolic products, (2) competition for vital substrates, (3) ATP depletion by rickettsiae leading to sodium pump failure and influx of water, and (4) cell-membrane damage related to multiple rickettsial penetration and later to massive rickettsial release. Vascular lesions are most prominent in small vessels of skin, myocardium, and brain and appear to account for the most common clinical manifestations, including rash. In contrast to other rickettsioses, *C. burnetii* is transmitted most frequently by inhalation of dust or animal hides contaminated by rickettsiae, leading to prominent respiratory tract manifestations. Rocky Mountain spotted fever has also been acquired via aerosol, particularly in laboratory settings.

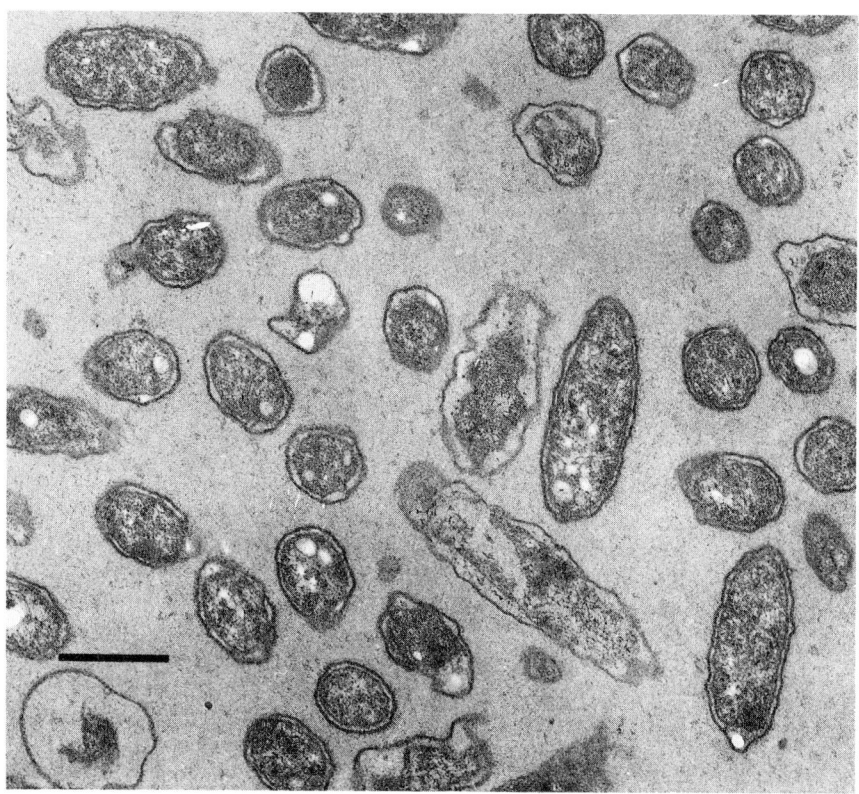

Figure 30–2. Ultrathin section through cells of Rickettsia prowazekii *typical of those seen in the lumen of the louse midgut (bar, 0.5 μm). (From Silverman, D. J., Boese, J. L., and Wisseman, C. L., Jr. Ultrastructural studies of* Rickettsia prowazekii *from louse midgut cells to feces: Search for "dormant" forms.* Infect. Immun. 10:257, 1974.)

The host response to rickettsiae is complex. Host defenses including antibody do not impair rickettsial replication within endothelial cells, and when released from endothelial cells, rickettsiae are phagocytosed by macrophages. In the absence of antibody, rickettsiae replicate well within macrophages (Fig. 30–1), passing from the phagolysosome into the cytoplasm, where replication occurs. However, in the presence of antibody, rickettsiae remain within the phagolysosome, perhaps because of neutralization of a rickettsial product or substrate, and are killed and degraded within that structure. In contrast, the killing of rickettsiae within endothelial or other target cells is antibody-independent and is most likely due to acquired T-cell immunity. Additionally, it can be shown *in vitro* that rickettsial-stimulated lymphocytes release lymphokines that can kill rickettsia within phagocytic or endothelial cells.

CLINICAL DISORDERS

The rickettsioses are divided into several groups, including spotted fevers, typhuslike fevers, scrub typhus group, Q fever, ehrlichiosis, and trench fever (Table 30–1).

Spotted Fevers

Rocky Mountain Spotted Fever

Rocky Mountain spotted fever (RMSF) is by far the most important and the most severe of the spotted fevers, which, except for rickettsialpox, are all tick-transmitted. RMSF has a fatality rate of 20–25% without specific therapy, and although early treatment is important to lower the mortality, diagnosis in the early stages is frequently very difficult. RMSF is caused by *R. rickettsii*, which is antigenetically and genetically closely related to other members of the spotted fever group. RMSF was first described in Idaho and Montana in the late 1800s but since the mid-1940s has almost completely disappeared from the Rocky Mountain region. Since 1931, RMSF has been recognized in the southeastern United States, and the vast majority of U.S. cases now occur in the region from Virginia to

TABLE 30–1. *Clinical Features of Rickettsial Diseases*

	Agent	Vector	Reservoir	Geography	Severity	Eschar	Unique Features
Spotted Fever Group RMSF	*Rickettsia rickettsii*	Tick	Ticks/Rodents	Western Hemisphere	Severe	0	Most important in U.S.
Tick typhuses Boutonneuse	*R. conorii*	Tick	Ticks/Rodents/ Dogs	Mediterranean, Africa, India	Moderate	+	
Queensland	*R. australis*	Tick	Marsupials	Queensland, Australia	Moderate	+	
Siberian	*R. sibirica*	Tick	Long-tailed suslik	China, Mongolia, Pakistan, USSR	Moderate	+	
Rickettsialpox	*R. akari*	Mite	Mites/Mice	U.S., USSR, Korea	Mild	+	Vesicular rash
Typhus Group Epidemic typhus	*R. prowazekii*	Louse	Man/Flying squirrel	Worldwide	Severe	0	Rash spares hands, feet
Brill-Zinsser disease	*R. prowazekii*	(Reactivation)	Humans	Worldwide	Mild	0	Occurs years after infection
Murine typhus	*R. typhi (mooseri)*	Flea	Rodents	Scattered foci worldwide	Moderate	0	
Scrub Typhus	*R. tsutsugamushi*	Chigger (mite larva)	Mites/Rodents	Japan, S.E. Asia, Southwestern Pacific	Variable (strain-dependent)	+	General adenopathy; immunity doesn't follow illness
Q Fever	*C. burnetii*	Ticks possibly	Ticks/Mammals	Worldwide	Mild (usually)	0	Inhalation transmission; no rash; hardy organism; reticuloendothelial system target
Ehrlichiosis	*E. sennetsu*	Unknown	Humans	Far East	Mild	0	Intraleukocytic parasites
	E. canis	Dog tick	Dogs	Worldwide	Not defined	0	Few cases documented to date
Trench Fever	*Rochalimaea quintana*	Louse	Humans	Eastern Europe, N. Africa, Mexico	Mild	0	

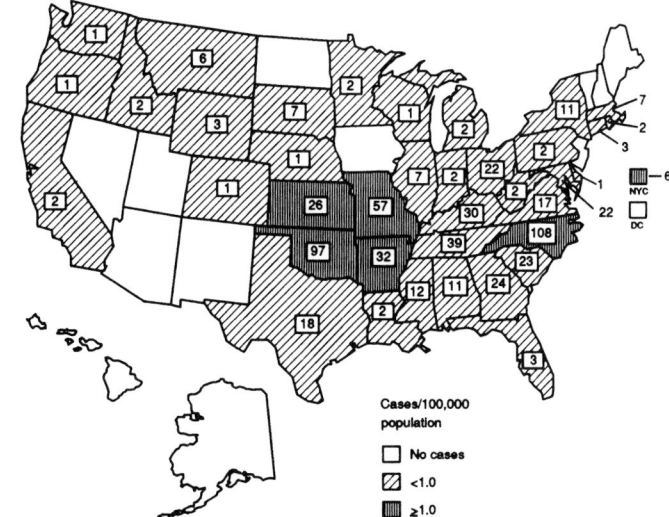

Figure 30–3. Incidence and rates of Rocky Mountain spotted fever, by state in the United States in 1988. (From Morbidity and Mortality Weekly Report, *July 28, 1989, p. 514.)*

Georgia, the Ohio River Valley, Tennessee, Arkansas, and Oklahoma (Figs. 30–3 and 30–4). At present, RMSF occurs to some degree throughout the Western Hemisphere.

The epidemiologic characteristics of RMSF are directly related to the ticks that serve as reservoir and vector (the dog tick, *Dermacentor variabilis,* in the eastern U.S.; the wood tick, *D. andersoni,* in the West; the Lone Star tick, *Amblyomma americanum,* in the Southwest; and others in Mexico and South America). *R. rickettsii* in ticks are passed transovarially to subsequent generations of ticks, and the ticks require a blood meal, usually from a dog, horse, or sheep, to proceed through their stages of development to maturity. Most cases occur from April to September, coinciding with tick prevalence. Humans are incidental hosts, with rick-ettsial transmission occurring from salivary secretions when an infected adult tick remains attached to humans for at least several hours. The rickettsiae disseminate widely and establish infection within vascular endothelial and smooth muscle cells, resulting in vascular damage.

The major clinical features of RMSF are high fever, headache, rash, toxicity, confusion, and myalgia. On average, RMSF is a fairly serious illness. The course is highly variable, with some patients manifesting only mild nonspecific symptoms but others with a fulminant course leading to death within a few days. The mean incubation period is 7 days (range is 2–14 days) after an infected tick bite, with the earliest symptoms being nonspecific. The classic triad of fever, rash, and history of tick bite is present in only 3% of patients by the third day of illness. Rash

*Figure 30–4. Rates of reported Rocky Mountain spotted fever cases in the south Atlantic states and all other states for 1970–1985, by year. *South Atlantic states include Delaware, Maryland, Virginia, West Virginia, North Carolina, South Carolina, Georgia, Florida, and the District of Columbia. (From* Morbidity and Mortality Weekly Report, *April 18, 1986, p. 248.)*

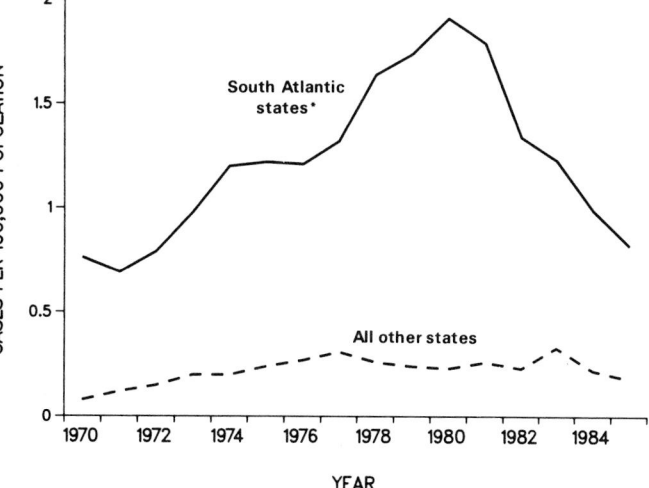

develops as late as the sixth day but is usually present on the third or fourth day, first appearing on the wrists and ankles and spreading within hours up the extremities to the trunk (Fig. 30–5). Rash on the palms and soles is highly characteristic. The rash initially consists of small red macules that blanch with pressure and that then progress to macular–papular, and ultimately, to petechial–purpuric lesions. Intense, persistent headache is common, and patients appear toxic. Signs of meningoencephalitis, such as lethargy, confusion, delirium, stupor, ataxia, coma, seizures, and focal neurologic findings, may develop, with CNS damage being a major factor in RMSF mortality. Fatality rates increase with age and are higher in males and in blacks. The diagnosis of early RMSF is difficult, especially prior to development of the skin rash, and must be suspected on the basis of symptoms, signs, and epidemiologic features in order to institute specific therapy sufficiently early to affect favorably the course of the illness.

Early nonspecific laboratory features include leukopenia, thrombocytopenia, and hyponatremia. In some hospitals, *R. rickettsii* can be demonstrated by immunofluorescence in biopsies of skin lesions. Culture of rickettsiae is difficult and generally impractical. Serologic tests are not useful early in the disease, but are very valuable for diagnosis in retrospect (Table 30–2). Rising titers to *Proteus* OX-19 or OX-2 are usually seen in the second week of illness, but it must be recognized that sera of some healthy individuals are positive for these Weil-Felix reactions. More specific antirickettsial antibodies can be detected in convalescent sera by complement-fixation or other methods, but again, they are only useful in retrospect and cannot be relied upon to facilitate early treatment decisions. Considerable cross-reactivity exists among rickettsiae.

The differential diagnosis of RMSF includes meningococcal infection, measles, enteroviral exanthems, toxic shock syndrome, leptospirosis, disseminated gonococcal infection, secondary syphilis, systemic lupus, thrombotic thrombocytopenic purpura, immune thrombocytopenia, and other rickettsioses.

Within the first week of illness, antibiotic therapy is highly effective in RMSF, but therapy instituted later may have little effect on the course of this potentially fatal disease. Effective agents are chloramphenicol, 50–100 mg/kg/day orally or intravenously divided into four doses, or tetracycline, 25–50 mg/kg/day orally or 15–25 mg/kg/day intravenously divided into four doses. Therapy is continued until the patient is completely afebrile for at least 48 h, usually about a 1-week course. Tetracycline is avoided in pregnancy and for children younger than 9 years old. Both chloramphenicol and tetracyclines are rickettsiostatic, not rickettsiocidal. The value of corticosteroids in severe RMSF has been suggested but not proved. The overall mortality from RMSF in the United States is 5–7%, primarily occurring in patients undiagnosed until the second week of illness. Death is usually related to vascular collapse, cardiac or renal failure, encephalitis, or thrombocytopenia. Solid immunity develops in those who recover. Prevention requires avoidance or reduction of tick exposure in endemic areas. Frequent deticking is useful since ticks must remain attached for at least 4–6 h to transmit RMSF. Although an RMSF vaccine was prepared as early as 1924, no effective vaccine is currently available.

Other Spotted Fevers

Tick-Borne Spotted Fevers

Three other tick-borne spotted fevers (also called *tick typhuses*) are widely distributed in Europe, Asia, Africa, and Australia and are

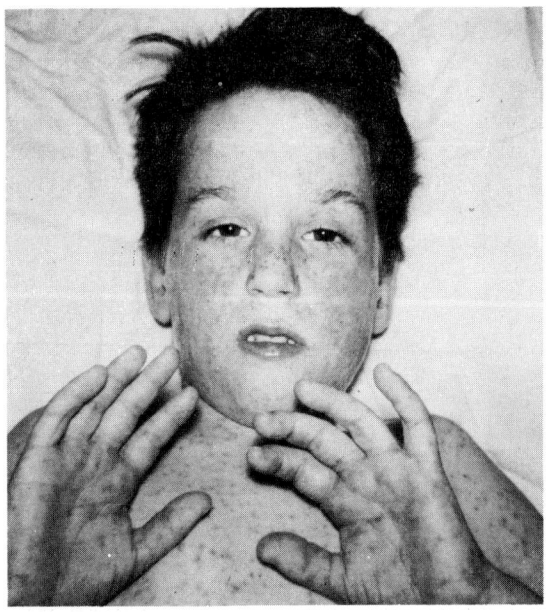

Figure 30–5. Rocky Mountain spotted fever. Typical rash occurring on the face and the palms. (From Hazard, G. W., et al. Rocky Mountain spotted fever in the eastern United States. (N. Engl. J. Med. 280:57, 1969. Reprinted by permission.)

TABLE 30–2. *Serologic Responses in Rickettsial Infections*

	Weil-Felix Reactions			Complement-Fixation Tests		
	OX-19	*OX-2*	*OX-K*	*Typhus*	*Spotted Fever*	*Q Fever*
Spotted Fevers						
RMSF	+ + +	+ + +	0	0	+ + +	0
Tick typhuses	+ + +	+ + +	0	0	+ + +	0
Rickettsialpox	0	0	0	0	+ + +	0
Typhus Fevers						
Epidemic louse-borne	+ + +	+	0	+ + +	0	0
Brill-Zinsser disease	+ + +/0	0	0	+ + +	0	0
Murine typhus	+ + +	+	0	+ + +	0	0
Scrub Typhus	0	0	+ + +	0	0	0
Q Fever	0	0	0	0	0	+ + +

caused by rickettsiae that share the same group antigen as *R. rickettsii* but have different type-specific antigens. These species include *R. conorii*, causing boutonneuse fever in India, Pakistan, Israel, Ethiopia, Kenya, South Africa, Morocco, and southern Europe; *R. australis*, causing Queensland tick typhus in Australia; and *R. sibirica*, causing Siberian tick typhus in China, Mongolia, Pakistan, and the Soviet Union.

Rickettsialpox

The second most common rickettsiosis of the spotted fever group in the United States is *rickettsialpox*, caused by *R. akari*. This benign infection was first recognized in New York City in 1946 and is seen primarily there and in other cities in the northeastern United States. Occasional cases are seen in other parts of the United States, the Soviet Union, and Korea. This disease is the result of disruption of the natural cycle between the mite vector and the house mouse, with humans infected when a paucity of mouse hosts leads mites to seek humans as alternative hosts. After an incubation period of 9–14 days, a red papule develops at the mite bite location and evolves to a papulovesicle and then to a black eschar. Concomitantly, regional lymph glands become enlarged and low to moderate fever (100–103°F) occurs, lasting up to 1 week, along with headache. A remarkable rash develops within a few days of the onset of fever, consisting of scattered macules that rapidly become firm maculopapules, and then vesicles develop on the papules. Lesions over the face, trunk, and extremities number from 5 to more than 100, and the rash is very similar to chickenpox, hence the name rickettsialpox. Weil-Felix reactions are negative. The illness is benign and self-limited. Therapy is not necessary although

chloramphenicol and tetracycline have been used.

Typhus Fevers

These are three illnesses that are caused by two rickettsial species, *R. prowazekii* and *R. typhi* (formerly *R. mooseri*). Although they are clinically and pathologically similar, these illnesses differ epidemiologically and in severity.

Classic Epidemic Typhus (Louse-Borne)

Classic epidemic typhus is an acute infection by *R. prowazekii* transmitted by the body louse *(Pediculus humanus corporis)*. Its existence has been well documented for at least five centuries. Lice are essential for typhus fever, and therefore it occurs in epidemics during famine, war, and other catastrophes associated with louse proliferation. For example, more than 30 million cases occurred in Eastern Europe following World War I, causing about 3 million deaths. In cases that still occur sporadically in the United States, the flying squirrel serves as the reservoir. *R. prowazekii* is antigenically distinct from the spotted fever agents and is more closely related to *R. typhi*. Clinically, 1–2 weeks after the bite of an infected louse, high fever (40°C), rash, myalgia, and headache appear abruptly. Untreated epidemic louse-borne typhus has a reported fatality rate of 60–70% in those older than 50 and about 10% in young adults. Small vessel vasculitis leads to protean clinical manifestations that may include renal failure, myocardial disease, CNS dysfunction, pneumonia, and gastrointestinal involvement, in addition to the fairly characteristic rash. Rash begins on the trunk and spreads in 1–2 days to the extremities (the opposite of RMSF), usually sparing the face, palms, and soles (unlike RMSF). The rash then produces lesions that progress from macules to papules to hemorrhagic or even necrotic lesions. Early diagnosis depends on clinical and epidemiologic features. Serologic tests are useful for confirmation of the diagnosis; *Proteus* OX-19 reactivity is generally positive in the second week of illness and more specific complement-fixation and ELISA tests are now available. Therapy is the same as for RMSF, and complete recovery is the rule when therapy is begun early. Premature discontinuation of therapy (before 5 days) is associated with recrudescence many years later (Brill-Zinsser disease, see below). Prevention is achieved by louse control.

Brill-Zinsser Disease

Brill-Zinsser disease is a relapse or recrudescence of louse-borne typhus years after the initial attack, first noted by Nathan Brill in 1898 in Russian and Polish immigrants living in New York. The organisms lie dormant, probably in the reticuloendothelial system, until reactivation occurs. Clinical manifestations are similar to epidemic louse-borne typhus. Probably because of partial immunity as a result of the initial infection, recrudescent disease is milder and of short duration. Tetracycline or chloramphenicol is the recommended therapy. Frequently, history of a previous episode of typhus can be elicited from patients with Brill-Zinsser disease. As predicted, an IgG (secondary) rather than IgM (primary) immune response can be demonstrated.

Murine (Endemic) Typhus

Murine typhus is a flea-borne disease caused by *R. typhi* (previously known as *R. mooseri*), and is transmitted worldwide by rats by the oriental rat flea *(Xenopsylla cheopis)*. Humans are incidentally infected from the bite of an infected flea. Once the flea is infected asymptomatically with *R. typhi* from feeding on an acutely ill rat, the organism multiplies in the flea gut and is excreted in feces. When feeding on humans, the flea defecates and rickettsia-contaminated feces can be inoculated into skin abrasions or bites, leading to human infection. As recently as the 1940s, 2000–5000 cases of murine typhus occurred yearly in the United States, particularly in the southeastern and Gulf Coast areas. Recently, with rat control programs, only 40–80 cases have been reported yearly, mostly in Texas

(Fig. 30–6). The clinical features are similar to those for louse-borne typhus, but are milder and of shorter duration. Fever is up to 39°C and regresses after about 10 days. Headache and rash are less severe and of shorter duration than in louse-borne typhus. Complications are rare and mortality is less than 1%. The serologic responses in murine typhus are very similar to those in louse-borne typhus, although *R. typhi* antigens should be used for CF and ELISA tests. Therapy is as outlined for other rickettsioses. Prevention obviously depends upon rat and flea control measures.

Scrub Typhus

Scrub typhus is a mite-borne rickettsiosis indigenous to Southeast Asia, Japan, and the southwestern Pacific. The etiologic agent is *R. tsutsugamushi*; the illness is also known as tsutsugamushi fever. There is marked antigenic heterogenicity among strains of *R. tsutsugamushi* that appear to correlate with striking differences in severity. This disease was first described in Japan by Hashimoto in 1810. It was early noted that this illness was confined to farmers in river valleys in July and August and that they developed a characteristic eschar linked to the bite of a mite. Trombiculid mites, such as the red mite serve as both vector and reservoir, with transmission occurring transovarially; there is a wild rodent reservoir as well. Humans that intrude upon the low vegetation or scrub areas may become incidentally infected from larval mite bites. Clinically, scrub typhus is a potentially very serious disease, although its severity is quite variable. A necrotic eschar develops in 50% of individuals during the 6–21-day incubation period. High fever, headache, maculopapular rash, and (unlike any other rickettsiosis) generalized adenopathy develop. Splenomegaly and conjunctivitis are common. Scrub typhus among western troops in endemic areas during World War II was associated with pneumonitis, myocarditis, shock, seizures, and hemorrhagic phenomena. Preantibiotic era mortality ranged from 1 to 60%, but fatalities are rare in the antibiotic era. Diagnosis is facilitated by *Proteus* OX-K agglutinins in about 60% of patients and by specific CF or immunofluorescent assays. The latter are difficult because of the great degree of strain variability. Treatment is the same as for other rickettsioses. Reinfections are relatively common in scrub typhus, in contrast to other rickettsial infections.

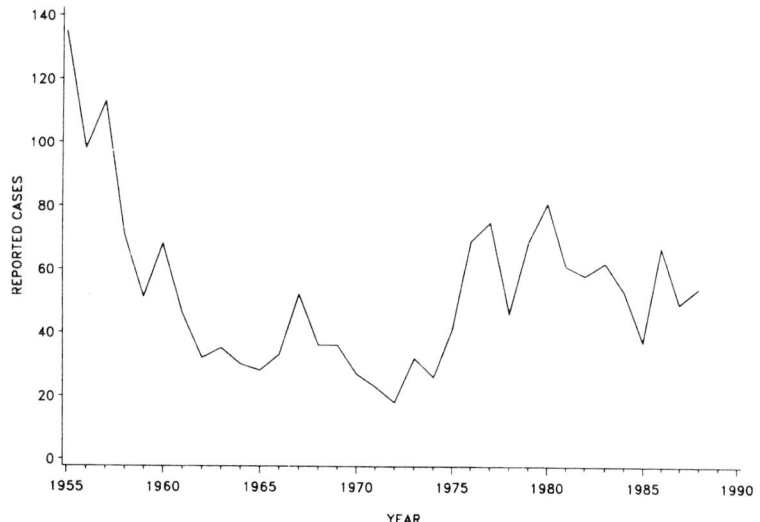

TYPHUS FEVER, FLEA-BORNE (endemic, murine) — By year, United States, 1955-1988

Figure 30–6. Incidence of flea-borne typhus fever (endemic, murine) from 1955 to 1988 (by year) in the United States. (From Morbidity and Mortality Weekly Report, Summary of notifiable disease. *October 6, 1989, p. 45.)*

Q Fever

Q (or query) fever is a worldwide acute rickettsiosis caused by *C. burnetti* that is unique by being transmitted to humans primarily by inhalation rather than by an arthropod bite. Q fever was first recognized in 1937 by Frank Burnet in Australia and Harold Cox in the United States. Cattle, sheep, goats, and ticks are the major reservoirs for *C. burnetii*, and infection is usually subclinical in animals, with transmission occurring as a result of excretion of rickettsiae in milk, urine, and feces. *C. burnetii* is uniquely highly resistant to desiccation, heat, and physical and chemical agents, and is extremely infectious for humans and animals. Q fever is unique among the rickettsioses in that it is most often acquired by inhalation of contaminated aerosols; arthropods are unimportant in spread, and the clinical illness is not associated with rash. In domestic livestock the infection is usually inapparent until an event like parturition leads to reactivation, with contamination of soil with infected milk, urine, feces, placental tissues, and fluids. Dried dust particles containing *C. burnetii* remain potential sources of infection for many months. The incubation period averages 20 days (range is 14–39 days), and the illness begins abruptly with rigors, high fever, severe headache, retrobulbar pain, and myalgia, but no rash. Respiratory symptoms (cough, chest pain) are common, with multiple round lesions or patchy pulmonary infiltrates seen in about 50%. Hepatosplenomegaly is frequent with only minimal liver dysfunction and only occasional icterus. Gastroenteritis and hemolytic anemia are also seen. Q fever endocarditis is a rare, but severe and often fatal, complication in patients with preexisting cardiac disease. Q fever is generally a mild, self-limited disease lasting only 1–2 weeks and associated with less than 1% mortality. No Weil-Felix reaction develops in Q fever, but highly specific ELISA, complement fixation, and immunofluorescence assays allow confirmation of the diagnosis from convalescent sera. Attempts to isolate the organism may be dangerous and should be avoided if possible. Q fever responds promptly to tetracyclines or chloramphenicol, and relapses are rare. Treated patients appear to recover somewhat more quickly than those who do not receive treatment. Endocarditis has required very prolonged therapy (12 months or more), probably because the effective agents are rickettsiostatic rather than rickettsiocidal. Attempted preventive measures include development of a vaccine (not yet available) and control of infected herds and of aerosol in laboratories.

Ehrlichiosis

Ehrlichia, a genus of the family Rickettsiaceae, are intraleukocytic parasites that infect humans and a variety of animals. The primary human pathogen is *E. sennetsu,* which has been reported to cause an infectious mononucleosis-like illness in the Far East, particularly in Kyushu, Japan. This has been termed sennetsu rickettsiosis, and is probably transmitted by the bite of an unknown vector in swampy coastal areas of southeast Kyushu, Japan. Patients manifest fever, myalgia, headache, sore throat, and generalized lymphadenopathy; rash and eschar are very rare. More recently, human infection by *E. canis,* the worldwide agent of tropical canine pancytopenia, has been reported. The vector is the brown dog tick, and a few humans with illnesses resembling RMSF but without rash have been shown to have *E. canis* infection. It has been suggested that human infection should be suspected in those with seronegative RMSF-like illnesses and perhaps in some with pancytopenias. Confirmation includes identifying intraleukocytic inclusions and observing a specific serologic response.

Trench Fever

Endemic in Mexico, North Africa, and Eastern Europe, trench fever is a mild louse-borne disease caused by the rickettsia *Rochalimaea quintana.* Humans are thought to be the reservoir. This infection emerges when louse-infected humans are gathered in unhygienic circumstances (e.g., prisons, refugee camps). Tetracycline is a highly effective treatment. An organism thought to be related to *R. quintana* has recently been associated with bacillary angiomatosis, an infectious disease of immunocompromised hosts that is characterized by proliferation of small blood vessels in skin and viscera.

CASE HISTORY

An 11-year-old boy from North Carolina was admitted to the hospital in June with severe headache, fever, and rash. Three days earlier he had complained of not feeling well. The next day a rash appeared on his wrists and ankles and his temperature was 103.5°F (39.7°C). The next day rash had spread to the arms and was noted on the soles and palms. His temperature remained high, a severe frontal headache developed, and marked tenderness of the calves and swelling of the ankles appeared. Headache was not relieved by aspirin. At this time he was brought to the hospital.

Upon admission the boy appeared acutely ill, with temperature of 103.6°F (39.8°C), pulse 115/min, respirations 34/min, and blood pressure 128/66 mm Hg. Confluent erythematous macular lesions were present on the palms and soles and over the distal parts of all four extremities. The lesions extended to the proximal part of the extremities with a few lesions on the abdomen and chest. In some areas, the lesions were papular, but none blanched upon pressure. Lymphadenopathy and nuchal rigidity were not noted. There was marked tenderness when pressure was exerted on both gastrocnemius muscles.

Examination of the urine revealed no abnormalities. The white blood cell count was 11,500/mm³, with 65% segmented neutrophils, 5% band forms, 20% lymphocytes, and 10% monocytes. A chest roentgenogram and an electrocardiogram revealed normal findings. Spinal fluid obtained by lumbar puncture was clear; the pressure was 300 mm Hg. The spinal fluid contained 20 WBC/mm³, mostly mononuclear cells. No microorganisms were seen.

Because of the typical distribution and appearance of the rash, the severe frontal headache, and the muscle tenderness, Rocky Mountain spotted fever was suspected. It was learned that on the previous weekend the patient had taken an overnight camping trip with several friends in an area known to be infested with ticks. Three campers, including the patient, had tick bites. Because of the high probability that the patient had Rocky Mountain spotted fever, tetracycline was started immediately. Symptoms promptly abated and the patient made an uneventful recovery. He was discharged on the fifth hospital day.

Serum collected on the first hospital day (3 days after the onset of illness) was negative in both the Weil-Felix and complement-fixation tests for Rocky Mountain spotted fever. However, a second serum 2 weeks later had an OX-19 titer of 1:640. The specific complement-fixation test was strongly positive. Thus, the diagnosis of Rocky Mountain spotted fever was confirmed.

REFERENCES
Books

Manson-Bahr, P. E. C., and Bell, D. R., eds. *Manson's Tropical Diseases,* 19th ed. London: Bailliere Tindall, 1987:213–245.

Walker, D. H., ed. *Biology of Rickettsial Diseases*. Boca Raton, FL: CRC Press, 1988.

Zinsser, H., ed. *Rats, Lice and History*. Boston: Little Brown and Co., 1935.

Review Articles

Brettman, C. R., Lewin, S., Holymein, R. S., et al. Rickettsialpox: Report of an outbreak and a contemporary review. *Medicine 60*:363–372, 1981.

Font-Creus, B., Bella-Cueto, F., Espejo-Arenas, E., et al. Mediterranean spotted fever. *Rev. Infect. Dis. 7*:635–643, 1985.

Hase, T. Developmental sequence and surface membrane assembly of rickettsiae. *Annu. Rev. Microbiol. 39*:69–88, 1985.

Helmick, C. G., Bernard, K. W., and D'Angelo, L. J. Rocky Mountain spotted fever: Clinical, laboratory and epidemiological features of 262 cases. *J. Infect. Dis. 150*:480–488, 1984.

McDade, J. E., and Newhouse, V. F. Natural history of *Rickettsia rickettsii*. *Annu. Rev. Microbiol. 40*:287–309, 1986.

Sawyer, L. A., Fishbein, D. B., and McDade, J. E. Q fever: Current concepts. *Rev. Infect. Dis. 9*:935–946, 1987.

Weiss, E. The biology of the rickettsiae. *Annu. Rev. Microbiol. 32*:345–370, 1982.

Wisseman, C. L., Jr. Rickettsiae: Diversity in obligate intracellular parasitism. In: Schlessinger, D., ed., *Microbiology—1983*. Washington, D.C.: American Society of Microbiology, 1983:375–390.

Original Articles

Brill, N. E. An acute infectious disease. A clinical study based on 221 cases of unknown origin. *Am. J. Med. Sci. 139*:484, 1910.

Huebner, R. J., and Armstrong, C. Rickettsialpox—A newly recognized rickettsial disease. I. Isolation of the etiologic agent. *Public Health Rep. 61*:1605–1614, 1946.

McDade, J. E., Shepard, C. C., Redus, M. A., et al. Evidence of *Rickettsia prowazekii* infections in the U.S. *Am. J. Trop. Med. Hyg. 29*:277–284, 1980.

Maeda, K., Markowitz, N., Hawley, R. C., et al. Human infection with *Ehrlichia canis*, a leukocytic rickettsia. *N. Engl. J. Med. 316*:853–856, 1987.

Oster, C. N., Burke, D. S., Kenyon, R. M., et al. Laboratory-acquired Rocky Mountain spotted fever. *N. Engl. J. Med. 297*:859–863, 1977.

Ricketts, H. T. The study of Rocky Mountain spotted fever (tick fever?) by means of animal inoculations: A preliminary communication. *JAMA 47*:33–36, 1906.

Salgo, M. P., Telzak, E. E., Currie, B., et al. A focus of Rocky Mountain spotted fever within New York City. *N. Engl. J. Med. 318*:1345–1348, 1988.

Silverman, D. J., and Bond, S. B. Infection of human vascular endothelial cells by *Rickettsia rickettsii*. *J. Infect. Dis. 149*:201–206, 1984.

Wilfert, C. M., MacCormack, J. N., Kleeman, K., et al. Epidemiology of Rocky Mountain spotted fever as determined by active surveillence. *J. Infect Dis. 150*:469–479, 1984.

Woodward, T. E. A historical account of the rickettsial diseases with a discussion of unresolved problems. *J. Infect. Dis. 127*:583–594, 1973.

Woodward, T. E.: Rocky Mountain spotted fever: Epidemiological and early clinical signs are keys to treatment and reduced mortality. *J. Infect. Dis. 150*:465–468, 1984.

Zinsser, H. Varieties of typhus virus and epidemiology of American form of European typhus fever (Brill's disease). *Am. J. Hyg. 20*:513–532, 1934.

31 *A TODD DAVIS, M.D.*

Zoonoses

INTRODUCTION

Zoonoses are infectious diseases that occur principally in animals but which may spread to humans. Table 31–1 lists some, but certainly not all, of the diseases that fall under this category. Viruses, bacteria, fungi, and protozoans are all represented in zoonotic diseases. Given the large number of infectious agents and the animal hosts they infect, it is not surprising that the skin, digestive tract, and respiratory tract may serve as portals of entry for these diseases. For example, tularemia may be acquired transcutaneously by contact with infected animal tissue. Trichinosis is acquired by ingestion of infected meat. Psittacosis and plague may be acquired by the airborne route.

Control of zoonoses rests on diminishing the incidence of disease in the animal reservoir; animal vaccination when possible; preventing the importation of infected birds or animals; changing hygenic practices, such as preventing pigs from eating raw sewage; pasteurization of milk to reduce the likelihood of brucellosis or listeriosis; and control of vectors, such as eradication of fleas which may transmit plague from animal to animal.

BRUCELLOSIS

Sir David Bruce discovered the etiology of brucellosis while investigating an outbreak of Malta fever in the early part of the 20th century. Brucellosis, named after him, is caused by a fastidious, gram-negative, aerobic bacterium found throughout the world.

The animal reservoirs for this disease include cattle *(Brucella abortus)*, dogs *(B. canis)*, pigs *(B. suis)*, goats *(B. melitensis)*, and sheep *(B. ovis)*. Patterns of transmission include handling of infected carcasses during the slaughtering process in abattoirs, handling of infected animals or touching their secretions, or drinking contaminated (unpasteurized) milk.

The organism gains entry to the human host through broken skin, the conjunctivae, the lungs, and the gastrointestinal tract. Humans are terminal hosts, unable to transmit the infection to other humans. Adults, because of occupational exposure, are much more frequently infected than are children.

After gaining entry, the organisms are phagocytized by polymorphonuclear leukocytes (PMNs), but they are not effectively killed in the intraphagocytic vacuoles. As infected PMNs burst, macrophages and reticuloendothelial cells ingest the organisms which then may persist for weeks or months; this is the biologic basis for chronic human infections.

Clinical manifestations, whether in children or adults, may be acute or gradual in onset. Fever, shaking chills, weakness, lethargy, and weight loss occur. The nonspecific nature of the symptoms mimics other diseases, such as influenza, malaria, typhoid fever, tularemia, and miliary tuberculosis. On occasion, brucellosis has been confused with lymphoma. Physical findings are often limited to such reticuloendothelial signs as hepatosplenomegaly or lymphadenopathy. However, splenomegaly occurs less

TABLE 31–1. Selected Zoonoses

Disease	Etiology	Usual Reservoir	Usual Mode of Transmission	Disease in Nonhuman Host	Disease in Human	Human–Human Transmission
Anthrax	Bacillus anthracis	Cattle, sheep, goats	Infected animals or their products	Systemic illness, GI problems	Pneumonitis, malignant pustule	No
Brucellosis	Brucella sp.	Cattle, swine, goats	Milk or infected carcasses	Abortion, mastitis, lameness, abscesses	Fever, nodes, bacteremia, etc.	No
Campylobacteriosis	Campylobacter fetus, C. jejuni	Cattle, sheep, pets, wild mammals	Contaminated food and water	Usually none	Gastroenteritis	Yes (fecal–oral)
Leptospirosis	Leptospira sp.	Cattle, rodents, other mammals	Water contaminated by urine	Usually none	Nephritis, hepatitis, systemic disease	No
Tularemia	Francisella tularensis	Rabbits, other small mammals	Bite of fleas, deer flies, mosquitoes	Usually none	Pneumonia, skin lesion, adenitis	No
Psittacosis	Chlamydia psittaci	Birds (especially imported)	Contact with birds	Usually none	Pneumonia	No
Plague	Yersinia pestis	Rats and other rodents	Flea bite	Usually none	Bubonic, pneumonic, septicemic plague	Yes (respiratory droplet)
Listeriosis	Listeria monocytogenes	Mammals, birds	Ingestion of contaminated food (cheese, etc.)	Usually none	Meningitis, abortion	No
Relapsing fever	Borrelia sp.	Rodents	Tick bite	Usually none	Relapsing fevers, hemorrhage	Yes (body louse)
Salmonellosis	Salmonella sp.	Poultry, cattle	Ingestion of contaminated food	Usually none	Gastroenteritis, sepsis	Yes (fecal–oral)
Pasteurellosis	Pasteurella multocida	Animal oral cavities	Animal bites or scratches	Usually none	Wound infection	No
Orf	Parapoxvirus	Sheep, goats	Animal contact	Pustular lesions	Papulovesicular granulomatous skin lesions	No
Rabies	Rabiesvirus	Small mammals	Animal bite	None, or death with paralysis	Hydrophobia, excitation, paralysis, death	No
Yellow fever	Yellow fever virus	Nonhuman primates	Mosquito bites	Usually none	Hepatitis	Rare
Melioidosis	Pseudomonas pseudomallei	Rats, mice, rabbits, ruminants, primates	Inhalation or direct inoculation	Usually none	Lung abscess, septicemia	Very rare
Sleeping sickness	Trypanosoma brucei	Wild ungulates, humans	Tsetse fly	Usually none	Meningoencephalitis	Yes
Lyme disease	Borrelia burgdorferi	White-footed mouse	Bite of deer tick (Ixodes) nymphs	Usually none	Erythema chronicum migrans, arthritis, carditis, neuropathy	No

than 50% of the time and hepatomegaly in about 25% of bacteremic patients. Liver function tests are usually normal.

The diagnosis is largely dependent on clinical suspicion, particularly if there is no clear-cut history of exposure to a known source of brucellosis. Although the definitive diagnosis is made by recovering the organism from blood cultures, a strongly presumptive diagnosis can be made by obtaining a positive febrile agglutinin response, that is, demonstrating high titer of specific brucella agglutinins.

The principles underlying therapy are the use of at least one appropriate antibiotic for a sufficient time. Very low rates of relapse are associated with treatment with oral trimethoprim-sulfamethoxazole or, in those >8 years old, oral tetracycline for 3 weeks combined with IM gentamicin for the first 5 days.

TULAREMIA

Tularemia is a bacterial disease caused by *Francisella tularensis*, a pleomorphic, gram-negative, aerobic coccobacillus. The illness was first detected in Tulare County, California, hence the species name *tularensis*. The genus name, *Francisella*, is in honor of Dr. Edward Francis, who extensively studied the disease in the early part of the 20th century.

Rabbits, particularly snowshoe rabbits but also jackrabbits, muskrats, and occasionally beavers, can harbor the organism for a long time without becoming demonstrably ill. Fleas, deer flies, and ticks serve as vectors for transmitting the disease to other rodents and to human beings. Given the nature of the animal and insect reservoirs and the environments in which they live, there are a variety of ways in which humans become infected. The most frequent route may be through the bite of an insect, although the bite of an animal can transmit the organism if the animal has recently consumed infected flesh. Handlers of such wild game as rabbits are occasionally infected through undetected or visible breaks in the skin. Occasionally, when water becomes contaminated by beavers, the organism can enter through the conjunctivae. Airborne transmissions occur following harvesting in fields contaminated by small animals or in laboratory workers handling infected material or cultures.

All strains of *F. tularensis* appear to be antigenically identical. However, there are strain differences: the so-called Jellison type A strain causes severe and fulminant illness, whereas Jellison type B causes much milder disease in humans.

The typical infection begins after an incubation period of only 1–3 days. A maculoerythematous lesion develops at the inoculation site and soon evolves into a papule. As the papule continues to develop, the overlying skin becomes thinned and taut, ulcerating within 1–2 days. As the papule enlarges, fever, systemic symptoms, and regional lymphadenopathy develop. If the infection remains unrecognized, it may linger for 2–4 weeks. If infection occurs by airborne transmission, organisms may deposit anywhere along the respiratory tract, causing tracheitis, bronchitis, or pneumonia. The last is an extremely serious disease, with a mortality rate approaching 30%. As organisms escape the lung parenchyma, they may temporarily lodge in the hilar lymph nodes on their way to the bloodstream. As bloodstream invasion occurs, a typhoid-like septic illness develops. Ironically, *F. tularensis* seems unable to infect the gut as a prelude to sepsis.

Streptomycin remains the drug of choice for managing tularemia. The local lesion, systemic symptoms, and regional lymphadenopathy usually resolve within a few days of treatment. With adequate therapy, mortality is less than 1%, except in cases of pneumonic or typhoidal tularemia.

PLAGUE

Yersinia pestis, the causative agent of plague, is a small, pleomorphic, nonmotile, gram-negative bacillus. Staining with Wayson or Giemsa stains gives the cell a bipolar or "safety pin" morphology. Plague has caused large-scale epidemics throughout history, thereby altering history itself. Indeed, one third of the population of Europe died of plague during the 14th century. *Y. pestis* apparently entered the United States from shipboard rats in San Francisco in the early part of the 20th century.

Reservoirs include infected rodents and their fleas. Persistence of plague over the centuries probably depends on the organisms' surviving in hibernating animals over the winter, and on fleas which may harbor the organisms for 12–15 months after becoming infected from a rodent. In addition, *Y. pestis* may be able to survive in soil.

Humans invariably become infected by either the bite of a flea or handling an infected animal. Within 3–4 days, there is an abrupt onset of illness characterized by fever, malaise, weakness, and headache. The fever is frequently high and hectic. The organisms move from the initial site of inoculation to the regional lymph nodes, causing extremely tender and painful lymph glands—buboes (thus, bubonic plague). The nodes are typically large, fixed, edematous, and exquisitely tender. The most frequent site is in the groin, although the axillary or cervical glands may be involved. Usually only one set of regional glands is involved.

As the local defenses in regional nodes are overcome, the organisms quickly spread throughout the body. Many of the fulminant manifestations of the illness, such as coagulation disturbances, shock, and death, appear related to the release of endotoxin by the organisms.

Pulmonary involvement, either by direct inhalation of organisms or secondary to septicemic spread, results in rapidly progressive, highly fatal pneumonic plague. Plague should be considered in the face of a rapidly progressive febrile illness in the rural southwestern part of the United States where plague is endemic—an average of 18 cases per year have been documented in this region.

Rapid treatment is mandatory. A number of antibiotics are effective, including tetracycline, streptomycin, and chloramphenicol. Even with prompt, effective therapy, death still occurs in about 5% of cases. However, this rate is vastly different from the almost universal mortality for untreated pulmonic plague and the 40–70% mortality rate seen in other forms in the preantibiotic era.

TRICHINOSIS

Trichinosis differs in four ways from those diseases discussed previously in this chapter. First, it is not a bacterial disease; rather, the causative agent is a nematode parasite, *Trichinella spiralis*. Second, only occasionally does the illness have distinctive enough clinical features to allow a clinical diagnosis. Third, the disease is self-limiting and rarely fatal. Fourth, therapy is of uncertain benefit.

Trichinella spiralis is transmitted directly to wild carnivorous animals and to domesticated pigs through ingestion of infected meat. The latter occurred in the past when pigs were fed raw garbage which contained infected table scraps.

The disease in humans begins with the ingestion of raw or undercooked meat containing trichinella cysts. Upon reaching the small intestine, encysted organisms become sexually mature within 24–48 h. Larvae are produced within

5 days, and invasion across the mucosa occurs within another day or two. Accompanying symptoms consist of fever, diarrhea, and abdominal pain during the intestinal phase of the illness. Dissemination occurs during the second week following ingestion as parasites are carried throughout the body via the blood and lymphatic systems. Striated muscles, including those of the arms, legs, chest, and diaphragm, are the principal targets. The fourth week after ingestion, larval migration from the intestine to peripheral tissues diminishes, and the larvae already in the muscles begin to encyst. Symptoms during this phase include periorbital edema and muscle pain. Eosinophilia may be present in the peripheral blood.

It should be emphasized that infections are often mild in the United States and frequently remain undiagnosed. When trichinosis is suspected on the basis of ingestion of food, the aforementioned symptoms, the history of ingesting undercooked meat, in addition to eosinophilia and results from several tests may be helpful in diagnosing the disease. Serum levels of muscle enzymes, such as aldolase and creatine phosphokinase, may be elevated. A variety of serologic tests are available, with bentonite flocculation being the usual first test. However, it may take 3 or more weeks before sufficient antibodies are present for detection. Other methods include complement fixation, fluorescent antibody, latex agglutination, and immunoelectrophoresis. Because of insufficient sensitivity of any of these tests, two or more tests may be necessary to obtain a positive result.

The most definitive diagnostic technique is muscle biopsy. However, even this may be negative when the infestation is light. Fortunately, the overall prognosis is good in the majority of cases. However, occasionally myocarditis or meningitis may occur.

Treatment with an antihelminthic agent, thiabendazole, is often recommended, but its efficacy is unproven.

PSITTACOSIS

Psittacosis is caused by *Chlamydia psittaci*. Birds, particularly imported birds, are the major reservoir for this organism in the United States. The organisms may be excreted intermittently for long periods by either ill or healthy birds. Persons in close proximity to infected birds, such as pet shop employees and poultry workers, are at particular risk. This infection is quite uncommon in children.

The incubation period ranges from 7–14 days. The illness is characterized by high fever, chills, and pronounced cough. Initially, the cough may be dry, later becoming more productive. Auscultation often reveals a disproportionately slow heart rate, tachypnea, and diffuse fine rales. The patient may have constitutional symptoms similar to those of other illnesses discussed in this chapter, such as fatigue, malaise, anorexia, and myalgia. As expected, most patients with psittacosis demonstrate pulmonary infiltrates on chest roentgenograms.

The diagnosis depends on eliciting a history of bird exposure in the patient with fever, chills, and pneumonia. Because laboratory workers are at unusually high risk, isolation of the organism should *not* be attempted in most laboratories. Rather, a rising complement-fixation titer is the preferred diagnostic test.

Tetracycline is the drug of choice and should be continued for at least 3 weeks.

LYME DISEASE

Lyme disease (LD) is a multisystemic disease caused by the spirochete, *Borrelia burgdorferi,* transmitted to humans by *Ixodes* ticks, in the nymphal stage. LD occurs in the northeastern United States and Wisconsin, Minnesota, and California. Adult *Ixodes* mate on deer in the fall and winter and deposit eggs in the spring. In summer larvae obtain a blood meal from the white-footed mouse, the main reservoir of *B. burgdorferi,* and ingested spirochetes persist in the tick. The nymphal tick obtains a blood meal from a vertebrate such as a human the following spring or summer and thus may transmit *B. burgdorferi.* Engorged nymphs mature into adult ticks and complete their 2-year life cycle by parasitizing deer. LD does not occur in areas not inhabited by deer. Many other mammals (e.g., dogs) can be infected with *B. burgdorferi.* Infection usually occurs from May to September and is most common in children. LD is evidenced in one of three illness stages. The primary stage includes flulike symptoms of fever, muscle and joint aches, and headache or mild meningeal irritation; there is also a characteristic rash, *erythema chronicum migrans* (ECM). ECM begins as a small macule or papule at the tick bite site within 3–14 days and then expands to an annular lesion with a raised red border and central clearing. This slowly expands, and adjacent rings may form. Without treatment, ECM disappears after several weeks and constitutional symptoms appear after several months.

Weeks or months after resolution of ECM, the second stage may develop, involving the nervous system and/or the heart. Symptoms involving the nervous system include peripheral neuropathy, facial palsy, and fluctuating meningitis. Cardiac involvement includes atrioventricular block and/or acute myocarditis. These features may subside spontaneously within several months. The third stage of LD involves fluctuating arthritis of the large joints (i.e., the knees) weeks to years after infection. In some patients, chronic erosive arthritis develops. Because spirochetes are only rarely demonstrated in tissues after the first stage of LD, host immune responses are probably responsible for the cardiac, arthritic, and neurologic manifestations of the second and third stages.

Diagnosis of LD generally requires serologic evidence of infection, i.e., identification of IgG and/or IgM antibodies to *B. burgdorferi,* particularly by Western blot test. Standardization of assays is a serious problem. Demonstration or culture of spirochetes from tissues is very difficult.

Treatment of early LD is oral tetracycline or doxycycline for those older than 8 years old and oral penicillin V or amoxicillin for those younger than 8 years for 10–30 days. Isolated Bell's palsy, arthritis, or mild cardiac disease is treated with these same agents for 30 days. More serious neurologic or cardiac disease is treated with parenteral ceftriaxone or penicilin for 14–21 days. Measures to prevent LD include minimizing skin exposure in endemic areas, spraying of clothes with permethrin, and daily inspection and removal of ticks. Prophylactic antibiotics following tick bites are not warranted.

TOXOPLASMOSIS

Toxoplasmosis is a parasitic disease caused by a coccidian parasite, *Toxoplasma gondii*. The disease is worldwide in distribution, although more common in warmer climates than in cold ones. *Toxoplasma gondii* exists in three forms, leading to a variety of ways in which the disease is transmitted and varying pathogenesis. The tachyzoite form is a proliferative form seen during acute infections. The organism produces an enzyme that alters the host membrane, allowing entry into the cell. Subsequently, the bradyzoite form exists in tissue cysts. There is usually little inflammatory reaction surrounding the cysts, but organisms persist for a prolonged time. This characteristic allows for occasional reactivation of infection in body tissues. Finally, the oocyst form is found exclusively in the intestinal tract of cats. Oocysts become infectious after undergoing sporulation, which occurs from 1 to 21 days after defecation. Ingestion of the sporulated oocyst is probably the most frequent way in which humans become infected. However, some infections occur by the ingestion of undercooked meat or milk products containing encysted bradyzoites.

The vast majority of acquired toxoplasmosis is asymptomatic. Only about 10% of infected individuals develop signs or symptoms. Commonly, the patient develops lymphadenopathy, frequently around the head and neck, without fever. Occasionally, lymphadenopathy may be accompanied by fever, malaise, fatigue, sore throat, and myalgia, mimicking infectious mononucleosis. On occasion, toxoplasmosis has also been confused with lymphoma.

In immunocompromised adults and children, disseminated infection may develop, involving any body tissue including lungs, myocardium, liver, and central nervous system. In adult patients with AIDS, cerebral toxoplasmosis has been a particular problem (see Chapter 27).

Ocular toxoplasmosis is a troublesome, recurrent problem following usually congenital or occasionally acquired infection. Chorioretinitis may occur unilaterally or bilaterally. From time to time, these white or yellowish elevated foci may activate, presumably on the basis of reactivation of infection. Hypersensitivity accompanies reactivation, which may be a prominent cause of inflammation and sequelae. Following treatment of a reactivation, there often is some permanent loss of vision, which is particularly worrisome because of the perimacular location of many of these lesions.

Although the organisms can sometimes be seen in tissue, the diagnosis is usually made on the basis of rising antibody titers. Indirect immunofluorescent antibody (IFA) test is the most widely available. Reference laboratories continue to provide the Sabin-Feldman dye test, which is the most reliable test. Other tests that are sometimes used include complement fixation and enzyme-linked immunoabsorbent assays (ELISA).

The diagnosis of acute infection is based on a rising antibody titer. The presence of either cysts in tissue or a high titer cannot date the age or activity of a toxoplasma infection.

Treatment is not required for the vast majority of infections. In symptomatic patients, a combination of pyrimethamine and sulfadiazine is usually used. Other agents are sometimes used, including spiramycin, which is preferred in the treatment of pregnant women.

CASE HISTORY

A female mammalogist, after collecting small mammals near LaPaz, Bolivia, had the sudden onset of chills, fever, sweating, severe headache, pain and swelling of the right axilla, muscle pains in the lower back and hip, and anorexia. She was initially treated with amoxicillin without benefit. The pain and swelling in the axilla continued to increase. Within a day or two, she developed a dry cough. Upon her return to the United States a few days after the onset of her illness, her temperature was 101.3°F and she had a fluctuant 2.5-cm lymph node in the right axilla. These findings led to a presumptive diagnosis of bubonic plague. The diagnosis was subsequently confirmed by isolation of *Y. pestis* organisms from the node. She responded well to streptomycin.

During the collection of specimens in Bolivia, she had used Nembutal to euthanize the animals rather than chloroform. Chloroform kills fleas, but Nembutal does not. She had noted fleas on the animals, and had crushed some between her fingers. This was the probable mechanism of infection.

Adapted from *Morbidity and Mortality Weekly Report*, Vol. 39, No. 49, December 14, 1990.

REFERENCES

Books

Gould, S. E. ed. *Trichinosis in Man and Animals*. Springfield, IL: Charles C Thomas, 1970.

Hoeprich, P. D., and Jordan, M. C., eds. *Infectious Diseases: A Modern Treatise of Infectious Processes*. 4th ed. Philadelphia: J. B. Lippincott Co., 1989.

Mandell, G. L., Douglas, R. G., Jr., and Bennett, J. E., eds. *Principles and Practice of Infectious Diseases*. 3rd ed. New York: Churchill Livingstone, 1990.

Manson-Bahr, P. E. C., and Bell, D. R. *Manson's Tropical Diseases*. 19th ed. London: Ballière Tindall, 1987.

Spink, W. W. *The Nature of Brucellosis*. Minneapolis: University of Minnesota Press, 1956.

Review Articles

Christie, A. B. The clinical aspects of anthrax. *Postgrad. Med. J. 49*:565–570, 1973.

Foshay, L. Tularemia. *Annu. Rev. Microbiol. 4*:313–330, 1950.

Francis, E. A summary of the present knowledge of tularemia. *Medicine 7*:411–432, 1928.

Holliman, R. E. J. Toxoplasmosis and AIDS. *Infection 16*:121–128, 1988.

Yung, A. P., and Grayson, M. L. Psittacosis—a review of 135 cases. *Med. J. Aust. 148*:228–233, 1988.

Original Articles

Kaufmann, A. F., Boyce, J. M., and Martone, W. J. Trends in human plague in the United States. *J. Infect. Dis. 141*:522–524, 1980.

Malaria

INTRODUCTION

Malaria is a parasitic infection produced by one of four species of the genus *Plasmodium: P. vivax, P. falciparum, P. ovale*, and *P. malariae*. Humans become infected with one of these strains of *Plasmodium* following the bite of an infected female *Anopheles* mosquito. Rarely, infection may occur via other means: following transfusion of blood or blood components, *in*

utero as a result of malaria complicating pregnancy, or through the use of shared needles by drug addicts. Humans are the intermediate host of the malarial parasites in which the asexual forms develop. The *Anopheles* mosquito is the definitive host in which the sexual reproductive phase of the cycle takes place.

Malaria remains the most common serious infection of humankind. It has been estimated that worldwide there may be as many as 100 million cases of malaria per year and that in sub-Saharan Africa alone, a million children die of malaria each year.

In the United States malaria is an episodic illness occurring mostly in travelers returning from endemic areas or in foreign citizens who become ill while in residence in the United States. Anopheline species capable of transmitting malaria are present in southeastern and western sections of the United States. In fact an outbreak of 30 cases of *P. vivax* malaria occurred in San Diego County in 1988 and was the largest outbreak of introduced malaria in the United States since 1952, when 35 *P. vivax* infections were reported in members of a girls' club in California.

LIFE CYCLE

Infection in humans is initiated by the bite of the female *Anopheles* mosquito. In the process of feeding, sporozoites present in the saliva of the mosquito are injected into the blood of the human host. The sporozoites are cleared from the blood by the liver within 60 min. The mechanism by which the sporozoites bind to and penetrate the liver cells is poorly understood. The initial development of the malarial parasites occurs within the liver. This exoerythrocytic phase usually takes 6–16 days, depending upon the species of *Plasmodium* involved.

During the exoerythrocytic phase, the parasite undergoes growth and several nuclear divisions leading to the formation of tissue merozoites. The number of merozoites produced from a single sporozoite varies considerably with the infecting species. A single *P. falciparum* sporozoite may form as many as 40,000 merozoites, whereas sporozoites from the other species of *Plasmodium* produce only 2000–15,000 merozoites. Once formed, the tissue merozoites rupture the hepatocyte and enter the circulation. Many of the merozoites are quickly destroyed, but a significant number attach to specific receptor sites on the red blood cell. The merozoites then penetrate the red cell membrane, and development of the asexual, erythrocytic cycle begins (Fig. 32–1).

The earliest recognizable form of the parasite within the erythrocyte is the ring-stage trophozoite, which appears as a ring of blue cytoplasm with a dotlike nucleus of red chromatin as seen on Giemsa stain of the peripheral blood smear. With time, the trophozoites enlarge and appear ameboid or bandlike in shape. The nucleus of the trophozoite divides and, with nuclear division, the schizont stage is reached. Successive nuclear divisions occur, and each nucleus is surrounded by a small amount of cytoplasm. The merozoites thus produced rupture the erythrocyte and attach to unparasitized erythrocytes, starting the cycle again. The duration of the erythrocytic cycle is constant for each species of malaria. For *P. falciparum*, *P. vivax*, and *P. ovale*, the cycle length (ring trophozoite to blood merozoite) is 48 h. In *P. malariae* infection, the erythrocyte cycle requires 72 h for completion (Table 32–1); this translates to longer periods between cyclic recurrences of fever and can be helpful in differential diagnosis.

After initiation of the erythrocytic stage, hepatic parasites persist in *P. vivax* and *P. ovale* malaria. Relapse may thus occur months to years after the primary infection. There is no persistent exoerythrocytic stage of *P. falciparum* and *P. malariae*. Thus, no true relapse of infection occurs with these malarial species. In patients who acquire their infection because of blood or blood component transfusion, no exoerythrocytic stage develops because only the sporozoites that develop in the mosquito are capable of hepatic invasion.

A small number of merozoites that enter the red blood cell develop into male and female gametocytes. The gametocytes do not rupture the red blood cells but have to be ingested by the *Anopheles* mosquito for further develop-

ment. Fertilization of the gametocytes occurs within the stomach of the mosquito. Further maturation leads to the production of sporozoites that migrate through the body cavity of the mosquito to reach the salivary glands. When such a mosquito bites a person, a new cycle is initiated.

PATHOGENESIS OF INFECTION IN HUMANS

Erythrocyte Age and Susceptibility to Infection

There are a number of factors that govern the ability of the malarial parasite to invade the red blood cell. The age of the erythrocyte is a major determinant of its susceptibility to parasitism by all species of malaria except *P. falciparum*. Infection by *P. vivax* or *P. ovale* is limited to the reticulocyte or very young erythrocyte. *P. malariae* merozoites parasitize senescent erythrocytes. The selection of specific red blood cells for parasitism accounts in large part for the low percentage of erythrocytes parasitized by *P. vivax*, *P. ovale*, and *P. malariae*, a number that rarely exceeds 2%. *P. falciparum* merozoites are capable of invading red cells of all ages, although recent experimental evidence indicates that the rate of parasitic invasion was higher in young compared with old erythrocytes. The resulting parasitemia may approach 60% of the circulating erythrocytes. When this occurs, infection is life-threatening, and this condition has been termed *malignant tertian malaria*.

Erythrocyte Receptor Sites

It has been recently discovered that the merozoite attaches to a specific receptor site on the surface of the red blood cell. It has been known for many years that the majority of Africans and African Americans are resistant to *P. vivax* infection. This inherent resistance is related to blood types. The majority of people of African ancestry are Duffy blood group–negative; that is, they are *FyFy* and lack both the Fy^a and Fy^b alleles. When such individuals are deliberately exposed to the bite of a vivax-infected mosquito, infection does not occur. People of African heritage who are Duffy blood group–positive and who are exposed in a similar manner do develop infection. This specificity of the merozoite–RBC antigen binding is highly suggestive of a classic receptor–ligand interaction.

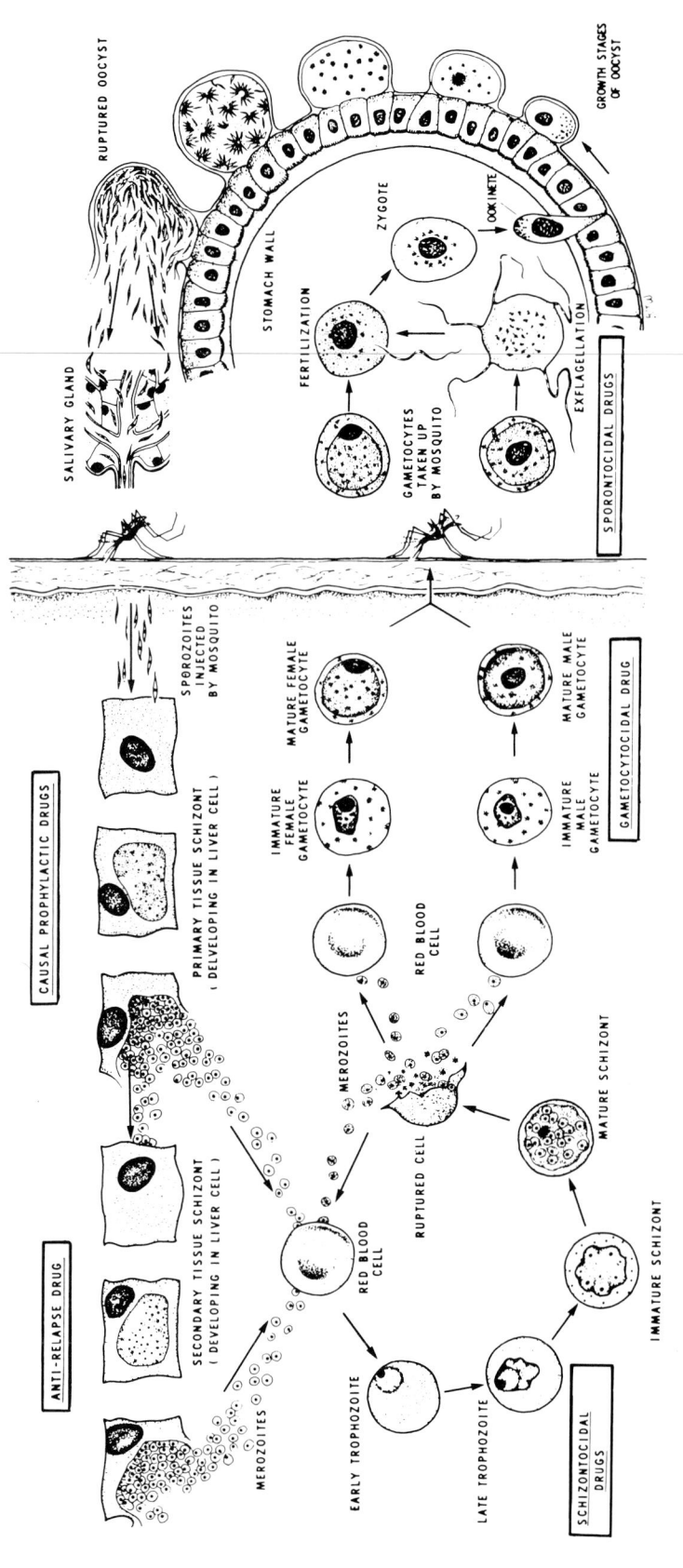

CYCLE IN MOSQUITO

CYCLE IN MAN

Figure 32–1. Life cycle of Plasmodium. (Modified from Bruce-Chwatt and Alvarado. Courtesy of the University of Florida College of Medicine. Gainesville. From Hunter, G. W., III, Swartzwelder, J. C., and Clyde, D. F. Tropical Medicine. 5th ed. Philadelphia, W. B. Saunders Co., 1976.)

TABLE 32–1. *Comparison of the Life Cycles of Malarial Species That Infect Humans*

	P. falciparum	**P. vivax**	**P. ovale**	**P. malariae**
Incubation period (days)	10–14	12–15	12–15	18–30
Persistence of exoerythrocytic parasites	No	Yes	Yes	Probably not
Stage of erythrocyte parasitized	All	Reticulocyte	Reticulocyte	Senescent
Duration (hours) of erythrocytic cycle	48	48	48	72
Magnitude of RBC parasitemia	High (Up to 60%)	Low (<2%)	Low (<2%)	Low (<1%)

Determinants other than blood types per se influence the capacity of erythrocytes of persons of diverse racial backgrounds to be invaded by plasmodia. For example, the receptor for *P. falciparum* attachment appears to be glycophorin A, the principal membrane sialoglycoprotein of red cells. Red blood cells that are blood group En(a−) are resistant to invasion of *P. falciparum* merozoites. En(a−) cells are totally deficient in glycophorin A. In addition, antibody against glycophorin A blocks invasion of normal En(a+) erythrocytes. Even though there is a marked resistance to invasion by *P. falciparum* merozoites, once inside a susceptible cell, parasitic maturation occurs normally. The specific receptor sites for *P. ovale* and *P. malariae* have not yet been determined.

Invasion

The merozoites attach themselves to the red cell membrane at their apical pole, which contains specialized organelles. Next, there are waves of marked deformation of the erythrocyte surface, producing a small invagination at the site of attachment. The invagination deepens, encasing the entire merozoite in an erythrocyte, membrane-lined vacuole. At the end of this process, the red cell membrane is resealed. This process of interiorization is rapid, taking about 20 s, and requires major alterations in the surface structure of the erythrocyte.

Intracellular Growth of the Malarial Parasite

Once inside the erythrocyte, the developing malarial parasite ingests from 25 to 75% of the red blood cell hemoglobin content by endocytosis. In the process of growth and development, the malarial parasite also alters the structure of the parasitized red cell and its biologic properties. Schüffner's dots, or granules, found on the cell wall of red cells parasitized by *P. vivax* or *P. ovale* have been shown by electron micros-

copy to be small invaginations surrounded by vesicles. Red cells parasitized by *P. falciparum* and *P. malariae* develop small electron-dense protrusions at the cell surface, called knobs. The knobs found on the surface of *P. falciparum*–infected red cells have been found to promote the adherence of these cells to the surface of endothelial cells. This phenomenon of endothelial adherence probably is responsible for the sequestration of parasitized erythrocytes in the capillary beds of vital organs and is directly involved in the pathogenesis of multiple organ dysfunction seen in *P. falciparum* malaria.

Certain variant hemoglobins affect the growth and development of malarial parasites. Red cells that contain fetal hemoglobin (Hb F) retard the intracellular growth of *P. falciparum*. Interestingly, attachment and invasion of the erythrocyte are not inhibited, but because of the retardation in intracellular growth, clinical infection in the first 6 months of life is extremely uncommon.

Under aerobic conditions, erythrocytes from persons with sickle cell trait (AS) support the normal development and maturation of *P. falciparum* parasites. Under reduced oxygen tension, however, the intracellular parasites are damaged. Electron-microscopic studies of these reduced Hb S–containing cells reveal needlelike aggregates of deoxyhemoglobin S, producing disruption of the parasites. Reduced oxygen tension also leads to intracellular loss of potassium, and this may lead to the death of the parasite. Hemoglobin C also retards invasion and intracellular growth of malarial parasites. Heterozygotic (AC) red cells reduce invasion and growth only minimally. Less clear is the effect of red cells that are deficient in glucose-6-phosphate dehydrogenase (G6PD) and those containing thalassemia (A_2) hemoglobin.

EPIDEMIOLOGY

Malaria occurs mostly in the tropical areas of the world, where the climate is warm and moist. This region includes parts of Mexico, Haiti, Central America, South America, Africa, the

Middle East, the Indian subcontinent, Southeast Asia, Korea, Indonesia, and Oceania (Fig. 32–2). More than 1 billion people live in these areas. In the United States, malaria was endemic until the early 1950s.

Much has been done to eradicate malaria in many parts of the world, but any hope of total elimination of the disease is still in the distant future. Eradication has been impeded by the emergence of mosquitos resistant to residual insecticides, especially DDT. A more pressing clinical problem, however, has been the emergence of strains of *P. falciparum* that are resistant to chemotherapeutic agents. There have also been social and political impediments to the implementation of eradication procedures.

Of the four species of malarial parasites that infect humans, *P. vivax* and *P. falciparum* are the species most frequently responsible for producing disease. Infection with *P. malariae* is uncommon, and *P. ovale* infection, which is confined to Africa, is quite rare.

Very rarely, malaria is acquired through blood transfusion. During the period 1927–1981, 26 cases of transfusion-acquired malaria were reported to the Centers for Disease Control in Atlanta, Georgia. Nine patients developed malaria with *P. malariae*; eight developed infection with *P. falciparum* and eight with *P. vivax*; and one case was due to *P. ovale*. The estimated risk was 1 case of malaria for every 4 million units of blood collected.

CLINICAL MANIFESTATIONS

The initial symptoms of malaria often are nonspecific and are similar to those occurring in patients with systemic viral illness. Thus arthralgias, myalgias, headache, back or abdominal pain, and low-grade fever are frequently the first symptoms experienced by patients. With time, typical paroxysms of chills and fever commonly develop.

The typical paroxysm of malaria is initiated by a violent rigor that lasts from a few minutes to an hour. At times the associated vasoconstriction is so intense that the patient appears cyanotic. The rigor is followed by a rapidly rising temperature that reaches 104–106°F (40–41°C). The fever usually lasts 3–8 h, and with defervescence, marked sweating occurs. At this point, the patient usually feels drained and exhausted and may even fall asleep. These successive stages have been respectively referred to as the cold phase, hot phase, and wet phase of the typical malarial paroxysm. The patient experiencing periodic fevers may feel fairly well between paroxysms. The paroxysm of chills and fever is related to the synchronization of the erythrocytic cycle and is initiated by the liberation of merozoites from the erythrocyte.

Thus, *P. falciparum*, *P. vivax*, and *P. ovale* malarias classically produce fever every 48 h, and *P. malariae* malaria produces fever every 72 h. Early in the course of most cases of malaria, erythrocytic schizogony does not occur in a synchronized fashion, and the fever tends to remain elevated or to be more than one spike per day. This pattern is especially true of *P. falciparum* malaria, which may never exhibit periodicity.

Gastrointestinal symptoms of nausea, vomiting, and diarrhea are fairly common in malaria. These symptoms, in association with high fever and chills, may be confused with bacillary dysentery or typhoid fever. Patients also frequently complain of headache, low back pain, arthralgia, and myalgia (Table 32–2).

Physical examination usually shows an elevated pulse rate and normal blood pressure. In patients with *P. falciparum* malaria, orthostatic hypotension, periorbital and facial edema are not uncommon. Herpes labialis is commonly present in patients with malaria. The lungs are usually clear to auscultation, but in severe *P. falciparum* malaria with pulmonary involvement, scattered rhonchi and rales may be heard. The spleen is palpable in 50% of patients with acute malaria and is often tender to palpation. The liver is less commonly enlarged.

Routine laboratory examination usually reveals a normal to low white blood cell count and a normal hematocrit and hemoglobin. In *P. falciparum* malaria, anemia is often seen, reflecting the severe hemolysis. Thrombocytopenia is not uncommon but again is most frequently seen with falciparum malaria. Hypoglycemia and increased lactic acid levels frequently occur in *P. falciparum* infections, especially in children and pregnant women. In approximately one third of patients, routine urinalysis demonstrates proteinuria and an increased number of white cells in the sediment. Tests of liver function reveal mild elevations of transaminases, and in patients with brisk hemolysis, the bilirubin level is elevated. Clinical jaundice is uncommon.

Plasmodium falciparum Malaria

The severity of falciparum malaria is directly related to the net mass of the parasitized red

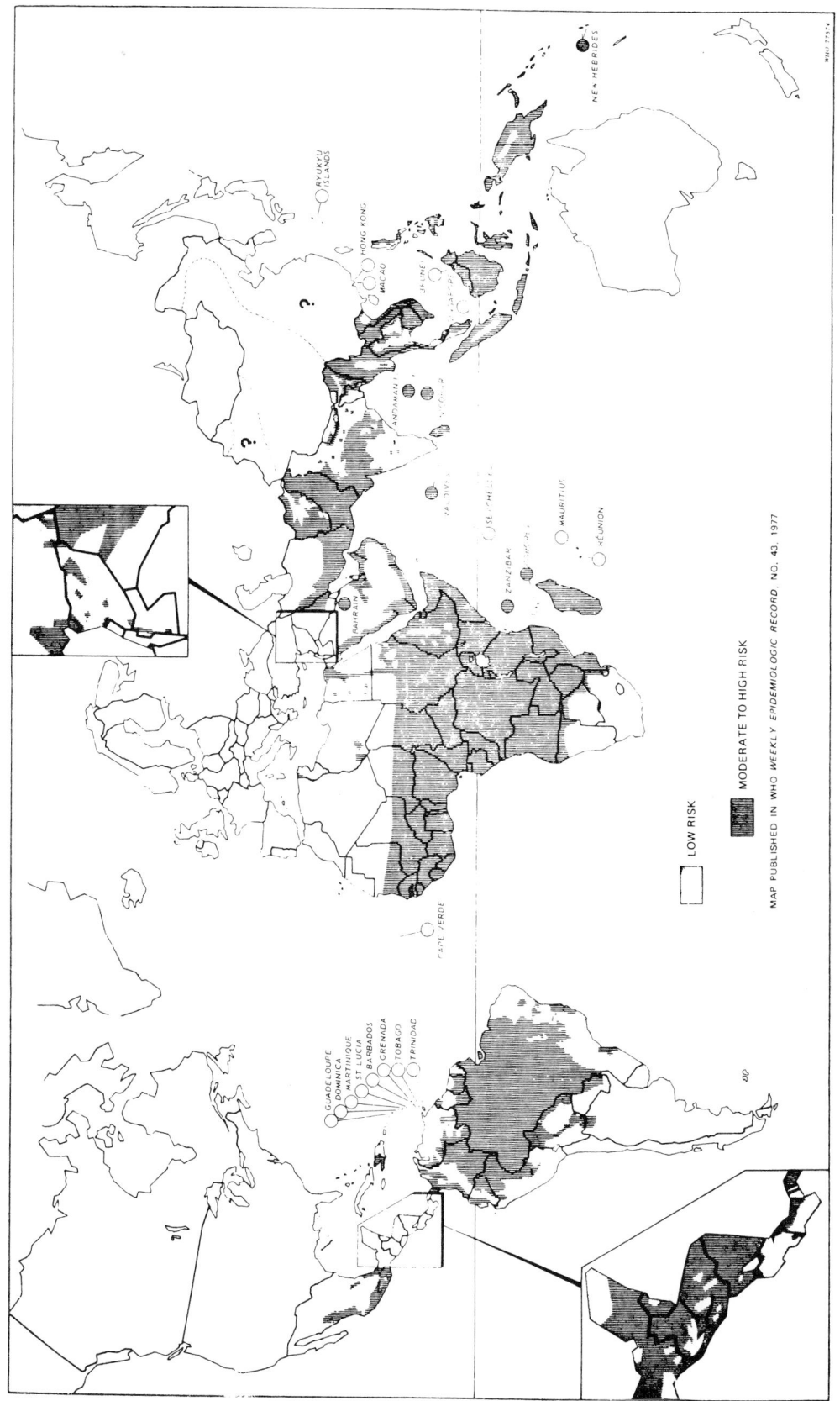

Figure 32–2. Areas of risk for malaria transmission, December 1976. (From Centers for Disease Control, U.S. Public Health Service, Annual Summary 1977, July 1978.)

TABLE 32–2. *Malaria: Common Symptoms*

Fever
Chills
Headache
Nausea, vomiting
Diarrhea
Low back pain
Arthralgia, myalgia
Anorexia
Fatigue

cells. On the surface membrane of these infected cells, excrescences, called knobs, are found that increase the adherence of these cells to endothelial surfaces. As a result, capillaries are occluded in many vital organs. The resultant tissue anoxia and edema, if severe enough, may lead to organ failure. Tissue anoxia may be further increased by a decrease in effective circulating blood volume. Finally, falciparum malaria may be complicated by severe intravascular hemolysis and disseminated intravascular coagulation, which also contribute to tissue anoxia.

Blackwater Fever

Hemolysis, associated with all four types of malaria, occurs primarily by splenic sequestration of parasitized erythrocytes. In some patients with falciparum malaria, especially individuals who have never been exposed to infection previously, massive intravascular hemolysis occurs. This massive hemolysis is accompanied by the development of jaundice, hemoglobinuria, hypotension, and acute renal failure. As a result of hemoglobinuria, the urine becomes very dark in color; this is the basis for the descriptive name of this clinical variant of malarial infection. Renal failure is a result of the decreased microcirculation within the kidney. In those patients who have died, postmortem examination reveals acute tubular necrosis and hemoglobin casts within the renal tubules.

Glomerular damage may also develop in falciparum malaria. The glomerulonephritis and nephrotic syndrome that occur after the first week of infection in some patients are thought to be produced by immunologic mechanisms. Kidney biopsies in such patients demonstrate deposition of immunoglobulins, mostly IgM and complement, on the glomerular basement membrane and within the mesangium. Malarial antigen is also found, though less often, in a similar distribution. These findings indicate immune-complex-mediated glomerular injury.

Cerebral Malaria

Clinical manifestations of central nervous system dysfunction in acute falciparum malaria are uncommon, occurring in only 1–2.5% of all cases. Although rare, cerebral malaria is often life-threatening, with mortality rates of 15–50% despite antimalarial therapy in modern medical facilities. Disturbances in consciousness, ranging from lethargy and stupor to frank coma, are the most frequently observed signs of cerebral malaria. Patients may also develop focal neurologic signs, such as disturbances in movement (myoclonus and chorea), acute changes in personality, and seizures. Lumbar puncture most frequently reveals an elevated opening pressure and clear spinal fluid. The CSF protein level ranges from normal to elevated, and the glucose concentration is normal. Usually there is no increase in inflammatory cells in the CSF. The basic pathologic process is anoxic damage secondary to capillary occlusion by parasitized red blood cells. This process leads to the development of cerebral edema, ring (perivascular) hemorrhages, and necrosis around central veins. If the patient survives, there is usually no residual neurologic disability.

Respiratory Failure

In a small number of patients with falciparum malaria, pulmonary edema may develop in the absence of fluid overload. These patients exhibit marked impairment of gas exchange and become hypoxic and cyanotic. Chest roentgenograms usually reveal bilateral, diffuse pulmonary infiltrates. Pulmonary involvement is a grave complication of falciparum malaria, since it does not respond to the therapy that is effective in clearing parasitemia.

Hepatic and Cardiac Involvement

In some patients with falciparum malaria, centrilobular necrosis of the liver is found. Usually liver dysfunction is not severe. Involvement of the heart, including cardiac failure, has been observed in cases of fatal falciparum malaria. At autopsy, plugging of myocardial capillaries and venules by parasitized erythrocytes has been observed, as well as petechial hemorrhages and edema of cardiac muscle.

Plasmodium vivax and Plasmodium ovale Malaria

In untreated vivax malaria, the primary attack lasts from 3 weeks to 2 months. Similar to falciparum infection, the initial febrile period for *P. vivax* and *P. ovale* infection is often irregular and the fever sustained. Early in the course of vivax malaria there may be two groups of parasites maturing on alternate days. When this occurs, the patient has a daily temperature spike (quotidian fever). Usually by the end of the first week, one of the two groups of parasites drops out, and the typical malarial paroxysms occur every 42–47 h (tertian fever). Complications are uncommon, and the prognosis, even without therapy, is good. Because of the persistence of parasites in the liver, relapse may occur as long as 3–5 years after the initial attack. Ovale malaria is similar to vivax infection but tends to be even milder.

Plasmodium malariae Malaria

Malaria produced by *P. malariae* (quartan malaria) is very similar to vivax infection except that the febrile period occurs every 72 h. The periodicity of the fever tends to be established early and may even be present from the onset of the infection. Recurrent infection with *P. malariae* has been implicated in the development of the nephrotic syndrome. It is thought that repeated antigenic stimulation by recurrent episodes of malariae malaria leads to the deposition of immune complexes on the glomerular capillary basement membrane. Renal biopsy in patients with malariae malaria who have the nephrotic syndrome has demonstrated the presence of IgG and IgM in 96% of the specimens examined. The third component of complement (C3) was present in over half the specimens, and *P. malariae* antigen was found in one quarter of the kidney biopsies studied. The resulting nephrotic syndrome unfortunately does not respond to corticosteroid therapy, and even aggressive antimalarial therapy has little effect on the clinical course.

HOST FACTORS IN MALARIAL INFECTION

Both humoral and cellular immunity serve to limit the extent and duration of malarial infection. In individuals living in highly endemic areas of malaria, a relative immunity to symptomatic infection develops. This immunity is associated with the development of tolerance to erythrocyte parasitemia. It is not unusual to find children living in holoendemic areas of Africa to be asymptomatic in spite of erythrocyte parasitemias as high as 20%.

Human beings and experimental animals can also be protected from malarial infection by the passive administration of immunoglobulin derived from individuals or animals who have recovered from malarial infection. Antibody may protect the red cell from invasion and prevent intracellular development of the malarial parasite. Red cells with parasitic antigen on their surfaces may also be opsonized by antibody, leading to accelerated destruction of the erythrocytes by the monocyte/macrophage reticuloendothelial system.

Malarial infection may be associated with generalized immunosuppression of the host. Infected children tend to have lower antibody responses to certain antigens, including tetanus toxoid and certain bacterial vaccines. Immunosuppression may also account for greater susceptibility to and severity of intercurrent viral infections.

Pregnant women, especially primigravidas, appear to be especially susceptible to malarial infection. In geographic areas endemic for *P. falciparum*, attack rates 4–12 times greater than those found in nonpregnant women have been observed. The higher attack rate in pregnant women may be due in part to a loss of acquired immunity during pregnancy. Not only is the woman's health jeopardized by malaria but the fetus may also become infected via the transplacental route. Infections during pregnancy have been associated with spontaneous abortion, still birth, and infants of lower than normal birth weight.

Recently, soluble monocyte mediators, such as tumor necrosis factor alpha (TNF-alpha) and interleukin 1 (IL-1), have been shown to play a role in the host response to malarial infection. In a recent study by Kern et al., 31 of 32 patients with severe falciparum malaria had elevated levels of TNF-alpha in their serum. TNF-alpha levels were proportional to the number of parasitized red blood cells, with the highest concentrations being found in patients with cerebral malaria and hypotension.

DIAGNOSIS

Malaria should be considered in any patient who develops fever and chills and who has visited, or is a citizen of, a country where malaria is known to exist (see Fig. 32–2). Malaria should also be considered in the differential diagnosis of patients who present with fever of undetermined origin and a history of transfusions of blood or blood components or of intravenous drug abuse.

The vast majority of travelers who develop malaria in the United States after having visited an endemic area become clinically ill within the first month of their return to the United States. A smaller number of patients develop symptoms 1–6 months after their return. Only rarely do patients (usually those with vivax or malariae infections) develop clinical illness after 1 year of their visit to a malarious area.

The definitive diagnosis of malaria is made by demonstrating the presence of parasites within the red blood cell. To do this, both thick and thin blood smears are stained with either Giemsa's or Wright's stain. If the initial smears are negative, additional smears should be obtained every 6–12 h for an additional 48 h. The thick smear is most useful when there is low-grade parasitemia, since in these cases parasites may be impossible to find in the thin smears. However, when parasites are present in sufficient numbers, as in most cases of malaria, they are most easily recognized by inexperienced personnel in the thin smear. The thin smear is also used for speciation of the infection. Monitoring of serial thick and thin smears is also useful in following the disappearance of parasitemia after the institution of chemotherapy.

There are several serologic tests that are useful in detecting the presence of malarial antibody. These include agar gel diffusion, passive hemagglutination, immunofluorescence, and the ELISA technique. Antibody is usually not detectable within the first week of a primary infection, and, therefore, attempting to determine its presence is not helpful when the patient first presents. A nonimmune person with a primary infection may develop only low antibody titers that persist only a few weeks to months if rapid and adequate chemotherapy is administered. On the other hand, individuals living in endemic areas with minimal or no treatment develop high levels of antibody with a broad spectrum of reactivity. These antibodies may persist for years even after the person has left an endemic area.

When blood smears are negative, serologic testing can establish a diagnosis of malaria in individuals returning from an endemic area with a fever of undetermined origin. The smears may be negative as a result of suppressive chemoprophylaxis taken by the patient, or they can be negative if obtained at the wrong time. Serologic testing has been useful for detecting individuals responsible for transmitting transfusion-related malaria. Such individuals, usually carriers of *P. vivax* or *P. malariae*, have such low-grade parasitemia that blood smears are often negative.

TREATMENT

In areas where malaria is known to exist, the traveler should take precautions to reduce exposure to mosquito bites. Use of insect repellent and protective clothing is strongly advised. Since the *Anopheles* mosquito feeds primarily from dusk to dawn, the traveler should limit outdoor exposure at those times and should sleep under mosquito netting.

Acute Infections

Patients with malaria generally should be treated initially in the hospital, with attention being given to fluid and electrolyte therapy; serious complications of falciparum malaria should be anticipated. Acute renal failure in falciparum malaria is best managed by peritoneal dialysis or hemodialysis.

In many institutions, medical personnel are not capable of making a species-specific diagnosis. In such cases, patients should be considered to have falciparum malaria and treated accordingly. This procedure should be followed especially when only ring trophozoites are seen in the thin smear and red cell parasitemias approach 5% or greater. Treatment of falciparum malaria must take into account the possibility of chloroquine resistance. At present, chloroquine-resistant strains of *P. falciparum* are found in Southeast Asia, South America, Africa, and India (Fig. 32–3).

In patients who have, or are suspected of having, chloroquine-resistant falciparum malaria, treatment should begin with oral quinine sulfate, 650 mg three times a day for 10 days. (For all medications listed, adult dosages are provided.) Patients who are seriously ill or who cannot tolerate oral medication can be given intravenous quinine dihydrochloride, 600 mg dissolved in normal saline. This dosage may be repeated in 8 h (maximum, 1800 mg/day) until the patient can take oral medication. Quinine therapy frequently produces nausea, vomiting, tinnitus, and vertigo. The presence of these side effects (cinchonism), although distressing, should not deter continuation of therapy. In addition to quinine, pyrimethamine (25 mg by mouth twice a day for 3 days) and sulfadiazine

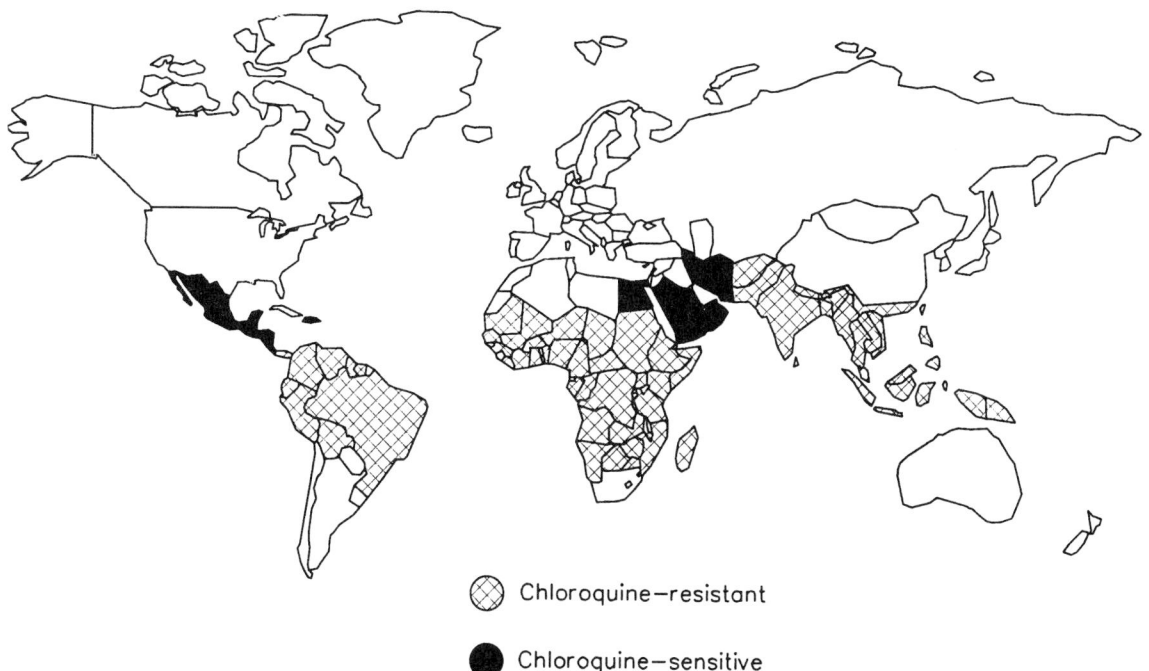

Figure 32–3. Malarious areas with Plasmodium falciparum *resistant and sensitive to chloroquine, 1990. (From* Morbidity and Mortality Weekly Report, *March 9, 1990, 39, pp. 140–142, No. 8.)*

(500 mg orally four times a day for 5 days) are given.

A new and very promising antimalarial agent is mefloquine. This agent has minimal side effects and is effective in the treatment of all known strains of human malaria, including chloroquine-resistant *P. falciparum*. In field trials in Thailand, cure rates of 100% were achieved after a single oral dose of 1500 mg of mefloquine.

Chloroquine phosphate is given to patients with *P. vivax, P. ovale, P. malariae,* and chloroquine-sensitive *P. falciparum* infections for the suppression of symptoms and the elimination of erythrocytic parasites. The initial adult dose for chloroquine phosphate (a 4-aminoquinoline) is 1000 mg orally, followed by an additional 500 mg in 6 h and a third dose of 500 mg 24 h after the initial dose. A final dose of 500 mg of chloroquine phosphate is given 48 h after the initial dose. In seriously ill patients who cannot tolerate oral medication, chloroquine can be given intramuscularly or intravenously. When given parenterally, 250 mg of chloroquine hydrochloride dissolved in normal saline is administered every 6 h until oral therapy is possible.

In infections caused by *P. vivax* and *P. ovale,* it is necessary to eliminate hepatic parasites to prevent future relapses. This can be accomplished by administration of primaquine phosphate, 26.3 mg (15 mg of the base) orally once a day for 14 days. Primaquine may be given concomitantly with chloroquine or started after chloroquine has been discontinued. The combination of chemotherapeutic agents effective against both erythrocytic and exoerythrocytic parasites is frequently referred to as a *radical cure.* Primaquine phosphate (an 8-aminoquinoline) can produce hemolysis in patients whose red blood cells lack G6PD. The anemia produced is of major consequence, primarily in Caucasians with the Mediterranean type of G6PD deficiency. Persons of African ancestry who are G6PD-deficient usually experience only mild hemolysis.

Prophylaxis

Individuals who are traveling to areas where malaria is endemic should receive chemoprophylactic treatment. Travelers to Africa are at the highest risk of developing malaria since, in most rural and many urban areas, infected anopheline mosquitoes are present. From 1980 to 1988, over 1500 cases of *P. falciparum* malaria occurred in U.S. travelers. Of these, 80% of the infections were acquired in sub-Saharan Africa. Travelers to South America and Asia are at less risk for developing malaria since most urban and resort areas have limited if any risk of exposure.

In areas where chloroquine-resistant *P. falciparum* is not a consideration, chloroquine phosphate, 500 mg (one tablet) once a week, starting 1 or 2 weeks before departure and continued for 4 weeks after return, is the drug of choice. Chloroquine is capable of suppressing the clinical symptoms of the disease and eliminating the erythrocytic parasites of all four forms of human malaria (except chloroquine-resistant *P. falciparum*).

Mefloquine is now considered the most effective prophylactic agent for travelers to areas endemic for chloroquine-resistant *P. falciparum* malaria. Mefloquine is recommended at a dosage of 250 mg started 1 week before departure, then one 250-mg tablet weekly while in an endemic area, and an additional weekly tablet for 4 weeks after returning to a malaria-free area. Mefloquine should not be given to travelers who have cardiac conduction defects or who are taking beta blockers. Because confusion, depression, anxiety, and psychotic manifestations have been reported rarely, patients with psychiatric disorders and individuals involved in tasks requiring fine coordination and spatial discrimination such as airline pilots and operators of heavy machinery should not take mefloquine prophylaxis.

Alternative prophylaxis for chloroquine-resistant *P. falciparum* is doxycycline, 100 mg by mouth once a day starting 1–2 days prior to departure, then taken daily while in an endemic area, and continued for 4 weeks after returning to a malaria-free area. Because of the potential for photosensitivity resulting in a severe sunburn reaction, persons taking doxycycline are advised to use an efficient sunscreen that absorbs ultraviolet light. Doxycycline, like all tetracyclines, cannot be given to pregnant women and young children under 8 years old.

Another alternative to mefloquine prophylaxis is 500 mg of chloroquine phosphate taken weekly, starting 1–2 weeks before departure and 4 weeks after returning along with a single-treatment dose (three tablets) of sulfadoxine and pyrimethamine (Fansidar). All three tablets of Fansidar (each tablet contains 25 mg pyrimethamine and 500 mg sulfadoxine) are to be taken at once if a febrile illness occurs during travel and prompt medical attention is unavailable. This regimen is only a temporary measure, and professional medical follow-up is imperative. Fansidar cannot be taken by individuals allergic to sulfa drugs.

The Centers for Disease Control has set up a malaria hotline where detailed recommendations for the prevention of malaria may be obtained 24 h a day. The CDC Malaria Hotline number is (404)332-4555.

Vaccine

Because of the ever-changing susceptibility of *P. falciparum* to the currently used antimalarial agents and the inability to eliminate the mosquito vector, the development of an effective vaccine is imperative. Most attention has been focused on the development of a vaccine directed against the surface protein of the sporozoite. This protein, designated the circumsporozoite, or CS protein, *is* species-specific and has been found to be nearly identical in strains of *P. falciparum* obtained from different parts of the world. In theory, if an effective immune response could be made to the CS protein, sporozoites injected by the bite of the mosquito would be prevented from ever reaching and entering the liver to initiate infection.

The initial sporozoite vaccine trials were carried out in 1987 on a small number of human volunteers. Although the antibody titers to the synthetic peptide used were low, the antibody produced recognized native *P. falciparum* circumsporozoite protein. When these volunteers were subsequently challenged by multiple bites from infected mosquitoes, only a few individuals with the highest titers were protected and did not develop active infection.

One of the problems recognized in these early attempts at producing a sporozoite vaccine was that there was no helper T-cell sensitization. This lack may be due in part to the fact that these early vaccines used tetanus toxoid as the carrier protein, and the T-cell response was directed against the tetanus toxoid rather than the CS peptide. If the T-cell limb of the immune system could also be sensitized by an appropriate vaccine, subsequent bites from infected mosquitoes would boost the host's antibody titer. Sensitized T cells may even recognize and eliminate any infected hepatocytes, thus giving the individual a second level of protection directed against sporozoites that make it through the initial barrier of circulating antibody. A vigorous search is in progress for epitopes present on the CS protein that will elicit an effective T-cell response. Part of the problem in finding a good T-cell inducer is that there is a great deal of variability of the T-cell epitopes on the CS protein of *P. falciparum*.

The ideal malaria vaccine of the future may contain multiple antigenic components directed against not only the sporozoite but also blood stage antigens and gametocytes.

REFERENCES

Book

Wyler, D. J. Plasmodium species (malaria). In: Mandell, G. L., Douglas, R. G., and Bennett, J. E., eds. *Principles and Practice of Infectious Diseases*. New York: Churchill Livingstone, Inc. 1990.

Original Articles

Cattani, J. A. Malaria vaccines: Results of human trials and directions of current research. *Exp. Parasitol. 68*:242–247, 1989.

Centers for Disease Control: Recommendations for the prevention of malaria among travelers. *MMWR 39*: No. PR-3, 1990.

Centers for Disease Control: Transmission of *Plasmodium vivax* malaria—San Diego County, California, 1988 and 1989. *MMWR 39*:91–94, 1990.

Gilles, H. M. Malaria—An overview. *J. Infect. 18*:11–23, 1989.

Gordon, S., Brennessel, D. J., Goldstein, J. A., et al. Malaria—A city hospital experience. *Arch. Intern. Med. 148*:1569–1571, 1988.

Hoffman, S. L., Rustama, D., Punjabi, N. H., et al. High-dose dexamethasone in quinine-treated patients with cerebral malaria: A double-blind, placebo-controlled trial. *J. Infect. Dis. 158*:325–331, 1988.

Kern, P., Josef Hemmer, C., Van Damma, J., et al. Elevated tumor necrosis factor alpha and Interleukin-6 serum levels as markers for complicated *Plasmodium falciparum* malaria. *Am. J. Med. 87*:139–143, 1989.

Nussenzweig, V., and Nussenzweig, R. S. Progress toward a malaria vaccine. *Hosp. Pract. 25*:45–57, 1990.

Ruebush, T. K., II, Breman, J. G., Kaiwer, R. L., et al. Selective primary health care. XXIV Malaria. *Rev. Infect. Dis. 8*:454–465, 1986.

33 *A TODD DAVIS, M.D.*

Exanthematous Diseases

INTRODUCTION

Viral exanthems, cutaneous manifestations of viral infection, have long fascinated physicians. Exanthems often challenge diagnostic acumen because they are associated with infections caused by herpes, pox, enteric, respiratory, and other viruses. Some viral exanthems are benign and self-limited, such as roseola (exanthem subitum) and erythema infectiosum (fifth disease). In contrast, rubeola (measles), rubella (German measles), and varicella (chickenpox), although usually self-limited, may be associated with serious disease. Measles virus can produce acute encephalitis and subacute sclerosing panencephalitis, and it may be etiologically linked to multiple sclerosis. Rubella has been a major contributor to congenital defects, and chickenpox is a potentially life-threatening illness in immunocompromised patients.

There are hundreds of diseases with cutaneous manifestations. Only a few are discussed here; they have been chosen because of their occurrence in the United States and for the lessons they teach about immunology, epidemiology, and immunization practices. Excellent color photographs illustrating the features of the exanthematous diseases discussed here can be found in the color atlas by Lambert and Farrar (see References).

RUBEOLA (MEASLES)

Measles virus is currently included in the genus Morbillivirus and the family Paramyxoviridiae. This is a relatively large virus, 150–300 nm in diameter, having helical capsid symmetry and containing ribonucleic acid (see Chapter 4 for overview and comparison with other viruses).

Measles can be thought of as a serious respiratory illness that happens to have an associated skin rash. The measles virus gains access to the respiratory tract, invades the lymphatic tissue, and then spills over into the bloodstream. As this occurs, respiratory symptoms and fever become manifest 2–3 days prior to the development of the skin rash. The early phase of the illness, the prodrome, consists of fever (with temperatures gradually rising to 103°–104°F), cough, coryza, and conjunctivitis. Within 2–3 days, a pathognomonic enanthem consisting of Koplik's spots begins on the buccal mucosa opposite the first and second molars, followed by an exanthem beginning on the head and neck. Koplik's spots are tiny white lesions on an erythematous base, whereas the exanthem consists of small, reddish, flat macules and papules. Within 24 h the Koplik's spots disappear and the rash begins to spread onto the arms, upper trunk, and back. Over the next 2–3 days, the fever remains elevated as the rash continues to spread caudally, ultimately involving the legs. Within a day or two of the appearance of the rash on any body site, the discrete maculopapular lesions begin to coalesce, forming large, reddish areas. During the healing phase of the exanthem, there may be a brownish discoloration of the skin.

Measles presents a particular problem because of the occasional associated occurrence of encephalitis. Approximately 1 in every 1000–2000 children with measles develops acute encephalitis; half of those so afflicted die and at least half of the survivors suffer serious neurologic impairments (see Chapter 24). Worldwide, measles encephalitis is the most common initiating cause of demyelinating inflammatory disease in human beings. In some other children with measles, subacute sclerosing panencephalitis develops months to years later (see Chapter 24). Fortunately, this occurs rarely, in approximately 1 per 100,000 cases. A search was begun in the early 1960s for an effective immunizing agent to prevent these serious sequelae.

Initial efforts focused on a *killed* virus vaccine. It was soon appreciated, however, that the vaccine was not highly protective and that some immunized children, upon contracting the wild virus, developed very serious measles. This same paradoxical situation (i.e., recipients of killed vaccine contracting disease more severe than that occurring in susceptible children) has also been seen in recipients of a killed respiratory syncytial virus vaccine. The first *live* measles virus vaccine, the Edmonston B vaccine, was highly protective but frequently caused side effects such as fever, which necessitated concomitant administration of gammaglobulin. The gammaglobulin dosage was carefully titrated to decrease the incidence of serious complications, while not impairing antigenic potency. By 1967, this burdensome procedure was supplanted by a further attenuated vaccine that could be used without gammaglobulin. The Schwarz vaccine, which is in current use, produces seroconversion in 95% of vaccinees and has few side effects.

The effectiveness of any vaccine can be tested in numerous ways. Seroconversion rates to the Schwarz vaccine are about 95%. This means that 95% of subjects who receive the vaccine at 15 months of age or older can be expected to produce a fourfold or higher rise in antibody titer. The effectiveness of measles vaccine, or vaccine efficacy, also has been measured in various studies in which a population sustaining a measles outbreak is thoroughly investigated. Attack rates are calculated for those children who have been vaccinated and for those who are susceptible. It is assumed that the attack rate among the members of the vaccinated group, had they not been immunized, would have been the same as the attack rate among those in the susceptible group. Accordingly, an equation can be generated to show the number of cases observed versus the number expected

in the vaccinated group. This reduction in cases experienced by the vaccinees is mathematically converted to a percentage called the vaccine efficacy. Multiple studies have revealed an efficacy of about 95% for measles vaccine.

The marked reduction in the number of children with measles in the United States further attests to the effectiveness of this vaccine. In the prevaccine era, about 500,000 cases of measles were reported annually. In 1982, only 1697 cases were reported, representing a reduction of 99.7%. This impressive control effort stemmed from two key immunization strategies: (1) the achievement and maintenance of high immunization levels, and (2) the rapid detection of new cases of measles with immunization of susceptible contacts as quickly as possible. This latter strategy was borrowed from the program that resulted in eradication of smallpox from the world in the late 1970s.

Unfortunately, the United States may never be totally free of measles. Indeed, several large American cities including Chicago, Los Angeles, Houston, New York, and others have experienced extensive outbreaks during the late 1980s and early 1990s. In 1989, for example, 17,850 measles cases were recorded. Unimmunized preschool children, most from impoverished neighborhoods, serve as major reservoirs for propagation of the outbreaks. Even when these epidemics are controlled, the United States will probably continue to experience occasional problems. First, there will likely continue to be pockets of endemic spread among certain social and ethnic groups with low vaccination rates in American cities. Second, measles continues to be highly epidemic and endemic throughout the world, including in European countries and underdeveloped nations. Accordingly, periodic importations can be expected into the continental United States.

There are a number of interesting immunologic and biologic questions that remain unanswered with respect to measles. What produces the rash? Why does the rash invariably begin on the head and spread downward in the susceptible host? Why does the rash go through a fixed progression—macules, confluence, and fading?

Immunofluorescence and electron-microscopy studies have demonstrated both measles antigen and viral particles in the exanthematous lesions. However, the precise mechanism or mechanisms directly leading to the individual cutaneous lesions that constitute the rash of rubeola are unknown. Possibilities include (1) host cell injury caused by the virus; (2) acute inflammation in response to the presence of the virus or injury caused by the virus, or both; (3) *in situ* binding of measles antibody to, or interaction of sensitized lymphocytes with, intact virus or residual viral antigens, with resulting immune injury; and (4) a combination of two or more of these pathogenetic sequences of events.

The fixed sequential body site distribution of the rash is probably caused by immunologic mechanisms. Evidence for this is derived from two clinical conditions. When gammaglobulin is administered to an exposed susceptible host, the intensity of the illness may be attenuated, but the same general features are present as in fully susceptible subjects. Atypical measles stands in marked contrast. This entity occurs in previously, but only partially, immunized children who lack measurable antibody titers. However, the cellular immune system obviously has been activated, as determined by *in vitro* T-lymphocyte studies. In atypical measles, there is no prodrome, Koplik's spots are absent, the rash begins on the ankles and wrists and spreads towards the trunk, and the rash may assume many different forms. These two examples suggest that the site and distribution of the rash are determined more by the cellular immune system than by the humoral system.

The preceding examples also illustrate the important role of antibodies in protection against measles. Protection is highly correlated with the presence of serum antibodies. Administration of serum globulin can modify the severity of naturally acquired infection. In atypical measles, serum antibody is unmeasurable at the beginning of the illness but subsequently develops. Although the role of the cellular immune system in protection against acquisition of measles is unknown, cellular immunity seems to be of key importance in eradicating measles virus from the host. Children who have hypogammaglobulinemia but intact cellular immunity recover from measles. In contrast, children with impaired cellular immunity do poorly with measles infection.

RUBELLA

Rubella virus is a member of the Rubivirus genus of the family Togaviridae. This virus is spherical, has a diameter of 50–60 nm, and contains single-stranded ribonucleic acid.

In contrast to measles, rubella is usually a mild disease. Young children rarely have prodromal symptoms. Adolescents and adults may have a variety of prodromal symptoms such as eye pain, headache, fever, and myalgia. When a rash occurs, discrete, pinkish maculopapular lesions begin on the head and spread downward over a 2–3-day period and then disappear. However, the distribution, appearance, and extent of the rash are highly variable. Indeed, one third to one half of patients with rubella never develop a rash. The absence of the characteristic rash in many individuals makes the clinical diagnosis of an isolated case quite difficult. When present, occipital adenopathy and joint pain suggest the diagnosis but are not pathognomonic. Accurate diagnosis depends on a significant rubella antibody titer rise between acute and convalescent sera.

The majority of children with rubella have a mild illness and suffer no sequelae. When questioned, as many as 25% of children will report mild joint pain. Rubella is a more serious illness in adults, with 25–40% complaining of short-lived joint pain. Permanent joint sequelae are quite rare. The most serious effects of rubella occur in the fetus whose susceptible mother becomes infected during the first trimester. Severely affected infants may have cataracts, sensorineural deafness, congenital heart disease, mental retardation, and other features.

Rubella vaccine was developed to interrupt or eliminate the usual 6–9-year cycle of major epidemics in the United States that had been observed in the first half of the 20th century and thereby to reduce the large number of resulting rubella-related congenital defects in affected infants. In the 1964 outbreak, it was estimated that about 20,000 infants were born with severe congenital rubella syndrome. Live attenuated rubella vaccine became commercially available in the United States in 1969. Since that time, efforts have been directed toward immunization of school-aged children. There were two major reasons for choosing this strategy. First, rubella usually begins in school-aged populations and spreads to infect preschool children, older adolescents, and young adults. Thus, it was postulated that creation of a large "immune herd" of school-aged children would effectively disrupt the previous patterns of transmission. Second, there were grave concerns about the possible teratogenic effects that could occur if the vaccine virus was inadvertently administered to a woman during the first trimester of pregnancy.

This strategy has effectively prevented any large-scale outbreak since introduction of the vaccine. As expected, there also has been a marked reduction in the number of children born with congenital rubella syndrome. However, there continue to be small outbreaks of rubella in adolescents and young adults that occasionally involve susceptible pregnant women, resulting in infants with congenital rubella syndrome.

In contrast to the United States, Great Britain chose to immunize preadolescent girls. This strategy is based on administration of the vaccine to the population at risk (each preadolescent female is assumed to be susceptible and about to become fertile). In addition, the risk of pregnancy is considered to be essentially nonexistent in prepubertal females. As one might expect, rubella has continued to be an endemic and epidemic problem in Great Britain; the incidence of congenital rubella syndrome has decreased, but not as markedly as in the United States.

Evidence accumulated since the 1970s shows that inadvertent administration of rubella virus to women in the first trimester rarely results in fetal damage. In fact, the risk to the fetus is so small that official advisory committees suggest that abortion is not indicated in such situations. This new knowledge about the extremely low risk of inadvertent vaccine immunization during early pregnancy may lead to additional public health measures in the United States. In particular, women of childbearing age (15–45 years) who have not been previously immunized should be strongly considered for immunization as long as they are reasonably sure that they are not pregnant or will not become pregnant around the time administration of the vaccine is planned. In the past, such women were immunized only when effective contraception for the three months subsequent to the vaccination could be assured. In addition, there may be immunization programs specifically aimed at girls who are just entering puberty.

Like measles vaccine, rubella vaccine results in seroconversion rates of at least 95%. Efficacy rates for rubella vaccine are thought to be approximately 95%, although remarkably few studies have been done. Moreover, rubella vaccine markedly diminishes the risk of infection in persons subsequently challenged experimentally with wild rubella virus.

CHICKENPOX (VARICELLA)

Chickenpox is usually a benign disease in normal children. This is not true, however, in children with primary compromise of their immune defenses from diseases such as AIDS or with secondary immunodeficiency in association with leukemia, lymphoma, and the immunosuppression therapy for such disorders. In the aforementioned settings, chickenpox can cause severe disease and death. This has led to both passive and active immunization strategies.

There is no prodrome in chickenpox. Rather, the first sign of the illness is the presence of small, clear, fluid-filled vesicles, often dimpled in the middle. The child may have fever as well as mild constitutional symptoms such as myalgia, irritability, and some fussiness. The first lesions may occur anywhere on the body. Subsequent vesicles occur without any discernible pattern of progression from one body area to another. During the first 3–4 days, vesicular lesions continue to appear on various body sites. New lesions are uncommon after 6 or 7 days. Some but not all of the vesicles progress to pustular lesions, resulting in dry, crusted lesions. All three kinds of lesions are usually present after the first or second day. Although the diagnosis is usually obvious on clinical grounds, a smear of epithelial cells from the base of a vesicle invariably demonstrates multinucleated cells and intranuclear inclusion bodies, suggesting the diagnosis. This test, in conjunction with electron-microscopic studies, may be essential for rapid differentiation of chickenpox from smallpox and rickettsialpox (see Chapter 30). These procedures as well as culture of the virus from vesicular fluids are described in Chapter 7.

The appearance and distribution of chickenpox, which so markedly differs from measles and rubella, suggests different mechanisms for cutaneous manifestations of these viral diseases. The skin lesions, heavily laden with virus, are almost certainly caused either by the virus itself, by an acute inflammatory reaction to the virus, or by both. The evolution from vesicle to pustule to crusted lesion is primarily due to an acute inflammatory reaction and not to a cellular immune response.

As with measles and rubella, the role of the immune system in protection against subsequent challenge by chickenpox is better understood than its role in controlling an established infection. Specific antibody seems to be of crucial importance in protection against disease. Newborn babies whose mothers had chickenpox are immune for the first few months of life. There is no reason to believe that such infants have received sensitized lymphocytes from their mothers. As maternally acquired antibody levels decline, the child becomes fully susceptible to chickenpox. Further evidence suggesting the importance of antibody for protection is seen in the efficacy of varicella–zoster hyperimmune globulin (VZIG) in protection of immunocompromised hosts (see Chapter 40). This regimen works very well either to prevent entirely or to attenuate significantly the severity of chickenpox.

The role of the cellular immune system in terminating the disease process can be extremely important, as evidenced by the lethality of chickenpox in immunosuppressed patients. Even in the face of an effective cell-mediated host immune system leading to uneventful clinical recovery, the virus has an uncanny propensity for establishing latent or persistent infection of spinal cord ganglia, analogous to herpesvirus infection. Decades later, in association with dwindling cell-mediated immune defense resulting from advancing years or subtle onset of an underlying malignant disorder, the virus becomes activated and produces vesicular lesions. These lesions are essentially identical to those of varicella except that the former are ordinarily restricted to the region of skin or dermatome innervated by the peripheral nerves originating from the ganglia that are harboring the virus. This disease, called herpes zoster, or shingles, at one time was thought to be distinct from varicella. It is now clear, however, that it is caused by the same virus. If cellular immunity is profoundly and persistently impaired, the localized form of herpes zoster may become disseminated and life-threatening (see Chapter 27).

ERYTHEMA INFECTIOSUM (FIFTH DISEASE)

Similar-appearing childhood rashes were numbered as they were described and differentiated. Thus, erythema infectiosum was named "fifth disease" because it was described after scarlet fever, rubeola, rubella, and epidemic pseudo-scarlatina. This disease is caused by the parvovirus B19. Erythema infectiosum is a benign childhood disease whose principal feature is an exanthem, with mild or absent systemic toxicity and fever. The condition is easily diagnosed when the child has the classic presentation which includes very red cheeks ("slapped cheeks") and an erythematous rash in a lacy distribution over the extensor surfaces of the arms and legs. The rash may recur for several weeks upon exposure to sunlight or changes in temperature.

A variety of other rashes have been found during documented outbreaks of erythema in-

fectiosum including vesicular, purpuric, and rubella-like rashes. None of these is sufficiently characteristic to make a clinical diagnosis.

Erythema infectiosum is a benign disease in the normal host. However, the propensity of the virus to affect red cell precursors in the bone marrow causes serious illness in two groups: the developing fetus and individuals with hemoglobinopathies. When *in utero* infections occur, particularly during the second trimester, there is high likelihood of severe anemia resulting in hydrops or fetal death secondary to heart failure. Fortunately, fetal infections occur infrequently. There are no known congenital anomalies associated with fetal B19 infection.

Children with hemoglobinopathies, such as sickle cell anemia, have circulating red cells with shortened lifespans. The transient interruption of red cell production by parvovirus B19 leads to a clinically significant anemia, the so-called aplastic crisis. Parvovirus B19 infection has occasionally caused long-lasting chronic anemia in individuals whose bone marrow has been damaged by chemotherapeutic agents or who have T-cell defects.

ROSEOLA (EXANTHEM SUBITUM)

Roseola is a benign, although frightening, disease of young children. The etiologic agent is a virus, human herpesvirus 6 (HHV-6). Most neonates have maternally acquired antibodies to this virus. By 5–6 months of age, this immunity has waned and the child becomes susceptible. Roseola is an extraordinarily frequent infection during infancy, with most infants having sustained a primary infection by age 2 years.

Roseola usually begins with a high spiking fever without any particular physical findings. The temperature is frequently high, 104°–105°F. After a few days, the fever abates, followed by a generalized maculopapular rash which lasts 24–36 h.

KAWASAKI DISEASE

This illness was described by Dr. Tomisaku Kawasaki in 1967. He noted the appearance of a previously unrecognized febrile, exanthematous disease in Japanese children. Subsequently, this disease has been found throughout the world.

Were it not for the complication of coronary

artery disease, Kawasaki syndrome would be but another curious viral exanthem. However, 20–25% of untreated patients develop aneurysms and subsequent stenosis of the coronary arteries, which may lead to death if left untreated. Accordingly, the early recognition and treatment of this entity is mandatory to prevent fatal myocardial infarction, which occurs in about 0.2% of untreated children.

Typically, the illness begins with the onset of a high fever for several days. Initially, there may be no associated findings, although soon bulbar conjunctival injection begins, mucous membranes of the mouth become inflamed, and the lips may become fissured and cracked. The dorsa of the hands and feet often become swollen and a rash with pleomorphic features may occur over a variety of body surfaces. Urticarial lesions on erythematous plaques, and morbilliform and scarlatiniform erythroderma have all been described. The above features are each present in about 90% of children with Kawasaki disease. Enlargement of one or more cervical lymph nodes is seen in 50–70% of affected children.

If left untreated, a subacute phase of the disease supervenes, characterized by anorexia, extreme irritability, persistent conjunctival injection, and desquamation of the fingers and toes. The desquamation typically begins in the periungal regions, usually involving only the distal parts of the fingers and toes, although on occasion more extensive desquamation of the hands and feet may occur. This phase of the illness lasts from about day 10 to day 25 after onset of the acute manifestations.

The third stage of the illness (convalescence) begins after all clinical signs of illness have abated, but an elevated erythrocyte sedimentation rate and thrombocytosis persist. It often takes 6–10 weeks for the sedimentation rate and platelet count to return to normal.

The fever of untreated Kawasaki disease frequently lasts 7–10 days. However, with the onset of the other clinical features mentioned above, the skillful physician will consider this diagnosis and institute intravenous gammaglobulin therapy. For unknown reasons, this treatment, when begun within 10 days of the onset of the fever, is highly effective in reducing coronary artery disease to about 3% of recipients.

The etiology of this condition is presently unknown. The epidemic characteristics, which lead to outbreaks with little intervening endemic spread, suggest an infectious etiology. However,

the search for the agent has been frustratingly difficult. Common bacterial and viral pathogens have been studied and excluded as possibilities. Similarly, retroviruses have been extensively looked for but unfortunately not found. The search for the agent causing this entity is currently one of the most fascinating challenges in infectious disease.

REFERENCES

Books

Feigin, R. D., and Cherry, J. D., eds. *Textbook of Pediatric Infectious Diseases*. 2nd ed. Philadelphia: W. B. Saunders Co., 1987.

Krugman, S., and Katz, S. L., eds. *Infectious Diseases of Children*. 8th ed. St. Louis: C. V. Mosby Co., 1985.

Lambert, H. P., and Farrar, W. E. *Infectious Diseases Illustrated. An Integrated Text and Color Atlas*. Philadelphia: W. B. Saunders Co., 1982.

Review Articles

American Academy of Pediatrics, Committee on Infectious Diseases: Measles: reassessment of the current immunization policy. *Pediatrics 84*:1110–1113, 1989.

Cherry, J. D. The "new" epidemiology of measles and rubella. *Hosp. Pract. 15*:49–57, 1980.

Rowley, A. H., Gonzalez-Crussi, F., and Shulman, S. T. Kawasaki syndrome. *Rev. Infect. Dis. 10*:1–15, 1988.

Ware, R. Human parvovirus infection. *J. Pediatr. 114*:343–348, 1989.

Original Articles

Asano, Y., Yoshikawa, T., Suga, S., et al. Viremia and neutralizing antibody response in infants with exanthem subitum. *J. Pediatr. 114*:535–539, 1989.

Brodsky, A. L. Atypical measles. Severe illness in recipients of killed measles virus vaccine upon exposure to natural infection. *JAMA 222*:1415–1416, 1972.

Centers for Disease Control. Current trends: Rubella vaccination during pregnancy—United States, 1971–1982. *MMWR 32*:429, August 26, 1983.

Centers for Disease Control. Rubella and congenital rubella—United States, 1984–1986. *MMWR 36*:664, October 16, 1987.

Centers for Disease Control. Risks associated with human parvovirus B19 infection. *MMWR 38*:81, February 17, 1989.

Cherry, J. D., Feigin, R. D., Lobes, L. A., Jr., et al. Atypical measles in children previously immunized with attenuated measles virus vaccines. *Pediatrics 50*:712–717, 1972.

Clark, M., Boustred, J., Schild, G. C., et al. Effect of rubella vaccination programme on serological status of young adults in United Kingdom. *Lancet 1*:1224–1226, 1979.

Frank, J. A., Jr., Orenstein, W. A., Bart, K. J., et al.

Major impediments to measles elimination. The modern epidemiology of an ancient disease. *Am. J. Dis. Child. 139*:881–888, 1985.

Hinman, A. R. Measles and rubella in adolescents and young adults. *Hosp Pract 17*:137–146, 1982.

Hinman, A. R., Orenstein, W. A., Bart, K., et al. Rational strategy for rubella vaccination. *Lancet 1*:39–41, 1983.

Kipps, A., Dick, G., and Moddie, J. W. Measles and the central nervous system. *Lancet 2*:1406–1410, 1983.

Markowitz, L. E., Sepulveda, J., Diaz-Ortega, J. L., et al. Immunization of six-month-old infants with different doses of Edmonston-Zagreb and Schwarz measles vaccines. *N. Engl. J. Med. 322*:580–587, 1990.

Marks, J. S., Halpin, T. J., and Orenstein, W. A. Measles vaccine efficacy in children previously vaccinated at 12 months of age. *Pediatrics 62*:955–960, 1978.

Suringa, D. W. R., Bank, L. J., and Ackerman, A. B. Role of measles virus in skin lesions and Koplik's spots. *N. Engl. J. Med. 283*:1139–1142, 1970.

Yamanishi, K., Shiraki, K., Kondo, T., et al. Identification of human Herpesvirus-6 as a causal agent for exanthem subitum. *Lancet 1*:1065–1067, May 14, 1988.

34 *JOHN WARREN, M.D.*

Sepsis

INTRODUCTION

The presence of bacteria or fungi in a patient's blood *(bacteremia* or *fungemia)* can be transient, intermittent, or continuous. *Transient bacteremia* clears within a few minutes, and occurs as a result of instrument probing of colonized mucosal surfaces, especially dental procedures or cystoscopy, and as a consequence of surgery involving infected tissue, such as drainage of an abscess. Transient bacteremia is not significant except in patients with underlying valvular heart disease, for whom bacterial seeding of thrombi present on diseased cardiac valves can cause infective endocarditis. *Intermittent bacteremia* is associated primarily with an extravascular source of infection in tissue, most notably pneumonia, meningitis, pyelonephritis, osteomyelitis, peritonitis, pyogenic arthritis, subcutaneous soft tissue infection, and undrained abscesses. This form of bacteremia results from failure of the host to contain tissue infection by allowing intermittent escape of bacteria or fungi into the circulation via lymphatic vessels. For patients with intermittent bacteremia, approximately 75–80% of blood cultures obtained in a series of several cultures are positive (Fig. 34–1). *Continuous bacteremia* is a cardinal feature of intravascular foci of infection, especially infective endocarditis and contaminated intravenous catheters, but also infected arteriovenous fistulae and vascular aneurysms *(mycotic aneurysms)*. When one blood culture from a patient with infective endocarditis is positive, the probability that subsequent blood cultures will be positive is 95–100% (Fig. 34–1) (see Chapter 35).

The signs and symptoms of bacteremia and fungemia *(sepsis)* include hyperventilation, altered mental status, fever, chills, and occasionally hypothermia. The earliest clinical findings in bacteremia are hyperventilation with respiratory alkalosis and apprehension. Fever and chills generally follow, but in markedly debilitated patients, or in the very young or the very old, euthermia (normal body temperature) or

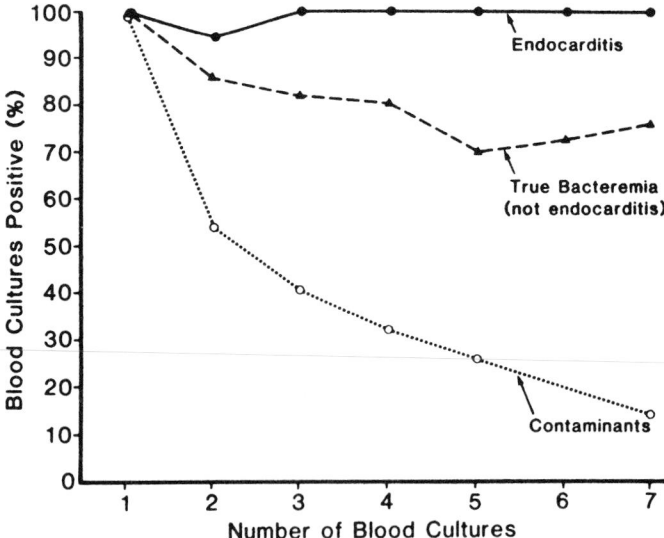

Figure 34–1. Patterns of positivity with successive blood cultures from patients with endocarditis, with other types of bloodstream infection (true bacteremia but not endocarditis), or with an initial culture contaminated by a skin commensal. The continuous bacteremia of endocarditis and intermittent bacteremia secondary to tissue infection (but not endocarditis) are indicated by the two top curves. With skin contaminants, the probability that subsequent blood cultures will be positive is very low. Also, if skin contaminants are detected in subsequent cultures, they are almost always different from the contaminants detected in the initial culture (for example, diphtheroids in the initial culture, followed by coagulase-negative staphylococci in a subsequent culture). (From Weinstein, M. P., Reller, L. B., Murphy, J. R., et al. The clinical significance of positive blood cultures: A comprehensive analysis of 500 episodes of bacteremia and fungemia in adults. I. Laboratory and epidemiologic observations. Rev. Infect. Dis. 5:35, 1983.)

hypothermia may be present. The mortality due to bacteremia and fungemia shows an inverse relationship with body temperature, with an increased risk of death among patients whose body temperature is low or normal during sepsis (Fig. 34–2). A serious complication of sepsis is the development of hypotension *(septic shock)*, which can progress to hypoperfusion of tissues and organ failure with oliguria, jaundice, congestive heart failure, and metabolic lactic acidosis. Once shock occurs in bacteremic patients, the mortality rate increases severalfold. To prevent septic shock, the bacterial or fungal cause of sepsis must be promptly identified using blood culture, and appropriate therapy must be initiated. Other complications of sepsis include adult respiratory distress syndrome (ARDS), bleeding due to disseminated intravascular coagulation (DIC), precipitous neutropenia, thrombocytopenia, and hemorrhagic (petechiae, purpura, ecchymoses) and ulcerative skin lesions.

Most septic patients demonstrate a focus of tissue infection as the source of their bacteremia, either intravascular or extravascular. This type of bacteremia is known as *secondary bacteremia*, and occurs most frequently in association with urinary and respiratory tract infection. Other important sources include intraabdominal infection (biliary tract, abscess, enteritis, peritonitis), and infections of wounds, the central nervous system, bone, soft tissue of skin, and intravascular catheters or heart valves. In a significant number of septic episodes, however, tissue or vascular sources of bacteremia are not

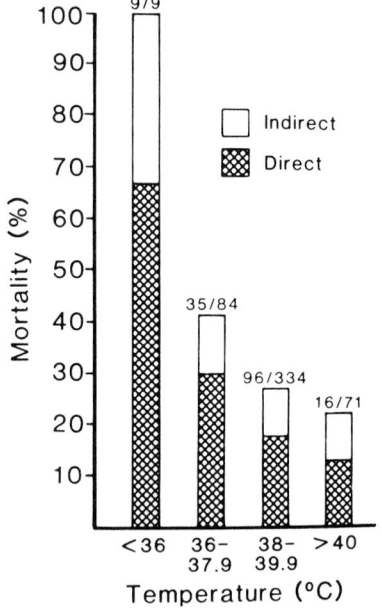

Figure 34–2. Outcome of bacteremia and fungemia in relation to body temperature. Two thirds of the hypothermic (<36°C) patients died from causes directly related to sepsis, and about one third of the euthermic (36–37.9°C) patients died as a direct result of sepsis. The lowest mortality was observed among patients with moderate (38–39.9°C) or marked (>40°C) temperature responses. The total number of patients who died (numerator) and the total number of patients with the indicated temperature response (denominator) are reported at the top of each data bar. (From Weinstein, M. P., Murphy, J. R., Reller, L. B., et al. The clinical significance of positive blood cultures: A comprehensive analysis of 500 episodes of bacteremia and fungemia in adults. II. Clinical observations, with special reference to factors influencing prognosis. Rev. Infect. Dis. 5:54, 1983.)

identified, a circumstance designated as *primary bacteremia*. Bacterial flora of the intestinal tract are recognized as major pathogens in primary bacteremia. It has been postulated that motile phagocytes ingest intestinal bacteria, fail to achieve intracellular killing, transport the phagocytosed bacteria to extraintestinal sites *(translocation)*, and liberate the bacteria to cause bacteremia. Primary bacteremia can also be caused by direct invasion of intestinal microorganisms across ulcers and necrotic tumors of the gastrointestinal tract. Etiologic agents in both primary and secondary sepsis include gram-negative bacteria, gram-positive bacteria, obligately anaerobic bacteria, or fungi, and sepsis can be due either to a single organism *(monomicrobial)* or to multiple organisms *(polymicrobial)*.

GRAM-NEGATIVE BACTEREMIA

Highly virulent gram-negative bacteria, especially *Neisseria meningitidis, Yersinia pestis,* and *Salmonella typhi,* can cause fulminant or persistent bacteremia in the normal host. However, most bacteremic episodes due to gram-negative organisms occur in individuals with an underlying debilitating disease, are acquired in the hospital *(nosocomial infection,* see Chapter 28), and are often caused by microorganisms present in the endogenous flora. Inflammatory mediators released in the bacteremic patient can result in life-threatening hemodynamic instability or pulmonary insufficiency.

Clinical Aspects

The development of septic shock and/or ARDS is of paramount importance in gram-negative bacteremia. Shock is observed in 20–35% of patients with gram-negative bacteremia, and in previously normotensive adults shock is clinically defined as systolic blood pressure less than 90 mm Hg and diastolic pressure less than 60 mm Hg. Peripheral vasodilatation with warm dry skin ("warm shock") is present initially, but if shock persists, skin and splanchnic vasoconstriction develops in an attempt to maintain blood flow to vital organs (brain, heart, kidneys), and the skin becomes pale and cool ("cold shock"). A moribund phase of shock with anuria reflects inability of compensatory mechanisms to maintain arterial perfusion of vital organs. A greatly increased mortality results from the development of shock in gram-negative bacteremia. ARDS is characterized by severe dyspnea, tachypnea, hypoxemia, and diffuse bilateral infiltrates on chest radiograph. The occurrence of ARDS reflects diffuse damage to both alveolar septal capillaries and alveolar lining epithelium of the lung, with fulminant interstitial and intraalveolar fibrinous exudation. ARDS usually occurs when shock has already complicated bacteremia. The mortality of ARDS due to gram-negative bacteremia is very high (50–80%).

A fulminant variant of gram-negative bacteremia is caused by the gram-negative diplococcus *Neisseria meningitidis* (meningococcus). Hematogenous dissemination follows nasopharyngeal colonization with *N. meningitidis.* Meningococcemia is accompanied by activation of the blood coagulation system, with coagulation proteins and platelets being consumed (and depleted). The consumption coagulopathy, in turn, results in hemorrhage with dramatic development of skin petechiae and ecchymoses. Bilateral adrenal gland hemorrhage (Fig. 34–3), shock, and meningococcemia were first described as a syndrome by Waterhouse and Friderichsen. Another fulminant variant of gram-negative bacteremia is *plague*, a bacteremic infection due to *Yersinia pestis* in which the mortality in untreated cases is greater than 50%. *Y. pestis* is a gram-negative coccobacillus transmitted to humans by contact with rodent fleas. A distinctive feature of plague is marked inflammatory enlargement of infected lymph nodes *(acute lymphadenitis)*, with large (1–10 cm) ovoid lymph node swellings *(buboes)* visible in the femoral, inguinal, axillary, and cervical regions. Patients with bubonic plague are typically febrile and hypotensive due to the *Y. pestis* bacteremia (see Chapter 31).

The sepsis of typhoid fever is a severe and prolonged disease, and *Salmonella typhi* is recovered from blood cultures in over 80% of patients during the first week of illness. The portal of entry for *S. typhi* is the small intestine. Following ingestion of organisms in contaminated food, the typhoid bacilli multiply in the small intestine, penetrate the mucosal barrier, infect mesenteric lymph nodes, and eventually enter the bloodstream through the thoracic duct to cause sepsis. The onset of typhoid fever is insidious. Fever is prominent, but the pulse is typically slow *(bradycardia)* relative to the temperature. Neutropenia due to bone marrow depression is almost uniformly present, following early transient leukocytosis. Bradycardia

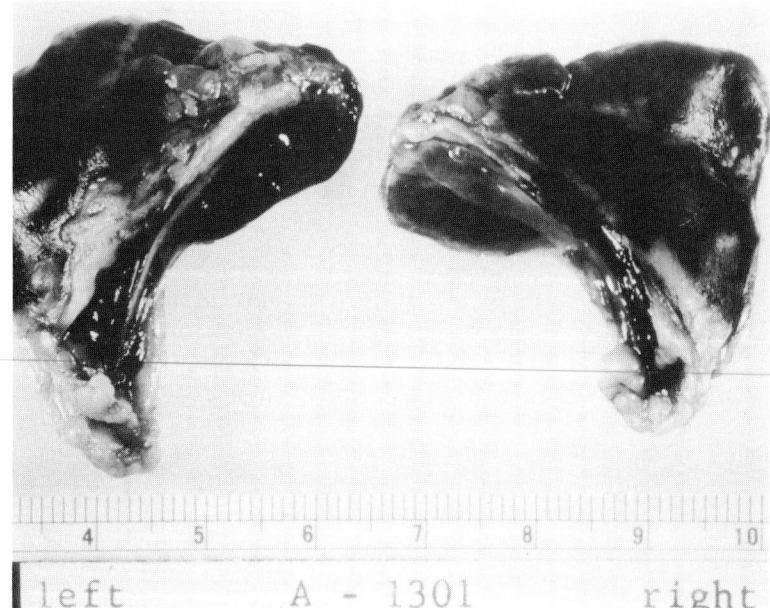

Figure 34–3. Adrenal gland hemorrhage in bacteremia due to Neisseria meningitidis *(Waterhouse-Friderichsen syndrome). Endotoxic lipopolysaccharide activates factor XII (Hageman factor), which in turn activates the intrinsic coagulation system with formation of fibrin microthrombi. In fulminant meningococcemia (or other forms of gram-negative bacteremia), a consumption coagulopathy (disseminated intravascular coagulation) can develop resulting in tissue hemorrhage. The consumption coagulopathy is a secondary reflection of severe gram-negative bacteremia and is not a primary cause of lethal shock. (From Warren, J. R., Scarpelli, D. G., Reddy, J. K., et al.* Essentials of General Pathology. *New York: Macmillan Publishing Company, 1987.)*

and neutropenia in a febrile septic patient strongly suggest *Salmonella* bacteremia. Complications of typhoid fever include toxic myocarditis, persistent and disseminated infection with *S. typhi* (arthritis, endocarditis, meningitis), gastrointestinal hemorrhage or perforation, and secondary bacterial pneumonia with an organism other than *S. typhi*. The mortality of untreated cases is 12–16% (see Chapter 19).

Microbiologic Aspects

Enterobacteriaceae

The most frequently observed organism in gram-negative bacteremia is *Escherichia coli* (Table 34–1) because of the prevalence of *E. coli* in pyelonephritis and abdominal infections. *Klebsiella pneumoniae* is also a common cause of gram-negative bacteremia. *K. pneumoniae* often replaces *E. coli* in the gastrointestinal tract of seriously ill patients, and causes life-threatening bacteremia from this reservoir. In addition, *K. pneumoniae* is a common etiologic agent of both urinary and respiratory tract infections. Other members of the family *Enterobacteriaceae* implicated in gram-negative bacteremia (although not as frequently) are *Enterobacter* and *Serratia* species, as well as *Proteus* and *Providencia* species. As is true for *E. coli* and *K. pneumoniae*, bacteremia due to these organisms is very frequently hospital-acquired. *Proteus* and *Providencia* bacteremia is especially associated with

urinary tract infection. *Salmonella* bacteremia, which often occurs in the normal host with enteric infection, is made worse by impairment of T-lymphocyte function, particularly in AIDS.

Nonfermentative and Oxidase-Positive Fermentative Gram-Negative Rods

The *nonfermentative gram-negative rods*, most notably the oxidative organism *Pseudomonas aeruginosa*, closely follow the *Enterobacteriaceae* as a frequent cause of bacteremia (Table 34–1). Infection with *P. aeruginosa* is nearly always nosocomial, and generally occurs among severely ill, neutropenic, or burn patients. Other nonfermentative gram-negative organisms that cause nosocomial bacteremia are *Xanthomonas maltophilia* and *Acinetobacter calcoaceticus*. *X. maltophilia* is a motile, oxidative bacillus closely related to *Pseudomonas* but lacks cytochrome oxidase. *A. calcoaceticus* is a nonmotile bacillus that also does not produce cytochrome oxidase. As with *P. aeruginosa*, resistance to multiple antimicrobial agents is an important aspect of bacteremia due to *X. maltophilia* and *A. calcoaceticus*. Yet a third group of gram-negative rods is emerging as an important cause of sepsis in debilitated individuals, the *oxidase-positive fermenters*, particularly *Aeromonas hydrophila* and *Vibrio vulnificus* (Table 34–1). The natural habitat of *A. hydrophila* is water, and soft tissue (wound) or gastrointestinal tract infection related to exposure to fresh or saltwater can result in bacteremia,

TABLE 34–1. *Etiologic Agents of Gram-Negative Bacteremia*

Group	Microorganisms
Oxidase-negative fermenters (Enterobacteriaceae)*	*Escherichia coli* *Klebsiella* *Enterobacter* *Serratia* *Proteus* *Providencia* *Salmonella* *Yersinia*
Oxidase-positive nonfermenters†	*Pseudomonas aeruginosa*
Oxidase-negative nonfermenters‡	*Xanthomonas maltophilia* *Acinetobacter calcoaceticus*
Oxidase-positive fermenters§	*Aeromonas hydrophila* *Vibrio vulnificus*
Fastidious species‖	*Neisseria meningitidis* and *N. gonorrhoeae* *Haemophilus influenzae,* *H. parainfluenzae,* *H. aphrophilus,* and *H. paraphrophilus* *Cardiobacterium hominis* *Actinobacillus actinomycetemcomitans*

*Fermentation is an oxidation–reduction process that utilizes a carbohydrate substrate to produce ATP, and for which an organic substrate serves as the final electron acceptor. Fermentation generates strong acids and CO_2, and is easily measured. Members of the family Enterobacteriaceae metabolize glucose fermentatively and lack the enzyme of aerobic respiration, cytochrome oxidase.

†*P. aeruginosa* is an oxidative organism that produces the respiratory enzyme, cytochrome oxidase, and is incapable of glucose fermentation.

‡ *X. maltophilia* and *A. calcoaceticus* are aerobic organisms that are cytochrome oxidase–negative. *X. maltophilia* oxidizes maltose, hence its species designation. There are two subspecies of *Acinetobacter calcoaceticus*, *A. anitratus*, which vigorously oxidizes a number of carbohydrates (including glucose), and *A. lwoffi*, which is metabolically inert.

§These organisms metabolize glucose fermentatively, but also produce cytochrome oxidase.

‖Fastidious bacteria require special nutritional media and ambient gases for their growth. Both *Neisseria* and *Haemophilus* species grow best on chocolate agar in the presence of CO_2. Likewise, increased CO_2 tension promotes the growth of *Cardiobacterium hominis* and *Actinobacillus actinomycetemcomitans*.

particularly among patients with cirrhosis or malignancy. *V. vulnificus* bacteremia characteristically occurs among individuals with underlying liver disease who have recently ingested raw oysters. However, as with *A. hydrophila*, wound infection related to water exposure can also serve as a portal of entry.

Fastidious Gram-Negative Bacteria

The fastidious gram-negative bacteria that cause sepsis in special settings are common and must be remembered (Table 34–1). *Neisseria meningitidis* can cause fulminant sepsis in normal individuals but can also cause chronic and re-

peated episodes of bloodstream infection in individuals deficient in the fifth, sixth, seventh, or eighth component of complement (as can *Neisseria gonorrhoeae*). Bacteremia due to *Haemophilus influenzae* type b is a scourge of children between ages 3 months and 6 years, after the disappearance of maternal *H. influenzae* antibody and before the appearance of the child's own protective antibody, as a consequence of colonization or immunization (see Chapter 23). Finally, several infrequently occurring, fastidious, and slow-growing gram-negative species can be associated with endocarditis and systemic embolization, including several *Haemophilus* species (*H. parainfluenzae, H. aphrophilus, H. paraphrophilus*), *Cardiobacterium hominis*, and *Actinobacillus actinomycetemcomitans*.

Pathophysiologic Mechanisms

Mechanisms of gram-negative sepsis operate in the dynamic context of host–parasite interaction and include both host defense factors and invasive and toxic properties of bacteria. On the host side of the equation, the nature and severity of underlying disease, the source of bacteremia, and the age of the host are critical determinants of outcome. The risk of death increases with age (older than 40 years), especially in individuals with neoplastic disease, asplenia, cirrhosis, granulocytopenia, renal failure, diabetes mellitus, or those undergoing corticosteroid therapy. Mortality is high for bacteremic patients with a primary infected focus in the respiratory tract, a surgical wound, or an abscess. Properties of bacteria that promote host invasion include adherence to mucosal surfaces via specific adhesin molecules in surface pili (Fig. 34–4), resistance to complement-dependent lysis in the absence of antibody, resistance to neutrophil phagocytosis due to surface encapsulation, and production by bacteria of protein enzymes and toxins that cause tissue necrosis and thereby facilitate spread of infection. *Pseudomonas aeruginosa*, for example, produces elastases, which degrade extracellular connective tissue matrix and blood vessel walls, and *exotoxin A*, which inhibits tissue protein synthesis by a mechanism analogous to that of diphtheria toxin (ADP-ribosylation of elongation factor 2).

The outer membrane antigens of gram-negative bacteria are of fundamental importance in determining host responses to bacteremia. Polysaccharide *O antigens* of the outer membrane are composed of long chains of repeating car-

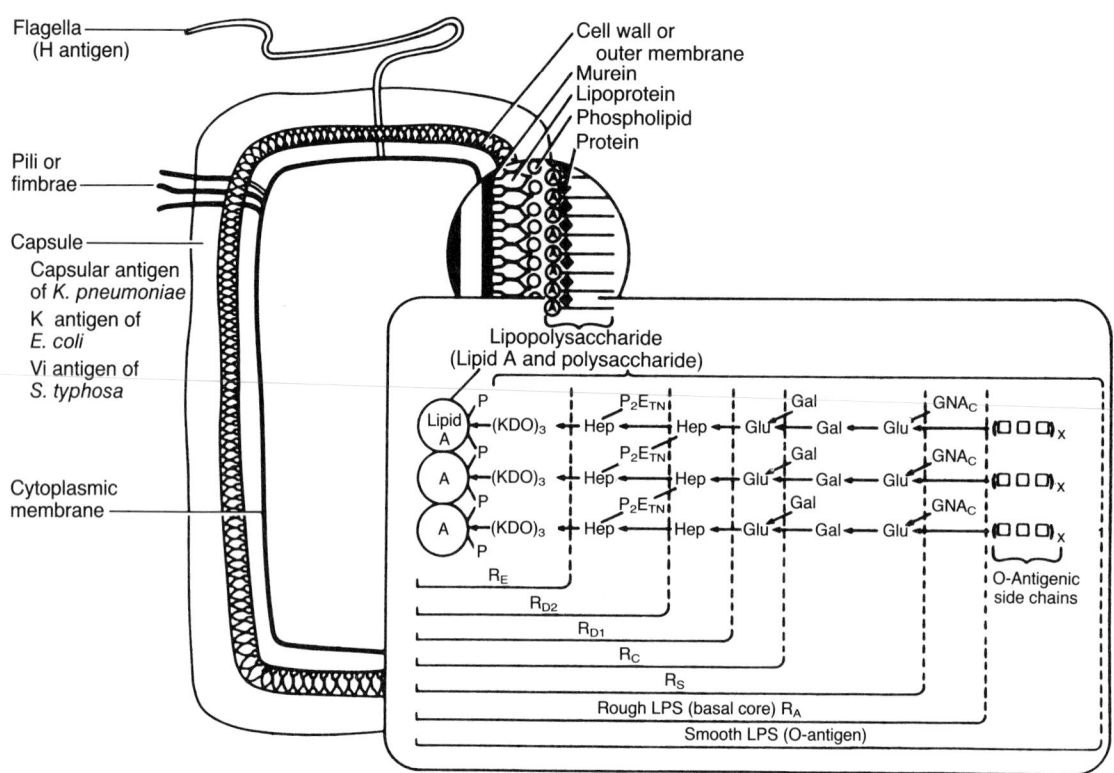

Figure 34–4. Schematic depiction of endotoxic lipopolysaccharide (LPS) and its position in the gram-negative bacterial cell wall. Lipid A (depicted as A) anchors LPS in the outer membrane, and core and O-antigen arise from lipid A as linear polysaccharides. The chemical structure of smooth wild-type (S) and rough (R) mutant strains of Salmonella *is shown in the insert. The R mutants R_A, R_B, R_C, R_{D1}, R_{D2}, and R_E are shown in order of increasing roughness, resulting from deletion of O-antigen and core polysaccharides. (GNA$_c$) N-acetylglucosamine, (Glu) glucose, (Gal) galactose, (Hep) heptose, and (P) phosphate. Lipid A is present in all pathogenic gram-negative bacteria, and the carbohydrate 2-keto-3-deoxyoctonate (KDO), which links lipid A to core antigen, is present in most, except for a few obligate anaerobes. Also depicted are the pili (or fimbriae), which contain adhesins, the antiphagocytic capsule, and the cytoplasmic membrane of the bacterial cell. The periplasmic space is located between the cytoplasmic membrane and the murein (peptidoglycan) layer. (From McCabe, W. R. Endotoxin: Microbiological, chemical, pathophysiologic and clinical correlations. In: Weinstein, L., and Fields, B. N., eds.* Seminars in Infectious Disease, *Vol. 3. New York: Thieme-Stratton, 1980, pp. 38–88.)*

bohydrate units exposed on the surface of bacterial cells (Fig. 34–4). The carbohydrate composition of O antigens shows strain variation within individual gram-negative species. For example, there are more than 160 different strains of *Escherichia coli*, each with a unique O antigen. O antigen chains are linked to a *core region*, which consists of an acidic oligosaccharide of *N*-acetylglucosamine, glucose, galactose, heptose phosphate, and 2-keto-3-deoxyoctonate (KDO). The KDO residues link the core polysaccharide to an acylated glucosamine disaccharide termed *lipid A* (Fig. 34–5). Lipid A is amphipathic because of the simultaneous presence of both a hydrophilic structure (phosphorylated glucosamine disaccharide) and lipophilic structures (long-chain fatty acids). This molecular composition is unique to lipid A and is highly conserved among diverse species of gram-negative bacteria. The macromolecular complex composed of O antigen, core oligosaccharide, and lipid A is called *endotoxic lipopolysaccharide (LPS)*. Endotoxic LPS is the dominant structure present in the gram-negative outer membrane and is held within the outer membrane by a combination of noncovalent hydrophobic and electrostatic bonds. Endotoxic LPS induces tissue inflammation, fever, and shock in the infected host, and lipid A structures carry the toxic conformations of LPS responsible for these host reactions. Highly ordered and rigidly packed structures of fatty acid chains and the charged functional groups of the phosphorylated diglucosamine are both essential for induction of host reactions. The hydrophilic polysaccharides of O and core-region antigen are needed to make lipid A soluble, thereby facilitating delivery of lipid A to cellular and plasma protein

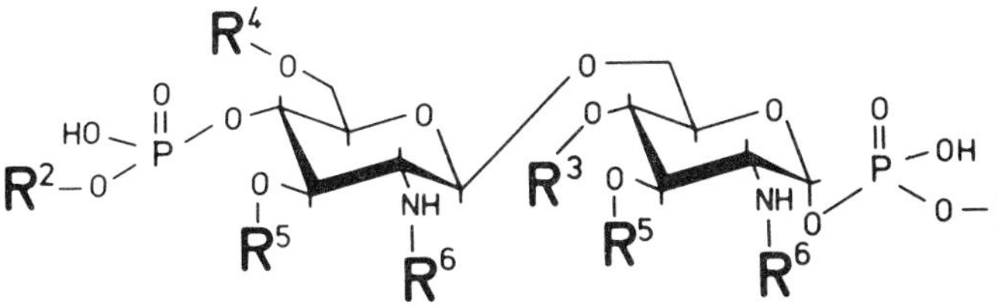

Figure 34–5. Structure of lipid A. The phosphorylated diglucosamine backbone possesses O-linked (at position R^5) and N-linked (at position R^6) 3-hydroxy long-chain fatty acids. Frequently, a second long-chain fatty acid is esterified to the 3-hydroxy group of the primary fatty acid chain. A variety of constituents can be linked to the phosphate groups at positions R^1 and R^2, including another phosphate group, phosphoryl ethanolamine, D-glucosamine, or furanosidic D-arabinose. Linkage to KDO occurs at position R^4 to the primary 6'-hydroxyl group. (From Rietschel., E. Th., Wollenweber, H.-W., Russa, R., et al. Concepts of the chemical structure of lipid A. Rev. Infect. Dis. 6:432, 1984.)

targets, but these hydrophilic polysaccharides do not play a direct role in LPS toxicity.

Endotoxic LPS initiates the pathophysiologic reactions of gram-negative sepsis, as demonstrated by the following observations:

1. LPS injection in humans and experimental animals induces chills, fever, and shock.
2. High plasma levels of LPS correlate with high mortality in septic patients.
3. Mortality due to shock can be reduced by lipid A antibodies.

However, LPS itself is not toxic. Instead, LPS stimulates production of humoral mediators, which in turn are responsible for the pathophysiologic manifestations of gram-negative sepsis. The macrophage-secreted polypeptides *tumor necrosis factor* (TNF) (cachectin) and *interleukin 1* (IL-1) are the key mediators, but kinins and complement factors play important roles as well. Transcription of macrophage TNF mRNA is rapidly increased in response to LPS, and TNF is released into the bloodstream, achieving peak serum levels within minutes after LPS injection. However, macrophages do not continuously secrete TNF, owing partly to the presence of the consensus octamer UUAUUUAU in untranslated regions of TNF mRNA, which destabilizes the mRNA. This consensus octamer is present in the mRNA that encodes a number of inflammatory mediators, and it is thought to ensure synthesis of these potent molecules only in discrete and efficient bursts when needed. IL-1, a cytokine structurally distinct from TNF, is also secreted by macrophages in response to LPS. Two forms of IL-1 exist, an acidic form with an isoelectric pH of 5 (IL-1 α), and a basic form with an isoelectric pH of 7 (IL-1 β). IL-1 β has been implicated as a mediator in host responses to gram-negative disease.

The biologic effects of TNF and IL-1 are expressed both locally in tissue (*autocrine effects*) and systemically. Autocrine effects are directed primarily to the vascular endothelium.

Increased expression of the endothelial surface glycoprotein, *intercellular adhesion molecule 1* (ICAM-1), occurs, enhancing the adherence of neutrophils to endothelium (Fig. 34–6). Also, endothelial membrane cyclooxygenase activity is stimulated, producing potent prostaglandin vasodilators. Vasodilatation with increased blood flow, and neutrophil adherence to vascular endothelium, strongly promote inflammation with exudation of plasma containing antibody and complement, and the emigration of phagocytic cells into infected tissue. The autocrine effects of TNF and IL-1 are enhanced by the ability of LPS to activate Hageman factor (factor XII), thereby generating kinins and complement fragments C3a and C5a, which increase blood vessel permeability and serve as chemotaxins. LPS can also activate complement directly in the absence of specific LPS antibody. These autocrine effects are of benefit to the host in containment and eradication of tissue infection.

Both TNF and IL-1 induce fever through their ability to stimulate hypothalamic prostaglandin synthesis. Elevated body temperature reduces the replication of many bacteria, and also augments helper T-cell activation and antibody synthesis by B cells. Consequently, fever as an acute-phase systemic reaction is beneficial to the host (see Fig. 34–2). However, bacteremia results from the release of millions of organisms from infected tissue into the circulation, even though the numbers of bacteria directly cultured from blood are relatively low because of reticuloendothelial clearance. Furthermore, since endotoxin is held in cell walls only by noncovalent forces, substantial amounts of free LPS escape from dead bacteria in tissue abscesses and enter the bloodstream via lymphatics. Thus, failure of the septic patient to prevent bacterial dissemination results in large circulating amounts of LPS and inflammatory mediators, especially TNF, resulting in "systemic activation" of vascular endothelium. Generalized vasodilatation and increased blood vessel permeability lead to reduction in the effective

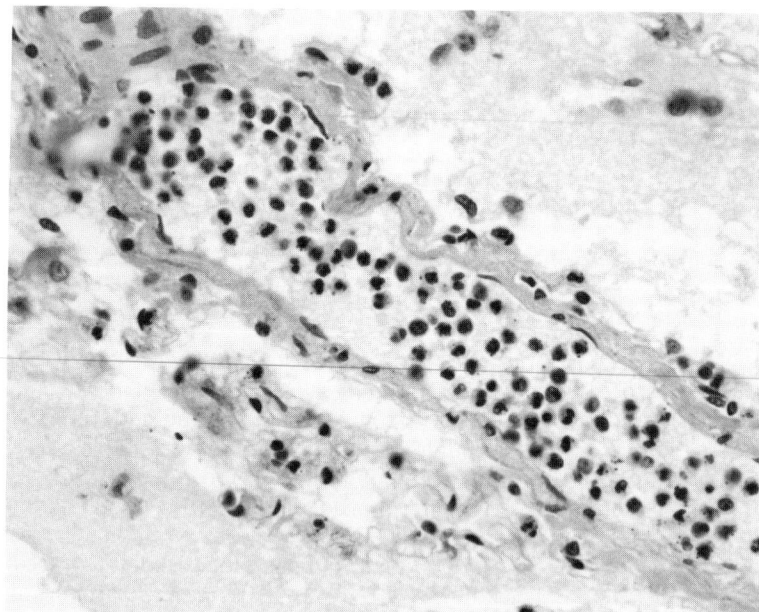

Figure 34–6. Leukostasis in ARDS caused by increased adherence of polymorphonuclear neutrophils to endothelium of pulmonary blood vessels. (Photomicrograph courtesy of Dr. Kenneth Haines, Department of Pathology, Northwestern University Medical School.)

blood volume and hypovolemic shock. Pulmonary leukostasis (Fig. 34–6), with its accompanying local neutrophilic release of oxygen radicals (especially hydroxyl radicals) and neutral proteases (especially elastase), causes endothelial and alveolar epithelial damage, effecting the development of ARDS. Clinical studies reveal higher plasma levels of IL-1 in patients who survive septic shock, whereas plasma levels of TNF tend to be higher in patients who do not survive septic shock. In addition, TNF lacks the immunopotentiating activity of IL-1. TNF markedly increases expression of neutrophil adherence glycoproteins causing hyperadherence, thereby making neutrophils incapable of detaching and emigrating into extravascular tissue. On balance, current evidence favors the concept that TNF is the most potent mediator of gram-negative shock and ARDS.

GRAM-POSITIVE BACTEREMIA

The occurrence of gram-positive bacteremia has become more frequent in recent years. This increase is due primarily to growing utilization of intravascular catheters, central nervous system (CNS) ventricular shunts, and surgical placement of prosthetic devices, all of which disrupt natural mucocutaneous barriers and introduce foreign bodies into tissue. Many blood isolates of gram-positive bacteria demonstrate resistance to multiple antibiotics. Consequently, prompt recognition of gram-positive bacteremia

is necessary to ensure effective antimicrobial therapy.

Clinical Aspects

Although shock and ARDS may develop, these complications are not as common as in gram-negative bacteremia. Patients typically present with signs and symptoms of local infection, such as pneumonia, meningitis, wound infection, skin abscess, or endocarditis. Two major concerns arise in gram-positive bacteremia. First, metastatic dissemination of infection is common. For example, during *Staphylococcus aureus* bacteremia, organisms can directly seed the kidneys from the bloodstream, causing acute pyelonephritis and numerous cortical abscesses. The recovery of *S. aureus* in urine culture is an important clue that the patient is bacteremic with *S. aureus*, as this organism rarely causes primary urinary tract infection. Second, many gram-positive bacteria can directly infect heart valves. Thus, patients bacteremic with these organisms must be carefully evaluated for endocarditis.

Microbiologic Aspects

Gram-Positive Cocci

Among the gram-positive cocci, the staphylococci, enterococci, and streptococci are

TABLE 34–2. *Etiologic Agents of Gram-Positive Bacteremia*

Group	Microorganisms
Gram-positive cocci	
Catalase-positive*	*Staphylococcus aureus* (coagulase-positive)
	Staphylococcus epidermidis (coagulase-negative)
Catalase-negative	*Enterococcus faecalis†*
	Streptococcus pneumoniae‡
	Viridans streptococci‡
Gram-positive rods§	
Nonhemolytic	*Corynebacterium* JK
Hemolytic	*Listeria monocytogenes*

*Catalase is an intracellular enzyme that decomposes hydrogen peroxide to water and O_2, and is uniformly present in staphylococci. Coagulase is a thrombin–like substance that causes visible clotting of plasma, and its presence identifies catalase-positive, gram-positive cocci as *Staphylococcus aureus*. Among the coagulase-negative species, *S. epidermidis* is most common, but *S. hominis*, *S. haemolyticus*, *S. simulans*, and others can cause bloodstream infection.

†Enterococcus was previously classified as a group D streptococcus, but nucleic acid hybridization measurements reveal little genetic relatedness of enterococci to the genus *Streptococcus*. *E. faecalis* is responsible for about 90% of enterococcal bloodstream infections, with occasional infections caused by *E. faecium*.

‡*S. pneumoniae* is an alpha-hemolytic *Streptococcus* that is bile-soluble and susceptible to lysis by the detergent optochin. The viridans streptococci are alpha-hemolytic (or rarely, nonhemolytic) and lack both bile solubility and optochin sensitivity. *S. mitior* and *S. sanguis* are the viridans streptococci most often associated with endocarditis.

§*Corynebacterium* JK grows as a nonhemolytic, penicillin-resistant, gram-positive bacillus on blood agar, whereas colonies of *L. monocytogenes* demonstrate distinct zones of beta-(clear) hemolysis on blood agar.

important causes of bacteremia (Table 34–2). Bacteremia with *Staphylococcus aureus* (coagulase-positive staphylococci) most often occurs in older hospitalized patients with underlying disease, children, patients with vascular access infections, or young adults who acquire their infection in the community by intravenous drug abuse. The overall incidence of endocarditis in adult *S. aureus* bacteremia is 5–20%. The coagulase-negative staphylococci have also been implicated in nosocomial bloodstream infections, especially *Staphylococcus epidermidis*. Emergence of coagulase-negative staphylococci as blood pathogens is due to their great numbers on the skin and their ability to adhere to surfaces of vascular catheters and prosthetic implants. Although endocarditis involving native heart valves is not often caused by *S. epidermidis*, coagulase-negative staphylococci frequently produce prosthetic valve endocarditis (see Chapter 35).

The enterococci (Table 34–2) are normally found in the feces, and bacteremia due to these organisms is almost always hospital-acquired. Prolonged hospitalization and the use of cephalosporins, which have little or no activity against the enterococci, are important risk factors for the development of enterococcal bacteremia. *Enterococcus* is unusual in that, unlike other gram-positive bacteria, bacteremia with this organism is associated with a high overall mortality (approximately 40%). Around 2–8% of patients with enterococcal bacteremia have endocarditis. The *viridans streptococci* (alpha-hemolytic, or green, streptococci) continue to account for the majority of cases of endocarditis (Table 34–2). Finally, the isolation of *Streptococcus pneumoniae* in blood culture always indicates bacteremia, which occurs most often in association with pneumococcal pneumonia or meningitis. Certain groups of patients are at increased risk of pneumococcal bacteremia, including *asplenic individuals* (autosplenectomy in sickle cell anemia, congenital, traumatic, surgical removal), patients with B-cell lymphoma or leukemia, and individuals with multiple myeloma. This increased risk reflects the importance of opsonizing antibody and splenic clearance in host defense against heavily encapsulated pneumococci.

Gram-Positive Rods

A number of gram-positive rods also produce bacteremia, most notably *Corynebacterium* JK diphtheroids and *Listeria monocytogenes*. Although diphtheroids are most often normal skin commensals, *Corynebacterium* JK causes nosocomial bacteremia in patients with indwelling catheters, in those with extended periods of granulocytopenia due to hematologic malignancy, or in those who have undergone bone marrow transplantation. As many as 20% of blood isolates of *Corynebacterium* JK are associated with serious nosocomial infection. *Corynebacterium* JK has been isolated also from patients with prosthetic valve endocarditis. *L. monocytogenes* is a facultative intracellular parasite whose dissemination is favored by impairment of T-lymphocyte function. Meningitis is most often present in listeriosis, but endocarditis also occurs.

Pathophysiologic Mechanisms

Shock and ARDS occur in gram-positive sepsis, presumably as a result of excessive inflammatory mediator production. But in contrast to gram-negative bacteria, a unique, highly conserved, and toxic cell-wall antigen analogous to LPS has not been discovered. Metastatic infection and a propensity to produce tissue abscesses are the dominant pathophysiologic determinants in gram-positive bacteremia.

ANAEROBIC BACTEREMIA

The obligately anaerobic bacteria fail to multiply when exposed to the oxygen tension of air (see Chapter 29). Many indigenous anaerobic bacteria grow on mucosal surfaces where local oxygen tension is sufficiently low. Large concentrations of anaerobic bacteria are thus found in gingival crevices of the oral cavity, the distal ileum and colon, and the endocervix and vagina. Anaerobic bacteremia in most instances represents infection related to these indigenous organisms.

Clinical Aspects

Anaerobic bacteremia is most often associated with intraabdominal abscess, infection of the female genital tract, or aspiration pneumonia. The development of hypotension is relatively common, especially with gram-negative species.

Microbiologic Aspects

The bacteriology of anaerobic bacteremia depends on the portal of entry. *Bacteroides fragilis*, an anaerobic, gram-negative bacillus, is the dominant isolate in intraabdominal sepsis. *Bacteroides* organisms, including *B. bivius* and other *Bacteroides* species, are commonly associated with bacteremic genital tract infections, along with the anaerobic, gram-positive *Peptostreptococcus*. *Bacteroides*, *Peptostreptococcus*, and anaerobic gram-negative *Fusobacterium nucleatum* are frequently recovered in patients with bacteremic aspiration pneumonia. The variable bacteriology reflects the indigenous flora at the different portals of entry.

Pathophysiologic Mechanisms

Isolation of anaerobic bacteria from blood cultures suggests a breach in a normal mucocutaneous barrier, such as occurs in colon carcinoma with obstruction or perforation, in inflammatory bowel disease, and in gynecologic surgery or obstetric procedures. Compromised conscious-

ness is a strong predisposing factor in the aspiration of colonized or infected material from the oral cavity, which leads to pleuropulmonary infection.

A number of virulence factors have been identified for anaerobic organisms. *Bacteroides fragilis* possesses a polysaccharide capsule that impedes phagocytosis and promotes abscess formation. Also, many anaerobic organisms produce succinic acid, which inhibits phagocytic killing at the low pH of abscesses. Anaerobic gram-negative bacteria contain LPS, but *Bacteroides* LPS lacks KDO and beta-hydroxymyristic acid and is without toxicity when injected into primates. However, *Fusobacterium* contains a biologically active LPS.

POLYMICROBIAL BACTEREMIA

Polymicrobial bacteremia is the isolation of more than one microorganism from blood culture in a single episode of sepsis. Polymicrobial bacteremia is detected in around 10% of bacteremic patients and in the vast majority of cases is hospital-acquired. Polymicrobial bacteremia most often arises from infections in sites contiguous to body surfaces normally colonized with bacteria, including the gastrointestinal and female genital tracts and the skin. Thus, intraabdominal infections (abscesses, cholangitis), pelvic abscesses, necrotizing fasciitis, decubitus ulcers, and subcutaneous soft tissue infections are common sources for polymicrobial bacteremia. The Enterobacteriaceae, enterococci, and anaerobic bacteria are disproportionately frequent in polymicrobial bacteremia, which reflects intestinal and genital tract colonization with these organisms. Polymicrobial bacteremia is often detected among patients with underlying malignant disease, especially acute leukemia, who have undergone immunosuppressive therapy and invasive procedures. Shock and death directly related to sepsis are more frequent in polymicrobial than in monomicrobial bacteremia.

FUNGEMIA

The presence of fungi in the bloodstream is known as *fungemia*. The incidence of fungemia has been rising in recent years, especially fungemia due to yeast forms. *Candida* species are the most common fungi isolated from blood. Ulceration of the normal gastrointestinal mucosa, usually due to a carcinoma or therapy for malignant disease with cytotoxic drugs, and overgrowth of the gastrointestinal flora with *Candida* after treatment with broad-spectrum antibiotics facilitate invasion of the bloodstream by gut *Candida*. Additionally, disruption of the skin by catheters and wounds predisposes to candidemia. Phagocytic neutrophils and T lymphocytes constitute the major host defense mechanism against invasion by *Candida*. As a consequence, illnesses or treatment modalities that cause neutropenia or loss of T lymphocytes are frequently complicated by candidemia. The clinical presentation of candidemia resembles bacteremia, with fever that can progress to hypotension, metabolic acidosis, and ARDS.

Cryptococcus neoformans is an encapsulated yeast that produces meningitis and fungemia. Appearance of cryptococci in the blood indicates suppression of host T-lymphocyte function, and cryptococcal infection occurs in approximately 10% of AIDS patients. CNS signs in cryptococcal meningitis are highly variable and may be minimal. Consequently, detection of *C. neoformans* in blood culture is often the first sign of cryptococcosis in an AIDS patient.

LABORATORY DIAGNOSIS OF SEPSIS

Most bacteremias and fungemias in adults are of a low order of magnitude, that is, relatively few organisms are present per milliliter of blood. Adult patients septic with Enterobacteriaceae, *Pseudomonas*, *Staphylococcus*, *Streptococcus*, anaerobic bacteria, or yeast are generally culture-positive for 10 or fewer organisms per milliliter of blood, and frequently fewer than 1 organism is detected per milliliter of blood. It is obvious that detection of bacteremia or fungemia requires at least one viable microorganism in the sample of blood cultured. Consequently, a blood sample smaller than 10 mL will miss many bacteremic episodes in adults, and at least 10 mL and preferably 20–30 mL of blood should be obtained for each blood culture. However, in infants and children, the magnitude of bacteremia is usually far greater, so that smaller volumes of blood (1–5 mL) are sufficient.

In addition to low intensity, most bacteremias are intermittent. To increase the probability of detecting bacteremia, two or three blood cultures should be obtained to evaluate each episode of sepsis, and if possible each blood culture should be obtained at 1-h intervals. The diagnosis of bacteremia can be established in 99%

of patients with three separate blood cultures (Fig. 34–7), and therefore in most instances it is not necessary to submit more than three cultures to the clinical microbiology laboratory. However, occasional patients have received antibiotics prior to admission, and concern may arise that the antibiotics might suppress growth of organisms in blood culture. In this setting, it is reasonable to obtain another two blood cultures on each of three successive days, if cultures from the previous days are negative. Three fourths of broth blood cultures are positive the first day of incubation, and 90–95% are positive by the third day (Table 34–3). Thus, it is advisable to obtain the results of previously submitted blood cultures each day before deciding whether additional blood cultures are necessary for antibiotic-treated patients.

Discrimination between Bacteremia and Contamination

The skin is heavily colonized with coagulase-negative staphylococci, *Corynebacterium* species, alpha-hemolytic streptococci, and the lipophilic anaerobic organism *Propionibacter-*

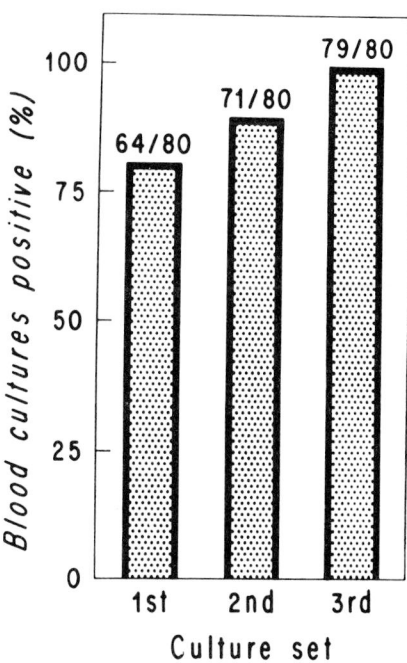

Figure 34–7. Cumulative rates of positivity in three blood culture sets obtained from bacteremic patients. A broth culture system was utilized in this study of 80 patients. The number of positive patients with one, two, and three culture sets is reported at the top of each data bar. (From Washington, J. A., II. Blood cultures: Principles and techniques. Mayo Clin. Proc 50:91, 1975.)

TABLE 34–3. *Recovery Rate of Microorganisms in Blood Culture*

	VA Lakeside Medical Center Chicago, IL	Methodist Medical Center St. Joseph, MO	St. Luke's Hospital Bethlehem, PA
Number of blood cultures	5464	2761	18,130
Length of study	19 months	12 months	39 months
Day 1+	71.4%	79.0%	72.7%
Day 2+	84.7%	89.0%	86.3%
Day 3+	89.8%	95.0%	92.0%

Day 1+, Day 2+, and Day 3+ = cumulative positive blood cultures after 1, 2, and 3 days of incubation, respectively. The radiometric broth culture method was utilized by all three medical centers. (Reproduced with permission of the *American Journal of Clinical Pathology*. From Robinson, P. G., Sulita, M. J., Matthews, E. K., et al: Failure of the Bactec® 460 radiometer to detect *Cryptococcus neoformans* fungemia in an AIDS patient. Am. J. Clin. Pathol. 87:783–786, 1987.)

ium acnes. Despite rigorous aseptic technique in the collection of blood, 2–3% of blood cultures are contaminated with these skin commensals. Because patients can develop true sepsis with these organisms, it is necessary to discriminate true bacteremia from contamination. If only one of multiple blood cultures is positive for coagulase-negative staphylococci, *Corynebacterium*, or alpha-hemolytic streptococci, the isolate is probably a skin contaminant (see Fig. 34–1). However, if the organism is recovered from two or more blood cultures, the isolate is a good candidate as the cause of a septic episode. Thus, not only are multiple blood cultures important for the detection of intermittent bacteremia, but they are needed to document true bacteremia due to gram-positive organisms generally regarded as skin contaminants. Presence of gram-negative bacteria or yeast in a single blood culture almost always indicates true bacteremia or fungemia.

Diagnostic Methods

The laboratory diagnosis of bacteremia and fungemia is accomplished using broth, lysis-concentration, and biphasic culture methods (Table 34–4). The responsibility of the clinical microbiology laboratory is to identify the species of bacteria and fungi responsible for sepsis and to assess the antimicrobial drug susceptibility of bacterial isolates. Direct communication between the clinical microbiology laboratory and the patient's physician is essential, since bacteremia is acute and life-threatening and the physician must have accurate and comprehensive information in order to recommend effective therapy.

Endotoxic LPS induces coagulation of extracts obtained from the pluripotential hematologic cell (amebocyte) of the horseshoe crab, *Limulus polyphemus*. This property forms the basis of the *in vitro Limulus gelation assay* (LGA), which is sensitive to trace quantities (0.1 pg/mL) of LPS. The LGA has found application in the screening of parenteral fluids for absence of LPS contamination and also in the laboratory testing of cerebrospinal fluid for the rapid diagnosis of gram-negative meningitis. Clinical research has revealed that high plasma LPS levels measured by LGA correlate with development of severe septic shock in systemic meningococcal disease. Also, plasma levels of free LPS are elevated after administration of bactericidal antibiotics to patients with gram-

TABLE 34–4. *Blood Culture Methods for the Laboratory Diagnosis of Bacteremia and Fungemia*

Blood Culture Method	Principle
Broth	Culture bottles containing nutrient broth (tryptic or trypticase soy, supplemented peptone, Columbia) are inoculated with blood. Each blood culture consists of at least two culture bottles, one of which is incubated under aerobic conditions and the other under anaerobic conditions. Blood cultures are monitored for bacterial and fungal growth by turbidity, gas, colony formation, hemolysis, and Gram stains of broth smears. Gas production is detected by appearance of bubbles in the broth or infrared measurement of released CO_2.
Lysis-centrifugation	Following lysis of red and white cells in blood, bacteria or fungi present are concentrated into a pellet by centrifugation. The pellet is then inoculated to solid growth media for recovery of microorganisms.
Biphasic	Culture bottles are designed to permit immersion of solid growth media in nutrient broth inoculated with blood by tilting or inverting the bottles. Microorganisms in blood can thus be recovered by growth in broth or on solid media.

negative bacteremia. Often, the clinical condition of such patients worsens despite bactericidal antibiotic therapy, perhaps due to free LPS released by antibiotic-induced bacterial cell lysis. The inflammatory mediators TNF and IL-1 can be detected by immunoassay in the blood of bacteremic patients. Some preliminary data indicate that plasma TNF levels correlate directly with the severity of illness for septic patients. Currently, laboratory measurement of plasma LPS and inflammatory mediators is not generally available, but it holds promise for use in assessment of patient prognosis.

THERAPY OF BACTEREMIA AND FUNGEMIA

Removal of infected catheters or other intravascular devices and drainage of infected tissue are generally necessary for the effective treatment of bloodstream infection. In addition, mortality is substantially reduced by the appropriate use of antimicrobial drugs and of supportive therapy with fluid replacement and vasopressor amines in patients who develop septic shock.

Antibiotic Therapy

Important and complex patterns of antibiotic resistance can develop for different groups of pathogens in the bacteremic patient. The production of beta-lactamase occurs in both gram-negative and gram-positive bacteria, and with gram-negative species can be either plasmid-mediated or chromosome-mediated. Plasmid-mediated beta-lactamase production is prevalent with *Klebsiella pneumoniae* and has recently appeared with *Haemophilus influenzae* and *Escherichia coli*. The plasmid-mediated beta-lactamase degrades the aminopenicillins and when present renders these species resistant to ampicillin and related drugs. Chromosome-mediated beta-lactamase involves spontaneous mutation of gram-negative bacteria to a stable derepressed state for beta-lactamase production. Derepression of the chromosomal beta-lactamase gene results in accumulation of large amounts of beta-lactamase in the periplasmic space (see Fig. 34–4) of bacterial cells. The beta-lactamase has a high affinity for second- and third-generation cephalosporins and extended-spectrum penicillins, and the enzyme renders these drugs inactive by hydrolysis or binding. Under the selective pressure of treatment with cephalosporins or extended-spectrum penicillins, emergence of derepressed, antibiotic-resistant bacteria commonly occurs in patients infected with *Enterobacter, Serratia,* indole-positive *Proteus, Providencia, Pseudomonas aeruginosa,* and *Acinetobacter*. A novel antimicrobial drug has been introduced, imipenem, which is unaffected by the chromosomally mediated beta-lactamase. However, mutants of *Pseudomonas aeruginosa* have recently been identified that are impermeable to imipenem, and hence demonstrate resistance to this drug.

The plasmid-mediated beta-lactamase of *Staphylococcus aureus* is well known. This beta-lactamase rapidly inactivates penicillin, and most episodes of hospital-acquired staphylococcal bacteremias are due to penicillin-resistant organisms. Semisynthetic penicillinase-resistant penicillin (PRP) is available, including methicillin (which is rarely used today), oxacillin, and nafcillin. Unfortunately, however, an altered penicillin-binding protein (PBP 2a) is associated with a low binding affinity for PRP, and the presence of PBP 2a results in PRP resistance. Vancomycin, a cell-wall-active peptidoglycan antibiotic, must be utilized to treat bacteremia due to methicillin (PRP)-resistant staphylococci (MRSA). Although rare, low-affinity penicillin-binding proteins also occur in *Streptococcus pneumoniae* and when present render pneumococci penicillin-resistant. *Corynebacterium* JK, unlike other diphtheroids, is uniformly penicillin-resistant. Vancomycin is indicated for bacteremia due to penicillin-resistant *S. pneumoniae* and *Corynebacterium* JK.

The principal mechanism of aminoglycoside resistance among bacteria is the presence of aminoglycoside-modifying enzymes, which inactivate by acetylation, phosphorylation, or adenylation of the aminoglycosides. Gentamicin continues to be the aminoglycoside of choice for bacteremia due to the Enterobacteriaceae and *Pseudomonas aeruginosa*. However, amikacin may be active against gentamicin-resistant gram-negative organisms and is the aminoglycoside of choice where gentamicin resistance is prevalent. The aminoglycosides are also useful in combined therapy with ampicillin or vancomycin for endocarditis due to *Enterococcus faecalis*. Unfortunately, however, highly aminoglycoside-resistant strains of *E. faecalis* are appearing in increasing numbers and are refractory to synergistic therapy with an aminoglycoside and a beta-lactam drug.

Presumptive (empiric) antimicrobial therapy is frequently provided prior to isolation of the causative microorganism and antibiotic susceptibility testing. Presumptive therapy must include broad-spectrum coverage, and imipenem approaches this ideal, although it lacks activity against MRSA. In hospitals with a high prevalence of MRSA, vancomycin should be included in empiric therapeutic regimens. However, once a causative organism(s) has been detected in blood culture and its antimicrobial susceptibility identified, chemotherapy should be based on the antimicrobial susceptibility patterns of the individual isolates.

The polyene antibiotic, amphotericin B, is the cornerstone of therapy for fungemia. The orally administered fluorinated pyrimidine drug, flucytosine, has an additive effect with amphotericin B for the treatment of cryptococcal meningitis and fungemia. Very recently, clinical evidence has emerged that the antifungal triazole drug, fluconazole, is effective in the long-term therapy of chronic cryptococcal infection.

Therapy of Septic Shock

Perfusion of vital organs, especially the brain and heart, must be maintained in the patient with septic shock. The first goal must be volume replacement with crystalloid solutions, in order to expand intravascular fluid volume. If aggressive volume replacement fails to maintain blood pressure, sympathomimetic amines should be considered, especially dopamine. At low doses dopamine exerts a positive inotropic effect on the myocardium while reducing regional arterial resistance in the kidneys, heart, and brain. The end result is an increase in systolic blood pressure and heart rate and an increased flow of blood to these vital organs. The administration of corticosteroids or anticoagulants is, in general, not indicated. The use of monoclonal antibody to prevent or terminate septic shock is currently under investigation, with encouraging early clinical experience. Human monoclonal IgM antibody reactive with lipid A can protect against lethal gram-negative bacteremia, presumably by binding of the antibody to lipid A. Whether antibody binds to lipid A in the cell wall of intact bacteria, to free endotoxin released upon bacterial cell lysis, or to both is uncertain at the present time. Regardless of exact binding sites, the mechanism of protection by lipid A antibody is probably that of an antitoxin, in which lipid A induction of host toxicity is blocked by antibody binding. Monoclonal antibodies directed against TNF improve survival in bacteremic shock in baboons and neutropenic rats. Therapeutic use of anti-TNF monoclonal antibodies might be particularly important in septic shock caused by gram-positive

bacteremia or fungemia. However, administration of anti-TNF antibody carries the risk of interfering with host-protective properties of this inflammatory mediator. Monoclonal antibodies hold promise in decreasing the mortality associated with septic shock, but more work is needed before they can be introduced into general clinical practice.

CASE HISTORY

The patient was a 65-year-old man who complained of abdominal pain, nausea, and vomiting. The patient had recently been diagnosed as having type II (non–insulin-dependent) diabetes mellitus. Physical examination revealed a temperature of 100.2°F, pulse rate of 86/min, respiration of 20/min, and blood pressure of 132/88 mm Hg. The abdomen was tender to palpation in the epigastric to right upper quadrant, but rebound tenderness or guarding was not evident. On the second hospital day, jaundice became apparent, and abdominal ultrasound revealed gallstones with dilatation of the hepatic ducts and gallbladder. Three sets of blood cultures were positive for *Klebsiella pneumoniae* and *Enterococcus faecalis*. Treatment was begun with intravenous ampicillin-sulbactam and gentamicin, and by the sixth hospital day the patient was afebrile, blood cultures were negative, and antimicrobial chemotherapy was discontinued. The patient underwent a cholecystectomy, and bile and peritoneal cultures obtained at the time of surgery were negative. However, a few days following surgery the patient again became febrile, and developed a neutrophilic leukocytosis with immature band forms. Laboratory evaluation showed elevated serum amylase and lipase levels, and three blood culture sets were positive for *Klebsiella pneumoniae*. Antimicrobial therapy was instituted with ampicillin-sulbactam, but the patient progressed to severe respiratory distress and hypoxemia, and became unresponsive with hypotension. Resuscitation efforts were unsuccessful.

At autopsy, the right ventricular cavity of the heart was filled with coils of an embolus, which extended into the large pulmonary arteries near the hilum of both lungs. Thus, the immediate cause of death in this patient

was acute pulmonary embolism. Microscopic examination of the lung showed marked leukostasis in pulmonary blood vessels and severe intraalveolar edema. Sections through the pancreas revealed a large intrapancreatic abscess in the junction between the head and body, and another abscess cavity immediately adjacent to the pancreatic tail. The peripancreatic fat demonstrated numerous gray to tan plaques of acute enzymic fat necrosis, and eight loculated abscesses were present in the retroperitoneal adipose tissue adjacent to the pancreas. Gram-staining of smears prepared from the pancreatic and peripancreatic abscesses revealed gram-negative rods and many neutrophils, and culture of aspirated pus was positive for *Klebsiella pneumoniae*. Enteric bacteria can reach the pancreas by reflux of contaminated bile, particularly in patients with biliary obstruction. It is likely that reflux of bacteria into the pancreas of this patient occurred secondary to his cholelithiasis, with accompanying development of pancreatic and retroperitoneal abscesses; gram-negative bacteremia was a complication of the abscesses. The presence of leukostasis and edema in the lung suggest early vascular injury due to gram-negative bacteremia.

REFERENCES

Review Articles

Bryan, C. S. Clinical implications of positive blood cultures. *Clin. Microbiol. Rev.* 2:329–353, 1989.

Burman, L. A., Norrby, R., and Trollfors, B. Invasive pneumococcal infections: Incidence, predisposing factors, and prognosis. *Rev. Infect. Dis.* 7:133–142, 1985.

Dinarello, C. A. Cytokines: Interleukin-1 and tumor necrosis factor (cachectin). In: Gallin, J. I., Goldstein, I. M., and Snyderman, R., eds. *Inflammation: Basic Principles and Clinical Correlates*. New York: Raven Press, 1988:195–208.

Murray, B. E. The life and times of the Enterococcus. *Clin. Microbiol. Rev.* 3:46–65, 1990.

Nowotny, A. Review of the molecular requirements of endotoxic actions. *Rev. Infect. Dis.* 9:S503–S511, 1987.

Pfaller, M. A., and Herwaldt, L. A. Laboratory, clinical, and epidemiological aspects of coagulase-negative staphylococci. *Clin. Microbiol. Rev.* 1:281–299, 1988.

Quinn, J. P., Studemeister, A. E., DiVincenzo, C. A., et al. Resistance to imipenem in *Pseudomonas aeruginosa*: Clinical experience and biochemical mechanisms. *Rev. Infect. Dis.* 10:892–898, 1988.

Reuben, A. G., Musher, D. M., Hamill, R. J., et al. Polymicrobial bacteremia: Clinical and microbiologic patterns. *Rev. Infect. Dis.* 11:161–183, 1989.

Rietschel, E. Th., Wollenweber, H.-W., Russa, R., et al. Concepts of the chemical structure of lipid A. *Rev. Infect. Dis.* 6:432–438, 1984.

Sanders, W. E., Jr., and Sanders, C. C. Inducible beta-lactamases: Clinical and epidemiologic implications for use of newer cephalosporins. *Rev. Infect. Dis.* 10:830–847, 1988.

Tracey, K. J., Lowry, S. F., and Cerami, A. Cachectin: A hormone that triggers acute shock and chronic cachexia. *J. Infect. Dis.* 157:413–420, 1988.

Washington, J. A., II, and Ilstrup, D. M. Blood cultures: Issues and controversies. *Rev. Infect. Dis.* 8:792–802, 1986.

Wells, C. L., Maddaus, M. A., and Simmons, R. L. Proposed mechanisms for translocation of intestinal bacteria. *Rev. Infect. Dis.* 10:958–979, 1988.

Young, L. S. Gram-negative sepsis. In: Mandell, G. L., ed. *Principles and Practice of Infectious Diseases*. 3rd ed. New York: Churchill Livingstone, 1990:611–636.

Ziegler, E. J. Protective antibody to endotoxin core: The emperor's new clothes? *J. Infect. Dis.* 158:286–290, 1988.

Original Articles

Beutler, B., Milsark, I. W., and Cerami, A. C. Passive immunization against cachectin/tumor necrosis factor protects mice from lethal effect of endotoxin. *Science* 229:869–871, 1985.

Brandtzaeg, P., Kierulf, P., Gaustad, P., et al. Plasma endotoxin as a predictor of multiple organ failure and death in systemic meningococcal disease. *J. Infect. Dis.* 159:195–204, 1989.

Calandra, T., Baumgartner, J.-D., Grau, G. E., et al. Prognostic values of tumor necrosis factor/cachectin, interleukin-1, interferon-alpha, and interferon-gamma in the serum of patients with septic shock. *J. Infect. Dis.* 161:982–987, 1990.

Cannon, J. G., Tompkins, R. G., Gelfand, J. A., et al. Circulating interleukin-1 and tumor necrosis factor in septic shock and experimental endotoxin fever. *J. Infect. Dis.* 161:79–84, 1990.

Kreger, B. E., Craven, D. E., Carling, P. C., et al. Gram-negative bacteremia. III. Reassessment of etiology, epidemiology and ecology in 612 patients. *Am. J. Med.* 68:332–343, 1980.

Kreger, B. E., Craven, D. E., and McCabe, W. R. Gram-negative bacteremia. IV. Re-evaluation of clinical features and treatment in 612 patients. *Am. J. Med.* 68:344–355, 1980.

McCabe, W. R., and Jackson, G. G. Gram-negative bacteremia. I. Etiology and ecology. II. Clinical, laboratory, and therapeutic observations. *Arch. Intern. Med.* 110:847–864, 1962.

Miller, P. J., and Wenzel, R. P. Etiologic organisms as independent predictors of death and morbidity associated with bloodstream infections. *J. Infect. Dis.* 156:471–477, 1987.

Opal, S. M., Cross, A. S., Kelly, N. M., et al. Efficacy of a monoclonal antibody directed against tumor necrosis factor in protecting neutropenic rats from lethal infection with *Pseudomonas aeruginosa*. *J. Infect. Dis.* 161:1148–1152, 1990.

Riebel, W., Frantz, N., Adelstein, D., et al. *Corynebacterium* JK: A cause of nosocomial device-related infection. *Rev. Infect. Dis.* 8:42–49, 1986.

Salyer, J. L., Bohnsack, J. F., Knape, W. A., et al. Mechanisms of tumor necrosis factor-alpha alteration of PMN adhesion and migration. *Am. J. Path.* 136:831–841, 1990.

Shenep, J. L., Flynn, P. M., Barrett, F. F., et al. Serial

quantitation of endotoxemia and bacteremia during therapy for gram-negative bacterial sepsis. *J. Infect. Dis. 157*:565–568, 1988.

Teng, N. N. H., Kaplan, H. S., Hebert, J. M., et al. Protection against Gram-negative bacteremia and endotoxemia with human monoclonal IgM antibodies. *Proc. Natl. Acad. Sci. U S A 82*:1790–1794, 1985.

Tracey, K. J., Fong, Y., Hesse, D. G., et al. Anti-cachectin/TNF monoclonal antibodies prevent septic shock during lethal bacteraemia. *Nature 330*:662–664, 1987.

Waage, A., Halstensen, A., and Espevik, T. Association between tumor necrosis factor in serum and fatal outcome in patients with meningococcal disease. *Lancet 1*:355–357, 1987.

Weinstein, M. P., Murphy, J. R., Reller, L. B., et al. The clinical significance of positive blood cultures: A comprehensive analysis of 500 episodes of bacteremia and fungemia in adults. II. Clinical observations, with special reference to factors influencing prognosis. *Rev. Infect. Dis. 5*:54–70, 1983.

Weinstein, M. P., Reller, L. B., Murphy, J. R., et al. The clinical significance of positive blood cultures: A comprehensive analysis of 500 episodes of bacteremia and fungemia in adults. I. Laboratory and epidemiologic observations. *Rev. Infect. Dis. 5*:35–53, 1983.

Ziegler, E. J., Fisher, C. J., Jr., Sprung, C. L., et al. Treatment of gram-negative bacteremia and septic shock with HA-1A human monoclonal antibody against endotoxin. *N. Engl. J. Med. 324*:429–436, 1991.

35

STANFORD T. SHULMAN, M.D. • JOHN P. PHAIR, M.D.

Infective Endocarditis

INTRODUCTION

Infective endocarditis (IE), a universally fatal disease before the introduction of antibiotics, represents a major triumph of "modern medicine" and a continuing challenge. Ninety-five percent of cases of endocarditis due to penicillin-susceptible streptococci can be bacteriologically cured. In contrast, management of fungal endocarditis is still inadequate. Other remaining concerns include effective prophylaxis, appropriate timing of surgical intervention, and intravenous drug abuse, a major source of cases of IE in urban centers.

Malignant endocarditis due to infection was not clearly distinguished from endocarditis secondary to rheumatic fever until the early 1900s, even though Sir William Osler had recognized in the 1880s that cocci were sometimes present in the vegetations of endocarditis. By the late 1930s, the potential of antibiotics for cure was beginning to be appreciated. Work since then has delineated the clinical forms, pathogenesis, principles of therapy, and hemodynamic, infectious, and immunologic complications of IE.

CLINICAL DESCRIPTION

Two basic forms of IE are recognized: acute and subacute, and this distinction remains useful clinically (Table 35–1). Many patients present typically, although features of acute and subacute disease may be combined. Thus, patients with valvular infection due to viridans (alpha-hemolytic) streptococci may lack classic features of subacute endocarditis. In contrast, patients infected with *Enterococcus faecalis* are often acutely ill with a fulminant infection that rapidly destroys the infected valve, mimicking acute endocarditis.

Acute Endocarditis

The patient with acute IE usually presents with signs and symptoms of severe fulminant infection (e.g., high fever, rigors, prostration, and significant leukocytosis) without history of chronic illness. Staphylococci are the most frequent etiologic agents. Commonly, there is no evidence of significant preexisting cardiac disease on a rheumatic or congenital basis; the organisms usually associated with acute IE can infect a normal valve. Acute staphylococcal endocarditis is rising in frequency among the elderly, who often have calcific sclerosis of the aortic or mitral valve, and is frequent in patients with prosthetic valves and in intravenous drug abusers.

491

TABLE 35–1. *Clinical–Etiologic Classification of Acute and Subacute Forms of Infective Endocarditis*

Features	Acute Form of Disease	Subacute Form of Disease
Duration of disease	Less than 6 weeks	6 weeks or longer
Cardiovascular status	Normal heart valve or prosthetic valve implant	Rheumatic or congenital heart disease; prosthetic valve implant
Most important causative microorganisms	*Staphylococcus aureus* and *S. epidermidis* *Streptococcus pneumoniae* Lancefield group A beta-hemolytic streptococci (*Streptococcus pyogenes*) *Neisseria gonorrhoeae* *Pseudomonas aeruginosa* *Candida* sp. *Aspergillus* sp.	Viridans (alpha-hemolytic) streptococci Lancefield group D enterococci (*Enterococcus faecalis*) Anaerobic or microaerophilic streptococci
Therapy	Penicillin class drug (plus an aminoglycoside for *P. aeruginosa* infections) Antifungal agents Surgery	Penicillin class drug plus aminoglycoside in combination

Initially, the patient with acute IE may have few signs to indicate a cardiac focus of infection. Murmurs may be absent and attention drawn to other organs, the sites of metastatic infection or immune-mediated vascular disease, that is, *hypersensitivity angiitis*. These organs are typically the central nervous system, joints, long bones, and kidneys. The skin may show evidence of embolic pustules or hemorrhage secondary to an intravascular coagulopathy. Occasionally, Janeway lesions—flat, painless, erythematous areas—are seen on the palms and soles. The typical patient with acute staphylococcal endocarditis is ill for 7 days or less before seeking medical attention. Mitral and aortic valves are most commonly involved, and a murmur is often of recent onset or develops under observation. In the preantibiotic era, acute gonococcal and pneumococcal endocarditis were common but are now only rarely seen. Acute IE due to gram-negative bacilli and fungi is clearly increasing in frequency.

Subacute Endocarditis

In contrast to acute IE, subacute disease presents either as a vague wasting illness, suggesting a malignancy, or as a fever of unknown origin. The patient feels unwell and often has anorexia and weight loss. The duration of the illness is unclear, or the patient may state that an episode of "flu" never completely resolved. A heart murmur, splenomegaly, and petechiae (usually restricted to the conjunctivae, head, neck, and upper thorax) represent typical physical findings. Osler nodes (red painful nodules on the fingertips) and Roth spots (pale lesions on an erythematous base in the retina) are uncommon in subacute IE. Splinter hemorrhages are common. Although a changing murmur is commonly cited as a major finding in IE, it usually occurs if an infected valve perforates or a papillary muscle ruptures. Laboratory evaluation may reveal a normal white cell count or slight leukocytosis, and normochromic normocytic anemia. Microscopic hematuria is frequent.

Culture-Negative Endocarditis

In older series, the frequency of blood culture–negative endocarditis ranged from 10 to 20%. Today, abacteremic endocarditis accounts for about 2%, if patients who received antibiotics prior to culture are excluded. Causes of abacteremic endocarditis include IE due to chlamydia, rickettsiae (Q fever), and certain fungi, notably *Aspergillus*. Occasionally, gram-positive cocci are demonstrated in vegetations at surgery or autopsy despite sterile blood cultures. Fastidious, nutritionally deficient streptococci that require supplementation with specific nutrients such as pyridoxine may account for such cases.

Culture-negative endocarditis should be suspected in any patient with signs of IE and an elevated sedimentation rate. IE is rarely proved in the absence of the latter finding. Established atrial fibrillation and congestive heart failure are uncommon antecedents for IE. Cardiac failure occurring after the onset of IE usually reflects compromised valvular function.

The differential diagnosis of a patient with suspected culture-negative IE includes those illnesses that cause prolonged and perplexing fevers including lymphoproliferative diseases, collagen vascular diseases, recurrent pulmonary emboli, hepatic disease, valvular myxoma, and neoplastic tumors. Following a negative investigation, a trial of antibiotic therapy may be warranted if no alternative diagnosis has been established.

Fungal Endocarditis

In contrast to abacteremic endocarditis, which with improved microbiologic techniques is less common, fungal endocarditis is increasing in frequency. Responsible factors include:

1. Use of central venous and arterial lines for therapy and for monitoring
2. Increasing numbers of immunocompromised patients who survive for extended periods
3. Increasing numbers of patients undergoing valve replacement
4. The rise in intravenous drug abuse

Fungal endocarditis represents a difficult diagnostic and therapeutic dilemma. Organisms such as aspergillus are infrequently isolated from blood cultures, and currently available medical therapy is ineffective. Treatment includes antifungal agents and surgery, but cures are uncommon. Patients with fungal endocarditis usually present with acute IE as described. A characteristic of fungal endocarditis is the presence of large vegetations that commonly embolize and occlude large arteries.

Endocarditis and Drug Abuse

Endocarditis as a result of intravenous drug abuse (IVDA) is increasingly diagnosed in urban centers. Patients may develop acute aortic or mitral valve infection; however, 30–40% of IVDA-associated endocarditis involves the tricuspid valve. Because right-sided endocarditis is otherwise uncommon, tricuspid endocarditis should suggest IVDA. The murmur of tricuspid insufficiency is often inaudible, and infection of this valve should be suspected with fever, sustained bacteremia, and multiple septic pulmonary emboli.

IE most frequently associated with IVDA involves *Staphylococcus aureus, Pseudomonas aeruginosa, Serratia marcescens,* and *Candida* species. These organisms demonstrate geographic variability (e.g., *P. aeruginosa* in Detroit) for unclear reasons. Methicillin-resistant staphylococci are increasingly found in IVDA-associated IE, although staphylococci are not readily cultured from street drugs or apparatus.

Abusers of intravenous drugs have heavy skin carriage of *S. aureus*, and the organisms infecting cardiac valves are of the same phage type as those colonizing the noses, axillae, and groins of these patients.

Prosthetic Valve Endocarditis

Infection of prosthetic cardiac valves is common and carries substantially greater mortality than other forms of IE. Two distinct forms of prosthetic valve endocarditis (PVE) are discernible: early (occurring within 60 days of valve implantation), and late (developing after the 60-day postoperative period). Early PVE must be differentiated from the postpericardiotomy syndrome, an immunologically mediated disease resulting from injury to the pericardium or myocardium. Fever is common to PVE and postpericardiotomy syndrome, and both may occur 2–3 weeks after surgery. Blood cultures are often positive in PVE and not in the latter illness. The postpericardiotomy syndrome commonly presents with signs and symptoms of pericarditis or pleuritis. It is usually self-limited or responds to antiinflammatory agents. If present, embolic events suggest PVE. Arterial lines used in cardiac surgery may be associated with petechiae or splinter hemorrhages.

Other causes of fever in the immediate postoperative period include urinary tract infection, postoperative pneumonia, and phlebitis or arteritis secondary to intravascular monitoring. Sternotomy wound infections are uncommon but can cause diagnostic difficulties.

Six weeks after surgery, fever due to cytomegalovirus mononucleosis transmitted by infected blood can be confused with PVE. This infection lacks many features of mononucleosis due to Epstein-Barr virus, such as pharyngitis and adenopathy, but it is associated with fever, splenomegaly, and occasionally hepatitis. Rarely, retinitis may be noted. Atypical lymphocytosis, which is not present with PVE, is common (see Chapter 10).

Although PVE may be obscured by prophylactic perioperative antibiotics, diagnosis is established by demonstrating sustained bacteremia. Staphylococcal species are the most common isolates. *S. epidermidis* in blood cultures in this clinical setting should not be dismissed as a skin contaminant. Gram-negative bacilli, diphtheroids, and fungi are also causes of early PVE. Late PVE is usually due to staphylococci; *S. aureus* predominates, but *S. epidermidis* still occurs. Organisms associated with acute and subacute IE on natural valves are commonly isolated in the late form of PVE.

Specific signs of PVE include obstruction by a vegetation, which is associated with changing sounds of valve closure and a narrowing pulse pressure if the aortic valve is involved, or valve ring dehiscence, demonstrated by the development of a regurgitant murmur. Finally, evidence of intravascular hemolysis is not uncommon in patients with PVE. Surgical therapy is commonly required (see below).

ETIOLOGY

The majority of cases of IE are due to infection with streptococci or staphylococci. Many other organisms, however, can produce IE. In community hospitals where IVDA is not seen, the classic causative agent of IE (i.e., viridans streptococci) accounts for 70–80% of cases. Viridans streptococci are particularly associated with IE in patients with poor dental hygiene, especially following dental manipulation, and in those with preexisting heart disease. *Enterococcus faecalis* endocarditis most often results from bacteremia due to manipulation of the genitourinary or gastrointestinal tracts. IE due to *Streptococcus bovis*, another group D streptococcal organism, is associated with colonic lesions. The prevalence of this organism in stool of patients with colonic carcinoma is five times greater than in patients without colon lesions.

The association of specific organisms with IE appears to be due to specific bacterial–valvular interaction resembling bacterial adherence (see Chapter 3). Streptococci that convert sucrose to dextran adhere better to the platelet–fibrin mesh produced by blood flow disturbances or endothelial damage, the primary lesion required for the development of IE. Staphylococci readily cause platelet aggregation and consequently also adhere well to this nidus. The most common overall blood culture isolates in modern hospitals, aerobic gram-negative bacilli, cause endocarditis only infrequently and adhere poorly to endothelial cells *in vitro*. Viruses have not been proved to cause IE despite intensive efforts to implicate them as causes of abacteremic endocarditis.

PATHOGENESIS

Infective endocarditis requires bloodstream invasion with an organism capable of colonizing an intravascular site, most commonly a previously damaged valve, a prosthetic valve, or an intracardiac shunt. Bacteremia with mouth organisms occurs following brushing of teeth, chewing hard candy, or dental manipulation. Positive blood cultures may also be found after certain endoscopic procedures or biopsies. These bacteremias are transient, rarely demonstrable 5 min after the procedure, and the inoculum is low. Generally, a sterile platelet–fibrin mesh serves as a nidus for IE to develop, and endothelial disruption predisposes to platelet–fibrin mesh formation. Anaerobic organisms are more uncommon causes of valvular infection, presumably lacking the ability to adhere to the fibrin–platelet mesh.

The importance of the fibrin–platelet mesh as the nidus of intravascular infection was established in Freedman's rabbit model of IE. Microscopic deposition of fibrin and platelets was established with placement of a plastic cannula across a valve, producing endothelial damage. Following catheter removal, intravenous inoculation of organisms, such as *Staphylococcus aureus, Enterococcus faecalis,* or *Streptococcus sanguis,* results in colonization and valvular infection. Earlier studies showed that vegetations occurred in areas of turbulence, which favor fibrin–platelet deposition. Thus, in a child with a ventricular septal defect and a left-to-right shunt, the vegetation occurs at the site where the jet stream hits the right ventricular wall or on the right ventricular side of the septum where maximum turbulence exists.

A unique feature of intravascular infection is that the platelet–fibrin mesh excludes neutrophils, the major host defense against most microorganisms associated with IE. In addition, antibody is not bactericidal for the usual organisms that cause IE. In contrast to streptococci and staphylococci, many gram-negative bacilli are lysed by complement. When *Pseudomonas* species and *Escherichia coli* cause IE, however, they are serum-resistant and produce experimental endocarditis easily in rabbits. Thus, it has been stated that IE is an opportunistic infection occurring in an immunocompromised site. The importance of the platelet–fibrin mesh in the pathogenesis of IE is perhaps best illustrated by the clinical observation that endocarditis is uncommon in thrombocytopenic leukemic patients, although bacteremia with pyogenic organisms occurs frequently in this setting.

PATHOLOGY

The majority of the clinical manifestations of IE are due to valvular infection, valve destruction or dysfunction, arrhythmias resulting from myocardial abscesses, metastatic infection, and embolic phenomena. Valvular destruction and myocardial involvement occur in acute endocarditis and can be fatal despite bacteriologic cure. Metastatic infection is also usually the consequence of infection by organisms causing the acute form of IE. Brain abscess; meningitis; infection of long bones or joints; and hepatic, renal, and splenic abscesses are frequent sequelae of staphylococcal endocarditis.

Mycotic aneurysms are vasculitic lesions resulting from intramural infection arising in the vaso vasorum; they occur in both acute and subacute IE. These aneurysms can result in arterial insufficiency or can rupture.

Embolic phenomena can be trivial, resulting in splinter hemorrhages, or devastating if a large piece of vegetation reaches the central nervous system or a major artery. Emboli occur in both the subacute and acute forms of IE and occasionally occur even after sterilization of the blood. Fungal endocarditis is frequently associated with large and friable vegetations that can occlude major arteries. Although Janeway lesions, Osler nodes, and Roth spots may be immune-mediated, several studies suggest that they result from emboli. Microscopic evaluation and culture sometimes demonstrate the infecting organism in peripheral lesions. The few histologic studies of retinal lesions indicate that they are due to embolic disease rather than to immune vasculitis.

IMMUNOPATHOLOGY

Persistent bacteremia, the hallmark of IE, has a profound impact on the immune system, including marked production of immunoglobulins, which are only partially directed at the infecting organism. Titers of antibody to non–cross-reacting antigens (a polyclonal gammopathy) also rise, rendering a diagnosis of the infecting organism that is based solely on serologic evaluation often inaccurate. Circulating immune complexes also are demonstrable. The components of these circulating complexes have not been well defined and may represent bacterial antigens plus antibody or complement components plus antibody directed against a wide range of endogenous or exogenous antigens.

Glomerulonephritis due to immune complex deposition represents a serious consequence of the immune response to endocardial infection. In untreated patients, uremia accounts for 10% of the deaths due to valvular infection. Anti-

biotic therapy renders IE a reversible cause of renal insufficiency. A second, much less common syndrome associated with circulating immune complexes is a form of thrombotic thrombocytopenic purpura. Thrombocytopenia and intravascular hemolysis are reversible with antibiotic treatment.

Among the well-studied serologic responses in IE is the development of antiglobulins—rheumatoid factors. Antiglobulins develop in about 50% of patients with IE of at least 6 weeks' duration, occur in people with no familial tendency toward collagen vascular disease, are independent of the infecting microorganism, and disappear following cure of IE. The role, if any, of antiglobulins in the clinical picture of IE is not defined. These anti-antibodies are not associated with glomerulonephritis. Antiglobulins bind to the Fc fragment of IgG and can block complement fixation, which could be deleterious to defense against bacterial infection. There is no evidence, however, that antiglobulin-positive patients have a poorer prognosis. Other autoantibodies are frequently noted in IE, including antimyocardial antibodies, but there is no evidence to indicate that they alter cardiac function during or following recovery from IE.

DIAGNOSIS

The diagnosis of IE is established in the appropriate clinical setting by documentation of sustained bacteremia or fungemia. Other laboratory tests may be helpful. The erythrocyte sedimentation rate is usually elevated. Leukocytosis is usually present, and anemia is frequent. Antiglobulins are present in 50% of people with subacute disease, usually with polyclonal hypergammaglobulinemia.

Three blood cultures per day for 2 days in subacute IE, and three cultures over 1–2 h before initiation of therapy in acute IE establish the presence of sustained bacteremia. In proven IE the first culture is positive in 95% of patients; fewer than 5% of patients require more than three cultures for confirmation of the diagnosis.

Bacteremia in endocarditis is continuous, and there is no need to wait for a chill or rising temperature to obtain blood cultures. Skin preparation is important to reducing the risk of contamination of the culture with skin flora. The skin should be cleaned with 70% alcohol and 1–2% iodine or povidone-iodine, which should be allowed to dry. Arterial blood provides no higher yield. Separate venipunctures must be used to document sustained bacteremia.

The echocardiogram is often helpful in the diagnosis and treatment of patients with IE. Unsuspected vegetations can be detected with the two-dimensional sector echocardiogram. In addition, this technique can detect signs of acute left-ventricular strain, such as early closure of the mitral valve, which accompany destruction of the aortic valve. Such findings represent indications for early surgical intervention. Echocardiography can determine the size of a vegetation, and larger vegetations may be associated with more frequent emboli, hemodynamic alterations, and difficulty in achieving bacteriologic cure.

Radionucleotide scanning with gallium has not proved useful in the management of IE. Experimental studies of platelets tagged with indium 111, however, suggest they can be detected in vegetations.

PRINCIPLES OF THERAPY

Rational therapy of IE is predicated on isolation, identification, and determination of antibiotic susceptibility of the infecting microorganism. Cure requires efficient antibiotic therapy and, in selected situations, surgical intervention. The antibiotics chosen must be rapidly bactericidal. With certain infections like those due to enterococci, two antibiotics are used to achieve synergistic killing of the infecting organisms. After the choice of antibiotics, treatment should be monitored closely. Blood cultures should be obtained after 3 and 6 days of therapy to confirm sterilization of the bloodstream. In addition, peak and trough serum should be assayed for bactericidal effect against the infecting organisms (see Chapter 38). Peak serum bactericidal titers should be maintained at 1:16 or greater. It may be difficult with some infections to maintain this titer without producing antibiotic toxicity. To be useful, the serum bactericidal assay must be carefully standardized (see Chapter 38).

One of the more vexing problems of endocarditis therapy relates to the optimal duration of treatment. A number of factors are relevant to the sterilization of a vegetation. First, the organism is a major determinant: highly penicillin-sensitive viridans streptococcal IE can be cured with 2 weeks of penicillin plus streptomycin; in contrast, 6 weeks of ticarcillin plus an aminoglycoside rarely cures aortic valve infection due to *Pseudomonas aeruginosa*. Second, the duration of disease influences results of

therapy. Patients infected with penicillin-susceptible streptococci for less than 2 months are easily cured with 2 weeks of therapy, but IE of longer duration due to the same organism requires 4 weeks of treatment. Finally, prolonged disease results in larger vegetations that contain metabolically inactive organisms deep in the fibrin–platelet mesh. Such organisms divide slowly and are less susceptible to penicillin, thus necessitating prolonged therapy for eradication of bacteria.

Right-sided IE is more easily cured than left-sided endocarditis in humans and in experimental animals. The intravenous drug abuser with staphylococcal tricuspid endocarditis often will not remain in the hospital to complete an optimal course of therapy (4–6 weeks); bacteriologic cure is achieved in most such patients with 3 weeks or less of therapy. In contrast, the presence of an intravascular prothesis necessitates prolonged antibiotics, even for late onset IE. Early prosthetic valve endocarditis often requires surgical replacement in addition to antibiotics.

IE provides one of the clearest examples of the value of antibacterial synergism. *Enterococcus faecalis* is much less susceptible to penicillin than other streptococci, with minimum inhibitory concentrations ranging from 0.8 to 25 μg/mL. In contrast, viridans streptococci are inhibited by 0.02 μg/mL penicillin or less. *Enterococcus faecalis* and the other group D enterococci, *E. faecium* and *E. durans*, also are resistant to cephalosporins and other cell-wall-active agents. Penicillin G or ampicillin alone is not successful in curing IE due to *E. faecalis*. Thus, treatment has required either penicillin G or ampicillin plus an aminoglycoside, for synergy.

The American Heart Association's recommended treatment regimens for streptococcal, enterococcal, and staphylococcal endocarditis are shown in Tables 35–2 through 35–4.

Penicillin-aminoglycoside synergism against enterococci is based on increased uptake of aminoglycoside by the organism in the presence of a cell-wall-active agent (Fig. 35–1). The actual killing of the organisms is due to the action of the aminoglycoside. Not all enterococci are killed synergistically by all penicillin-aminoglycoside combinations. Thus, *E. faecalis* with its high level of resistance to streptomycin (minimal inhibitory concentration or MIC >2000 μg/mL) is killed synergistically only by the combination of penicillin and gentamicin. Because high-level resistance is very common among blood isolates

TABLE 35–2. *Treatment of Streptococcal Infective Endocarditis (Non–Penicillin-Allergic)*

Highly penicillin-sensitive streptococci (MIC <0.1 μg/mL)
Penicillin G, IV 10–20 × 10^6 U/day for 4 weeks
OR
Penicillin G, IV 10–20 × 10^6 U/day for 2 weeks
plus gentamicin, 1.0 mg/kg/dose IM or IV (up to 80 mg) every 8 h for 2 weeks
OR
Penicillin G, IV 10–20 × 10^6 U/day for 4 weeks
plus gentamicin, 1.0 mg/kg/dose IM or IV (up to 80 mg) every 8 h for 2 weeks
Relatively penicillin-resistant streptococci (MIC >0.1 μg/mL, <0.5 μg/mL)
Penicillin G, IV 20 × 10^6 U/day for 4 weeks
plus gentamicin, 1.0 mg/kg/dose IM or IV (up to 80 mg) every 8 h for 2 weeks
Enterococci, or streptococci with penicillin MIC >0.5 μg/mL
Penicillin, IV 20–30 × 10^6 U/day for 4–6 weeks
plus gentamicin, 1.0 mg/kg/dose IM or IV (up to 80 mg) every 8 h for 4–6 weeks
OR
Ampicillin, 12 g/day IV for 4–6 weeks
plus gentamicin 1.0 mg/kg/dose IM or IV (up to 80 mg) every 8 h for 4–6 weeks

Adapted from Bisno, A. L., Dismukes, W. E., Durack, D. T., et al. Antimicrobial treatment of infective endocarditis due to viridans streptococci, enterococci, and staphylococci. *JAMA 261*:1471–1477, 1989.

of *E. faecalis*, penicillin and gentamicin is the treatment of choice unless susceptibility to streptomycin is determined. High-level gentamicin resistance has also been seen recently.

Enhanced killing of viridans streptococci in vegetations in the rabbit model of endocarditis by penicillin plus streptomycin confirms clinical results with this combination. This regimen has allowed shortening of therapy to 2 weeks in specific low-risk cases due to a penicillin-susceptible organism. Similar synergism both *in vitro* and in animal models has been demonstrated for *S. aureus* and *P. aeruginosa*. Clinical results in staphylococcal endocarditis with a beta-lactam antibiotic plus gentamicin, however, are disappointing. Treatment of pseudomonas endocarditis requires the combination of carbenicillin or ticarcillin plus an aminoglycoside.

One unresolved issue is the problem of tolerance of *S. aureus*. Tolerant staphylococci are inhibited by the usual concentrations of beta-lactam antibiotics, but require at least 32 times higher concentrations for killing. Although tolerant staphylococci have been isolated from blood of patients with IE, the clinical relevance of this phenomenon is not clear. The disparity between inhibitory and bactericidal concentrations is affected by a number of methodologic variables, and bacteriologic cure of rabbits infected with tolerant organisms is achieved with usual therapy. However, in patients with persistent bacteremia with tolerant staphylococci, combination of a penicillin and an aminoglycoside or rifampin is advocated.

Since the 1970s, surgery has become an extremely important therapeutic modality for IE. If necessary, an infected valve can be replaced safely before the vegetation is sterilized by antibiotic therapy. Indications for surgical intervention include failure to clear the bloodstream of the infecting microorganism with antibiotics. This frequently occurs with infection due to *Pseudomonas* species, fungi, or aerobic gram-negative bacilli when a large vegetation is

TABLE 35–3. *Treatment of Streptococcal Infective Endocarditis (Penicillin-Allergic)*

Highly penicillin-sensitive streptococci (MIC <0.1 μg/mL)
Cephalothin, 2 g IV every 4 h for 4 weeks
or cefazolin, 1 g IM or IV every 8 h for 4 weeks
OR
Vancomycin, 30 mg/kg/day IV in two or four divided doses (up to 2 g/day) for 4 weeks
Relatively penicillin-resistant streptococci (MIC >0.1 μg/mL, <0.5 μg/mL)
Cephalothin, 2 g IV every 4 h for 4 weeks
plus gentamicin, 1.0 mg/kg/dose IM or IV (up to 80 mg) every 8 h for 2 weeks
OR
Vancomycin, 30 mg/kg/day IV in two or four divided doses (up to 2 g/day) for 4 weeks
plus gentamicin, 1.0 mg/kg/dose IM or IV (up to 80 mg) every 8 h for 2 weeks
Enterococci, or streptococci with penicillin MIC >0.5 μg/mL
Vancomycin, 30 mg/kg/day IV in two or four divided doses (up to 2 g/day) for 4–6 weeks
plus gentamicin, 1.0 mg/kg/dose IM or IV (up to 80 mg) every 8 h for 4–6 weeks

Adapted from Bisno, A. L., Dismukes, W. E., Durack, D. T., et al. Antimicrobial treatment of infective endocarditis due to viridans streptococci, enterococci, and staphylococci. *JAMA 261*:1471–1477, 1989.

TABLE 35–4. *Treatment of Staphylococcal Infective Endocarditis*

Methicillin-susceptible staphylococci in absence of prosthetic valve or material
  Nafcillin or oxacillin, 2 g IV every 4 h for 4–6 weeks
    with or without gentamicin, 1.0 mg/kg IV (up to 80 mg) every 8 h for 5 days
      OR (for penicillin-allergic patients)
  Cefazolin or cephalothin, 2 g IV every 4 h for 4–6 weeks
    with or without gentamicin, 1.0 mg/kg IV (up to 80 mg) every 8 h for 5 days
      OR (for penicillin-allergic patients)
  Vancomycin, 30 mg/kg/day IV in two or four divided doses (up to 2 g/day) for 4–6 weeks
Methicillin-resistant staphylococci in absence of prosthetic valve or material
  Vancomycin, 30 mg/kg/day IV in two or four divided doses (up to 2 g/day) for 4–6 weeks
Methicillin-susceptible staphylococci in presence of prosthetic valve or material
  Nafcillin or oxacillin, 2 g IV every 4 h for 6–8 weeks
    plus rifampin, 300 mg every 8 h postoperatively for 6–8 weeks
    plus gentamicin, 1.0 mg/kg IV (up to 80 mg) every 8 h for 2 weeks
      OR (for penicillin-allergic patients)
  Vancomycin, 30 mg/kg/day IV in two or four divided doses (up to 2 g/day) for 6–8 weeks
    plus rifampin, 300 mg postoperatively for 6–8 weeks
    plus gentamicin, 1.0 mg/kg IV (up to 80 mg) every 8 h for 2 weeks
Methicillin-resistant staphylococci in presence of prosthetic valve or material
  Vancomycin, 30 mg/kg/day IV in two or four divided doses (up to 2 g/day) for 6–8 weeks
    plus rifampin, 320 mg postoperatively for 6–8 weeks
    plus gentamicin, 1.0 mg/kg IV (up to 80 mg) every 8 h for 2 weeks

Adapted from Bisno, A. L., Dismukes, W. E., Durack, D. T., et al. Antimicrobial treatment of infective endocarditis due to viridans streptococci, enterococci, and staphylococci. *JAMA* 261:1471–1477, 1989.

present, and in some cases of staphylococcal endocarditis. Another indication for valve replacement is destruction of the valve with resultant congestive heart failure. PVE occurring within 2 months of placement of the valve usually requires reoperation for bacteriologic cure. Dysfunction of a prosthetic valve, loosening of the ring, or obstruction of blood flow is an indication for surgical replacement. Embolization is the last major indication for surgical intervention because emboli remain major causes of morbidity and mortality since the introduction of effective antimicrobial therapy. Emboli to the brain, coronary arteries, the eye,

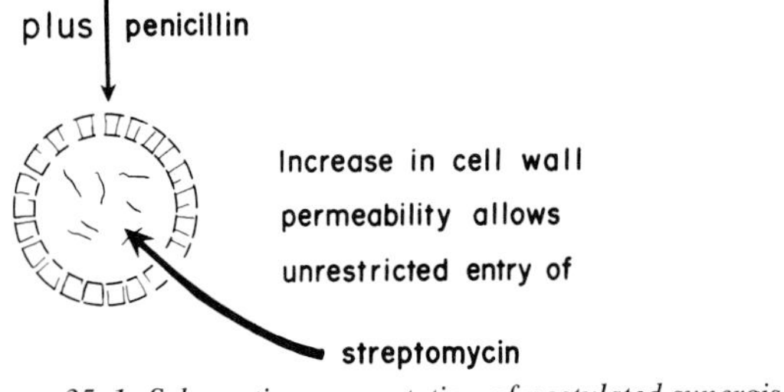

and the kidney can result in long-term disability or in death. A second major embolic event is a clear indication for the removal of the vegetation or replacement of the valve, but controversy continues as to whether a single major embolus or demonstration of large vegetation by echocardiography represents an indication for surgery.

Finally, it is imperative to monitor patients after completion of antibiotic therapy. The majority of relapses occur during the first 3 months of convalescence. Blood cultures may become positive prior to significant constitutional signs or symptoms. Therefore, a patient should be seen at least monthly for 3 months, at 6 months, and at 1 year following therapy. Occasionally, emboli occur after completion of antibiotic treatment. This does not necessarily indicate a bacteriologic relapse but requires thorough evaluation including blood cultures to ensure that infection has not recurred.

One of the major problems encountered in designing antibiotic therapy for IE is penicillin allergy. Penicillin G or a semisynthetic analog is the mainstay of treatment of most forms of endocarditis. Cephalosporins are adequate substitutes for penicillin for viridans streptococcal and staphylococcal but not for enterococcal endocarditis. Vancomycin can be substituted for penicillin in cases of endocarditis due to these three organisms. With endocarditis due to *Pseudomonas* species, ceftazidime and an aminoglycoside is probably adequate, but desensitization and treatment with either ticarcillin or pipera-

Bactericidal action of streptomycin requires

a) passage through restrictive bacterial cell wall

b) binding to 30S or 50S ribosomal subunits

plus | penicillin

Increase in cell wall permeability allows unrestricted entry of

streptomycin

Figure 35–1. Schematic representation of postulated synergistic bactericidal activity of penicillin plus streptomycin for enterococci.

cillin plus an aminoglycoside should be considered.

PROGNOSIS AND COMPLICATIONS

The prognosis of endocarditis patients infected with viridans streptococci is generally good except in the presence of valve destruction or perforation. Major complications include cerebral emboli and relapse. The latter event is most common in patients who have a prolonged illness, and retreatment usually results in cure. Infection with enterococci is associated with a higher frequency of relapse. With relapse, enterococcal susceptibility to the combinations of penicillin plus the various aminoglycosides should be investigated. The results of therapy of staphylococcal IE in patients who are not intravenous drug abusers are generally poor. The majority of nonaddicted patients are older, with a high rate of failure of medical therapy, sometimes associated with significant metastatic infection, such as meningitis.

Death during treatment is most common in patients with high fever that persists for more than 7 days into therapy and who have CNS involvement, gross hematuria, and marked leukocytosis. The long-term prognosis among survivors of such infection is poorer than that of the general population, with increased mortality due to heart failure related to the degree of valvular damage consequent to IE. Thus, cardiovascular surgery should be strongly considered with the development of congestive failure due to valvular incompetence. Another long-term complication is the development of reinfection, with a 5–10% reinfection rate in patients recovered from one episode of IE. The majority of these recurrences are due to penicillin-susceptible streptococci and require no more intensive therapy than did the initial infection.

PROPHYLAXIS

Attempts to prevent IE represent one of the most traditional forms of antibiotic prophylaxis. Principles of prophylaxis are based on recognition of the common causes of bacteremia and the identification of patients at risk (e.g., those with rheumatic valve disease, congenital heart disease, mitral valve prolapse with regurgitation, or prosthetic valves). Antibiotics should be administered to achieve adequate blood and tissue levels before, during, and for 8 h after the potential bacteremic episode. There are no controlled studies to prove that antibiotics prevent infection on a damaged valve, and a number of failures of prophylaxis have been reported. Despite these limitations, attempts to prevent this potentially fatal illness are justified. The American Heart Association periodically publishes guidelines for use of prophylactic antibiotics that should be followed (Table 35–5). Rheumatic fever patients receiving long-term oral penicillin to prevent recurrences harbor penicillin-resistant organisms in the oropharynx, and therefore endocarditis prophylaxis must be designed to deal with this problem. Monthly injections of benzathine penicillin for rheumatic prophylaxis obviate this problem, in that resistant mouth organisms are less common in patients receiving this form of penicillin.

CASE HISTORY 1

A 10-year-old boy with surgically corrected tetralogy of Fallot was admitted to the hospital with a 12-day history of fever and loss of appetite. Examination in his physician's office failed to document the cause of fever. At admission, the temperature was 38°C, the pulse 120/min, respirations normal, and blood pressure 120/80mm Hg. Examination revealed a murmur that was unchanged from previous examinations, splenomegaly, and petechiae over the thorax. The white blood cell count was 11,500/mm³ with 70% polymorphonuclear neutrophils and 20% band forms. The hemoglobin was 11 g/dL. The urine contained four to six erythrocytes per high-power field. Six blood cultures grew viridans streptococci after 24 h of incubation. The concentration of penicillin required to inhibit growth was 0.01 μg/mL. Therapy was begun with penicillin at 9.0 × 10⁶ U/day and gentamicin 80 mg every 8 h. The patient was afebrile within 36 h, his appetite returned, and he stated that he had not realized he had been feeling so poorly before coming to the hospital. The peak-and-trough serum bactericidal assay revealed killing of the infecting organism at titers of 1:512 and 1:256, respectively. Therapy was continued for 2 weeks. The patient was discharged and was well 1 year later. Close questioning during hospitalization revealed that the patient had been to the dentist for oral hygiene 1 week before the onset of the febrile illness, but no

TABLE 35–5. *Prevention of Infective Endocarditis*

Standard regimen for dental, oral, or upper respiratory tract procedures in patients at risk
  Amoxicillin, 3 g orally 1 h before procedure, then 1.5 g 6 h later
  For amoxicillin- or penicillin-allergic patients
    erythromycin ethylsuccinate, 800 mg or stearate 1 g orally 2 h before procedure, then ½ dose 6 h later
                              OR
  clindamycin, 300 mg orally 1 h before procedure, 150 mg 6 h later
Alternative regimens for dental, oral, or upper respiratory tract procedures
  For patients unable to take oral medications
    ampicillin, 2 g IV or IM, 30 min before procedure, then ampicillin, 1 g IV or IM, or amoxicillin, 1.5 g orally 6 h later
    For ampicillin- or penicillin-allergic patients: Clindamycin, 300 mg/IV 30 min before procedure and 150 mg IV or
      postoperatively 6 h later
  For patients considered at very high risk
    ampicillin, 2 g IV or IM *plus* gentamicin 1.5 mg/kg IV or IM (maximum = 80 mg) 30 min before procedure, then
      amoxicillin 1.5 g orally 6 h later *or* repeat parenteral drugs
    For ampicillin- or penicillin-allergic patients: Vancomycin, 1 g IV over 1 h starting 1 h before procedure
Regimens for genitourinary or gastrointestinal procedures
  Standard regimens:
    ampicillin, 2 g IV or IM, 30 min before procedure, then ampicillin, 1 g IV or IM, or amoxicillin, 1.5 g orally 6 h later
    For ampicillin- or penicillin-allergic patients: Vancomycin, 1 g IV over 1 h *plus* gentamicin 1.5 mg/kg IV or IM
      (maximum = 80 mg) 1 h before procedure. May be repeated once 8 h later.
Alternative oral regimen for low-risk patients
  Amoxicillin, 3 g postoperatively 1 h before procedure, then 1.5 g 6 h later
    Pediatric Initial Doses
    (not to exceed adult doses)

Amoxicillin or Ampicillin:	50 mg/kg
Erythromycin:	20 mg/kg
Clindamycin:	10 mg/kg
Gentamicin:	2.0 mg/kg
Vancomycin:	20 mg/kg

Adapted from Dajani, A. S., Bisno, A. L., Chung, K. J., Shulman, S. T., et al. Prevention of bacterial endocarditis. *JAMA 264*:2919–2922, 1990.

antibiotic prophylaxis had been administered. The patient's mother was informed that prophylaxis would be necessary for future dental treatments.

CASE HISTORY 2

A 65-year-old woman was admitted with a 2-day history of chills and fever. When she became confused and developed widespread bruising, she was brought to the emergency room. Purpura fulminans probably due to meningococcemia was suspected. Lumbar puncture revealed cloudy spinal fluid; the Gram's stain was nondiagnostic. Penicillin was begun, 2.0×10^6 U every 2 h. There was no improvement during the initial 24 h of hospitalization. The laboratory reported that all three blood cultures and the cerebrospinal fluid were growing *Staphylococcus aureus*.

Intravenous oxacillin (3 g every 6 h) and gentamicin (80 g every 8 h) were substituted for penicillin. Coagulation studies revealed prolonged prothrombin time, partial thromboplastin time, increased fibrin split products, and low fibrinogen. The white blood cell count was 20,000/mm³ with 50%

neutrophils, and 40% band forms. The platelet count was 80,000/mm³. The patient gradually awakened. An apical systolic murmur with radiation to the axilla was first noted on the third hospital day. Coagulation studies returned to normal. Serum bactericidal titers were 1:32, peak, and 1:16, trough. After the first week, gentamicin was discontinued. Oxacillin was continued for a total of 42 days. The patient's recovery was uneventful.

CASE HISTORY 3

A 24-year-old man attending a methadone clinic was admitted to an outside hospital with fever. No cause of the fever was ascertained upon admission, but six blood cultures grew *Pseudomonas aeruginosa*. Pseudomonas endocarditis was diagnosed, and ticarcillin and tobramycin begun. A diastolic blowing murmur was heard along the left side of the sternum on the second hospital day. Despite serum bactericidal titers of 1:8 or greater throughout a 6-week course of therapy, blood cultures remained positive. The patient was transferred to another hospital for valve replacement. On admission to the second hospital, the patient had a low-grade fever, leukocytosis, anemia, an aortic regurgitant murmur, and splenomegaly. Blood cultures were positive, and the aortic valve was replaced with a porcine prosthesis. Following surgery, blood cultures became sterile. Ticarcillin and tobramycin were continued for 1 month. Following discharge the patient was afebrile for 2 weeks, but fever recurred, and he was readmitted. Blood cultures grew *Pseudomonas aeruginosa* with the same antibiotic susceptibilities as the original isolate. Following reinstitution of antibiotics, the patient had a grand mal seizure, became comatose, and died. Postmortem examination revealed a ruptured intracerebral mycotic aneurysm. Culture of the prosthesis grew *Pseudomonas aeruginosa*.

REFERENCES

Books

Bisno, A. L., ed. *Treatment of Infective Endocarditis.* New York: Grune & Stratton, 1981.

Freedman, L. R. *Infective Endocarditis and Other Intravascular Infections.* New York: Plenum, 1982.

Kaplan, E. L., and Taranta, A. V., eds. *Infective Endocarditis.* American Heart Association. Monograph No. 52, American Heart Association, 1977.

Sande, M. A., Kaye, D., and Root, R. K., eds. *Endocarditis: Contemporary Issues in Infectious Diseases Series.* Vol. 2. New York: Churchill Livingstone Inc. 1984.

Original Articles

Beeson, P. B., Brannon, E. S., and Warren, J. V. Observations on the sites of removal of bacteria from the blood in patients with bacterial endocarditis. *J. Exp. Med. 81*:9–23, 1945.

Bisno, A. L., Dismukes, W. E., Durack, D. T., et al. Antimicrobial treatment of infective endocarditis due to viridans streptococci, enterococci, and staphylococci. *JAMA 261*:1471–1477, 1989.

Dajani, A. S., Bisno, A. L., Chung, K. J., et al. Prevention of bacterial endocarditis. *JAMA 264*:2919–2933, 1990.

Gutman, R. A., Striker, G. E., Gilliland, B. C., et al. The immune complex glomerulonephritis of bacterial endocarditis. *Medicine 51*:1–25, 1972.

Kauffmann, R. H., Thompson, J. Valentijn, R. M., et al. The clinical implications and pathogenetic significance of circulating immune complexes in infective endocarditis. *Am. J. Med. 71*:17–25, 1981.

Klein, R. S., Recco, R. A. Cotalona, M. T., et al. Association of *Streptococcus bovis* with carcinoma of the colon. *N. Engl. J. Med. 297*:800–802, 1977.

Okell, C. C., and Elliott, S. D. Bacteremia and oral sepsis with special reference to the etiology of subacute endocarditis. *Lancet 2*:869–872, 1935.

Osler, W. The Gulstonian lectures on malignant endocarditis. *Br. Med. J. 7*:467, 1885.

Reid, C. L., Chandraratna P. A. N., Rahimtoola, S. H. Infective endocarditis: Improved diagnosis and treatment. *Curr. Probl. Cardiol. 10*:1–10, 1985.

Scheld, W. M., Zak, O., Vasbeck, K., et al. Bacterial adhesion in the pathogenesis of infective endocarditis. Effect of subinhibitory antibiotic concentration on streptococcal adhesion *in vitro* and the development of endocarditis in rabbits. *J. Clin. Invest. 68*:1381–1384, 1981.

Wilson, W. R., Wilkowske, C. J., Wright, A. J., et al. Treatment of streptomycin-susceptible and streptomycin-resistant enterococcal endocarditis. *Ann. Intern. Med. 100*:816–823, 1984.

Staphylococci, Staphylococcal Disease, and Toxic Shock Syndrome

INTRODUCTION

Staphylococci are very important bacterial causes of human disease. They normally inhabit the human upper respiratory tract, skin, intestinal tract, and vagina and are particularly likely to produce infection when host resistance is lowered, such as by an antecedent viral infection or a foreign body. These microorganisms are remarkable for the production of many exotoxins and other extracellular substances. Precisely how these extracellular products are involved in disease production remains somewhat obscure.

CLASSIFICATION

Staphylococci are nonflagellate, nonmotile, gram-positive, catalase-positive cocci, approximately 0.5–1.5 μm in diameter. Cells divide in more than one plane and as a result form irregular masses resembling clusters of grapes.

Only 3 of the 12 species in the genus *Staphylococcus* that colonize humans are of major medical importance. These are conveniently divided into coagulase-positive *(S. aureus)* and coagulase-negative (all others, including *S. epidermidis* and *S. saprophyticus*) staphylococci (Table 36–1), which differ very substantially in their disease-producing capacity. *S. aureus* is highly pathogenic, producing serious infections in previously healthy individuals, whereas coagulase-negative species generally produce infection in those whose host defenses are compromised or in those with an implanted foreign body.

GROWTH

Staphylococci are aerobes and facultative anaerobes that grow well on ordinary media. Colonies are fairly large, smooth, and glistening after 24–48 h of incubation on agar plates. *S. aureus* colonies are usually pigmented, from a light yellow to a deep orange or lemon yellow color, resulting from carotenoid pigments elaborated by the microorganism. *Aureus* means "gold" in Greek. Colonies of coagulase-negative staphylococci are white, lacking carotenoid pigments. Because *S. aureus* produces hemolysins, colonies are usually surrounded by a variable zone of beta hemolysis on blood agar. Colonies of staphylococci on blood agar plates are much larger than those of *Streptococcus, Neisseria,* or *Haemophilus* species and are easily recognized.

Staphylococcal cells grow over a wide range of temperatures, from 5° to 46°C, with the optimum temperature for growth between 30°

TABLE 36–1. *Differential Characteristics of Species of Staphylococci*

Characteristic	S. aureus	Coagulase-negative Staphylococci
Coagulase	+	−
Mannitol		
Acid aerobically	+	+ or −
Acid anaerobically	+	−
Alpha toxin	+	−
Heat-resistant endonucleases	+	−
Biotin for growth	−	+
Cell wall		
Ribitol	+	−
Glycerol	−	+
Protein A	+	−
Salt resistance	+	−

+ : 90% or more strains positive.
− : 90% or more strains negative.

and 37°C. Two other growth characteristics are of importance. Most strains of *S. aureus*, but not coagulase-negative staphylococci, grow in high concentrations of sodium chloride (10–15%) and are resistant to the action of bile salts, since they grow well in up to 40% bile.

HABITAT

Because *S. aureus* and coagulase-negative staphylococci are members of the indigenous microbial flora of humans (see Chapter 2), many persons are asymptomatic carriers of staphylococci and thus may serve as a source of infection for themselves as well as for others. This situation is analogous to that for infections with *S. pyogenes, S. pneumoniae, H. influenzae,* and *N. meningitidis.* Epidemics of staphylococcal disease may occur, especially with so-called epidemic types of *S. aureus* in hospitals or other institutions. Generally, staphylococcal disease occurs sporadically in the community, since it is usually a disease of carriers.

In contrast to the microorganisms mentioned above, which colonize primarily the upper respiratory tract, staphylococci are also found in other regions of the body. Skin is frequently inhabited, and staphylococci are commonly found in the umbilicus, axilla, perineum, face, hands, hair, and vagina.

In the upper respiratory tract, staphylococci colonize the oropharynx and nasopharynx, but they occur in greatest numbers in the anterior nares. Colonization of the anterior nares by *S. aureus* provides a convenient source for colonization of the skin.

It is estimated that 20–75% of all persons at any given time harbor *S. aureus* in or on one of the sites referred to above. Hospital employees demonstrate rates at the higher end of this range. Asymptomatic staphylococcal carriers can be divided into several types: *persistent carriers,* who harbor a specific strain of *S. aureus* for prolonged periods; *occasional carriers,* who sporadically harbor pathogenic staphylococci; and *intermittent,* or *transient, carriers,* who harbor one staphylococcal type for a period and then a different type.

When outbreaks of *S. aureus* infections occur, it is essential to identify the responsible strain in order to characterize those who have been infected or colonized by that strain. Determination of the antibiogram (pattern of antibiotic resistance) and phage typing are important epidemiologic tools. Phage typing assesses the pattern of susceptibility of a strain of *S. aureus* to lysis by an international set of more than 20 bacteriophages after overnight incubation.

DISSEMINATION

Figure 36–1 indicates the epidemiologic cycle of staphylococci in the hospital and in the community. Staphylococci harbored by either asymptomatic carriers or by a person with an infection can be disseminated in a number of ways to others or to the environment. Staphylococci may be expelled from the upper respiratory tract during sneezing. Inanimate objects and even the dust on the floors and walls of rooms may be contaminated in this manner and then may serve as sources of spread to others. Staphylococci can also be transmitted to others by the hands of an asymptomatic carrier. Hands are readily contaminated by staphylococci that have colonized the anterior nares, and *S. aureus,* therefore, can be transmitted directly to others. Hospital personnel are particularly apt to spread staphylococci in this manner. The asymptomatic carrier can also transmit staphylococci to his or her own skin and clothing by sneezing or by contaminated hands.

A number of studies have examined the spread of strains of *S. aureus* in neonatal nurseries. The upper respiratory tract and skin of newborns become colonized with staphylococci within a few hours after birth. Impetigo, conjunctivitis, omphalitis (infection of the umbilical stump), and even pneumonia or septicemia may develop. The staphylococcal strain may originate from another colonized infant in the nursery or from carriers among the nurses or other

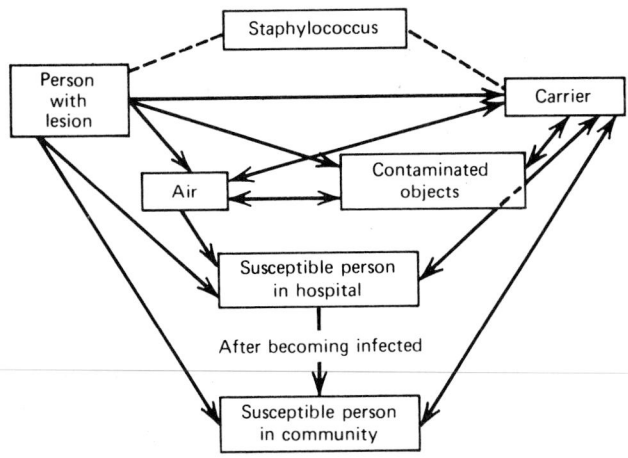

Figure 36–1. Epidemiologic cycle of staphylococci in the hospital and in the community. (From Nahmias, A. J., and Schulman, J. A. Epidemiologic aspects and control methods. In: Cohen, J. O., ed. The Staphylococci. New York: John Wiley & Sons, 1972.)

hospital personnel. The major mode of transmission to the newborn is by the hands of health professionals who handle the infants. Fomites such as diapers, undershirts, sheets, and blankets, if heavily contaminated with staphylococci, may also serve as vectors.

Staphylococcal disease occurs more frequently in patients in hospitals (nosocomially) than in individuals in the nonhospital population. The major reason for this higher incidence is that staphylococcal infection occurs more commonly in persons with lowered host resistance. Asymptomatic carriers of pathogenic staphylococci only rarely develop staphylococcal disease while their resistance to this microorganism is high; however, if there is a reduction in host resistance, resident staphylococci may cause infection. Table 36–2 lists factors known to predispose to disease by *S. aureus*, readily explaining why *S. aureus* infections are more common in hospital patients.

PATHOGENESIS

Staphylococci may produce disease in almost every organ and tissue. The skin is particularly prone to infection, and staphylococcal skin infections are probably among the most common of infectious diseases. For example, over 1.5 million cases of furunculosis occur in the United States each year. The spread of staphylococcal infection and the major organs and tissues in which infections occur are shown in Figure 36–2. This figure demonstrates that *S. aureus* infections may spread by direct extension to contiguous tissues or by way of lymphatics and then blood. Metastatic infections are produced in a wide variety of tissues.

The disease process is initially localized with

an acute inflammatory response and an accumulation of enormous numbers of segmented neutrophils. Lesions tend to be walled off, owing to the deposition of fibrin. Subsequently, central necrosis appears, and an abscess is formed. Thus, staphylococcal infections are characterized by abscess formation. Dissemination as outlined in Figure 36–2 may occur from an initial abscess, appearing most often in compromised hosts.

The enormous influence of foreign bodies on susceptibility to staphylococcal infection was dramatically shown by Elek and Conan. These investigators found that it was necessary to inject 5×10^6 viable *S. aureus* into the skin of human volunteers in order to produce infection. However, as few as 100 viable *S. aureus* were

TABLE 36–2. *Factors Predisposing to Staphylococcus aureus Infection**

Injury to normal skin, e.g., traumatic abrasions and wounds, surgical incisions, burns, primary skin diseases
Prior viral infections, e.g., influenza, measles
Leukocyte defects
  Decreased numbers of leukocytes, e.g., congenital or acquired leukopenia, immunosuppressive drugs
  Defects in chemotaxis
  Defects in phagocytosis or facilitation of this process by serum opsonins or other serum factors
  Defects in intracellular killing, e.g., chronic granulomatous disease
Deficiencies in humoral immunity
Presence of foreign bodies, e.g., intravenous catheters, sutures, prosthetic cardiac valves, tampons
Prior prophylactic or therapeutic use of antibiotics to which the infecting *S. aureus* is not susceptible
Miscellaneous illnesses with less well understood defects in host resistance, e.g., diabetes mellitus, alcoholism, cystic fibrosis, coronary artery disease, various malignant tumors, uremia

*From Schulman, J. A., and Nahmias, A. J. Staphylococcal infections: Clinical aspects. In: Cohen, J. O., ed. *The Staphylococcus.* New York: John Wiley & Sons, 1972.

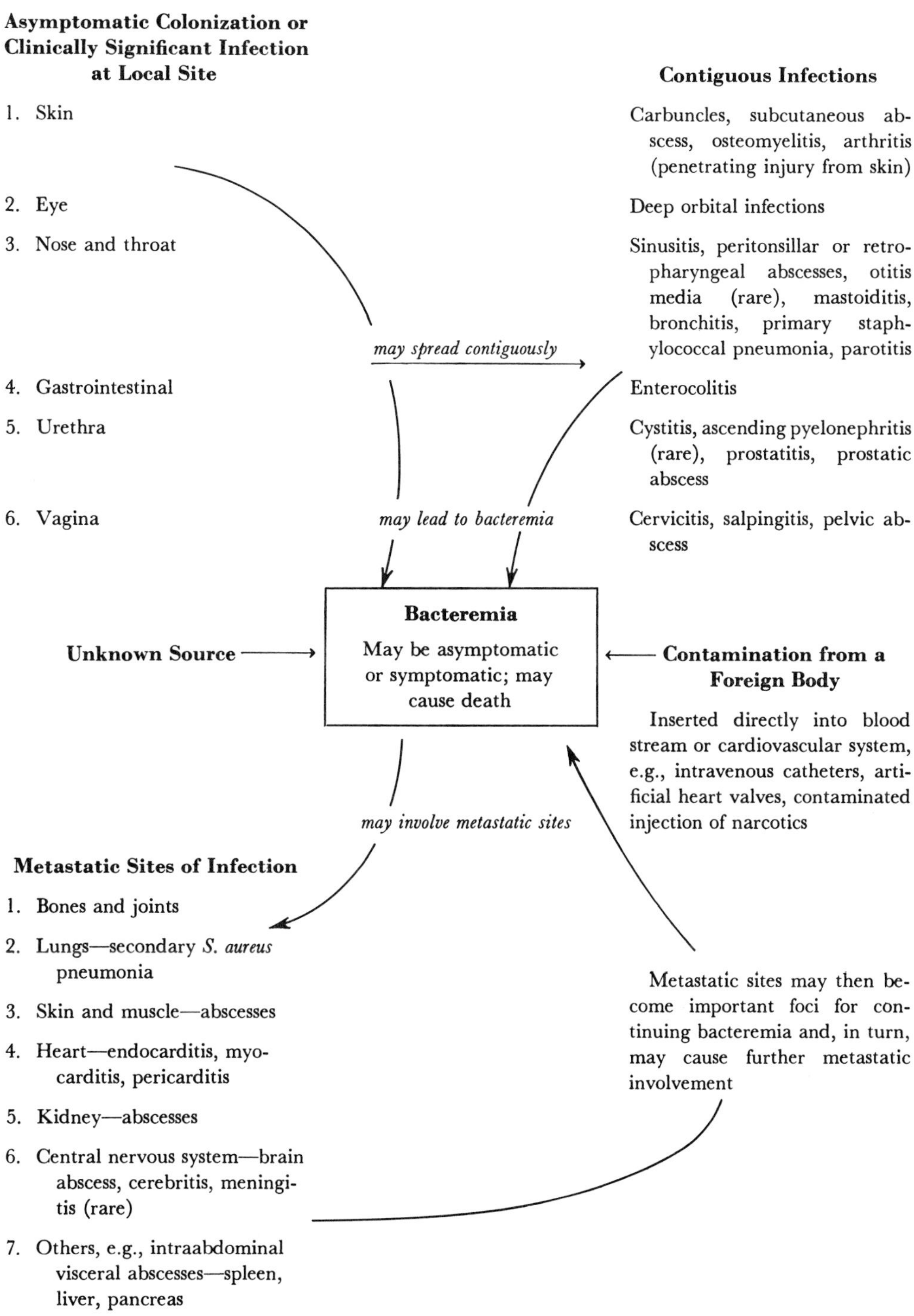

**Asymptomatic Colonization or
Clinically Significant Infection
at Local Site**

                                    Contiguous Infections

1. Skin

Carbuncles, subcutaneous abscess, osteomyelitis, arthritis (penetrating injury from skin)

2. Eye

Deep orbital infections

3. Nose and throat

Sinusitis, peritonsillar or retropharyngeal abscesses, otitis media (rare), mastoiditis, bronchitis, primary staphylococcal pneumonia, parotitis

may spread contiguously

4. Gastrointestinal

Enterocolitis

5. Urethra

Cystitis, ascending pyelonephritis (rare), prostatitis, prostatic abscess

6. Vagina

may lead to bacteremia

Cervicitis, salpingitis, pelvic abscess

Bacteremia

May be asymptomatic or symptomatic; may cause death

Unknown Source ———→

←—— **Contamination from a Foreign Body**

Inserted directly into blood stream or cardiovascular system, e.g., intravenous catheters, artificial heart valves, contaminated injection of narcotics

may involve metastatic sites

Metastatic Sites of Infection

1. Bones and joints

2. Lungs—secondary *S. aureus* pneumonia

Metastatic sites may then become important foci for continuing bacteremia and, in turn, may cause further metastatic involvement

3. Skin and muscle—abscesses

4. Heart—endocarditis, myocarditis, pericarditis

5. Kidney—abscesses

6. Central nervous system—brain abscess, cerebritis, meningitis (rare)

7. Others, e.g., intraabdominal visceral abscesses—spleen, liver, pancreas

Figure 36–2. Pathogenic sequence of Staphylococcus aureus *infection. (From Schulman, J. A., and Nahmias, A. J. Staphylococcal infections: Clinical aspects. In: Cohen, J. O., ed.* The Staphylococci. *New York: John Wiley & Sons, 1972.)*

required if the microorganisms were impregnated on a silk suture and tied into the skin. It is no wonder that cardiac prostheses, indwelling venous catheters, and other foreign bodies are so frequently colonized by staphylococci, even by low-virulence, coagulase-negative staphylococci.

VIRULENCE FACTORS

S. aureus probably elaborates more extracellular toxins, hemolysins, enzymes, and cellular components than any other bacterium, and all of these factors at one time or another have been thought to be responsible for virulence. Table 36–3 shows a partial list of these bacterial constituents and products. At present, it is not clear that any one or any combination of these factors accounts for the virulence of *S. aureus*. It is likely that many of them play some role in the pathogenesis of staphylococcal disease, but it is more likely that no one factor is essential for pathogenicity.

Some of these substances are, however, of particular interest. *Coagulase*, a protein which promotes the clotting of plasma, is thought by some to be largely responsible for the virulence of *S. aureus*. There is a high correlation between the presence of coagulase and virulence, because most strains isolated from infectious processes in humans are coagulase-positive (see Table 36–1). A simple procedure has been developed for detecting the presence of coagulase—the slide coagulase test.

The hemolysins of *S. aureus* are of interest, particularly the *alpha hemolysin*, or alpha toxin. This was the first staphylococcal hemolysin to be investigated. It is a chromosomally encoded protein exotoxin that not only lyses red cells and destroys other cells but also kills rabbits

TABLE 36–3. *Potential Virulence Factors*

Enzymes	Enterotoxins
Coagulase	Leukocidin
Hyaluronidase	Exfoliatin
Phosphatase	Cellular Antigens
DNAse	Polysaccharide A
Penicillinase	Polysaccharide 263
Proteases	Protein A
Lipases	Protein B
Lysozyme	Antigen D
Lactate dehydrogenase	Capsular antigen (SSA,
Hemolysins	SPA)
Alpha toxin	Teichoic acids
Beta toxin	
Gamma toxin	
Delta toxin	

when injected intravenously in sufficient amount (lethal action). If injected into the skin of rabbits or guinea pigs, alpha toxin also produces acute inflammation and necrosis (dermonecrosis). On sheep blood agar plates, colonies of *S. aureus* are surrounded by a large zone of beta-type hemolysis due to the lysis of the red cells by this and other hemolysins.

It seems clear that although alpha hemolysin may play some role in the pathogenesis of staphylococcal disease (since it may be responsible for some of the extensive necrosis that occurs), it does not appear to be a major factor in disease production. Antitoxin directed against alpha hemolysin has no protective effect against staphylococcal infection, even though the toxin is effectively neutralized in this manner. None of the other hemolysins appears to play an important role in virulence.

The enterotoxins of *S. aureus* are clearly responsible for a syndrome known as *staphylococcal food poisoning*. There are four antigenically distinct enterotoxins. Staphylococcal food poisoning occurs when food becomes contaminated with an enterotoxin-producing strain of *S. aureus*. If such food is left at room temperature, staphylococci multiply rapidly and produce toxin, which is excreted into the food; when the food is ingested, acute gastroenteritis results. Rather than acting directly on the gastrointestinal tract, the toxin is absorbed and reaches the central nervous system via the systemic circulation. It is the action of the toxin on selected areas of the nervous system that results in the often violent gastrointestinal tract manifestations of this disease. Not infrequently, there is marked malaise and sometimes prostration. Normally, the acute phase is self-limited, lasting no longer than 24 h. Rarely, prostration and dehydration are severe enough to warrant hospitalization.

S. aureus is the most common cause of food poisoning in the Western World. The disease frequently occurs in epidemics, when contaminated food is ingested by large groups of people. (An example of such an epidemic is given at the end of this chapter.) The disease can also occur sporadically and be limited to members of a household.

Food is usually contaminated by an infected person or by an asymptomatic carrier. A person with a staphylococcal lesion on the hand may infect food directly. Food may also be contaminated by the hands of a noninfected person if he or she is carrying an enterotoxin-producing strain of staphylococci on the skin. Regardless of the manner in which the food is contaminated, all staphylococcal food poisoning cases have one characteristic in common. Following contamination with staphylococci, there must be a period of several hours in which the food is maintained at a temperature high enough to permit multiplication of staphylococci and the elaboration of enterotoxin. Therefore, staphylococcal food poisoning can best be prevented by refrigerating prepared foods at all times. Ham is a very common source of staphylococcal enterotoxin. Because of the use of a high salt concentration for curing ham, the meat does not readily support bacterial growth. However, since staphylococci grow readily in high concentrations of sodium chloride, ham is an excellent medium for the growth of these particular microorganisms. It is wise to avoid ingestion of ham and other foods preserved in this manner when it cannot be ascertained that the food has been kept refrigerated until served.

Certain *S. aureus* strains produce *exfoliatins,* two distinct exotoxins (one chromosome-mediated and the other plasmid-mediated). Exfoliatin produces separation and loss of the most superficial layers of the epidermis, apparently by selectively destroying cells of the stratum granulosum of the epidermis. Exfoliatin produced locally can cause marked exfoliation at distant sites, resulting in Ritter's disease in neonates and scalded skin syndrome in older individuals. Circulating antiexfoliatin confers protection.

Only polysaccharide capsular antigens of certain strains of *S. aureus* are antiphagocytic and thus are definite virulence factors. Antibody against the antiphagocytic capsular material serves as opsonin. The exact role of capsular antigens in the virulence of these strains for humans has not been ascertained, but in experimental animals they act as antiphagocytic factors and their antiphagocytic action is neutralized by specific antibody.

Penicillinase results in resistance of almost all staphylococcal strains to penicillin. Resistant strains appeared rapidly after the introduction of therapy. Now both community-acquired and hospital-acquired staphylococci must be considered to be penicillin-resistant unless proved otherwise. Plasmid-encoded penicillinase (beta-lactamase) production is the basis of this penicillin resistance. Antibiotics such as methicillin, oxacillin, cephalosporins, and vancomycin have been developed that are not susceptible to the degradative action of staphylococcal penicillinase. However, staphylococci can rapidly develop resistance to these beta-lactamase-resistant penicillins by means of transduction between *S. aureus* strains, or conjugative transfer of plasmids from other *S. aureus*, coagulase-negative staphylococci or enterococci. An exception is vancomycin, to which resistance is very rare.

Recent epidemics of hospital-acquired infections have called attention to the increasing occurrence of multiresistant staphylococcal strains that are also resistant to the penicillinase-resistant penicillins and cephalosporins. These are commonly termed *methicillin-resistant S. aureus* (MRSA). They are considered to be *heteroresistant* in that most staphylococcal cells are fairly sensitive to penicillinase-resistant antibiotics, but a small proportion are quite resistant to high concentrations of these agents. This resistance is chromosomally mediated and involves production of penicillin-binding protein PBP-2', a peptidoglycan transpeptidase with low affinity for beta-lactams. MRSA strains are very important clinically and should be considered resistant to all penicillinase-resistant penicillins and cephalosporins. Fortunately, vancomycin remains effective against these organisms.

Penicillinase-producing strains of staphylococci have been found in the absence of known exposure to penicillin. Hopps and colleagues found that some staphylococcal isolates collected in late 1951–1952 from natives of the interior of Borneo, where medical care including penicillin therapy had never existed, proved to be highly resistant to penicillin. These strains may have been induced to produce penicillinase by contact in nature with *Penicillium notatum*.

IMMUNITY

There is remarkably little information not only on the role of specific products of *S. aureus* in the genesis of staphylococcal disease but also on the host factors that specifically work to prevent staphylococcal infection. *S. aureus* is an extracellular parasite and therefore is ordinarily killed following phagocytosis, which appears to be primarily responsible for resolution of infection. Although most humans, particularly adults, have fairly high levels of circulating antibody to staphylococci, the relative roles of humoral and cellular immunity are unclear. Efforts to induce specific antistaphylococcal immunity have been unsuccessful.

LABORATORY DIAGNOSIS

The definitive diagnosis of staphylococcal disease is made by isolation and identification of the species of staphylococcus involved. Material such as sputum or purulent drainage can be plated on appropriate media, and the size and the pigmentation of colonies of *S. aureus* surrounded by a zone of beta hemolysis usually make recognition of staphylococci on the plate fairly easy. Once a staphylococcus has been identified, *S. aureus* must be differentiated from coagulase-negative staphylococci. The latter frequently show little pigmentation, but the most important differential characteristic is the demonstration of coagulase production. There is a high correlation between production of coagulase and pathogenicity. Coagulase-negative staphylococci rarely produce alpha toxin (see Table 36–1).

Coagulase-positive strains can be differentiated into groups and types by bacteriophage typing. Phage typing for coagulase-negative strains is only beginning to be developed. Phage typing is not essential for identification of staphylococci but is very useful epidemiologically. Many strains of *S. aureus* are susceptible to more than one phage and can be placed into a phage group by their typing pattern. Bacteriophage typing is particularly useful when investigating epidemics of staphylococcal disease in hospitals. The source of such hospital infections can sometimes be traced to a diseased patient or a carrier among hospital personnel.

Antibody to cell-wall teichoic acid antigens in serum has been studied for usefulness as a diagnostic test for staphylococcal infection. However, these assays are insufficiently specific to be of much use clinically.

PREVENTION

No specific prevention for staphylococcal disease is available. Immunization with products of the staphylococcus, although producing some increase in resistance in experimental animals, has not been particularly useful in humans.

In those with recurrent staphylococcal infection, prevention is directed toward controlling reinfection and, if possible, eradicating carriage. Use of chlorhexidine soaps and high-temperature laundering may be useful in reducing risk of reinfection. Application of creams containing antistaphylococcal antibiotics (neomycin, bacitracin, mupirocin) to the anterior nares, with or without oral agents such as rifampin or ciprofloxacin, is sometimes helpful. To prevent infection of surgical implants (e.g., prosthetic valves or joints), a short-term systemic perioperative antistaphylococcal antibiotic is used.

The most important prevention of nosocomial staphylococcal infections is *careful handwashing* by hospital personnel between patients.

TOXIC SHOCK SYNDROME

It has long been known that *S. aureus* infections could rarely be accompanied by a scarlatiniform rash that desquamated—a clinical syndrome known as *staphylococcal scarlet fever*. This infection was thought to reflect production of an erythrogenic toxin by *S. aureus*, which was biologically similar to the extracellular product of group A streptococci responsible for the classic form of scarlet fever (see Chapter 9). In 1978, Todd and coworkers reported a group of children with an acute multisystemic illness that they designated as *toxic shock syndrome* (TSS). This syndrome is characterized by high fever, rash, vomiting, diarrhea, myalgia, hypotension (shock), and eventual desquamation. By 1980, it was realized that the persons at greatest risk of developing TSS were young menstruating women who used highly absorbent tampons.

S. aureus was isolated from these cases and is now established as the etiologic agent responsible for TSS. It is now known that TSS may develop in persons of any age, race, or sex who have staphylococcal infection or colonization with a strain that elaborates TSST-1 (toxic shock syndrome toxin 1). Regardless of the type of infection, the clinical and laboratory findings are the same as those found in menstruating women. Unless recognized and treated vigorously, the case fatality rate of TSS may be as high as 10–15%.

In tampon-associated TSS, *S. aureus* grows in large numbers adjacent to the tampon and releases TSST-1. Toxin release seems to be facilitated by binding of magnesium to fibers of certain high-absorbency tampons. Magnesium deficiency slows bacterial growth and increases toxin release. The toxin is absorbed from the site of infection and acts upon distant tissues and organs in individuals who lack antibody to TSST-1. Thus, the classic pattern seen in diphtheria, tetanus, and some other infectious diseases is followed. Repeated attacks of TSS have occurred, reflecting the fact that many do not develop antibody to TSST-1 after infection. Since the removal of certain high-absorbency tampons, such as Rely, from the market, the incidence of TSS has fallen sharply.

The pathologic manifestations found in TSS are numerous and widespread; many tissues and organs may be involved, including disseminated intravascular coagulation, inflammation and desquamation of the skin, periportal inflammation in the liver, hyaline membrane formation in the lung, and acute tubular necrosis in the kidney. Late sequelae may include chronic renal failure, prolonged neuromuscular disorders, late onset rash, cyanotic extremities, and neuropsychologic abnormalities. The diagnosis of TSS must be made on clinical grounds, relying on major manifestations of the clinical setting; there are few laboratory tests of diagnostic help, other than documenting multiorgan system involvement.

Treatment of TSS should be prompt and vigorous, including removal, or reduction, of the nidus of infection. The need for removal of tampons when present is obvious. Other sites of focal infection may require surgery and drainage. Intravenous antibiotic therapy against *S. aureus* is essential. Fluids, electrolytes, and drugs to combat shock are part of the overall treatment of patients with TSS.

STAPHYLOCOCCAL FOOD POISONING (A TYPICAL OUTBREAK)

Staphylococcal food poisoning is an intoxication rather than an infection: as noted above, it results from ingestion of food that contains preformed staphylococcal enterotoxin at the time of ingestion. Typically, the food is moist, most often potato salad or other creamy dishes. After the food has been contaminated by toxin-producing *S. aureus* by an infected (or rarely by a carrier) food preparer and has been inadequately refrigerated, *S. aureus* can multiply to greater than 10^5 organisms/g with enterotoxin elaboration. Since the toxin is heat-resistant, toxicity persists even if the food is subsequently heated to boiling. After ingestion of the contaminated food, acute vomiting and diarrhea without fever develop within 1–10 h. Except in the elderly or in debilitated individuals, recovery occurs rapidly. A description of a typical epidemic follows.

On July 26–27, approximately 725 incoming freshmen, 475 parents, and 150 faculty and staff members attended summer preregistration activities at a large state university. On July 27, several hours after a box lunch was served between 12:00 and 1:00 P.M., an estimated 300 persons experienced the onset of vomiting and diarrhea, and 84 were subsequently admitted to a nearby emergency room. Two adults and one student had documented hypotension respon-

sive to intravenous fluids. All but four patients were released the same evening.

A sample of 198 students (27%) and their families was randomly chosen for a telephone survey; 22 students and 45 parents reported gastrointestinal symptoms. For those eating the box lunch, the attack rate was 27.5% for students and 50.6% for parents. For those not eating the box lunch, the attack rate was 0%. Symptoms included nausea (76%), cramps (71%), diarrhea (67%), vomiting (44%), chills (25%), fever (25%), and collapse (9%). The incubation period in 98% of cases was between 1 and 10 h; the median was 4.5 h. Those whose symptoms included nausea and vomiting had shorter incubation periods than those with only diarrhea. Forty percent of those ill sought medical attention. The median duration of illness was 5 h for students and 7.5 h for parents. Of the 150 faculty members who were given free tickets for the box lunch, 84 ate the lunch and 47.7% of those but none who did not eat the lunch became ill.

Food-specific attack rates implicated the macaroni salad. Chicken could not be excluded as a vehicle of transmission, because all but one of the individuals also ate chicken. No other foods were significantly associated with illness.

The macaroni was cooked and rinsed on July 25 and refrigerated overnight. On July 26, between 10 A.M. and 2 P.M., celery, fresh green peppers, onions, and canned red peppers were hand sliced, chopped mechanically, and hand mixed with the macaroni and commercial dressing, which did not contain egg. The salad was placed into 30-lb closed plastic containers in a walk-in cellar overnight. At 6:00 A.M. on July 27, it was taken out of storage, and from 6:30 A.M. to 12:20 P.M. individual portions were put into Styrofoam boxes, which were transported in large groups to eating areas. The lunches were kept at room temperature during this time.

Examination of the macaroni salad from unused trays left at room temperature until 7 or 8 P.M. revealed 10^4–10^5 coagulase-positive staphylococci per gram and 10^6–10^9 enterococci per gram and contained type C staphylococcal enterotoxin. The chicken contained small numbers of coagulase-positive staphylococci. The staphylococci isolated from these foods were nontypeable.

Twenty-four kitchen workers were interviewed, and cultures from anterior nares, back of wrist, and rectum were obtained on August 2. Four workers had nontypeable staphylococci isolated from wrists or nares. Antibiotic sensitivity testing of nontypeable organisms from two workers and from the macaroni salad revealed them to be identical. One of the workers was directly involved in the preparation and serving of the macaroni salad and was the probable source of contamination.

REFERENCES

Book

Easmon, C. S. F., ed. *Staphylococci and Staphylococcal Disease.* New York: Academic Press, 1983.

Review Articles

Arbuthnott, J., and Bergdoll, M. S., eds. Toxic shock syndrome. *Rev. Infect. Dis. 11* (suppl. 1):S1–S333, 1989.

Lyon, B. R., and Skurray, R. Antimicrobial resistance of *Staphylococcus aureus*: Genetic basis. *Microbiol. Rev. 51*:88–134, 1987.

Sheagren, J. N. *Staphylococcus aureus*. The persistent pathogen. *N. Engl. J. Med. 310*:1368–1373; 1437–1442, 1984.

Original Articles

Chow, A. W., Bartlett, K. H., and Goldring, A. M. Quantitative vaginal microflora in women convalescent from toxic shock syndrome and in healthy controls. *Infect. Immun. 44*:650–652, 1984.

Davis, J. P., Chesney, P. J., Wand, P. J., et al. Toxic shock syndrome: Epidemiologic features, recurrence, risk factors, and prevention. *N. Engl. J. Med. 303*:1429–1435, 1980.

Elek, S. D., and Conan, P. E. The virulence of *Staphylococcus pyogenes* for man. A study of the problems of wound infections. *Br. J. Exp. Pathol. 38*:573–577, 1957.

Hopps, H. E., Wisseman, C. L., Jr., and Wheland, J. Relation of antibiotic resistance of staphylococci to prevalence of antibiotic therapy in diverse geographic areas. *Antibiot. Chemother. 4*:270–276, 1953.

Kass, E. H. Toxic shock syndrome: A reprise. *Ann. Intern. Med. 97*:608–610, 1982.

Kushnaryov, V. M., MacDonald, H. S., Reiser, R., et al. Staphylococcal toxic shock toxin specifically binds to cultured human epithelial cells and is rapidly internalized. *Infect. Immun. 45*:566–571, 1984.

Levine, D. P., Cushing, R. D., Jui, J., et al. Community-acquired methicillin-resistant *Staphylococcus aureus* endocarditis in the Detroit Medical Center. *Ann. Intern. Med. 97*:330–338, 1982.

Melish, M. E., Glasgow, L. A., and Turner, M. D. The staphylococcal scalded-skin syndrome. Isolation and partial characterization of the exfoliative agent. *J. Infect. Dis. 125*:129–140, 1972.

Peters, G. New considerations in the pathogenesis of coagulase-negative staphylococcal foreign body infections. *J. Antimicrob. Chemother. 21*(suppl. C):139–148, 1988.

Pfaller, M. A., and Herwaldt, L. A. Laboratory, clinical and epidemological aspects of coagulase-negative staphylococci. *Clin. Microbiol. Rev. 1*:281–290, 1988.

Shands, K. N., Schmid, G. P., Dan, B. R., et al. Toxic shock syndrome in menstruating women: Its association with tampon use and *Staphylococcus aureus* and the clinical features in 52 cases. *N. Engl. J. Med. 303*:1436–1442, 1980.

Todd, J., and Fishaut, M. Toxic shock syndrome associated with phage-group-I staphylococci. *Lancet 2*:1116–1118, 1978.

X

Treatment and Prevention of Infectious Diseases

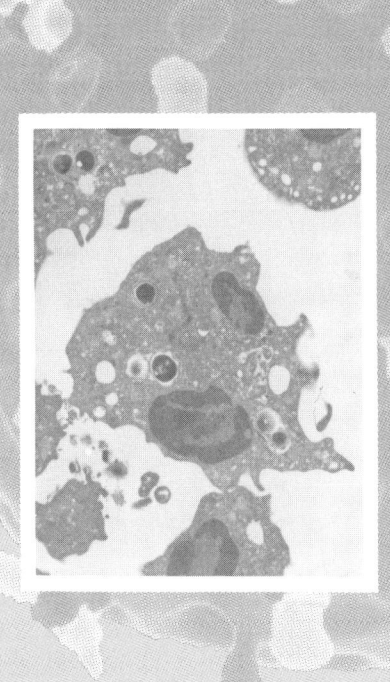

Molecular Biology of Sensitivity and Resistance to Antimicrobial Agents

INTRODUCTION

Just prior to the outbreak of World War I, Paul Ehrlich stated that the two essential qualities of a useful chemotherapeutic drug were: (1) an *affinity* between some part of the drug and a receptor possessed by the parasite, and (2) a *toxic potential* of the drug, which is capable of destroying the (viability of the) parasite once the binding has occurred. Although the language used by Ehrlich is somewhat old-fashioned, his analysis is as fresh and compatible with current biology as anything now being written.

The treatment of infectious diseases with antibiotics has been one of the major miracles of modern medicine. History has seen incredible ravages caused by relatively few infectious agents, with whole populations nearly eliminated or suddenly greatly reduced, victims of cholera, typhus, plague, and other diseases caused by infectious agents. These diseases are now treatable with antimicrobial agents or preventable by immunization.

BASIC PRINCIPLES

Before an antibiotic can act, it must first interact with a pathogenic microorganism. This interaction may be less specific than the binding implied by Ehrlich's definition. The interaction may be initiated by a specific active transport process of the cell that serves to increase the intracellular "free" concentration of the antibiotic above that which would be achieved by passive diffusion. The intracellular concentration of the antibiotic is determined by the balance of influx and efflux, and no specific binding of the drug to any intracellular components needs to be assumed. The consequence of the high intracellular concentration of the antibiotic is eventually expressed by a specific interaction of the drug molecule with an enzyme or a subcellular component of the cell.

The explanation of how any given antibiotic acts ultimately involves one or more very specific biochemical or biophysical events within the invading bacterial or fungal cell. Successful chemotherapy requires that the metabolic process to be attacked in the microorganism be as different as possible from that of the animal host. Obviously it is a clinical failure to kill or inhibit the growth of the microorganism at the cost of the patient's life or continued well-being. Some antibiotics (e.g., aminoglycosidic antibiotics, chloramphenicol) are toxic to the host as well as to the microorganism, and the real damage that may be done to the patient by the antimicrobial agent must be balanced against the degree of danger to his life posed by the microorganism.

A discussion of the biochemical basis of the *mode of action* of the clinically used antibiotics depends on understanding some fundamental processes in the human host. *Resistance* to the effect of an antibiotic, either as a constitutive property of the microorganism before it infects

a host or as a complication that appears during a course of therapy with an antibiotic, is also explicable in highly specific biochemical terms.

The purpose of this chapter is to discuss the biochemical basis of susceptibility (sensitivity) and resistance to some commonly used antibiotics. There are a variety of specific ways by which an antimicrobial agent may inhibit a microorganism. However, there are only four general ways by which a microorganism can *resist* an antibiotic.

1. The antibiotic may be unable to reach the potential target site of its action. This usually is related to decreased permeability of the organism to the antibiotic.

2. The pathogenic organism may possess some biochemical mechanism (enzyme) that acts to reduce or eliminate the antibiotic. In a mutant, an increased level of enzymatic activity or even a new mechanism for inactivating the drug may develop. Examples are (1) beta-lactamases that cleave penicillins and cephalosporins to inactive components, (2) acetylases that *acetyl*ate chloramphenicol to yield inactive derivatives, and (3) enzymes that inactivate aminoglycosides by phosphorylation, adenylation, or acetylation.

3. The pathogenic agent may have evolved biochemically in such a way that the target site for the antibiotic no longer accommodates the drug, and no drug–target interaction occurs. In the mutant cell this change in the biochemistry of the target site occurs during the treatment of the patient. Examples are cells that become resistant to erythromycin, clindamycin, streptomycin, and other agents during therapy.

4. The organism may have developed the ability to increase the synthesis of an essential metabolite that is antagonistic to the antibiotic, that is, that bypasses the antibiotic's effect.

All four mechanisms for blocking the action of an otherwise active antibiotic or for acquiring resistance to it are known. These are discussed in more detail at the end of this chapter. To understand them it is necessary to know the biochemical basis for the mode of action of the drug. This is particularly essential if resistance is related to a change of the cellular target of the antibiotic. A number of salient features of some of the antibiotics currently useful in medicine are discussed in the remaining portion of this chapter. The general organization follows the known (or presumed) major biochemical target for each antibiotic or class of antibiotic if a large number of chemically related drugs have the same or similar targets. The ways in which an antibiotic may disturb the physiology of a parasitic or pathogenic agent are almost infinite. Any enzyme or structure in the living cell can potentially be rendered incapable of fulfilling its normal function. Despite this tremendous range of potential target sites, antibiotics most used in human and veterinary medicine fall into well-defined categories and only a few critical areas of microbial physiology are affected. These include genetic replication of the cell (transcription), the expression of that genetic information into functional proteins (translation), and the assembly or function of critical cell components such as the bacterial cell wall and membranes.

A major difference between human eukaryotic cells and the usual bacteria or fungus is that the human cell possesses mitochondria, semiautonomous organelles that have many characteristics of bacteria. Their nonchromosomal genetic material and their apparatus for transcription and translation of mitochondrial DNA and RNA are similar to those of bacteria. Thus, although many useful antibiotics attack some part of the bacterial or fungal cell that is fundamentally different from anything in the human host, there is real potential for some damage to the mitochondria of human cells. The toxic action of chloramphenicol on mammalian cells is perhaps related to its ability to permeate the mitochondrial membrane and interfere with mitochondrial protein synthesis. A chemically unrelated drug, erythromycin, which has a very similar target site and mode of action, is unable to cross the mitochondrial membrane and thus shows little, if any, toxicity for human cells. Factors of this sort account for many of the anomalies connected with the practical use of antibiotics.

MODE OF ACTION OF MAJOR ANTIMICROBIAL AGENTS USED IN CLINICAL MEDICINE

Thousands of antimicrobial agents have been derived either from natural selection procedures or from chemical routes. Of these many agents, a large number have been tested for potential clinical application. Unfortunately, the vast majority have not proved useful, often because the agent is too toxic to be employed as a selective chemotherapeutic agent. In pharmacologic terms, this means that the therapeutic index (ratio of the curative to the toxic dose) is unfavorable. Many toxic antibiotics have been thoroughly studied by those interested in the mechanisms of microbial physiology and chemotherapy. Detailed chapters on some of these clinically ineffective drugs are to be found in the references.

This chapter focuses on a limited number of examples of drugs used today in clinical practice. In cases in which a large variety of agents with the same basic structure and mode of action are available to the physician (e.g., semisynthetic penicillins, cephalosporins, and aminoglycosides), only a few representative examples are discussed.

The presence of a drug causes both primary and secondary biochemical changes in a microbial cell, and it is often difficult to separate one group of changes from the other. Perhaps the best example of confusion regarding a primary mode of action for a clinically important antibiotic group is that seen with streptomycin and the other aminoglycosides. A tremendous amount of work now suggests strongly that the primary effect of streptomycin is to inhibit and to distort ribosomal-dependent protein synthesis.

Inhibitors of Bacterial Cell Function

An antimicrobial agent may affect either the function or the structure of a bacterial cell. Although the function of a structurally normal cell may be inhibited in an almost infinite number of ways, it is convenient to categorize inhibitors as (1) inhibitors of nucleic acid synthesis or function, (2) inhibitors of protein synthesis, (3) inhibitors of the normal functioning of the plasma membrane, (4) inhibitors of the function of a specific microbial enzyme or enzyme system, or (5) inhibitors of cell-wall formation. Useful antimicrobial agents fit into each of these five categories.

Antimicrobial Agents That Affect DNA and RNA

Many drugs are potent inhibitors of some phase of transcription and translation, the complex series of reactions by which the DNA of a parent cell is copied prior to cell division and directs the formation of RNA species needed for the synthesis of cellular proteins, cofactors, and substrates. A number of potent antibiotics inhibit transcription. However, relatively few antibiotics of this type are in clinical use, probably because the biochemistry of transcription in bacteria is not sufficiently different from that in the human host cells to permit a very favorable therapeutic index with this class of drug. Agents such as the actinomycins are too toxic to be of use as antimicrobial drugs in humans, although they are used occasionally as antitumor agents. In clinical medicine, the most useful antibiotics that affect DNA transcription are the rifamycins (rifampin) and nalidixic acid and its newer analogues, the fluorinated quinolones. Rifampin is an inhibitor of bacterial, but not eukaryotic, DNA-dependent RNA polymerase. The quinolones inhibit bacterial DNA replication and repair without seriously affecting mammalian cells by blocking bacterial DNA gyrase.

Rifamycins (Rifampin, Ansamacrolides)

There are a large number of rifamycin antibiotics, mostly of semisynthetic origin. The original rifamycins isolated from *Streptomyces mediterranei* were not well absorbed and were not very active. Chemical modification of the structures has led to several series of semisynthetic derivatives with high antimicrobial potency and excellent therapeutic indices. The most useful and best known derivative, rifampin, is a potent inhibitor of *Mycobacterium tuberculosis* and many other microbes. Therapy for tuberculosis has been greatly improved by the availability of rifampin (see Chapter 15).

The rifamycins (rifampin) are very specific inhibitors of bacterial DNA-dependent RNA polymerase. They inhibit neither DNA-dependent DNA synthesis in bacteria nor nuclear DNA-dependent RNA synthesis by eukaryotic cells. The specific method by which rifamycins inhibit RNA explains the selective toxicity of rifampin toward bacterial cells. Rifampin can inhibit RNA synthesis in the mitochondria of human cells, but the mitochondrion is relatively impermeable to the drug. Rifampin occasionally causes hepatotoxicity, which may be related to an effect on mitochondrial RNA replication.

Quinolones

Nalidixic acid (Fig. 37–1), a rather simple synthetic compound, is an inhibitor of DNA replication in bacterial mammalian cells by blocking bacterial DNA gyrase, an enzyme that is important for DNA repair and replication. The usefulness of nalidixic acid is confined to urinary tract infections because of its narrow microbial spectrum and concentration in urine. Many years after introduction of nalidixic acid, fluor-

oquinolones were found to have much greater potency and a much broader antibacterial spectrum. These DNA gyrase inhibitors, such as ciprofloxacin, have become widely used antibacterial agents in recent years.

Inhibitors of Protein Synthesis

A large group of clinically important antimicrobial agents interfere with protein synthesis in bacteria. Because this process differs in some essential details from that in eukaryotic (mammalian) cells, it is a good target for chemotherapy. In particular, the ribosomal subunits involved in messenger RNA translation in bacterial systems are smaller (30S and 50S) than those involved in mammalian translation (40S and 60S, respectively). Although most antibiotics that act upon the ribosome are *bacteriostatic*, the aminoglycosides are *bactericidal*.

Aminoglycosidic Antibiotics (Streptomycin, Amikacin, Kanamycin, Gentamicin)

A large number of antibiotics are included in the category known as aminoglycosides (Table 37–1). Their common structure is a cyclohexane ring with basic (amino or guanidino) groups in positions 1 and 3. In naturally occurring structures, other positions have hydroxyl groups to which are attached two or more sugars, including at least one amino sugar. Thus, a great variation in overall structure is possible. The mode of action of the aminoglycosides is believed to be roughly similar and is discussed here in terms of streptomycin, the oldest aminoglycoside and the substance whose action has been the most intensely studied. Streptomycin is one of the oldest antibiotics known, and it is still used occasionally. It has a broad spectrum of action, but resistance in bacteria readily develops, as will be discussed. In addition, this and other aminoglycosidic antibiotics are selectively toxic to the eighth cranial nerve, which is responsible for hearing and equilibrium, and are nephrotoxic.

The various actions of streptomycin on both *in vivo* and *in vitro* protein synthesis in bacteria have been well described. A large number (10 or more) of rather different effects of streptomycin have been noted, and the problem is distinguishing between primary and secondary actions. The major effects of aminoglycosides include induction of bacterial cell-membrane leakage, inhibition of protein synthesis, and

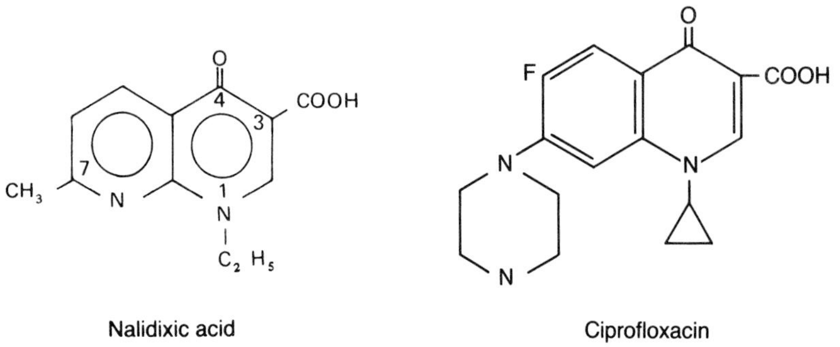

Figure 37–1. Structure of nalidixic acid and ciprofloxacin.

Nalidixic acid   Ciprofloxacin

misreading of protein synthesis messages. An important effect of streptomycin is interference with 30S ribosomal unit function and the ability of the ribosome to form an initiation complex with messenger RNA, an aminoacyl transfer RNA species, and the various initiation factors. Another property of streptomycin and most other aminoglycosides is the ability to induce misreading of the codons in messenger RNA, producing mistakes in the translated product. A protein component in the 30S ribosomal unit determines the degree of sensitivity to streptomycin, and mutants that lack this protein are resistant to streptomycin. Similar mechanisms exist for the more widely used aminoglycosides: gentamicin, tobramycin, and amikacin.

Tetracycline Antibiotics

Aureomycin (7-chlorotetracycline) was isolated in 1948, and oxytetracycline (Terramycin) was isolated 2 years later. Since then, several other clinically useful tetracyclines have been developed (Table 37–2), all containing four fused rings. All the tetracyclines are amphoteric substances that tend to form insoluble complexes with many anions (Ca^{2+}, Mg^{2+}, etc.).

The mode of action of the tetracyclines has been studied extensively, and many metabolic effects have been observed. The primary effect of the tetracyclines is produced by the binding of the antibiotic to the 30S ribosomal subunit. This binding, which is nearly stoichiometric (1:1), causes inhibition of the subsequent binding of an aminoacyl-tRNA moiety to the 30S

subunit. The normal further binding of an aminoacyl-tRNA species to the 70S or 80S functional ribosome is not specifically affected. Also, the bound tetracycline molecule does not interfere with the hydrolysis of guanosine triphosphate that accompanies the binding of this second aminoacyl-tRNA molecule, and it does not specifically affect peptide bond formation between the two differently substituted aminoacyl-tRNA species.

Resistance to the tetracyclines is quite common and is often associated with the acquisition of plasmids (see below). A major factor in inherent or acquired resistance to tetracyclines is bacterial cell-membrane function. Naturally resistant bacteria may accumulate insufficient intracellular tetracycline to lead to bacteriostatic or bactericidal action. After acquisition of a plasmid with new genetic information, a naturally susceptible bacterium also may exhibit reduced accumulation of tetracycline. Other types of resistance to the tetracyclines (often resulting from chromosomal mutations) are related to an alteration in a protein moiety of the 30S ribosomal subunit, with reduced binding affinity between the antibiotic and the ribosomal subunit.

Macrolide Antibiotics

The so-called macrolides are a very large group of antibiotics produced primarily by the genus *Streptomyces*. Their common structure is a large lactone ring with no *N* and with one or more amino-sugar and sugar substituents. The 14- and

TABLE 37–1. *Aminoglycoside Antibiotics Used in Chemotherapy*

Amikacin (Amikin)
Gentamicin (Garamycin)
Kanamycin (Kantrex)
Neomycin
Spectinomycin (Trobicin)
Streptomycin
Tobramycin (Nebcin)

TABLE 37–2. *Clinically Useful Tetracycline Antibiotics*

Chlortetracycline (Aureomycin, etc.)
Demeclocycline (Declomycin)
Doxycycline (Vibramycin)
Methacycline (Rondomycin)
Minocycline (Minocin)
Oxytetracycline (Terramycin)
Tetracycline (Achromycin, etc.)

16-member macrolide antibiotics are the most studied and used in both human and veterinary antibacterial chemotherapy. Erythromycin and oleandomycin, which are quite similar in structure, are examples of the 14-member group. The 16-member macrolides have lactones different from the 14-member macrolides, and, although their sugars are similar to those of the erythromycin type, the mode of structural attachment is different. Currently, the 16-member macrolide antibiotics are not used in clinical practice in the United States but are used for the treatment of humans in Japan and the Orient and for veterinary infections in the United States. Therefore, one should be aware of their existence and of the possibility that exposure of the microbial population to these agents, even if in animals used for food, may increase resistance to erythromycin.

Another quite different type of antimicrobial agent is also classified with the macrolides. These are antifungal agents that have no antibacterial effects. They are structurally quite different from erythromycin and have a very different mode of action. Two of them, amphotericin B and nystatin, are used in human chemotherapy and are discussed below.

Erythromycin. Erythromycin A is one of four closely related macrolide antibiotics produced by *Streptomyces erythreus*. Erythromycin has been in clinical use since the 1950s. It is a relatively nontoxic antibiotic effective mainly against gram-positive bacteria, mycoplasma, and some gram-negative bacteria.

All studies on the mode of action of erythromycin lead to the conclusion that its primary action is to inhibit RNA-dependent protein synthesis in bacteria. Protein synthesis in resistant bacteria (e.g., *Escherichia coli*) is also sensitive to erythromycin, but these bacteria are limited in their ability to accumulate erythromycin at the target site of action. Erythromycin inhibits protein synthesis in a very specific way. It first binds to a 50S ribosomal subunit and then remains attached to this subunit when the functional 70S monosome is formed (including the polysomes in which many monosomes are simultaneously translating a molecule of messenger RNA). A single molecule of erythromycin binds to each 50S subunit; this same stoichiometry occurs with all macrolide antibiotics. Bound erythromycin blocks synthesis only after a short polypeptide has been formed. The blocked peptide is not released by puromycin, implying a block either in peptidyl transfer or in translocation. The net effect is a slowdown

in the translation of messenger RNA into functional protein molecules. The effect of erythromycin is reversible; thus, if the concentration of the drug is low and the duration of contact with the bacterium is short, bacteriostasis occurs. In contrast, the bacterial cell will be killed if contact is prolonged and the concentration of erythromycin is high.

Lincomycin and Clindamycin

First reported in 1962, lincomycin is an antibiotic with an unusual structure. Other so-called lincosaminides have been prepared by chemical partial synthesis, and one in particular, the 7-chloro derivative known as clindamycin, is an important chemotherapeutic agent. The spectrum of action of lincomycin and clindamycin is similar to that of erythromycin, although clindamycin is noteworthy for its anaerobic potency in particular. In its action, lincomycin binds to the 50S ribosomal subunit or to free ribosomes but not to polysomal ribosomes, and both biochemical and genetic evidence strongly suggests that the binding site overlaps but is not identical with that of erythromycin. Lincomycin does not bind to the ribosome as tightly as does erythromycin, but once bound it may be a more potent inhibitor of bacterial protein synthesis. There is an antagonism between erythromycin and lincomycin that is explained by the fact that erythromycin can displace the more potent lincomycin from its binding site on the ribosome.

Although originally believed to be as nontoxic as erythromycin, the lincosaminides (especially clindamycin) occasionally are associated with pseudomembranous colitis.

Chloramphenicol

Chloramphenicol is a broad-spectrum antibiotic produced by *Streptomyces venezuelae* and, more practically, by chemical synthesis. It has a simple structure (Fig. 37–2) but possesses two relatively unusual features: an aromatic nitro group and a dichloroacetyl side chain. Of four possible stereoisomers, only one possesses antibacterial activity. Both the nitro group and the dichloroace-

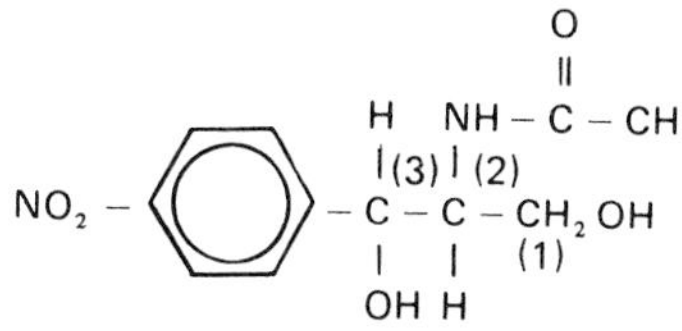

Figure 37–2. Structure of chloramphenicol.

tyl residue may be replaced by some other groupings with substantial retention of biologic activity.

Chloramphenicol, one of the first broad-spectrum agents, still is used in selected circumstances. It can produce highly toxic symptoms, including rare idiosyncratic aplastic anemia, and common dose-dependent depression of bone marrow function. These dangers must be balanced against the broad spectrum of activity of chloramphenicol and its ability to inhibit the growth of most bacteria, rickettsiae, and chlamydiae. It should be used with caution, and most physicians believe that it should be administered only with adequate supervision.

Of all the known inhibitors of bacterial protein synthesis, chloramphenicol has most likely been studied in the greatest detail. Nonetheless, its precise mode of action remains in doubt. It binds to the large ribosomal subunit and blocks peptidyl transfer on chain-elongating ribosomes. The binding is quite weak when compared with that of either erythromycin or lincomycin. There may be some overlap of the binding sites for these three antimicrobial agents, although studies performed with clinically significant concentrations of the drugs suggest that the binding of erythromycin and chloramphenicol is additive. At higher concentrations, mutual interference between erythromycin and chloramphenicol occurs.

The toxicity of chloramphenicol is probably due to its ability to penetrate the eukaryotic cell and in particular, the mitochondria. Here it probably inhibits mitochondrial protein synthesis and thus is toxic to the host as well as to the infectious microorganism.

ANTIMICROBIAL AGENTS THAT AFFECT FUNCTION OF THE BACTERIAL CYTOPLASMIC MEMBRANE

A large number of antimicrobial agents affect the function of the cytoplasmic membrane of bacteria. Most of these drugs are toxic because they also affect erythrocyte membranes and the membranes of other cells in the human host. Thus, for the most part, these agents are of little clinical use. A few are used when the mode of application is topical.

Polymyxins

These cyclic polypeptides resemble cationic detergents, binding to cell membranes and damaging the outer membrane, and are the only antibiotics that are bactericidal to nongrowing cells. Nephrotoxicity limits the systemic use of these agents.

Imidazole Antifungal (Antiprotozoal) Agents

A number of clinically useful antifungal agents possess imidazole rings as partial structures. Of these, miconazole and ketoconazole are used clinically. Among the many effects of these imidazole derivatives, leakage of cations across the fungal cell membrane may be related to their antifungal effect. The mechanism of this effect is not known. An important antianaerobic and antiprotozoal agent, metronidazole (Flagyl), also possesses a substituted imidazole ring, and the possibility exists of a similar biologic effect on membrane function.

Amphotericin B and Nystatin

These antimicrobial agents are also members of the macrolide groups, but they are chemically quite different from erythromycin. Structurally, they have a lactone ring much larger than the 14-membered ring of erythromycin, and their mode of action is completely different from that of erythromycin. Neither amphotericin B nor nystatin is an antibacterial agent. They demonstrate instead antifungal activity and are among the few systemic antifungal agents available for clinical use; however, these two agents are toxic and must be used with care (see Chapter 16). The methyl ester of amphotericin B is currently under study as a possibly less toxic and better absorbed form of this antibiotic.

The biologically active antifungal macrolides, such as amphotericin B and nystatin, possess a number of conjugated carbon-carbon double bonds and are quite unstable to both ultraviolet light and mild chemical reagents. The *polyene* agents, such as amphotericin B, selectively inhibit organisms whose cell membranes contain sterols. The antibiotic–sterol interaction results in cells becoming selectively permeable particularly to potassium and small vital metabolites. These agents bind particularly well to ergosterol (an essential component of fungal but not of bacterial or eukaryotic cell membranes) and less well to cholesterol (an essential component of mammalian membranes). This binding preference explains the selective action of these agents against human and fungal cells.

INHIBITORS OF MICROBIAL ENZYME SYSTEMS

There are many individual enzymes and complexes of enzymes in bacterial cells. Only relatively recently has systematic screening for inhibitors of many of these enzymes begun. Many such inhibitors are too toxic to be useful as antimicrobial agents, but a few inhibitors of this type have been very useful. Perhaps the most important example is the sulfonamide group.

Sulfonamides

Introduced in the mid-1930s, the sulfa drugs were the first useful antimicrobial agents. They were found to be active against a wide range of bacteria, but their main success was in the treatment of streptococcal infections and pneumococcal pneumonia. The agents developed since then have greater value because of their higher potency and the fact that bacteria readily develop resistance to sulfonamides. However, sulfonamides are still widely used in the treatment of urinary tract infections and in veterinary medicine. Many derivatives of the sulfonamides have been developed, and a few are employed in the treatment of highly selective infections; for example, 4,4'-diaminodiphenyl sulfone (dapsone) is used in the treatment of leprosy.

The mode of action of sulfonamides is rather clearly defined. Para-aminobenzoic acid (PAB) is a component of tetrahydrofolic acid, the carrier of one-carbon units in metabolism. The structure and shape of the sulfonamides closely resemble those of PAB. These drugs inhibit the incorporation of PAB into the pteridine moeity of folic acid (the nonreduced form of tetrahydrofolic acid) because they are competitive inhibitors of the PAB moiety that must be incorporated into the tetrahydrofolate structure if an active cofactor is to be made (Fig. 37–3).

Trimethoprim

This substance has a potent synergistic effect with sulfonamides and some inhibitors of cell-wall formation such as vancomycin (discussed later in this chapter). Trimethoprim, like the sulfonamides, is a drug that inhibits a step in folic acid metabolism (Fig. 37–3), in this case the activity of dihydrofolate reductase, which converts the inactive folic acid into the biologically active tetrahydro form. The combination of trimethoprim and sulfamethoxazole is widely used for many bacterial infections and for prevention and treatment of *Pneumocystis carinii* pneumonitis.

Isonicotinic Acid Hydrazide (Isoniazid)

Isoniazid (INH) is the most important drug used in the chemotherapy of tuberculosis. It is usually given in combination with rifampin (see Chapter 15). INH has a very limited antimicrobial spectrum with activity only against certain mycobacteria and related nocardiae. Its limited activity appears to relate to the effect of INH to inhibit synthesis of the very long chain fatty acids (mycolic acids) unique to the waxy cell walls of these organisms.

ANTIMICROBIAL AGENTS THAT AFFECT BACTERIAL CELL-WALL SYNTHESIS

Perhaps the best known antibiotics that selectively inhibit bacterial cells without harming the human host are some of those that interfere with synthesis of the bacterial cell wall. Mammalian cells completely lack a cell wall, the semirigid structure possessed by most bacteria. Thus, agents that prevent normal synthesis of the bacterial cell wall should not directly inhibit or affect the human host. The natural and semisynthetic penicillins (penams) and cephalosporins (cephams), bacitracin, and vancomycin are examples of remarkably effective antibiotics, and they act in this way. They selectively inhibit bacterial cell-wall formation without an appreciable concomitant toxic effect on the human host (vancomycin, for instance, may be toxic but for reasons not related to its direct mode of action).

It is important to note that antibiotics that act by inhibiting cell-wall formation should be effective only on growing populations of bacteria. Mature cells are not inhibited. Fortunately, however, in most clinical infections the causative bacteria must multiply in order to endanger the host; thus, the possibility that only mature cells would be present is not a real concern. The antibiotics in this group are therefore highly effective in preventing rapid or uncontrolled proliferation of the pathogenic bacteria.

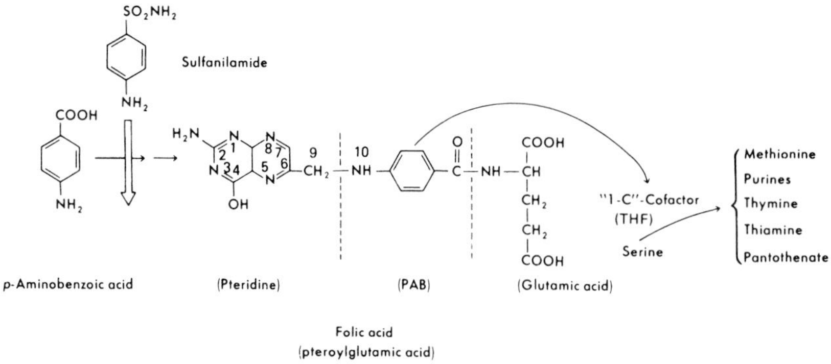

SO₂NH₂

Sulfanilamide

Figure 37–3. Metabolism affected by structural sulfonamides. (From Davis, B. D., et al. Microbiology. 2nd ed. Hagerstown, MD: Harper & Row, 1973.) Note the similarity between PAB and sulfonamides and the block induced in folic acid synthesis (large arrow).

BIOSYNTHESIS OF BACTERIAL CELL WALLS AND INHIBITION BY ANTIBIOTICS

A number of antibiotics with widely differing chemical structures have as the basis of their mode of action a three-dimensional structural similarity to either D-alanine (Fig. 37–4) or the simple dipeptide D-alanyl-D-alanine. A D-alanyl-D-alanine moiety is found in a developing monomer whose eventual extracellular polymerization leads to peptidoglycan, the insoluble, semirigid, basketlike structure that provides both rigidity to the cell wall and an osmotic barrier. In addition, numerous other morphologic features of bacteria (e.g., septum formation) are determined by polymers derived from the same monomeric building block. The biogenesis of this monomer starts within the cytoplasm (cytosol) of the developing bacterial cell (Fig. 37–5). In *Staphylococcus aureus*, activated uridine diphosphate (UDP) *N*-acetyl-lactyl-glucosamine (muramic acid) is linked via the lactyl group to a pentapeptide chain whose *C*-terminus is a D-alanyl-D-alanine residue. At the cytosol–bacterial membrane interface, this unit is transferred from its UDP carrier to a lipid-soluble undecaprenyl phosphate carrier, and it enters the membrane (Fig. 37–6). During passage through the lipid-rich membrane, the monomer is enlarged by attachment of an *N*-acetyl-glucosamine residue and the resultant disaccharide is modified further in its pendant polypeptide chain (amidation, attachment of a pentaglycine moiety, etc.). Finally, the mature monomer is discharged on the extracellular side of the bacterial membrane, where it participates as the substrate for the development of the peptidoglycan structure that imparts rigidity to the cell wall.

All members of the chemically disparate antibiotics that inhibit the biosynthesis and use of the cell-wall-forming monomer are structural analogs of either D-alanine or D-alanyl-D-alanine. They behave as inhibitors of the normal substrates used by the numerous enzyme systems involved in this complex biosynthetic pathway. As such, they may act as true competitive inhibitors and reduce the rate of a given enzymatic step or they may completely block an enzyme system by forming extremely tight complexes with it. These complexes may be potentially reversible or irreversible, covalently linked species. A number of different sites in the pathway leading to cell-wall synthesis are sensitive to inhibition by antibiotics, and since this pathway is not operative in eukaryotic cells, the antibiotics have the potential for effective chemotherapy without damage to the host. Several are toxic, but by mechanisms not directly related to their mode of action.

Among the clinically useful inhibitors of cell-wall formation, the penicillins and cephalosporins interfere with numerous reactions involved in the polymerization and fashioning of the peptidoglycan portion of the mature cell wall (Fig. 37–6); cycloserine interferes with formation of the pentapeptide chain in the cytosol;

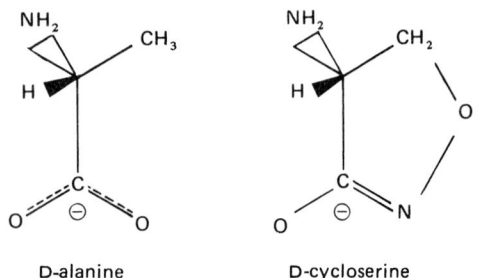

Figure 37–4. Structure of D-alanine and comparison with D-cycloserine.

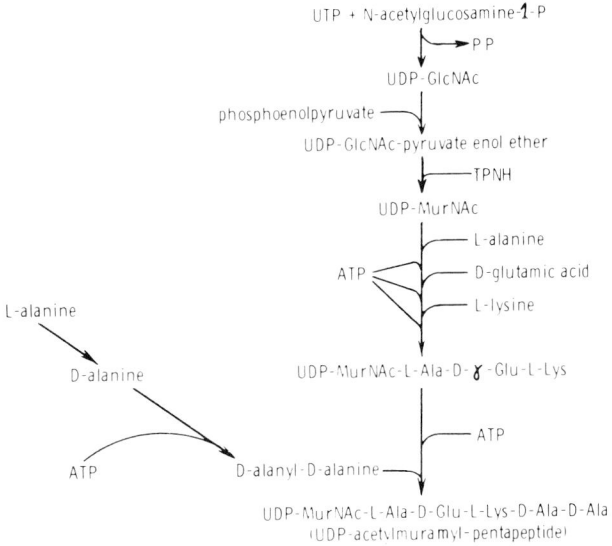

Figure 37–5. The first stage of cell-wall synthesis: formation of UDP-N-acetylmuramyl pentapeptide (structure shown at bottom). (From Strominger, Jack L. The actions of penicillin and other antibiotics on bacterial cell wall synthesis. Johns Hopkins Med. J. *133:63, 1973. Copyright © 1973, The Johns Hopkins University Press.)*

bacitracin blocks formation of the undecaprenyl phosphate carrier from its diphosphate precursor; and vancomycin inhibits modifications of the pentapeptide chain and attachment of the glycine polymer.

It is beyond the scope of this chapter to present complete evidence to support each of the preceding conclusions. Nonetheless, a few important observations may be mentioned. A large and species-dependent number of penicillin-binding proteins (PBPs) have been defined (at least seven in *E. coli*), and each apparently has an enzymatic function related to the later steps in peptidoglycan synthesis. The PBPs are located in the periplasmic space between the outer membrane and the cell wall, and defects in these PBPs lead to morphologic abnormalities. At least one is involved in the cross-linking between a pentapeptide chain on one peptidoglycan (nascent) strand and one a second, different strand. This reaction is an exchange of a peptide link between the D-alanyl-D-alanine moiety (*C*-terminus) of one and an amide on the second pentapeptide chain. A molecule of free D-alanine is released during this transpep-

tidation reaction. A second PBP is a D-carboxypeptidase that salvages D-alanine from D-alanyl-D-alanine units that do not participate in cross-linking. Other PBPs seem to be involved in septum formation and determination of length versus diameter ratios of the mature *E. coli*. The steps are all potentially inhibited by the beta-lactam antibiotics, but considerable variation in sensitivity is noted. Clearly, some of the clinical differences among the various penicillins and cephalosporins are related to their differential action on the various PBPs.

Beta-Lactam Antibiotics (Penicillins, Cephalosporins)

The discovery of penicillin marked a milestone in the history of chemotherapy. The detailed story of the original finding of penicillin by Alexander Fleming in 1929 is well known. By 1942, the work on the determination of its structure was begun at Oxford and developed into a giant Anglo-American joint effort soon thereafter. By the end of World War II, peni-

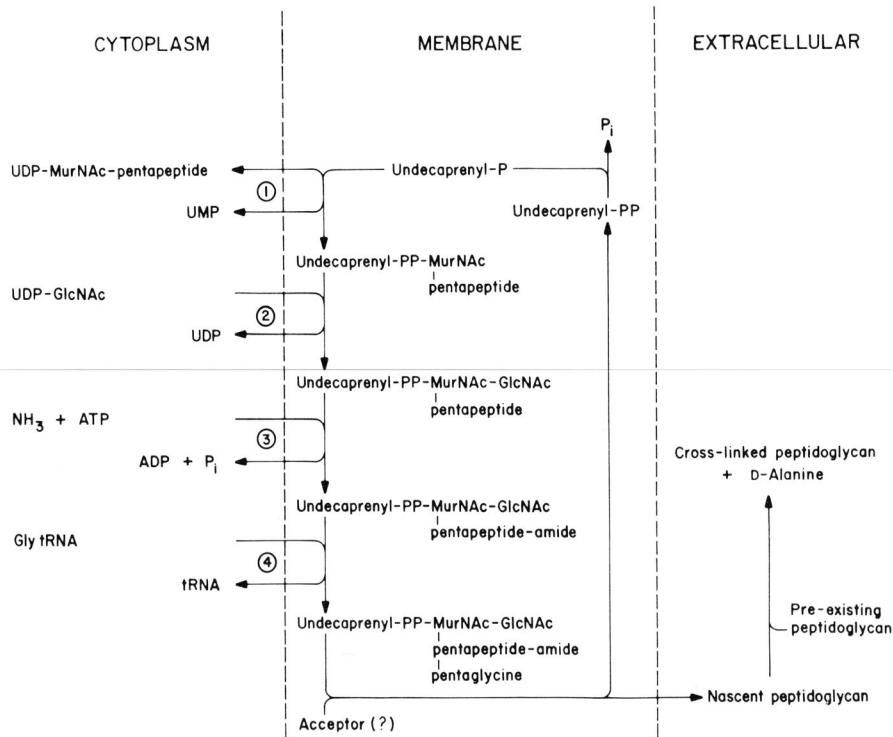

CYTOPLASM   MEMBRANE   EXTRACELLULAR

Figure 37–6. Biosynthesis of the bacterial cell wall, with emphasis on the steps taking place in the bacterial plasma membrane (reactions 1 to 4) where a lipid carrier (undecaprenyl alcohol) is involved. Reaction 1 is prevented by bacitracin, whereas vancomycin affects a step later in the scheme. (Diagram prepared by Francis C. Neuhaus, Department of Biochemistry and Molecular Biology, Northwestern University, Evanston, IL.)

cillin was used for chemotherapy, and the basic structure of its beta-lactam nucleus was established (Fig. 37–6). The fermentation of the producing *Penicillium* species was affected by the composition of the growth medium employed, and various penicillins were obtained following supplementation of the medium with certain organic acids. In the search for additional natural antibiotics of the penicillin type, a new substance known as cephalosporin C was discovered. It proved to have a beta-lactam moiety fused onto a sulfur-containing ring different from that of the penicillins (Fig. 37–7).

The resistance of cephalosporin C to inactivation by beta-lactamases brought much attention to this antibiotic in spite of its inherently low activity.

Semisynthetic Beta-Lactam Antibiotics

The naturally occurring penicillins and cephalosporins (e.g., penicillin G and cephalosporin C) have several handicaps as useful chemotherapeutic agents. Although penicillin G is the drug of choice when an infectious agent is susceptible to it, such is often not the case. Many gram-

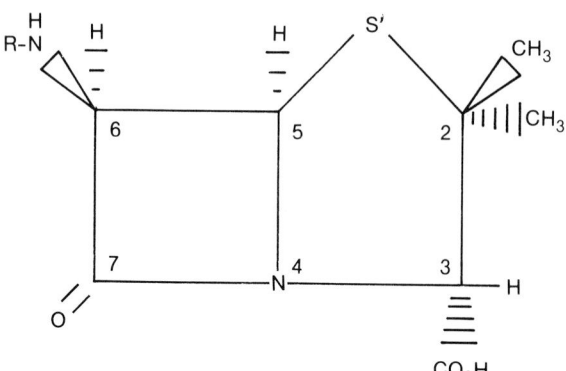

Figure 37–7. Structure of the penicillins. The four-member ring is the beta-lactam structure.

positive bacteria produce hydrolases (beta-lactamases) that destroy penicillin, and most gram-negative organisms are not susceptible to penicillin G. Although cephalosporin C has a much greater inherent resistance to inactivation by beta-lactamases than does penicillin G and has a broader spectrum of antibacterial action, it is not potent enough to be of clinical value. Useful alterations in these two antibiotics must yield one or more of the following: (1) increased resistance to the inactivating effect of beta-lactamases; (2) broader spectrum of activity, mainly in the direction of gram-negative organisms; and (3) increased potency of action or improved distribution into the tissues following oral administration. All semisynthetic penicillins and cephalosporins developed in recent years have at least one of these desired properties.

Semisynthetic Penicillins. Essentially all useful modifications of the penicillin structure (Table 37–3) have resulted from acylation of the side-chain–free nucleus of 6-aminopenicillanic acid (6-APA). This intermediate (Fig. 37–7, R=H) is available in bulk at reasonable prices as a result of the commercial enzymatic deacylation of naturally occurring penicillins that are produced at low cost by fermentation. Depending on the newly added acyl side chain, two types of altered penicillin result (Table 37–3). In one, typified by methicillin, increased resistance to beta-lactamase degradation is seen. In the other (e.g., ampicillin), increased activity against gram-negative organisms is noted, an attribute that is usually somewhat selective and differs among the semisynthetic penicillins in this group. Also, as the spectrum widens, the gram-positive activity of semisynthetic penicillins usually decreases.

Semisynthetic Cephalosporins. Modified cephalosporins (Table 37–4) have been derived either by acylation of the side-chain–free inter-

TABLE 37–3. *Semisynthetic Penicillins*

Altered spectrum of antimicrobial action
  Ampicillin (Polycillin, etc.)
  Amoxicillin (Amoxil)
  Azlocillin (Azlin)
  Carbenicillin (Geopen)
  Mezlocillin (Mezlin)
  Piperacillin (Piperacil)
  Ticarcillin (Ticar)

Resistant to penicillinase-producing staphylococci, etc.
  Cloxacillin (Tegopen)
  Dicloxacillin (Dynapen)
  Methicillin (Staphcillin)
  Nafcillin (Unipen)

TABLE 37–4. *Semisynthetic Cephalosporins*

First generation (similar to cephalosporin C but more potent)
  Cefadroxil (Duricef)
  Cefazolin (Ancef, Kefzol)
  Cephalexin (Keflex)
  Cephalothin (Keflin)
  Cephaprin (Cefadyl)
  Cephradine (Anspor, Velosef)

Second generation (wider gram-negative activity)
  Cefamandole (Mandol)
  Cefoxitin (Mefoxin)
  Cefuroxime (Zinacef)

Third generation (more resistant to beta-lactamase and greater gram-negative activity)
  Cefoperazone (Cefobid)
  Cefotaxime (Claforan)
  Ceftazidine (Fortaz)
  Ceftizoxime (Ceftizox)
  Ceftriaxone (Rocephin)

mediate 7-aminocephalosporanic acid (7-ACA) (Fig. 37–8, R_1=H) or, unlike the penicillins, as the result of discovery of new members of the group in fermentation broths of new microbial isolates. The intermediate 7-ACA is also available in bulk (Fig. 37–8). With two readily substituted positions, the structural variety of the semisynthetic cephalosporins is greater than that of the penicillins. As indicated in Table 37–4, these derivatives can be separated into three groups. The so-called *first-generation* agents have a spectrum of activity similar to that of cephalosporin C but with a much greater potency. The *second-generation* cephalosporins have a wider spectrum of activity, especially for gram-negative organisms. The *third-generation* agents demonstrate greater resistance to beta-lactamase degradation and substantially greater activity against selected gram-negative bacterial strains.

New Naturally Occurring Beta-Lactam Antibiotics

An intensive search has resulted in the discovery of several additional natural beta-lactam antibiotics. Their structures are novel, and their antibacterial activity is not always easily correlated with structure. Among these new beta-lactam structures are some with a 7-alpha-methoxy moiety, another natural substance with an alpha-aminoadipyl side chain, and a semisynthetic derivative, cefoxitin, with a side chain that contains a thiazole ring. Examples of other, even more unusual, structures are clavulanic acid (a weak antibiotic that is a potent inhibitor of beta-lactamases and is used in combination

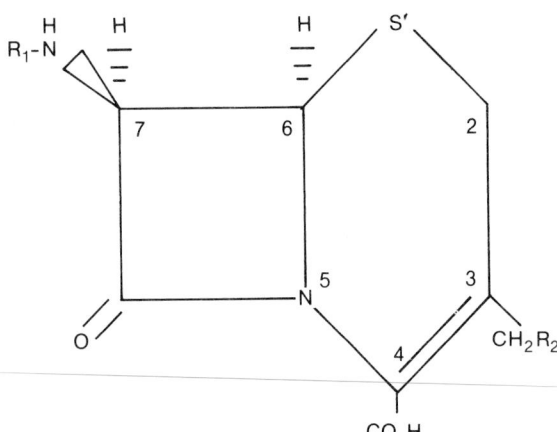

Figure 37–8. Structure of the cephalosporins. Note the four-member beta-lactam ring attached to the six-member ring.

with ampicillin or ticarcillin); thienamycin (Fig. 37–9), a carbapenem that contains the beta-lactam ring attached to a 5-member ring in which carbon substitutes for the sulfur of penicillin, and which is used clinically as imipenem, an extremely broad-spectrum agent; and aztreonam, a monobactam that has a monocyclic nucleus and has excellent gram-negative activity. Note that some of these structures lack the fused beta-lactam-thiolidine/dihydrothiazine nuclei of the penicillins and cephalosporins and that the simple beta-lactam ring itself is compatible with high antibacterial activity.

D-CYCLOSERINE

This is a broad-spectrum antibiotic with a very simple structure resembling that of D-alanine (Fig. 37–4). It is used clinically only for treatment of infection with *M. tuberculosis* or other mycobacteria. The action of D-cycloserine is specifically aimed at interference with the synthesis of the D-alanyl-D-alanine dipeptide, a necessary step of the biosynthesis of the UDP-muramylpentapeptide involved in the formation of the cell wall of bacteria (Fig. 37–5). Both of

the enzymes involved, L-alanine racemase and D-alanyl-D-alanine synthetase, are competitively inhibited by cycloserine.

BACITRACIN

The bacitracins are antimicrobial agents produced by *Bacillus licheniformis*. They are a mixture of peptides, and the A form of bacitracin is the most important. Bacitracin A inhibits the growth of many gram-positive bacteria and *Neisseria*. Bacitracin prevents the formation of the bacterial cell wall by inhibiting one of the steps occurring within the plasma membrane of the bacteria (see below). Bacitracin is used only as a topical antibiotic.

VANCOMYCIN

This agent is a complex glycopeptide that is being increasingly used in human chemotherapy, particularly for treatment of infections due to staphylococci resistant to beta-lactam agents. Its toxicity, when noted, is quite variable and includes nephrotoxicity and, if higher than nor-

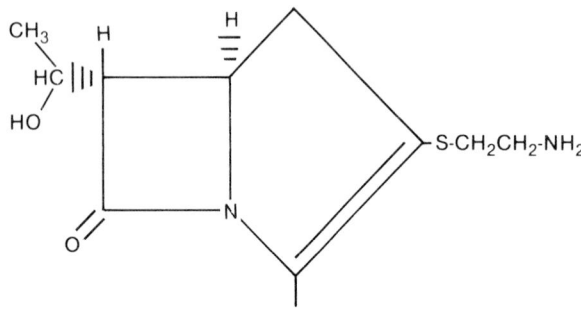

Figure 37–9. Structure of thienamycin. Note the presence of the beta-lactam ring.

mal serum levels of the drug occur, damage to the eighth cranial nerve (ototoxicity). Vancomycin is an inhibitor of peptidoglycan synthesis of the normal bacterial cell wall. Its specific target is quite different from that of the penicillins and cephalosporins.

EFFECTS OF TWO OR MORE ANTIMICROBIAL AGENTS IN COMBINATION

Considered from a theoretical viewpoint, chemotherapy with combinations of two or more antibiotics could have a substantial advantage over treatment with a single agent. The spectrum of inhibitory action might be broadened. Mixed infections might be more efficiently suppressed, the emergence of resistant strains might be inhibited, and bactericidal action may increase as compared with bacteriostatic effects. Some or all of these potential advantages are sometimes realized by judicious use of two or more antibiotics in combination. However, it is also possible that the desired additive or synergistic effect may not be realized, and sometimes antagonistic effects may be observed. Therefore, caution is imperative when combinations are being used.

The theoretical case for the advantageous use of combinations of antibiotics rests on a number of known examples. The sequential inhibition of a common biochemical pathway is an attractive target, as illustrated by the bacterial synthesis of the folate coenzymes (Fig. 37–3) and their reductive activation to the tetrahydro state (Fig. 37–10), as discussed above. Combinations of sulfamethoxazole and trimethoprim (Bactrim, Septra) often synergistically inhibit bacterial growth, and the biosynthesis of thymidine (an essential methylated pyrimidine base) is possibly the critical inhibition resulting from this effect (Fig. 37–3).

Another case in which two antibiotics with different modes of action may act synergistically is that of the aminoglycosides and the beta-lactams. The latter cause defects in cell-wall structure that permit increased entry of the aminoglycosides, resulting in increased inhibition of ribosome-dependent protein synthesis. Another example relates to inactivation of enzymes that destroy penicillins and cephalosporins (beta-lactamases) by beta-lactamase-resistant structures capable of binding tightly to these enzymes. For instance, cloxacillin potentiates the activity of beta-lactamase-sensitive penicillins.

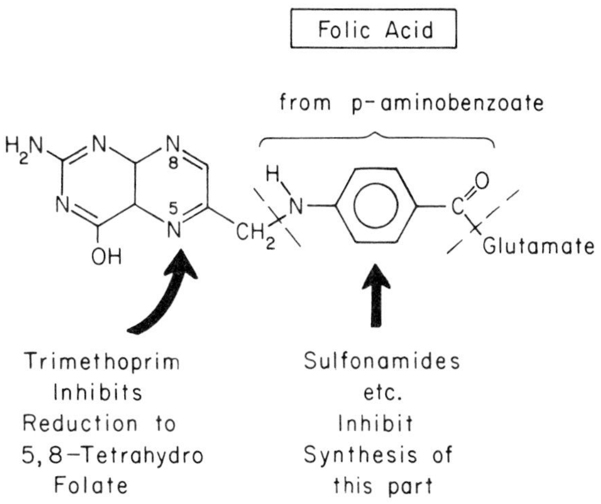

Figure 37–10. *Biosynthesis of tetrahydrofolate in bacteria with an indication of the sites of inhibition produced by sulfonamides and trimethoprim. (From Burroughs Wellcome Co. Bulletin SE-19R 5M, November, 1973.)*

As noted above, antagonism is occasionally noted between antibiotics. One example is penicillin and chlortetracycline when used together in treatment of pneumococcal meningitis. Much higher mortality was noted when both antibiotics were used in combination than with penicillin alone. The explanation may be that bacteriostatic agents like tetracycline produce reduced cell growth and division and penicillin thus has reduced target as less cell wall formation occurs. A second example of antagonism has already been mentioned—that of antibiotics with different potencies but affecting the same or similar biochemical target (e.g., the effect of erythromycin and lincomycin on 50S ribosomal function).

BIOCHEMICAL MECHANISMS OF RESISTANCE TO ANTIMICROBIAL AGENTS

It was discovered very early that microorganisms could develop resistance to previously effective antibiotics. The continued ability of many microbes to develop resistance to antimicrobial agents leads to the need for continued development of new agents. A bacterial strain may become resistant by two quite different genetic mechanisms: *mutation in a chromosomal gene*, and *infection by a plasmid*.

Mutation or Natural Selection

That resistance to chemotherapeutic drugs occurs has been known since the time of Ehrlich.

The current view of how resistance may develop in a large population of microbial cells exposed to an antimicrobial agent is rather simple: If, in that large population of cells, there are a few genotypically resistant cells (possessing constitutive resistance to the drug in question), the ability of those cells to grow in the presence of the antibiotic leads to a new population of progeny that are mostly of the resistant genotype. How the few genotypically resistant cells arise is related to microbial mutagenesis. With many agents (e.g., radiation and ultraviolet light), a more or less spontaneous genetic change in chromosomal DNA takes place. These mutational changes may occur either in the presence or absence of an antimicrobial agent, and single-point mutations occur (e.g., in *E. coli* at about the rate of 1 per 10^5–10^7 cell divisions). If such a change leads to resistance to an antimicrobial agent, the resistance may appear in either of two ways:

1. If the change is specifically related to the drug (e.g., if it increases the amount of an enzyme such as beta-lactamase, which hydrolyzes penicillin), high-level resistance may suddenly occur.
2. Alternatively, if the genetic change is only indirectly related to the biochemical action of the antibiotic, small increases in resistance may occur. However, if such small increases appear several times in the same microbial population, step-wise development of much greater resistance to the drug is seen.

Both types of changes occur with most common antibiotics.

Transformation, Transduction, or R Factor (Plasmid) Transfer

In contrast to the relatively simple single-point mutation of bacterial chromosomal DNA in which a single nucleotide base is altered, there are several ways in which larger pieces of new or foreign DNA may be introduced into a microbial cell. If these DNA segments encode for enzymes that affect antibiotic sensitivity, resistance may result.

Transformation

Exposure of a microbial cell to DNA isolated from a different species affords the possibility that some of this DNA will be incorporated into its chromosomes. This process is relatively in-

efficient, and the foreign DNA must be derived from a strain of microorganism with which it has something in common. This mechanism is not of great clinical importance, although it has been used often by research workers in the laboratory.

Transduction

Phage particles of both gram-positive and gram-negative cells may enter receptive phage-sensitive cells of related microbial strains. The DNA of the infectious phage can be inserted into the bacterial genome and can then replicate with the bacterial DNA. If the phage DNA encodes for proteins that confer drug resistance, this may be a mechanism by which the infected cell suddenly acquires resistance to an antimicrobial agent. Such phage DNA simultaneously may carry resistance determinants for more than one antibiotic, explaining the sudden appearance of resistance to two or more antibiotics, often some that are unrelated to each other in terms of structure or mode of action.

The foreign DNA that enters a recipient cell by direct means (transformation) or via a bacteriophage (transduction) is believed to exert its effect on that cell only after being integrated into the cell's chromosomal DNA. For this to occur there needs to be a considerable degree of homology between the exogenous DNA (or at least a substantial part of it) and some region in the chromosome of the recipient. The insertion of the homologous portion of the foreign DNA into the chromosome is rather efficient, depending on the degree of similarity, and the size of the resultant modified chromosome is not much different from what it was before the exchange took place.

R Factor (Plasmid) Transfer

As dramatic as the effects of chromosome modification by transformation or transduction are, a far more complex set of mechanisms for the introduction of foreign DNA into recipient cells is now recognized. Following epidemics of bacterial dysentery in Japan in the 1950s, it became known that the pattern of antibiotic resistance in the causative *Shigella* species was very similar to that of nonpathogenic *E. coli* strains from the same patients. Study of these mixed bacterial populations (*E. coli* and *Shigella*) led to the realization that an "infective" process occurred by which some genetic characteristics of the *E. coli* (measured as antibiotic resistance determinants) were being transferred to *Shigella* strains in a rapid and direct manner. The mechanism was found to be direct movement of extrachromosomal DNA from *E. coli* to *Shigella* by conjugation during which a physical mating of *E. coli* and *Shigella* cells occurs. A narrow tube, or *pilus*, connects the two mating cells, and the extrachromosomal DNA passes through the tube from donor to recipient. This DNA is termed a plasmid, an episome, or an R factor (for resistance factor).

R-factor-mediated transfer of genetic information between two often quite different bacterial strains is now recognized as a general bacteriologic phenomenon. The R factor DNA is usually quite large (10^6–10^8 d) and consists of covalently linked closed circles of deoxynucleotide bases. They do not become incorporated into the chromosomal material of the host, but rather reproduce as independent extrachromosomal elements. R factor reproduction is temporally related to that of chromosomal replication or other events in the cell cycle of the host bacterium. The number of R plasmids per bacterial cell is carefully regulated by an unknown mechanism.

When foreign DNA sequences are introduced into the chromosomes of the host by transformation or transduction, roughly the same number of nucleotide bases are deleted as are introduced, and there must be some degree of homology between the foreign and native DNA sections. With plasmids, however, it is known that their nucleotide base composition is extremely unstable and their size is subject to great variation. R plasmids consist of two distinct components: (1) a resistance transfer factor (RTF), which initiates and controls the conjugation process, and (2) an r determinant, a series of genes that confer resistance to specific antimicrobials. These components replicate separately in the bacterial cell, with r determinants conferring resistance only in the cells that possess them unless RTF is also present to initiate conjugation. The R plasmid in *E. coli* has a composite structure with a gene for tetracycline resistance plus an r determinant with genes for resistance to other drugs. In *Salmonella* species, the similar R factor shows rapid loss with selective retention of the tetracycline-resistant gene. *Proteus* species are similar to *E. coli* when cultured in the absence of the drugs corresponding to their resistance genes, but when grown in the presence of the appropriate drugs the R plasmid becomes much larger and possesses multiple tandem sequences of the r determinants

attached to a single copy of the gene sequence determining resistance to tetracyclines. This phenomenon reflects amplification, dissociation, and reassociation of composite R plasmid DNA. The mechanism might involve the effect of restriction endonucleases that remove certain sequences of deoxynucleotides, starting with certain initiation patterns specific for different endonucleases upon the circular R plasmid DNA followed by covalent linking of new DNA to the resultant ends by ligases. The result would be a regeneration of the circular DNA structure, but possibly with a very different size. Because little or no homology is required, except for recognition of the sequences at the termini where the endonucleases had acted, this mechanism can explain the addition of variable amounts of foreign DNA to an R plasmid. Such a process may be involved in the "evolution" of plasmids, and seems to be involved in the phenomenon of acquiring or losing resistance to antibiotics.

The role of R factors in resistance to antibiotics and their importance to chemotherapy are obvious. Because the R factors carry genetic information that by definition is not required for the survival of the bacterium, it follows that the presence of an R factor in a cell or its retention over many generations of cell division can be related to the bacterial environment. If the antibiotics are present and the R factor carries determinants that confer resistance to the antibiotic, the retention of the R factor is favored because it permits bacterial survival. However, growth of the same bacterial cell in the absence of the antibiotic may lead to physical loss of the R factor during a cell division cycle because there would be no selective advantage to favor survival of progeny carrying the R factor. Bacterial strains resistant to groups of antibiotics because of R factors may appear after initiation of antibiotic therapy, and often they rapidly disappear from the human host when antibiotic treatment is discontinued.

BIOCHEMICAL MECHANISMS OF ANTIBIOTIC RESISTANCE

Among the biochemical mechanisms of bacterial resistance to specific antibiotics are (1) decreased permeability to an antibiotic, (2) enzymatic inactivation of the antibiotic, (3) modification of the properties of the drug receptor site, and (4) increased synthesis of a metabolite antagonistic for the antibiotic.

Permeability Changes

Altered permeability to an antibiotic may reflect a change in a specific cell-surface receptor, loss of ability for active transport across the cell membrane, or structural changes that nonspecifically affect permeability. Gram-negative bacteria have a lipid outer membrane outside the cell-wall layer, and this outer membrane is traversed by water-filled channels made of porin proteins that facilitate entry by hydrophilic compounds. Changes in porins may occur, resulting in decreased permeability of a specific antibiotic, such as the newer beta-lactam agents, limiting the amount of these agents delivered to the periplasmic space where beta-lactamases function. Tetracycline resistance and some sulfonamide resistance also reflect permeability changes.

Enzymatic Inactivation

Many specific examples of enzymatic inactivation of antibiotics are known. The two most widely studied groups of antibiotics subject to this inactivation are the beta-lactams and the aminoglycosides.

Beta-lactam antibiotics are subject to the action of *beta-lactamases*, enzymes that catalyze the hydrolysis of the beta-lactam rings of the penicillins and cephalosporins to inactive penicilloic or cephalosporic acid derivatives (Fig. 37–11). Important clinical problems reflect beta-lactamases produced by staphylococci, those of *Bacteroides fragilis*, and the enzymes produced by gram-negative aerobic bacilli. The latter include chromosomally encoded cephalosporinases and more than 30 plasmid-mediated enzymes. Many of these enzymes are similar, with an active-site serine, but others are metalloenzymes requiring zinc for activity.

The aminoglycosides also are particularly susceptible to the action of inactivating enzymes. The conversion of streptomycin into phosphoryl and adenylyl derivatives is well known. Similar degradation of other aminoglycosides also occurs and, in addition, acetylation (dependent on acetylcoenzyme A) is common. The position of the attachment of the phosphate, adenylate, or acetate groups varies from one aminoglycoside to another. Amikacin is much less susceptible to these enzymatic inactivation mechanisms than are the other aminoglycosides. Thus, research and development in this field continues to be heavily oriented toward finding new aminoglycosides that are incapable of serving as good substrates for inactivating enzymes.

Another antibiotic that is readily inactivated by enzyme action is chloramphenicol (Fig. 37–2). An acetyltransferase that leads first to the 3-acetyl and then to the 1,3-diacetyl derivative is well known. This enzyme is either constitutive in certain resistant microbial strains or it is acquired by one of the mechanisms described previously. Both of the acetylated forms of chloramphenicol are inactive.

The chemical modification of antibiotics by bacterial enzymes is one of the most serious problems affecting the use of antibiotics in chemotherapy. This problem probably affects many more antibiotics than those mentioned here.

Modification of Target Site

Modification of the target site is another common mechanism for the acquisition of resistance to an antibiotic. The best studied example is that seen with streptomycin. The S12 protein of the 30S ribosomal subunit is the specific binding site of streptomycin, and a single amino acid mutation in this protein leads to impaired binding of streptomycin to the 30S subunit, resulting in markedly reduced sensitivity to streptomycin.

A similar situation exists with respect to erythromycin. Two kinds of changes in the structure of the 50S ribosomal subunit correlate with reduced sensitivity to the drug. Dimethylation of a specific adenine sequence in the 23S ribosomal RNA in *Staphylococcus aureus*, as well as alteration in a specific protein of the 50S ribosomal subunit in *E. coli*, are associated with

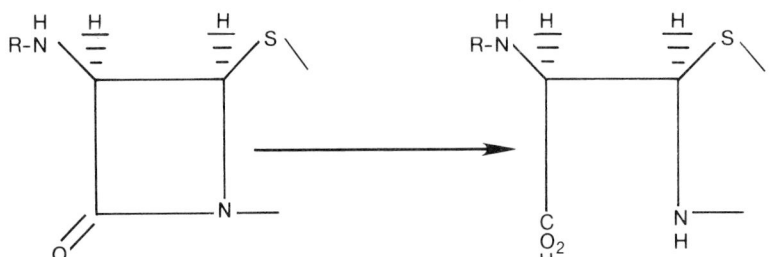

Figure 37–11. Inactivation of beta-lactam ring by beta-lactamases, with opening of the four-member beta-lactam ring.

reduced sensitivity to erythromycin. The *S. aureus* change may be introduced into the cell by a plasmid in a quite novel fashion, by induction of an enzyme system caused by subinhibitory concentrations of erythromycin itself. The induced methylase persists only as long as erythromycin is present. In its absence, the cells lose the methylase and revert to their original sensitive state.

Rifampin-resistant mutants have an RNA polymerase with an altered B subunit that fails to bind to rifampin. Penicillin-resistant strains of *Streptococcus pneumoniae* or *Neisseria gonorrhoeae*, as well as methicillin-resistant strains of *S. aureus* (MRSA), all of which are responsible for serious medical problems, result from altered penicillin-binding proteins (PBPs). In MRSA strains, synthesis of PBP-2a or PBP-2′, which has very low affinity for beta-lactam agents, is present, thus accounting for insensitivity to the antibiotic. MRSA organisms are now responsible for numerous nosocomial infections (see Chapter 28), and generally require vancomycin therapy.

Increased Synthesis of a Resistant Pathway

Resistance to sulfonamides is mediated by a plasmid that leads to production of an altered dihydropteroate synthetase, which is 1000 times less sensitive to sulfonamides than the wild-type enzyme. Similarly, trimethoprim resistance is due to a plasmid encoding a dihydrofolate reductase that is several thousand times more resistant to trimethoprim than the wild enzyme. Thus, organisms with these plasmids are provided a mechanism by which the drug-blocked reaction can be bypassed.

REFERENCES

Books and Monographs

Bryan, L. E., ed. *Antimicrobial Drug Resistance.* New York: Academic Press, 1984.

Corcoran, J. W., and Hahn, F. E., eds. *Antibiotics.* Volume III. *Mechanism of Action of Antimicrobial and Anti-Tumor Agents.* New York: Springer-Verlag, 1975.

Davis, B. D., Dulbecco, R., Eisen, H. N., et al. *Microbiology.* 4th ed. Hagerstown, MD: Harper & Row, 1990.

Gale, E. F., Cundliffe, E., Reynolds, P. E., et al. *The Molecular Basis of Antibiotic Action.* 2nd ed. New York: Wiley Interscience, 1981.

Review Articles

Bryan, L. E. General mechanisms of resistance to antibiotics. *J. Antimicrob. Chemother.* 22(Suppl A):1–15, 1988.

Davis, B. D. The mechanism of the bacterial action of aminoglycosides. *Microbiol. Rev.* 51:341–350, 1987.

Foster, T. J. Plasmid determined resistance to antimicrobial drugs. *Microbiol Rev.* 47:361–409, 1983.

Kerridge, D. Mode of action of clinically important antifungal drugs. *Adv. Microb. Physiol.* 27:1–72, 1986.

Murray, B. E. Problems and mechanisms of antimicrobial resistance. *Infect. Dis. Clin. North Am.* 3:423–439, 1989.

Neu, H. C. Overview of mechanisms of bacterial resistance. *Diagn. Microbiol. Infect. Dis.* 12:109S–116S, 1989.

Nikaido, H. Outer membrane barriers as a mechanism of antimicrobial resistance. *Antimicrob. Agents Chemother.* 33:1831–1836, 1989.

Waxman, D. J. Penicillin-binding proteins. *Annu. Rev. Biochem.* 52:825–869, 1983.

38 *HERBERT M. SOMMERS, M.D.*

Drug Susceptibility Testing *in Vitro* and Monitoring of Antimicrobial Therapy

INTRODUCTION

The discovery of the sulfonamide compounds in the 1930s opened a new and highly successful approach to the control of bacterial and fungal infections. The ability to predict a favorable clinical response to the use of an antimicrobial agent by *in vitro* testing is of great help in treating serious infections. Valuable guidance in the selection and monitoring of antimicrobial therapy can often be gained through *in vitro* testing.

The susceptibility of many microorganisms to penicillin (e.g., group A beta-hemolytic streptococci) is well known and need not be tested. By contrast, microorganisms that do not have a known, stable antimicrobial susceptibility pattern should usually be tested to save time that might otherwise be wasted awaiting the patient's clinical response. Variation in susceptibility of microorganisms to different antimicrobial agents may be caused by mutation, by transmissible episomes coding for drug resistance, or by induction of beta-lactamase enzymes. The use of *in vitro* antimicrobial susceptibility testing can rapidly separate resistant from susceptible organisms, facilitating the selection of effective antimicrobial agents.

The selection of an antimicrobial agent for treatment of an infection depends on several factors, including the mode of action of the agent, the optimal method of administration, penetration into specific tissues, and the rate of excretion. The microorganism involved and the site of infection are also significant factors. It should be emphasized that the most important factor in recovery from infection is the status of the patient's immune system (see Chapter 3).

METHODS FOR ANTIMICROBIAL SUSCEPTIBILITY TESTING

Antimicrobial susceptibility testing is directed toward correlating *in vitro* susceptibility of a microorganism to clinically achievable concentrations of antimicrobial agents. This can be determined by incorporating antimicrobial agents into a culture medium and then seeing whether the microorganism is inhibited from growing or is killed at different concentrations

TABLE 38–1. *Antimicrobial Susceptibility Tests*

	Type of Susceptibility Test			
	Dilution			
	Broth			Agar-Disc Diffusion
Property	(Tube)	(Micro)*	Agar	(Kirby-Bauer)
Gives minimum inhibitory concentration	+	+	+	–
Can be used to determine lethal action of antimicrobial agent	+	+	–	–
Accurate to within ±1 dilution	+	+	+	–
Requires relatively little effort (cost)	–	+	+†	+
Information about a large number of microorganisms easily obtainable	–	+	+	+
Contamination easily recognized	–	–	+	+

*Microdilution performed in microtiter dilution plates.
†Will depend on number of isolates.

of the test agent. Although there are a number of variations on this principle, most susceptibility testing is carried out either by one of several "dilution" methods or by measuring a zone of growth inhibition of the test microorganism surrounding a paper disc containing varying amounts of the antimicrobial agent. Some of the advantages and disadvantages of these procedures are listed in Table 38–1.

Broth and Agar Dilution

Quantitative susceptibility testing is performed by making twofold dilutions of the test antimicrobial agent in a culture medium, either broth or agar, inoculating a standard number of microorganisms, and incubating for 18 h. The amount of the test agent that will inhibit visible growth of the microorganism is called the *minimum inhibitory concentration (MIC)*. If the culture medium is a broth, subcultures from tubes showing inhibition of growth after 18 h are made to a medium free of antimicrobial agents and reincubated for an additional 18 h to determine the minimum lethal concentration. The *minimum bactericidal concentration (MBC)* is defined as the lowest concentration of antimicrobial agent that on subculture either fails to show growth or results in a 99.9% decrease of the initial inoculum. General usage terms antimicrobial agents that have an MBC the same as, or within one dilution of, the MIC as *lethal* or *bactericidal* agents, whereas antimicrobial agents showing more than a one or two dilution difference between the MIC and the MBC are called *bacteriostatic*. The distinction between bactericidal and bacteriostatic effects of antimicrobial drugs often is relevant clinically (see Chapter 39). Bacteriostatic agents particularly

should be avoided in those who are immune-compromised.

Although both the broth and agar dilution methods of susceptibility testing of antimicrobial agents provide the MICs of agents, only the broth dilution test can be used to determine the MBC. Broth dilution studies have traditionally been carried out by serial twofold dilutions of a single antimicrobial agent to provide 8–10 separate concentrations of the agent. The large degree of technical effort necessary to assess MIC and MBC by this technique has limited its use to special problems, such as susceptibility testing of isolates from patients with infective endocarditis, where such information may be essential for successful antimicrobial drug therapy (see Chapter 35).

A modification of the broth dilution test carried out in small plastic microdilution plates has become increasingly popular in clinical laboratories. The tests are usually performed in volumes of 0.1 mL in each well of microdilution trays. These wells may be filled by an instrument designed for this purpose in the user's laboratory or purchased prefilled in a frozen or lyophilized state. Results obtained by this method are comparable to those obtained by the conventional broth dilution method using culture tubes or by the agar dilution method. The endpoints among the different methods are usually within one doubling dilution. The low cost and ease with which microdilution trays can be used have made discrete antibiotic susceptibility information available for widespread clinical use. A microdilution plate adapted to determine the antibiotic susceptibility pattern and identification characteristics of anaerobic bacteria is shown with the accompanying template in Figure 38–1.

In order to standardize results from one lab-

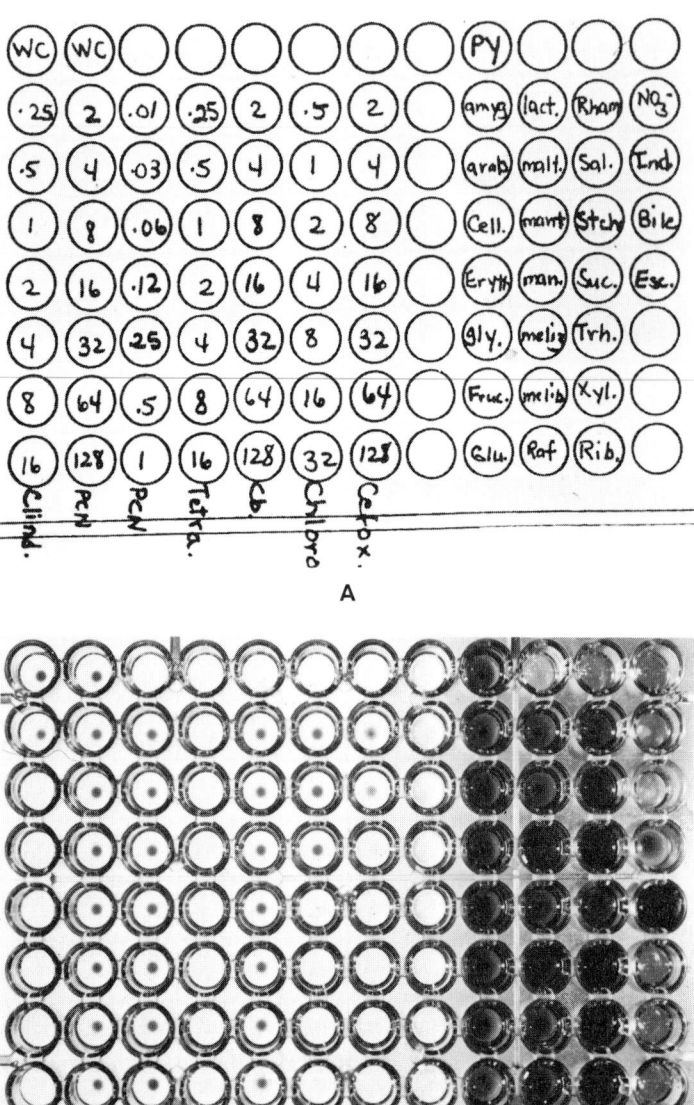

A

B

Figure 38–1. A. Template of microdilution plate containing antimicrobial agents and biochemical identification characteristics for anaerobic bacteria. The numbers above the abbreviations of the antimicrobial agents are concentrations of the agent in micrograms per milliliter. Drugs tested are (left to right), clindamycin, penicillin (2 columns), tetracycline, carbenicillin, chloramphenicol, and cefoxitin. B. Microdilution plate combining antimicrobial susceptibility tests and identification characteristics for Bacteroides fragilis. *The minimal inhibitory concentrations (MIC) in micrograms per milliliter are: clindamycin, 0.5; penicillin, > 128; tetracycline, ≤ 0.25; carbenicillin, > 128; chloramphenicol, 4; and cefoxitin, 8.*

oratory to another, it is recommended that the broth and microbroth dilution susceptibility testing be performed with Mueller-Hinton medium that is supplemented with Ca^{2+} and Mg^{2+} ions at the physiologic concentrations found in serum. When susceptibility tests are performed in this manner, it is thought that the result more closely reflects the *in vivo* response of the bacterium to the antibiotic tested than if no ions were added. This relationship is most apparent between *Pseudomonas aeruginosa* and the aminoglycoside antibiotics, in that supplementation of the medium to physiologic concentrations of Ca^{2+} and Mg^{2+} results in significantly higher MICs. When Mueller-Hinton agar is used, supplementation with Ca^{2+} and Mg^{2+} is not necessary since varying amounts of inorganic ions

are normally present in the agar because of its derivation from seaweed. Removal of all the various ions from the processed agar is not practical.

Agar dilution susceptibility testing is easily adapted to multiple bacterial or fungal isolates by use of a replicator device. This device, called the Steer's replicator, can inoculate 32–36 cultures to a single culture plate (Figs. 38–2 and 38–3). Although serial twofold dilutions of the antimicrobial agent can be made with agar in the same manner as with broth culture medium, it is more economical in terms of time and materials to test only several concentrations of drug that bracket the clinically useful range. Meaningful information on the MICs of a large number of microorganisms can be determined

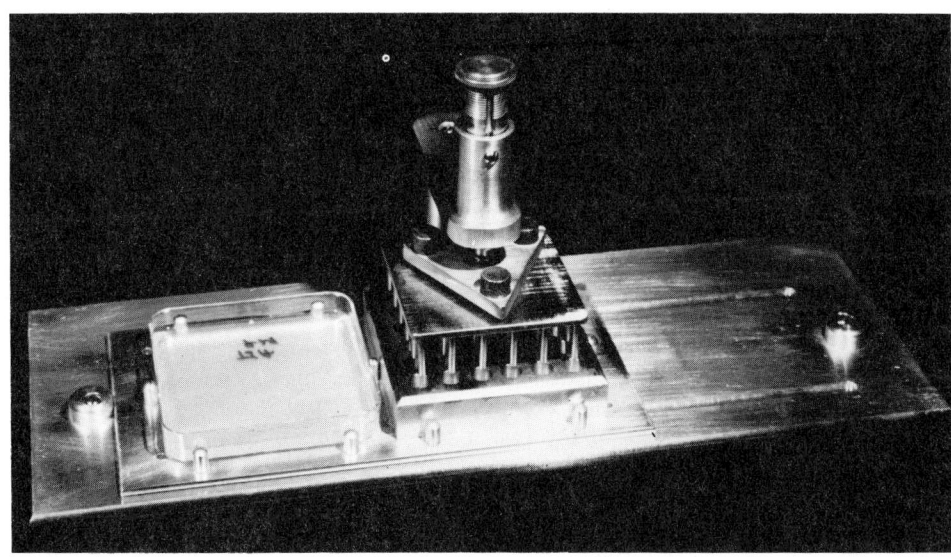

Figure 38–2. Steer's replicator. Standardized broth suspensions of microorganisms are placed in wells beneath the inoculating pins. The inoculation head is dipped into the wells and the agar plate moved to the right beneath the inoculation head. The inoculation head is lowered so that the pins touch the culture medium and deliver a defined number of microorganisms to the medium.

with use of only two to five concentrations of the test agent. Inadvertent contamination of the test inoculum, an error that may produce a misleading result, is more easily recognized with agar than with broth dilution tests.

Disc-Agar Diffusion

A very widely used method for antimicrobial susceptibility testing is disc-agar diffusion, also known as the Kirby-Bauer agar diffusion test.

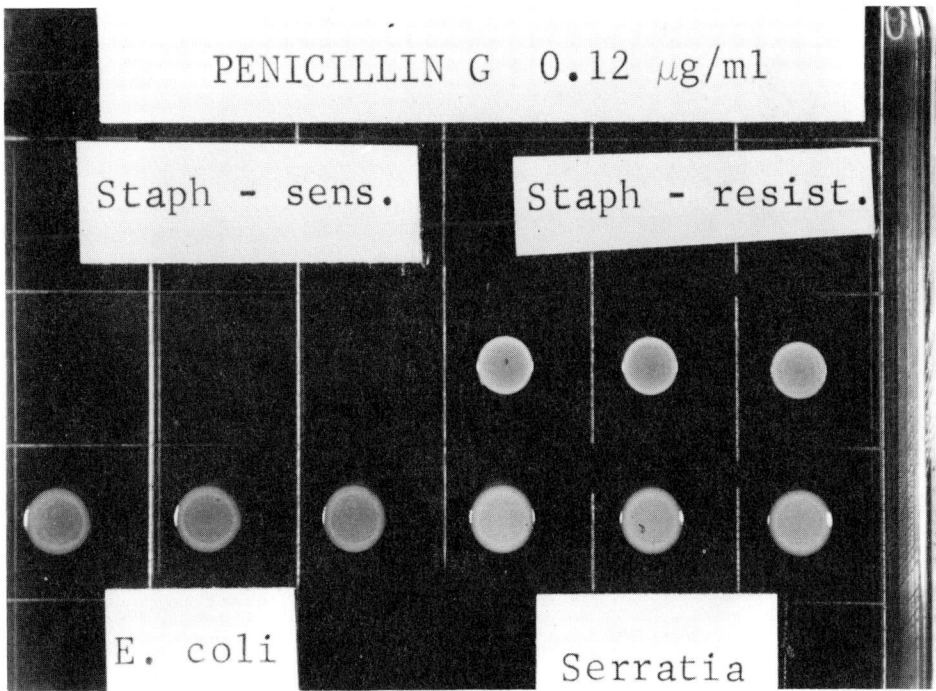

Figure 38–3. Four different bacterial strains inoculated in triplicate to a culture medium containing 0.12 μg per mL of penicillin G. Growth, indicating resistance to the concentration of penicillin, is seen for all strains except a penicillin-sensitive Staphylococcus aureus.

Susceptibility testing by this method consists of exposure of a pure culture of the test microorganism on an agar culture medium to a filter paper disc containing a known amount of an antimicrobial agent. Once the antimicrobial disc has been placed on the agar, diffusion of the agent from the disc produces a concentration gradient of the agent, which in turn inhibits susceptible microorganisms until a critical population is reached. At this point, further bacterial multiplication is no longer inhibited. Variations in the lag phase of growth, generation time of the test microorganism, molecular weight, electric charge and diffusion rate of the antimicrobial agent, and size of the test inoculum all contribute to the size of the zone of growth inhibition surrounding the disc (Fig. 38–4).

Criteria have been established to relate the diameter of the zone of growth inhibition found on disc-agar diffusion susceptibility tests to the MIC as determined by either broth or agar dilution. An inverse linear relationship exists between the MIC and the zone of inhibition from antimicrobial agents and rapidly growing bacteria. The larger the inhibitory zone, the lower the corresponding MIC. This inverse relationship has made possible the construction of regression lines and the correlation of zones of inhibition with the MIC (Fig. 38–5). When clinically achievable levels of the test antimicrobial agent are correlated with MICs, broad

guides of clinical susceptibility or resistance can be deduced. Information of this type is available for a large number of antimicrobial agents. Recommendations for performing the disc-agar dilution test in a standardized manner have resulted in significant improvement in intra- and interlaboratory precision and reproducibility.

Automated Susceptibility Testing

Instrumentation for automated susceptibility testing has undergone rapid development for several years. The principle used in most instruments is quantitation of light scattering associated with increasing numbers of microorganisms indicating growth or, conversely, lack of growth. Cultures are monitored in small cuvettes or wells, and some instruments provide an interpretation within 6 h. Most instruments are not able to produce results in MICs, but provision for this modification can be made on some. At present, intensive evaluation studies are underway. Further modifications have resulted in improved performance.

Interpretation of Results

The interpretation of *in vitro* susceptibility tests is usually based on the assumption that the administration of an antimicrobial agent will

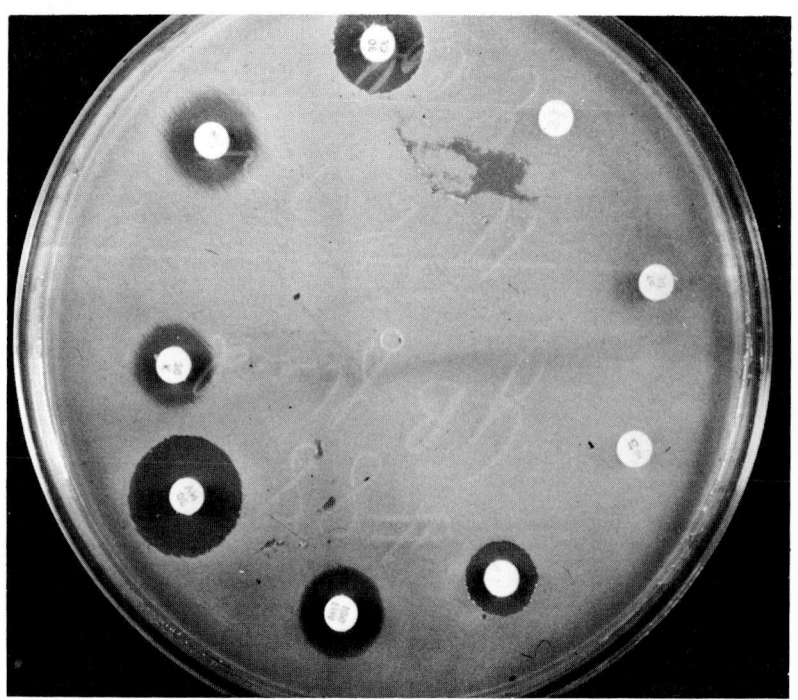

Figure 38–4. An agar plate inoculated with Escherichia coli *shows a series of paper discs containing different antimicrobial agents. The size of the zone of growth inhibition is measured and the susceptibility of the microorganism is determined by reference to an interpretive chart.*

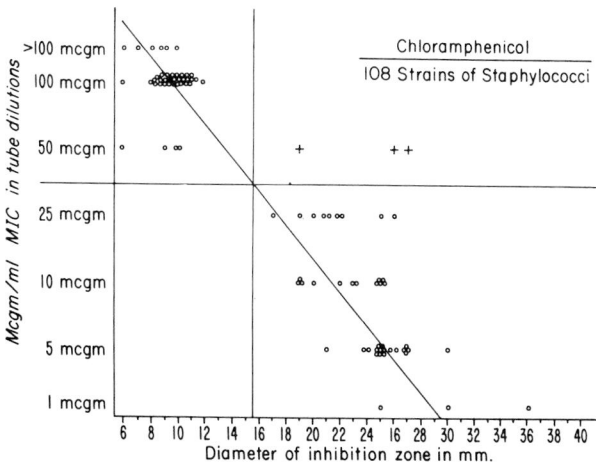

Figure 38–5. Results of tube-dilution and single-disc tests of 108 strains of staphylococci. The correlation was good in 105 instances. (From Bauer, A. W., et al. Single-disc antibiotic sensitivity testing of staphylococci. Arch. Intern. Med. 104:208, 1959. Copyright © 1959, American Medical Association.)

achieve a serum level from one- to fivefold greater than the MIC. In reporting the results of susceptibility tests by disc-agar diffusion, three terms are used—*susceptible, intermediate or indeterminate susceptibility*, and *resistant*. *Susceptible* indicates that an infection with the test microorganism will likely respond to the usual dose of an antimicrobial agent recommended for that microorganism. The term *resistant* is used for those agents that do not inhibit the test microorganism within the range of achievable blood levels. The term *intermediate or indeterminate susceptibility* is reserved for microorganisms that may respond to an agent if large doses are used or when other measures are taken to optimize the mode of treatment. The term *indeterminate susceptibility* is best used in the interpretation of small differences in zone sizes that may result from technical variability.

A somewhat similar set of interpretative categories was recommended in 1971 by an international collaborative study on antimicrobial susceptibility testing. This report recommended

a fourth category to include the situation in which a favorable *in vivo* response was probable in the treatment of localized infections at sites where the agent could be concentrated by physiologic processes or local application (Table 38–2). This would include the concentration of antimicrobial agents in the urine, which achieves levels many times the levels found in serum. Such a category would also include antimicrobial agents in ointments that can be employed in local skin infections.

The standardized Kirby-Bauer disc susceptibility test is a simple procedure widely used by many clinical laboratories. Although disc-agar diffusion susceptibility testing provides good reproducibility in separating susceptible from resistant microorganisms, the zones of inhibition for many microorganisms fall into the narrow indeterminate zone where results often produce interpretations different from those of dilution tests. One study has indicated that comparison of zones of inhibition against a number of aminoglycosides did not show good regression

TABLE 38–2. *Categorization of Antimicrobial Susceptibility*

Group 1
    Should include high degrees of bacterial susceptibility that make *in vivo* response probable when patients with mild to moderately severe systemic infections are treated with the usual dosage of antimicrobial agent. This would be the oral route when applicable (e.g., ampicillin). Group 1 can be defined as "sensitive" without further qualification.

Group 2
    Should include degrees of susceptibility that make *in vivo* response probable in systemic infections when the antimicrobial agent is given in high dosage or up to the limits of toxicity.

Group 3
    Should include degrees of susceptibility that make *in vivo* response probable in the treatment of localized infections at sites where the agent can be concentrated by physiologic processes or local application, e.g., the urinary tract or application of an ointment to a local skin infection.

Group 4
    Should include microorganisms of a degree of resistance that makes *in vivo* response improbable. This group can be designated "resistant."

(Adapted from Ericsson, H. M., and Sherris, J. C. Antibiotic sensitivity testing. Report of an international collaborative study. *Acta Pathol. Microbiol. Scand.* [B] *217*(Suppl. 217):1, 1971.)

curves between disc-agar diffusion and dilution studies for determination of *susceptibility*, although the ability to detect *resistance* was good.

INDICATIONS FOR SUSCEPTIBILITY TESTING

Testing of all bacterial isolates for antimicrobial susceptibility is neither necessary nor desirable. Alpha-hemolytic streptococci, normally present in the throat, should not be tested for drug susceptibility, unless they represent blood culture isolates and are implicated etiologically in infective endocarditis (see Chapter 35). Similarly, there is no reason to test the susceptibility of group A beta-hemolytic streptococci to penicillin.

All staphylococci should be tested for susceptibility to antimicrobial agents. Resistance to penicillin and other antimicrobial agents is of therapeutic importance. Members of the family Enterobacteriaceae show wide variation of susceptibility and resistance, partially due to the presence of transferable episomes. Occasionally, susceptibility studies should be repeated on microorganisms isolated during therapy to monitor for the induction of resistance. The appearance of an episome-carrying variant of the infecting microorganism or replacement by a similar but drug-resistant strain can rapidly alter the course of an infection.

The Kirby-Bauer disc-agar diffusion susceptibility test has been standardized only for rapidly growing microorganisms, such as those of the family Enterobacteriaceae and staphylococci. The determination of antimicrobial susceptibility of more fastidious and slowly growing bacteria, including *Haemophilus influenzae, Neisseria gonorrhoeae*, and anaerobic bacteria, requires more exacting test conditions than are provided by the Kirby-Bauer method.

The appearance of ampicillin-resistant strains of *H. influenzae* and penicillin-resistant strains of *N. gonorrhoeae* and *Streptococcus pneumoniae* has resulted in the development of several rapid, easily performed procedures to detect beta-lactamase (penicillinase). In most instances, the demonstration of beta-lactamase in these organisms is all that is required to establish the need for chemotherapy with alternative antimicrobial agents. Susceptibility testing of these and other fastidious bacteria is usually performed by tube dilution with a broth medium containing certain supplements to stimulate or support growth. In certain organisms (e.g., *H. influenzae*) the number of organisms used in the inoculum can play a significant part in determining the MIC. Failure to standardize the inoculum to 10^5 organisms/mL may result in a report suggesting false resistance.

SELECTION OF ANTIMICROBIAL AGENTS FOR SUSCEPTIBILITY TESTING

During the past 30 years, there have been numerous antimicrobial agents introduced that differ from the original member of a class of drugs by only slight chemical modifications. The modified forms may provide certain improvements in pharmacologic characteristics, such as superior resistance to degradation by gastric acid, improved gastrointestinal absorption, or slower renal excretion. *In vitro* testing of microorganisms for susceptibility to closely related antimicrobial agents is usually not affected by the chemical modifications. For this reason, it is not usually necessary to test microorganisms against more than one tetracycline or one penicillinase-resistant penicillin. A similar situation formerly existed with the cephalosporin antibiotics. Susceptibility of six to eight cephalosporins was determined by the use of a single agent, cephalothin. The release of cephamandole and cefoxitin (a cephalosporin and a cephamycin, respectively, showing resistance to beta-lactamase enzymes produced by certain Enterobacteriaceae and anaerobic bacteria) has resulted in change of this practice. In general, the beta-lactamase–resistant cephalosporins and cephamycins are not as effective against the gram-positive bacteria as are the earlier cephalosporins. Cefoxitin is quite active *in vitro* against the penicillin-resistant strains of *Bacteroides* and other anaerobic bacteria. It is now clear that in some instances more than one member of a family or class of antibiotics may have to be incorporated into the screening selection to determine the most effective agent for certain bacterial species.

With the release of a large number of second- and third-generation cephalosporins, many of which show significantly different microbiologic and pharmacologic characteristics, it is no longer possible to select a single agent as representative of the entire group of cephalosporins for routine susceptibility testing. As a result, there is wide variation among clinical microbiology laboratories in the number and types of cephalosporin antibiotics tested against different bacteria isolated from various sources. Many hospitals restrict the use of certain antibiotics, permitting the administration of certain agents only on approval of a designated local authority (e.g., the Infectious Diseases Service). For this reason, the laboratory may test the more recently introduced antibiotics only against bacteria isolated from sites of serious infection (e.g., blood or cerebrospinal fluid), testing other isolates only on request. The considerable expense of many of the newly released antibiotics requires their careful use when less expensive antibiotics do not perform as well.

The recognition of genetic and inducible beta-lactamase production to cephamandole by certain species of the *Enterobacter* genus has shown that current methods for susceptibility testing may not be sufficiently sensitive to detect such resistance. It has been estimated that beta-lactamase–producing genetic mutants of *Enterobacter* species resistant to cephamandole occur in low numbers, 1 in every 10^6–10^8 organisms. Current methods of *in vitro* susceptibility testing, particularly the microdilution and automated or rapid testing procedures, use smaller numbers of organisms, usually 10^4–10^5 bacteria. This is an inadequate number of organisms to detect the rare stable genetic mutants and might result in a major error in reporting of the test as susceptible when therapy with cephamandole might result in clinical failure. This problem is currently under study.

The number of different types of antimicrobial agents necessary for susceptibility testing of either gram-negative or gram-positive bacteria can usually be reduced to no more than 10 or 12. Additional agents can be added for microorganisms isolated from the urinary tract when concentration of the agent in the urine makes it active at this site but not elsewhere in the body (e.g., nalidixic acid). Because nalidixic acid is not present in therapeutic levels until it is concentrated and excreted by the kidney, it is meaningless to report the susceptibility of a microorganism to this agent unless it is isolated from the urinary tract.

IN VITRO *STUDIES OF ANTIMICROBIAL SYNERGISM*

Occasionally, it is appropriate to determine the susceptibility of bacteria or fungi to the synergistic action of two or more antimicrobial agents. For example, the determination of synergism is particularly useful in the treatment of patients with endocarditis caused by *Enterococcus faecalis*. Optimal treatment of endocarditis

caused by this microorganism requires the use of cell-wall active antimicrobial agents, such as penicillin or vancomycin, with an aminoglycoside, usually either streptomycin or gentamicin, to inhibit protein synthesis. The method for studying synergism by *in vitro* tests involves a cross-titration of tube-dilution susceptibility tests. This gives the minimum combination of both agents resulting in the inhibition and killing of the microorganism. The endpoint may then be reported either as minimum inhibitory or lethal concentrations of the different combinations or as the log decrease in viable microorganisms plotted against time. Based on the assumption that no host defect in cellular phagocytic or immune mechanisms exists, combinations of agents sufficient to result in a 99.9% decrease in the number of inoculated microorganisms are considered sufficient to bring about a prompt clinical response. Note in Figure 38–6 that counts of viable bacteria drop significantly at 3 and 7 h with 0.5 μg/mL of ampicillin, 4 μg/mL of gentamicin, or the combination of 0.5 μg/mL ampicillin and 2 μg/mL of gentamicin. In each test, there was a significant decrease in the number of viable organisms detected by counts within the first 8 h with a rebound to at least the inoculated number by 22 h. In contrast, the combination of 0.5 μg/mL ampicillin and 4 μg/mL of gentamicin appeared highly effective.

PROTEIN BINDING OF ANTIBIOTICS

Many antimicrobial agents bind reversibly to serum proteins in varying amounts, resulting in free and bound components that make up the total serum level. Binding of most antimicrobial agents occurs to albumin, but erythromycin binds to alpha$_1$ globulin. Protein binding is of clinical significance because only the unbound portion of the drug is available for antimicrobial effect and diffusion into the interstitial tissues. The free and bound portions of an antimicrobial agent are in equilibrium, and in this manner binding fulfills a storage function, preventing rapid excretion by glomerular filtration. Because the degree of protein binding with individual antimicrobial agents varies among sera of different species, studies of protein binding for drugs used in humans can be performed only with human serum free of antimicrobial activity. The degree of protein binding of antimicrobial agents influences its partition among blood, interstitial tissue, and the site of infection, because the gradient of drug concentration is related to the amount of free agent in the serum.

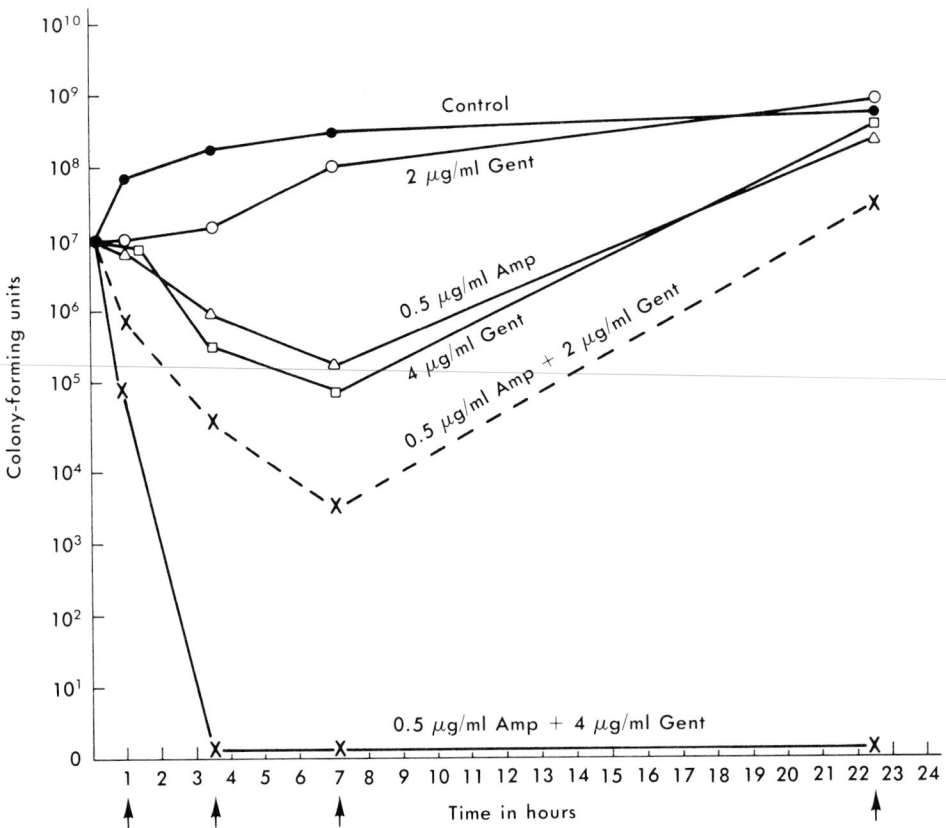

Figure 38–6. Test for antimicrobial synergism of ampicillin with gentamicin for Enterococcus faecalis *from a patient with endocarditis. See p. 537 for interpretation.*

The peak level of the drug at the site of infection rarely exceeds the peak level of free drug in the blood and usually reaches a maximum sometime later than the peak in the serum. The effective delivery of an antimicrobial agent to the site of an infection depends on the presence of an intact blood supply. The presence of necrosis with interruption of the capillary network (abscess) may inhibit this delivery and the diffusion of the agent, offering the invading microorganism protection from effective levels of the drug. Conversely, the active inflammatory process with vascular dilation and increased permeability can aid in the accumulation of agents at sites of infection (e.g., meningitis). Data from these experiments are summarized in Table 38–3, confirming *in vivo* the *in vitro* test results of protein binding for ampicillin and nafcillin.

ASSAY OF ANTIMICROBIAL AGENTS IN SERUM AND OTHER BODY FLUIDS

Occasionally, it is helpful to determine the total amount of antimicrobial agent in serum, cere-brospinal fluid, urine, or another clinical specimen. Requests to assay the total amount of an antimicrobial agent in serum are usually related to those drugs exerting a significant nephrotoxic or other toxic action, such as gentamicin. Assay for antimicrobial agents can be done by chemical, biologic, enzymatic, or immunologic procedures. Sulfonamide compounds are the only antimicrobial agents readily measured by chemical means.

TABLE 38–3. *Relationship between Binding to Protein and the Ratio of Antibiotics in Skin-Window Interstitial Fluid to Those in Serum*

Antibiotic	Skin-Window to Serum Ratio				Bound to Protein (%)
	1 hr	**2 hr**	**3 hr**	**4 hr**	
Ampicillin	—*	0.17	0.39	0.46	18–29
Penicillin G	0.093	0.174	0.209	0.212	59–65
Penicillin V	0.071	0.24	0.21	—	80
Nafcillin	0.016	0.035	0.045	0.042	89–90

(Modified from Tan, J. S., Trott, A., Phair, J. P., et al. A method for measurement of antibiotics in human interstitial fluid. *J. Infect. Dis.* 126:492, 1972.)

*No detectable antibiotic activities in the majority of skin-window fluid specimens.

The simplest and, in the past, most commonly used method for measuring antibiotic concentrations is a biologic assay based on the principle of inhibition of bacterial growth by various concentrations of test agent. A microorganism susceptible to the antibiotic to be assayed is incorporated in an agar culture plate. A series of small metal cups is placed on the surface of the agar and filled with measured amounts of the test specimen to be assayed. Because of the variation of protein binding and other factors that can influence the activity of antimicrobial agents, standard concentrations of the test agent are prepared in a medium similar to the test material but known to be free of antimicrobial activity (e.g., serum or cerebrospinal fluid). The known amounts of test agent, along with the clinical specimen to be tested, are then placed in similar metal cups. During incubation, the antimicrobial agent diffuses from the cup, resulting in a zone of growth inhibition proportional to the concentration of the test agent in the cup. Zones of inhibition for the reference standards are measured and plotted on semilogarithmic graph paper. The zone of inhibition surrounding the test specimen is then measured and the concentration of antimicrobial agent in the specimen is read from the curve. This procedure has been a standard method of measuring drug levels for many years and is known as the *cup-plate method.* Modifications of this procedure include the use of paper discs instead of metal cups, preincubated seed plates, and rapidly growing strains of microorganisms that yield

results within 4–6 h (Figs. 38–7 and 38–8). The accuracy of these biologic assays is approximately ±10%, well within the limits necessary for clinical usefulness.

Occasionally, the patient may be treated with several antimicrobial agents, but a serum level is needed for only one. It may be possible to inactivate some agents by adding enzymes such as penicillinase or cephalosporinase. When enzymatic inactivation is not practical, a test organism may be used that is sensitive only to the agent to be measured but resistant to all other antimicrobial agents, for example, a strain of *Staphylococcus epidermidis* resistant to all antimicrobial agents but gentamicin. The biologic assay for antimicrobial agents can best be applied to infrequently requested agents. The assay is inexpensive, not technically demanding, and relatively easy to adapt to most antimicrobial agents.

The development of competitive binding immunoassay procedures for aminoglycosides, such as gentamicin, offers another approach for assay of antimicrobial agents. Rapid and specific, the simplicity and ease of immunoassay have made it a popular method for measuring serum levels of gentamicin, tobramycin, amikacin, vancomycin, and other agents.

In addition to the biologic method and immunoassays for measurement of antibiotics, a number of other methods have been developed. Liquid chromatography has been adapted to the assay of a large variety of antimicrobial agents and is rapid and specific. Instrumentation can

Figure 38–7. Serum assay for gentamicin. Serum from the patient is placed on the center disc while control serum containing 1, 2, 4, and 5 μg/mL of gentamicin is placed peripherally. The zone of inhibition around each disc is measured after incubation. Owing to small differences in the size of zones, the test is run in quadruplicate and the mean zone plotted (see Fig. 38–8).

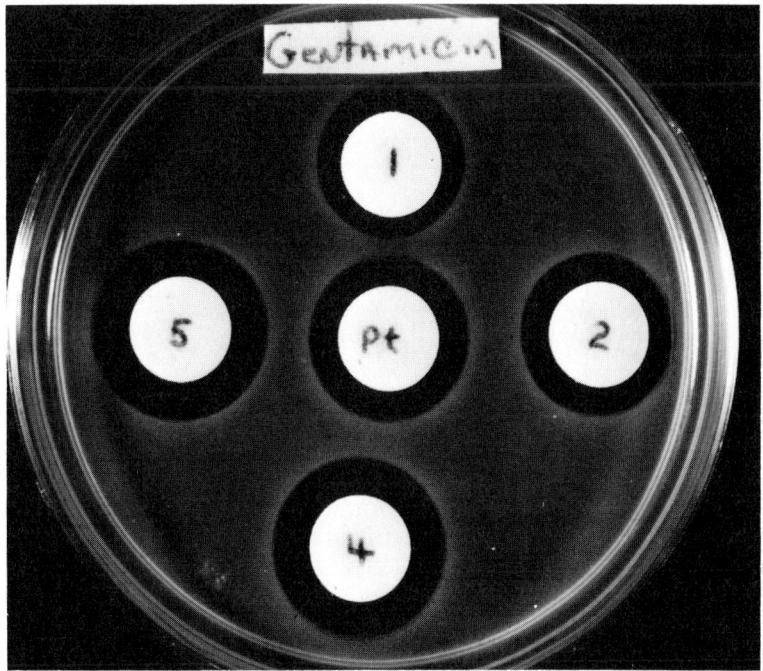

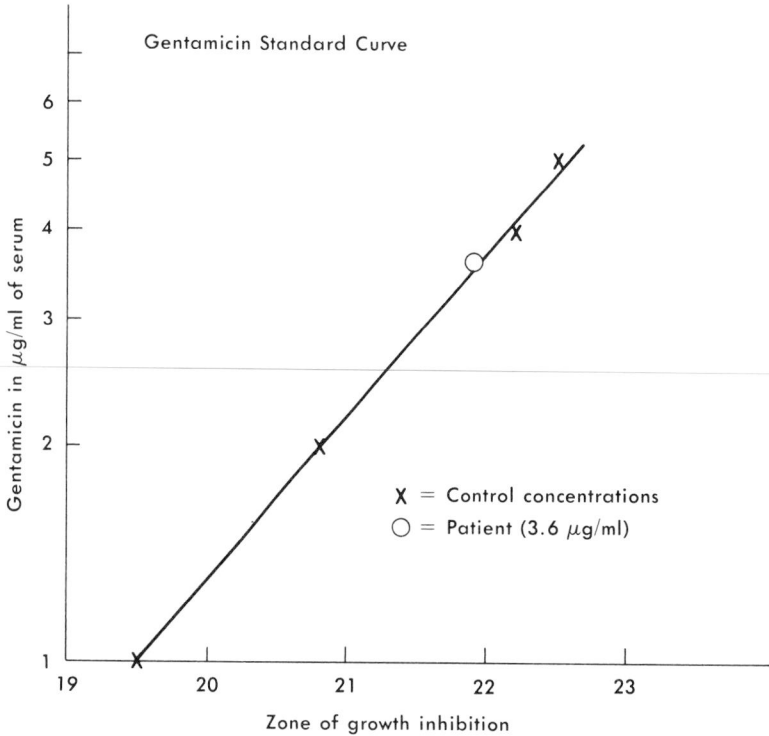

Gentamicin Standard Curve

X = Control concentrations
○ = Patient (3.6 μg/ml)

Figure 38–8. The mean inhibitory zones determined from quadruplicate control concentrations in serum are plotted to establish a standard curve. The test serum concentration is then read from this curve.

be expensive and requires special technical expertise, but once established, chromatographic assays are easily performed, are accurate, and can be internally standardized, thereby reducing costs and time per assay. Fluorescence polarization has been successfully applied to the assay of serum for antibiotics. Most assay procedures are directed toward vancomycin and the aminoglycoside antibiotics because of potential renal toxicity and ototoxicity.

DETERMINATION OF ANTIMICROBIAL ACTIVITY

The use of the assay procedures mentioned above for measuring the total amount of penicillin or other highly protein-bound antimicrobial agents in serum is usually inappropriate. Measurement of the actual free and protein-bound portions of antimicrobial agents is a research procedure. Whereas the determination of the serum concentration of the unbound portion of an antimicrobial agent may allow the physician to determine whether he has achieved a level consistent with the MIC for the infecting microorganism, the correlation of total serum levels of highly protein-bound agents with MICs may be grossly misleading. In addition to an antibiotic, there are numerous other antibacterial substances in the blood, including opsonins, specific antibody, lysozyme, beta-lysin, and other poorly defined components, that contribute to the total antimicrobial effect of the serum. For these reasons, the determination of serum levels of antimicrobial agents as a means of determining the adequacy of therapy is not always appropriate.

A more useful test to monitor patients with severe infection who are receiving antimicrobial therapy is to measure the inhibitory or lethal action of serial twofold dilutions of the patient's serum, CSF, urine, or other specimen against a standard inoculum of the microorganism causing the infection. This test is sometimes called the *bactericidal,* or *antimicrobial, activity test* since it can be used against both bacteria and fungi. The purpose of this test is to measure the net effect of all factors in the test specimen, such as serum or CSF, against the infecting microorganism.

Serum antimicrobial activity has been used most often to monitor the treatment of patients with infective endocarditis (see Chapter 35). Empirically, it has been found that serum bactericidal levels of 1:8 or greater are usually associated with favorable outcomes, whereas levels lower than 1:8 may be associated with less favorable results. The test is also useful in determining the effectiveness of therapy for

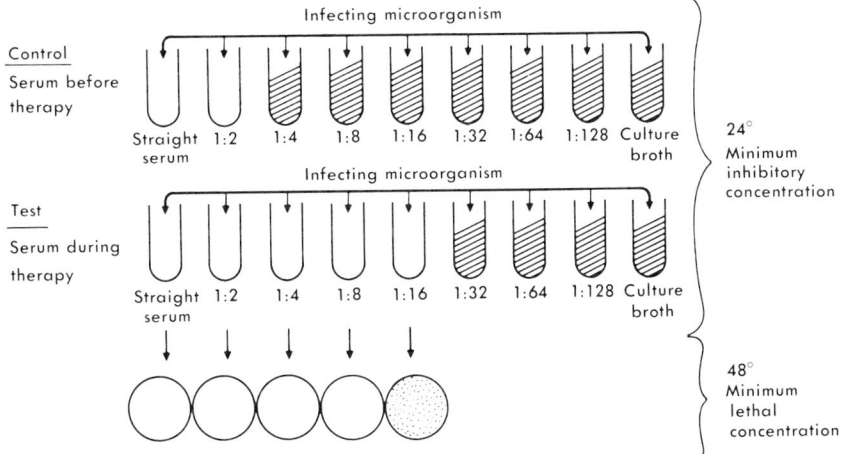

Figure 38–9. Serum antimicrobial activity. Principle*: The test determines the maximum dilution of serum that shows bacteriostatic or lethal activity against an infecting microorganism. Serum taken before and during antimicrobial therapy defines the* in vivo *effect of an agent against the infecting microorganism. (The test can also be used with cerebrospinal fluid, urine, or other types of clinical specimens.)* Interpretation*: Serum minimum inhibitory activity = 1:16; serum minimum lethal activity = 1:8.*

other types of infection. Response of patients with urinary tract infections also is directly correlated with the level of antimicrobial activity in the urine (see Chapter 17).

When performing the antimicrobial activity test, one should remember that normal serum contains antimicrobial substances and may have a lethal activity in dilutions of 1:4–1:6. To perform the test, one draws two serum samples—one within 30–60 min following the administration of the antimicrobial agent and another just prior to the dose. This provides a "peak" and a "trough" level, presumably reflecting the full therapeutic range. The test sera are diluted in human serum free of antimicrobial activity to compensate for protein binding. A standard number of the patient's microorganisms are added to the diluted sera, and the inhibitory levels are determined after 18–20 h of incubation. The serum lethal levels are determined 18–20 h later by subculture (Fig. 38–9).

It must be emphasized that serum assay and antimicrobial activity levels are not the only considerations when one is choosing an antimicrobial agent. The selection of any antimicrobial agent should be based on careful evaluation of the patient's needs and the characteristics of individual antimicrobial agents, but the significance of all factors should be carefully placed in perspective.

REFERENCES

Books

Anhalt, J. P. Special tests of antimicrobial activity. In: Washington, J. A., ed. *Laboratory Procedures in Clinical Microbiology*. New York: Springer-Verlag, 1981.

Grove, D. C., and Randall, W. A. *Assay Methods of Antibiotics. A Laboratory Manual*. New York: Medical Encyclopedia, 1955.

Koneman, E. W., Allen, S. D., Dowell, V. R., et al., eds. *Color Atlas and Textbook of Diagnostic Microbiology*. 2nd ed. (chapter on antibiotic susceptibility testing). Philadelphia: J. B. Lippincott Co., 1983.

Lorian, V., ed. *Antibiotics in Laboratory Medicine*. 2nd ed. Baltimore: Williams & Wilkins, 1986.

Sherris, J. C. Laboratory tests in chemotherapy. In: Lennette, E. H., et al., eds. *Manual of Clinical Microbiology*. 4th ed. Washington, D.C.: American Society for Microbiology, 1985.

Technical Manual

National Committee on Clinical Laboratory Standards. *Performance Standards for Antimicrobial Disc Susceptibility Tests. Approved Standard, M2-A3*. Villanova, PA: 1983.

Original Articles

Bauer, A. W., Kirby, W. M., and Sherris, J. C. Antibiotic susceptibility testing by a standardized single disc method. *Am. J. Clin. Pathol.* 45:493, 1966.

Dutcher, B. S., Reynard, A. M., Beck, M. E., et al. Potentiation of antibiotic bactericidal activity by normal human serum. *Antimicrob. Agents Chemother.* 13:820, 1978.

Eisenstein, B. I., Beachey, E. H., and Ofek, I. Influence of sublethal concentrations of antibiotics on the expression of the mannose-specific ligand of *Escherichia coli. Infect. Immun.* 28:154, 1980.

Jones, R. M. Antimicrobial susceptibility testing (AST): A review of changing trends, quality control guidelines, test accuracy and recommendations for the testing of β-lactam drugs. *Diagn. Microbiol. Infect. Dis. 1*:1, 1983.

Krogstad, D. J., Moellering, R. C., Jr. Antimicrobial combinations. In Lorian, V., ed. *Antibiotics in Laboratory Medicine*, 2nd ed. Baltimore: Williams & Wilkins, 1986.

Reller, L. B. The serium bactericidal test. *Rev. Inf. Dis.* 8:803, 1986.

Root, R. J., et al. Interaction between antibiotics and human neutrophils in the killing of staphylococci. *J. Clin. Invest.* 67:249, 1981.

Schlichter, J. G., and MacLenn, H. A method of determining the effective therapeutic level in the treatment of subacute bacterial endocarditis with penicillin. *Am. Heart J.* 34:209, 1947.

Thornsberry, C. Automated procedures for antimicrobial susceptibility tests. In Lennette, E. H., ed. *Manual of Clinical Microbiology*. Washington, D.C.: American Society of Microbiology, 1985:1015.

Vaisanen, V., Lounatmaa, K., and Korhonen, T. K. Effects of sublethal concentrations of antimicrobial agents on the hemagglutination, adhesion, and ultrastructure of pyelonephritogenic *Escherichia coli* strains. *Antimicrob. Agents Chemother.* 22:120, 1982.

Wolfson, J. S., and Swartz, M. N. Serum bactericidal activity as a monitor of antibiotic therapy. *N. Engl. J. Med.* 312:968, 1985.

39

STANFORD T. SHULMAN, M.D. • *JOHN P. PHAIR, M.D.*

Antimicrobial Therapy

INTRODUCTION

This chapter deals primarily with the treatment of bacterial infections, although drugs used in the systemic treatment of fungal and viral diseases are also discussed briefly.

An antimicrobial agent should be used when there is clinical or cultural evidence of infection and there are data indicating that treatment produces a shorter duration of discomfort or illness or a lower incidence of complications. Not all bacterial infections need specific treatment, such as minor skin infections or gastrointestinal salmonellosis, in which host defense mechanisms effect a cure. However, even these infections may require specific treatment if they occur in compromised hosts or if local or systemic complications develop.

`Unnecessary use of antibiotic agents should be avoided for several reasons, including side effects, allergic reactions, cost, effects upon endogenous normal flora, and induction of antibiotic resistance (relevant to the patient and to society as a whole). As with any medication the risk-benefit ratio should be favorable to justify use of an antibiotic.

INITIAL MICROBIOLOGIC EVALUATION

Some infections can be treated without Gram's stain or culture of the site of infection. In these instances the physician makes a diagnosis of infection at a particular site by clinical criteria and institutes *empiric* therapy based upon the most likely bacterial etiology (Table 39–1).

In contrast, efforts to make an accurate microbiologic diagnosis should be performed if the host is compromised and in serious or potentially serious infections, when the infecting bacterium and its susceptibility pattern cannot be predicted with a fair degree of accuracy. If a clinical specimen (e.g., exudate or CSF) can be examined directly, the correlation between bacteria seen on Gram's stain and the cause of the infection is excellent. When the exudate must pass through a normally colonized area before examination, as with expectorated sputum, the Gram's stain must be evaluated cautiously. Blood cultures should always be obtained when signs and symptoms suggest possible systemic spread of infection.

INTERPRETATION OF BACTERIAL CULTURE REPORTS

Potential limitations of culture reports include the possible contamination of the specimen with indigenous bacterial flora and consideration of the pathogenic potential of the isolated organism. Positive cultures from normally sterile fluids—such as blood, CSF, synovial fluid—should be considered accurate unless there is strong evidence to the contrary. Certain bacteria (e.g., *Streptococcus pneumoniae* and *Haemophilus influenzae*) are almost never contaminants at these sites, and Enterobacteriaceae are rarely contaminants. However, when normal flora, such as alpha streptococci, *Propionibacterium acnes*, or coagulase-negative staphylococci, are isolated, the clinical picture must be reviewed carefully. Specimens frequently contaminated by normal flora of the sample site or of a contiguous site are more difficult to evaluate, including wound and sputum specimens. Culture results must be correlated with clinical evidence to decide whether the isolated bacteria are indeed pathogens.

CORRELATION BETWEEN RESULTS OF ANTIBACTERIAL SUSCEPTIBILITY TESTING AND CURE OF INFECTION

The designation of a bacterium as *susceptible* or *resistant* to a particular antibacterial agent relates to an amount of the drug that corresponds to achievable serum concentration with ordinary dosage. The assumption is made that a similar level of antibacterial activity is achievable at the site of infection. Whether this actually occurs depends on dosage level, pharmacologic properties of the individual drug, site of infection and host factors (see below and Chapter 38).

With these limitations, data correlation between *in vitro* susceptibility and eradication of infection in patients is surprisingly good, although there are exceptions; for example, systemic *Salmonella* infections do not respond uniformly to antibiotics other than chloramphenicol, ampicillin, quinolones, or trimethoprim-sulfamethoxazole, although salmonellae are susceptible *in vitro* to other agents, including aminoglycosides. Because of the critical role of host defenses in recovery, the use of an appropriate antibacterial agent does not always lead to clinical cure.

The terms *bactericidal* and *bacteriostatic* are best defined in terms of the activity of an antibacterial agent *in vitro*, and *in vitro* results cannot be directly translated to clinical effectiveness (see Chapter 38). For example, in endocarditis bactericidal activity is necessary for eradication of infection, but in meningitis bacteriostatic agents may be curative.

TABLE 39–1. *Most Frequent Causes of Infection at Selected Body Sites and Suggested Initial Antimicrobial Treatment**

Site	Microorganism(s)	Antimicrobial Agents
Upper Respiratory Tract and Oropharyngeal Infections		
Tonsillitis and pharyngitis	*Streptococcus pyogenes*	Penicillin
Sinusitis and otitis		
Acute		
Adults	*S. pneumoniae* or *S. pyogenes*	Penicillin
		Penicillin
Children <12 years	*Haemophilus influenzae*	Ampicillin or ampicillin/clavulanic acid
Chronic	*S. pneumoniae*, *S. pyogenes*, plus oropharyngeal anaerobes	Penicillin
Epiglottitis	*H. influenzae*	Ampicillin/chloramphenicol or ceftriaxone
Lower Respiratory Tract Infections		
Pneumonia and bronchitis		
Adults	*S. pneumoniae* or anaerobes from oropharynx	Penicillin
	Legionella pneumophila	Erythromycin
Young adults	*Mycoplasma pneumoniae*	Erythromycin or tetracycline
Children <6 years and adults with chronic lung disease	*H. influenzae*	Ampicillin/chloramphenicol or cefuroxime
Cardiovascular Infections		
Endocarditis	Streptococci, enterococci, or	Penicillin with or without aminoglycoside
	Staphylococcus aureus	Penicillinase-resistant penicillin
Postoperative endocarditis (immediate postoperative period)	*S. aureus* or coagulase-negative staphylococcus or diphtheroids	Vancomycin plus aminoglycoside
Gastrointestinal Infections		
Salmonellosis†		
Adults	*Salmonella* sp.	Quinolones
Children		Trimethoprim-sulfamethoxazole
Shigellosis		
Adults	*Shigella* sp.	Quinolones
Children		Trimethoprim-sulfamethoxazole
Infections (abscess, peritonitis, etc.) originating from gastrointestinal, biliary, or female genital tract	Facultative gram-negative enteric bacilli plus anaerobes from gastrointestinal tract	Cefoxitin, imipenem, or aminoglycoside *plus* clindamycin or metronidazole
Genital Infections		
Syphilis	*Treponema pallidum*	Penicillin
Gonorrhea	*Neisseria gonorrhoeae*	Ceftriaxone
Nongonococcal urethritis or pelvic inflammatory disease	*Chlamydia* sp.	Tetracycline
Central Nervous System Infections		
Meningitis		
Adults	*N. meningitidis* or *S. pneumoniae*	Penicillin
Children <6 years	Above two organisms or *H. influenzae*	Third-generation cephalosporin or ampicillin and chloramphenicol
Brain abscess	Anaerobes	Penicillin and/or metronidazole
Bone Infections		
Osteomyelitis	*S. aureus*	Penicillinase-resistant penicillin or cephalosporin
Joint Infections		
Adults	*N. gonorrhoeae*	Penicillin or ceftriaxone
	or *S. aureus*	Penicillinase-resistant penicillin
Children <6 years	*S. aureus* or *H. influenzae*	Chloramphenicol/ampicillin or cefuroxime
Skin Infections	*S. aureus*	Penicillinase-resistant penicillin or first-generation cephalosporin
	S. pyogenes	Penicillin

Table continued on following page

TABLE 39–1. *Most Frequent Causes of Infection at Selected Body Sites and Suggested Initial Antimicrobial Treatment** Continued

Site	Microorganism(s)	Antimicrobial Agents
Urinary Tract Infections and Prostatitis		
Simple	Facultative enteric gram-negative bacilli	Sulfonamide, ampicillin, trimethoprim-sulfamethoxazole. Aminoglycoside (if sepsis suspected)
Complicated‡		Trimethoprim-sulfamethoxazole, aminoglycoside, or quinolone
Blood Infections		
Presumed gram-negative bacteremia	Facultative enteric gram-negative bacilli or *Pseudomonas aeruginosa*	Aminoglycoside.§ Extended-spectrum cephalosporin in children or in those with compromised renal function
Presumed gram-positive bacteremia	*S. aureus* or penicillin-susceptible streptococci and pneumococci	Penicillinase-resistant penicillin, or first-generation cephalosporin, or vancomycin

*Prior antimicrobial therapy or hospital acquisition of infection may alter expected organism or antimicrobial susceptibility or both. The bacterial etiology of infections in newborn infants is not considered here. Drug allergy may necessitate alternative therapy.

†Antimicrobial treatment generally not required for disease limited to gastrointestinal tract except in the elderly and the very young.

‡By anatomic or neurogenic obstruction or multiple previous episodes or nosocomial acquisition.

§In the treatment of patients with severe granulocytopenia, an extended-spectrum penicillin active against *P. aeruginosa* should be added.

CHOICE OF ANTIBACTERIAL AGENT AND TREATMENT COURSE

The optimal antibacterial agent for treatment of an infection is one with the narrowest possible spectrum of antibacterial activity (including the infecting bacterium, of course), the fewest side effects, and the lowest toxicity. The agent should be administered in a dosage form by a schedule that achieves an antibacterial level at the site of infection at least equal to (preferably, several times higher than) the level of that agent required to inhibit bacterial growth *in vitro*.

When, as often happens, therapy for a bacterial infection is begun empirically prior to identification of the causative organism, the choice of an agent is based on the following: (1) the bacteria most likely to cause the particular infection (Table 39–1), (2) the bacteria presumptively identified by Gram's stain of exudate, (3) predicted susceptibility of the organism, (4) pharmacologic properties of the antibacterial agents, (5) cost, and (6) knowledge that the agent chosen has been successful in treating similar infections. Accurate clinical diagnosis of the site and extent of infection is a critical initial step.

The host's immune status clearly influences the likelihood that serious infection may occur, the likely organisms, and the course of the infection (see Chapter 3). The generally poorer results of treatment of infection in compromised hosts reflects not less activity by the antibacterial agent but rather the limited contribution of the host defenses.

Allergy to Antibacterial Agents

Although allergic manifestations do not invariably recur on readministration of a drug to which a patient has demonstrated allergy, such history should be considered a contraindication to treatment with an antibiotic. Anaphylactic-type hypersensitivity reactions are a particularly important type of drug allergy. Effective alternative antibiotics are available for virtually all infections (Table 39–2). Rarely, a life-threatening infection that is very difficult to treat with an alternative agent may require administration of an antibacterial agent to which the patient is allergic. One example is enterococcal endocarditis in a patient with penicillin allergy. In this situation the patient may undergo desensitization so that penicillin is tolerated.

TABLE 39–2. *Alternatives to Penicillin for the Penicillin-Allergic Patient*

Bacteria	Antibacterial Agent
Streptococci, including *S. pneumoniae*, but excluding enterococci	Erythromcyin
Enterococci	Vancomycin
Staphylococcus aureus	Cephalosporin, clindamycin, vancomycin
Anaerobic bacteria	Clindamycin, metronidazole
Neisseria meningitidis	Chloramphenicol
N. gonorrhoeae	Spectinomycin (genital disease)
	Tetracycline (systemic or articular disease)
Treponema pallidum	Erythromycin, tetracycline

Treatment with More Than One Antibacterial Agent

The indications for using more than one agent in the treatment of a single infection are somewhat limited. The most frequent situations include: (1) treatment of infection due to more than one organism, if the organisms are not susceptible to the same drug; (2) presumptive treatment of life-threatening infection when the causative bacterium is unknown; (3) treatment of difficult organisms for which synergism of agents has been demonstrated or is postulated; (4) prevention of emergence of resistance to antibiotics. This last indication is particularly important in the chemotherapy of tuberculosis. The treatment of gram-negative sepsis in patients with severe granulocytopenia with a combination of an aminoglycoside and an extended-spectrum penicillin is an example of indication 3, whereas combination therapy for fever and neutropenia relates to indication 2.

Colonization and Superinfection

Antibiotic therapy leads to alteration in colonizing flora, with antibiotic-resistant bacteria and fungi becoming more dominant. Gram-positive flora tend to be replaced by gram-negative organisms as the colonizing surface flora. In contrast to this *colonization*, the term *superinfection* refers to a second clinical infection that occurs during or after an earlier course of therapy.

Although colonization occurs to some extent in everyone treated with antibiotics, clinical superinfection is unusual in treated outpatients, with the exception of superficial *Candida* infection. In contrast, superinfection is quite frequent in hospitalized patients with severe infections and in patients with granulocytopenia or other host defense impairment.

Follow-Up Treatment of Infection

Most patients with infection are best followed clinically rather than bacteriologically. Repeated cultures are usually unnecessary if the patient has a good therapeutic response, as in uncomplicated pneumonia. However, if the infection is one for which bacteriologic cure (eradication of the causative agent) is known to be difficult, follow-up cultures are indicated. Examples are the treatment of endocarditis and infections treated with a drug with less than optimal efficacy against the infecting bacterium.

The appropriate duration of antibacterial treatment is defined as the shortest period necessary to prevent bacteriologic or clinical relapse, that is, to produce a cure. The duration of treatment varies with the site and extent of infection, the bacterium, and the host response. A standard duration of treatment is established for reliable cure of some infections, such as streptococcal pharyngitis, but has not been rigorously determined for many other infections. Occasionally, assessing the optimal duration of treatment is complicated by difficulty in determining the exact site of infection by routine means. For example, cystitis requires a shorter course of treatment for bacteriologic cure than do renal infections, but it is often difficult to determine the exact site of a urinary tract infection.

Failure of Antibacterial Treatment

When a patient appears not to respond to antibacterial treatment, it must be determined whether true antibacterial failure has occurred. Treatment may be considered unsuccessful prematurely if the physician is unfamiliar with the expected rate of clinical and bacteriologic response of a particular infection to effective therapy. A common error is to focus on a single clinical sign, such as fever, rather than to consider the patient's overall response. Bacteriologic failure is the persistence of a bacterium beyond its expected time of clearance and is usually accompanied by clinical failure to respond.

When review of the clinical and bacteriologic findings indicates that the patient has not improved, it is important to determine whether antibacterial treatment was actually indicated for the illness by reexamining the initial diagnosis and subsequent confirmatory data. Of course, antibiotics cannot be expected to affect nonbacterial diseases. If antibacterial therapy had been indicated, details of the regimen should be examined, such as susceptibility of the bacterium, dosage, route of administration, interval between doses, possible drug incompatibilities, and penetration of the drug to the site of infection. When there is a closed collection of inflammatory fluid (e.g., an abscess), drainage is more important than antibacterial treatment in resolving the infection. Among the most common reasons for antibacterial treatment failure, and the most difficult to correct, are deficiencies in specific host defense mechanisms as well as more general host problems, such as poor nutrition, inability to clear respiratory secretions, and poor tissue perfusion. Development of drug resistance by an initially susceptible bacterium during treatment is uncommon.

Occasionally, complications of antibacterial therapy are superimposed on the acute bacterial illness and are difficult to distinguish from antibacterial failure. The antibacterial agent itself may be the cause of symptoms, particularly allergic symptoms or drug fever. Penicillin allergy is more frequent than recurrent disease as a cause of recurrent fever in patients treated for pneumococcal pneumonia. Superinfection with another microbe may cause persistent or recurrent symptoms during antibacterial treatment. In the hospital, the most frequent sites for superinfection are the urinary tract (particularly in catheterized patients), the lower respiratory tract, and intravenous sites (phlebitis). (See Chapter 28.)

Cost of Antibacterial Treatment

Some newer antibiotics are among the most costly drugs. Frequently, any of several agents could be used for treatment of a given infection, with approximately the same efficacy and risk. Table 39–3 illustrates the widely differing costs of several oral agents commonly used for treatment of urinary tract infection.

In the hospital, the cost of an antibacterial agent is further increased by the cost of drug administration. A large private metropolitan hospital uses the following formula to calculate patient charges for intravenous antibiotic administration: cost of drug to hospital × 2.8 (mark-up) + $28.50 administration fee × doses/day. Thus, each day of an intravenous antibiotic costing only $5 per dose and given every 6 h costs the patient $170. Most antibiotics are substantially more expensive, resulting in much higher patient costs. Those agents that require monitoring of serum drug levels or periodic renal or hepatic function testing have those added costs. Use of the intramuscular or oral route of administration rather than the intravenous route, and use of drugs permitting longer dosage intervals may result in lower costs.

ANTIBACTERIAL PROPHYLAXIS

Use of antibacterial agents to prevent infection is termed *antibiotic prophylaxis*. Prophylaxis is most efficacious when attempting to prevent infection by a single bacterium for a relatively brief period, and it is least effective in attempting to prevent infections in an immunologically compromised host. Penicillin G has been proved to prevent infection by group A streptococci and recurrence of rheumatic fever in persons with history of rheumatic fever (see Chapter 9). Another well-established, but not proven, indication for antibacterial prophylaxis is prevention of infective endocarditis by administration of antibiotics to patients with cardiac valvular disease before specific medical, surgical, or dental procedures (see Chapter 35).

The administration of antibiotics to prevent postoperative wound infections is now well accepted. There is good evidence that prophylaxis reduces postoperative wound infection rates after procedures involving areas that are heavily contaminated with bacteria, such as head and neck, gynecologic, and colonic surgery. The evidence that antibiotics prevent wound infections is less compelling for clean procedures in less heavily contaminated areas. Factors such as long duration of surgery or placement of a foreign body such as a prosthetic device (hip joint, cardiac valve) are associated with unacceptable infections which are difficult to treat

TABLE 39–3. *Comparative Drug Costs for a 10-Day Course of Oral Therapy for Urinary Tract Infection*

Antibacterial Agent	Dose	Cost* ($)
Ampicillin	250 mg q 6 h	3.25
Carbenicillin	2 tab q 6 h†	111.75
Cephalexin	250 mg q 6 h	41.25 (generic = 20.00)
Ciprofloxacin	750 mg q 12 h	91.15
Sulfamethoxazole	1 g q 12 h	7.50 (generic = 3.30)
Trimethoprim-sulfamethoxazole	1 DS tab q 12 h	17.10 (generic = 3.00)
Tetracycline	250 mg q 6 h	1.05

*Average wholesale price
†Recommended dose for *P. aeruginosa* infections.

and, therefore, warrant use of prophylactic antibiotics. When antibacterial prophylaxis is used, a single agent active against the bacteria most frequently isolated from postoperative infections at that site should be employed. The risk of contamination of a wound occurs as the operation begins. Therefore, administration of an antibacterial agent must be initiated immediately before the operation, and an effective blood and tissue level must be maintained during the procedure. Generally, prolonged administration of prophylactic antibiotics beyond 8–12 h is associated with an increased incidence of adverse effects, as well as with colonization and infection due to antibiotic-resistant organisms. In specific situations, such as cardiac surgery or placement of an orthopedic prosthesis, however, prophylactic antibiotics are frequently continued for 2–5 days.

CLINICAL PHARMACOLOGY OF ANTIMICROBIAL AGENTS

Absorption

Many antimicrobial agents are absorbed very well after oral administration. Others are either so poorly absorbed (e.g., vancomycin, aminoglycosides) or so rapidly degraded in the intestinal tract that they must be administered parenterally to treat systemic infection. With few exceptions, antimicrobial agents are only partially absorbed after oral administration, and serum concentrations are much lower after oral than after identical parenteral dosing. Major exceptions are chloramphenicol and metronidazole, which reach serum levels that are as high or higher after oral administration as after intravenous infusion. The serum concentrations achieved by the usual oral doses of such agents as ampicillin, the cephalosporins, and the tetracyclines are generally not high enough to inhibit the gram-negative enteric bacilli that are susceptible to these drugs. However, preparations of these agents are useful for enterobacterial infections when urinary antibacterial activity alone is sufficient because they are concentrated in urine.

In hospitalized patients with severe infection, antimicrobial therapy generally should be administered parenterally because inadequate intestinal absorption can then be excluded as a cause if there is a subsequent failure to respond to therapy.

Distribution

After absorption from the intestine or parenteral site, antimicrobial agents are bound by plasma proteins to varying degrees. The initial rapid rise in blood concentration soon after intravenous administration and more slowly after intramuscular or oral administration is followed by a decrease as the drug is distributed to body tissues. The subsequent rate of decline relates to excretion and inactivation. The most frequently used measure of this decline is the serum half-life (the time required for a 50% decrease in serum concentration), a measure of the duration of pharmacologic effect. Serum half-life is an important determinant of dosage interval, both for normal patients and for those in whom the half-life is prolonged because of decreased drug excretion or metabolism.

The extravascular concentration of an antibiotic depends on the degree of protein binding, the concentration gradient from blood to tissue fluid, and the drug diffusibility. Diffusibility is affected by molecular size, dissociation constant, and lipid solubility of the drug. Lipid solubility of certain antimicrobial agents accounts for their penetration into those body compartments into which water-soluble agents penetrate poorly. Most antibiotics penetrate well into pleural, peritoneal, pericardial, and synovial fluids. Penetration into the brain, CSF, eye, placenta, and prostatic fluid is more variable. In general, penetration of a body compartment increases in the presence of inflammation. For example, penicillins enter the CSF much more readily in inflammatory states.

Inactivation and Excretion

Several mechanisms of excretion and inactivation of antimicrobial agents exist. An antibiotic may be secreted into bile, removed by the kidney, inactivated by the liver, or inactivated by other, unknown means. A single agent may be handled by more than one of these mechanisms. Inactivation of a few antimicrobials by a secondary means occurs when primary inactivation or excretion does not occur because of organ failure.

Renal excretion is the major means of clearance of most antimicrobials. Chloramphenicol, erythromycin, clindamycin, doxycycline, ceftazidime and metronidazole are the major exceptions. Some agents are at least partially inactivated by the liver. Renal failure results in accumulation of antimicrobials normally excreted by the kidney, and hepatic failure causes accumulation of drugs inactivated primarily by that organ unless the dose is reduced. Renal function decreases with aging, renal clearance being about one third less in the elderly, a degree of impairment not apparent by routine renal function tests. Dosage adjustment is essential for agents, such as the aminoglycosides or vancomycin, which have a low therapeutic-toxic ratio (ratio of the concentration of the agent required to inhibit an infecting microorganism and the concentration at which toxic reactions occur) and a single means of excretion or inactivation.

Many antimicrobial agents are secreted into bile, and a few (e.g., erythromycin, tetracycline, and some cephalosporins) reach high concentration. However, biliary secretion is generally reduced by the obstructive processes that almost always precede or accompany biliary tract infection.

CLASSES OF ANTIMICROBIAL AGENTS

The following discussion of antimicrobials is an introduction to their use in the treatment of common infectious diseases, those that an American physician is likely to encounter in practice. Only more frequent and serious side effects and toxicities are noted.

Penicillins

Penicillin G and its semisynthetic derivatives constitute the single most useful class of antimicrobial agents because of their high therapeutic-toxic ratio. The penicillins are discussed here in groups based on their antibacterial spectra.

Penicillins G and V

Penicillin G and V are active against some bacteria at low concentrations and against others at significantly higher concentrations. The very susceptible group of bacteria includes most aerobic and anaerobic gram-positive streptococci but not staphylococci. *Neisseria meningitidis, Treponema pallidum,* and many anaerobic gram-positive and gram-negative bacilli, other than *Bacteroides fragilis,* are also very susceptible. The less susceptible group of bacteria includes many strains of enterococci, *Listeria*

monocytogenes, Neisseria gonorrhoeae, Proteus mirabilis, and *H. influenzae.*

Preparations. The most common parenteral penicillins, in order of increasing half-life and decreasing peak serum concentrations, are aqueous crystalline, aqueous procaine, and benzathine (Bicillin) penicillin G. Oral preparations include potassium penicillin G and penicillin V. Penicillin V is a more acid-stable analogue of penicillin G that is better absorbed orally; its antibacterial activity is similar to that of penicillin G.

The level of penicillin G or V achieved after oral dosage or by intramuscular aqueous procaine penicillin G is adequate for treatment of most infections due to the very susceptible bacteria listed. Benzathine penicillin G is used for treatment (and prevention) of infections such as streptococcal pharyngitis, in which the low but sustained concentration of penicillin achieved by a single injection is sufficient. Certain infections, such as endocarditis and meningitis—as well as most infections caused by the less penicillin-susceptible group of bacteria—require the higher penicillin concentrations attainable by crystalline penicillin G or, as in the case of gonococcal infection, an unusually high dose of procaine penicillin. Crystalline penicillin G is usually combined with an aminoglycoside in treating systemic enterococcal infection.

Distribution, Inactivation, and Excretion. The concentration of penicillins in body fluids and tissues is usually measured in the presence of inflammation, and at appropriate dosages these concentrations are adequate in most tissues. The penicillins do not enter the CSF well in the absence of inflammation, but they penetrate well enough in its presence that therapeutic CSF levels are achieved at high dosages.

Most of a dose of penicillin G is rapidly eliminated by the kidney, primarily by tubular excretion. The serum level is raised and the half-life prolonged by renal failure or by the administration of probenecid (Benemid), which partially blocks tubular secretion of penicillin.

Side Effects and Toxicity. Penicillin G is relatively nontoxic; interstitial nephritis occurs rarely. Neurotoxicity occurs rarely in patients with renal failure given inappropriately high intravenous doses.

Allergy to penicillin is frequent. It is estimated that 5–7% of the general population claims to be allergic to penicillin. A pruritic, erythematous rash occurring after several days of therapy is by far the most frequent allergic manifestation. Other manifestations of hypersensitivity (drug fever, serum sickness, and immediate hypersensitivity reactions such as anaphylaxis, angioedema, and urticaria) occur less frequently. An individual allergic to one penicillin should be presumed to be allergic to other penicillins. Cross-allergenicity between penicillins and cephalosporins is such that 10% of those with penicillin allergy do not tolerate cephalosporins. Alternatives to penicillin G for treatment of specific infections are listed in Table 39–3.

Indications. Penicillin G is the preferred antimicrobial agent for treatment of infections by very susceptible organisms (see above).

Penicillinase-Resistant Penicillins

These semisynthetic penicillins are active against penicillinase-producing staphylococci. They are also active, although less so than penicillin G, against most other aerobic gram-positive cocci, except enterococci. The activity of penicillinase-resistant penicillins against bacteria other than gram-positive cocci is significantly less than that of penicillin G.

Preparations. Several penicillinase-resistant penicillins are available. Despite significant pharmacologic differences, these drugs are of essentially equal efficacy at equivalent dosage. Methicillin (Staphcillin) is not absorbed orally, and is available only parenterally. Nafcillin (Unipen), cloxacillin (Tegopen), and oxacillin (Prostaphlin) are available in both parenteral and oral forms. Dicloxacillin (Dynapen) is available only as an oral preparation. Cloxacillin or dicloxacillin is preferred for oral use because the other preparations are less reliably absorbed.

Inactivation and Excretion. Most of an absorbed dose of a penicillinase-resistant penicillin is excreted unchanged by the kidney, primarily by tubular secretion, with a small amount secreted in bile. Some inactivation occurs, probably in the liver. Oxacillin is the agent in this group most readily inactivated by extrarenal mechanisms.

Side Effects and Toxicity. Mild gastrointestinal symptoms occasionally occur with oral therapy. Abnormal liver function tests and reversible granulocytopenia occur occasionally.

Interstitial nephritis occurs more rarely. Allergic reactions are similar to those seen with penicillin G.

Indications. The penicillinase-resistant penicillins are preferred for treatment of staphylococcal infections because of their excellent activity, low toxicity, and relatively narrow antibacterial spectrum.

Extended-Spectrum Penicillins

This class of semisynthetic penicillins includes two groups of penicillins with activity against many gram-negative bacteria at an ordinary dosage level, but they are not active against penicillinase-producing staphylococci.

Ampicillin and Amoxicillin. Ampicillin and amoxicillin have activity similar to that of penicillin G against other aerobic gram-positive cocci and anaerobic bacteria. These drugs have generally good activity against *N. meningitidis*, many *H. influenzae*, most strains of *P. mirabilis* and *Salmonella*, many strains of *Escherichia coli*, and some strains of *Shigella*. Beta-lactamase-producing *H. influenzae* represent up to 25% of the isolates in many areas, and their recognition has changed the initial presumptive treatment of life-threatening *H. influenzae* infection. These agents have relatively little activity against other common gram-negative bacteria (e.g., *Klebsiella* and *Pseudomonas*). Amoxicillin is somewhat less active *in vitro* than ampicillin against *Shigella*. Its major advantage over ampicillin is better oral absorption and less drug-related diarrhea.

PREPARATIONS. Ampicillin is available for oral, intravenous, and intramuscular use. In the United States amoxicillin is available for oral use only. The concentration of these agents required to inhibit susceptible Enterobacteriaceae, with the possible exception of *P. mirabilis* strains, is generally higher than the peak concentrations achieved by standard oral dosage. Thus, oral ampicillin and amoxicillin are useful for gram-negative enteric infections primarily localized to the urinary tract.

INACTIVATION AND EXCRETION. These semisynthetic penicillins are partially (about 50%) inactivated, primarily in the liver, and partially secreted as active antibacterial agents in the urine.

SIDE EFFECTS AND TOXICITY. Diarrhea is frequent but does not usually require cessation of treatment. Significant toxicity due to ampicillin and amoxicillin is rare. Reversible hematologic and liver function test abnormalities have been reported. Rash suggestive of an allergic reaction is a frequent problem with ampicillin and amoxicillin, and other allergic reactions may occur.

INDICATIONS. Ampicillin and amoxicillin are ordinarily the preferred drugs for treatment of infections due to susceptible gram-negative bacilli.

Carbenicillin, Ticarcillin, Mezlocillin, Piperacillin, and Azlocillin. Carbenicillin (Geopen), ticarcillin (Ticar), mezlocillin (Mezlin), piperacillin (Pipracil), and azlocillin (Azlin) are active (but less so than ampicillin) against ampicillin-susceptible gram-positive bacteria. Exceptions are enterococci, which are susceptible to mezlocillin, piperacillin, and azlocillin but resistant to carbenicillin and ticarcillin. Penicillinase-producing *Staphylococcus aureus* is resistant to all these agents. In addition, these antibiotics are active against many strains of *Pseudomonas aeruginosa, Proteus,* and some *Enterobacter* and *Serratia.* They are generally active against *B. fragilis* as well as against ampicillin-sensitive anaerobes.

Clavulanic acid, an effective inhibitor of beta-lactamases, has been combined with amoxicillin (Augmentin) and with ticarcillin (Timentin). Although plasmid-mediated beta-lactamases are bound by clavulanic acid, chromosomally mediated, inducible enzymes, such as those produced by *P. aeruginosa,* are not.

PHARMACOLOGY AND PREPARATIONS. Even though the protein-binding of these penicillins is somewhat variable, their half-lives and achievable serum concentrations with a given dose are similar within the group. These penicillins are available as sodium salts to be administered intramuscularly or intravenously, but the high concentration required for inhibition of susceptible gram-negative bacteria, especially *P. aeruginosa,* generally restricts them to the intravenous route. Carbenicillin is available as the sodium indanyl salt for oral use (Geopen), and it is useful only for treatment of urinary tract infection because the high concentration required for inhibition of susceptible gram-negative bacilli cannot be reached in the serum.

INACTIVATION AND EXCRETION. These penicillins are excreted primarily unchanged in the urine, although some inactivation occurs in the liver.

SIDE EFFECTS AND TOXICITY. Administration of these penicillins is occasionally associated with a dose-related bleeding disorder. Reversible neutropenia has been reported rarely. The sodium content of these drugs may contribute to sodium overload in patients receiving large dosages. Similarly, if electrolytes are not monitored, hypokalemia can occur with large dosages, presumably because the penicillin acts as a nonreabsorbable anion, leading to increased excretion of potassium. These electrolyte effects may be less common with mezlocillin, piperacillin, and azlocillin because their 1–2 mEq/g sodium content is less than the 5–6 mEq/g sodium content of carbenicillin and ticarcillin. Allergic reactions are similar to those observed with other penicillins.

INDICATIONS. These penicillins are used for the treatment of *P. aeruginosa* infections, gram-negative enteric infections not susceptible to ampicillin, and infections due to *B. fragilis.* Because *P. aeruginosa* causes a significant minority of infections in granulocytopenic patients, these agents have found wide use in combination with an aminoglycoside for the febrile, granulocytopenic patient.

Cephalosporins

The cephalosporins are semisynthetic antibiotics active against gram-positive cocci, including penicillinase-producing *S. aureus* (but not methicillin-resistant *S. aureus*) and against many gram-negative bacilli. Enterococci are not included in the cephalosporin spectrum.

First-Generation Cephalosporins

The spectrum of activity of the *first-generation cephalosporins* includes most of the gram-positive bacteria susceptible to penicillin G as well as penicillinase-producing *S. aureus* and *S. epidermidis.* Among gram-negative bacteria, some strains of *E. coli, Klebsiella pneumoniae,* and *P. mirabilis* are susceptible. *P. aeruginosa* is resistant. The parenteral preparations include cephalothin (Keflin), cefazolin (Ancef, Kefzol), and cephapirin (Cefadyl). The oral preparations include cephalexin (Keflex), cephradine (Anspor, Velosef), and cefadroxil (Duricef). The first-generation cephalosporins have better activity against gram-positive bacteria than do other cephalosporins.

Second-Generation Cephalosporins

Cefoxitin (Mefoxin), cefuroxime (Zinacef), cefonicid (Monocid), ceforanide (Precef), and the oral preparation cefaclor (Ceclor) are called *second-generation cephalosporins* because they have a somewhat wider range of activity against gram-negative bacteria compared with the first-generation agents. The second-generation cephalosporins differ among themselves in pharmacologic properties. They have about the same level of activity as the earlier cephalosporins against the gram-negative enteric genera that are susceptible to the first-generation drugs. All have good activity against *H. influenzae*. Cefoxitin is often active against *Proteus* species. Gram-positive anaerobes (excluding *Clostridium difficile*) are generally susceptible to the second-generation cephalosporins, but *B. fragilis* is susceptible only to cefoxitin.

Third-Generation Cephalosporins

Those cephalosporins with at least some activity against *P. aeruginosa* are the *third-generation cephalosporins*. In this group are cefotaxime (Claforan), ceftizoxime (Cefizox), cefoperazone (Cefobid), ceftriaxone (Rocephin) and ceftazidime (Fortaz, Tazidime). The third-generation cephalosporins have increased activity *in vitro* against gram-negative enteric bacilli. Ceftazidime has the best *in vitro* activity against *P. aeruginosa* and is the only cephalosporin with activity similar to that of the extended-spectrum penicillins against this bacterium. Ceftriaxone has relatively poor activity against *B. fragilis*; the activity of the other third-generation cephalosporins against *B. fragilis* is similar to that of cefoxitin, a second-generation cephalosporin.

Pharmacology and Preparations

Half-life, protein binding, and volume of distribution vary considerably among the cephalosporins. Consequently, the appropriate doses and dosage intervals differ considerably. The parenteral cephalosporins are usually used intravenously because of the large doses required for treatment of systemic infections. Those agents with longer half-lives such as ceftriaxone may be given intramuscularly for relatively susceptible infections. Oral cephalosporins, in ordinary dosages, reach therapeutic levels in the serum against susceptible gram-negative bacteria only transiently, if at all. Thus, they are useful against gram-negative bacteria only in the treatment of urinary tract infections, although they are useful in pulmonary and soft tissue infections due to gram-positive bacteria.

Distribution, Inactivation, and Excretion

The cephalosporins are widely distributed to body tissues and fluids. Penetration into the CSF in amounts sufficient for treatment of meningitis occurs only with the third-generation cephalosporins.

The cephalosporins are primarily excreted unchanged in the urine. Cephalothin, cephapirin, and cefotaxime also undergo significant inactivation in the liver. Some cephalosporins are secreted into the bile.

Side Effects and Toxicity

Particularly with the parenteral cephalosporins, eosinophilia is relatively common, as is a positive direct Coombs' test, only rarely associated with hemolytic anemia. Other hematologic and transient liver-function test abnormalities occur rarely. The presence of the thiomethyltetrazole group in cephalosporins has been linked to two undesirable effects: (1) bleeding disorders due to hypoprothrombinemia, and (2) a disulfiram (Antabuse)-like reaction if alcohol is ingested during administration of the antibiotic. Cefamandole and cefoperazone, have this thiomethyltetrazole group, but bleeding disorders are not common.

Indications

First-Generation Cephalosporins. These antibiotics are useful for the treatment of systemic infections and oral treatment of urinary tract infections due to susceptible gram-negative bacilli. They are useful as alternatives to penicillin and to penicillinase-resistant penicillins for gram-positive infections, particularly those due to staphylococci. They are useful in prophylaxis against surgical wound infections in those circumstances when a cephalosporin may be indicated (e.g., insertion of a foreign body or gynecologic surgery).

Second-Generation Cephalosporins. These antibiotics are indicated for the treatment of infections due to susceptible bacteria that are *not* susceptible to the first-generation cephalosporins. Cefoxitin is used in disease presumed or known to be due to *B. fragilis*. All are alternative drugs for the treatment of nonmeningitic *H. influenzae* infections.

Third-Generation Cephalosporins. These agents are indicated in the treatment of those gram-negative enteric bacterial infections that are not susceptible to earlier cephalosporins or to broad-spectrum penicillins. Ceftazidime is the most active agent against *P. aeruginosa* infections and is often given with an aminoglycoside in granulocytopenic patients. Because of beta-lactamase–producing *H. influenzae*, for presumptive initial treatment of meningitis in the pediatric (not newborn) age group, one of the third-generation cephalosporins (cefotaxime, ceftazidime, or ceftriaxone) is appropriate. A third-generation cephalosporin is indicated in the treatment of gram-negative enteric meningitis in adults or children.

Other Beta-Lactam Agents

Monobactams

This is a new class of beta-lactam agents that possess a monocyclic basic structure. The first of these agents is aztreonam (Azactam). The spectrum of aztreonam is limited to aerobic gram-negative bacteria, including neisseria, haemophilus, most Enterobacteriaceae, and *P. aeruginosa*. It is particularly well tolerated by individuals allergic to other beta-lactams.

Preparations. Aztreonam must be given parenterally (intramuscularly or intravenously) as it is not absorbed following oral administration.

Distribution, Inactivation, and Excretion. Aztreonam is widely distributed in tissues, including bone, bile, bronchial secretions, prostate, and CSF, and high concentrations are achieved in urine. About 70% is excreted unchanged in the urine, with only about 7% metabolized and then excreted in urine.

Side Effects and Toxicity. This agent, like other beta-lactams, is generally well tolerated. Phlebitis related to the intravenous site occurs occasionally, and rash and gastrointestinal upset are rarely observed. No cross-allergenicity with penicillins or cephalosporins is observed, a very important feature.

Indications. Indications for these drugs are being developed at this time. Aztreonam appears to be a less toxic alternative to the aminoglycosides for serious aerobic gram-negative infections, particularly in those with renal impairment or at high risk of aminoglycoside toxicity. Its role in the febrile neutropenic patient and in those with gram-negative meningitis remains to be clarified.

Carbapenems

This is another new class of beta-lactam agents in which the dicyclic ring has been modified with substitution of carbon for sulfur. The first agent of this class is imipenem-cilastatin (Primaxin). Imipenem has the broadest antibacterial spectrum of all available beta-lactams, with activity against most gram-positives (including enterococci and listeria), against most gram-negatives (including *P. aeruginosa*), and against most anaerobes (including *B. fragilis*).

Preparations. Imipenem is not absorbed orally and must be given parenterally. It is administered in a 1:1 fixed ratio with cilastatin, a specific inhibitor of dehydropeptidase 1, an enzyme located in the brush border of renal proximal tubular cells that extensively degrades imipenem.

Distribution, Inactivation, and Excretion. The drug is well distributed into most tissues and body fluids, including CSF. Little drug is excreted in bile, but urinary concentrations are high. When given with cilastatin, about 70% of imipenem is excreted unchanged in urine and the remainder is nonrenally eliminated by metabolic inactivation.

Side Effects and Toxicity. Imipenem is generally well tolerated, like other beta-lactams. Rash and gastrointestinal side effects occur occasionally. Cross-allergenicity with other beta-lactams is well-documented. A potentially worrisome toxic effect has been seizure activity, particularly in elderly patients and those with renal insufficiency.

Indications. Like aztreonam, the precise niche for this agent has yet to be firmly established. It may be quite useful in those circumstances associated with polymicrobial infections, such as peritonitis due to a ruptured viscus.

Macrolides (Erythromycin)

Erythromycin is active against many gram-positive bacteria and against *T. pallidum*, *Legionella pneumophila*, and *Mycoplasma pneumoniae*. Most strains of *S. aureus* are susceptible initially, but resistance may develop during treatment. Several new macrolides including clarithromycin will soon be available.

Preparations

Erythromycin is available in oral and intravenous preparations. Among the oral preparations, the parent compound and its stearate are less well absorbed than the estolate (Ilosone).

Distribution, Inactivation, and Excretion

Erythromycin is widely distributed in tissues. Most erythromycin is inactivated, probably by the liver, some is secreted in the bile, and relatively little is excreted in the urine.

Side Effects and Toxicity

Mild gastrointestinal symptoms, such as abdominal cramping, occur very frequently with erythromycin. Erythromycin estolate, but not other forms, is a rare cause of intrahepatic cholestasis. This reaction is usually reversible when the drug is stopped.

Indications

Erythromycin is indicated for the treatment of legionnaire's disease and *M. pneumoniae* infections, and is used for otitis media and for penicillin-susceptible infections in penicillin-allergic patients. Although its antibacterial activity against susceptible bacteria is less than that of penicillin G, erythromycin is usually an effective alternative. It should not be used for severe *S. aureus* infections.

Tetracyclines

Tetracyclines are active against some, but not nearly all, streptococcal and staphylococcal strains, both aerobic and anaerobic. Tetracyclines are active against many *Escherichia, Enterobacter,* and *Klebsiella* strains, as well as many *H. influenzae* and *N. meningitidis* and *N. gonorrhoeae* strains. Tetracycline has some gram-negative anaerobic activity and is active against *T. pallidum, M. pneumoniae, Rickettsia,* and *Chlamydia.*

Preparations

Numerous tetracycline preparations exist. The newer derivatives—demeclocycline (Declomycin), methacycline (Rondomycin), doxycycline (Vibramycin), and minocycline (Minocin)—are generally better absorbed orally. Peak serum concentrations achieved by recommended dosages of newer tetracycline derivatives are lower.

The level of tetracyclines required to inhibit most Enterobacteriaceae, as well as some *Haemophilus* species, exceeds that obtained in serum by ordinary dosage. Thus, in therapy of gram-negative infection, tetracyclines are considered useful primarily in the urinary tract.

Distribution, Inactivation, and Excretion

Tetracyclines are widely distributed, but tissue levels vary with the derivative used. Minocycline, a more lipid-soluble drug, penetrates the subarachnoid space in normal patients better than other tetracyclines, but all penetrate well in the presence of inflammation.

Inactivation and excretion of the tetracycline derivatives vary, with all being secreted into bile. About half of a doxycycline dose is inactivated by the liver, and some is excreted by nonrenal mechanisms. There is relatively little inactivation of other tetracyclines, and they are excreted unchanged by the kidney, accumulating in patients with renal failure.

Side Effects and Toxicity

Gastrointestinal side effects—nausea, epigastric distress, and occasional vomiting and diarrhea—are relatively common with tetracyclines, but may be less frequent with the newer, better absorbed derivatives. Photosensitivity, manifested by rash on exposed skin, occasionally occurs with doxycycline and is rare with other tetracyclines. All tetracyclines may be deposited in calcifying areas of bones and teeth, causing yellowish discoloration. Although obvious tooth discoloration is usually apparent only after prolonged or repeated usage, tetracyclines should be avoided in pregnant women during the last 24 weeks of pregnancy and in children younger than 7 years of age.

Hepatotoxicity (acute fatty liver) was reported after large doses of intravenous tetracycline, particularly in pregnant women, and has also been reported occasionally in individuals with renal insufficiency who were given standard dosages. Further deterioration in abnormal renal function tests may be observed after tetracyclines. Reversible vestibular disturbance, usually with dizziness, weakness, nausea, and vertigo, has been observed with minocycline but not with other tetracyclines.

Indications

Tetracyclines are useful in exacerbations of chronic bronchitis and for urinary tract infection due to susceptible bacteria. They are indicated in rickettsial and chlamydial infections and are effective in the treatment of *M. pneumoniae* infections.

Clindamycin

Clindamycin (Cleocin) has replaced its parent drug, lincomycin (Lincocin). Clindamycin is active against aerobic gram-positive cocci, and against most gram-positive and gram-negative anaerobes, including *B. fragilis*.

Preparations

Clindamycin is available in parenteral and oral preparations.

Distribution, Inactivation, and Excretion

Clindamycin is widely distributed to body tissues and achieves a relatively high bone to serum ratio whether measured in normal or infected bone. Clindamycin is largely inactivated, probably by the liver. It is secreted in the bile, and a relatively small amount is excreted in the urine.

Side Effects and Toxicity

Diarrhea may occur with use of clindamycin, particularly when administered orally. Diarrhea after clindamycin use does not necessarily indicate pseudomembranous colitis, but the possibility should be considered.

Indications

Clindamycin is indicated for the treatment of disease due to anaerobes, including *B. fragilis*. It is also useful as an alternative to penicillin and penicillinase-resistant penicillins in the treatment of staphylococcal infections and occasionally other gram-positive infections. This is particularly important in penicillin-allergic individuals.

Chloramphenicol

Chloramphenicol (Chloromycetin) is active against gram-positive and gram-negative cocci and against *H. influenzae* and *Salmonella*. It is active against *E. coli*, *K. pneumoniae*, and *P. mirabilis*, and against many anaerobes.

Preparations

Chloramphenicol is available as an oral preparation. The sodium succinate salt may be used intravenously or intramuscularly, but absorption from intramuscular sites may be problematic. In marked contrast to other antibacterial agents, oral chloramphenicol achieves higher serum levels than an equivalent intravenous dose.

Distribution, Inactivation, and Excretion

Chloramphenicol is very widely distributed in tissues, including normal CSF, brain, and eye, which are not well penetrated by many antimicrobial agents. A small amount of chloramphenicol is excreted in an active form in the urine. Most of the drug is inactivated by the liver, and its metabolites are excreted in the urine.

Side Effects and Toxicity

Chloramphenicol is associated with bone marrow depression of two distinct types. The first is a common dose-related, reversible depression that is a pharmacologic property of the drug. Bone marrow depression is usual at ordinary dose levels of 2–4 g daily. The second type is a very rare, non–dosage-related (idiosyncratic) aplastic anemia, associated with a high mortality rate, usually occurring weeks to months after completion of therapy. Neonates with immature hepatic glucuronide function can develop the potentially fatal "gray baby syndrome" unless dosages are reduced.

Indications

Because of chloramphenicol's potential for irreversible toxicity, its indications are limited. Chloramphenicol is indicated for the initial treatment of systemic *Salmonella* infections, unless the isolate is demonstrated to be susceptible to ampicillin. Chloramphenicol is often indicated in the initial treatment of serious *H. influenzae* infections, such as meningitis and bacteremia, until susceptibility to ampicillin has been established. Because of its excellent penetration of the blood-brain barrier with or without inflammation, chloramphenicol is also indicated for treatment of meningitis due to bacteria susceptible to it but not to the penicillins or in penicillin-allergic individuals. Chloramphenicol is also effective in treatment of brain abscess.

Aminoglycoside Antibiotics

The aminoglycosides are active against a wide variety of aerobic and facultatively anaerobic gram-positive and gram-negative bacteria. They are inactive against anaerobes and *Haemophilus*. They are clinically important primarily because of their activity against gram-negative enteric bacilli and *P. aeruginosa*. The aminoglycosides currently in clinical use for systemic disease include streptomycin, gentamicin (Garamycin), tobramycin (Nebcin), and amikacin (Amikin). Other aminoglycosides are generally compared with gentamicin, the agent with the most extensive clinical history. Two areas of particular comparative interest are (1) activity against bacteria that have acquired resistance against an aminoglycoside, usually gentamicin, and (2) the frequency of ototoxicity and nephrotoxicity at equivalent dosage levels.

Gentamicin and Tobramycin

Gentamicin and tobramycin are active against most enteric bacilli and most strains of *P. aeruginosa*. Tobramycin is somewhat more active *in vitro* against many strains of *P. aeruginosa* than is gentamicin and is slightly less active against some strains of Enterobacteriaceae, particularly *Serratia marcescens*.

Amikacin

The spectrum of amikacin is similar to that of gentamicin and tobramycin, although its relative activity against *P. aeruginosa* is often poorer than that of gentamicin and tobramycin. As discussed in Chapter 37, however, amikacin has fewer chemical linkages susceptible to bacterial aminoglycoside-inactivating enzymes. Bacteria that produce enzymes inactivating other aminoglycosides are frequently susceptible to amikacin. However, bacteria resistant to aminoglycosides because of failure to transport the antibiotic intracellularly also transport amikacin poorly, and resistance is likely.

Streptomycin

Streptomycin is no longer used for the treatment of enteric bacterial disease because resistance develops rapidly during treatment and safer agents are available. Streptomycin is used in the treatment of some uncommon infections such as brucellosis and plague, as an adjunct to penicillin in streptococcal endocarditis, and in tuberculosis.

Kanamycin and Neomycin

Kanamycin and neomycin are active against most enteric bacilli but not against *P. aeruginosa*. Kanamycin is used only infrequently. Neomycin is a poorly absorbed local intestinal antibiotic when given orally or used topically.

Preparations

Because none of the aminoglycosides is absorbed significantly orally, these drugs are given intramuscularly or intravenously. Oral neomycin and kanamycin are available for their local effect on facultative intestinal bacteria. Gentamicin and tobramycin are pharmacologically very similar, and amikacin has a longer half-life.

Distribution, Inactivation, and Excretion

The aminoglycosides are well distributed in most tissues and body fluids. However, they do not achieve therapeutic CSF levels in children (except in neonates) or adults, even in the presence of inflammation. All available aminoglycosides are excreted essentially unchanged in the urine. Dosage reduction is essential in patients whose renal function is even mildly abnormal.

Side Effects and Toxicity

The aminoglycosides have the lowest therapeutic-toxic ratio of the commonly used antimicrobial agents. The eighth cranial nerve and the kidney are the major sites for drug toxicity, with the incidence of toxicity generally related to the intensity and duration of administration. Although any of the aminoglycosides may cause damage to either the auditory or the vestibular portion of the eighth cranial nerve, the auditory portion appears to be the primary site of toxicity from amikacin, kanamycin, and, at a lower order of magnitude, tobramycin. The vestibular portion is the most frequent site for gentamicin and streptomycin toxicity. Improvement in vestibular toxicity occurs frequently, but ototoxicity rarely disappears after discontinuation of therapy.

Audiometric testing before and during prolonged treatment may alert the physician to ototoxic effects before clinical hearing loss occurs. High-frequency hearing loss that is not appreciated clinically usually precedes hearing loss in the audible range. The baseline audiogram is important because asymptomatic high-frequency hearing abnormalities unrelated to aminoglycoside usage are fairly common, particularly in the elderly.

Renal function should be monitored because renal dysfunction may occur during aminoglycoside therapy, particularly in older people. Renal function generally returns to or near baseline level after the antibiotic is discontinued. Clinical studies have not shown consistent differences in nephrotoxicity among the various aminoglycosides currently used. Determination of serum antibiotic concentration is the best way to guide dosage levels. Antibiotic levels should be measured on the second full day of therapy and repeated periodically. Formulas and nomograms are available to calculate aminoglycoside dosage on the basis of body weight and renal function. Certain diuretics such as ethacrynic acid and furosemide potentiate aminoglycoside ototoxicity, and their concurrent use should be avoided.

Indications

Aminoglycosides should be restricted to the treatment of infections not susceptible to other antimicrobial agents and to the initial treatment of serious presumptive gram-negative bacillary infections in which, because of nosocomial acquisition or other circumstances, resistance to other agents is likely.

Vancomycin

Vancomycin (Vancocin) is active against many gram-positive bacteria, including *S. aureus*, enterococci, and toxin-producing *C. difficile*, the agent of antibiotic-associated (pseudomembranous) colitis. Gram-negative bacteria are generally resistant.

Preparations

For systemic use, vancomycin is available only as an intravenous preparation. The drug is not absorbed after oral administration, and the oral preparation is useful only for intraluminal intestinal disease.

Distribution, Inactivation, and Excretion

Vancomycin diffuses readily into most body fluids except CSF, although there is some penetration in the presence of inflammation. A small percentage of the drug is inactivated, but 90% or more is excreted unchanged into the urine.

Side Effects and Toxicity

Vancomycin must be administered intravenously over at least 1 h to avoid hypotension or other side effects ("red man syndrome") of rapid administration. Thrombophlebitis at the administration site is frequent. Auditory nerve toxicity may occur. Measurement of the serum vancomycin concentration is desirable because of the variability in levels achieved after a given dose to different individuals and because of the effect of renal insufficiency on excretion. Allergic reactions to vancomycin may occur.

Indications

Vancomycin is the drug of choice for methicillin-resistant *S. aureus* (MRSA) infections and is useful as an alternative drug to penicillins in the treatment of serious *S. aureus*, *S. epidermidis*, and enterococcal infections when the bacterium is resistant to the penicillins or when allergy precludes their use. When vancomycin is used for enterococcal endocarditis, it should be given in combination with an aminoglycoside. Oral vancomycin is used in the treatment of antibiotic-associated pseudomembranous colitis.

Metronidazole

Metronidazole (Flagyl) has been used in the treatment of trichomoniasis since the early 1960s. More recently, its excellent activity against obligate anaerobes, including *Entamoeba histolytica* and particularly anaerobic bacteria, has been recognized. The drug is effective against gram-negative anaerobic bacilli, including *B. fragilis*, anaerobic gram-positive and gram-negative cocci, and *Clostridia*. Facultative bacteria are resistant.

Preparations

Metronidazole is available in oral and intravenous preparations. It is well absorbed after oral administration, with serum levels similar to those achieved by equivalent intravenous administration. Metronidazole is metabolized in the liver and excreted primarily as an active metabolite in the urine. The drug is minimally protein-bound and is widely distributed in body compartments, including CSF.

Side Effects and Toxicity

Anorexia, a metallic taste, and occasionally nausea and vomiting may be observed with metronidazole. Phlebitis after intravenous administration, reversible neutropenia, and rash occur. Peripheral neuropathy and central nervous system toxicity have been observed, primarily after high-dose intravenous administration. Long-term administration of metronidazole is carcinogenic in rats and mice, and the drug is mutagenic in bacteria. Approximately 10-year epidemiologic follow-up studies of patients who had received metronidazole for treatment of trichomoniasis failed to suggest an increased incidence of malignancy in these individuals.

Indications

Metronidazole is indicated for the treatment of trichomoniasis in the United States. Metronidazole is bactericidal *in vitro*, unlike other drugs available for the treatment of *B. fragilis*, and thus is indicated for treatment of *B. fragilis* endocarditis. Its excellent penetration into the CSF makes it the primary choice for *B. fragilis* meningitis. The efficacy of metronidazole in the treatment of other anaerobic infections is probably equal to that of other appropriate antibiotics. It is commonly used for the treatment of brain or liver abscess. Because of metronidazole's lack of activity against facultative or microaerophilic bacteria, it should not be used alone in infections in which these bacteria may be implicated.

Sulfonamides

Many of the strains of both gram-positive and gram-negative bacteria originally susceptible to the sulfonamides (the first available antibiotics) have become resistant. Many strains of Enterobacteriaceae remain susceptible, however, to concentrations of sulfonamides generally achieved in the urine.

The sulfonamides are divided into three groups on the basis of their duration of pharmacologic effect. Only the more widely used compounds are mentioned here.

Short-Acting Sulfonamides

These drugs are rapidly excreted and must be administered every 4–8 h. Sulfadiazine reaches high systemic levels with intravenous administration but is poorly soluble in the urine. It is used occasionally for treatment of systemic disease. Sulfisoxazole (Gantrisin), which is highly soluble in the urine, is administered orally for urinary tract infections, and is combined with erythromycin ethylsuccinate (Pediazole) for otitis media.

Intermediate-Acting Sulfonamides

These sulfonamides are more slowly excreted and may be administered at 12-h intervals. Sulfamethoxazole (Gantanol) is used for the treatment of urinary tract infections. Sulfamethoxazole is the sulfonamide in the trimethoprim-sulfonamide preparations (Bactrim, Septra) used in the United States.

Long-Acting Sulfonamides

These sulfonamides are no longer available in the United States because of their association with severe hypersensitivity reactions (the Stevens-Johnson syndrome). This reaction is less common with other sulfonamides.

Distribution, Inactivation, and Excretion

The sulfonamides are widely distributed. Sulfadiazine and sulfisoxazole penetrate uninflamed meninges to some extent but penetrate much better in the presence of inflammation.

A portion of absorbed sulfonamide drugs is acetylated in the liver to inactive conjugates. The proportion of drug thus inactivated varies with the individual and with the particular sulfonamide. Both the free and the conjugated forms of the short- and intermediate-acting sulfonamides are excreted in the urine, primarily by glomerular filtration.

Side Effects and Toxicity

Hematologic toxicity is uncommon but most frequently manifests as agranulocytosis, which is usually reversible. Thrombocytopenia and acute hemolytic anemia are less common. Side effects such as renal damage from crystalluria and hepatotoxicity, which were reported with older sulfonamide preparations, are rarely seen today. Hemolysis occurs in G6PD-deficiency. Allergy to sulfonamides is relatively frequent, including cutaneous reactions.

Indications

Sulfonamides are useful for acute urinary tract infection, nocardiosis, in combination with trimethoprim for urinary tract and certain other infections, and in otitis media in combination with erythromycin.

Trimethoprim and Trimethoprim-Sulfamethoxazole

Trimethoprim is a synthetic antimicrobial active against many gram-positive and gram-negative bacteria, excluding *P. aeruginosa*. It is available as a single drug but is usually combined with a sulfonamide because the two drugs interrupt bacterial purine synthesis at sequential stages, resulting in synergistic activity against certain bacteria. The combination is effective against the opportunistic fungus *Pneumocystis carinii*.

Preparations

Trimethoprim is available alone as an oral preparation (Trimpex) and in combination with sulfamethoxazole in a 1:5 trimethoprim-sulfamethoxazole ratio, both as oral and intravenous preparations (Bactrim, Septra).

Distribution, Inactivation, and Excretion

Trimethoprim is widely distributed in body tissues and fluids, including the normal CSF and prostatic fluid. A variable amount, usually about one half of a trimethoprim dose, is excreted unchanged in the urine, primarily by glomerular filtration. Another major portion of the drug is inactivated in the liver, and a small amount is secreted in the bile.

Side Effects and Toxicity

Gastrointestinal side effects are unusual with lower doses of trimethoprim-sulfamethoxazole. Reversible hematologic toxicity includes hemolysis in G6PD-deficient individuals as well as depression of any of the formed elements of the blood or megaloblastic erythropoiesis. Nephrotoxicity has been reported rarely. Allergy, particularly with rash, is relatively frequent. It is usually unclear which of the components of the combination is responsible for adverse reactions.

Indications

Trimethoprim-sulfamethoxazole is indicated for the treatment of susceptible urinary tract infection that is resistant to less toxic, cheaper drugs.

It may be more effective than other agents for the suppression of chronic prostatitis. Trimethoprim-sulfamethoxazole is indicated for the treatment of shigellosis and, in high doses, for the treatment of *P. carinii* pneumonia. Trimethoprim-sulfamethoxazole is an alternative to ampicillin for treatment of *H. influenzae* otitis media and for treatment of bronchitis in adults.

Quinolones

Nalidixic acid (NegGram), the first of a promising group of antibiotics called quinolones, was introduced in 1962 and because of low serum and high urinary concentrations following oral administration is still used for treatment of urinary tract infections. Over the two decades following its introduction, additional quinolones were developed through molecular modification of the basic nucleus, and this recently has led to introduction into clinical practice of agents with an extremely broad spectrum of activity, good absorption after oral administration, and effectiveness many times that of nalidixic acid. These agents interfere with DNA gyrase activity.

Preparations

Nalidixic acid is available only as an oral agent. Norfloxacin (Noroxin) also is poorly absorbed, provides low serum levels after oral administration and is used for treatment of urinary tract infections. It has, however, an enhanced spectrum and is a much more useful agent than nalidixic acid. Ciprofloxacin (Cipro) is better absorbed than the other quinolone antibiotics and currently is the only quinolone available for use in treatment of systemic infections. Many newer agents have activity for Enterobacteriaceae, *P. aeruginosa*, *Salmonella*, *Shigella*, *Staphylococcus aureus*, and *Moraxella catarrhalis*. Ciprofloxacin also has marked activity for *H. influenzae*, *N. gonorrheae*, *L. pneumophila*, *Chlamydia trachomatis*, the majority of streptococci, mycoplasma, and many mycobacteria.

Distribution, Inactivation, and Excretion

The distribution of each of the quinolones differs. Ciprofloxacin does not enter cerebrospinal fluid well, but newer agents under development, such as ofloxacin and pefloxacin, do cross the blood–brain barrier. Tissue levels achieved with the newer quinolones are excellent, but nalidixic acid is poorly distributed in tissues other than the kidney. These agents are metabolized by the liver and excreted by the kidney. Biliary excretion of ciprofloxacin is high; concentrations achieved are several times that of serum. Administration of some of the newer quinolones leads to increased serum theophylline concentrations. This type of drug interaction is less apparent with ciprofloxacin.

Side Effects and Toxicity

Nalidixic acid produces occasional gastrointestinal effects. Pruritus and rash are also relatively common adverse effects. Central nervous system reactions, including seizures and toxic psychosis, have been reported, and the drug should not be administered to persons with convulsive disorders. Adverse effects reported with use of the newer agents are similar. The central nervous system effects are second only to gastrointestinal reactions in frequency. Generally, central nervous system effects are mild and include headache, dizziness, restlessness, and insomnia. Seizures and psychotic reactions have been reported. Dermatologic effects, including photosensitization, are also common, and thus should be noted since quinolones are used in treatment and prevention of traveler's diarrhea.

Indications

Use of quinolones as primary treatment is indicated for complicated urinary tract and enteric infections. The newer agents also have proved effective in therapy of infections of the respiratory tract, skin, soft tissues, bone, and joint, and those associated with sexual transmission. Currently treatment of mycobacterial infections, in combination with other antituberculous drugs, is being evaluated. The newer quinolones have also been employed successfully as prophylactic agents in granulocytopenic patients, but there is limited information relevant to treatment of established infections in the compromised host. Nalidixic acid is primarily used for chronic suppression of bacteriuria. Quinolones other than nalidixic acid are not approved for use in children under 16 years because of possible damage to developing cartilage.

Nitrofurantoin

Nitrofurantoin achieves therapeutic antibacterial levels in the urine and is used only for urinary tract infections. Many strains of *E. coli* and gram-positive cocci, such as enterococci, are quite susceptible to nitrofurantoin. Other Enterobacteriaceae are much less susceptible.

Preparations

Nitrofurantoin is available in the standard oral form (Furadantin) and in a macrocrystalline form (Macrodantin).

Distribution, Inactivation, and Excretion

Therapeutic levels of nitrofurantoin are achieved only in the urine and, perhaps, in renal tissue. Nitrofurantoin is well absorbed orally. About one third of an administered dose is excreted in therapeutically active form in the urine; the rest is inactivated.

Side Effects and Toxicity

Nausea and vomiting are frequent dosage-related side effects. These effects may be related to the rate of absorption of the drug and may be less severe with the less rapidly absorbed macrocrystalline form. Nitrofurantoin may precipitate acute hemolysis in patients with G6PD-deficient red blood cells. Peripheral neuritis may occur, usually in patients with decreased renal function; the drug should be stopped if paresthesias occur. Pulmonary infiltration of an acute or chronic nature is rare. Nitrofurantoin should not be used in patients with significant renal impairment. Its therapeutic activity is less, and the incidence of toxicity is high in such patients.

Indications

Nitrofurantoin is useful in the treatment and suppression of infections limited to the lower urinary tract due to susceptible bacteria, particularly *E. coli* and enterococci.

Spectinomycin

Spectinomycin (Trobicin) is active *in vitro* against a number of gram-positive and gram-negative bacteria, but it is used now solely for the treatment of *N. gonorrhoeae*. Spectinomycin is administered intramuscularly, and the single dose usually used for gonorrhea is well tolerated.

Indications

Spectinomycin is indicated for the treatment of genital gonorrhea in penicillin-allergic patients, in those in whom treatment with standard penicillin or ampicillin plus probenecid regimens have failed, and in patients with genital or systemic disease due to penicillinase-producing *N. gonorrhoeae*. Spectinomycin-resistant gonococci have become prevalent in certain areas, making ceftriaxone the drug of choice in those situations.

Rifampin

Rifampin is active against many mycobacteria, against *Neisseria* species, and against many gram-positive bacteria. The possible synergistic activity of rifampin in combination with other antibiotics and with antifungal agents is being investigated in certain refractory infections. Rifampin is not indicated for the treatment of meningococcal disease but is useful for prophylaxis of meningococcus and haemophilus. Emergence of resistance occurs frequently when it is used as a single agent. Therefore, when rifampin is used to treat established infection, it should be in conjunction with another agent.

ANTIFUNGAL AGENTS

Many circumstances in which fungi are isolated do not require therapy. When therapy is indicated, however, there are only a relatively few available agents. Antimicrobial susceptibility testing of fungi is technically difficult and is available only in specialized laboratories. Susceptibility testing is most useful when susceptibility to an antifungal agent cannot be predicted with a fair degree of accuracy.

Amphotericin B

Amphotericin B (Fungizone) is active against most fungi that cause human disease. Intrinsic resistance to the drug is uncommon. Amphotericin B binds to fungi in two ways, a reversible binding at lower drug concentrations that causes increased permeability of fungal membranes and irreversible binding only at higher drug concentrations that accounts for fungicidal activity by the drug.

Investigators have attempted to exploit the membrane-altering properties of low-dose amphotericin B to allow passage of other antibiotics into fungi. Synergistic antifungal activity has been demonstrated *in vitro* by the combination of amphotericin B with several different antifungal drugs. Increased efficacy has been demonstrated clinically in cryptococcal meningitis by the combination of amphotericin B with flucytosine. In addition, amphotericin B acts as an immunoadjuvant and thus may enhance host resistance.

Pharmacology and Preparation

Amphotericin B is administered intravenously as a colloidal suspension. Neither its tissue distribution nor its metabolism is well understood. The drug is excreted in the urine over a period of weeks following a single dose. Serum levels are unaffected by renal function, and dosage need not be adjusted in patients with initially poor renal function. Treatment for refractory meningitis, such as that due to coccidioidomycosis, is given intrathecally. Amphotericin B may be used intraarticularly in joint infections. Liposomal amphotericin preparations may be associated with improved therapeutic ratio and should be available in the near future.

Side Effects and Toxicity

Caution is indicated with amphotericin B, the most toxic antimicrobial in common use today. Major toxic effects include tubular and glomerular renal dysfunction, anemia, and hypokalemia. Side effects include chills, fever, nausea, vomiting, and myalgias with the infusion, as well as phlebitis at the site of administration. The side effects appear to be ameliorated by administration of a small initial test dose with gradual increase in the daily dosage to therapeutic levels. Toxicity is less if the daily dosage is kept relatively low. Renal function, serum potassium, and hemoglobin must be monitored during therapy.

Indications

Amphotericin B is the standard therapy for most deep tissue fungal infections. It should be given in combination with flucytosine (5-FC) for cryptococcal meningitis.

Flucytosine (5-Fluorocytosine)

Flucytosine (Ancobon) is active *in vitro* against most *Cryptococcus neoformans*, against about half of *Candida* species, and against some other opportunistic fungi. Increasing resistance during treatment of both cryptococcal and candidal infections is frequent when 5-FC is used alone.

Pharmacology and Preparations

Flucytosine is available as an oral preparation. The drug is very widely distributed in body compartments, including the CSF. The drug is excreted unchanged in the urine.

Side Effects and Toxcity

The major side effects are gastrointestinal, including nausea, vomiting, and diarrhea. Thrombocytopenia, leukopenia, and anemia occur infrequently and appear to be dose-related. Careful evaluation of initial renal function and monitoring during treatment, particularly when amphotericin B is used concurrently, is necessary to avoid overdosage.

Indications

Flucytosine is indicated in combination with amphotericin B in the treatment of cryptococcal meningitis and occasionally in the treatment of other cryptococcal or candidal infections. 5-FC is usually given in combination with amphotericin B.

Imidazole Antifungal Agents

Miconazole (Monostat), now primarily a topical agent used for dermatophyte and superficial candidal infections, was the first in a promising series of new antifungal agents, the imidazoles. Ketoconazole (Nizoral) is active against dermatophytes and has been used effectively in many systemic mycoses, including those due to *Blastomyces dermatitidis, Histoplasma capsulatum, Coccidioides immitis, Cryptococcus neoformans,* and *Candida* species. Fluconazole (Diflucan), the newest available imidazole, has been used in therapy of cryptococcal meningitis and severe candidal infections. None of these agents is active against aspergillus infections, for which amphotericin B is the most effective agent.

Preparations and Distribution

Ketoconazole is well absorbed from the gastrointestinal tract in the presence of gastric acid and is available as an oral preparation. It does not enter CSF in therapeutic concentration. Fluconazole is well absorbed from the gastrointestinal tract, independent of acidity, and achieves effective CSF levels in acute therapy and for maintenance therapy of cryptococcal meningitis.

Inactivation and Excretion

Ketoconazole is largely metabolized by the liver, and excretion in the urine is minimal. Fluconazole is excreted largely unchanged in the urine.

Side Effects and Toxicity

Ketoconazole has been associated with rare serious hepatocellular toxicity but is more often associated with anorexia, nausea, vomiting, and rash. The drug is not absorbed in the absence of gastric acid. It also causes a dose-dependent depression of serum testosterone and inhibited cortisol responses to ACTH. Fluconazole is associated with allergic responses, does not inhibit testosterone or cortisol synthesis, and has not been associated with severe hepatitis.

ANTIVIRAL AGENTS

The close metabolic relationship between viruses and their host cells makes it challenging to develop specific antiviral agents. Antiviral agents are available to treat relatively few viral diseases.

Amantadine

Amantadine hydrochloride (Symmetrel) is active against influenza A virus but not against other respiratory viruses, including influenza B. The drug inhibits viral uncoating.

Pharmacokinetics

Amantadine is well absorbed after oral administration and is excreted unchanged in the urine.

Side Effects and Toxicity

The drug may cause reversible neuropsychiatric symptoms such as confusion, anxiety, insomnia and hallucinations, particularly in the elderly.

Indications

Amantadine may be used as a supplement to an influenza immunization program for the prevention of influenza in those who are most susceptible to its complications—the elderly and those with chronic illnesses. Amantadine is administered for the duration of an outbreak of influenza in the community. Amantadine has been demonstrated to decrease airway resistance and to shorten the course of clinical influenza if given within 48 h after the onset of symptoms. Its use should be limited to high-risk individuals.

Acyclovir (Acycloguanosine)

Acyclovir (Zovirax) is a purine that is selectively phosphorylated by a virus-coded thymidine kinase and converted to a triphosphorylated derivative that inhibits viral DNA polymerase. Host cell DNA polymerase is affected only at much higher levels. Low levels of acyclovir are effective against herpes simplex (HSV) type 1, with somewhat higher concentrations required against herpes simplex type 2, and higher yet concentrations required against varicella-zoster virus (VZV). The activity of acyclovir against cytomegalovirus (CMV) is much less, and the drug is not clinically useful in treating CMV infections.

Clinical studies suggest that although acyclovir does not eradicate latent herpesvirus infections, it may be effective in controlling acute episodes. Resistance to acyclovir occurs when the virus does not code for thymidine kinase or when the viral DNA polymerase is not inhibited by the drug. Herpes simplex mutants resistant by the first mechanism occur naturally and may be induced by the drug.

Pharmacology and Preparations

Acyclovir is available in intravenous, oral, and topical forms. Serum concentrations of the systemic preparations are increased by renal failure. Serum levels are found to be much higher after intravenous administration than after ingestion of the oral preparation. With either preparation, the dose should be reduced and the dosage interval increased in individuals with impaired renal function.

Toxicity and Side Effects

Acyclovir has caused decreased spermatogenesis and mutagenesis at high dosage levels in experimental animals in some studies.

Indications

Intravenous acyclovir is indicated for presumptive or definite herpes simplex encephalitis and for HSV and VZV infections in immunocompromised hosts. Oral acyclovir may be useful in suppressing frequent HSV recurrences but is not very effective in treating recurrences. It may be useful in treating zoster in the normal host.

Ribavirin

Ribavirin, 1-beta-D ribofuranosyl-1H-1,2,4-triazole-3-carboxamide, is a broad spectrum antiviral drug with an unclear mechanism of action. *In vitro*, ribavirin (Virazole) is active against both DNA and RNA viruses. Its clinical indications, however, are quite limited at present.

Preparations

Ribavirin is available as an aerosol requiring special nebulization equipment for treatment of certain respiratory viral agents and as an intravenous drug for Lassa fever, an arenavirus infection.

Distribution, Inactivation, and Excretion

Following aerosol administration, ribavirin is absorbed systemically to some degree, and accumulation in RBCs has been documented. Metabolism and excretion are poorly understood.

Side Effects and Toxicity

Use of aerosolized ribavirin with a respirator can lead to malfunction secondary to drug precipitation. A normochronic, normocytic anemia can occur, and rash and conjunctivitis are reported after aerosol exposure. In animals, ribavirin is mutagenic, teratogenic, tumor-promoting, and toxic to the reproductive system. It is contraindicated in pregnancy and some recommend that pregnant health care workers be excluded from caring for patients being treated.

Indications

Aerosolized ribavirin is indicated for seriously ill infants or for those with underlying cardiac or pulmonary disease who develop respiratory syncytial virus (RSV) infection. Intravenous ribavirin is used for Lassa fever and other hemorrhagic viral fevers.

Ganciclovir

This analog of acyclovir inhibits all human herpesviruses, including CMV, and is used in the latter infection.

Preparations

Ganciclovir (Cytovene) is administered intravenously.

Distribution, Inactivation, and Excretion

Ganciclovir enters host cells where CMV induces one or more cellular kinases that phosphorylate ganciclovir to its triphosphate, the active form. The triphosphated drug remains in infected cells for at least 18 h. The drug is excreted renally without further metabolism.

Side Effects and Toxicity

Ganciclovir causes granulocytopenia and thrombocytopenia which are usually reversible. Other side effects have included rash, fever, phlebitis, CNS symptoms, and abnormal liver-function tests. Ganciclovir is teratogenic, carcinogenic, and causes aspermatogenesis in animals.

Indications

This agent is used to treat sight- or life-threatening CMV infections and CMV retinitis in immunocompromised patients. Ganciclovir with intravenous gammaglobulin may have some efficacy in CMV pneumonitis in marrow transplant recipients, and it has been found to prevent CMV pneumonitis in CMV-infected marrow recipients.

Zidovudine

Zidovudine, formerly termed azidothymidine, or AZT, is the therapy of choice for HIV-1 infections. Zidovudine (Retrovir) is a thymidine analog which is phosphorylated to a triphosphate which interferes with HIV viral reverse transcriptase and thus with viral replication.

Preparations

Zidovudine is usually administered orally, although an intravenous preparation is also used.

Distribution, Inactivation, and Excretion

Zidovidine is well-absorbed and is rapidly glucuronidated. Both the native drug and the glucuronide are excreted in urine. The drug is widely distributed and penetrates CSF.

Side Effects and Toxicity

The usual dose-limiting toxicities are anemia and neutropenia, usually occurring with higher doses and in those with advanced HIV disease. Recombinant erythropoietin has decreased the need for transfusions. Long-term zidovudine use may cause a toxic myopathy. Initial adverse effects include headache, myalgia, anorexia, nausea, vomiting, and insomnia. Zidovudine is carcinogenic in rodents, and its safety in pregnancy is unknown.

Indications

Zidovudine decreases the frequency of opportunistic infections and prolongs survival in patients with HIV infection. It also delays progression of disease in HIV-infected adults with CD4 lymphocyte counts of less than $500/mm^3$ and few or no symptoms. The value of postexposure prophylaxis (as following a needle-stick injury) with zidovudine is uncertain.

Other Nucleoside Analogs. Two investigational agents for treatment of HIV infection are dideoxyinosine (DDI) and dideoxycytidine (DDC), oral drugs that inhibit HIV reverse transcriptase. DDI has led to increased CD4 counts, decreased p24 antigen levels, and decreased symptoms in HIV infection. DDI can cause painful peripheral neuropathy and sometimes fatal pancreatitis, as well as diarrhea and other symptoms. DDC has also been used to treat AIDS and advanced ARC patients and can cause rash, fever, and stomatitis in the first month and painful peripheral neuropathy later. Another agent, foscarnet (Foscavir), is not a nucleoside analog but a pyrophosphate analog with activity against herpesviruses and HIV-1. It has activity in CMV retinitis and in acyclovir-resistant HSV infections.

REFERENCES

Books

Davis, B. D., et al. *Microbiology*. 4th ed. Philadelphia: Lippincott, 1990.

Galasso, G. J., Whitley, R. J., and Merigan, T. C. *Antiviral Agents and Viral Diseases of Man*. 3rd ed. New York: Raven Press, 1990.

Sherris, J. C. *Medical Microbiology*. 2nd ed. New York: Elsevier Science Publ., 1990.

Wilson, G., Miles, A., and Parker, M. T. *Topley and Wilson's Principles of Bacteriology, Virology, and Immunity*. 7th ed. Baltimore: Williams & Wilkins Co., 1984.

Review Articles

Abramowicz, M., ed. The choice of antimicrobial drugs. *Med. Lett. 32*:41, 1990.

Abramowicz, M., ed. Drugs for viral infections. *Med. Lett. 32*:73, 1990.

Baley, J. E. Pharmacokinetics, outcome of treatment, and toxic effects of amphotericin B and 5-fluorocytosine in neonates. *J. Pediatr. 116*:791, 1990.

Bryan, L. E. General mechanisms of resistance to antibiotics. *J. Antimicrob. Chemother.* 22(Suppl. A):1–15, 1988.

Finegold, S. M.: Mechanisms of resistance in anaerobes and new developments in testing. *Diag. Microbiol. Infect. Dis.* 12:117S, 1989.

Murray, B. E. Problems and mechanisms of antimicrobial resistance. *Infect. Dis. Clin. North. Am.* 3:423, 1989.

Neu, H. C. Overview of mechanisms of bacterial resistance. *Diagn. Microbiol. Infect. Dis.* 12:109S, 1989.

Neu, H. C. Bacterial resistance to fluoroquinolones. *Rev. Infect. Dis.* 10(Suppl.):57, 1988.

Nikando, H. Outer membrane barrier as a mechanism of antimicrobial resistance. *Antimicrob. Agents Chemother.* 33:1831, 1989.

Robinson, P. A. Fluconazole for life-threatening fungal infections. *Rev. Infect. Dis.* 12(Suppl. 3): S349, 1990.

Walsh, T. J. Experimental basis for use of fluconazole for preventive or early therapy of disseminated candidiasis in granulocytopenic hosts. *Rev. Infect. Dis.* 12(Suppl. 3):S307, 1990.

Wolfson, J. S., and Hooper, D. C. Bacterial resistance to quinolones: Mechanisms and clinical importance. *Rev. Infect. Dis.* 11(Suppl. 5):S960, 1989.

Wood, M. J., and Geddes, A. M. Antiviral therapy. *Lancet* 2:1189, 1987.

40 *STANFORD T. SHULMAN, M.D.*

Principles of Immunization

INTRODUCTION

My inquiry into the nature of the cowpox commenced upwards of 25 years ago. My attention to this singular disease was first excited by observing, that among those whom in the country I was frequently called upon to inoculate many resisted every effort to give them the smallpox. These patients I found had undergone a disease they called the cowpox, contracted by milking cows affected with a peculiar eruption on their teats. On inquiry, it appeared that it had been known among the dairies time immemorial, and that a vague opinion prevailed that it was preventive of the smallpox. This opinion I found was comparatively new among them, for all the older families declared they had no such idea in their early days.

During the investigation of the casual cowpox, I was struck with the idea that it might be practicable

to propagate the disease by inoculation, after the manner of the smallpox, first from the cow, and finally from one human being to another. I anxiously waited some time for an opportunity of putting this theory to the test. At length the period arrived, and the first experiment was made upon a lad of the name of Phipps, in whose arm a little vaccine virus was inserted, taken from the hand of a young woman who had been accidentally infected by a cow. Notwithstanding the resemblance, which the pustule, this excited on the boy's arm, bore to variolous inoculation, yet as the indisposition attending it was barely perceptible, I could scarcely persuade myself the patient was secure from the smallpox. However, on his being inoculated some months afterwards, it proved that he was secure. The case inspired me with confidence; and as soon as I could again furnish myself with virus from the cow, I made an arrangement for a series of inoculations. A number of children were inoculated in succession, one from the other; and after several months they were exposed to the infection of smallpox—some by inoculation, others by variolous effluvia, and some in both ways, but they all resisted it. The result of these trials gradually led me into a wider field of experiment, which I went over not only with great attention, but with painful solicitude.

Edward Jenner, 1801

Jenner's experiments in Gloucestershire in 1796, in which he showed that infection with attenuated material (cowpox) induced immunity to the dread scourge, smallpox, replaced the previous, more dangerous and less effective practices of deliberate dermal inoculation with smallpox material. This experiment marked the experimental foundation of immunology and infectious diseases and served as a pivotal event in the history of medicine, as it was based upon solid scientific demonstration of efficacy. The subsequent achievements, including the ultimate eradication of smallpox from the face of the earth in 1977 and the development of effective immunization reagents against a wide range of infectious agents, have had astounding effects upon mankind. The very impressive decline in age-specific mortality rates since 1900 is a result, in large part, of the successful prevention of many infectious diseases by widespread immunization programs. However, it is estimated (World Health Organization, 1990) that about 3 million children die each year (8000 each day) in the world from vaccine-preventable illness and that an additional 4 million are permanently disabled (Table 40–1). Neonatal tetanus, preventable by natural immunization and by hygienic umbilical cord care, kills about 775,000 infants yearly despite the availability of an effective tetanus toxoid vaccine for many years. Measles causes 1,500,000 deaths yearly, and pertussis another 500,000 annually. Much needs to be done to improve delivery of vaccine in the field, among both children and adults, who are very undervaccinated, even in the United States. Table 40–2 shows the low cost of vaccines used in the WHO's Expanded Program on Immunization. Clearly cost of the vaccines per se is not the limiting factor. However, Table 40–3 shows the actual percentages of infants surviving to their first birthday in the largest developing countries who have received immunizations.

GENERAL CONCEPTS

Natural versus Deliberate Immunization

Following many infections, whether symptomatic or subclinical, solid long-lived natural protection against subsequent infection develops. Hepatitis A is an excellent example of an infection that is very commonly subclinical but which induces life-long natural immunity. In contrast, deliberate immunization, of course, refers to the medical practice of intentionally either exposing individuals (as Jenner did) to a modified

TABLE 40–1. *Global Deaths from Vaccine-Preventable Diseases*

Infection	Annual Deaths
Tuberculosis	3,000,000
Measles	1,500,000
Hepatitis B	1,000,000–2,000,000
Neonatal tetanus	775,000
Pertussis	500,000
Rabies	35,000
Typhoid	25,000
Yellow fever	25,000

Source: Data from World Health Organization, 1990.

TABLE 40–2. *Cost of Vaccines in the Expanded Program on Immunization (WHO)*

Vaccine	Cost/Dose ($)
Bacille Calmette-Guérin	0.05
DPT	0.01–0.05
Measles	0.13
Oral polio	0.04
Tetanus toxoid	0.02

Source: Hayden, G. F. Cost of vaccines. *J. Pediatr. 114*:520, 1989.

infecting agent (or component thereof) for the express purpose of inducing active immunity or, alternatively, providing presynthesized antibody for purposes of protecting passively against infection.

Active and Passive Immunization

Active immunization refers to the stimulation of an individual to produce an immune response (usually antibody) by the deliberate administration of an antigen (or antigens), usually prior to natural exposure to the agent. Protection is not present immediately but is usually of long duration. In contrast, passive immunization refers to the administration of preformed antibodies, obtained from an immune individual, to a nonimmune subject in order to provide temporary protection against an infecting agent or toxin. In this instance, protection is immediate but short-lived. The distinction between active and passive immunity was established in 1890 by the studies of Emil von Behring and Shibasaburo Kitasato related to protection against tetanus and diphtheria toxins. For this work, in 1901 von Behring was awarded the first Nobel Prize in Medicine.

Adjuvants

Materials such as aluminum salts are included in certain vaccines for the purpose of promoting a depot effect at the vaccine site to retain the immunogen and to delay degradation and elimination, thus producing a prolonged stimulus to the immune system. This is most important for achieving optimal immune responses to vaccines that contain killed microorganisms or their products.

Local and Systemic Immunity

Systemic immunity is reflected by circulating serum antibody and is distinguished from local

TABLE 40–3. *Estimated Immunization Coverage Rates in Developing Countries (1978)*

Country	Millions of Infants Surviving to 1 Year	Immunization Coverage (% infants <1 year)				Mothers
		BCG	Measles	3 DPTs	3 OPVs	2 Tetanus
India	23.1	29	1	53	45	40
China	18.1	70	63	62	68	NA
Indonesia	4.9	67	47	48	46	26
Nigeria	4.4	42	32	21	22	13
Pakistan	3.8	69	41	56	56	5
Bangladesh	3.2	5	3	5	4	5
Mexico	2.6	54	60	34	96	NA
Brazil	2.5	56	55	52	89	NA
TOTAL	103.2	51	37	49	50	19

From Hayden G. F., et al. Progress in worldwide control and elimination of disease through immunization. *J. Pediatr. 114*:521–527, 1989.
NA: Not available.

mucosal (secretory IgA) immunity. Inactivated Salk polio vaccine induces systemic immunity only, whereas live-attenuated Sabin polio vaccine administered orally induces local gastrointestinal antibody as well as systemic antibody. Mucosal antibody is important in preventing gastrointestinal infection by wild poliovirus.

Replicative and Nonreplicative Immunogens

Replicative vaccines are those live-attenuated agents (oral polio, measles, mumps, rubella, oral typhoid) that induce a subclinical infection that results in an active immune response. Nonreplicative immunogens are either killed whole organisms (pertussis, killed polio vaccine), inactivated toxins (diphtheria, tetanus toxoids), or cellular constituents (pneumococcal, haemophilus polysaccharides) that induce protective immune responses.

PASSIVE IMMUNIZATION

The most universal and physiologic form of passive immunity is the transplacental passage of IgG from mother to fetus. This is the result of an active transport process that occurs particularly during the last 2 months of gestation, resulting in IgG concentrations in full-term infants that are 100–110% of the maternal concentrations. Depending upon their gestational age, preterm infants are mildly to severely deficient in serum IgG, as compared with adult levels, because they missed some or all of the latter stage of gestation, and this contributes to their enhanced susceptibility to infection. Much transplacental IgG is protective, such as against *Haemophilus influenzae* b, rubeola, or varicella, whereas other IgG antibodies are clearly not protective, such as anti-HIV. The half-life of transplacental IgG is 3–4 weeks, and traces are still detectable at 12 months or later. Sufficient transplacental antirubeola antibody is still present in serum at 12–14 months of age to interfere with the active immune response to live-attenuated measles vaccine in a substantial fraction of infants, necessitating delay of vaccine administration in routine (nonepidemic) circumstances to infants 15 months of age.

In general, passive immunization is used to achieve temporary immunity in an unimmunized exposed individual when active immunization is not available (e.g., hepatitis A), or when time does not permit active immunization after an exposure has occurred (e.g., rabies). It is also employed in toxin-mediated disorders (e.g., diphtheria, tetanus), certain bites (spider, snake), or as an immunomodulator (anti-D [Rh$_o$], antilymphocyte sera). In addition, patients who are incapable of active antibody responses to immunization (e.g., B-cell deficiency) benefit from passive immunization. The forms of passive immunologic agents utilized include: (1) standard human immune serum globulin (ISG) available for intramuscular or in deaggregated preparations for intravenous use; (2) specific high-titered human globulins used in defined circumstances; and (3) antisera and antitoxins prepared in immunized animals, usually horses or rabbits. The use of reagents prepared in species other than humans is associated with a risk of hypersensitivity (serum sickness) reactions; these are related to development of antibody against the injected foreign protein. A negative scratch test or eye test followed by negative intradermal skin tests is essential before injection of an animal serum. Specific human and animal sera and antitoxins currently available are listed in Table 40–4.

Standard ISG, consisting almost exclusively of IgG (Cohn alcohol fraction II) pooled from large groups of adult donors, is used for the prevention of the following illnesses: (1) hepatitis A; (2) hepatitis B (when HBIG is unavailable); (3) non-A, non-B hepatitis (of unproved value); (4) measles; (5) varicella (when VZIG is unavailable); (6) rubella (only in pregnancy, of unproved value), and (7) poliomyelitis (rarely indicated). Thus, common usage relates to hepatitis A and measles prevention. ISG is also administered intramuscularly as replacement therapy in individuals with humoral immune deficiency states.

Intravenous gamma globulin (IVGG) is similar to ISG but is chemically treated to ensure deaggregation of IgG, thus obviating the complement-mediated reactions that occur when ISG is inadvertently administered intravenously. IVGG is utilized in the treatment of humoral immune deficiency states, idiopathic thrombocytopenic purpura, and Kawasaki disease (see Chapter 33), and studies have shown its usefulness in some patients with pediatric AIDS.

Specific high-titered human globulin preparations are available and are recommended for selected situations. The use of hepatitis B immune globulin (HBIG) is discussed in Chapter 21. Varicella-zoster immune globulin (VZIG) prepared from individuals convalescent from zoster (shingles) is used to prevent or ameliorate varicella in immunocompromised hosts with recent (within 96 h) exposure (see Chapter 27). Rabies immune globulin (RIG) is effective as prophylaxis when combined with active rabies immunization. RIG should be given within 24 h of exposure, infiltrated in and around the bite sites as well as intramuscularly (not in the same site as rabies vaccine). Tetanus immune globulin (TIG) contains a high concentration of tetanus antitoxin and is highly effective in prevention of tetanus when administered soon after an injury. Its value in established tetanus is unproved. Pertussis immune globulin is of little or no value in treatment or prevention of pertussis. $Rh_o(D)$ immune globulin (Rho-GAM) is highly effective in prevention of Rh hemolytic disease of the neonate and is indicated for Rh-negative women who have delivered an Rh-positive baby or have aborted and for Rh-negative inadvertent recipients of Rh-positive blood.

Animal serum and globulins are utilized infrequently and with the precautions noted above. Serum sickness reactions are common, including the development of rash, arthralgia or arthritis, and glomerulonephritis. Such reactions represent immune-complex–mediated events resulting from antibody produced after receipt of globulins from a nonhuman species. Tetanus antitoxin (equine) and rabies immune globulin (equine) are used only when the corresponding human preparations are unavailable. Diphtheria antitoxin (equine) is effective in neutralizing non–tissue-fixed diphtheria toxin even after clinical disease is apparent; efficacy is maximal early in the disease. Similarly, equine trivalent (A,

TABLE 40–4. *Passive Immunization in Prevention of Infection*

Human Immunoglobulin
　Standard immune serum globulin (ISG)
　　Hepatitis A postexposure prophylaxis: 0.02 mL/kg
　　Hepatitis B prophylaxis or attenuation (only when HBIG is unavailable): 0.06 mL/kg
　　Non-A, non-B hepatitis (unproved value): 0.06 mL/kg
　　Measles prophylaxis or attenuation: 0.25 mL/kg (0.5 mL/kg for immunocompromised) with maximum of 15 mL
　　Varicella prophylaxis or attenuation (only when VZIG is unavailable and only for individuals at high risk of serious
　　　disease): 0.06 mL/kg
　　Rubella in pregnancy (unproved value): 0.55 mL/kg
　　Polio prophylaxis (rarely indicated)
　Special immune globulins (all post-exposure)
　　Hepatitis B immune globulin (HBIG): 0.06 mL/kg (maximum: 5 mL)
　　Varicella-zoster immune globulin (VZIG): one vial (125 U/10 kg; maximum: 5 vials)
　　Rabies immune globulin (HRIG): 20 IU/kg (half locally, half IM)
　　Tetanus immune globulin (TIG): for treatment 500–3000 U, for prevention 250–500 U

Animal Immunoglobulins
　For use only when human product is unavailable
　　Equine tetanus antitoxin (TAT): 50,000–100,000 U (after safety testing) in single dose
　　Equine antirabies serum (ARS): 40 IU/kg (half locally, half IM) in single dose (after safety testing)
　Only available preparations
　　Equine diphtheria antitoxin: 20,000–100,000 units IV (after safety testing)
　　Equine trivalent (ABE) botulinum antitoxin (after safety testing)
　　Equine gas gangrene polyvalent antitoxin: no longer used or available in the U.S.

B, E) botulism antitoxin is effective in treatment of this very serious disorder by neutralizing unbound toxin. In contrast, equine gas gangrene antitoxin is of unproved value. Crotalidae antivenin is utilized in treatment of snake bites from certain poisonous species and is infiltrated locally as well as given systemically. Similarly, black widow spider antivenin is occasionally utilized. Antilymphocyte or antithymocyte antisera (ALG, ALS, ATG, ATS) usually raised in horses are increasingly utilized for prevention of organ transplant rejection, with murine monoclonal antibodies directed against T-cell populations (e.g., OKT3) also now being used to reverse rejection.

ACTIVE IMMUNIZATION

Active immunization programs are highly efficient in preventing viral illnesses and toxin-mediated bacterial disorders. They are clearly cost-effective and save lives. However, in certain developing areas of the world, vaccine delivery continues to be a major challenge. Contributing to the problem of delivery of vaccines is the problem of maintaining the *cold chain*, which refers to the fact that many vaccines must be maintained at refrigerator or freezer temperature until just prior to administration to retain immunogenicity. Vaccines composed of whole bacterial cells, rickettsiae, or mycoplasmas are only moderately effective immunogens. The goal of active immunization is to induce long-lived responses that provide protection against clinical disease. Clearly, there is a latent period between immunization and achievement of protective levels of antibody, and many vaccines require several doses to induce lasting responses. Primary immune responses are generally mostly IgM and transient. However, secondary responses are usually predominantly IgG and long-lived. Vaccines may contain trace amounts of constituents derived from the media in which the vaccine was prepared, including tissue-culture–derived antigens, egg antigens, or serum proteins, or the vaccines may contain preservatives or stabilizers. These contaminants may serve as inciting agents for hypersensitivity reactions. The most common component responsible for hypersensitivity is egg protein in vaccines prepared in embryonated chicken eggs or chicken embryo cell culture (yellow fever, mumps, measles, and influenza vaccines). Generally, those who can safely eat eggs or egg products can receive these vaccines, but those with history of anaphylaxis to eggs should not.

The formulation of vaccine schedules by public health authorities is based upon epidemiologic characteristics of the disease, age-dependent immune responses, age-specific complication risks of vaccine or of the natural disease, and duration of induced immunity, that is, upon careful risk-benefit assessments. In general, vaccines are recommended for the youngest age group both at risk and known to develop an acceptable response to vaccination. Usually, vaccine schedules call for simultaneous administration of several vaccines albeit in different sites. Complications that occur at even very low frequency are significant when one deals with millions of vaccine doses yearly. An example of this is the whole-cell pertussis vaccine which may be associated with serious adverse neurologic reactions with a frequency of approximately 1:300,000 doses. The cost associated with resultant litigation concerning alleged vaccine complications has led to great increases in the cost of vaccines in the United States over the past decade and has driven certain vaccine manufacturers out of the field. General contraindications to active immunization include (1) acute febrile illnesses of a nontrivial nature, (2) immunocompromised state (live vaccines should be avoided), (3) recent ISG, IVGG, whole blood, or plasma administration, (4) pregnancy, and (5) hypersensitivity to a vaccine component.

Vaccine efficacy is established from studies of relative attack rates for a disease in vaccinated and nonvaccinated populations. For example, if 10 per 1000 vaccinated and 900 per 1000 unvaccinated exposed individuals develop infection during an epidemic, the vaccine efficacy is .90 − .01/.90 = .99, or 99% effective.

Poliomyelitis Immunization

Vaccination against poliomyelitis has almost completely eradicated this disorder from the United States and other developed areas. It is estimated that about 5 million cases of paralytic polio were prevented by oral vaccine in the past two decades. Only 335 confirmed cases of paralytic polio were reported in the entire Western Hemisphere in 1988 and only 29 in the first half of 1989. The 1988 data represented a 64% decrease from 2 years earlier. Regionwide oral vaccine coverage of children by 1 year of age had reached 82% in Latin America in 1988, mainly through efforts by the Pan American Health Organization. However, worldwide it is estimated that about 250,000 cases of paralytic polio occur annually, with India now the greatest contributor of cases, 80% of whom are under 2 years old. Infants in the United States are now immunized routinely with Sabin trivalent, live-attenuated, oral vaccine (OPV) at 2 and 4 months of age, with booster doses administered at 18 months and at 4–6 years, just before entry into school. The oral vaccine replaced the Salk trivalent, inactivated, parenteral vaccine in the United States because of the former's ability to induce intestinal immunity, its ease of administration, its high acceptance, and its ability to immunize some contacts of fecally excreting vaccine recipients. It is a unique vaccine in that it multiplies extensively in the intestinal tract, is widely disseminated in the family and community, and immunizes a large proportion of the unvaccinated population. OPV is associated with rare instances of paralysis in vaccinees and in their contacts (now 2–8 per year in the U.S.), the estimated risks being 1 per 7.8 million doses of OPV for immunologically normal vaccine recipients, and 1 per 5.5 million doses for household and community contacts. The maximal risk of paralysis occurs with the first dose of OPV (1 case of paralysis per 520,000 first doses and 1 case per 12.3 million subsequent doses), and rates are slightly greater for adults compared with children. Immunocompromised persons who are exposed to OPV virus by vaccination or by exposure to a vaccinee are at somewhat higher risk of acquiring paralytic disease.

Inactivated poliovirus vaccine (IPV), containing the three formalin-inactivated poliovirus strains, has recently been licensed in the United States as an enhanced-potency inactivated polio (E-IPV) vaccine developed in human diploid cell culture. IPV, which was responsible for the initial sharp decline from 20,000–25,000 cases yearly of paralytic polio in the United States in the 1950s, is now indicated for individuals who refuse OPV or who have a contraindication to OPV, including those with compromised immunity including AIDS, household contacts of an immunodeficient individual, partially immunized adult household contacts of children who will receive OPV, and immunized or partially immunized adults at future risk of exposure to polio. It is recommended that IPV recipients receive boosters every 5 years after their primary series of immunization at 2, 3–4, and 10–16 months of age. A full series of IPV is recommended for immunizing previously unimmunized adults. Within the next few years, it is likely that a vaccine strategy in which initial DTP-coupled–E-IPV vaccination followed by OPV will be recommended, thereby reducing the risk of vaccine-related paralytic disease by deferring live virus vaccine until individuals have received at least one initial immunization.

Diphtheria, Tetanus, Pertussis Immunization

Diphtheria, tetanus, pertussis (DTP) vaccine is composed of purified diphtheria and tetanus toxoids and whole killed pertussis organisms. Efforts to develop a more effective but less reactogenic pertussis vaccine have focused on purified cell-free pertussis toxoids that are currently being developed and tested as possible vaccines. The toxoids are either chemically detoxified or, more recently, genetically engineered to be nontoxic by replacement of one or two key amino acids within the important S1 toxin subunit that harbors ADP-ribosyltransferase activity. These efforts are the result of the fact that pertussis whole-organism vaccines are associated with relatively low efficacy and relatively common adverse reactions. These reactions include frequent development of mild to moderate fever, local discomfort, local redness and swelling, drowsiness, fretfulness, and anorexia or vomiting occurring within several hours of vaccination and with spontaneous resolution. More significant adverse reactions include the following: about 1%, persistent crying lasting at least 3 h; 0.3%, very high fever (≥40.5°C); 0.1%, high-pitched cry; 0.06%, seizures; and 0.06%, collapse for several hours with a peculiar hypotonic, hyporesponsive state. Because many alleged vaccine reactions can be caused by other factors, a temporal association with immunization does not establish a causal relationship. This has been shown to be the case with regard to the onset of infantile spasms and with sudden infant death syndrome (SIDS), both of which are relatively common in the first 6 months of life but for which a causal relationship to immunization has not been demonstrated clearly.

Absolute contraindications to subsequent readministration of pertussis vaccine are: (1) encephalopathy occurring within 7 days of immunization (with severe alterations of consciousness and focal neurologic findings), with estimated frequency of 1:140,000; (2) seizure within 72 h; (3) persistent screaming or high-pitched cry within 48 h; (4) hypotonic-hyporesponsive episode within 48 h; (5) fever greater than or equal to 40.5°C within 48 h, without other cause; and (6) anaphylactic reaction to vaccine (extremely rare). The risk of administering subsequent vaccine doses to children with these reactions is not known, but prudence should prevail. In addition, DTP vaccine is deferred for children with progressive neurologic conditions or progressive developmental delay, personal past history of seizures, and those with known or suspected neurologic conditions that predispose to seizures or neurologic deterioration. A family history, but not personal history, of seizures is *not* a contraindication to pertussis immunization, even though data suggest that such children are at some increased risk for simple febrile convulsions which are considered generally benign.

Universal immunization of children is essential for control of pertussis since there is continuing risk of pertussis in the United States. Experiences in other countries have demonstrated repeatedly that falling vaccine rates are associated with dramatic epidemic occurrence of pertussis, associated with fatalities and significant morbidity. Approximately 500,000 preventable pertussis deaths occur each year worldwide among infants. Encephalopathy and seizures complicate the pertussis illness much more frequently than they result from pertussis immunization. DTP is recommended for infants and children at 2, 4, and 6 months of age, at 18 months, and at 4–6 years. After the seventh birthday DTP is replaced by Td, a vaccine that omits the pertussis component and contains a lower concentration of diphtheria toxoid to reduce reactogenicity. Boosters with Td should be given every 10 years. Children for whom pertussis immunization is deferred or contraindicated should receive DT if younger than 7 years old, and should receive four or preferably five immunizations by the time of school entry. A booster of tetanus toxoid should be given every 10 years. Since neither tetanus nor diphtheria infection necessarily confers immunity, individuals convalescent from these illnesses should receive active immunization.

Measles, Mumps, Rubella Immunization

Universal immunization with combined live-attenuated virus vaccines against rubeola, mumps, and rubella is recommended at 15 months of age in routine circumstances. Use of these vaccines has resulted in dramatic decreases in the frequencies of these illnesses, with concomitant decreases in the frequencies of the serious sequelae of measles, encephalitis, and pneumonitis, and of congenital rubella syndrome. However, the World Health Organization indicates that almost 1.5 million children die annually from measles.

Measles vaccine produces a subclinical or very mild noncommunicable infection, with approximately 95% of vaccine recipients immunized at 15 months developing long-lived immunity. Vaccination in the United States between 1963 and 1967 utilized killed measles vaccine and that from 1968 to 1979 utilized attenuated-live vaccine strains (sometimes given with ISG) or contained a less effective stabilizer than current vaccine, a procedure that resulted in relatively frequent lack of sustained immune responses. This vaccination problem accounts for recent outbreaks of measles among teenage and young adult populations, such as on college campuses. New recommendations call for reimmunization of children immunized at 15 months of age or older either upon entrance to middle school (junior high) or upon entrance to school (4–6 years). Immunization before 15 months of age, which is indicated only in epidemic or highly endemic circumstances, frequently results in relatively short-lived antibody responses as a result of the suppressive effect of residual transplacentally acquired maternal antibody. Such children require reimmunization at approximately 15 months of age.

Measles vaccine can provide some degree of protection even up to 72 h after exposure, so that vaccine is indicated following known exposure. Adverse reactions occur in about 5–15% of measles vaccine recipients, with fever as high as 103°F for 1–2 days, beginning 5–12 days after immunization and sometimes accompanied by a mild rash. Approximately 50% of prior recipients of the killed measles vaccine used in 1963–1967 develop reactions after revaccination with live measles vaccine, usually mild local swelling and redness, sometimes with low-grade fever for 1–2 days. Rarely, more serious reactions with prolonged fever, lymphadenopathy, extensive local reactions, and rash resembling rickettsial rashes (maximal on distal extremities) may occur. However, such individuals are more likely to develop severe reactions following exposure to wild measles virus than after live vaccine and therefore should be reimmunized.

Live-attenuated *mumps vaccine* (Jeryl-Lynn strain) is usually given with the initial measles vaccine at 15 months and results in antibody in more than 95% of recipients. Vaccination results in very long lasting immunity, and adverse reactions to this vaccine are very rare. Postexposure mumps vaccine has not been shown to be effective.

Live *rubella vaccine* (RA 27/3 strain), also given at 15 months, induces serum antibody in more than 98% of recipients and confers long-term (perhaps lifelong) immunity (see Chapter 33). This vaccine is also recommended for susceptible adolescent and adult females to decrease the risk of the congenital rubella syndrome resulting from rubella infection early in pregnancy. Although there is no evidence of teratogenic effects of live rubella vaccine, it is recommended that this vaccine, as well as the mumps and measles vaccines, not be given during pregnancy. Adverse reactions to primary rubella immunization include mild rash, lymphadenopathy, and arthralgias or arthritis, particularly in adult females. Postexposure immunization with rubella vaccine is not effective in preventing disease.

Haemophilus Influenzae B Immunization

A vaccine composed of purified *H. influenzae* type b (HIB) capsular polysaccharide was licensed in April, 1985 for children 24 months and over to prevent invasive infection by this organism. Younger children, who are at highest risk for HIB infection, are incapable of mounting an antibody response to this T-independent antigen. Therefore, conjugate vaccines, containing HIB polysaccharide (polyribose phosphate) covalently linked to a protein carrier such as diphtheria toxoid, have been developed and initially licensed in the United States for children 18 months and older in December, 1987. The latter vaccines are T-dependent and are associated with much improved immunogenicity, particularly in infancy, with recent data indicating that they are immunogenic in infants as young as 2–3 months of age (see Chapter 23). Two conjugate vaccines were recently approved in the United States. FDA for infants beginning at 2 months of age.

It is currently recommended that all children receive conjugate HIB vaccine at 2, 4, 6, and 15 months (Lederle-Praxis) or at 2, 4, and 12 months (Merck) and that children who received the unconjugated HIB vaccine at 18–23 months be reimmunized with conjugate vaccine.

Pneumococcal Vaccine

At least 83 serotypes of pneumococci are known, distinguished by the antigenicity of their capsular polysaccharides, which serve as antiphagocytic virulence factors. Anticapsular antibody is opsonic and protects against invasive infection with the homologous serotype. Active immunization against pneumococci is possible because (1) a relatively limited number of serotypes account for most pneumococcal disease of humans, (2) multiple purified polysaccharides can be combined into a single injection, and (3) type-specific antibody persists for years. The current pneumococcal vaccine in the United States contains 25 µg of each capsular polysaccharide of the 23 types responsible for 87% of bacteremic pneumococcal infections in the United States. Children younger than 24 months do not respond well to these purified polysaccharides. Pneumococcal vaccine efficacy is estimated to be about 60% in high-risk populations. Pneumococcal vaccine is currently recommended for children older than 24 months with asplenia, sickle cell disease, functional asplenia, nephrosis, HIV infection, and other illnesses associated with increased risk of pneumococcal infection, and for adults 65 years or older, and adults with chronic cardiac or pulmonary disease, lymphatic malignancies, or chronic liver disease.

Typhoid Fever Vaccine

Salmonella typhi has been estimated to result in 33 million infections and more than 500,000 deaths annually worldwide, particularly in areas with poor sanitation. Parenterally administered killed whole-cell vaccines (inactivated by heat and phenol or by acetone treatment) have been available since the 1960s. However, these vaccines have afforded only about 50–80% protection and are associated with a high frequency of adverse effects, including substantial fever and local reactions. Killed whole-cell vaccines administered orally are well tolerated but do not result in protection.

Two new typhoid vaccines have been developed recently and found to be safe, immunogenic, and protective in clinical trials. They include an attenuated strain of *S. typhi* (Ty21a) administered orally, and purified *S. typhi* capsular polysaccharide (Vi) administered parenterally. The Ty21a strain of *S. typhi* is completely deficient in the enzyme uridine diphosphoglucose-4-epimerase and harbors other mutations as well, including lacking Vi polysaccharide. Large field trials of three oral doses of Ty21a administered within 1 week demonstrated 86% efficacy in Egypt and 66% efficacy in Chile. Vi polysaccharide, a capsular material of *S. typhi* clinical isolates, serves as a virulence factor and has been highly purified and field-tested as a parenteral vaccine. Trials in Nepal and South Africa have demonstrated 72% and 64% protection against culture-proved typhoid fever. Both Ty21a and Vi vaccines have been licensed recently for usage in several countries. Further efforts to develop more effective typhoid vaccines are continuing, including creation of other *S. typhi* strains with enzymatic mutations for use as attenuated-live agents, and preparation of protein-polysaccharide conjugates that include Vi conjugated to tetanus or diphtheria toxoids for enhanced immunogenicity.

Other Vaccines

A large number of additional vaccines are available (Table 40–5), most being utilized for the rather selected indications outlined in the table. Hepatitis B vaccine is discussed in Chapter 21.

Current Recommendations

The schedule for routine immunizations of healthy children is shown in Table 40–6. Official vaccine recommendations are established in the United States by the Committee on Infectious Diseases of the American Academy of Pediatrics and by the Immunization Practices Advisory Committee of the Centers for Disease Control.

Six vaccines are currently recommended for routine use for adults in the United States. These include:

1. tetanus-diphtheria toxoid booster every 10 years (after a primary series)
2. influenza vaccine, particularly for those with chronic cardiac or pulmonary disease, those in chronic care facilities, those with diabetes or other metabolic disorders, renal disease, severe anemia, immunosuppressed patients, and all persons over 65 years old (see Chapter 14).
3. pneumococcal vaccine, for those with chronic cardiac or lung disease, cirrhosis, alcoholism, diabetes, Hodgkin's, nephrosis, renal failure, CSF leaks, immunosuppression, sickle cell, and asplenism
4. hepatitis B vaccine for the groups discussed in Chapter 21
5. measles vaccine for young adults (born after 1957) who have received only one dose of vaccine since their first birthday, particularly on enrolling in college, traveling to a foreign country, or entering a health care field
6. rubella vaccine for previously unimmunized women of childbearing age and susceptible health care personnel

Recommended immunizations for travelers to

TABLE 40–5. *Active Immunization Agents Used Selectively*

Vaccine	Type	Age	Indications	Comment
Influenza	Killed virus, whole or split virus	>6 mo.	Chronic lung, cardiac conditions	Yearly immunization required with current vaccine
Hepatitis B	Purified HBsAg	Any	See Chapter 21	Now recombinant vaccine
Yellow fever	Live-attenuated	>9 mo.	Residence or travel to endemic area	Avoid in egg-sensitive individuals
Smallpox	Live-attenuated	>6 mo.	None	U.S. military
Rabies	Inactivated virus grown in human diploid cells	Any	Animal handlers or postexposure	Use with rabies immune globulin
Tuberculosis	BCG, attenuated-live *M. bovis* strain	Any	See Chapter 15	Preparations vary in efficacy
Typhoid	Heat-killed *S. typhi*	>6 mo.	See Chapter 19	Relatively ineffective in prevention
Cholera	Phenol-killed *Vibrio cholerae*	>6 mo.	See Chapter 19	Marginally protective, for short period
Anthrax	Cell-free protein antigen	>6 mo.	Anticipated exposure (usually occupational)	Safe and highly effective
Meningococcal	Four capsular polysaccharides (A, C, Y, W-135)	>2 yr.	High-risk patients, to control epidemics	Children <2 yr. respond variably to individual components
Tularemia	Live-attenuated	>6 yr.	Anticipated exposure (e.g., lab techs)	Available from CDC
Plague	Killed, whole bacteria	>6 mo.	Occupational exposure	Not recommended for those living in plague-endemic areas

TABLE 40–6. *Schedule of Immunizations of Normal Children*

Age	Immunization(s)
2 mo.	DTP, OPV, HIB (conjugated)
4 mo.	DTP, OPV, HIB (conjugated)
6 mo.	DTP, HIB (conjugated)
15 mo.	MMR,* HIB (conjugated)
18 mo.	DTP, OPV
4–6 yr.	DTP, OPV
14–16 yr.	Td

*Repeat measles vaccination is recommended either at entrance to primary school (kindergarten) or to middle school (junior high).
DTP: diphtheria and tetanus toxoids with pertussis
OPV: oral poliovirus vaccine
MMR: measles, mumps, and rubella
HIB-conjugated: *H. influenzae* B conjugated to protein carrier
Td: Tetanus toxoid and reduced dose diphtheria toxoid

foreign countries are shown in Table 40–7. Note that more than one vaccine can be given at the same time, but that cholera and yellow fever vaccines should be given at least 3 weeks apart. Pregnancy and immunosuppression are contraindications for live virus vaccines.

Future Vaccines

Efforts to develop new vaccines that are safe and effective are continuing. In addition to an acellular pertussis vaccine (see above), work is progressing with respect to (1) live-attenuated varicella vaccine, which has been demonstrated to be safe and effective in leukemic children; (2) attenuated rotavirus vaccine; (3) herpes simplex vaccine; (4) malaria sporozoite vaccines; (5) HIV vaccine; (6) cytomegalovirus vaccine; and (7) group B streptococcal vaccine, among others.

Rotavirus deserves mention as the single most important etiologic agent of severe diarrhea in infants and young children, accounting for one third to one half of the 5–10 million deaths each year worldwide from severe diarrhea in children under 2 years of age. Attenuated rotaviruses of bovine and rhesus origin are undergoing evaluation as orally administered vaccines to prevent rotavirus diarrhea in infants.

Much current vaccine development is focused upon the preparation of protein-polysaccharide conjugates that result in enhanced immune responses to the polysaccharide component, particularly in young infants. It is probable that a number of such conjugates will be demonstrated to be effective immunogens and to result in protection against infections. Molecular biology has led to a number of new approaches to vaccine development, including synthesis of peptides or polypeptides by recombinant DNA techniques or gene insertion, attenuation of pathogens by gene-segment reassortment or mutations (gene deletions or missense), and production of anti-idiotypes. These and other approaches should result in improved agents for use as vaccines in the future.

CASE HISTORY

D.R. is a 5-year-old white male admitted to the pediatric intensive care unit following a

TABLE 40–7. *Vaccines for Foreign Travelers*

Vaccine	Type	Efficacy	When Indicated	Dose*
Cholera	Killed bacteria	Low	Rarely, but required by certain countries	0.5 mL SC or IM in 2 doses 1 wk–1 mo apart
Hepatitis A	Immune serum globulin	Moderate	Travel to areas with poor hygiene	2 mL (5 mL for longer stay, repeated every 5 mo)
Hepatitis B	Purified HbsAg	High	For medical personnel or those anticipating sexual contact	3 1.0 mL doses
Japanese encephalitis	Inactivated virus	Moderate	Travel to rural Asia in summer	3 doses, 1 wk apart
Measles	Live-attenuated	High	For those born after 1956 and who have not received 2 doses	1 dose (should precede ISG by ≥2 wk)
Meningococcal	Polysaccharide	Moderate	For travel to epidemic areas (e.g., sub-Saharan Africa)	0.5 mL SC (1 dose)
Polio	IPV or OPV	High	For travel to developing countries	1 booster of OPV or IPV; IPV if no 1° series; DT booster every 10 years
Tetanus/Diphtheria	Toxoids	High	If none in 10 years	DT booster every 10 years
Typhoid	Live oral bacteria	Moderate	Travel to rural areas of tropical countries or where an epidemic exists	One capsule QOD × 4 doses, at least 2 wk before departure
Yellow fever	Live-attenuated	Moderate	Travel to rural tropical S. America or Africa	0.5 mL SC (1 dose)

*For children's doses, consult Report of the Committee on Infectious Diseases of the American Academy of Pediatrics, the *Red Book*.

rattlesnake bite on the dorsum of the right foot. This boy lives in a tent in an isolated wooded area. Neither he nor his siblings have ever seen a physician, received an immunization, or attended school. He arrived in an emergency room 15 min after the bite with rapidly progressing local inflammatory changes of the foot. He was stabilized and received (among other agents): (1) 0.5 cc tetanus toxoid intramuscularly, (2) 1.0 cc human tetanus immune globulin, (3) 140 cc horse antisnake venom intravenously and around the snakebite, and (4) 0.5 cc trivalent oral polio vaccine. The patient steadily improved in the hospital, and, although there was initial concern about possible loss of some or all of the foot, all tissue remained viable. Twelve days after admission, he developed transient painful swelling of the knees and was found to have hematuria. These findings resolved after several days.

CASE DISCUSSION

This boy received both active and passive tetanus immunization, which is necessary to protect previously unimmunized individuals promptly. He received passive immunity in the form of human and equine globulins, and also was given active immunogens in the form of live-attenuated oral polio vaccine and a purified protein (tetanus toxoid). The symptoms of arthritis of the knees together with hematuria noted 12 days after a large dose of equine antiserum clearly represents classic serum sickness.

REFERENCES

Books

Committee on Infectious Diseases of the American Academy of Pediatrics. *Red Book*. 22nd ed. Elk Grove Village, IL: American Academy of Pediatrics, 1991.

Plotkin, S. A., and Mortimer, E. A., eds. *Vaccines*. Philadelphia: W. B. Saunders, 1988.

Articles

Anderson, D. C., Givner, L. B., and Shearer, W. T.: Active and passive immunization in the prevention of infectious diseases. In: Stiehm, E. R., ed. *Immunologic Disorders in Infants and Children*. 3rd ed. Philadelphia: W. B. Saunders, 1989.

Hayden, G. F., Sato, P. A., Wright, P. F., et al. Progress in worldwide control/elimination of disease through immunization. *J. Pediatr. 114*:520–527, 1989.

Hone, D., and Hackett, J. Vaccination against enteric bacterial diseases. *Rev. Infect. Dis. 11*:853–876, 1989.

Immunization Practices Advisory Committee. General recommendations on immunization. *MMWR 38*:205–227, 1989. Also, *Am. J. Dis. Child. 143*:1013–1019, 1989.

Livengood, J. R., Mullen, J. R., White, J. W., et al. Family history of convulsions and use of pertussis vaccine. *J. Pediatr. 115*:527–531, 1989.

Murphy, K. R., and Strunk, R. C. Safe administration of influenzae vaccine in asthmatic children hypersensitive to egg proteins. *J. Pediatr. 106*:931–933, 1985.

Rev. Infect. Dis. Vaccines, *11* (Suppl. 3), 1989.

Sabin, A. B. Oral poliovirus vaccine: History of its development and use and current challenge to eliminate poliomyelitis from the world. *J. Infect. Dis. 115*:420–436, 1985.

Index

Note: Page numbers in *italics* refer to illustrations; page numbers followed by t refer to tables.